Pulmonary Circulation

Pulmonary Circulation: Diseases and their Treatment

THIRD EDITION

Andrew J Peacock
Professor of Medicine, Consultant Respiratory
Physician and Director, Scottish Pulmonary Vascular Unit,
Regional Heart and Lung Centre, Golden Jubilee National Hospital,
Glasgow, UK

Robert Naeije
Professor of Physiology and Medicine and Consultant,
Department of Cardiology, Erasme Academic Hospital,
The Free University of Brussels, Belgium

Lewis J Rubin
Emeritus Professor of Medicine and Emeritus Director,
Division of Pulmonary and Critical Care Medicine,
University of California, San Diego School of Medicine,
La Jolla, California, USA

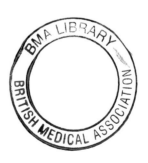

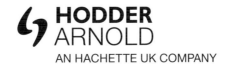

HODDER
ARNOLD
AN HACHETTE UK COMPANY

First published in Great Britain in 2004 by Hodder Arnold.
Second edition 2004.
This third edition published in 2011 by Hodder Arnold, an imprint of
Hodder Education, Hodder and Stoughton Ltd, a division of Hachette UK
338 Euston Road, London NW1 3BH

http://www.hodderarnold.com

Hachette UK's policy is to use papers that are natural, renewable and
recyclable products and made from wood grown in sustainable forests.
The logging and manufacturing processes are expected to conform to the
environmental regulations of the country of origin.

Whilst the advice and information in this book are believed to be true
and accurate at the date of going to press, neither the author[s] nor the
publisher can accept any legal responsibility or liability for any errors or
omissions that may be made. In particular (but without limiting the
generality of the preceding disclaimer) every effort has been made to
check drug dosages; however it is still possible that errors have been
missed. Furthermore, dosage schedules are constantly being revised and
new side-effects recognized. For these reasons the reader is strongly
urged to consult the drug companies' printed instructions before
administering any of the drugs recommended in this book.

British Library Cataloguing in Publication Data
A catalogue record for this book is available from the British Library

Library of Congress Cataloging-in-Publication Data
A catalog record for this book is available from the Library of Congress

ISBN-13   978-0-340-981-924

2 3 4 5 6 7 8 9 10

Commissioning Editor: Caroline Makepeace
Project Editor: Sarah Penny
Production Controller: Kate Harris
Cover Designer: Helen Townson

Typeset in India by MPS Limited, a Macmillan Company
Printed and bound in the UK by MPG Books, Bodmin, Cornwall
Text printed on FSC accredited material

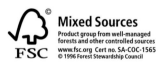

What do you think about this book? Or any other Hodder Arnold
title? Please visit our website: **www.hodderarnold.com**

Dedication

To my wife Jila and my children Leila, Johnnie and Vita who have put up with so much over the years and never questioned my love for science and medicine even though their own interests lay elsewhere.

Andrew Peacock

To my family for their support, and to our patients, who serve as a constant reminder of the importance of our commitment.

Lewis Rubin

We would like to thank our colleagues from around the world who have been an inspiration to this book and in many cases contributors to it. Whether we work in Respiratory Medicine or Cardiology, we all share the view that the connection between the heart and lungs is important.

Contents

Contributors

Vahitha Banu Abdul-Salam, BPharm (Hon), PhD
Research Associate, Burlington Danes Building
Centre for Pharmacology & Therapeutics
Imperial College London
London, UK

Steven H Abman, MD
Professor of Pediatric Pulmonary and Critical Care Medicine
Director, Pediatric Heart Lung Center
Department of Pediatrics
University of Colorado Denver School of Medicine
Colorado, USA

Eric D Austin, MD, MSCI
Department of Pediatrics
Vanderbilt University School of Medicine
Nashville, TN, USA

David B Badesch, MD
Professor of Medicine
Divisions of Pulmonary Sciences and Critical Care Medicine, and Cardiology
Clinical Director, Pulmonary Hypertension Center
University of Colorado
Denver, CO, USA

Joan Albert Barberà, MD, PHD
Servei de Pneumologia
Hospital Clínic, Universitat de Barcelona
Spain

Peter Bärtsch, MD
Professor of Medicine and Head of Division VII: Sports Medicine
Department of Internal Medicine
University Hospital
Heidelberg, Germany

Professor Maurice Beghetti
Pediatric Cardiology Unit
Department of the Child and Adolescent
Hôpital des Enfants
Geneva, Switzerland

Isabel Blanco, MD
Servei de Pneumologia
Hospital Clínic
Universitat de Barcelona
Spain

Diana Bonderman
Department of Internal Medicine II
Division of Cardiology
The Medical University of Vienna
Vienna, Austria

Henri Bounameaux, MD
Division of Angiology and Hemostasis
Department of Internal Medicine
Geneva University Hospital
Geneva, Switzerland

Todd M Bull, MD, FACP
Associate Professor of Medicine
Pulmonary Hypertension Center
Division of Pulmonary Sciences and Critical Care Medicine
University of Colorado
Denver, USA

Matthieu Canuet, MD
Département de Pneumologie
CHRU Strasbourg
Novel Hôpital Civil
Strasbourg, France

François Chabot, MD, PhD
Professor of Respiratory Medicine
Service des Maladies Respiratoires et Réanimation Respiratoire
CHRU Nancy
Hôpital de Brabois
Vandoeuvre-lès-Nancy, France

Hunter C Champion, MD, PhD
Assistant Professor
Division of Cardiology
Johns Hopkins University School of Medicine
Baltimore, MD, USA

Richard N Channick, MD
Pulmonary Unit, UCSD Medical Center,
University of California,
La Jolla, California, USA

Ari Chaouat, MD, PhD
Professor of Respiratory Medicine
Service des Maladies Respiratoires et Réanimation Respiratoire
CHRU Nancy, Hôpital de Brabois
Vandoeuvre-lès-Nancy, France

Kelly Chin, MD
Assistant Professor
University of Texas
Southwestern Medical Center
Dallas, TX, USA

Colin Church, BSc(Hons), MBChB, MRCP
Wellcome Trust Clinical Research Fellow
Scottish Pulmonary Vascular Unit and Institute of Cardiovascular
Sciences
University of Glasgow
Glasgow, Scotland

David W Courtman, PhD
Scientist, Regenerative Medicine
Ottawa Health Research Institute
Ontario, Canada

Barbara A Cockrill, MD
Assistant Professor of Medicine
Pulmonary and Critical Care Unit
Massachusetts General Hospital
Harvard Medical School
Boston, MA, USA

Paul A Corris, FRCP
Professor of Thoracic Medicine
Director National Pulmonary Hypertension Service (Newcastle)
Director of the Cardiopulmonary Transplantation Institute of
Cellular Medicine
Newcastle University and Newcastle Upon Tyne Hospitals
NHS Trust
Newcastle, UK

Peter Dorfmüller, MD, PhD
Hypertension Artérielle Pulmonaire: Physiopathologie et
Innovation Thérapeutique
Department of Pathology
Marie Lannelongue Hospital
Paris South University
Paris, France

Daniel Dumitrescu, MD
Centre National de Référence de l'Hypertension Artérielle
Pulmonaire
Hôpital Antoine-Béclère, Université Paris
Paris, France

TW Evans, PhD, MD, DSc, FRCP, FMedSci, FRCA
Adult Intensive Care Unit
Royal Brompton Hospital
London, UK

Caio Júlio César dos Santos Fernandes, MD
Pulmonary Department, The Heart Institute
University of Sao Paulo Medical School
Sao Paulo, Brazil

Robert P Frantz, MD
Associate Professor of Medicine
Department of Cardiovascular Diseases, Mayo Clinic
Rochester, MN, USA

Sean P Gaine, MD, PhD
Department of Respiratory Medicine
Mater Misericordiae Hospital, University College Dublin
Ireland

Nazzareno Galiè, MD
Associate Professor of Cardiology
Istituto di Cardiologia, Universita di Bologna
Italy

Jorge Gaspar MD, FACC
Chief
Interventional Cardiology Department
Ignacio Chávez National Institute of Cardiology
Mexico City, Mexico

Mark T Gladwin, MD
Division Chief
Pulmonary, Allergy and Critical Care Medicine
University of Pittsburgh Medical Center
Pittsburgh, PA, USA

Emmanuel Gomez, MD
Service des Maladies Respiratoires et Réanimation Respiratoire
CHRU Nancy, Hôpital de Brabois
Vandoeuvre-lès-Nancy, France

Friedrich Grimminger
Department of Internal Medicine
University Hospital Giessen and Marburg GmbH
Giessen, Germany

Bertram Groves, MD
Professor of Medicine
Pulmonary Hypertension Center
Division of Pulmonary Sciences and Critical Care Medicine
University of Colorado
Boulder, CO, USA

Marco Guazzi, MD, PhD
Associate Professor of Cardiology
Cardiopulmonary Unit
University of Milano, San Paolo Hospital
Italy

Charles A Hales, MD
Professor of Medicine, Pulmonary and Critical Care Unit
Massachusetts General Hospital
Harvard Medical School
Boston, MA, USA

Paul M Hassoun, MD
Professor
Division of Pulmonary and Critical Care Medicine
Johns Hopkins University
Baltimore, MD, USA

Anna R Hemnes, MD
Instructor
Division of Allergy, Pulmonary and Critical Care Medicine
Vanderbilt University School of Medicine
Nashville, TN, USA

Philippe Hervé
Service de Pneumologie et Réanimation Respiratoire
Hôpital Antoine Béclère
Université Paris Sud
Clamart, France

Marius Hoeper, MD
Professor, Deptartment of Respiratory Medicine
Hannover Medical School
Germany

André Hovnanian, MD
Pulmonary Department, Heart Institute
University of Sao Paulo Medical School
Sao Paulo, Brazil

Marc Humbert, MD, PhD
Service de Pneumologie et Réanimation Respiratoire
Hôpital Antoine Béclère
Université Paris Sud
Clamart, France

Dunbar Ivy, MD
Professor of Pediatrics
Chief and Selby's Chair of Pediatric Cardiology
Director, Pediatric Pulmonary Hypertension Program
University of Colorado
Denver School of Medicine
Denver, CO, USA

James E Jackson, MD
NHLI Cardiovascular Sciences, Imaging
Imperial College London
London, UK

Xavier Jaïs, MD
Service de Pneumologie et Réanimation Respiratoire
Hôpital Antoine Béclère
Université Paris Sud
Clamart, France

Carlos Viana Poyares Jardim, MD, PhD
Pulmonary Department, Heart Institute
University of Sao Paulo Medical School
Sao Paulo, Brazil

Steven M Kawut, MD, MS
Associate Professor of Medicine
Center for Clinical Epidemiology and Biostatistics
University of Pennsylvania School of Medicine
Philadelphia, PA, USA

Karina Keogh, MD
Division of Pulmonary and Critical Care Medicine
Mayo Clinic
Rochester, MN, USA

Kim M Kerr, MD
Clinical Professor of Medicine
Division of Pulmonary & Critical Care
University of California at San Diego
La Jolla, CA, USA

Michael J Krowka, MD
Professor of Medicine and Vice-Chair
Division of Pulmonary and Critical Care Medicine
Mayo Clinic
Rochester, MN, USA

Marcin Kurzyna, MD, PhD
Department of Chest Medicine
Institute of Tuberculosis and Lung Diseases
Warsaw, Poland

Irene M Lang, MD
Department of Internal Medicine II
Division of Cardiology, The Medical University of Vienna
Vienna, Austria

David Langleben, MD, FRCPC
Professor of Medicine, McGill University
Director, Center for Pulmonary Vascular Disease
Jewish General Hospital
Montreal, QC, Canada

James E Lloyd, MD
Professor, Department of Medicine
Vanderbilt University School of Medicine
Nashville, TN, USA

Roberto F Machado, MD
Associate Professor of Medicine
Section of Pulmonary, Critical Care Medicine
Sleep and Allergy University of Illinois at Chicago
Chicago, IL, USA

Marco Maggiorini
University of Zurich Hospital
Zurich Switzerland

Alessandra Manes, MD
Istituto di Cardiologia, Università di Bologna
Italy

Eckhard Mayer, MD
Professor, Department of Thoracic Surgery
Catholic Academic Hospital SHK
Germany

Michael D McGoon, MD
Department of Cardiovascular Diseases
Mayo Clinic
Rochester, MN, USA

Vallerie V McLaughlin, MD
Professor of Medicine, Department of Internal Medicine
Division of Cardiovascular Medicine
Director, Pulmonary Hypertension Program University of
Michigan Health System
Ann Arbor, MI, USA

David Montani, MD
Service de Pneumologie et Réanimation respiratoire
Centre National de Référence de l'Hypertension
Artérielle Pulmonaire, Hôpital Antoine-Béclère
Université Paris
Paris, France

Nicholas W Morrell, MD, FRCP
Professor, Department of Medicine
University of Cambridge School of Clinical Medicine
Cambridge, UK

Claudia R Morris, MD
Department of Emergency Medicine
Children's Hospital and Research Center Oakland
Oakland, CA, USA

Robert Naeije, MD, PhD
Professor of Physiology and Medicine and Consultant
Department of Cardiology
Erasme Academic Hospital
The Free University of Brussels
Belgium

John H Newman, MD
Professor, Department of Medicine
Vanderbilt University School of Medicine
Nashville, TN, USA

Andrea Olschewski, MD, PhD
Professor, Department of Anaesthesiology
University Clinic of Anaesthesia and Intensive Care Medicine
Medical University of Graz
Austria

Horst Olschewski, MD
Director, Division of Pulmonology
Department of Internal Medicine
Medical University of Graz
Graz, Austria

Mark L Ormiston
Terrence Donnelly Cardiovascular Research Laboratories
St. Michael's Hospital
Toronto, ON, Canada

Ronald J Oudiz, MD
Professor of Medicine, David Geffen School of Medicine at UCLA
Director, Liu Center for Pulmonary Hypertension
LA Biomedical Research Institute at Harbor, UCLA Medical Center
Torrance, CA, USA

Massimiliano Palazzini, MD
Istituto di Cardiologia,
Università di Bologna
Italy

Harold I Palevsky, MD
Pulmonary, Allergy, and Critical Care Division
Department of Medicine, Penn Cardiovascular Institute
University of Pennsylvania School of Medicine
Philadelphia, PA, USA

Andrew J Peacock MPhil, MD, FRCP
Professor of Medicine, Consultant Respiratory Physician and
Director, Scottish Pulmonary Vascular Unit
Regional Heart and Lung Centre
Golden Jubilee National Hospital
Glasgow, UK

Dante Penaloza, MD, FACC, FCCP
Professor Emeritus
University Cayetano Heredia
Lima, Peru

Arnaud Perrier, MD
Division of General Internal Medicine
Geneva University Hospital
Geneva, Switzerland

Michael R Pinsky, MD, Dr hc
Professor of Critical Care Medicine, Bioengineering,
Anesthesiology and Cardiovascular Disease
Department of Critical Care Medicine
University of Pittsburgh Medical Center
PA, USA

Sandra Pizarro, MD
Servei de Pneumologia
Hospital Clínic, Universitat de Barcelona
Spain

Laura Price, BSc, MBChB
Clinical Research Fellow, Adult Intensive Care Unit
Royal Brompton Hospital
London, UK

Soni Savai Pullamsetti
Department of Lung Development and Remodelling
Max-Planck-Institute for Heart and Lung Research
Department of Internal Medicine
University Hospital Giessen and Marburg GmbH
Giessen, Germany

Christopher Rhodes, BA
PhD Student
Centre for Pharmacology & Therapeutics
Department of Medicine, Imperial College London
London, UK

Melvyn Rubenfire, MD, FACC, FACCP, FAHA
Professor of Internal Medicine
University of Michigan
Ann Arbor, MI, USA

Lewis J Rubin, MD
Emeritus Professor of Medicine and Emeritus Director
Division of Pulmonary and Critical Care Medicine
University of California
San Diego School of Medicine
La Jolla, California, USA

Julio Sandoval, MD, FACC
Chief, Cardiopulmonary Department
Ignacio Chávez National Institute of Cardiology
Mexico City, Mexico

Laurent Savale, MD
Service de Pneumologie et Réanimation Respiratoire
Hôpital Antoine Béclère
Université Paris Sud
Clamart, France

Steven M Scharf, MD, PhD
Professor of Medicine
Division of Pulmonary and Critical Care Medicine
University of Maryland
Baltimore, MD

Ralph Theo Schermuly, MD
Department of Lung Development and Remodelling
Max-Planck-Institute for Heart and Lung Research;
Department of Internal Medicine
University Hospital Giessen and Marburg GmbH
Giessen, Germany

Christine Selton-Suty, MD
Département de Cardiologie Médicale
CHRU Nancy
Hôpital de Brabois
Vandoeuvre-lès-Nancy, France

Claire L Shovlin, PhD, FRCP, BA(Hons)
Senior Lecturer, Respiratory Medicine and Imaging
Imperial College Healthcare NHS Trust
Hammersmith Hospital
London, UK

Gérald Simonneau, MD
Service de Pneumologie et Réanimation respiratoire
Centre National de Référence de l'Hypertension Artérielle
Pulmonaire, Hôpital Antoine-Béclère
Université Paris Sud
Clamart, France

Olivier Sitbon, MD
Service de Pneumologie et Réanimation Respiratoire
Hôpital Antoine Béclère
Université Paris Sud
Clamart, France

Rogerio Souza, MD, PhD
Pulmonary Department, Heart Institute
University of Sao Paulo Medical School
Sao Paulo, Brazil

Rudolf Speich, MD
Department of Internal Medicine
University Hospital
Zurich, Switzerland

Michael William Sproule, MBChB (Edin), MRCP (UK), FRCR
Consultant Radiologist, Western Infirmary
Glasgow, United Kingdom

Robin H Steinhorn, MD
Professor and Head, Neonatology, Department of Pediatrics
Northwestern University Medical School
Chicago, IL

Duncan J Stewart, BSc, MASc, PhD
Canadian Institutes of Health Research Postdoctoral Fellow
University of Cambridge
Department of Medicine
Addenbrooke's Hospital
Cambridge, UK

Victor F Tapson, MD, FCCP, FRCP
Professor of Medicine and Director
Center for Pulmonary Vascular Disease
Duke University Medical Center
Durham, NC, USA

Adam Torbicki, MD, PhD
Head, Department of Chest Medicine
Institute of Tuberculosis and Lung Diseases
Warsaw, Poland

Fernando Torres, MD
Associate Professor
University of Texas
Southwestern Medical Center, USA

Anton Vonk-Noordegraaf, MD, PhD
Department of Pulmonology
VU University Medical Center
Amsterdam

Stephen J Watt BSc, MBBS, FRCPEd, Hon. FFOM
Consultant in Respiratory and Hyperbaric Medicine
NHS Grampian, Aberdeen Royal Infirmary
Aberdeen, Scotland

Emmanuel Weitzenblum, MD
Professor of Respiratory Medicine
Département de Pneumologie
CHRU Strasbourg
Nouvel Hôpital Civil
Strasbourg, France

John Wharton, BSc, PhD
Honorary Senior lecturer
Centre for Pharmacology & Therapeutics
Department of Medicine
Imperial College London
London, UK

Martin R Wilkins
Head, Division of Experimental Medicine and Toxicology
Imperial College
London, UK

S John Wort, BSc, MBChB, PhD
Adult Intensive Care Unit
Royal Brompton Hospital
London, UK

Foreword

As advances continue to evolve in understanding the pulmonary circulation, its role in pulmonary hypertension becomes increasingly more important. Pulmonary hypertension is not a disease; it is a hemodynamic condition reflecting an elevation in pulmonary artery pressure seen in a myriad of diseases. As there are important differences in the various forms of pulmonary hypertension with significant differences in treatment approaches and outcomes, delving further into understanding the pulmonary circulation and the right heart is necessary to further improve outcomes for patients with pulmonary hypertension. Few areas in cardiopulmonary medicine have been as successful in improving outcomes as those made in pulmonary hypertension. Prior to 1995, there were no therapies approved for pulmonary arterial hypertension; today, there are eight drugs approved worldwide providing physicians with evidence-based treatment guidelines. Technical advances have permitted us to diagnose patients earlier and assess their disease more thoroughly on an individual basis. Yet, despite these achievements, pulmonary hypertension remains incurable and treatment responses are often partial, at best – underscoring the need for identifying new therapeutic targets and developing new treatment strategies. The third edition of *Pulmonary Circulation*, edited by Professors Peacock, Rubin and Naeije and written by the experts in the field, confirms the progress that has been made over the past two decades.

In its third edition, *Pulmonary Circulation* has become a classic in its field. The contributors are the global experts. From basic science to clinical approaches, it provides an authoritative and comprehensive reference for all physicians interested in the pulmonary circulation and in pulmonary hypertension. It is a reminder of how far we have come yet how much farther we need to go. We need to remain cognizant that "A long habit of not thinking a thing wrong gives it superficial appearance of being right" (Thomas Paine). Professors Peacock, Rubin and Naeije continue to illuminate a field where there was all too often only the sound of cursing the darkness. They remind us "It is better to light a candle…."

As a physician who has been privileged to know many of these outstanding investigators, I am indebted to Professors Peacock, Rubin and Naeije, and to their colleagues for their contributions. I am certain that this 3rd edition of *Pulmonary Circulation* will serve as the premier source for understanding pulmonary physiology and pathophysiology and its roles in all pulmonary hypertension disorders.

Robyn J Barst, MD
Professor Emeritus of Pediatrics (in Medicine)
Columbia University College of Physicians & Surgeons
New York NY
USA

Preface

The consequences of disturbed function of the pulmonary circulation remain an enigma to most clinicians. There is disturbance of pulmonary circulatory function in nearly all cardiac and pulmonary disease, yet this is rarely recognized or treated. The reasons for this relative obscurity when compared, for example, with the systemic circulation, are clear. The pulmonary circulation is difficult to examine clinically and the tools we have for pulmonary circulatory measurement are either crude or invasive, or both. Even when we make invasive measurements with a cardiac catheter we only learn about the circulation in artificial surroundings (the catheter laboratory), in an unrepresentative position (supine on the table) and in a state of artificially restricted activity. Clearly, we need clinical measurement techniques that will allow us to pursue pulmonary circulatory function in all states of human activity both in normal people and those with cardiorespiratory disease. These are coming, but even now we know much about the pulmonary circulation that can help us in looking after patients in the ward and in the intensive care unit. Fortunately, there has been a great deal of research into the structure and function of the pulmonary circulation. We already understand much of its physiology and pathophysiology and, recently, a number of effective therapies have been developed, tested and put into clinical use with great effect. In this book, a distinguished group of authors, most of whom have a clinical background, have presented what is known about the pulmonary circulation in a readable and, more importantly, clinically relevant fashion, so that it can be understood by practising physicians. This is the third edition, with many completely new sections but a similar though more clinically orientated format. The book has been written especially with the busy clinician in mind, particularly those in respiratory medicine, cardiology, pediatrics and intensive care. It has been deliberately structured so that a subject can be appreciated at any level from the purely clinical right down to the biochemical. This allows the reader to start with a chapter about a particular clinical issue but, if interested, to pursue that subject from clinical to physiological to biochemical level as he or she desires. Each chapter stands alone, so some repetition is inevitable, for which we make no apology, but this hierarchy of structure will, we hope, make the book accessible without diminishing the quality of the information that is presented.

For the 3rd edition of *Pulmonary Circulation* we have included the latest clinical, pathophysiological and pathological research on pulmonary circulatory disorders. We have also included the new classification and all the recommendations from the World Conference on Pulmonary Circulation at Dana Point California in 2008 and the latest guidelines from the ESC/ERS published in 2009.

We hope that *Pulmonary Circulation* will remain, in this third edition, a useful reference for the pulmonary hypertension specialist as well as Pulmonologists, Cardiologists and Intensive Care physicians.

Andrew J Peacock
Robert Naeije
Lewis J Rubin

Preface to the second edition

The consequences of disturbed function of the pulmonary circulation remain an enigma to most clinicians. There is disturbance of pulmonary circulatory function in nearly all cardiac and pulmonary disease, yet this is rarely recognised or treated. The reasons for this relative obscurity when compared, for example, with the systemic circulation, are clear. The pulmonary circulation is difficult to examine clinically and the tools we have for pulmonary circulatory measurement are either crude or invasive, or both. Even when we make invasive measurements with a cardiac catheter we only learn about the circulation in artificial surroundings (the catheter laboratory), in an unrepresentative position (supine on the table) and in a state of artificially restricted activity. Clearly, we need clinical measurement techniques that will allow us to pursue pulmonary circulatory function in all states of human activity both in normal people and those with cardiorespiratory disease. These are coming, but even now we know much about the pulmonary circulation that can help us in looking after patients in the ward and in the intensive care unit. Fortunately, there has been a great deal of research into the structure and function of the pulmonary circulation. We already understand much of its physiology and pathophysiology and, recently a number of effective therapies have been developed, tested and put into clinical use with great effect. In this book, a distinguished group of authors, most of whom have a clinical background, have presented what is known about the pulmonary circulation in a readable and, more importantly, clinically relevant fashion, so that it can be understood by practising physicians.

This is the second edition, with many completely new sections but a similar though more clinically orientated format. The book has been written especially with the busy clinician in mind, particularly those in respiratory medicine, cardiology, paediatrics and intensive care. It has been deliberately structured so that a subject can be appreciated at any level from the purely clinical right down to the biochemical. This allows the reader to start with a chapter about a particular clinical issue but, if interested, to pursue that subject from clinical to physiological to biochemical level as he or she desires. Each chapter stands alone, so some repetition is inevitable, for which we make no apology, but this hierarchy of structure will, we hope, make the book accessible without diminishing the quality of the information that is presented.

Andrew J Peacock
Lewis J Rubin

Abbreviations

5-HETE	5-hydroxyeicosotetraenoic acid	CDH	congenital diaphragmatic hernia
5-HT	5-hydroxytryptamine; serotonin	CDMP1	cartilage-derived morphogenetic protein-1
5-HTT	5-HT transporter	CEMRA	contrast-enhanced magnetic resonance
5-LO	5-lipoxygenase		angiography
6MWT	6-minute walk test	CGD	chronic granulomatous disease
8-Br-GMP	8-bromo-guanosine monophosphate	cGMP	cyclic guanosine monophosphate
99mTcMAA	technetium-99 macroaggregated albumin	CI	cardiac index; confidence interval
ACE	angiotensin converting enzyme	CK	coefficient of kinship
ACS	acute chest syndrome	CK-MB	creative kinase-myocardial band
AcT	acceleration time	CMS	chronic mountain sickness
AEC	American-European Consensus	CMV	cytomegalovirus
aECA	anti-endothelial antibodies	CNS	central nervous system
aFGF	acidic fibroblast growth factor	CO	cardiac output
AIDS	acquired immunodeficiency syndrome	COPD	chronic obstructive pulmonary disease
ALI	acute lung injury	CPAP	continuous positive airway pressure
ALK1	activin receptor-like kinase 1	CPS	carbamoyl-phosphate synthetase
ALT	alanine aminotransferase	CREB	cAMP response element-binding protein
AMS	acute mountain sickness	CREST	calcinosis, Raynaud's, sclerodactyly and
ANA	antinuclear antibody		telangectasia
ANCA	antineutrophil cytoplasmic antibody	CSS	Churg–Strauss syndrome
ARDS	acute respiratory distress syndrome	CT	computed tomography
ARNT	aryl hydrocarbon receptor nuclear translocator	CTD	connective tissue disease
AS	atrial septostomy	CTE	chronic thromboembolic
ASD	atrial septal defect	CTEPH	chronic thromboembolic pulmonary
AST	aspartate aminotransferase		hypertension
AVF	atrioventricular fibrillation	CTPA	computed tomography pulmonary angiography
AVM	arteriovenous malformation	CTR	cardiothoracic ratio
AVP	arginine vasopressin	CVA	cerebrovascular accident
AVSD	atrioventricular septal defect	CvO_2	mixed venous oxygen content
BAL	bronchoalveolar lavage	CVP	central venous pressure
BBAS	blade balloon atrial septostomy	DA	ductus arteriosus
BCPA	bidirectional cavopulmonary anastomosis	DCO	diffusing capacity for carbon monoxide
BDAS	balloon dilation atrial septostomy	DLCO	diffusing capacity for carbon monoxide
bFGF	basic fibroblast growth factor	DLT	double lung transplant
BLT	bilateral sequential single lung transplant	DPI	diphenylene iodonium
BMI	body mass index	DTPA	ethylenediaminepentaacetic acid
BMP	bone morphogenetic protein	DVT	deep venous (vein) thrombus (thrombosis)
BMPR2	bone morphogenetic protein receptor 2	EBCT	electron beam computed tomography
BNP	brain natriuretic protein	ECE-1	endothelin-1 converting enzyme
BPI	bactericidal permeability-increasing protein	ECG	electrocardiogram
CADD	continuous ambulatory drug delivery	ECHO	echocardiography
cAMP	cyclic adenine monophosphate	ECMO	extracorporeal membrane oxygenation
cANCA	cytoplasmic ANCA	EGF	endothelial growth factor; epidermal growth
CcO2	oxygen content of end-capillary blood		factor

EGTA	ethyleneglycotetraacetic acid
EI	eccentricity index
ELISA	enzyme-linked immunoadsorbent assay
ENG	endoglin
eNOS	endothelial nitric oxide synthase
ENT	ear, nose and throat
ERK1	extracellular regulated kinase-1
ET	endothelin
ET-1 (2) (3)	endothelin-1 (-2) (-3)
ET_A receptor	endothelin receptor A
ET_B receptor	endothelin receptor B
EVE	endogenous vascular elastase
FAK	focal adhesion kinase
FDA	Federal Drug Administration
FDG-PET	fluorine-18-2-fluoro-2-deoxy-D-glucose positron emission tomography
FDP	fibrin degradation products
FEF	forced expiratory flow
FEV_1	forced expiratory volume in 1 second
FGN	fibrinogen
FIO_2	fraction of inspired oxygen
FLAP	5-lipoxygenase-activating protein
FO	foramen ovale
FPPH	familial primary pulmonary hypertension
FRC	functional residual capacity
FVC	forced vital capacity
G protein	guanine-nucleotide-binding protein
Gd-DTPA	gadolinium-diethylenetriamine pentaacetic acid
GDF	growth and differentiation factor
GI	gastrointestinal
GRE	gradient refocused echo
HAART	highly active antiretroviral therapy
HACE	high-altitude cerebral edema
HAPE	high-altitude pulmonary edema
HFOV	high-frequency oscillatory ventilation
HHT	hereditary hemorrhagic telangiectasia
HHV-8	human herpes virus
HIF	hypoxia-inducible factor
HIV	human immunodeficiency virus
HLT	heart/lung transplant
HOX	homeobox
HPS	hepatopulmonary syndrome
HPV	hypoxic pulmonary vasoconstriction
HPVR	hypoxic pulmonary vascular response
HRCT	high-resolution computed tomography
HSP	Henoch–Schönlein purpura
HVOD	hepatic veno-occlusive disease
HVR	hypoxic ventilatory response
ICAM	intracellular adhesion molecule
ICU	intensive care unit
IGF-1	insulin-like growth factor
IL	interleukin
IMV	intermittent mandatory ventilation
iNO	inhaled nitric oxide
INR	international normalized ratio
IP_3	inositol triphosphate; 1,4,5-inositol triphosphate
IPF	idiopathic pulmonary fibrosis
IPPHS	international primary pulmonary hypertension study
ITP	intrathoracic pressure
IVC	inferior vena cava
IVCCI	inferior vena cava collapsibility index
IVS	interventricular septal
IVUS	intravascular ultrasound
JVP	jugular venous pressure
K_{Ca}	calcium-sensitive potassium channel
KCO	specific gas transfer
KDR VEGF	receptor II
KSV	Kaposi's sarcoma virus
L-Arg	L-arginine
LA	left atrium
LAO	left anterior oblique
LAP	latency-associated protein; left atrial pressure
L-LAMMA	L-monomethylargine
LMWH	low molecular weight heparin
L-NNA	N-nitro-L-arginine
LPA	left pulmonary artery
LTOT	long-term oxygen therapy
LV	left ventricle; left ventricular
LVEDP	left ventricular end-diastolic pressure
LVEF	left ventricular ejection fraction
LVRS	lung volume reduction surgery
MAA	macroaggregates of human serum albumin
MAP	mitogen-activated protein
MCT	monocrotaline
MCTD	mixed connective tissue disease
MIGET	multiple inert gas elimination technique
mLAP	mean left atrial pressure
MMP	matrix metalloproteinase
MPA	microscopic polyangiitis
mPAP	mean pulmonary artery pressure
MRA	magnetic resonance angiography
mRAP	mean right atrial pressure
MRI	magnetic resonance imaging
mRNA	messenger ribonucleic acid
MSI	microsatellite instability
NANC	non-adrenergic, non-cholinergic
NEB	neuroepithelial body
NIH	National Institutes of Health
NMPG	N-mercaptopropionylglycine
NO	nitric oxide
NOS	nitric oxide synthase
NPR-A	atrial natriuretic peptide type A receptor
NYHA	New York Heart Association
OB	obliterative bronchiolitis
OI	oxygenation index
OLT	orthotopic liver transplantation
OSA	obstructive sleep apnea
OSAS	obstructive sleep apnea syndrome
P_A	alveolar pressure

PA	pulmonary artery	RANTES	regulated upon activation normal T-expressed and secreted
$PaCO_2$	arterial PCO_2	RAP	right atrial pressure
PADP	pulmonary artery diastolic pressure	RDS	respiratory distress syndrome
PAH	pulmonary arterial hypertension	REM	rapid eye movement
PAHRH	pulmonary arterial hypertension related to HIV infection	RHC	right heart catheterization
PAI	protein accumulation index	RHF	right heart failure
PAN	polyarteritis nodosa	RIJ	right internal jugular
pANCA	perinuclear ANCA	RNS	reactive nitrogen species
P_AO_2	alveolar PO_2	ROC	receptor-operated non-selective cation channel
PaO_2	partial pressure of arterial oxygen		
PAOP	pulmonary artery occlusion pressure	ROS	reactive oxygen species
PAP	pulmonary artery pressure	RP	Raynaud's phenomenon
PAR	pulmonary arterial resistance	RSV	respiratory syncytial virus
PASP	pulmonary artery systolic pressure	RV	right ventricle; right ventricular
PAVM	pulmonary arteriovenous malformation	RVD	right ventricular dysfunction
Paw	airway pressure	RVEDP	right ventricular end-diastolic pressure
PAWP	pulmonary artery wedge pressure	RVEF	right ventricular ejection fraction
PC	phase contrast	RVF	right ventricular failure
Pc	pulmonary capillary pressure	RVH	right ventricular hypertrophy
PCH	pulmonary capillary hemangiomatosis	RVP	right ventricular pressure
PCO_2	partial pressure of carbon dioxide	RVSP	right ventricular systolic pressure
PCP	pulmonary capillary pressure	SAC	stretch-activated cation channel
PCWP	pulmonary capillary wedge pressure	SaO_2	arterial oxygen saturation
PDA	patent ductus arteriosus	SAP	systemic artery pressure
PDE5	phosphodiesterase type 5	SD	standard deviation
PDGF	platelet-derived growth factor	SE	spin echo
PE	pulmonary embolism; pleural effusion	SEE	standard error of estimate
PEEP	positive end-expiratory pressure	SEM	standard error of mean
PG	pressure gradient; posterior gutter	SIRS	systemic inflammatory response syndrome
PG	prostaglandin	SIV	simian immunodeficiency virus
PGI_2	prostacyclin	SLE	systemic lupus erythematosus
PGI_2-R	prostacyclin receptor	SLT	single lung transplant
PGI_2-S	prostacyclin synthase	SM	smooth muscle
PH	pulmonary hypertension	SMC	smooth muscle cell
pHi	intramucosal pH	SO_2T	systemic oxygen transport
PKC	protein kinase C	SOD	superoxide dismutase
PKG	protein kinase G	SPH	scleroderma-associated pulmonary hypertension; secondary/severe pulmonary hypertension
PO_2	partial pressure of oxygen		
POPH	portopulmonary hypertension		
PPAR-γ	peroxisome proliferator-activated receptor-γ		
Ppc	pericardial pressure	SSLT	single sequential lung transplantation
PPET-1	preproendothelin-1	SVC	superior vena cava
PPH	primary pulmonary hypertension	SvO_2	mixed venous O_2 saturation
PPHN	persistent pulmonary hypertension of the newborn	SVR	systemic vascular resistance
		SVT	supraventricular tachycardia
Ppl	pleural pressure	TEE	transesophageal echocardiography
PTCER	pulmonary transcapillary escape route	TF	tissue factor
PTE	pulmonary thromboendarterectomy	TGA	transposition of the great arteries
PVOD	pulmonary vascular obstructive disease	TGF-β	transforming growth factor-β
PVP	pulmonary venous pressure	TIA	transient ischemic attack
PVR	pulmonary vascular resistance	TIMP	tissue inhibitor of matrix metalloproteinases
PVZ	pulmonary vascular impedance	TIPG	tricuspid insufficiency pressure gradient
Q	blood flow	TIPS	transjugular intrahepatic portosystemic shunting
QP	pulmonary blood flow		
QS	systemic blood flow	TLC	total lung capacity
RA	rheumatoid arthritis; right atrium	tPA	tissue-type plasminogen activator
		TPR	total pulmonary vascular resistance

TUNEL	terminal deoxynucleotidyl transferase (TdT) mediated dUTP nick end labeling	VILI	ventilator-induced lung injury
US	lower limb venous compression ultrasonography	VO_2	oxygen consumption
V/Q	ventilation/perfusion	VSD	ventricular septal defect
VA	alveolar ventilation	Vt	tidal volume
VC	vital capacity	VTE	venous thromboembolism
VEGF	vascular endothelial growth factor	WG	Wegener's granulomatosis
		Z_0	pulmonary vascular impedance at zero Hz
		Zc	pulmonary vascular characteristic impedance

A note on references

The reference lists are annotated, where appropriate, to guide readers to key primary papers and major review articles as follows:

Key primary papers are indicated by a bullet (●)
Major review articles are indicated by a diamond (◆)
Papers that represent the first formal publication of a management guideline are indicated by an asterisk (★).

We hope that this feature will render extensive lists of references more useful to the reader and will help to encourage self-directed learning among both trainees and practicing physicians.

PART 1

THE FUNCTION OF THE NORMAL PULMONARY CIRCULATION & RIGHT HEART

Pulmonary vascular function

ROBERT NAEIJE

INTRODUCTION

The pulmonary circulation is a high flow and low pressure circuit, which favors pulmonary gas exchange by preventing fluid moving out of the pulmonary vessels into the interstitial space, and allows the right ventricle to operate at a low energy cost. However, because of the low pressures, the pulmonary circulation is very sensitive to mechanical influences, and the "flow generator" right ventricle is thin-walled, poorly prepared to rapid changes in loading conditions. In addition, the pulsatility of the pulmonary circulation is more important than that of the systemic circulation, which affects the energy transmission from the right ventricle to the pulmonary arteries.

Many cardiac and pulmonary diseases are associated with an abnormal increase in pulmonary artery pressures. Pulmonary hypertension is the third most common cardiovascular condition, after coronary heart disease and systemic hypertension. As the pulmonary circulation is entirely within the thorax, relatively hidden from clinical examination, and symptoms of abnormal pulmonary vascular function are late, a sound physiological approach is essential for the diagnosis and treatment of pulmonary hypertension.

NORMAL PRESSURES AND FLOWS

Vascular function is defined by a pressure–flow relationship. Pulmonary vascular pressures and flows are usually measured with a triple lumen balloon-tipped thermodilution fluid-filled catheter. The catheter is inserted into a central vein and floated through the right heart chambers into the pulmonary artery under constant pressure wave monitoring (1) (Figure 1.1). The 1 mL balloon at the tip of the catheter allows for the placement into the pulmonary artery without fluoroscopic control, and the estimation of *left* ventricular filling pressures while catheterizing the *right* side of the heart. Thus, the pulmonary artery catheter provides successive measurements of a right atrial pressure (RAP), a right ventricular pressure (RVP), a pulmonary artery pressure (PAP), and an occluded PAP (PAOP).

A PAOP is a satisfactory estimate of left atrial pressure (LAP) provided the pulmonary vessels are fully recruited with a pulmonary capillary pressure (PCP) higher than surrounding alveolar pressure (P_A). A PCP higher than P_A defines a Zone 3 condition according to West's terminology (2). Lungs of a recumbent normovolemic healthy subject are normally completely in a Zone 3 condition.

With the catheter in place, a proximal lumen located 30 cm from the tip serves to the measurement of RAP, a distal lumen at the tip the measurement of PAP, and an air-filled lumen serves allows to inflate the balloon. A thermistor located 4 cm from the catheter tip records small temperature changes in the pulmonary artery induced by the injection of bolus of cold saline into the right atrium, allowing to calculate a mean pulmonary blood flow (Q) from a thermodilution curve.

To minimize the influence of intra-thoracic pressure and volume changes associated with respiratory movements, pulmonary vascular pressures are measured at end-expiration, when the lungs are at functional residual capacity.

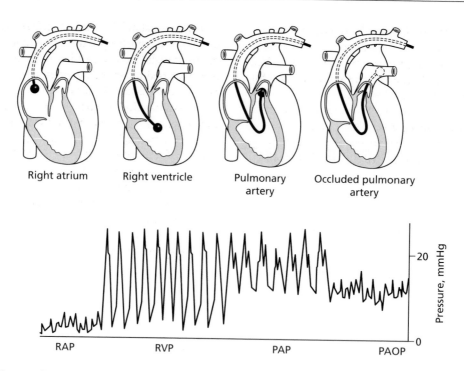

Figure 1.1 Right heart catheterization with flow-directed balloon-tipped catheter with successive measurements of right atrial pressure (RAP), right ventricular pressure (RVP), pulmonary artery pressure (PAP) and occluded PAP (PAOP).

The pressures are zero leveled at the so-called hydrostatic indifference point, assumed unaffected by body position, situated at the tricuspid valve. In a supine subject, this is at mid-chest, or 5 cm below the Louis angle of the sternum. In an upright subject, the zero is leveled at the junction of antero-posterior mid-chest and the lower third of the thorax.

In the pulmonary circulation, it is possible to calculate a pulmonary vascular resistance (PVR) by the difference between mean PAP taken as the inflow pressure, and mean LAP taken as the outflow pressure, divided by Q:

$$PVR = \frac{PAP - LAP}{Q}$$

Sometimes a measurement of LAP or PAOP cannot be obtained, and a *total* PVR (TPVR) is calculated as:

$$TPVR = \frac{PAP}{Q}$$

The absence of a measurement of an outflow pressure leads to an overestimation of PVR of unpredictable magnitude. Therefore, the use of total TPVR calculations is not recommended.

A resistance calculation derives from a simple physical law that governs laminar flows of Newtonian fluids through thin, non-distensible circular tubes. This law, initially enounced by the French physicist Poiseuille, states that resistance R to flow, defined as a pressure drop ΔP to flow Q ratio, is equal to the product of the length l of the tube by a viscosity constant η divided by the product of fourth power of the internal radius r by π:

$$R = \frac{\Delta P}{Q} = \frac{8l\eta}{\pi r^4}$$

The fact that r in the equation is at the fourth power explains why R is exquisitely sensitive to small changes in caliber radius. Accordingly, PVR is a good indicator of the state of constriction or dilatation of pulmonary resistive vessels, and helpful to monitor disease-induced pulmonary vascular remodeling and/or changes in tone.

The limits of normal of resting pulmonary vascular pressures and flows as derived from measurements obtained in a total of 55 healthy resting supine young adult healthy volunteers (3–5) are shown in Table 1.1. In that study population there were no gender differences in pulmonary hemodynamics after a correction of flow for body dimensions (Table 1.2).

Earlier studies have shown that aging is associated with an increase in PAP and a decrease in Q, leading to a doubling of PVR over a five decades life span (Table 1.3) (6–9).

EFFECTS OF EXERCISE

Supine exercise is associated with proportional increases in cardiac output and pulmonary vascular pressure gradient, with slightly decreased PVR (10). This is explained by the fact that the extrapolated pressure intercept of (PAP–PAOP)–Q relationships is often slightly positive, by a few mmHg, due to a slight curvilinearity of pulmonary vascular pressure–Q relationships and possibly also a closing pressure higher than LAP. Upright exercise is associated with an initial hyperbolic decrease in PVR. This is related to the fact that the upright position is associated with pulmonary vascular de-recruitment, with increased gradients between closing pressure and LAP, allowing for pre-exercise higher PVR. At moderate to high levels of exercise, PVR is identical for in upright or supine positions (Figure 1.2).

High levels of exercise markedly increase pulmonary vascular pressures. In athletes able to increase their cardiac output to 25–35 L/min, PAP may increase to 40–45 mmHg, together with PAOP of 25–35 mmHg (10). This is illustrated in Figure 1.3 by pulmonary hemodynamic measurements in six triathletes (11).

Table 1.1 Limits of normal of pulmonary blood flow and vascular pressures

Variables	Mean	Limits of normal
Q (L/min)	6.4	4.4–8.4
Heart rate (bpm)	67	41–93
PAP systolic (mmHg)	19	13–26
PAP diastolic (mmHg)	10	6–16
PAP, mean (mmHg)	13	7–19
PAOP (mmHg)	9	5–13
PCP (mmHg)	10	8–12
RAP (mmHg)	5	1–9
PVR (dyne s cm^{-5})	55	11–99
SAP, mean (mmHg)	91	71–110

Q, cardiac output; PAP, pulmonary artery pressure; PAOP, occluded PAP; PCP, pulmonary capillary pressure; RAP, right atrial pressure; PVR, pulmonary vascular resistance; SAP, systemic arterial pressure; limits of normal: from mean − 2 SD to mean + 2 SD; n = 55 healthy resting volunteers (n = 14 for the measurement of PCP). From refs 3–5.

Table 1.2 Influence of gender on pulmonary blood flow and vascular pressures

Variables (mean + SE)	Men (n = 34)	Women (n = 21)
Q (L/min)	6.7 ± 0.9	6.0 ± 1.2*
Q (L/min/m^2)	3.5 ± 0.5	3.6 ± 0.6
PAP (mmHg)	13 ± 3	13 ± 3
PAOP (mmHg)	9 ± 2	9 ± 2
RAP (mmHg)	5 ± 2	5 ± 1

Abbreviations: see Table 1.1. Values are means ± SD, *P < 0.05. From refs 3–5.

Table 1.3 Influence of age on pulmonary blood flow and vascular pressures

Age (years)	16–28	61–83
n	22	16
Q (L/min)	7.6 ± 0.3	5.6 ± 0.3
PAP (mmHg)	13 ± 1	16 ± 1
PAOP (mmHg)	8 ± 1	9 ± 1
PVR (dyne s cm^{-5})	54 ± 6	96 ± 7

Abbreviations: see Table 1.1. From refs 6–9.

For understandable ethical and technical limitations, none of the reported pulmonary hemodynamic measurements at high levels of exercise in normal subjects (10,11) have included direct measurements of LAP through a left heart catheterization. However, PAOP at exercise is unlikely to overestimate LAP. High levels of cardiac output are associated with a complete recruitment of the pulmonary capillary network, which is the condition for the valid estimation of LAP by a PAOP (Figure 1.4). On the other hand, the filling pressures of both ventricles, as assessed by directly measured RAP and indirectly measured LAP, rise at exercise and are related to stroke volume and exercise capacity (12). This suggests that the left ventricle tends to over-use the Frank Starling mechanism (increase stroke volume by an increased preload, or end-diastolic ventricular

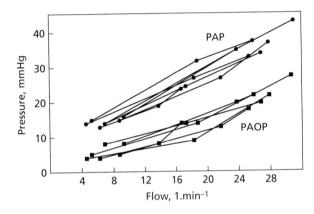

Figure 1.2 Mean ± SD values of pulmonary vascular resistance (PVR) during upright (triangles) versus supine exercise (circles) at progressively increased workloads. PVR is higher in the upright position at rest. PVR decreases slightly during exercise. (From refs 6–10.)

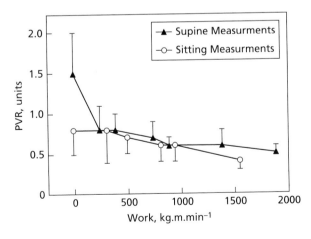

Figure 1.3 Pulmonary artery pressure (PAP) (circles) and occluded PAP (PAOP) (squares) as a function of pulmonary blood flow in athletes at rest and at two levels of exercise. High levels of exercise are associated with marked increases in PAP and PAOP. The slope of PAP–Q is approximately equal to 1 mmHg/L/min. (From ref 11.)

volume/pressure) to maximize cardiac output at the highest levels of exercise (12).

On the other hand, PCP has to be between PAP and LAP or PAOP. A PCP > 20–25 mmHg is associated with an increased extravascular lung water content because of an increased capillary filtration (13). Strenuous exercise may be associated with a decrease in arterial PO_2 and an increase in the alveolar to arterial PO_2 gradient, which may be a cause of maximum oxygen consumption limitation (14). Exercise-induced hypoxemia is at least in part explained by exercise-induced pulmonary capillary hypertension.

As mentioned above, PVR increases with aging, so that the average slope of PAP–Q plots during exercise is 1 mmHg/L/min in young adults, but more than doubles, up to 2.5 mmHg/L/min in old subjects. Much of the slope of PAP–Q is caused by an increase in PAOP (or LAP) (7,8,10,11). Earlier increase in LAP in older subjects at exercise could be explained by age-related decreased diastolic compliance of the left ventricle (8).

While PAP–Q relationships at exercise are generally best described by a linear approximation (10), a sufficient number of measurements at high levels of exercise, above the anaerobic threshold, may disclose an increased slope causing a biphasic "take-off" pattern on log PAP–log VO_2 (15). Because of the tight relationship between Q and VO_2, this is to be interpreted as a high level of exercise-induced pulmonary vasoconstriction, caused by sympathetic nervous system activation, acidosis and decreased mixed venous oxygenation (15). Increased slope of PAP–Q plots above the anaerobic threshold may also be related to an increase in LAP. It is intriguing that the take-off pattern of PAP–VO_2 plots at exercise is not observed in patients with pulmonary vascular disease, who rather show a "plateau" pattern (15). The reason for decreased slope of PAP–VO_2 relationships at high levels of exercise in patients with pulmonary vascular diseases is not clearly understood.

CAPILLARY PRESSURE

Arterial occlusion creates a stop–flow condition that extends the catheter lumen down to same diameter veins, so that an increase in small vein resistance can conceivably increase pulmonary artery wedge pressure (PAWP) but not PAOP (Figure 1.4). While in normal subjects, PAWP is indistinguishable from PAOP, it has been shown that PAWP may exceed PAOP by an average of 3–4 mmHg in patients with various lung diseases. This is explained by an increase in medium to large vein resistance (16).

Because of the resistance of the smallest veins, which do not contribute to PAWP as being of smaller diameter than the pulmonary artery catheter, and a low but significant capillary resistance, pulmonary capillary pressure (PCP) is necessarily higher than PAWP. A measurement of PCP can be obtained by the analysis of a PAP decay curve after balloon occlusion (17). As shown in Figure 1.5, such a pressure decay curve is made of a first fast component,

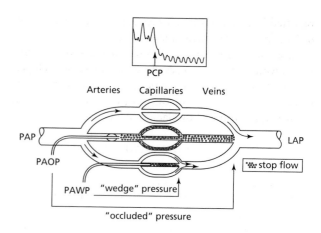

Figure 1.4   Schematic representation of the pulmonary circulation with successive arterial and venous branching pattern, to show stop–flow phenomenon downstream of balloon occlusion for a measurement of occluded pulmonary artery pressure (PAOP) and catheter tip occlusion for a measurement of pulmonary artery wedge pressure (PAWP). Both measurements differ from pulmonary capillary pressure (PCP) calculated from a PAP decay curve after occlusion. Stippled areas indicate stop–flow.

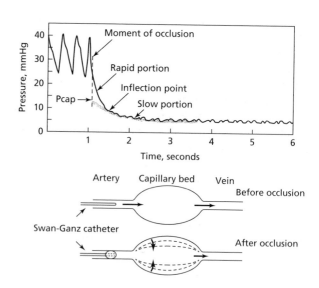

Figure 1.5   Analysis of the pressure transient after pulmonary arterial occlusion for the estimation of pulmonary capillary pressure (PCP) either by the intersection of the fast and the slow components of the pressure decay curve, or by the extrapolation of the exponential fitting of the slow component of the pressure decay curve to the moment of occlusion.

which corresponds to the stop of flow through an arterial resistance, and a slower component, which corresponds to the emptying of the compliant capillaries through a venous resistance. The intersection between the two components of the PAP decay curve offers an estimate of PCP that is in good agreement with the reference isogravimetric method (17).

Measurements of PCP from the analysis of the PAP decay curve after balloon occlusion have recently been reported in young adult volunteers, yielding a mean value of 10, range 6–14 mmHg (Table 1.1) (5).

Based on a normal longitudinal distribution of resistances within the pulmonary circulation, ascribing 60 percent PVR to the arterial segment and 40 percent to the capillary-venous segment, the normal PCP can also be calculated as proposed by Gaar *et al.* (13) as:

$$PCP = PAOP + 0.4\,(PAP - PAOP)$$

The Gaar equation is invalid in disease states associated with increases of the arterial or the venous components of PVR.

Pulmonary capillary pressure increases with cardiac output and pulmonary venous pressure. Hypoxia increases PCP, albeit normally slightly (5), probably because of a small venous participation to hypoxic pulmonary vasoconstriction (18). In a study on 14 healthy volunteers at rest, inspiratory hypoxia increased PAP from 13 ± 3 to 22 ± 3 and PCP from $10 = 2$ to 12 ± 2 mmHg (5).

In the early stages of high altitude pulmonary edema, PCP is higher than 20 mmHg, suggesting a hydrostatic mechanism (5). Variable increases in PCP have been reported in acute respiratory distress syndrome (19,20). An increase in PCP may be recorded in pulmonary arterial hypertension, which is explained either by small vein resistance, or by the fact the measurement actually captures resistance of the smallest arterioles (21). The occlusion method to determine PCP has been used to partition PVR and to detect peripheral small vessel disease in chronic thrombo-embolic pulmonary hypertension (22). In pulmonary hypertension in pulmonary veno-occlusive disease, PCP is increased but PAOP and PAWP are normal, which indicates that the disease process is exclusively located in the smallest pulmonary veins (21).

PRESSURE–FLOW RELATIONSHIPS

The inherent assumption of a PVR calculation is that the PAP–Q relationship is linear and crosses the pressure axis at a value equal to PAOP, allowing PVR to be constant whatever the absolute level of pressure of flow. While the (PAP–PAOP)–Q relationship has indeed been shown to be reasonably well described by a linear approximation over a limited range of physiological flows, the zero crossing assumption may be true only in case of well-oxygenated lungs in supine resting subjects, suggesting complete recruitment and minimal distension. Hypoxia, and a number of cardiac and respiratory diseases, increase both the slope and the extrapolated intercepts of multipoint (PAP–PAOP)–Q plots (23).

While an increase in the slope of a PAP–Q plots is easily understood as being caused by an decreased cumulated surface section area of pulmonary resistive vessels, the positive extrapolated pressure intercept has inspired various explanatory models. Permutt *et al.* conceived a vascular waterfall model made of parallel collapsible vessels with

a distribution of closing pressures (24). At low flow, these vessels would be progressively de-recruited, accounting for a low flow PAP–Q curve that is concave to the flow axis, and intercepts the pressure axis at the lowest closing pressure to be overcome to generate a flow. At higher flow, completed recruitment and negligible distension account for a linear PAP–Q curve with an extrapolated pressure intercept representing a weighted mean of closing pressures. In this model, the mean closing pressure is the effective outflow pressure of the pulmonary circulation. A left atrial pressure lower than the mean closing pressure is then an only apparent downstream pressure, irrelevant to flow as is the height of a waterfall. Resistance calculations remain applicable to evaluate the functional state of the pulmonary circulation provided the apparent downstream pressure is replaced by the effective one (24).

However, distensible vessel models have been developed which explain the shape of PAP–Q curves by changes in resistance and compliance (25,26). In fact, as illustrated in Figure 1.6, PAP–Q curves can always be shown to be curvilinear with concavity to flow axis provided a large enough number of PAP–Q coordinates are generated and submitted to adequate fitting procedure. On the other hand, derecruitment can be directly observed at low pressures and flows (27).

Both recruitment and distension probably explain most PAP–Q curves (28). According to this integrated view, at low inflow pressure, many pulmonary vessels are closed as an effect of their intrinsic tone and surrounding alveolar pressure, and those that are open are relatively narrow. As inflow pressure increases, previously closed vessels progressively open (recruitment), and previously narrow vessels progressively dilate (distension). Both mechanisms explain a progressive decrease in the slope of pulmonary vascular pressure/flow relationships with increasing flow or pressure.

The practical consequence is that single PVR determinations cannot be reliable for the evaluation of the functional state of the pulmonary circulation at variable flow (Figure 1.6). A better description of the resistive properties of the pulmonary circulation requires measurements of pulmonary vascular pressure at several levels of flow. The problem is to alter flow without affecting vascular tone. As already mentioned, exercise to alter flow may spuriously increase slopes of PAP–Q plots, in normal subjects (15) as well as in patients with cardiac or pulmonary diseases, leading to linear fitting of PAP–Q plots with negative extrapolated pressure intercepts (29,30). An infusion of low-dose dobutamine might be preferable to generate purely passive PAP–Q relationships (30).

PASSIVE REGULATION

Left atrial pressure and cardiac output

At a given Q, an increase in LAP is transmitted upstream to PAP in a less than one for one proportion, depending on

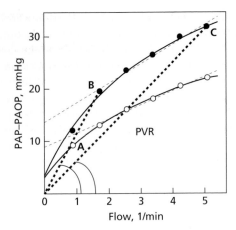

Figure 1.6 Pulmonary artery pressure versus flow coordinates at two levels of pulmonary hypertension are correctly described by a linear approximation over a physiological range of flows. The extrapolated pressure intercepts of these linearized pressure/flow relationships are positive, suggesting a closing pressure higher than left atrial pressure. However, the pressure/flow coordinates are better described by a curvilinear fitting, which takes more adequately into account the natural distensibility of the pulmonary vessels. In both situations, pulmonary vascular resistance (PVR) calculations are misleading: from A to B, PVR does not change, and from B to C, PVR decreases, in the presence of aggravated pulmonary hypertension as assessed by higher pressures at a given flow.

the state of arterial distension and the presence or not of a closing pressure higher than LAP (28). In a fully distended and recruited pulmonary circulation, a $\Delta PAP/\Delta LAP$ is close to the unity.

Lung volume

An increase in lung volume above functional residual capacity increases the resistance of alveolar vessels, that are the vessels exposed to alveolar pressure, but decreases the resistance of extra-alveolar vessels, that are the vessels exposed to interstitial pressure. A decrease in lung volume below functional residual capacity has the opposite effects. It has been shown that the combination of alveolar and extra-alveolar vessel resistance that gives the lowest resultant PVR is observed at functional residual capacity (31).

Gravity

Pulmonary blood flow increases almost linearly from non-dependent to dependent lung regions. This inequality of pulmonary perfusion is best demonstrated in an upright lung (2). The vertical height of a lung is on average about 30 cm. The difference in pressure between the extremities of a vertical column of blood of the same size amounts to 23 mmHg, which is quite large compared to the mean perfusion pressure of the pulmonary circulation. Accordingly,

the physiologic inequality of the distribution of perfusion of a normal lung can be explained by a gravity-dependent interplay between arterial, venous and alveolar pressures (2). At the top of the lung, alveolar pressure (P_A) is higher than mean PAP and pulmonary venous pressure (PVP). In this *Zone 1*, flow may be present only during systole, or not at all. Zone 1 is extended in clinical situations of low flow, such as hypovolemic shock, or increased alveolar pressure such as during ventilation with a positive end expiratory pressure (PEEP). Further down the lung there is a *Zone 2* where $PAP > P_A > PVP$. In this Zone 2, alveolar pressure is an effective closing pressure, and the driving pressure for flow is the gradient between mean PAP and P_A. As mentioned above, such a flow condition can be likened to a waterfall since PVP, the apparent outflow pressure, is irrelevant to flow as is the height of a waterfall. In *Zone 3*, PVP is higher than P_A, so that the driving pressure for flow is PAP–PVP.

At the most dependent regions of upright lung, there is an additional region where flow decreases (32). This Zone 4 has been attributed to an increase in the resistance of extra-alveolar vessels, because it expands when lung volume is reduced or in the presence of lung edema. Active tone may be an additional explanation for Zone 4 as it is also reduced by the administration of vasodilators.

The vertical height of lung tissue in a supine subject is of course much reduced compared to the upright position, and accordingly, the lung is then normally almost completely in Zone 3, with however persistence of a still measurable increase in flow from non-dependent to dependent lung regions.

Three-dimensional reconstructions using single-photon-emission computed tomography have shown that there is also a decrease in blood flow from the center of the lung to the periphery (33). High resolution methods and fractal modeling of the pulmonary circulation have actually led to the notion of a predominantly non-gravity-dependent distribution of pulmonary blood flow (34). Subtle differences in arterial branching ratios may indeed influence flow distribution with increased heterogeneity as the scale of the inquiry narrows, corresponding to the "what is the length of the coastline" effect (35). However, the overwhelming evidence remains in favor of the thesis that gravity is the single most important determinant of pulmonary blood flow distribution (35). Vascular geometry related small unit heterogeneity of pulmonary blood flow distribution has not been shown to be relevant to gas exchange.

ACTIVE HYPOXIC REGULATION

There is an active intrapulmonary control mechanism able to some extent to correct the passive gravity-dependent distribution of pulmonary blood flow: a decrease in PO_2 increases pulmonary vascular tone. Hypoxic pulmonary vasoconstriction was first reported by von Euler and Liljestrand (36), who proposed a functional interpretation that can still be considered valid. In lung tissue, PO_2 is determined by a ratio between O_2 carried to the lung by alveolar ventilation (V_A) and O_2 carried away from the lung by blood flow (Q):

$$PO_2 = \frac{VA}{Q}$$

In contrast with hypoxic vasodilation in systemic tissue, where local PO_2 is accordingly determined by a ratio flow of O_2 carried to the tissues (Q) and local O_2 consumption (VO_2):

$$PO_2 = \frac{Q}{VO_2}$$

The hypoxic pulmonary pressor response is universal in mammals and in birds, but with considerable inter-species and inter-individual variability (37). The attributes of hypoxic pulmonary vasoconstriction can be summarized as follows (37,38). The response is vigorous in cattle and in pigs, moderate in humans, dogs and camelids (including the llama), and almost absent in guinea pigs and rabbits. It is turned on in a few seconds, fully developed after 1 to 3 minutes, and more or less stable thereafter according to the experimental conditions. It is reversed in less than a minute. It is observed in lungs devoid of nervous connections, and indeed also in isolated pulmonary arterial smooth muscle cells. Hypoxic pulmonary vasoconstriction is enhanced by acidosis, a decrease in mixed venous PO_2, repeated hypoxic exposure (in some experimental models), perinatal hypoxia, decreased lung segment size, cyclooxygenase inhibition, nitric oxide inhibition, and certain drugs or mediators which include almitrine and low-dose serotonin. Hypoxic pulmonary vasoconstriction is inhibited by alkalosis, hypercapnia, an increase in

pulmonary vascular or alveolar pressures, vasodilating prostaglandins, nitric oxide, complement activation, low-dose endotoxin, calcium channel blockers, β_2 stimulants, nitroprusside, and, paradoxically, by peripheral chemoreceptor stimulation. The hypoxic pressor response is biphasic, with a progressive increase as PO_2 is progressively decreased to approximately 35 to 40 mmHg, followed by a decrease ("hypoxic vasodilatation") in more profound hypoxia.

The hypoxia-induced increase in PVR is mainly caused by a constriction of pre-capillary small arterioles (37,38). Small pulmonary veins also constrict in response to hypoxia, but this should not normally contribute to more than 20–30 percent of the total change in PVR (18). An exaggerated hypoxic constriction of small pulmonary veins could explain high altitude pulmonary edema (5).

While hypoxic pulmonary vasoconstriction has been shown to be an only moderately efficient feedback mechanism (4,39), it may still produce substantial improvements in arterial oxygenation of patients with inhomogenous lungs such as in chronic obstructive pulmonary disease (hypoxemia mainly explained by low V_A/Q ratios) or in the acute respiratory distress syndrome (hypoxemia mainly explained by V_A/Q ratios equal to zero, or shunt) (40). Topographical blood flow distribution (PET scan) and arterial PO_2 can be shown to conform to the expected functional effects of hypoxic pulmonary vasoconstriction in experimental acute lung injury models, as an inhibition of the response prevents redistribution of blood flow to non-dependent lung regions and markedly aggravates shunt and arterial hypoxemia (41). This is illustrated in Figure 1.7, in an experiment which also shows the predominant effects of gravity on the distribution of pulmonary blood flow and its relevance to gas exchange.

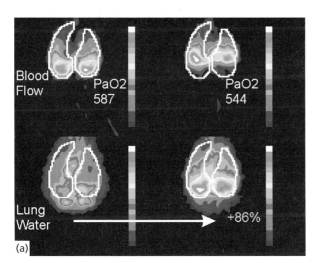
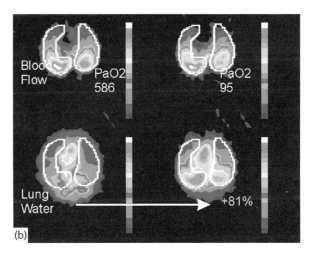

Figure 1.7   Positron emission tomography measurements of regional blood flow and lung water in a supine dog ventilated with pure oxygen, before and after induction of oleic acid lung injury, with intact (left) or ablated (right) hypoxic pulmonary vasoconstriction. Lung injury is associated with a significant increase in lung water. Pulmonary blood flow shows a gravity-dependent increase to the dependent lung regions. Hypoxic vasoconstriction redistributes blood flow upwards, and this is associated with preserved arterial PO_2. (From ref 41.)

The biochemical mechanism of hypoxic pulmonary vasoconstriction remains incompletely understood (42). Current thought is that a decrease in PO_2 inhibits smooth muscle cell voltage-gated potassium channels, resulting in membrane depolarization, influx of calcium, and cell shortening. However, the nature of the low PO_2 sensing mechanism remains elusive. Mitochondria and nicotinamide adenine dinucleotide phosphate oxidases are discussed as oxygen sensors. Reactive oxygen species, redox couples and adenosine monophosphate-activated kinases are candidate mediators. Whether H_2O and other reactive oxygen species are increased or decreased in hypoxia is a matter of on-going controversy (43,44). The reversal of hypoxic vasoconstriction by profound hypoxia is due to an activation of ATP-dependent potassium channels (38).

The normal as well as the abnormal pulmonary vascular tone has been shown to be modulated by a series of endothelium-derived and circulating mediators (45). Endothelium-derived relaxing factors include nitric oxide, prostacyclin, and the endothelium-derived hyperpolarizing factor. The major endothelium-derived contracting factor is endothelin. These observations have been at the basis of efficient treatments of pulmonary arterial hypertension with prostacyclin derivatives, phosphodiesterase-5 inhibitors to enhance nitric oxide signaling and endothelin receptor blockers (46).

The pulmonary circulation is richly innerved by the autonomic nervous system, which includes adrenergic, cholinergic, and nonadrenergic noncholinergic (NANC) (37,47). However, the role played by the autonomic nervous system in the control of pulmonary vascular tone appears to be minor. In fact, autonomic innervation of the pulmonary arterial tree is predominantly proximal, suggesting a more important effect in the modulation of proximal compliance (47).

PULSATILE FLOW HEMODYNAMICS

The study of the pulmonary circulation as a steady flow system is a simplification, since pulmonary arterial pulse pressure, or the difference between systolic and diastolic Ppa, is in the order of 40 to 50 percent of mean pressure, and instantaneous flow varies from a maximum at midsystole to around zero in diastole (37,48).

While pulmonary artery pressure and flow waves are superposable in normal subjects, they become markedly different in aspect and desynchronized in patients with pulmonary hypertension (48). In patients with severe pulmonary hypertension, the right ventricular pressure wave is characterized by a sharp initial upstroke, followed by a short plateau, and by a late systolic peaking, and the pulmonary artery pressure wave is characterized by a huge pulse pressure and a late systolic peaking as well. In the most severe forms of pulmonary hypertension the pulmonary artery pressure wave looks "ventricularized". On the other hand, the pulmonary blood flow wave presents with a late systolic deceleration, or even a midsystolic deceleration.

These morphological aspects of pulmonary artery pressure and flow waves in pulmonary hypertension are explained by decreases in pulmonary arterial compliance and by earlier return of reflected waves on forward waves (49,50). It can be shown experimentally that right ventricular output decreases because of an increased afterload if, at a given resistance, pulmonary arterial compliance decreases and/or wave reflection increases (49).

Pulmonary artery pressure and flow waves can be decomposed into their constituent harmonic oscillations by an application of the Fourier theorem (48). This analysis is possible because the pulmonary circulation acts as a linear system, that is that a purely sinusoidal flow oscillation produces a purely sinusoidal pressure oscillation of the same frequency. From the spectral analysis of the pulmonary arterial pressure and flow waves, one calculates pulmonary arterial impedance (PVZ) (48). PVZ is the ratio of pressure oscillations to flow oscillations. It is graphically represented as a pressure/flow ratio and a phase angle, both as a function of frequency. A typical PVZ spectrum is illustrated in Figure 1.8.

PVZ at zero Hz (Zo) corresponds to PVR calculated as Ppa/Q. Normally, the ratio of pressure and flow decreases rapidly to a first minimum at 2–3 Hz and increases again to a first maximum at 5–6 Hz. At low frequencies, the phase angle is negative, indicating that flow leads pressure.

An increase in the pressure/flow ratio at all frequencies indicates a decreased pulmonary arterial distensibility. A shift of the first minimum and maximum to higher frequencies indicates an increased wave velocity or a change in the dominant reflection site.

The PVZ spectrum allows the quantification of characteristic impedance (Zc) defined as PVZ without wave reflection. Characteristic impedance is measured as the average pressure/flow ratio at the highest frequencies. It can also be measured as the linearized slope of the early systolic pulmonary artery pressure/flow relationship (Figure 1.8).

Characteristic impedance is dependent on the ratio of inertia and compliance of the pulmonary circulation, and can be approximated by the equation:

$$Zc = \frac{\rho/\pi r^4}{\Delta \pi r^2/\Delta P}$$

Where ρ is the density of blood, r the mean internal radius, $\rho/\pi r^4$ the inertance and $\Delta \pi r^2/\Delta P$ the compliance of the pulmonary arterial tree.

The extent of the difference between Zo and Zc can be used to calculate an index of wave reflection as:

$$Rc = \frac{1 - Zc/Zo}{1 + Zc/Zo}$$

The pulsatile hydraulic power is most important in the proximal pulmonary arterial tree (48), and accordingly PVZ calculations are relatively insensitive to peripheral

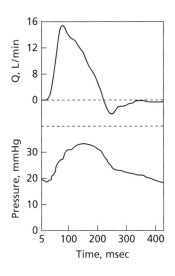
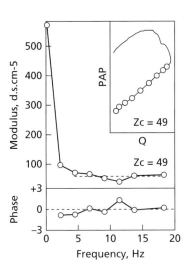

Figure 1.8 Pulmonary artery pressure (PAP) and flow (Q) waves and derived pulmonary arterial impedance (PVZ) spectrum in experimental embolic pulmonary hypertension. Pressure and flow waves are desynchronized, there is a shift of the first minimum of the pressure/flow ratio to higher frequencies, and phase angle is negative at low frequencies, indicating that flow leads pressure. There is a good agreement between characteristic impedance (Zc) measured at the average ratio of pressure and flow moduli at the highest frequencies, and as the early systolic slope of PAP as a function of Q.

physiologic or pathologic changes. The spectrum of PVZ is little affected by normal breathing (51), or by disease processes limited to alveolar or juxta-alveolar vessels (49). In contrast, proximal pulmonary arterial obstruction markedly affects pressure and flow wave morphology, the PVZ spectrum, and at any given PVR, has more important depressant effect on right ventricular output (52).

PVZ determinations have been reported until now in a few studies on patients with pulmonary hypertension secondary to mitral stenosis, congenital cardiac defects, congestive heart failure and COPD, and idiopathic pulmonary arterial hypertension (53). The general pattern has been that of an upwards shift of PVZ spectra, with the first minima and maxima of pressure/flow moduli shifted to higher frequencies. The limited number of available data has not allowed to identify specific patterns, and even less so the effects of therapeutic interventions. Semi-invasive approaches for the determination of PVZ with fluid-filled catheters and trans-thoracic Doppler have been reported in patients with idiopathic pulmonary arterial hypertension (54) and the results agree with those reported using high-fidelity technology (55). However, the method has not gained acceptance because of perceived mathematical complexity and reluctance of clinicians to give in to frequency-domain analysis.

A lately discovered characteristic of pulmonary vascular function has been the tight correlation between systolic, diastolic and mean PAP, which persists in pulmonary hypertension of all possible etiologies (56,57). Mean PAP (MPAP) can actually be calculated from systolic PAP (SPAP) using a simple formula (56):

$$MPAP = 0.6 \times SPAP + 2$$

This notion is of practical relevance as non-invasive evaluations of the pulmonary circulation in clinical practice often rely on the measurement of a maximum velocity of tricuspid regurgitation (TR) to calculate a SPAP using the

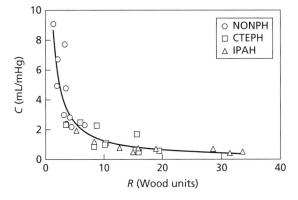

Figure 1.9 Hyperbolic relationship between pulmonary arterial resistance and compliance in patients with a normal pulmonary circulation (NONPH), with chronic thrombo-embolic pulmonary hypertension (CTEPH) and with idiopathic pulmonary arterial hypertension (IPAH). (From ref 59.)

simplified form of the Bernouilli equation and a measurement of RAP (58):

$$SPAP = (TR^2 + 4) + RAP$$

Tight relationships between pulmonary arterial pressures imply that the response of the pulmonary circulation to insults and diseases is more monotonous than previously assumed. Recent studies have indeed shown that the product of PVR by pulmonary arterial compliance (stroke volume divided by pulse pressure), or the time constant of the pulmonary circulation, remains constant at approximately 0.7 s in all circumstances (59,60). This is illustrated in Figure 1.9, which represents PVR and pulmonary artery compliance values from patients with pulmonary vasculopathies of various severities and origins. The hyperbolic relationship between compliance and resistance within the pulmonary circulation allows for the understanding that mild increases in PVR may already markedly increase right ventricular (RV) afterload because of associated proportionally more important decrease in compliance. Pharmacological decrease of mildly increased PVR may markedly improve RV flow output because of proportionally larger increase in compliance.

RIGHT VENTRICULO–ARTERIAL COUPLING

Instead of trying to quantify RV afterload by an estimate of hydraulic load from spectral analysis of pulmonary pressure and flow waves, it might be more realistic to quantify the coupling of RV function to the pulmonary circulation. Sunagawa *et al.* showed that this can be done graphically using a ventricular pressure–volume diagram (61). The diagram allows for the determination of maximal ventricular elastance (Emax), which is the best possible load-independent measurement of contractility, and of arterial elastance Ea as a measurement of afterload as it is "seen" by the ventricle, and the calculation of an Emax/Ea ratio as a measurement of the coupling of ventricular to arterial function. Complex mathematical modeling shows that the optimal matching of systolic ventricular and arterial elastances occurs at an Emax/Ea ratio around 1.5. Isolated increase in Ea, or decrease in Emax, decrease the Emax/Ea ratio, indicating uncoupling of the ventricle from its arterial system. Everything else being the same, a decrease in Emax/Ea is necessarily accompanied by a decrease in stroke volume. On the other hand, an isolated increase in preload is associated with an increase in stroke volume with unaltered ventriculo-arterial coupling.

However, the complex geometry of the RV makes functional evaluations with measurement of instantaneous volume changes technically difficult, and the determination of Emax may be unreliable because of the particular shape of the RV pressure–volume loop and non coincidence of end-ejection and end-systole. This problem can be overcome by measuring pressure–volume loops at several levels of preload (62), but bedside manipulations of venous return are too invasive to be ethically acceptable. In addition, when applied to intact beings, changes in venous return are associated with reflex sympathetic nervous system activation, which affects the ventricular function that is measured. These concerns have been addressed by a most recently reported single beat method allowing for a direct quantification of the coupling of the RV to the pulmonary circulation (63). The approach had been initially proposed for the left ventricle (64). In its principle, the method avoids absolute volume measurements and related technical complexities, to calculate Emax and Ea from instantaneous RV pressure and flow output measurements. As shown in Figure 1.10, a Pmax is estimated from a nonlinear extrapolation of the early and late systolic isovolumic portions of the right ventricular pressure curve. This estimated Pmax has been shown to be tightly correlated with Pmax directly measured during a non-ejecting beat (63). A straight line drawn from Pmax to the RV pressure

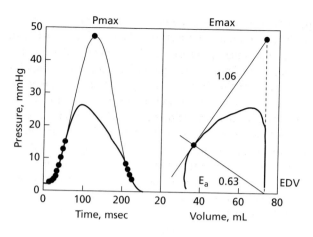

Figure 1.10 Single beat method to measure right ventriculo-arterial coupling. A maximum pressure (Pmax) is calculated from nonlinear extrapolation of early and late isovolemic portions of the right ventricular pressure curve. A straight line is drawn from the Pmax and end-diastolic volume (EDV) coordinate tangent to the pressure–volume curve to determine maximum, or end-systolic elastance (Ees), and from there, by a straight line to the zero pressure-EDV coordinate, arterial elastance (Ea).

versus relative change in volume curve allows for the determination of Emax. A straight line drawn from the Emax point to the end-diastolic relative volume point determines Ea.

The Emax/Ea ratio determined by this single beat method is around 1.5, which is similar to values reported for left ventricular-aortic coupling, and compatible with an optimal ratio of mechanical work to oxygen consumption (63). The Emax/Ea ratio is decreased by propranolol and increased by dobutamine, and maintained in the presence of increased Ea due to hypoxic pulmonary vasoconstriction. In fact, Emax increases adaptedly to increased Ea in hypoxia, even in the presence of adrenergic blockade, which is compatible with the notion of homeometric adaptation of right ventricular contractility. On the other hand, the approach allows for the demonstration that clinically relevant doses of dobutamine do not affect pulmonary arterial hydraulic load (63). The single beat approach has been used to show the superiority of dobutamine over norepinephrine to restore right ventriculo-arterial coupling in acute right heart failure produced by a brisk increase in pulmonary artery pressure (65), and the profound decoupling effects of inhaled anesthetics in the same setting (66), this being due to the devastating effects of both negative inotropy and pulmonary vasoconstriction. The method also showed that prostacyclin, at clinically relevant doses, has no intrinsic positive inotropic effect on the right ventricle (67).

Practically, all that is needed to determine single beat Emax/Ea ratios is measurements of instantaneous pulmonary blood flow and right ventricular pressure. This is feasible by echocardiography. Doppler pulmonary flow measurements synchronized to invasively measured pulmonary artery pressures have been reported to allow for realistic pulmonary arterial impedance calculations (54). Right ventricular pressure can be recalculated from the envelope of tricuspid regurgitant jets and point-by-point application of the simplified form of the Bernouilli equation (68). However, the entirely noninvasive Doppler echocardiographic determination of Emax/Ea ratios in patients has not yet been validated. Most recently, Kuehne *et al.* used magnetic resonance imaging (MRI) together with RV pressure measurements to generate pressure–volume loops and Emax and Ea determinations in patients with PAH (69). As compared to controls, RV Emax was increased from 5.2 ± 0.9 to $9.2 \pm 1.2\,\text{mmHg/mL/100\,g}$, $P < 0.05$, but RV Emax/Ea was decreased from 1.9 ± 0.4 to 1.1 ± 0.3, $P < 0.05$, indicating an increased RV contractility in response to increased afterload that was however insufficiently coupled to its hydraulic load, with inefficient mechanical work production.

KEY POINTS

- Pulmonary artery pressures are normally low, but increase passively with left atrial pressure and with pulmonary blood flow.
- There are no gender differences in pulmonary hemodynamics, provided pulmonary blood flow is corrected for body size.
- Pulmonary vascular resistance increases at high and at low pulmonary volumes, is minimal at functional residual capacity, and approximately doubles with aging.
- Pulmonary hypertension may be associated with an increase in pulmonary capillary filtration pressure, which is estimated from the analysis of the pulmonary arterial pressure decay curve after balloon occlusion.
- Gravity determines an increase in pulmonary blood flow from non-dependent to dependent lung regions.
- Hypoxic pulmonary vasoconstriction redistributes blood flow to better aerated lung areas, thereby limiting the hypoxemic effects of local decreases in ventilation/perfusion relationships.
- Right ventricular afterload can be calculated from a spectral analysis of pulmonary arterial pressure and flow waves.
- Pulmonary arterial resistance and compliance remain invariably coupled.
- The adequacy of the functional coupling of the right ventricle to the pulmonary circulation can be estimated by a ratio of end-systolic to arterial elastances.

REFERENCES

● = Key primary paper

●1. Swan HJC, Ganz W, Forrester JS, Marcus H, Diamond G, Chonette D. Catheterization of the heart in man with use of a flow-directed catheter. N Engl J Med 1970;283:447–51.
●2. West JB, Dollery CT, Naimark A. Distribution of blood flow in isolated lung: relation to vascular and alveolar pressures. J Appl Physiol 1964;19:713–24.
3. Naeije R, Mélot C, Mols P, Hallemans R. Effects of vasodilators on hypoxic pulmonary vasoconstriction in normal man. Chest 1982;82:404–10.
4. Mélot C, Naeije R, Hallemans R, Lejeune P, Mols P. Hypoxic pulmonary vasoconstriction and pulmonary gas exchange in normal man. Respir Physiol 1987;68:11–27.
5. Maggiorini M, Mélot C, Pierre S, Pfeiffer F, Greve I, Sartori C, Lepori M, Hauser M, Scherrer U, Naeije R. High altitude pulmonary edema is initially caused by an increased capillary pressure. Circulation 2001;103:2078–83.
6. Holmgren A, Jonsson B, Sjostrand T. Circulatory data in normal subjects at rest and during exercise in the recumbent position, with special reference to the stroke volume at different working intensities. Acta Physiol Scand 1960;49:343–63.
7. Granath A, Strandell T. Relationships between cardiac output, stroke volume, and intracardiac pressures at rest and during exercise in supine position and some anthropometric data in healthy old men. Acta Med Scand 1964;176:447–66.
8. Granath A, Jonsson B, Strandell T. Circulation in healthy old men, studied by right heart catheterization at rest and during exercise in supine and sitting position. Acta Med Scand 1964;176:425–46.
9. Bevegaard S, Holmgren A, Jonsson B. Circulatory studies in well trained athletes at rest and during heavy exercise, with special reference to stroke volume and the influence of body position. Acta Physiol Scand 1963;57:26–50.
●10. Reeves JT, Dempsey JA, Grover RF. Pulmonary circulation during exercise. In: Pulmonary Vascular Physiology and Physiopathology. Weir EK, Reeves JT, eds. New York: Marcel Dekker, 1989:107–133.
11. Naeije R, Mélot C, Niset G, Delcroix M, Wagner PD. Improved arterial oxygenation by a pharmacological increase in chemosensitivity during hypoxic exercise in normal subjects. J Appl Physiol 1993;74:1666–71.
12. Reeves JT, Groves BM, Cymerman A, Sutton JR, Wagner PD, Turkevich D, Houston CS. Operation Everest II: cardiac filling pressures during cycle exercise at sea level. Respir Physiol 1990;80:147–54.
●13. Gaar Jr KA, Taylor AE, Owens LJ, Guyton AC. Pulmonary capillary pressure and filtration coefficient in the isolated perfused lung. Am J Physiol 1967;213:910–914.
14. Dempsey JA, Wagner PD. Exercise-induced arterial hypoxemia. J Appl Physiol 1999;87:1997–2006.

15. Tolle JJ, Tolle JJ, Waxman AB, Van Horn TL, Pappagianopoulos PP, Systrom DM. Exercise-induced pulmonary arterial hypertension. Circulation 2008;118:2183–9.

●16. Zidulka A, Hakim TS. Wedge pressure in large vs small pulmonary arteries to detect pulmonary venoconstriction. J Appl Physiol 1985;59:1329–32.

●17. Cope DK, Grimbert F, Downey JM, Taylor AE. Pulmonary capillary pressure: a review. Crit Care Med 1992;20: 1043–56.

18. Hillier SC, Graham JA, Hanger CC, Godbey P, Glenny RW, Wagner WW. Hypoxic vasoconstriction in pulmonary arterioles and venules. J Appl Physiol 1997;82:1084–90.

19. Collee CG, Lynch KE, Hill D, Zapol WM. Bedside measurements of pulmonary capillary pressure in patients with acute respiratory failure. Anesthesiology 1987; 66:614–20.

20. Rossetti M, Guenard H, Gabinski C. Effects of nitric oxide on pulmonary serial resistances in ARDS. Am J Respir Crit Care Med 1996;154:1375–81.

21. Fesler P, Pagnamenta A, Vachiéry JL, Brimioulle S, Abdel Kafi S, Boonstra A, Delcroix M, Channink R, Rubin LJ, Naeije R. The occlusion method for the partitioning of pulmonary vascular resistance in severe pulmonary hypertension. Eur Respir 2003;21:1–7.

22. Kim NH, Fesler P, Channick RN, Knowlton KU, Ben-Yehuda O, Lee SH, Naeije R, Rubin LJ. Pre-operative partitioning of pulmonary vascular resistance correlates with early outcome following thromboendarterectomy for chronic thromboembolic pulmonary hypertension. Circulation 2004;109:18–22.

●23. Naeije R. Pulmonary vascular resistance: a meaningless variable? Intens Care Med 2003;29:526–9.

●24. Permutt S, Bromberger-Barnea B, Bane HN. Alveolar pressure, pulmonary venous pressure and the vascular waterfall. Med Thorac 1962;19:239–60.

25. Zhuang FY, Fung YC, Yen RT. Analysis of blood flow in cat's lung with detailed anatomical and elasticity data. J Appl Physiol 1983;55:1341–8.

26. Nelin LD, Krenz GS, Rickaby DA, Linehan JH, Dawson CA. A distensible vessel model applied to hypoxic pulmonary vasoconstriction in the neonatal pig. J Appl Physiol 1992;73:987–94.

27. Glazier JB, Hughes JMB, Maloney JE, West JB. Measurements of capillary dimensions and blood volume in rapidly frozen lungs. J Appl Physiol 1969;26:65–76.

●28. Mélot C, Delcroix M, Lejeune P, Leeman M, Naeije R. Starling resistor versus viscoelastic models for embolic pulmonary hypertension. Am J Physiol 1995;267 (Heart Circ Physiol 36):H817–27.

29. Janicki JS, Weber KT, Likoff MJ, Fishman AP. The pressure–flow response of the pulmonary circulation in patients with heart failure and pulmonary vascular disease. Circulation 1985;72:1270–78.

30. Kafi AS, Mélot C, Vachiéry JL, Brimioulle S, Naeije R. Partitioning of pulmonary vascular resistance in primary pulmonary hypertension. J Am Coll Cardiol 1998;31:1372–6.

31. Howell JBL, Permutt S, Proctor DF, Riley RL. Effect of inflation of the lung on different parts of the pulmonary vascular bed. J Appl Physiol 1961;16:71–76.

32. Hughes JM, Glazier JB, Maloney JR, West JB. Effect of lung volume on the distribution of pulmonary blood flow in man. Respir Physiol 1968;4:58–72.

33. Hakim TS, Lisbona R, Michel RP, Dean GW. Role of vasoconstriction in gravity-nondependent central-peripheral gradient in pulmonary blood flow. J Appl Physiol 1993;63:1114–21.

34. Glenny R. Counterpoint: gravity is not the major factor determining the distribution of blood flow in the healthy human lung. J Appl Physiol 2008;104:1533–5.

●35. Hughes M, West JB. Point: counterpoint: gravity is/is not the major factor determining the distribution of blood flow in the human lung. J Appl Physiol 2008;104: 1531–3.

●36. von Euler US, Liljestrand G. Observations on the pulmonary arterial blood pressure in the cat. Acta Physiol Scand 1946;12:301–20.

●37. Grover RF, Wagner WW, McMurtry IF, Reeves JT. Pulmonary Circulation. In: Handbook of Physiology. The Cardiovascular System. Peripheral Circulation and Organ Blood Flow. Bethesda MD: Am Physiol Soc, 1983, sect 2, vol III, part 1, Chap 4, pp. 103–36.

●38. Weir EK, Archer SL. The mechanism of acute hypoxic pulmonary vasoconstriction: the tale of two channels. FASEB J 1995;9:183–9.

39. Grant BJB. Effect of local pulmonary blood flow control on gas exchange: theory. J Appl Physiol: Respirat Environ Exercise Physiol 1982;53:1100–9.

●40. Brimioulle S, Lejeune P, Naeije R. Effects of hypoxic pulmonary vasoconstriction on gas exchange. J Appl Physiol 1996;81:1535–43.

41. Naeije R, Brimioulle S. Physiology in medicine: the importance of hypoxic pulmonary vasoconstriction in maintaining arterial oxygenation during acute lung injury. Crit Care 2001;5:67–71.

42. Sommer N, Dietrich A, Schermuly RT, Ghofrani HA, Gudermann T, Schulz R, Seeger W, Grimminger F, Weissmann N. Regulation of hypoxic pulmonary vasoconstriction: basic mechanisms. Eur Respir J 2008;32:1639–51.

43. Moudgil R, Michelakis ED, Archer SL. Hypoxic pulmonary vasoconstriction. J Appl Physiol 2005;98:390–403.

44. Waypa GB, Schumacker PT. Hypoxic pulmonary vasoconstriction: redox events in oxygen sensing. J Appl Physiol 2005;98:404–14.

45. Barnes PJ, Liu SF. Regulation of pulmonary vascular tone. Pharmacol Rev 1995;47:87–131.

46. Humbert M, Sitbon O, Simonneau G. Treatment of pulmonary arterial hypertension. N Engl J Med 2004; 351:1425–36.

●47. Downing SE, Lee JC. Nervous control of the pulmonary circulation. Ann Rev Physiol 1980;42:199–210.

48. Nichols WW, O'Rourke MF. In: McDonald's Blood Flow in Arteries, 4th edn, London: Edward Arnold, 1998.

•49. Elzinga G, Piene H, de Jong J.P. Left and right ventricular pump function and consequences of having two pumps in one heart. Circ Res 1980;46:564–74.

50. Furuno Y, Nagamoto Y, Fujita M, Kaku T, Sakurai S, Kuroiwa A. Reflection as a cause of mid-systolic deceleration of pulmonary flow wave in dogs with acute pulmonary hypertension: comparison of pulmonary artery constriction with pulmonary embolisation. Cardiovasc Res 1991;25:118–24.

51. Murgo JP, Westerhof N. Input impedance of the pulmonary arterial system in normal man: effects of respiration and comparison to systemic impedance. Circ Res 1984;54: 666–73.

52. Fitzpatrick JM, Grant BJB. Effects of pulmonary vascular obstruction on right ventricular afterload. Am Rev Respir Dis 1990;141:944–52.

53. Kussmaul WG, Noordergraaf A, Laskey WK. Right ventricular pulmonary arterial interactions. Ann Biomed Eng 1992;20:63–80.

54. Huez S, Brimioulle S, Naeije R, Vachiery JL. Feasibility of routine pulmonary arterial impedance measurements in pulmonary hypertension. Chest 2004;125:2121–8.

55. Laskey W, Ferrari V, Palevsky H, Kussmaul W. Pulmonary artery hemodynamics in primary pulmonary hypertension. J Am Coll Cardiol 1993;21:406–12.

•56. Chemla D, Castelain V, Humbert M, Hébert JL, Simonneau G, Lecarpentier Y, Hervé P. New formula for predicting mean pulmonary artery pressure using systolic pulmonary artery pressure. Chest 2004;126:1313–7.

57. Syyed R, Reeves JT, Welsh D, Raeside D, Johnson MK, Peacock AJ. The relationship between the components of pulmonary artery pressure remains constant under all conditions in both health and disease. Chest 2008; 133:633–9.

58. Yock P, Popp R. Noninvasive estimation of right ventricular systolic pressure by Doppler ultrasound in patients with tricuspid regurgitation. Circulation 1984;70:657–62.

•59. Lankhaar JW, Westerhof N, Faes TJ, Marques KM, Marcus JT, Postmus PE, Vonk-Noordegraaf A. Quantification of right ventricular afterload in patients with and without pulmonary hypertension. Am J Physiol Heart Circ Physiol 2006;291:H1731–7.

60. Lankhaar JW, Westerhof N, Faes TJ, Gan CT, Marques KM, Boonstra A, van den Berg FG, Postmus PE, Vonk-Noordegraaf A. Pulmonary vascular resistance and compliance stay inversely related during treatment of pulmonary hypertension. Eur Heart J 2008;29:1688–95.

61. Sagawa K, Maughan L, Suga H, Sunagawa K. Cardiac Contraction and the Pressure-volume Relationship. New York: Oxford University Press, 1988.

62. Maughan WL. Shoukas AA, Sagawa K, Weisfeldt ML. Instantaneous pressure–volume relationship of the canine right ventricle. Circ Res 1979;44:309–315.

•63. Brimioulle S, Wauthy P, Ewalenko P, Rondelet B, Vermeulen F, Kerbaul F, Naeije R. Single-beat estimation of right ventricular end-systolic pressure–volume relationship. Am J Physiol Heart Circ Physiol 2003;284:H1625–30.

64. Sunagawa K, Yamada A, Senda Y, Kikuchi Y, Nakamura M, Shibahara T. Estimation of the hydromotive source pressure from ejecting beats of the left ventricle. IEEE Trans Biomed Eng 1980;57:299–305.

65. Kerbaul F, Rondelet B, Motte S, Fesler P, Hubloue I, Ewalenko P, Brimioulle S, Naeije R. Effects of norepinephrine and dobutamine on pressure load-induced right ventricular failure. Crit Care Med 2004;32:1035–40.

66. Kerbaul F, Rondelet B, Motte S, Fesler P, Hubloue I, Ewalenko P, Naeije R, Brimioulle SI. Isoflurane and desflurane impair right ventricular–pulmonary arterial coupling in dogs. Anesthesiology 2004;101:1357–61.

67. Kerbaul F, Brimioulle S, Rondelet B, Dewachter C, Hubloue I, Naeije R. How prostacyclin improves cardiac output in right heart failure in conjunction with pulmonary hypertension. Am J Respir Crit Care Med 2007;175: 846–50.

68. Ensing G, Seward J, Darragh R, Caldwell R. Feasibility of generating hemodynamic pressure curves from noninvasive Doppler echocardiographic signals. J Am Coll Cardiol 1994;23:434–42.

•69. Kuehne T, Yilmaz S, Steendijk P, Moore P, Groenink M, Saaed M, Weber O, Higgins CB, Ewert P, Fleck E, Nagel E, Schulze-Neick I, Lange P. Magnetic resonance imaging analysis of right ventricular pressure–volume loops: in vivo validation and clinical application in patients with pulmonary hypertension. Circulation 2004;110:2010–6.

2

Right heart function

ANNA R HEMNES AND HUNTER C CHAMPION

INTRODUCTION

Sir William Harvey deduced the purpose of the right ventricle in his seminal treatise published in 1628, "the right ventricle may be said to be made for the sake of transmitting blood through the lungs, not for nourishing them" (1). Since his remarkable observation, much research has focused on the pulmonary vasculature to which the right heart is inextricably linked, the right ventricle's response to stress, ventricular interdependence and, more recently, the unique anatomy, physiology and molecular biology that facilitate this critical function. Advances in treatment of pulmonary hypertension have brought about increased interest in understanding the function or dysfunction of the right heart in health and disease, which has in turn led to an upsurge in research in this pump for the "lesser circulation."

Although pulmonary hypertension (PH) is defined by pulmonary artery pressure, it is characterized by right heart failure in its advanced stages. Indeed, the most important predictors of mortality from pulmonary arterial hypertension (PAH) include right atrial pressure and cardiac output (2), not merely pulmonary artery pressure alone. Furthermore, several of the drugs commonly used to treat PAH appear to affect the right ventricle (RV) as well as the pulmonary vasculature, suggesting that direct myocardial effects of pharmacologic intervention are likely a critical force behind the clinical improvements seen after drug administration (3–5). While much attention has been paid to the pulmonary vasculature and basic mechanisms underlying pulmonary arterial dysfunction in PAH, relatively little is known about the RV in health or in disease

(6,7). In this chapter we will review the normal structure and function of the right heart, discuss clinical presentation of right ventricular dysfunction as well as evaluation and management of right heart failure.

DEFINITIONS

Normal right ventricle

Long considered merely a conduit for blood flow to the left ventricle, the RV has recently been noted to be an important component of normal cardiopulmonary function. Understanding the pathology of the RV requires consideration of the normal structure and unique capacities of this cardiac structure. Both cardiac chambers have the same cardiac output – thus the same flow occurs in the pulmonary and systemic circulations. The RV has the capacity to accommodate marked increases in flow without substantial morphologic changes or afterload increases due to pulmonary vascular recruitment and distention (8,9). However, in contrast to the left ventricle where the primary goal of systole is to generate sufficient pressure to perfuse the high resistance circuit of the systemic vasculature, the RV has a much lower afterload in the normal state, as pulmonary vascular resistance is approximately one tenth that of the systemic bed and thus force generation is less important (10). This observation suggests the underlying explanation for the most obvious difference between right and left ventricles – their size. The free wall of the RV is a thin-walled triangular structure, compared with the more muscularized left ventricle (Figure 2.1).

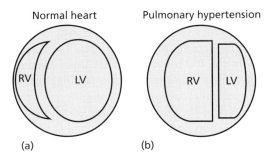

Figure 2.1 Structural relationship of right and left ventricle. Geometric shape of the left ventricle (LV) and right ventricle (RV) under conditions of normal RV pressures (a) and in pulmonary hypertension (b) in the short axis view. Schematic depicts the difference in the shape of the RV under normal RV pressures and with pulmonary hypertension such that the overall shape of the RV is more conductive to traditional measures of Ees and Ea.

In addition, unlike the cylindrical left ventricle, the RV is crescent shaped in cross-section under normal conditions with a concave septum. These anatomic differences translate into a much greater compliance in the RV. The volume of the right ventricle is larger than that of the left ventricle in the adult, though the muscle mass is only approximately one sixth the mass of the left ventricle (11). RV contraction occurs through muscle fiber shortening along the longitudinal axis with inward movement of the free wall and traction at the insertion of the RV free wall to the LV (12). Twisting and rotation movements are not as important to the RV contraction when compared to the left ventricle (12). Despite these important differences, the right and left ventricles share a pericardial sac and the interventricular septum, thus pathology in one ventricle not infrequently influences the function and hemodynamics of the other given the appropriate conditions.

Right ventricular chamber function is determined by preload, afterload and contractility. Preload, or the load present before contraction, is a measure of right ventricular filling. Under normal filling conditions, an increase in preload results in improved contractility and increased cardiac output (12). Because of its thin wall and connection to the systemic veins, RV filling is influenced to a greater degree by the negative pressure of normal inspiration than is the left ventricle. Other factors important to RV filling are ventricular chamber compliance which is much greater than the LV, heart rate, LV filling and the pericardium (13). RV afterload is primarily a function of pulmonary vascular resistance, though it can be substantially affected by valvular or intracardiac lesions. As described below, the RV has a limited ability to compensate for increased afterload. Finally, contractility in the RV can be studied using the same pressure volume loops used to understand left ventricular contractility and it has been shown that the RV also follows a time-varying elastance model (14,15). The relationship of these three variables is the primary determinant of right ventricular function in any given circumstance.

Right ventricular failure

The right ventricle's interaction with the pulmonary circulation is the primary determinant of right ventricular function or dysfunction. Right heart failure can be simply defined by an inability for the ventricle to pump sufficient blood to meet the needs of the systemic circulation; this can occur as a result of an inability to fill or to eject blood (12). As cardiac output is the same in both left and right ventricles, right heart failure necessarily causes left heart failure and, if advanced, can result in insufficient oxygen delivery to systemic beds. In general, chronic right heart failure is characterized by progressive enlargement of the right ventricle with hypertrophy, dilation or both, diminished ejection fraction and associated tricuspid enlargement and regurgitation (7,16). Right ventricular dysfunction refers to abnormal function of the right ventricle without requirement for symptoms or signs of heart failure (12). Specific pathophysiologies and their accompanying anatomic and physiologic changes will be discussed below.

INCIDENCE AND EPIDEMIOLOGY

While right heart dysfunction is nearly universal in significant pulmonary hypertension, right heart failure is not. Not all patients with pulmonary hypertension develop RV failure and mild PAH may not have yet resulted in RV dysfunction. For example, often patients with Eisenmenger's syndrome have preserved cardiac function despite sustained increases in pulmonary resistance compared with patients with idiopathic PAH (17). Alternatively, underlying diseases, such as scleroderma or sarcoidosis, that predispose to PAH might also affect the heart itself and diminish cardiac compensation thereby predisposing to earlier and more severe heart failure (18). Nonetheless, right heart failure nearly always accompanies advanced PAH (2) and it is a common finding in end-stage left heart failure, affecting 25–50 percent of patients (19,20). Research is ongoing to determine further risk factors for RV failure.

ETIOLOGY

Right heart failure commonly occurs in the context of pulmonary vascular pathology as this bed is the primary determinant of right ventricular afterload. However, primary right ventricular dysfunction and failure can occur without pulmonary vascular disease, e.g. primary cardiomyopathies (idiopathic, amyloidosis, myocarditis, etc.) may affect right ventricular myocardium either in isolation or in addition to the left ventricle, right ventricular ischemia can cause isolated right heart failure and severe pulmonic stenosis can result in right ventricular dysfunction. We will focus on right heart failure in association with pulmonary vascular disease. The right heart's response to pulmonary vascular disease is determined by the tempo of load stress development.

Acute pulmonary hypertension

An acute increase in afterload, as exemplified by a large pulmonary embolism, causes dilation in the compliant RV. Indeed, this acutely challenged structure is only capable of generating a maximum pressure of approximately 40–60 mmHg (21). Despite any further obstruction of the vascular bed, i.e. increased afterload from further thromboembolism, the RV cannot increase systolic pressure further, subsequently fails and cardiac output drops (22) (Figure 2.2). In addition, during the initial rise in afterload, increased RV end diastolic volume preserves cardiac output, as predicted by the Frank–Starling relationship. However, remembering the shared pericardial sac and interventricular septum, there is limited space for the RV and right atrium to dilate without impinging on the left ventricle and left atrium, respectively. Thus, ultimately, further increases in the right heart volume can result in diminished left ventricular filling and further drops in cardiac output (21). In patients with pulmonary hypertension and an absence of intrinsic left heart disease, diminished LV filling and a subsequent increase in pulmonary capillary wedge pressure is secondary to impingement of the left atrium by the right atrium. This phenomenon is not often observed clinically outside the intensive care unit when RV failure is a primary mode of death.

Chronic pulmonary hypertension

Given the extended period during which PAH arises, the chronic increase in RV afterload results in right-sided hypertrophy (23). Over time contractile dysfunction ensues and

preload must increase, along with ventricular end diastolic volume, in order to maintain cardiac output according to the Frank–Starling relationship (24). These structural changes in the RV contribute to tricuspid regurgitation through annular dilatation and the resulting inability of the tricuspid leaflets to coapt appropriately. As a final common pathway of these changes, filling pressures rise, diastolic dysfunction develops in the RV, and cardiac output drops, characterizing right heart failure (25).

These structural and functional changes in the RV translate into measurable differences on right heart catheterization. While pulmonary hypertension is defined by a mean pulmonary artery pressure of > 25 mmHg at rest and PAH requires the same findings with a normal (< 15 mmHg) pulmonary artery occlusion pressure, right heart dysfunction may have varying findings on right heart catheterization. While diminished cardiac output and cardiac index are the hallmark of right heart dysfunction, a drop in pulmonary arterial saturation is often found. Additionally, when heart failure advances, rising central venous pressure is frequently noted. Occasionally, the massively volume overloaded right heart can impinge on left ventricular filling as described above (Figure 2.3). In this circumstance, an elevated pulmonary artery occlusion pressure is a rare finding most often observed under conditions of severe right heart failure. This increase in PCW must be discriminated from the more common reason of elevation of pulmonary capillary wedge pressure, i.e. left-sided valvular lesions or systolic or diastolic dysfunction.

Underlying molecular mechanisms driving pathologic remodeling and hemodynamic dysfunction are beginning to be studied in right heart failure. In addition to well-described roles in left heart failure, sympathetic adrenergic stimulation and the rennin–angiotensin–aldosterone system have been shown to play a role in experimental models of right heart failure (26,27). More recent work suggests a role for the nitric oxide pathway and PDE5 inhibition in

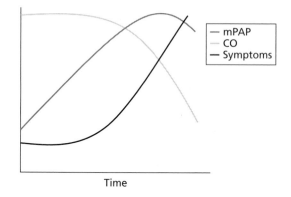

Figure 2.2 Relationship of right ventricular output reserve and symptoms in pulmonary vascular disease. Cardiac output shown in resting state (solid line) and in exercise (broken dash line) showing the inability to increase cardiac output in exercise, thereby diminishing physiologic capacity, ultimately to below life sustaining levels. In PAH, cardiac reserve, represented by the difference between the solid and the broken dashed lines, diminishes as disease progresses and symptoms become more prominent with lower activity levels such that ultimately patients are symptomatic at rest prior to reaching the lowest life-sustaining cardiac output (dotted line).

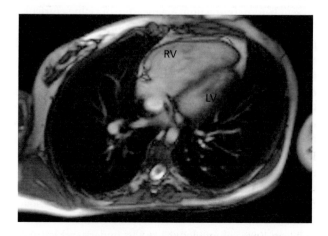

Figure 2.3 Cardiac MR image in a patient with idiopathic PAH. The right ventricle (RV) is enlarged and impinging on the underfilled left ventricle (LV). The septum appears bowed toward the LV, suggesting pressure overload of the RV.

attenuation of right ventricular dysfunction associated with load stress (5,28).

CLINICAL PRESENTATION

Right heart failure has a fairly stereotypical clinical presentation, however, the history and physical examination can also provide important clues as to the underlying etiology of this ailment. Regardless of the cause of right heart failure, symptoms of dyspnea, exertional syncope and palpitations often suggest decreased cardiac output, while lower extremity edema and ascites imply increased preload and right heart failure. The presence of orthopnea and paroxysms of nocturnal dyspnea should raise the suspicion for elevated left heart filling pressures. Rheumatologic history or symptoms or predisposing drug exposure may point the clinician in the direction of PAH, while a history of childhood murmur or activity limitation may suggest structural heart disease. Finally, exertional chest pain in the predisposed individual may prompt concern for ischemic heart disease, although increases in left atrial pressure with exertion can also lead to anginal symptoms. History and physical examination in PH evaluation is reviewed elsewhere. Physical examination may show RV heave or right-sided gallop with or without elevated jugular venous pressure, ascites, peripheral edema, or evidence of poor systemic perfusion with cool extremities and decreased pulse volume (29). Again, clues to etiology can be found by the presence of crackles that may suggest either parenchymal lung disease or elevated left heart filling pressures. A pulmonic ejection sound may suggest a stenotic valve. In advanced right heart failure, cardiogenic shock ensues which may be difficult to differentiate at the bedside from advanced left heart failure.

INVESTIGATIONS

While chest radiography, either computed tomogram or plain radiograph, may show right heat size in addition to visualization of the pulmonary arteries, neither allows functional assessment of the RV. Echocardiography and, more recently, cardiac MRI have been used to confirm the clinical suspicion of RV dysfunction. Both imaging modalities are non-invasive, however they each have unique assets that may make them more suitable to different clinical presentations.

Echocardiography

Echocardiography is the most commonly used assessment of RV structure and function, primarily due to its widespread availability and ease of viewing the right ventricle in most patients. In right heart dysfunction and failure regardless of cause, echocardiography frequently shows an enlarged right atrium and ventricle with tricuspid regurgitation. The tricuspid regurgitant jet is generally used to estimate RV systolic pressure via the Bernoulli equation, and formulae for estimating mean pulmonary artery pressure from the RV systolic pressure have been developed (30,31). When investigating potential etiologies of right heart dysfunction through echocardiography it is critical to consider the pitfalls in estimated systolic pressure. There are conflicting data as to the strength of correlation of RV systolic pressure and mean pulmonary artery pressure when measured via right heart catheterization. When RV and pulmonary artery pressures are estimated via echocardiography they more often are higher than the pressures measured directly by catheterization. Therefore, it cannot be recommended for use as the gold standard for diagnosis of pulmonary hypertension, but remains an excellent screening modality (32–34). Furthermore, the degree of regurgitation or jet velocity have not been shown to correlate with survival as invasive hemodynamic data have (35–38), which could be predicted from the clinical observation that a severely compromised RV is incapable of generating high systolic pressure. This finding in advanced disease could not be differentiated by tricuspid jet velocity from mild pulmonary hypertension when the RV systolic pressure alone is used to evaluate the possible presence of pulmonary hypertension. Evaluation of the position and curvature of the interventricular septum can provide important information on RV afterload, as it generally bows into the left ventricle during diastole when afterload is increased (39).

RV dysfunction and hypertrophy may be difficult to quantitate on echocardiography (40) because of the operator and acoustic window differences that determine image quality. However, when present, these findings can provide important information about cardiac effects of chronic pressure overload. Three-dimensional echocardiography can give accurate estimates of RV ejection fraction as well as structure and function, however, this technique is not currently widely available at this time (41). Great attention has recently been paid to alternative measures of RV function. The Tei index yields a computed value that combines Doppler-derived RV systolic and diastolic function to assess quantitatively RV function (42). However, this method requires a complex calculation and is not generally available to clinicians. More recently, tricuspid annular plane systolic excursion (TAPSE), as a marker of RV ejection fraction, has been shown to be an important prognostic marker in pulmonary arterial hypertension (43). This measurement can be made on standard echocardiography using either M-mode or 2D echo and is therefore widely available. Given the ready availability of M-mode and 2D echo, TAPSE may prove to be the most useful marker of RV function that is available to the broadest population of practitioners.

In addition to giving clues about pulmonary artery pressure, echocardiography can be useful in evaluating other structural lesions that may be associated with right heart failure. Contrast-enhanced echocardiography is critical for evaluating potential intracardiac shunt and may suggest congenital heart disease (39). Similarly, pulmonic stenosis is easily visualized on echocardiography and transvalvular gradients may be calculated. When right ventricular systolic pressure is not elevated and structural disease is not identified, consideration for a primary disorder of the right heart should be given.

Cardiac MR

There have been major advances in cardiac magnetic resonance (CMR) techniques in the last several years that have contributed significantly to knowledge of and care for patients with right heart dysfunction. In particular, ECG gating and respiratory suppression have markedly diminished imaging artifacts and allowed for computations of stroke volume and RV wall structure and function. Active research in CMR is underway that will undoubtedly change how we understand and image the RV in the next decade. Currently, limited availability of the technology and few cardiologists trained in its interpretation restrict widespread use of this imaging technique. CMR is safe, with the primary challenge being claustrophobia (44), however other implanted devices may also not be MR compatible thereby limiting its use. Currently pumps for chronic infusion of PAH medications (e.g. epoprostenol and treprostenil) are not MR compatible (45). Tubing for infusion pumps can be extended to allow for CMR in specialized centers, but this should only be handled by those well trained in PH therapy and the use of infusion pumps.

Because it allows visualization of cardiac structures along with flow, CMR is particularly well suited to evaluate suspected or known congenital heart disease with suspected associated pulmonary arterial hypertension. However, other applications have been studied. Given the challenges with RV free wall visualization and right ventricular ejection fraction measurement on echocardiography, this has been an area of intense interest in CMR. There has been conflicting data on the value of RV mass as a predictor of mean pulmonary artery pressure, with the largest and most recent trial showing a modest correlation between RV mass and mean pulmonary artery pressure (46). The complex endocardial structure of the RV can be well visualized in CMR and, when combined with ECG gating, RV ejection fraction can be calculated by subtracting the RV end diastolic volume from the RV end systolic volume. However, interstudy reproducibility of this calculation has been questioned and the calculated value often is markedly higher than the measured (47). This discrepancy between CMR-based RV ejection fraction and stroke volume when compared to catheter-based measures often rests in the difference between stroke volume and effective forward stroke volume. As tricuspid regurgitation increases relative hypercontractility of the RV ensues with more of the stroke volume being ejected into the RA. This is analogous to the left ventricle under conditions of mitral regurgitation in which the left ventricular ejection fraction may be very high, but the effective stroke volume that crosses the aortic valve is greatly reduced since much of the stroke volume is flowing retrograde into the left atrium (48). Finally, CMR measurements of the RV have not been used routinely as trial endpoints or studied as predictors of mortality in PAH and there is limited data regarding the effects of drug therapy on CMR parameters (46,49,50).

Like echocardiography, CMR may suggest underlying etiology of right heart failure including when pulmonary artery pressures are not evidently elevated. RV fibrosis via CMR in Eisenmenger's syndrome has been shown, suggesting this may be an important marker of RV remodeling and dysfunction in the setting of elevated pulmonary artery pressures (51). In arrhythmogenic cardiomyopathy CMR findings can include myocardial fat accumulation, ectasia of the RV outflow tract and regional RV wall motion abnormalities in addition to RV dilation (52–54). Overall, the cost and limited availability of CMR combined with the insufficient data using CMR as an endpoint in clinical trials of PAH, make this imaging modality an important research tool that is not yet ready as routine recommendation in PAH evaluation or management. However, it plays an important clinical role in evaluating unconfirmed cases of structural heart disease and in arrhythmogenic right ventricular cardiomyopathy. As the technique continues to improve, it does hold promise for future general clinical utility and may reduce the number of invasive procedures in which a patient must participate.

Right heart catheterization

Despite advances in imaging techniques, cardiac catheterization remains the gold standard for diagnosing pulmonary hypertension, assessing disease severity and determining prognosis and response to therapy. The persistence of this technique is in part due to its ability to measure RV function. By directly measuring pressures and indirectly measuring flow, right heart catheterization allows for determination of prognostic markers such as right atrial pressure, cardiac output and mean pulmonary artery pressure (2). Importantly, this procedure has been shown to be safe, with no deaths reported in the NIH registry study (2) and a recent study showing a procedure related mortality of 0.055 percent (55). Specifics of right heart catheterization will be discussed in a separate chapter.

Aside from differentiating PAH from PVH and establishing the presence of pulmonary hypertension, the right heart catheterization can provide essential information regarding patient prognosis through measurement of right heart function. In the original NIH registry, an mPAP > 55 mmHg, right atrial pressure > 20 mmHg or a cardiac index < 2.0 L/min/m^2 has the poorest survival, generally less than 12 months (2). Additionally, pulmonary arterial oxygen saturation has been shown to be a strong predictor of poor outcomes (56). Right atrial pressure, cardiac index and pulmonary arterial saturation measure right heart function, and these data clearly show that it is primarily the response of the RV to afterload that determines prognosis in this disease. It is important to note that in advanced PAH, the mPAP may in fact fall as the right heart fails and is unable to generate a stroke volume to maintain the mPAP. When this occurs, the cardiac index and pulmonary artery saturation invariably fall as well. This finding highlights the importance of RV functional assessment, not just assessment of mPAP on right heart catheterization.

MANAGEMENT

Treatment of right heart failure

Despite its critical role in determining morbidity and survival in pulmonary hypertension from many causes, the RV has not been a pharmaceutical target in this disease and there has been little research on therapies aimed at improving right ventricular function. In advanced left heart failure, there is a good body of literature regarding inotropic stimulation and improvements in right ventricular function; however, discussion of this is outside the scope of this chapter.

The RV in pulmonary hypertension has been an afterthought, at best, in pharmaceutical targeting for this disease. Nonetheless, several of the medications routinely used in the management of pulmonary hypertension have effects on the RV, whose alteration may account for at least part of the therapeutic benefit. Of note, intravenous epoprostenol has been shown to improve RV function (3,57). Similarly, bosentan, an oral endothelin receptor antagonist, has been shown to improve RV systolic function and left ventricular diastolic function in patients with pulmonary arterial hypertension (4). Sildenafil, a phosphodiesterase 5 inhibitor, has been shown in patients with pulmonary arterial hypertension to decrease RV mass and cardiac index (58). Moreover, there is a mounting basic science body of evidence to support this observation (5,59–61). Additionally, calcium channel blockers have shown improvements in cardiac index in patients with long-term response to these medications (62). Improvement in the Frank–Starling relationship can also be achieved with simple diuresis of the severely volume-overloaded RV. In end-stage disease, pericardial effusions may occur which have a poor prognosis. Large, hemodynamically significant effusions have been reported and drainage of these effusions has been associated with a high mortality. Simple diuresis may optimize RV function as described above and limit left ventricular impingement without excess risk exposure (63). Finally, surgical therapy for RV failure, including pulmonary thromboendarterectomy, correction of congenital lesions and lung transplantation, have been shown to improve cardiac function and may eliminate tricuspid insufficiency (64–67).

There has been some interest in using inotropes to augment RV function in advanced PAH and in end-stage left heart failure. There is minimal data on traditional inotropes such as dobutamine and dopamine in treatment of advanced PAH-associated right heart failure (68–73). The acute effects of dopamine have been shown to increase cardiac output without an increase in pulmonary vascular resistance in humans with PAH (73). Similar findings are reported with dobutamine (69,70), though the total number of patients described with either of these drug therapies is 11 and 28, respectively. Chronic inotrope infusion is not yet reported to our knowledge, though in our experience a more prolonged infusion of dopamine may be useful as a bridge to lung transplantation in patients with refractory right heart failure in PAH. Recently, levosimendan, a calcium channel sensitizer that acts as an inotrope, has been studied in animal models of RV failure where it has been shown that RV-pulmonary artery coupling was improved by levosimendan more than dobutamine via improvements in RV contractility (68,73). While this drug shows promise, human data are needed before its use can be recommended.

Follow-up evaluation of the RV

Despite the importance of the RV in determining survival in PAH, there are no current recommendations regarding frequency or modality of follow-up assessment after initiation of treatment. For patients doing well, general recommendations include annual right heart catheterization to objectively confirm this clinical impression and to determine if right heart performance could be optimized by more aggressive therapy. Patients who are doing poorly may require right heart catheterization sooner, often in conjunction with echocardiography. An incremental improvement in six-minute walk test has not been shown to correlate with a specific hemodynamic improvement yet and therefore this exercise test should not be the only functional assessment of the patient undergoing treatment for PAH.

COMPLICATIONS

Right heart failure is characterized by progressive dyspnea and eventually as cardiac output falls, by exertional syncope. Fluid accumulation with ascites and peripheral edema is nearly universal in end-stage right heart failure. Eventually, if treatment of underlying conditions is not successful, progressive right heart failure is generally fatal. Most commonly progressive hypotension proves to be the mode of exit, though sudden death is not uncommon and, as described above, hypoxemia due to left ventricular impingement and impaired pulmonary venous drainage may also prove fatal (2).

FUTURE DIRECTIONS

Pulmonary vascular impedance

In addition to the static data that is available on right heart catheterization, there is active research measuring the pulsatile properties of this vascular bed and how they are affected by PAH and interact with right heart function. Pulmonary hypertension affects the proximal, or elastic, pulmonary arteries as well as the distal, or resistive, pulmonary vasculature. Pulmonary afterload comprises resistance both to steady and pulsatile flow and can be represented by the pulmonary artery input impedance spectrum. In addition to the steady state standard hemodynamics, this function incorporates data about the effects of pulse wave reflection and may be able to aid in understanding the determinants of RV failure in PAH. Pulmonary artery impedance has been studied in patients with PAH where it was found to be elevated compared with controls at rest and the extent of wave reflection was greater in PAH patients than controls (74). Previously, difficulty in obtaining instantaneous pressure and flow measurements by a high-fidelity, manometer tipped catheter limited study in this area (74,75), however modern technical advances have made such catheters available now, sparking new interest in this area. Recently, the feasibility of obtaining these measurements during routine right heart catheterization has been shown and it has been found that impedance can be altered with standard PAH medication administration (76,77). Others have studied pulmonary vascular impedance in the pediatric population where it was found to predict outcomes better than pulmonary vascular resistance (78). Impedance, in combination with compliance and resistance have been studied using MR technology and shown that these techniques may differentiate different types of pulmonary hypertension (79). The study of pulmonary vascular impedance will hopefully yield important information about the RV response to stress in pulmonary hypertension and may prove to be a more predictive measure of prognosis and response to treatment than current standards.

Pressure–volume loops and PET

Other areas that hold promise for better measures of RV function in the future include pressure–volume loop analysis and PET scan of the RV (80–82). Pressure–volume loops have long been used to evaluate left ventricular function, but recently they have been explored both by classic *in vivo* hemodynamics and by CMR as a marker of RV contractility where feasibility has been shown in both modalities (80). This may prove to be an important mode of assessing RV function. Animal models have shown that [^{18}F]Fluorodeoxyglucose uptake is altered in left ventricular dysfunction (81). Recently the RV has been explored in humans, where it has been found that [^{18}F]Fluorodeoxyglucose uptake is increased in correlation with RV load

severity and that this can be decreased with epoprostenol administration (82).

KEY POINTS

- The RV under normal circumstances is a high flow conduit for blood into the low resistance pulmonary circulation.
- The RV has a limited ability to compensate for acute rises in afterload, but chronically can achieve near systemic systolic pressure through hypertrophy and conformational changes.
- Right heart failure presents with symptoms of fluid accumulation such as edema and ascites often in combination with symptoms of poor flow, such as exertional dyspnea and syncope.
- Functional assessment of the RV with imaging including echocardiography and possibly CMR is greatly enhanced by the right heart catheterization.
- Future study of impedance catheters and PET scanning may aid in care of patients with right heart failure in the future.
- Many of the medications currently used to treat pulmonary arterial hypertension may have direct effects on the right ventricle and account, at least in part, for the improvement seen with these medications.

REFERENCES

♦ = Major review article

1. Harvey W. Exercitatio Anatomica de Motu Cordis et Sanguinis in Animalibus, 1628.
2. D'Alonzo GE, Barst RJ, Ayres SM *et al.* Survival in patients with primary pulmonary hypertension. Results from a national prospective registry. Ann Intern Med 1991;115(5):343–9.
3. Kisch-Wedel H, Kemming G, Meisner F *et al.* The prostaglandins epoprostenol and iloprost increase left ventricular contractility in vivo. Intensive Care Med 2003;29(9):1574–83.
4. Galie N, Hinderliter AL, Torbicki A *et al.* Effects of the oral endothelin-receptor antagonist bosentan on echocardiographic and Doppler measures in patients with pulmonary arterial hypertension. J Am Coll Cardiol 2003;41(8):1380–6.
5. Hemnes AR, Zaiman A, Champion HC. PDE5A inhibition attenuates bleomycin-induced pulmonary fibrosis and pulmonary hypertension through inhibition of ROS generation and RhoA/Rho kinase activation. Am J Physiol Lung Cell Mol Physiol 2008;294(1):L24–33.
6. Bristow MR, Zisman LS, Lowes BD *et al.* The pressure-overloaded right ventricle in pulmonary hypertension. Chest 1998;114(1 Suppl):101S–106S.

◆7. Voelkel NF, Quaife RA, Leinwand LA *et al.* Right ventricular function and failure: report of a National Heart, Lung, and Blood Institute working group on cellular and molecular mechanisms of right heart failure. Circulation 2006; 114(17):1883–91.

8. Epstein SE, Beiser GD, Stampfer M, Robinson BF, Braunwald E. Characterization of the circulatory response to maximal upright exercise in normal subjects and patients with heart disease. Circulation 1967;35(6):1049–62.

9. Damato AN, Galante JG, Smith WM. Hemodynamic response to treadmill exercise in normal subjects. J Appl Physiol 1966;21(3):959–66.

10. Grossman WBE. Pulmonary Hypertension, 3 edn. Philadelphia: Saunders, 1988. (E B, ed. Heart Disease: A Textbook of Cardiovascular Medicine).

11. Lorenz CH, Walker ES, Morgan VL, Klein SS, Graham TP, Jr. Normal human right and left ventricular mass, systolic function, and gender differences by cine magnetic resonance imaging. J Cardiovasc Magn Reson 1999;1(1):7–21.

◆12. Haddad F, Doyle R, Murphy DJ, Hunt SA. Right ventricular function in cardiovascular disease, part II: pathophysiology, clinical importance, and management of right ventricular failure. Circulation 2008;117(13):1717–31.

13. Burgess MI, Mogulkoc N, Bright-Thomas RJ, Bishop P, Egan JJ, Ray SG. Comparison of echocardiographic markers of right ventricular function in determining prognosis in chronic pulmonary disease. J Am Soc Echocardiogr 2002;15(6):633–9.

14. Brown KA, Ditchey RV. Human right ventricular end-systolic pressure–volume relation defined by maximal elastance. Circulation 1988;78(1):81–91.

15. Dell'Italia LJ, Walsh RA. Application of a time varying elastance model to right ventricular performance in man. Cardiovasc Res 1988;22(12):864–74.

16. Quaife RA, Lynch D, Badesch DB *et al.* Right ventricular phenotypic characteristics in subjects with primary pulmonary hypertension or idiopathic dilated cardiomyopathy. J Card Fail 1999;5(1):46–54.

17. Hopkins WE, Ochoa LL, Richardson GW, Trulock EP. Comparison of the hemodynamics and survival of adults with severe primary pulmonary hypertension or Eisenmenger syndrome. J Heart Lung Transplant 1996; 15(1 Pt 1):100–5.

18. Champion HC. The heart in scleroderma. Rheum Dis Clin North Am 2008;34(1):181–90; viii.

19. Abramson SV, Burke JF, Kelly JJ, Jr. *et al.* Pulmonary hypertension predicts mortality and morbidity in patients with dilated cardiomyopathy. Ann Intern Med 1992;116(11): 888–95.

20. Enriquez-Sarano M, Rossi A, Seward JB, Bailey KR, Tajik AJ. Determinants of pulmonary hypertension in left ventricular dysfunction. J Am Coll Cardiol 1997;29(1):153–9.

21. Molloy WD, Lee KY, Girling L, Schick U, Prewitt RM. Treatment of shock in a canine model of pulmonary embolism. Am Rev Respir Dis 1984;130(5):870–4.

22. Schulman DS, Matthy RA. The right ventricle in pulmonary disease. Cardiol Clin 1992;10(1):111–35.

23. Dias CA, Assad RS, Caneo LF *et al.* Reversible pulmonary trunk banding. II. An experimental model for rapid pulmonary ventricular hypertrophy. J Thorac Cardiovasc Surg 2002;124(5):999–1006.

24. Spann JF, Jr., Covell JW, Eckberg DL, Sonnenblick EH, Ross J, Jr., Braunwald E. Contractile performance of the hypertrophied and chronically failing cat ventricle. Am J Physiol 1972;223(5):1150–7.

25. Chen EP, Craig DM, Bittner HB, Davis RD, Van Trigt P. Pharmacological strategies for improving diastolic dysfunction in the setting of chronic pulmonary hypertension. Circulation 1998;97(16):1606–12.

26. Rouleau JL, Kapuku G, Pelletier S *et al.* Cardioprotective effects of ramipril and losartan in right ventricular pressure overload in the rabbit: importance of kinins and influence on angiotensin II type 1 receptor signaling pathway. Circulation 2001;104(8):939–44.

27. Fan TH, Liang CS, Kawashima S, Banerjee SP. Alterations in cardiac beta-adrenoceptor responsiveness and adenylate cyclase system by congestive heart failure in dogs. Eur J Pharmacol 1987;140(2):123–32.

28. Hemnes AR HA, Mahmoud M, Champion HC. Right ventricular hypertrophy due to afterload stress is prevented by PDE5 inhibition and involves the Rho kinase pathway. American Thoracic Society, International Conference, 2007.

29. Gaine SP, Rubin LJ. Primary pulmonary hypertension. Lancet 1998;352(9129):719–25.

30. Syyed R, Reeves JT, Welsh D, Raeside D, Johnson MK, Peacock AJ. The relationship between the components of pulmonary artery pressure remains constant under all conditions in both health and disease. Chest 2008; 133(3):633–9.

31. Chemla D, Castelain V, Humbert M *et al.* New formula for predicting mean pulmonary artery pressure using systolic pulmonary artery pressure. Chest 2004;126(4):1313–7.

32. Denton CP, Cailes JB, Phillips GD, Wells AU, Black CM, Bois RM. Comparison of Doppler echocardiography and right heart catheterization to assess pulmonary hypertension in systemic sclerosis. Br J Rheumatol 1997;36(2):239–43.

33. Hinderliter AL, Willis PWt, Barst RJ *et al.* Effects of long-term infusion of prostacyclin (epoprostenol) on echocardiographic measures of right ventricular structure and function in primary pulmonary hypertension. Primary Pulmonary Hypertension Study Group. Circulation 1997;95(6):1479–86.

34. Berger M, Haimowitz A, Van Tosh A, Berdoff RL, Goldberg E. Quantitative assessment of pulmonary hypertension in patients with tricuspid regurgitation using continuous wave Doppler ultrasound. J Am Coll Cardiol 1985;6(2):359–65.

35. Raymond RJ, Hinderliter AL, Willis PW *et al.* Echocardiographic predictors of adverse outcomes in primary pulmonary hypertension. J Am Coll Cardiol 2002;39(7):1214–9.

36. Bustamante-Labarta M, Perrone S, De La Fuente RL *et al.* Right atrial size and tricuspid regurgitation severity predict

mortality or transplantation in primary pulmonary hypertension. J Am Soc Echocardiogr 2002;15(10 Pt 2): 1160–4.

37. Yeo TC, Dujardin KS, Tei C, Mahoney DW, McGoon MD, Seward JB. Value of a Doppler-derived index combining systolic and diastolic time intervals in predicting outcome in primary pulmonary hypertension. Am J Cardiol 1998;81(9):1157–61.

38. Fisher MR, Forfia PR, Chamera E et al. Accuracy of Doppler Echocardiography in the Hemodynamic Assessment of Pulmonary Hypertension. Am J Respir Crit Care Med 2009;179(7):615–21.

◆39. Barst RJ, McGoon M, Torbicki A et al. Diagnosis and differential assessment of pulmonary arterial hypertension. J Am Coll Cardiol 2004;43(12 Suppl S):40S–47S.

40. Rich SaMV. Pulmonary hypertension. In: Braunwald E, ed. Libby: Braunwald's Heart Disease: A Textbook of Cardiovascular Medicine, 8 edn. Philadelphia: Saunders Elsevier, 2007:1883–913.

41. Apfel HD, Shen Z, Gopal AS et al. Quantitative three dimensional echocardiography in patients with pulmonary hypertension and compressed left ventricles: comparison with cross sectional echocardiography and magnetic resonance imaging. Heart 1996;76(4):350–4.

42. Tei C, Dujardin KS, Hodge DO et al. Doppler echocardiographic index for assessment of global right ventricular function. J Am Soc Echocardiogr 1996;9(6): 838–47.

43. Forfia PR, Fisher MR, Mathai SC et al. Tricuspid annular displacement predicts survival in pulmonary hypertension. Am J Respir Crit Care Med 2006;174(9):1034–41.

44. Kuijpers D, Janssen CH, van Dijkman PR, Oudkerk M. Dobutamine stress MRI. Part I. Safety and feasibility of dobutamine cardiovascular magnetic resonance in patients suspected of myocardial ischemia. Eur Radiol 2004;14(10):1823–8.

45. McLure LE, Peacock AJ. Imaging of the heart in pulmonary hypertension. Int J Clin Pract Suppl 2007(156):15–26.

46. Roeleveld RJ, Marcus JT, Boonstra A et al. A comparison of noninvasive MRI-based methods of estimating pulmonary artery pressure in pulmonary hypertension. J Magn Reson Imaging 2005;22(1):67–72.

47. Grothues F, Moon JC, Bellenger NG, Smith GS, Klein HU, Pennell DJ. Interstudy reproducibility of right ventricular volumes, function, and mass with cardiovascular magnetic resonance. Am Heart J 2004;147(2):218–23.

48. Pennell D. Cardiovascular magnetic resonance. In: Braunwald E, ed. Libby: Braunwald's Heart Disease, 8th edn. Philadelphia: Saunders, 2008:393–412.

49. Gan CT, Holverda S, Marcus JT et al. Right ventricular diastolic dysfunction and the acute effects of sildenafil in pulmonary hypertension patients. Chest 2007;132(1):11–7.

50. Allanore Y, Meune C, Vignaux O, Weber S, Legmann P, Kahan A. Bosentan increases myocardial perfusion and function in systemic sclerosis: a magnetic resonance imaging and tissue-Doppler echography study. J Rheumatol 2006;33(12):2464–9.

51. Hartke LP, Gilkeson RC, O'Riordan MA, Siwik ES. Evaluation of right ventricular fibrosis in adult congenital heart disease using gadolinium-enhanced magnetic resonance imaging: initial experience in patients with right ventricular loading conditions. Congenit Heart Dis 2006;1(5):192–201.

52. Bluemke DA, Krupinski EA, Ovitt T et al. MR imaging of arrhythmogenic right ventricular cardiomyopathy: morphologic findings and interobserver reliability. Cardiology 2003;99(3):153–62.

53. Boxt LM, Rozenshtein A. MR imaging of arrhythmogenic right ventricular dysplasia. Magn Reson Imaging Clin N Am 2003;11(1):163–71.

54. Midiri M, Finazzo M, Brancato M et al. Arrhythmogenic right ventricular dysplasia: MR features. Eur Radiol 1997; 7(3):307–12.

55. Hoeper MM, Lee SH, Voswinckel R et al. Complications of right heart catheterization procedures in patients with pulmonary hypertension in experienced centers. J Am Coll Cardiol 2006;48(12):2546–52.

56. Sandoval J, Bauerle O, Palomar A et al. Survival in primary pulmonary hypertension. Validation of a prognostic equation. Circulation 1994;89(4):1733–44.

57. Montalescot G, Drobinski G, Meurin P et al. Effects of prostacyclin on the pulmonary vascular tone and cardiac contractility of patients with pulmonary hypertension secondary to end-stage heart failure. Am J Cardiol 1998;82(6):749–55.

58. Wilkins MR, Paul GA, Strange JW et al. Sildenafil versus Endothelin Receptor Antagonist for Pulmonary Hypertension (SERAPH) study. Am J Respir Crit Care Med 2005;171(11):1292–7.

59. Takimoto E, Belardi D, Tocchetti CG et al. Compartmentalization of cardiac beta-adrenergic inotropy modulation by phosphodiesterase type 5. Circulation 2007;115(16): 2159–67.

60. Takimoto E, Champion HC, Li M et al. Chronic inhibition of cyclic GMP phosphodiesterase 5A prevents and reverses cardiac hypertrophy. Nat Med 2005;11(2):214–22.

61. Nagendran J, Archer SL, Soliman D et al. Phosphodiesterase type 5 is highly expressed in the hypertrophied human right ventricle, and acute inhibition of phosphodiesterase type 5 improves contractility. Circulation 2007;116(3): 238–48.

62. Sitbon O, Humbert M, Jais X et al. Long-term response to calcium channel blockers in idiopathic pulmonary arterial hypertension. Circulation 2005;111(23):3105–11.

63. Hemnes AR, Gaine SP, Wiener CM. Poor outcomes associated with drainage of pericardial effusions in patients with pulmonary arterial hypertension. South Med J 2008;101(5):490–4.

64. Schulman LL, Leibowitz DW, Anandarangam T et al. Variability of right ventricular functional recovery after lung transplantation. Transplantation 1996;62(5):622–5.

65. Kasimir MT, Seebacher G, Jaksch P et al. Reverse cardiac remodelling in patients with primary pulmonary hypertension after isolated lung transplantation. Eur J Cardiothorac Surg 2004;26(4):776–81.

66. D'Armini AM, Zanotti G, Ghio S *et al.* Reverse right ventricular remodeling after pulmonary endarterectomy. J Thorac Cardiovasc Surg 2007;133(1):162–8.

67. Reesink HJ, Marcus JT, Tulevski, II *et al.* Reverse right ventricular remodeling after pulmonary endarterectomy in patients with chronic thromboembolic pulmonary hypertension: utility of magnetic resonance imaging to demonstrate restoration of the right ventricle. J Thorac Cardiovasc Surg 2007;133(1):58–64.

68. Kerbaul F, Rondelet B, Demester JP *et al.* Effects of levosimendan versus dobutamine on pressure load-induced right ventricular failure. Crit Care Med 2006;34(11): 2814–9.

69. Kerbaul F, Rondelet B, Motte S *et al.* Effects of norepinephrine and dobutamine on pressure load–induced right ventricular failure. Crit Care Med 2004;32(4):1035–40.

70. Vizza CD, Rocca GD, Roma AD *et al.* Acute hemodynamic effects of inhaled nitric oxide, dobutamine and a combination of the two in patients with mild to moderate secondary pulmonary hypertension. Crit Care 2001;5(6):355–61.

71. Zamanian RT, Haddad F, Doyle RL, Weinacker AB. Management strategies for patients with pulmonary hypertension in the intensive care unit. Crit Care Med 2007;35(9):2037–50.

72. Holloway EL, Polumbo RA, Harrison DC. Acute circulatory effects of dopamine in patients with pulmonary hypertension. Br Heart J 1975;37(5):482–5.

73. Missant C, Rex S, Segers P, Wouters PF. Levosimendan improves right ventriculovascular coupling in a porcine model of right ventricular dysfunction. Crit Care Med 2007;35(3):707–15.

74. Laskey WK, Ferrari VA, Palevsky HI, Kussmaul WG. Pulmonary artery hemodynamics in primary pulmonary hypertension. J Am Coll Cardiol 1993;21(2):406–12.

75. Haneda T, Nakajima T, Shirato K, Onodera S, Takishima T. Effects of oxygen breathing on pulmonary vascular input impedance in patients with pulmonary hypertension. Chest 1983;83(3):520–7.

76. Huez S, Brimioulle S, Naeije R, Vachiery JL. Feasibility of routine pulmonary arterial impedance measurements in pulmonary hypertension. Chest 2004;125(6):2121–8.

77. Lankhaar JW, Westerhof N, Faes TJ *et al.* Pulmonary vascular resistance and compliance stay inversely related during treatment of pulmonary hypertension. Eur Heart J 2008;29:1688–95.

78. Hunter KS, Lee PF, Lanning CJ *et al.* Pulmonary vascular input impedance is a combined measure of pulmonary vascular resistance and stiffness and predicts clinical outcomes better than pulmonary vascular resistance alone in pediatric patients with pulmonary hypertension. Am Heart J 2008;155(1):166–74.

79. Lankhaar JW, Westerhof N, Faes TJ *et al.* Quantification of right ventricular afterload in patients with and without pulmonary hypertension. Am J Physiol Heart Circ Physiol 2006;291(4):H1731–7.

80. Kuehne T, Yilmaz S, Steendijk P *et al.* Magnetic resonance imaging analysis of right ventricular pressure–volume loops: in vivo validation and clinical application in patients with pulmonary hypertension. Circulation 2004;110(14): 2010–6.

81. Kagaya Y, Kanno Y, Takeyama D *et al.* Effects of long-term pressure overload on regional myocardial glucose and free fatty acid uptake in rats. A quantitative autoradiographic study. Circulation 1990;81(4):1353–61.

82. Oikawa M, Kagaya Y, Otani H *et al.* Increased [^{18}F]fluorodeoxyglucose accumulation in right ventricular free wall in patients with pulmonary hypertension and the effect of epoprostenol. J Am Coll Cardiol 2005;45(11): 1849–55.

PART **2**

PATHOPHYSIOLOGY & PATHOLOGY OF PULMONARY VASCULAR DISEASE

3

Pathology of pulmonary vascular diseases

PETER DORFMÜLLER

MORPHOLOGY OF TYPICAL VASCULAR LESIONS IN LUNGS OF PATIENTS WITH PULMONARY HYPERTENSION

Vascular lesions found in lungs of patients suffering from pulmonary hypertension are classically being considered as responsible for the increase of pulmonary arterial pressures and share some characteristic peculiarities, but should not be regarded as specific or even pathognomonic. These fibrotic and proliferative lesions concern the small lung vessels; arterial lesions are typically located in muscular arteries less than 500 μm diameter in patients with pulmonary arterial hypertension (PAH), while predominantly septal veins and preseptal venules are affected in patients suffering from pulmonary veno-occlusive disease (PVOD). The exceptional entity known as pulmonary capillary hemangiomatosis (PCH) concerns alveolar septal capillaries within the lung-parenchyma. Once included in Group 1 of pulmonary hypertension during the consensus meeting in Venice in 2003, the latter two entities have now been attributed to a novel category of pulmonary venous hypertension (Group 1′) after the fourth World-Symposium in Dana Point, California, in 2008 (1,2).

PATHOLOGY OF PULMONARY HYPERTENSION IN TIME

Pulmonary hypertension due to pulmonary arterial "sclerosis" was described for the first time in 1891 by Ernst von Romberg, a German internal medicine physician (3). After several case reports, it was only in 1951 that a larger study, with clinical and hemodynamical data of 39 patients displaying severe precapillary pulmonary hypertension of unknown cause, was published by Dresdale and colleagues, and the term primary pulmonary hypertension was introduced (4). The first histological classification of hypertensive pulmonary vascular disease referred to patients with congenital heart disease and was proposed by Heath and Edwards in 1958 (5). The grading relies on six different grades of "severity": the authors designate arterial muscular hypertrophy, arteriolar muscularization and subintimal fibrosis into a category of potentially reversible lesions, as confronted to irreversible forms presenting with additional angiomatoid lesions, plexiform lesions and necrotizing arteritis. However, this classification addresses a subgroup of patients with pulmonary hypertension and comprises some peculiarities, e.g. necrotizing arteritis, a lesion less frequently found in other forms of PH. In 1970 Waagenvoort and Waagenvoort reported a retrospective inventory of histological lesions in 156 patients from 51 medical centers with a first diagnosis of primary pulmonary hypertension (6). In 1973, the World Health Organization (WHO) presented a first definition of the disease, which relied on morphological and etiological criteria (7). Since then, some retrospective studies have been published, often with a very limited number of patients. It was only in 1987 that the National Institutes of Health (NIH) initiated a large prospective study (American National Register), in order to focus better on the epidemiology, pathogenesis and possible therapy of the disease (8). In 1997, Pietra proposed a revised histological classification, roughly based on the observations made by the Wagenvoorts (9). This assessment of typical pathological lesions in pulmonary hypertension was the foundation for expert meetings within the pathobiology group during three World Symposia held in Evian (France, 1998), Venice (Italy, 2003) and Dana Point (US, 2008) and will be introduced in the present chapter.

ARTERIAL LESIONS

As mentioned above, characteristic lesions in lungs of patients with PAH do not concern the larger pulmonary arteries of the elastic type; intimal and medial lesions on this level may be found in patients with chronically increased pulmonary arterial pressures, but mainly correspond to non-obstructing atherosclerotic lesions as they are typically found in the systemic vasculature (9). Typical obliterating PAH-lesions are found in pre- and intra-acinar arteries with a muscular medial layer. Different vessel wall compartments may contribute to the thickening of the arterial wall, and hence various histological patterns may occur. They are described below.

Isolated medial hypertrophy

This abnormality of the vessel wall can be observed in all subgroups of PAH and may even be encountered in other forms of pulmonary hypertension, e.g. in mitral valve stenosis. The lesion corresponds to a proliferation of smooth muscle cells within the tunica media; the histological criterion of medial hypertrophy (which corresponds more precisely to hypertrophy and hyperplasia, that is, increase in volume and number of smooth muscle cells, respectively) is fulfilled. This occurs when the diameter of a single medial layer, delimited by its internal and external elastic lamina, exceeds 10 percent of the arteries' cross-sectional diameter. An isolated hypertrophy of the medial layer may be considered as an early and even reversible event, as has been shown for pulmonary hypertension due to hypoxia at high altitude (10). However, medial hypertrophy is usually associated with other PAH-lesions. See Figure 3.1.

Concentric and eccentric non–laminar intimal fibrosis

Fibrotic lesions of the intimal layer are frequent in PAH-diseased lungs. The intima may be thickened by proliferation and recruitment of fibroblasts, myofibroblasts and other connective tissue cells, and consequently by the interstitial deposition of collagen. In a purely descriptive approach, this thickening may be uniform and concentric, or focally predominating and eccentric. Both forms can lead to a complete occlusion of the artery. In fact, the eccentric intimal thickening is frequently observed in cases with thrombotic events and probably represents residues of wall-adherent, organized thrombi. Thrombotic lesions, or so called *in situ* thrombosis, are a frequent pattern in different PAH-subgroups: organization and recanalization of totally occluding thrombotic material may lead to bizarre, fibrotic multi-channel lesions (so-called "colander-like" lesions) which can easily be confused with proliferative complex lesions (see below). Nonetheless, thrombotic or thrombo-embolic events are not a necessary precondition of intimal fibrosis; the gain in intimal cellularity is generally understood as a reaction of the inner arterial layer to a luminal stimulus, e.g. chronic pressure and shear stress (11). In many cases, intimal thickening is associated with adventitial fibrosis, but it remains difficult to evaluate, due to the lack of a clear anatomical delimitation. See Figure 3.2.

Concentric laminar intimal fibrosis

This morphologically conspicuous phenotype of intimal fibrosis is also known as "onion-skin" or "onion-bulb" lesion. Numerous concentrically arranged fibrotic layers occlude the arterial lumen of small (diameter: 100–200 μm) arteries. The cell-lacking morphology of this lesion may be found in lungs of patients suffering from all different forms of PAH, including PAH associated with connective tissue disease (12). Nevertheless, the observation that intimal thickening proximal to plexiform lesions in supernumerary arteries usually displays a concentric laminar phenotype seems to closely associate these two lesions (see below). Immunohistochemical analysis reveals fibroblasts, myofibroblasts and smooth muscle cells. See Figure 3.3.

Complex lesions

The pathological classification of the World Symposium meeting in Venice comprises three lesion entities:

- The *plexiform lesion* probably represents the most illustrious form of vascular lesions in PAH: it was considered for a long time as a pathognomonic pattern of idiopathic PAH (formerly known as primary pulmonary hypertension) (6). Hitherto, this presumption has been revised, as plexiform lesions have been shown to occur in other PAH-subgroups like congenital heart disease associated PAH or porto-pulmonary hypertension. The peculiar lesion affects various vascular compartments: a focal intimal thickening of small pulmonary arteries, preferably beyond branching points, is followed by an exuberant endothelial cell proliferation, leading to the formation of capillary-like, sinusoidal channels on a smooth muscle cell and collagen-rich matrix within the native arterial lumen and resulting in obstruction (1,13). This glomerulum-like arterial zone feeds into dilated,

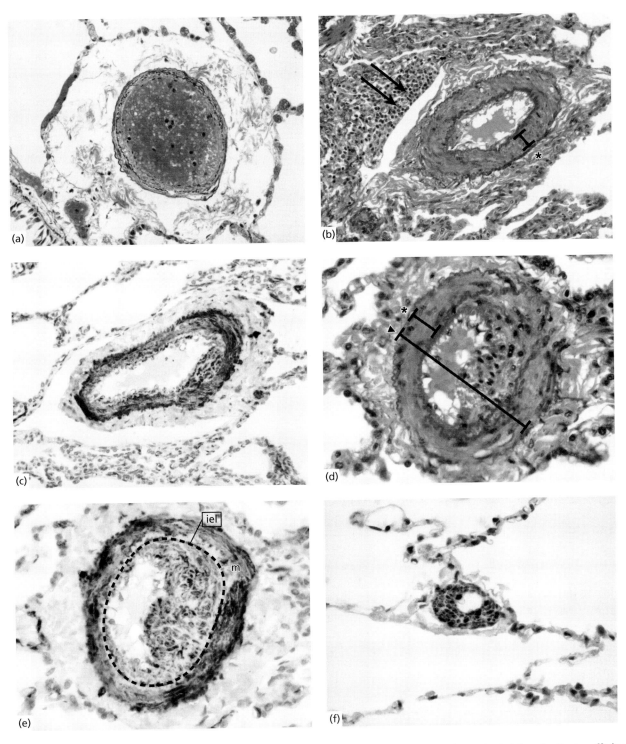

Figure 3.1   Remodeling of the media with proliferation of smooth muscle cells in pulmonary arteries and arterioles of patients suffering from IPAH. (a) Unaffected, slender medial layer in a congestive pulmonary artery. WHPS (Weigert-hematoxylin-phloxin-saffron) staining, magnification ×100. (b) Medial hypertrophy of a pulmonary artery: the medial thickness is defined as the distance between internal and external elastic lamina (asterisk). Note the peri-arterial lymphocytic infiltrate, frequently present in affected vessels (arrows). WHPS staining, magnification ×100. (c) Same artery after immunohistochemical reaction with an antibody directed against smooth muscle cell actin highlighting the tunica media. Magnification ×100. (d) Pulmonary artery with hypertrophy of the tunica media, defined as the exceeding of 10 percent of the arterial cross-sectional diameter (asterisk: medial thickness; triangle: cross-sectional diameter). WHPS staining, magnification ×200. (e) Same artery after immunohistochemical staining with anti-smooth muscle cell actin: note recruitment of smooth muscle cells/myofibroblasts into the intimal layer: medial and intimal thickening (iel: internal elastic lamina, separating media and intima). Magnification ×200. (f) Muscularized arteriole (< 100 μm) with anti-smooth muscle cell actin staining. Magnification ×200.

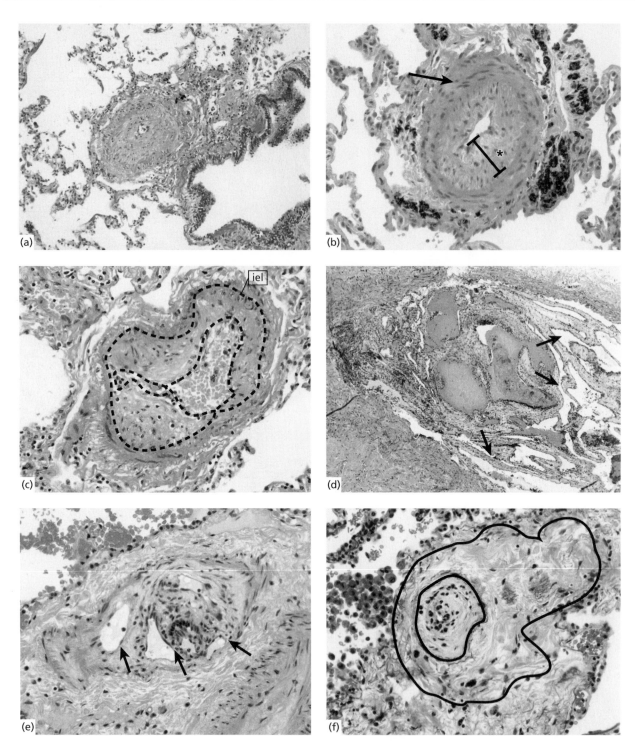

Figure 3.2   Concentric and eccentric remodeling, thrombotic lesions and adventitial fibrosis in pulmonary arteries of patients suffering from IPAH. (a) Pulmonary artery and its adjacent bronchiole: the arterial lumen is narrowed by intimal concentric non-laminar fibrosis. HES (hematoxylin-eosin-saffron) staining, magnification ×40. (b) Another artery with intimal concentric non-laminar fibrosis: note the extensive intimal thickening (asterisk), as compared to the discrete medial hypertrophy (arrow). HES staining, magnification ×100. (c) Pulmonary artery with eccentric intimal fibrosis: note the uneven thickening of the intimal layer (i) which is delimited by the internal elastic lamina (iel) and by the lumen (l). HES staining, magnification ×100. (d) Large pulmonary artery with remodeled thrombus/embolus in a patient with thrombo-embolic disease: note the wide lumina of newly developed vessels within the occlusion (arrows) in an attempt to recanalize the obstructed artery. WHPS staining, magnification ×40. (e) Small pulmonary artery with thrombotic lesion, or "colander lesion" in a patient with IPAH: same recanalization phenomenon (arrows) leading sometimes to confusion with plexiform lesions (see beneath). WHPS staining, magnification ×100. (f) Pulmonary artery with occluding intimal fibrosis and associated excessive adventitial fibrosis (dashed lining: external elastic lamina, inner boundary of the adventitial layer; continuous lining: approximate outer boundary of the adventitial layer). WHPS staining, magnification ×100.

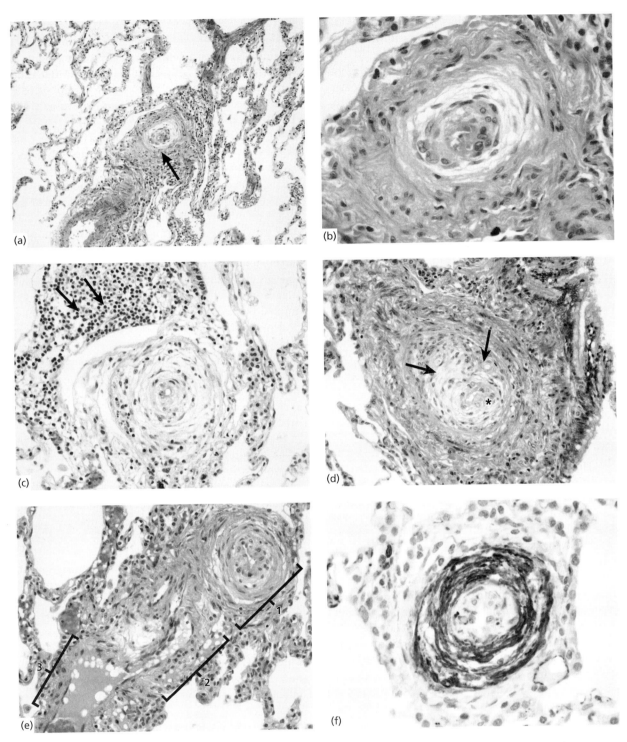

Figure 3.3 Concentric laminar remodeling and complex lesions in pulmonary arteries of patients suffering from IPAH. (a) Pulmonary artery displaying concentric laminar fibrosis (arrow) with its adjacent bronchiole (arrowhead). HES staining, magnification ×40. (b) Magnification of same arterial lesion: note the concentric and laminar arrangement of fibrous layers with a decrease of cellular density in the periphery of the lesion. HES staining, magnification ×200. (c) "Onion-skin" lesion with near arterial occlusion. Note the adjacent perivascular lymphocytic infiltrate (arrows). HES staining, magnification ×100. (d) Combined concentric laminar and plexiform lesion: central laminar fibrotic arrangement (asterisk) and peripheral endothelial cell proliferation with small channels developing within/from the intima (arrows). HES staining, magnification ×100. (e) Typical constellation of a complex lesion with three segments: 1 = concentric intimal fibrosis; 2 = plexiform lesion with exuberant endothelial cell proliferation; 3 = dilation lesion. HES staining, magnification ×100. (f) Smooth muscle cell staining in a concentric laminar fibrosis: smooth muscle elements are present within this intimal lesion. Note negativity of the inner, endothelial layer. Magnification ×200.

vein-like congestive vessels, which are perceivable at low magnification and may be helpful as sentinel lesions when tracing plexiform lesions.

- The latter vein-like congestive pulmonary vessels, also known as *dilation lesions,* may predominate the histological pattern, but are most frequently associated with plexiform lesions. Pulmonary hemorrhage in PAH patients could be a consequence of the unstable aneurysm-like vessel wall structure.

- Classical *arteritis* with transmural inflammation and fibrinoid necrosis, as first described by Heath and Edwards, has become a rather infrequent phenomenon in PAH, possibly due to the prolonged survival of patients (5). Nevertheless, perivascular inflammatory infiltrates of diseased pulmonary arteries in PAH patients can be found regularly. Infiltrates mainly consisting of T-lymphocytes and macrophages, as well as scattered mast-cells are frequently associated with plexiform or other intimal lesions. This inflammatory phenotype, in most cases, is histologically assessed as "mild" to "moderate".

See Figures 3.3 and 3.4.

VENOUS AND VENULAR LESIONS

During the Dana Point meeting in 2008 a consensus was reached, formally separating Group 1 (pulmonary arterial hypertension) of the classification of pulmonary hypertension from the rare entities of PVOD and PCH, now categorized as the new Group 1' (one prime): pulmonary venous hypertension. This differentiation seemed necessary because of particularities regarding therapeutic strategies and the cautious, if not restrictive use of potent vasodilating drugs, such as intravenous epoprostenol, in the case of pulmonary venous involvement. From the pathologist's point of view, this separation is comprehensible, but not ideal: in fact some cases of PAH (Group 1) show PVOD-like pattern (see below), and the vast majority of PVOD and PCH cases (Group 1') present at least mild arterial alteration. The frequent occurrence of mixed vascular involvement seems to demand a less absolute evaluation into pulmonary vascular lesions either predominating the arterial or the venous system.

Pulmonary veno–occlusive disease

PVOD is a rare pulmonary vascular disease causing pulmonary hypertension and has been considered together with pulmonary capillary hemangiomatosis (PCH) a subgroup of pulmonary arterial hypertension (PAH) until recently, according to the Venice classification of 2003. It shows an estimated prevalence of 0.1 to 0.2 per million (14). Historical reports and large case studies have extrapolated a proportion of PVOD in PAH ranging from 5 percent to 25 percent (14,9). In PVOD as in PCH, vascular lesions predominate on the postcapillary level of pulmonary vasculature. However, lesions frequently concern both veins *and* arteries in lungs of patients with PVOD. Interestingly, a recent report indicates that certain subgroups of PAH regarded as precapillary forms simultaneously display a PVOD-like pattern (see below).

In PVOD the observed postcapillary lesions concern septal veins and preseptal venules and frequently consist of loose, fibrous remodeling of the intima, that may totally occlude the lumen. The involvement of preseptal venules should be considered as necessary for the histological diagnosis of PVOD; fibrous occlusion of large septal veins may be seen in many forms of pulmonary venous hypertension, including a frequently reported obstruction of large pulmonary veins following catheter ablation for cardiac atrial fibrillation (15). While septal veins usually display a pauci-cellular, cushion-like fibrous obstruction, intimal thickening of preseptal venules can present with a dense pattern and increased cellularity. Anti-α-actin staining may reveal involvement of smooth muscle cells and/or myofibroblasts within such venular lesions. Also, thrombotic occlusion of small postcapillary microvessels has been observed, corresponding to "colander-like" lesions, which can be seen otherwise in small pulmonary arteries.

The tunica media may be muscularized in both septal veins and preseptal venules. Pleural and pulmonary lymphatic vessels are usually dilated (5). The presence of calcium-encrusting elastic fibers in the vessel-wall or the perivascular space, and consecutive inflammatory activation through a foreign body giant-cell response is considered as an argument in favor of PVOD as confronted to secondary venous hypertension (1).

Importantly, occult pulmonary hemorrhage regularly occurs in patients displaying PVOD. This is certainly due to the postcapillary bloc, and is of particular diagnostic interest, as broncho-alveolar lavage can reveal an occult hemorrhage. The degree of hemorrhage can be evaluated semi-quantitatively and qualitatively using the Golde Score, which takes number and staining degree of intra-alveolar siderin-laden macrophages (Perls-Prussian Blue staining) into consideration (16,17). In addition to an increased number of siderophages, large amounts of hemosiderin can be found in type II pneumocytes, as well as within the interstitial space. Moreover, postcapillary obstruction may frequently lead to capillary angiectasia and even capillary angioproliferation; in PVOD cases, doubling and trebling of the alveolar septal capillary layers may be focally present. Lately, this histological peculiarity has raised questions concerning a possible overlap between PVOD and cases of PCH, a disease classically characterized by an aggressive patch-like angioproliferation of capillaries; indeed, Lantuejoul and co-workers have recently reported 35 cases of PVOD and PCH with more or less similar pattern and evoke the possibility of a same disease entity (18). See Figures 3.5 and 3.6.

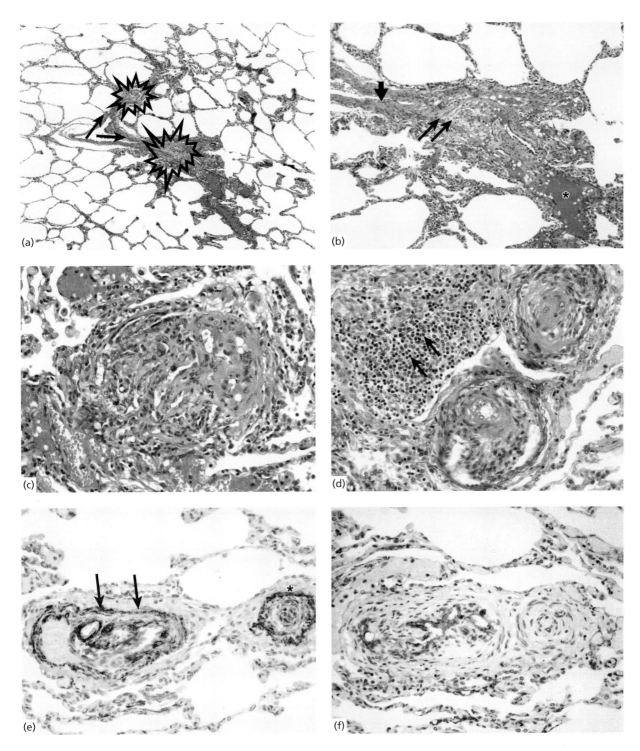

Figure 3.4 Complex lesions in pulmonary arteries of patients suffering from IPAH. (a) Branching point of a pulmonary artery (bold arrows) with two complex lesions developing on each of the successive branches (explosions). Note the "normal" aspect of the surrounding pulmonary alveolar parenchyma. WHPS staining, magnification ×20. (b) Magnification of the lower lesion: note the successive steps of stenosis (arrowhead), plexiform lesion (arrows) and dilation lesion (asterisk). WHPS staining, magnification ×40. (c) "Glomeruloid" aspect of a plexiform lesion with small endothelium-lined channels building into the lumen of a distended pulmonary artery. WHPS staining, magnification ×100. (d) Concentric laminar (above) and "beginning" of a plexiform lesion (below) surrounded by inflammatory, round cells, corresponding to lymphocytes. WHPS staining, magnification ×100. (e) Smooth muscle cell staining on another complex lesion: smooth muscle cells/myofibroblasts are present in the plexiform segment (arrows), as well as in the concentric fibrotic segment. Magnification ×100. (f) Endothelial staining with an anti-CD31 antibody on a serial section, highlighting the sinusoid-like channels in the plexiform segment. Note the absence of endothelial cell proliferation within the concentric fibrotic segment. Magnification ×100.

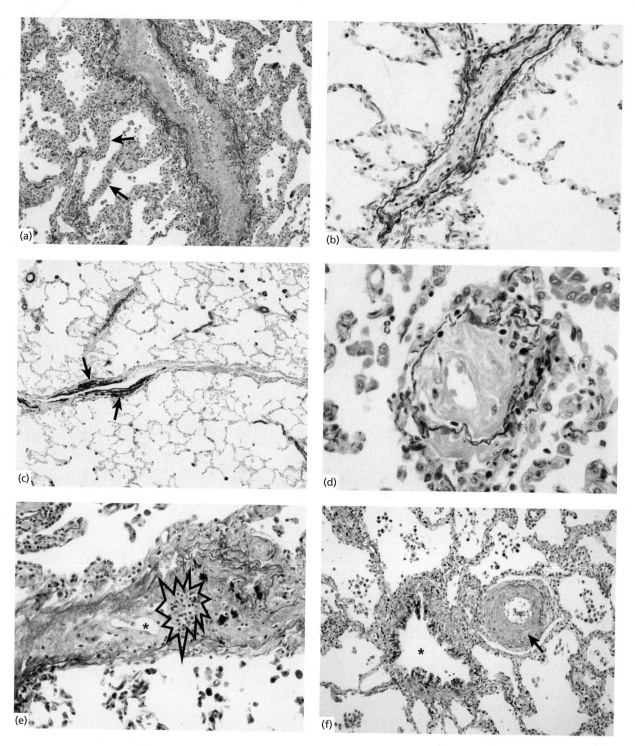

Figure 3.5   Remodeling of pulmonary septal veins and preseptal venules in patients suffering from PVOD. (a) Fibrous intimal thickening in a large septal vein. Note the adjacent broad alveolar septa with capillary multiplication (arrows). WHPS staining, magnification ×40. (b) Smaller septal vein with loose intimal fibrosis, partially occluding the lumen. WHPS staining, magnification ×100. (c) Smooth muscle cell staining highlighting partially muscularized pulmonary septal veins (arrows). Magnification ×20. (d) Small preseptal venule displaying occlusive intimal fibrosis. Note the pauci-cellular aspect of the occluded venule. WHPS staining, magnification ×200. (e) Small pulmonary vein with near occlusion (asterisk: narrowed lumen) and inflammatory lymphocytic infiltrate (explosion). WHPS staining, magnification ×100. (f) Pulmonary artery and adjacent bronchiole (asterisk) in a patient with PVOD: note the intimal concentric non-laminar fibrosis and the broadening of alveolar septa due to congestion and capillary proliferation. HE (hematoxylin-eosin) staining, magnification ×40.

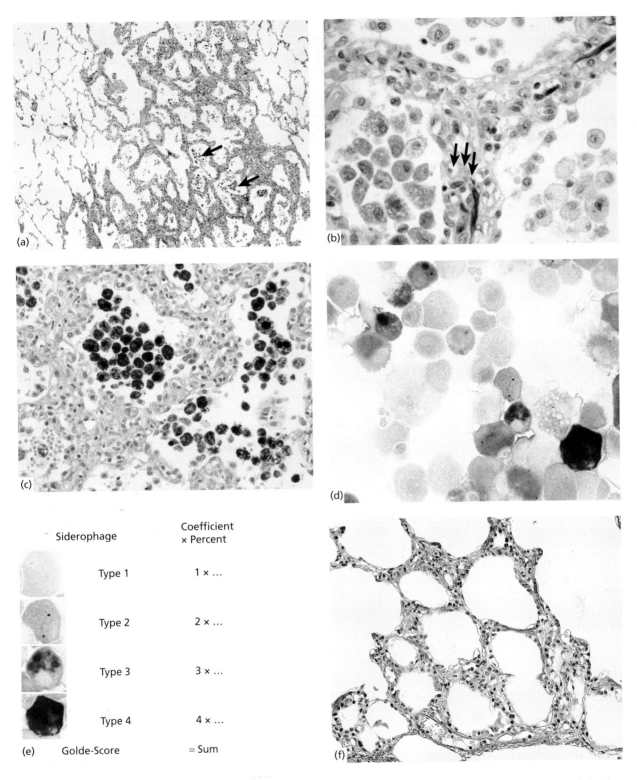

Figure 3.6   Remodeling of alveolar septa and alveolar hemorrhage in patients suffering from PVOD. (a) Patchy distribution of alveolar septal thickening. Alveoli within this remodeled area contain numerous macrophages (arrows). HES staining, magnification ×20. (b) Capillary multiplication leading to alveolar septal thickening with doubling or even trebling of the capillary lumina (arrows). Note the pigment-rich macrophages to the left of the marked alveolar septum. HES staining, magnification ×400. (c) Same area with Perls–Prussian Blue staining, revealing siderin-laden macrophages within the alveoli, the morphologic equivalent of persistent hemorrhage. Magnification ×200. (d) Broncho-alveolar lavage: numerous siderin-laden macrophages (or siderophages) are present, displaying different degrees of Prussian Blue staining. Magnification ×400. (e) Siderophages isolated from part D: typing of macrophagic Prussian Blue staining is performed in order to assess the degree of alveolar hemorrhage: a Golde score above 100 is considered as occult alveolar hemorrhage. (f) Pulmonary parenchyma of a patient suffering from PCH: note the capillary proliferation within the alveolar septa leading to a histological pattern very similar to PVOD. HE staining, magnification ×40.

Pulmonary capillary hemangiomatosis

Wagenvoort and colleagues were the first to describe this lesion as an entity of its own, within the pulmonary capillary bed in a 71-year-old woman with progressive dyspnea, hemoptysis, and hemorrhagic pleural effusions. They found a distinctive "atypical proliferation of capillary-like channels" in the lung tissue and compared it to angiomatous growth (19). This rare cause of pulmonary hypertension has recently been regrouped into Group 1' (pulmonary venous hypertension). Histologically, an aggressive capillary proliferation with patchy to nodular distribution can be observed in the pulmonary parenchyma: early lesions demonstrate several rows of capillaries along alveolar walls. Eventually, this feature progresses to nodules and sheets of back-to-back capillaries in advanced lesions (20). Alveolar septa are thickened by three to four capillary layers and this multiplication leads to the histological appearance of densely cellular alveolar walls. A malignant disorder is unlikely as cytological atypia and mitoses are usually absent. Proliferating capillaries surround and compress walls of pulmonary venules and veins, causing intimal fibrosis and secondary vein occlusion. An infiltration of bronchiolar structures has also been described. It is thought that a clinically relevant postcapillary bloc is the result of this angiomatoid expansion. Occult hemorrhage or hemosiderosis, therefore, is frequently found (19). As in PVOD, these characteristics lead to compensatory muscularization of arterioles and medial hypertrophy. As mentioned above, the similarities in clinical and histological presentation have recently led to the assumption that PVOD and PCH might be the same disease entity with a vein- or a capillary-predominating phenotype (18). See Figure 3.6.

FORMS OF PULMONARY HYPERTENSION WITH SIGNIFICANT ARTERIAL AND VENOUS REMODELING

PAH associated with connective tissue disease

Connective tissue diseases (CTD) such as systemic sclerosis and systemic lupus erythematosus can be complicated by severe pulmonary hypertension, a condition worsening the patient's prognosis dramatically (21). Indeed, systemic sclerosis represents one of the leading pathological conditions associated with pulmonary hypertension and CTD-associated pulmonary hypertension belongs to Group 1 (pulmonary arterial hypertension) as defined by the World Symposium in Dana Point. Prevalence of PAH in certain forms of CTD has been estimated in up to 50 percent of cases (22). In a recent cross-sectional national screening it has been observed that at least 8 percent of scleroderma patients displayed moderate to severe PAH (23). In patients with CTD, PAH is the first cause of mortality and necessitates intensive medical treatment, which frequently proves difficult and with mixed results (24). Treatment with vasodilators such as continuous intravenous epoprostenol has

shown improvement of exercise capacity and cardiopulmonary hemodynamics, but is less effective than in IPAH, and survival remains poor among patients with associated CTD (25,26). Endothelin receptor antagonists may be less effective in systemic sclerosis patients than in other forms of PAH (27). In addition, adverse effects of vasoactive treatment in PAH associated with CTD can occur and may lead to severe pulmonary edema (28). Noteworthy, in small groups of patients suffering from systemic lupus erythematosus (SLE) with PAH, beneficial effects of immunosuppressive therapy have been reported (29,30) highlighting a possible link between systemic inflammatory condition and pulmonary vascular disease.

Until now, lesions of the pulmonary arterial system, more or less similar to those occurring in idiopathic PAH, have been held responsible for pulmonary hypertension in these patients. In a recent published analysis of eight patients suffering from CTD-associated PAH, we observed that six out of eight patients (75 percent) presented occlusive lesions of pulmonary veins and venules, as can be typically seen in PVOD. In contrast, only five out of 29 reviewed non-CTD control patients with the primary diagnosis PAH presented some venous involvement (17.2 percent). Though all investigated CTD-PAH patients displayed pulmonary arterial changes, venous and venular fibrous remodeling, when present, was more pronounced than arterial changes, concerning the quantity of affected vessels. All cases of CTD-associated PAH revealed pulmonary arterial lesions, involving small muscular vessels on the pre- and intra-acinar level. The vessel wall remodeling corresponded to arterial changes found in PAH, ranging from intimal constrictive and non-constrictive lesions to associated medial hypertrophy and adventitial thickening. Inflammatory infiltrates were observed in six patients. Besides interstitial involvement, immunostaining experiments revealed the importance of perivascular lymphocytic infiltrates concerning both pulmonary arteries and veins. The role of inflammatory cells and their mediators in the evolution of PAH has been widely discussed in the past, and it seems particular noteworthy in PAH associated with systemic inflammatory disease (31–33). However, the described findings of a PVOD-like setting in CTD-associated PAH highlight the important hemodynamic effect of postcapillary occlusion on pulmonary vasculature. Resistance of CTD-associated PAH to common vasodilative therapies and complications like pulmonary edema could be the mere consequence of a higher prevalence of veno-occlusive remodeling in these patients, as compared with other forms of PAH. See Figure 3.7.

INTERPRETATION OF PECULIAR VASCULAR LESION TYPES AND PARALLELS TO OTHER PULMONARY PATHOLOGIES

The pathobiology of the disease will be addressed in Chapter 5 of this book, but a few remarks on the question

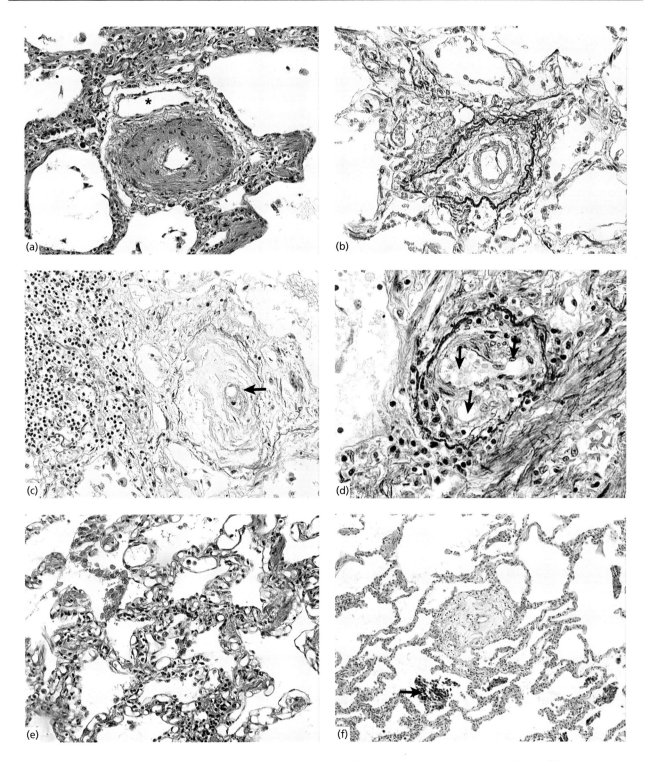

Figure 3.7   Pulmonary vascular lesions found in patients suffering from PAH associated to connective tissue disease. (a) Intimal concentric non-laminar fibrosis of a small pulmonary artery. Note the dilated lymphatic vessel adjacent to the artery (asterisk). HE staining, magnification ×100. (b) Preseptal venule with loose occlusive intimal fibrosis. WHPS staining, magnification ×100. (c) Occlusive loose fibrotic remodeling of a preseptal venule (arrow) with peri-vascular lymphocytic infiltrate. WHPS staining, magnification ×100. (d) Thrombotic lesion of a preseptal venule with recanalization channels within the occluded vessel (arrows). WHPS staining, magnification ×200. (e) Capillary angiectasia and alveolar septal thickening similar to the histological pattern seen in PVOD (see above). HE staining, magnification ×100. (f) Occluded vein (center) and signs of occult alveolar hemorrhage: note the stained siderin-laden macrophages within the adjacent alveoli. Perls-Prussian Blue staining, magnification ×40.

of what all this diversity of vascular lesions means, should be made. The descriptive approach to pulmonary arteries in PAH and their histological phenotype is based on the different vascular compartments affected by alteration, and consequently by different cell types involved in this pathological anatomy. As we lack longitudinal temporary information of histological changes in most cases, observations and hypothesis are based on transverse time points of different subjects. In addition, most PAH cases will have early clinical diagnosis, but only preterminal histological confirmation, either through analysis of lung explants, or through autopsy. In the actual diagnostic setting, lung biopsy is contraindicated for the vast majority of patients suffering from PAH and so the morphological correlate will be a tardy one, possibly skipping important levels of disease evolution.

Medial hypertrophy is reversible in high altitude pulmonary hypertension

It is widely accepted that an early phase of pulmonary arterial pressure elevation of PAH patients is reflected by the thickening of the medial layer through hyperplasia and hypertrophy of smooth muscle cells; this process is present in reversible forms of pulmonary hypertension, e.g. high altitude pulmonary hypertension and chronic mountain sickness. In a recent study and review of the literature Penazola and Arias-Stella explained that healthy natives of high altitude regions over 3500 meters above sea level have pulmonary hypertension, right ventricular hypertrophy and an increased amount of smooth muscle cells in the distal pulmonary arterial branches. Their results obtained after clinical and histological comparison of 30 healthy high altitude natives with 30 sea level natives indicate that the main factor responsible for pulmonary hypertension in healthy highlanders is the increased amount of smooth muscle cells in the distal pulmonary arteries and arterioles, which increases pulmonary vascular resistance. Vasoconstriction is a secondary factor because the administration of oxygen decreases the pulmonary arterial pressure only by 15 to 20 percent. This adaptive increase in cardiac and smooth muscle cell mass is reversed after a prolonged residence at sea level (34).

Intimal fibrosis in idiopathic spontaneous pneumothorax and idiopathic pulmonary fibrosis

However, medial thickening is not the major hallmark of PAH, as mentioned above. During histological examination of lung tissue in severe forms of PAH, intimal thickening with concentric laminar and/or non-laminar fibrosis is a more striking abnormality. Interestingly, alterations of the tunica intima, which physiologically consists of a single endothelial layer and a basal membrane, can be observed in other pulmonary diseases without pulmonary hypertension. Cyr and Co-workers have described medial and intimal thickening in 20 cases of idiopathic spontaneous pneumothorax. They identified pulmonary vasculopathy in 18 out of 20 cases (90 percent). The most frequent lesion was intimal fibrosis of the small pulmonary arteries and veins. In six cases (30 percent), pulmonary arterial intimal fibrosis was graded as severe because the mean intimal thickness exceeded 20 percent of the internal diameter (distance from one elastic internal lamina to the diametrically opposite elastic internal lamina). In 19 cases (95 percent), the lungs presented some histological features of fibrosis and chronic inflammation, with a significant positive correlation between mean pulmonary artery medial thickness and lung fibrosis/chronic inflammation scores, linking arterial remodeling and inflammatory activity in the absence of elevated pulmonary arterial pressures (35).

Another frequent lung disease combining alterations of different vascular compartments is idiopathic pulmonary fibrosis (IPF) (synonym: usual interstitial pneumonia). This condition is marked by interstitial collagen deposition and so called fibroblastic foci, probably the stigma of an ongoing aggressive fibrosing process. Moreover, interstitial smooth muscle proliferation may be observed. Typically, fibrotic remodeled areas within the pulmonary parenchyma closely alternate with unremodeled areas in a patchy pattern. Pulmonary arterial adventitial thickening can be seen and is due to an increase of fibroblasts, myofibroblasts, and extracellular matrix deposition. Smooth muscle cell hypertrophy and proliferation and collagen accumulation occur in the media of the small muscular pulmonary arteries, and distal pulmonary arterioles become muscularized. In addition, there may be extensive intimal hyperplasia, fibrosis, and reduplication of the inner elastic lamina in the small muscular pulmonary arteries in IPF (36). Vascular changes may occur in unaffected parenchyma, but are more consistently confined to the patchy fibrotic areas, frequently displaying inflammatory pattern with lymphocytic infiltration. However, pulmonary hypertension in these patients is only present in 20 to 40 percent before lung transplantation, hence in a terminal phase. This lack of correlation between quality of vascular lesions and hemodynamic changes could be explained by the typical persistence of non-fibrotic areas in IPF: it underscores that the installation of high pulmonary arterial pressures probably requires a more or less constant fraction of obstructed lung vessels, or in other words a threshold in vascular overall diameter reduction.

Recently, Colombat and co-workers have documented intimal proliferation and fibrosis in the pulmonary veins and venules of patients with IPF. Arterial lesions and occlusive veins were observed in fibrotic areas, but venular lesions were equally present in architecturally preserved lung zones in 65 percent of the patients, as compared to only mild changes of muscular pulmonary arteries in normal areas (37). Interestingly, the authors found a significant positive correlation between the macroscopic extent of lung fibrosis and mean pulmonary artery pressure, supporting the concept of a quantitative threshold in arterial obstruction leading to relevant pulmonary hypertension. See Figure 3.8 A–D.

Inflammation is frequently observed in the range of vascular lesions in PH

It has not been elucidated until now, whether the inflammatory pattern seen in plexiform lesions and other intimal lesions is of pathogenetic importance, or if it represents a pure epiphenomenon within disease evolution. The reported evidence of proinflammatory mediators, so called chemokines, released by altered endothelial cells of PAH-lungs strongly indicates a self-supporting and self-amplifying process (38,39). As elements of inflammation seem to be present in affected arteries of patients displaying PAH in various associated disease conditions, as well as in idiopathic pulmonary arterial hypertension, the specific role of immune cells within installation and/or maintenance of

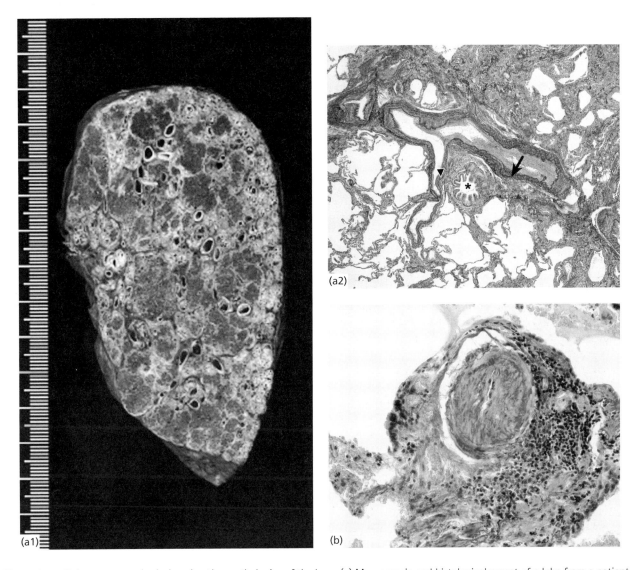

Figure 3.8 Pulmonary vascular lesions in other pathologies of the lung. (a) Macroscopic and histological aspect of a lobe from a patient with interstitial pulmonary fibrosis (IPF). Note the patchy distribution of parenchymal fibrotic lesions (macroscopy, left). Histological aspect of the transition zone between diseased and preserved pulmonary parenchyma (microscopy, right). Note the pulmonary artery and the adjacent bronchiole (asterisk): Arterial intimal thickening is present within the zone of IPF typical parenchymal remodeling (arrow), while absent in the arterial branch leaving the main artery into the preserved area (arrowhead). Elastica van Gieson staining (EvG), magnification ×20. (b) Small pulmonary artery of the same lung displaying concentric intimal fibrosis. Note the close association to inflammatory cells mainly consisting of lymphocytes. EvG staining, magnification ×100. (c) Same lung with smooth muscle actin staining: Smooth muscle cell hyperplasia is present in a remodeled artery (arrowhead) and in the pulmonary interstitium (arrows). Magnification ×40. (d) Pulmonary artery in a lung resection specimen of a patient with spontaneous idiopathic pneumothorax: intimal thickening is present in the absence of pulmonary hypertension. HES staining, magnification ×100. (e) Pulmonary arterial remodeling in a patient with pulmonary hypertension associated with sarcoidosis. The arterial wall displays intense inflammatory infiltrate and numerous epitheloid granulomas with giant cells (arrows), narrowing the arterial lumen considerably. Smooth muscle actin stain, magnification ×40.

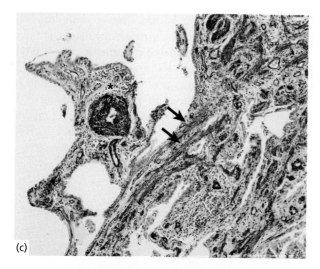

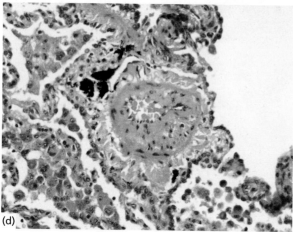

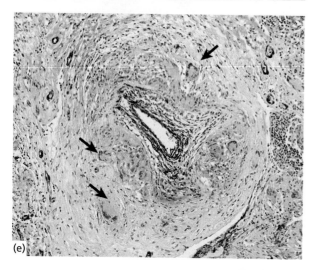

Figure 3.8   (*Continued*)

obstructive lesions remains still unclear. It seems unlikely that intimal proliferation and medial hypertrophy of pulmonary arteries could be the sole result of "scarring" vasculitis-like lesions, because lymphocytic and macrophagic infiltrates being observed in the setting of PAH remain perivascular and are less abundant than in pulmonary forms of vasculitis,

as seen, e.g. in Wegener's granulomatosis (40). Nonetheless, Waagenvoort and co-workers had discussed such a possibility 40 years ago, and it cannot be excluded that a phase of intense inflammatory activity precedes a clinically symptomatic arterial remodeling with proliferation and recruitment of smooth muscle cells, endothelial cells and fibroblasts/myofibroblasts. This straight inflammatory involvement can be observed in cases of pulmonary hypertension due to sarcoidosis, with typical epitheloid and histiocytic granulomas directly participating in vessel wall remodeling (see Figure 3.8E). In fact, latest investigations provide evidence that chemokines with specific chemotactic activity on T-lymphocytes and macrophages can increase smooth muscle proliferation (41). A link between inflammatory components and growth-stimulating factors would be of great interest in inflammatory diseases with vast proliferation of fibrotic and myofibroblastic elements, as can be seen in highly active forms of, for example, idiopathic pulmonary fibrosis (see above), presenting fibroblastic foci and interstitial smooth muscle proliferation (42).

Plexiform lesions – an intriguing phenomenon and still a matter of interpretation

A more peculiar, if not unique lesion occurring in PAH is the complex lesion. It was first described in patients with congenital cardiac left-to-right shunts (5), and eventually in other forms of PAH, all belonging to the Group 1 of the Venice and Dana Point classification. A study from 1993 reporting plexiform lesions in 20 out of 31 patients with confirmed chronic major vessel thromboembolic pulmonary hypertension remains isolated until today, but raises the possibility of a relationship between organizing thromboembolic and complex lesions, which in fact mirrors an old theory first inspired by Harrison in 1958 (43). Another historic hypothesis explaining the pathogenesis of the glomerulum-like exuberant endothelial cell proliferation within the affected pulmonary artery is the formation of arteriovenous shunts (44). Waagenvoort and Waagenvoort explain the generation of plexiform lesions in cardiac left-to-right shunting by an increased blood flow eliciting reflective vasoconstriction with subsequent development of endothelial alteration (6). More interestingly, they speculate that vascular necrosis with arteritis might result from intense vasospasm, as seen in the systemic circulation. The pathogenetic plot, here, is that plexiform lesions develop in the focal areas of fibrinoid necrosis by active cellular reorganization and recanalization of the thrombus composed of fibrin and platelets, usually present in this setting and observed within plexiform lesions. In fact, the only animal model leading to obvious plexiform lesions has been achieved by producing necrosis of pulmonary arterioles in dogs after 2 weeks of severe pulmonary hypertension due to the creation of a shunt between pulmonary and systemic circulations (45). This explanation would take into consideration that elements of inflammation are consistently present in the range of plexiform and other vascular lesions in PAH (31,33).

On the other hand, Tuder and co-workers have proposed a neoplastic approach to the hardly understandable proliferation of intra-luminal neovessels at the core of plexiform lesions: they found that a large proportion of the endothelial cells in this area show monoclonality, raising the question of a possible tumor-like growth (46). These different observations of arterial wall alteration within plexiform lesions are probably connected in a temporary line. However they could feed into a broader concept of pathogenesis, first mentioned by Waagenvoort, but interestingly developed by Yaginuma and co-workers: they submitted histological data from 11 patients with pulmonary hypertension due to congenital heart disease to a computer-based three-dimensional image reconstruction and found that plexiform lesions mostly occurred in supernumerary arteries branching apart from larger pulmonary arteries, proximal to arterial lesions with intimal fibrosis and medial hypertrophy. They also gathered evidence for generation of indirect anastomoses between the post-plexiform arterial segment to bronchial arteries running along the close bronchiole, passing via arterioles and the capillary bed and thereby creating the thin-walled congestive dilation lesions (47). In this view, the generation of proximal complex lesions might be the mere attempt of the pulmonary vasculature to bypass the primary downstream obstruction and to ensure capillary oxygenation through overt contact with arterial blood from proximal pulmonary and distal bronchial arteries. On the other hand, plexiform lesions are not restricted to supernumerary branching and can be observed after distal dichotomous branching of pulmonary arteries.

Cool and co-workers have come to different conclusions after a computerized three-dimensional study on five patients with severe pulmonary hypertension from a different cause. In their view plexiform lesions are functionally important because blood flow is severely obstructed along the entire length of a vessel affected by a single lesion (48). This, in fact, puts at least a working shunt concept into question. They hypothesize that the plexiform lesion could be an early vascular alteration in severe pulmonary hypertension, independent of a component of medial smooth muscle cell hypertrophy. At a later time-point in disease evolution, the plexiform lesion could transform into an intraluminal concentric obstruction composed of endothelial cells and recruited myofibroblasts, following the path of the plexiform lesion and thus representing a fibrous scar of the latter (48). The close association that can be observed between concentric laminar intimal fibrosis and plexiform lesions in lungs of patients suffering from PAH, makes this thought a tempting assumption. Nevertheless, a shunt hypothesis would not be contradictory if seen in the light of a failed attempt to shortcut other correlates of obstruction such as medial hypertrophy, intimal non-laminar fibrosis and thrombotic lesions.

KEY POINTS

- Characteristic vascular lesions in pulmonary hypertension may concern the lung vasculature and microvasculature from the pre- to the post-capillary level.
- In addition to clinical differentiation, histological resemblance or difference has led to the categorization of pulmonary hypertension into different groups, now summed up under the Dana Point Classification.
- It is important to stress that the differentiation of lesions and their localization might be of significant importance considering the outcome and therapeutic strategies.
- A clear cut separation of different forms of pulmonary hypertension through recognition of a histological phenotype will always be difficult or even impossible: different etiological factors (e.g. hypoxia versus anorexigen intake) may trigger a final common step in the cascade of pathologic events (e.g. oxidative stress and consecutive growth factor expression) and finally lead to the same morphologic pattern (e.g. medial hypertrophy).
- The correct interpretation of the pathological vascular anatomy remains an important tool in the successful interplay of clinical, biological, and pharmaceutical research dedicated to pulmonary hypertension.

REFERENCES

1. Pietra GG, Capron F, Stewart S, Leone O, Humbert M, Robbins IM, Reid LM, Tuder RM. Pathological assessment of vasculopathies in pulmonary hypertension. J Am Coll Cardiol 2004;43:25S–32S.
2. Simonnean G, Robbins IM, Beghetti M et al. Updated clinical classification of pulmonary hypertension. J Am Coll Cardiol 2009;54:543–54.
3. Romberg E. Über die Sklerose der Lungenarterien. Dtsch Arch Klin Med 1891;48:197.
4. Dresdale DT, Schultz M, Mitchom RJ. Primary pulmonary hypertension: clinical and hemodynamic study. Am J Med 1951;11:686–94.
5. Heath D, Edwards JE. The pathology of hypertensive pulmonary vascular disease. Circulation 1958;18:533–47.
6. Waagenvoort CA, Waagenvoort N. Primary pulmonary hypertension: a pathological study of the lung vessels in 156 clinically diagnosed cases. Circulation 1970;42: 1163–84.
7. Hatano S, Strasser T, eds. Primary pulmonary hypertension. Report on a WHO-meeting October 15–17 1975; Geneva, WHO.

8. Rich S, Dantzer DR, Ayres SM *et al.* Primary pulmonary hypertension: a national prospective study. Ann Int Med 1987;107:216–23.

9. Pietra, G.G. The pathology of primary pulmonary hypertension. In: Rubin L, Rich S, eds. Primary Pulmonary Hypertension. New York: Marcel Dekker, 1997;19–61.

10. Heath D, Williams DR. High-altitude Medicine and Pathology. London: Butterworths, 1989:102–14.

11. Voelkel NF, Tuder RM. Cellular and molecular mechanisms in the pathogenesis of severe pulmonary hypertension. Eur Respir J 1995;8:2129–38.

12. Cool CD, Kennedy D, Voelkel NF, Tuder RF. Pathogenesis and evolution of plexiform lesions in pulmonary hypertension associated with scleroderma and human immunodeficiency virus infection. Human Pathol 1997;28:434–42.

13. Bjornsson J, Edwards WD. Primary pulmonary hypertension: a histopathologic study of 80 cases. Mayo Clin Proc 1985;60:16–25.

14. Mandel J, Mark EJ, Hales CA. Pulmonary veno-occlusive disease. Am J Respir Crit Care Med 2000;162:1964–73.

15. Di Biase L, Fahmy TS, Wazni OM *et al.* Pulmonary vein total occlusion following catheter ablation for atrial fibrillation: clinical implications after long-term follow-up. J Am Coll Cardiol 2006;48:2493–9.

16. Golde DW, Drew WL, Klein HZ, Finley TN, Cline MJ. Occult pulmonary haemorrhage in leukaemia. Br Med J 1975;2:166–8.

17. Capron F. Bronchoalveolar lavage and alveolar hemorrhage. Ann Pathol 1999;19:395–400.

18. Lantuejoul S, Sheppard MN, Corrin B, Burke MM, Nicholson AG. Pulmonary veno-occlusive disease and pulmonary capillary hemangiomatosis: a clinicopathologic study of 35 cases. Am J Surg Pathol 2006;30:850–7.

19. Wagenvoort CA, Beetstra A, Spijker J. Capillary haemangiomatosis of the lungs. Histopathology 1978;2:401–6.

20. Tron V, Magee F, Wright JL, Colby T, Churg A. Pulmonary capillary hemangiomatosis. Hum Pathol 1986;17:1144–50.

21. Simonneau G, Galie N, Rubin LJ *et al.* Clinical classification of pulmonary hypertension. J Am Coll Cardiol 2004;43:5S–12S.

22. Ungerer RG, Tashkin DP, Furst D *et al.* Prevalence and clinical correlates of pulmonary arterial hypertension in progressive systemic sclerosis. Am J Med 1983;75:65–74.

23. Hachulla E, Gressin V, Guillevin L *et al.* Early detection of pulmonary arterial hypertension in systemic sclerosis: a French nationwide prospective multicenter study. Arthritis Rheum 2005;52:3792–800.

24. Sanchez O, Humbert M, Sitbon O, Simonneau G. Treatment of pulmonary hypertension secondary to connective tissue diseases. Thorax 1999;54:273–77.

25. Badesch DB, Tapson VF, McGoon MD *et al.* Continuous intravenous epoprostenol for pulmonary hypertension due to the scleroderma spectrum of disease. Ann Intern Med 2000;132:425–34.

26. Ramirez A, Varga J. Pulmonary arterial hypertension in systemic sclerosis: clinical manifestations, pathophysiology, evaluation, and management. Treat Respir Med 2004; 3:339–52.

27. Humbert M, Simonneau G. Drug insight: endothelin-receptor antagonists for pulmonal arterial hypertension in systemic rheumatic diseases. Nat Clin Pract Rheum 2005;1:93–101.

28. Humbert M, Sanchez O, Fartoukh M *et al.* Short-term and long-term epoprostenol (prostacyclin) therapy in pulmonary hypertension secondary to connective tissue diseases: results of a pilot study. Eur Respir J 1999; 13:1351–6.

29. Tanaka E, Harigai M, Tanaka M, Kawaguchi Y, Hara M, Kamatani N. Pulmonary hypertension in systemic lupus erythematosus: evaluation of clinical characteristics and response to immunosuppressive treatment. J Rheumatol 2002;29:282–7.

30. Sanchez O, Sitbon O, Jaïs X, Simonneau G, Humbert M. Immunosuppressive therapy in connective tissue diseases-associated pulmonary arterial hypertension. Chest 2006;130:182–9.

31. Tuder RM, Groves B, Badesch DB, Voelkel NF. Exuberant endothelial cell growth and elements of inflammation are present in plexiform lesions of pulmonary hypertension. Am J Pathol 1994;144:275–85.

32. Humbert M, Monti G, Brenot F *et al.* Increased interleukin-1 and interleukin-6 serum concentrations in severe primary pulmonary hypertension. Am J Respir Crit Care Med 1995;151:1628–31.

33. Dorfmüller P, Perros F, Balabanian K, Humbert M. Inflammation in pulmonary arterial hypertension. Eur Respir J 2003;22:358–63.

34. Penaloza D, Arias-Stella J. The heart and pulmonary circulation at high altitudes: healthy highlanders and chronic mountain sickness. Circulation 2007;115:1132–46.

35. Cyr PV, Vincic L, Kay M. Pulmonary vasculopathy in idiopathic spontaneous pneumothorax in young subjects. Arch Pathol Lab Med 2000;124:717–20.

36. Patel NM, Lederer DJ, Borczuk AC, Kawut SM. Pulmonary hypertension in idiopathic pulmonary fibrosis. Chest 2007;132:998–1006.

37. Colombat M, Mal H, Groussard O *et al.* Pulmonary vascular lesions in end-stage idiopathic pulmonary fibrosis: histopathologic study on lung explant specimens and correlations with pulmonary hemodynamics. Hum Pathol 2007;38:60–5.

38. Dorfmüller P, Zarka V, Durand-Gasselin I *et al.* Chemokine RANTES in severe pulmonary arterial hypertension. Am J Respir Crit Care Med 2002;165:534–9.

39. Balabanian K, Foussat A, Dorfmüller P *et al.* CX_3C chemokine fractalkine in pulmonary arterial hypertension. Am J Respir Crit Care Med 2002;165:1419–25.

40. Dorfmüller P, Humbert M, Capron F, Müller KM. Pathology and aspects of pathogenesis in pulmonary arterial hypertension. Sarcoidosis Vasc Diffuse Lung Dis 2003;20:9–19.

41. Perros F, Dorfmüller P, Souza R *et al.* Fraktalkine-induced smooth muscle cell proliferation in pulmonary hypertension. Eur Respir J 2007;29:937–43.

42. Ohta K, Mortenson RL, Clark RA, Hirose N, King TE Jr. Immunohistochemical identification and characterization of smooth-muscle-like cells in idiopathic pulmonary fibrosis. Am J Respir Crit Care Med 1995;152:1659–65.

43. Harrison CV. The pathology of the pulmonary vessels in pulmonary hypertension. Br J Radiol 1958;31:217–26.

44. Kucsko L. Arteriovenous communications in the human lung and their functional significance. Frankf Z Pathol 1953;64:54–83.

45. Saldana ME, Harley RA, Liebow AA, Carrington CB. Experimental extreme pulmonary hypertension and vascular disease in relation to polycythemia. Am J Pathol 1968;52:935–81.

46. Lee SD, Shroyer KR, Markham NE, Cool CD, Voelkel NF, Tuder RM. Monoclonal endothelial cell proliferation is present in primary but not secondary pulmonary hypertension. J Clin Invest 1998;101:927–34.

47. Yaginuma GY, Mohri H, Takahashi T. Distribution of arterial lesions and collateral pathways in the pulmonary hypertension of congenital heart disease: a computer aided reconstruction study. Thorax 1990; 45:586–90.

48. Cool CD, Stewart JS, Werahera P, Miller GJ, Williams RL, Voelkel NF, Tuder RM. Three-dimensional reconstruction of pulmonary arteries in plexiform pulmonary hypertension using cell-specific markers. Am J Pathol 1999;155:411–19.

4

Hypoxic pulmonary vasoconstriction and hypertension

ANDREA OLSCHEWSKI

INTRODUCTION

Hypoxic pulmonary vasoconstriction (HPV) is a physiological response of small pulmonary arteries that diverts mixed venous blood away from hypoxic alveoli, thus optimizing the matching of perfusion and ventilation and preventing arterial hypoxemia. The pulmonary vascular bed is unique compared with most studied systemic vascular beds. During normoxic conditions, the pulmonary circulation is at low pressure – that is, vasodilated – compared with the high-pressure systemic circulation. In the systemic circulation, hypoxemia elicits vasodilatation that increases O_2 delivery to the tissues. In contrast, small resistance arteries in the pulmonary circulation constrict in response to hypoxia. HPV has been an area of intensive investigation since it was reported over a hundred years ago (1) and was more precisely described in 1946 by von Euler and Liljestrand (2). Although the responses to hypoxia are relatively well characterized, the molecular mechanisms of O_2 signaling and how changes in environmental O_2 are translated into signals recognizable by the cell are just beginning to be understood.

HYPOXIC PULMONARY VASOCONSTRICTION

In the developing fetus, pulmonary vascular resistance is high. The oxygenated blood from the placenta flows through the foramen ovale and ductus arteriosus, largely bypassing the lungs. If the oxygen level in the fetus is raised by increasing maternal oxygenation, the fetal pulmonary vascular resistance falls, demonstrating that normally in the fetus active hypoxia-induced vasoconstriction contributes to the high resistance (3). At birth, lung expansion and rising oxygen levels cause a rapid drop in pulmonary vascular resistance and subsequent remodeling of the resistance pulmonary arteries. Thus, from the ontogenetic point of view HPV can be also regarded as the other side of the coin to "normoxic pulmonary vasodilation" (4).

Once out of the uterus, the lung displays HPV in response to alveolar hypoxia. In humans, hypoxic vasoconstriction can be defined as a rapid, monophasic, reversible increase in pulmonary vascular resistance, due to the contraction of small muscular pulmonary arteries with an internal diameter of approximately 200 to 600 μm and in response to physiological levels of hypoxia (5). The considerable individual variability in the magnitude of HPV between individuals might be based on genetics and adaptive mechanisms. HPV is a conserved response, found in most mammals (6) as well as in reptiles (7). Hypoxic vasoconstriction depends largely on the alveolar and not on the mixed venous pO_2 (8,9) and starts within seconds of the onset of airway hypoxia; by a decrease in alveolar O_2 tension below a threshold fractional inspired O_2 concentration of ~10 percent (9,10). Subsequently, a fall in the alveolar oxygen partial pressure below 50 mmHg doubles pulmonary vascular resistance (11).

In intact dogs (12), rabbits (13), isolated ferret lungs (14), rabbit lungs (9) as well as in isolated pulmonary arteries (15,16) the response to alveolar hypoxia shows a biphasic character, with an early pulmonary arterial pressure peak and a more protracted secondary pressure elevation. The acute, initial transient vasoconstrictor phase I is independent of the endothelium. For the slowly developing increase in vascular tone (phase II) both, endothelium and calcium sensitization possibly via activation of Rho-kinase, are required. Hypoxia appears to activate mechanisms intrinsic to the pulmonary vasculature, independent of blood-borne factors or influences that require the central nervous system, as HPV can be demonstrated in isolated perfused lungs and isolated pulmonary arteries (9,17,18). According to current knowledge, neither angiotensin, prostaglandins, thromboxane nor arachidonic acid lipoxygenase products directly mediate the mechanism of acute HPV. In contrast, hypoxic vasoconstriction is blocked by calcium antagonists, reduced by endothelin antagonists and α-adrenergic antagonists and modulated by serotonin, suggesting not only involvement of voltage-dependent calcium channels and extracellular calcium but also the participation of the serotonin and endothelin pathways and possibly the contribution of catecholamines. Administration of exogenous vasodilatators such as NO and prostacyclin are able to override HPV, which does not necessarily suggest an endogenous role of these substances in the mechanism.

If only a small region of the lung is hypoxic, HPV can occur without a significant effect on pulmonary arterial pressure (19). However, if the critical mass of the lung becomes hypoxic, as seen in many lung diseases (e.g. widespread atelectasis) and in high-altitude exposure, the subsequent pulmonary vasoconstriction contributes to pulmonary hypertension, heart failure and finally death.

Superimposed effects of acidosis, alkalosis and hyperventilation

Hypoxia stimulates ventilation and ventilation per se can affect the pulmonary vascular tone. Hyperventilation has been demonstrated to reduce the elevated pulmonary arterial pressure in different animal models, and is applied during anesthesia for treatment of children with pulmonary hypertensive disorders. The induction of hypocapnic alkalosis is thought to play an important role in these vasodilatory effects (20,21), alkalosis and not hypocapnia being the crucial factor (22). Among the many potential pH-sensitive molecular targets that could contribute, the ion channels that are active at or near resting membrane potentials have been recently emphasized as potential key regulators. Acid-sensitive two-pore domain K^+-selective channels such as TASK-1 are unique among those ion channels cloned to date that generate an open-rectifier 'leak' K^+ current regulated by the physiological extracullar pH. Thus, alkalosis would lead to a facilitation of TASK-1 resulting in hyperpolarization of the pulmonary arterial smooth muscle membrane and consequently, in vasodilation. The molecular site underlying the pH sensitivity of TASK-1 has been extensively investigated by Morton et al. (23).

MECHANISM OF ACUTE HYPOXIC VASOCONSTRICTION: HYPOXIC SIGNALING

Knowledge of the mechanism of O_2 sensing and the signaling pathways that mediate the cellular response to hypoxia has developed rapidly in the last decade (Figure 4.1).

The oxygen sensing system

There are a variety of tissues that sense the oxygen level in different strategic locations in the body. These include the type I cells of the carotid body, neuroepithelial bodies in the lung, chromaffin cells of the fetal adrenal medulla, as well as smooth muscle cells of the resistance pulmonary arteries (PASMCs), fetoplacental arteries, systemic arteries, and the ductus arteriosus (24). Together, they constitute a specialized homeostatic oxygen-sensing system which is able to sense deviations from the optimum. For more details see refs 25–30.

HEME OXYGENASES AND CYTOCHROMES

Iron-containing heme proteins, including heme oxygenases, cytochromes and NADPH oxidases, were proposed long ago as potential O_2 sensors in a variety of cellular systems. Heme oxygenase degrades heme to CO, biliverdin and Fe(II) in the presence of O_2 and NADPH (31). The heme protein in the deoxy conformation could activate effectors either directly or through a signaling cascade. Some native (32,33) and recombinant ion channels (34,35) have been reported to retain O_2 sensitivity in excised membrane patches in the absence of intracellular mediators, which could suggest a direct interaction between channels and O_2 sensors. See refs 36–42 for more details.

ROLE OF REACTIVE OXYGEN SPECIES (ROS)

Two principal systems have been recognized to produce ROS, the NAD(P)H oxidases and the mitochondria. ROS, including superoxide anion (O_2^-), hydroxyl radical ($OH^·$) and hydrogen peroxide (H_2O_2), are produced in the lung in proportion to the ambient O_2 tension. Superoxide anion formed by the one electron reduction of molecular oxygen (O_2), is converted by SOD enzymatically into hydrogen peroxide. In the presence of reduced transition metals, hydrogen peroxide can be converted into the highly reactive hydroxyl radical or alternatively into water by the enzymes catalase or glutathione peroxidase. Several studies have shown that hypoxia decreases production and tissue levels of ROS, although this is still disputed as summarized in Table 4.1.

NADPH OXIDASE

NADPH oxidase, a flavocytochrome, is expressed in a variety of O_2-sensitive tissues, including neuroepithelial bodies

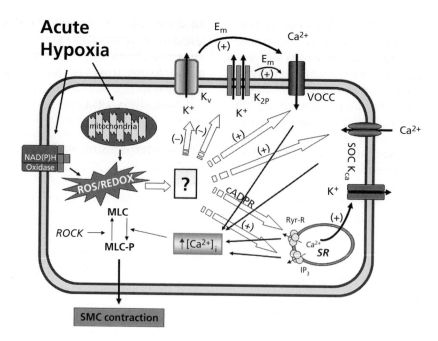

Figure 4.1   Proposed schematic presentation of acute HPV in pulmonary artery smooth muscle cells (PASMCs). In PASMC hypoxia, in part due to altered release of reactive oxygen species (ROS) and/or changes in redox status inhibits voltage-gated K^+ channels (K_v) and two-pore domain K^+ channels (K_{2P}), leading to the depolarization of the membrane (E_m) and activation of voltage-operated L-type Ca^{2+} channels (VOCC). Depletion of Ca^{2+} from the sarcoplasmic reticulum opening of SOC allows for Ca^{2+} influx, termed capacitative calcium entry. Intracellular $[Ca^{2+}]$ is also increased by hypoxia through the activation of store-operated (SOC) or receptor-operated (ROC) Ca^{2+} channels. The hypoxia-induced rise in $[Ca^{2+}]$ then triggers PASMC contraction. ETC electron transport chain, NAD(P)H oxidase; SR sarcoplasmic reticulum; Ryr-R ryanodine receptors, IP3 inositol-1,4,5-triphosphate receptor; K_{Ca} Ca^{2+}-sensitive K^+ channels.

Table 4.1   Effect of acute hypoxia on reactive oxygen species (ROS) production in the lung

Tissue	Hypoxia	ROS	Techniques	Reference
PASMCs (human)	5 percent	↓	DCFH fluorescence, DHE; Amplex Red	178
Isolated Pas (rat)	40 mmHg pO_2	↓	lucigenin-enhanced chemiluminescence, Amplex Red and DCFH assay	179
Isolated PA (rat)	1 percent	↓	luminol analogue (L-012)-enhanced chemiluminescence, Amplex Red	180
Isolated perfused lung (rat)	0–10 percent	↓	luminol- and lucigenin-enhanced chemiluminescence	181
Isolated perfused lung (rabbit)	0 percent	↓	lucigenin-enhanced chemiluminescence	182
Isolated perfused lung (rat)	2.5 percent	↓	luminol-enhanced chemiluminescence	73
Isolated perfused lung (rabbit)	1 percent	↓	horseradish peroxidase and DCF assay for H_2O_2 measurement in exhaled air	183
Isolated perfused lung (rabbit and mouse)	1–10 percent	↓	cyclic hydroxylamine spin probe CPH and ESR spectroscopy	184
PASMC (calf)	40 mmHg pO_2	↑	lucigenin-enhanced chemiluminescence	46
PASMCs (rat)	25 mmHg pO_2	↑	DCFH fluorescence	185
PASMCs (rat)	2 percent	↑	DCFH fluorescence	81
PA and PASMCs (porcine)	4 percent	↑	DCFH fluorescence, lucigenin-enhanced chemiluminescence, ESR	186
PASMCs (mouse)	1.5 percent	↑	FRET	187
Lung tissue slices and PASMCs (mouse)	1 percent	↑	DCFH fluorescence	188
Isolated perfused lung (rabbit and mouse)	5 percent	↑	cyclic hydroxylamine spin probe CPH and ESR spectroscopy after PMA	184

in the lung (NEBs) (43), smooth muscle cells of the pulmonary arteries (44–46), endothelial cells (47) and carotid bodies (48). The classical form of this enzyme (leukocytic NADPH oxidase) is comprised of a membrane-bound flavocytochrome containing two subunits, gp91[phox] and p22[phox], and the cytosolic proteins p47[phox] and p67[phox] (49,50); for detailed review see Bedard & Krause (51), also refs 52–55.

There is a support for the central role of an NADPH oxidase in O_2 sensing in lung NEBs and the H-146 cell line (56,57), and see refs 58–62. Several studies report evidence against the involvement of an NADPH oxidase in O_2 sensing. See refs 56, 63 and 64 for more details.

MITOCHONDRIA

Depletion of high-energy phosphates, a shift toward the reduced form of redox couples, or cytochromes with an unusually low affinity for pO_2 could act as a sensor for hypoxia. In the mitochondria throughout the cytoplasm, ROS are produced in the form of superoxide by electrons that traverse the electron transport chain, primarily from reduced flavins in complex I and ubisemiquinone of complex III. The superoxide is rapidly changed to H_2O_2 by superoxide dismutase 2 (SOD2), an intramitochondrial antioxidant enzyme. The model of O_2 sensing based on the mitochondria came from observations on the carotid body. A cytochrome with an unusually low affinity for O_2 was reported 30 years ago in carotid body mitochondria (65). Duchen and Biscoe have described a graded increase in NAD(P)H autofluorescence in type I cells in response to decreasing levels of pO_2 over a physiologically significant range (below a pO_2 of about 60 mmHg), reflecting a rise in NAD(P)H/NAD(P) ratio (66,67). In similarly isolated chromaffin cells and dorsal root ganglion neurons no measurable change in autofluorescence was seen until the pO_2 fell close to zero. They interpreted these results to suggest that specialized mitochondrial electron transport might confer the unusual oxygen sensitivity in type I cells.

The exact role of mitochondria has been the basis for debate for many years and was recently reviewed by Ward and Weir and Archer in detail (24,68,69). (See also refs 18, 70–80 for further details.) These data suggest that changes in the redox status of the cytoplasm might alter the gating of K^+ channels, such that hypoxia (more reduced status) closes channels in PA and opens them in DASMCs.

In direct contrast, the ROS hypothesis developed by Schumacker proposes that generation of ROS from complex III of the ETC increases during hypoxia. Studies showing that inhibition of the proximal ETC prevents the rise in ROS production and blocks the response to hypoxia are consistent with this hypothesis (64,81,82). Oxygen sensing does not occur in mutant pulmonary artery myocytes that lack a functioning ETC81. Leach et al. have shown that rotenone and myxothiazol block the rise in intracellular [Ca2+] during hypoxia and HPV, and succinate, substrate

for complex II, can overcome the effect of rotenone and restore HPV without altering the rise in NADH/NAD ratio. These experiments suggest a critical role of complex III of the electron transport chain as an oxygen sensor for HPV (83).

Investigations using mitochondrial inhibitors provide arguments for both concepts, although in general their specificity should be considered carefully, similar to those used for inhibiting NADPH-oxidase function. Additionally, besides being a possible trigger organelle, mitochondria can be a modulator of HPV as mitochondria affect calcium buffering (84,85) and regulate capacitative calcium entry (86,87).

Effector mechanisms (intracellular and extracellular sources of Ca^{2+})

The most widely distributed structures mediating the effect of changes in pO_2 are ion channels. They can be considered the executive limb of the response. Several studies have provided direct evidence that hypoxic vasoconstriction of PASMCs is mediated, at least in part, by the inhibition of one or several K^+ channels leading to cell depolarization, opening of voltage-gated Ca^{2+} channels, and myocyte contraction (18,88–91). See also refs 2, 92–97 for more details.

Potassium channels

The potassium current in PASMCs is an ensemble, reflecting activity of many different channels. At least four classes of K^+ channels have been identified in PASMCs: voltage-dependent K^+ channels (Kv) (89,93,98), calcium-activated K^+ channels (K_{Ca}) (99,100), ATP-sensitive K^+ channels (K_{ATP}) (101) and the more recently identified family of two-pore domain K^+ (K_{2p}) channels. See refs 34, 61, 102–111 for more details.

Multiple pathways may exist for hypoxia-induced Kv channel inhibition. Hypoxic signaling may be related to (a) a conformational change of a membrane-bound heme-linked protein closely associated with the channel, secondary to the binding of O_2; (b) a change in cellular (sarcoplasmic or cytoplasmic) redox status, secondary to altered NAD(P)H oxidase- and/or mitochondrial-dependent oxygen radical formation; or (c) a decrease in the ratios of the cytosolic redox couples (NAD/NADH; NADP/NADPH; GSH/GSSG), secondary to slowing of mitochondrial electron transfer; or (d) release of intracellularly stored Ca^{2+}.

Sources of calcium

An increase of the cytosolic Ca^{2+} concentration ($[Ca^{2+}]_i$) is necessary to elicit constriction of the vessels. In excitable cells, $[Ca^{2+}]_i$ is increased by Ca^{2+} influx through Ca^{2+}-permeable channels and/or by Ca^{2+} mobilization from intracellular Ca^{2+} stores (e.g., endoplasmic/sarcoplasmic reticulum). There are three main pathways by which extracellular Ca^{2+} can enter into the PASMCs: (1) voltage-dependent Ca^{2+}-channels and nonspecific cation channels consisting of (2) receptor-activated Ca^{2+}-channels and (3) store-operated Ca^{2+}-channels. However store-operated Ca^{2+}-channels are frequently defined as a major subfamily of receptor-activated Ca^{2+}-channels. See refs 88 and 113–123 for more details.

The findings suggest that the mechanisms that are necessary for sensing and responding acutely to hypoxia are intrinsic to the PASMCs and that both intracellular and extracellular Ca^{2+} are important.

CHRONIC HYPOXIC VASOCONSTRICTION: HYPOXIC PULMONARY HYPERTENSION

Chronic hypoxia related to a number of primary lung diseases or a prolonged stay at high altitude, results in both structural changes in the PA and a sustained increase in pulmonary vascular tone contributing to a morbidity and mortality of pediatric and adult patients. The feature of the changes depends on the species affected (nearly universally in the PAs of mammals), the gender and the developmental stage at which the exposure to hypoxia occurred (124,125). See also refs 126, 127.

Proinflammatory and vasoactive substances

Chronic hypoxia is associated with changes in the production and release of proinflammatory and potent vasoactive substances by the endothelium. These proinflammatory responses include increased interleukin (IL)-1 and IL-6 mRNA levels and an enhanced IL-1α production, probably due to the nuclear factor κB (NF-κB) or NF-IL-6 (128,129). In addition, hypoxia can also rise the expression of endothelial leukocyte molecule (ELAM)-1, intracellular adhesion molecule (ICAM)-1, and vascular cell adhesion molecule (VCAM)-1 on endothelial cells (130).

Endothelin-1 (ET-1) is considered to be a major player within the pathological mechanisms involved in pulmonary arterial hypertension (131,132) and specific antagonists of ET-1 receptors represent an important pillar of modern therapy of this devastating disease (133,134).

Several studies have shown the role of vasoactive serotonin (5-HT) in the regulation of chronic hypoxic responses. In an animal model, increases of plasma 5-HT have been observed under hypoxia (142), and see refs 143–148. Furthermore decreased production and activity of prostacyclin (149) and NO (150) have been reported. Finally, changes in endothelial permeability, coagulant, inflammatory, and protein synthetic capabilities are observed in response to hypoxic exposure. All these alterations can exert significant effects not only on the contractile state of SMCs but on their proliferative and synthetic state as well (151).

Ion balance and calcium homeostasis

The precise control of the balance between proliferation and apoptosis is important for adaptation to changed oxygenation, flow and pressure conditions within the resistance vessels of the lung. In chronic hypoxia this balance seems to be disturbed. The maladaptive response, increased PASMC proliferation and decreased apoptosis, results in vessel wall thickening, vascular remodeling and consequently in sustained pulmonary hypertension (Figure 4.2). If enhanced proliferation in combination with inhibited apoptosis leads to vascular remodeling, how might they occur?

K⁺ channels in chronic hypoxic pulmonary hypertension

Since K^+ channels are important determinants of vascular tone control and the proliferative status of vascular smooth muscle cells, the impact of K^+ channels and membrane potential has been investigated in several animal models of chronic pulmonary hypertension. Shortly after the first reports about the effect of acute hypoxia on K^+ channels, Smirnov et al. demonstrated that PASMCs of rats raised for four weeks in an hypoxic environment have reduced voltage-gated K^+ (Kv) current compared to normoxic rats (152). The resting potential of PASMCs from chronically hypoxic animals was significantly more positive (152). It was proposed that the observed reduction in Kv current amplitude was as a result of decreased channel expression (153). The first proof of the chronic hypoxia-induced transcriptional and translational changes of K^+ channels genes in PASMCs was provided by Wang et al. (107). Decreased mRNA expression of Kv1.1, Kv1.5, Kv2.1, Kv4.3 and Kv9.3 α-subunits in cultured rat PASMCs under hypoxia was confirmed by other groups (154,155), whereas no appreciable change in expression is seen in mesenteric arterial SMCs (154,155). These observations suggest that the response is specific to PASMCs and therefore, selective for the pulmonary circulation. Two animal models emphasize the importance of Kv channels in the pulmonary vascular response, the chronically hypoxic animal model and the Kv1.5 knockout mouse model. Most studies that focus on changes in protein expression and function of Kv α-subunits show a downregulation of Kv1.2, Kv1.5 and Kv2.1 with consequent membrane depolarization and increased $[Ca^{2+}]_i$ in chronically hypoxic rats (156,157). A recent study by Pozeg and co-workers indicates that enhancing expression of Kv1.5 via Kv1.5 adenoviral gene transfer, restores Kv expression, O_2-sensitive K^+ current, and HPV (158). Finally, Kv1.5 knockout mice show impaired HPV and reduced O_2-sensitive K^+ current in PASMCs (110). These data provide evidence for the role of Kv channels in the chronic pulmonary vascular response to hypoxia. In PASMCs, the reduction of the Kv channel activity and the consequent membrane depolarization appears to be involved in the development of chronic hypoxic pulmonary hypertension by mediating pulmonary vasoconstriction and vascular remodeling through increased $[Ca^{2+}]_i$.

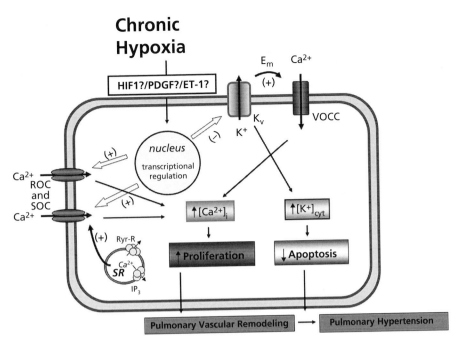

Figure 4.2   Roles of multiple ion channels in chronic hypoxia-induced pulmonary vascular remodeling. Chronic hypoxia downregulates K_v channel expression and upregulates canonical transient receptor potential (TRPC) channel expression in PASMC. The resultant decrease in K_v currents causes E_m depolarization, opens VOCC, and increases $[Ca^{2+}]_{cyt}$, whereas the increase in SOC and ROC activity enhances voltage-independent CCE and raises $[Ca^{2+}]_{cyt}$, causing sustained pulmonary vasoconstriction and stimulating PASMC proliferation. The selective loss of sarcolemmal K^+ channels like K_v decreases transmembrane K^+ efflux, which then increases cytosolic K^+ $[K^+]_{cyt}$ and thus reduces apoptosis. The increased PASMC proliferation and decreased apoptosis, results in pulmonary vascular remodeling and consequently in sustained pulmonary hypertension. ET-1 endothelin-1; HIF1 hypoxia-inducible factor-1; PDGF platelet-derived growth factor.

Many hypotheses have been put forth to explain the chronic hypoxia-induced inhibition of Kv channels in PASMCs (see refs 159–161).

In the last decade the knowledge of the mechanism behind the decreased apoptosis in vascular remodeling and the signaling pathways that mediate this cellular response to sustained hypoxia has rapidly developed. In PASMCs, any changes in K^+ efflux or influx via ion channels and transport mechanisms will influence the regulation of the cellular volume and the extent of apoptosis. Several studies have proposed that apoptosis is mediated, at least in part, by loss of K^+ through one or several K^+ channels (165–167). In PASMCs, the selective loss of sarcolemmal K^+ channels such as Kv during chronic hypoxia decreases transmembrane K^+ efflux, which in turn increases the cytosolic K^+ and thus reduces apoptosis. In contrast, increased transmembrane K^+ efflux (K^+ channels open and/or the number of functional K^+ channels increased due to upregulation of K^+ channel gene expression) enhances cell volume decrease and causes apoptosis.

Ca²⁺ and Ca²⁺ sensitization in chronic hypoxia induced PAH

An increase in intracellular Ca^{2+} plays an obligatory role in the pulmonary pressor response to hypoxia. Although the precise mechanisms involved in sustained hypoxia-induced Ca^{2+} influx across the plasma membrane are still unclear, it is now apparent that voltage-independent Ca^{2+} channels are most affected in vascular smooth muscle cells. In the pulmonary vasculature, Ca^{2+} influx through voltage independent cation entry pathways involve: (1) store-operated Ca^{2+} channels (SOC) activated by depletion of Ca^{2+} from intracellular stores; and (2) receptor-operated Ca^{2+} channels (ROC) activated by interaction of agonist with membrane receptors. The characterization of the canonical transient receptor potential (TRPC) family of cation channel proteins has given fresh impetus to the molecular identification of membrane potential-independent Ca^{2+} influx in cells involved in the pulmonary hypoxic response. In PASMCs, the first evidence for role of the Ca^{2+} influx due to SOCs and ROCs in chronic pulmonary vasoconstriction, was provided by Hong *et al.*, Lin *et al.* and Wang *et al.* (168–170). See also refs 171–177 for more details.

Upregulation of TRPC channels, in conjunction with elevated circulating levels of vasoconstrictors, growth factors and increased agonist receptors in PASMCs as well as changes in Rho/Rho kinase signaling have an important impact on the development of chronic hypoxia-induced pulmonary hypertension by increasing and maintaining vascular tone.

KEY POINTS

- Hypoxic pulmonary vasoconstriction (HPV) is a physiological response of pulmonary arteries that diverts mixed venous blood away from hypoxic alveoli, thus optimizing the matching of perfusion and ventilation and preventing arterial hypoxemia.
- HPV depends largely on the alveolar and not on the mixed venous pO_2 and starts within seconds of the onset of airway hypoxia by a decrease in alveolar O_2 tension below a threshold fractional inspired O_2 concentration of ~10 percent.
- Oxygen sensing could be achieved through conformational changes of the effectors or through production of reactive oxygen species (ROS), thus altering the redox status of signaling molecules and the function of effectors.
- Mitochondria and nicotinamid adenine dinucleotide phosphate (NADPH) oxidases are discussed as oxygen sensors.
- The effector pathways include potassium channels and both influx of calcium and intracellular release of calcium in pulmonary artery smooth muscle cells.

ACKNOWLEDGEMENTS

The author would like to thank Ken Weir for his endless support and inspiring discussions.

REFERENCES

• = Key primary paper
♦ = Major review article

1. Bradford JR, Dean HP. The pulmonary circulation. J Physiol 1894;16:34–96.
2. Euler v US, Liljestrand G. Observations on the pulmonary arterial blood pressure in the cat. Acta Physiol Scand 1946;12:301–20.
3. Cornfield DN, Reeve HL, Tolarova S, Weir EK, Archer S. Oxygen causes fetal pulmonary vasodilation through activation of a calcium-dependent potassium channel. Proc Natl Acad Sci USA 1996;93:8089–94.
4. Weir EK. Does normoxic pulmonary vasodilatation rather than hypoxic vasoconstriction account for the pulmonary pressor response to hypoxia? Lancet 1978;1:476–7.
5. Shirai M, Sada K, Ninomiya I. Effects of regional alveolar hypoxia and hypercapnia on small pulmonary vessels in cats. J Appl Physiol 1986;61:440–8.
6. Peake MD, Harabin AL, Brennan NJ, Sylvester JT. Steady-state vascular responses to graded hypoxia in isolated lungs of five species. J Appl Physiol 1981;51:1214–9.
7. Skovgaard N, Abe AS, Andrade DV, Wang T. Hypoxic pulmonary vasoconstriction in reptiles: a comparative study of four species with different lung structures and pulmonary blood pressures. Am J Physiol Regul Integr Comp Physiol 2005;289:R1280–8.
•8. Marshall C, Marshall BE. Influence of perfusate pO_2 on hypoxic pulmonary vasoconstriction in rats. Circ Res 1983;52:691–6.
9. Weissmann N, Grimminger F, Walmrath D, Seeger W. Hypoxic vasoconstriction in buffer-perfused rabbit lungs. Respir Physiol 1995;100:159–69.
10. Jensen KS, Micco AJ, Czartolomna J, Latham L, Voelkel NF. Rapid onset of hypoxic vasoconstriction in isolated lungs. J Appl Physiol 1992;72:2018–23.
11. Riley RL, Himmelstein A. Studies of the pulmonary circulation at rest and during exercise in normal individuals and in patients with chronic pulmonary disease. Am J Physiol 1948;152:372–82.
12. Welling KL, Sanchez R, Ravn JB, Larsen B, Amtorp O. Effect of prolonged alveolar hypoxia on pulmonary arterial pressure and segmental vascular resistance. J Appl Physiol 1993;75:1194–1200.
13. Vejlstrup NG, Dorrington KL. Intense slow hypoxic pulmonary vasoconstriction in gas-filled and liquid-filled lungs: an in vivo study in the rabbit. Acta Physiol Scand 1993;148:305–13.
14. Wiener CM, Sylvester JT. Effects of glucose on hypoxic vasoconstriction in isolated ferret lungs. J Appl Physiol 1991;70:439–46.
15. Bennie RE, Packer CS, Powell DR, Jin N, Rhoades RA. Biphasic contractile response of pulmonary artery to hypoxia. Am J Physiol 1991;261:L156–63.
16. Robertson TP, Aaronson PI, Ward JP. Hypoxic vasoconstriction and intracellular Ca^{2+} in pulmonary arteries: evidence for PKC-independent Ca^{2+} sensitization. Am J Physiol 1995;268:H301–7.
17. Barnes PJ, Liu SF. Regulation of pulmonary vascular tone. Pharmacol Rev 1995;47:87–131.
♦18. Weir EK, Archer SL. The mechanism of acute hypoxic pulmonary vasoconstriction: the tale of two channels. FASEB J 1995;9:183–9.
19. Nakanishi K, Tajima F, Osada H et al. Pulmonary, vascular responses in rats exposed to chronic hypobaric hypoxia at two different altitude levels. Pathol Res Pract 1996;192:1057–67.
20. Fineman JR, Wong J, Soifer SJ. Hyperoxia and alkalosis produce pulmonary vasodilation independent of endothelium-derived nitric oxide in newborn lambs. Pediatr Res 1993;33:341–6.
21. Yamaguchi K, Takasugi T, Fujita H et al. Endothelial modulation of pH-dependent pressor response in isolated perfused rabbit lungs. Am J Physiol 1996;270:H252–8.
22. Schreiber MD, Heymann MA, Soifer SJ. Increased arterial pH, not decreased $PaCO_2$, attenuates hypoxia-induced pulmonary vasoconstriction in newborn lambs. Pediatr Res 1986;20:113–7.

23. Morton MJ, O'Connell AD, Sivaprasadarao A, Hunter M. Determinants of pH sensing in the two-pore domain K(+) channels TASK-1 and -2. Pflugers Arch 2003;445:577–83.

◆24. Weir EK, Lopez-Barneo J, Buckler KJ, Archer SL. Acute oxygen-sensing mechanisms. N Engl J Med 2005;353: 2042–55.

25. Kato M, Staub NC. Response of small pulmonary arteries to unilobar hypoxia and hypercapnia. Circ Res 1966; 19:426–40.

26. Harder DR, Madden JA, Dawson C. Hypoxic induction of Ca^{2+}-dependent action potentials in small pulmonary arteries of the cat. J Appl Physiol 1985;59:1389–93.

27. Madden JA, Dawson CA, Harder DR. Hypoxia-induced activation in small isolated pulmonary arteries from the cat. J Appl Physiol 1985;59:113–8.

●28. Yuan XJ, Tod ML, Rubin LJ, Blaustein MP. Contrasting effects of hypoxia on tension in rat pulmonary and mesenteric arteries. Am J Physiol 1990;259:H281–9.

29. Jin N, Packer CS, Rhoades RA. Pulmonary arterial hypoxic contraction: signal transduction. Am J Physiol 1992;263: L73–8.

30. Madden JA, Vadula MS, Kurup VP. Effects of hypoxia and other vasoactive agents on pulmonary and cerebral artery smooth muscle cells. Am J Physiol 1992;263:L384–93.

31. Migita CT, Fujii H, Mansfield MK, Takahashi S, Zhou H, Yoshida T. Molecular oxygen oxidizes the porphyrin ring of the ferric alpha-hydroxyheme in heme oxygenase in the absence of reducing equivalent. Biochim Biophys Acta 1999;1432:203–13.

32. Ganfornina MD, Lopez-Barneo J. Single K^+ channels in membrane patches of arterial chemoreceptor cells are modulated by O_2 tension. Proc Natl Acad Sci USA 1991;88:2927–30.

33. Jiang C, Haddad GG. A direct mechanism for sensing low oxygen levels by central neurons. Proc Natl Acad Sci USA 1994;91:7198–201.

34. Perez-Garcia MT, Lopez-Lopez JR, Gonzalez C. Kvβ1.2 subunit coexpression in HEK293 cells confers O_2 sensitivity to Kv4.2 but not to Shaker channels. J Gen Physiol 1999;113:897–907.

35. Osipenko ON, Tate RJ, Gurney AM. Potential role for kv3.1b channels as oxygen sensors. Circ Res 2000;86:534–40.

●36. Williams SE, Wootton P, Mason HS et al. Hemoxygenase-2 is an oxygen sensor for a calcium-sensitive potassium channel. Science 2004;306:2093–7.

37. Kemp PJ. Hemeoxygenase-2 as an O_2 sensor in K^+ channel-dependent chemotransduction. Biochem Biophys Res Commun 2005;338:648–52.

38. Riesco-Fagundo AM, Perez-Garcia MT, Gonzalez C, Lopez-Lopez JR. O(2) modulates large-conductance Ca(2+)-dependent K(+) channels of rat chemoreceptor cells by a membrane-restricted and CO-sensitive mechanism. Circ Res 2001;89:430–6.

39. Adachi T, Ishikawa K, Hida W et al. Hypoxemia and blunted hypoxic ventilatory responses in mice lacking heme oxygenase-2. Biochem Biophys Res Commun 2004;320:514–22.

40. Ortega-Saenz P, Pascual A, Gomez-Diaz R, Lopez-Barneo J. Acute oxygen sensing in heme oxygenase-2 null mice. J Gen Physiol 2006;128:405–11.

41. Zhang F, Kaide JI, Yang L et al. CO modulates pulmonary vascular response to acute hypoxia: relation to endothelin. Am J Physiol Heart Circ Physiol 2004;286:H137–44.

42. Keseru B, Barbosa-Sicard E, Popp R et al. Epoxyeicosatrienoic acids and the soluble epoxide hydrolase are determinants of pulmonary artery pressure and the acute hypoxic pulmonary vasoconstrictor response. FASEB J 2008;22:4306–15.

43. Youngson C, Nurse C, Yeger H, Cutz E. Oxygen sensing in airway chemoreceptors. Nature 1993;365:153–5.

44. Mohazzab KM, Wolin MS. Properties of a superoxide anion-generating microsomal NADH oxidoreductase, a potential pulmonary artery PO_2 sensor. Am J Physiol 1994;267:L823–31.

45. Mohazzab KM, Fayngersh RP, Kaminski PM, Wolin MS. Potential role of NADH oxidoreductase-derived reactive O_2 species in calf pulmonary arterial PO_2-elicited responses. Am J Physiol 1995;269:L637–44.

●46. Marshall C, Mamary AJ, Verhoeven AJ, Marshall BE. Pulmonary artery NADPH-oxidase is activated in hypoxic pulmonary vasoconstriction. Am J Respir Cell Mol Biol 1996;15:633–44.

47. Zulueta JJ, Yu FS, Hertig IA, Thannickal VJ, Hassoun PM. Release of hydrogen peroxide in response to hypoxia-reoxygenation: role of an NAD(P)H oxidase-like enzyme in endothelial cell plasma membrane. Am J Respir Cell Mol Biol 1995;12:41–9.

48. Kummer W, Acker H. Immunohistochemical demonstration of four subunits of neutrophil NAD(P)H oxidase in type I cells of carotid body. J Appl Physiol 1995;78:1904–9.

49. Jones SA, Hancock JT, Jones OT, Neubauer A, Topley N. The expression of NADPH oxidase components in human glomerular mesangial cells: detection of protein and mRNA for p47phox, p67phox, and p22phox. J Am Soc Nephrol 1995;5:1483–91.

50. Umeki S. Activation factors of neutrophil NADPH oxidase complex. Life Sci 1994;55:1–13.

◆51. Bedard K, Krause KH. The NOX family of ROS-generating NADPH oxidases: physiology and pathophysiology. Physiol Rev 2007;87:245–313.

52. Matsuzaki I, Chatterjee S, Debolt K, Manevich Y, Zhang Q, Fisher AB. Membrane depolarization and NADPH oxidase activation in aortic endothelium during ischemia reflect altered mechanotransduction. Am J Physiol Heart Circ Physiol 2005;288:H336–43.

53. Diebold BA, Bokoch GM. Molecular basis for Rac2 regulation of phagocyte NADPH oxidase. Nat Immunol 2001;2:211–5.

54. Shmelzer Z, Haddad N, Admon E et al. Unique targeting of cytosolic phospholipase A2 to plasma membranes mediated by the NADPH oxidase in phagocytes. J Cell Biol 2003;162:683–92.

55. Weissmann N, Voswinckel R, Hardebusch T et al. Evidence for a role of protein kinase C in hypoxic pulmonary vasoconstriction. Am J Physiol 1999;276:L90–5.

56. Wang D, Youngson C, Wong V et al. NADPH-oxidase and a hydrogen peroxide-sensitive K$^+$ channel may function as an oxygen sensor complex in airway chemoreceptors and small cell lung carcinoma cell lines. Proc Natl Acad Sci USA 1996;93:13182–7.

57. O'Kelly I, Lewis A, Peers C, Kemp PJ. O$_2$ sensing by airway chemoreceptor-derived cells. Protein kinase c activation reveals functional evidence for involvement of NADPH oxidase. J Biol Chem 2000;275:7684–92.

58. Fu XW, Wang D, Nurse CA, Dinauer MC, Cutz E. NADPH oxidase is an O$_2$ sensor in airway chemoreceptors: evidence from K$^+$ current modulation in wild-type and oxidase-deficient mice. Proc Natl Acad Sci USA 2000;97:4374–9.

59. Wolin MS, Burke-Wolin TM, Mohazzab H. Roles for NAD(P)H oxidases and reactive oxygen species in vascular oxygen sensing mechanisms. Respir Physiol 1999;115:229–38.

60. Lee YM, Kim BJ, Chun YS et al. NOX4 as an oxygen sensor to regulate TASK-1 activity. Cell Signal 2006; 18:499–507.

•61. Gurney AM, Osipenko ON, Macmillan D, McFarlane KM, Tate RJ, Kempsill FE. Two-pore domain K channel, TASK-1, in pulmonary artery smooth muscle cells. Circ Res 2003;93:957–64.

62. Olschewski A, Li Y, Tang B et al. Impact of TASK-1 in human pulmonary artery smooth muscle cells. Circ Res 2006;98:1072–80.

63. Archer SL, Reeve HL, Michelakis E et al. O$_2$ sensing is preserved in mice lacking the gp91 phox subunit of NADPH oxidase. Proc Natl Acad Sci USA 1999;96:7944–9.

64. Weissmann N, Zeller S, Schafer RU et al. Impact of mitochondria and NADPH oxidases on acute and sustained hypoxic pulmonary vasoconstriction. Am J Respir Cell Mol Biol 2006;34:505–13.

65. Mills E, Jobsis FF. Mitochondrial respiratory chain of carotid body and chemoreceptor response to changes in oxygen tension. J Neurophysiol 1972;35:405–28.

66. Duchen MR, Biscoe TJ. Mitochondrial function in type I cells isolated from rabbit arterial chemoreceptors. J Physiol 1992;450:13–31.

67. Duchen MR, Biscoe TJ. Relative mitochondrial membrane potential and [Ca^{2+}]$_i$ in type I cells isolated from the rabbit carotid body. J Physiol 1992;450:33–61.

♦68. Ward JP. Curiouser and curiouser: the perplexing conundrum of reactive oxygen species and hypoxic pulmonary vasoconstriction. Exp Physiol 2007;92:819–20.

69. Archer SL, Gomberg-Maitland M, Maitland ML, Rich S, Garcia JG, Weir EK. Mitochondrial metabolism, redox signaling, and fusion: a mitochondria-ROS-HIF-1alpha-Kv1.5 O$_2$-sensing pathway at the intersection of pulmonary hypertension and cancer. Am J Physiol Heart Circ Physiol 2008;294:H570–8.

70. Archer SL, Will JA, Weir EK. Redox status in the control of pulmonary vascular tone. Herz 1986;11:127–41.

71. Weir EK, Hong Z, Porter VA, Reeve HL. Redox signaling in oxygen sensing by vessels. Respir Physiol Neurobiol 2002;132:121–30.

72. Chander A, Dhariwal KR, Viswanathan R, Venkitasubramanian TA. Pyridine nucleotides in lung and liver of hypoxic rats. Life Sci 1980;26:1935–45.

73. Archer SL, Huang J, Henry T, Peterson D, Weir EK. A redox-based O$_2$ sensor in rat pulmonary vasculature. Circ Res 1993;73:1100–12.

74. Shigemori K, Ishizaki T, Matsukawa S, Sakai A, Nakai T, Miyabo S. Adenine nucleotides via activation of ATP-sensitive K$^+$ channels modulate hypoxic response in rat pulmonary arteries. Am J Physiol 1996;270:L803–9.

75. Park MK, Bae YM, Lee SH, Ho WK, Earm YE. Modulation of voltage-dependent K$^+$ channel by redox potential in pulmonary and ear arterial smooth muscle cells of the rabbit. Pflügers Arch 1997;434:764–71.

76. Schach C, Xu M, Platoshyn O, Keller SH, Yuan JX. Thiol oxidation causes pulmonary vasodilation by activating K$^+$ channels and inhibiting store-operated Ca^{2+} channels. Am J Physiol Lung Cell Mol Physiol 2007;292:L685–98.

77. Yuan XJ, Tod ML, Rubin LJ, Blaustein MP. Deoxyglucose and reduced glutathione mimic effects of hypoxia on K$^+$ and Ca^{2+} conductances in pulmonary artery cells. Am J Physiol 1994;267:L52–63.

78. Reeve HL, Weir EK, Nelson DP, Peterson DA, Archer SL. Opposing effects of oxidants and antioxidants on K$^+$ channel activity and tone in rat vascular tissue. Exp Physiol 1995;80:825–34.

79. Reeve HL, Tolarova S, Nelson DP, Archer S, Weir EK. Redox control of oxygen sensing in the rabbit ductus arteriosus. J Physiol 2001;533:253–61.

•80. Olschewski A, Hong Z, Peterson DA, Nelson DP, Porter VA, Weir EK. Opposite effects of redox status on membrane potential, cytosolic calcium, and tone in pulmonary arteries and ductus arteriosus. Am J Physiol Lung Cell Mol Physiol 2004;286:L15–22.

•81. Waypa GB, Chandel NS, Schumacker PT. Model for hypoxic pulmonary vasoconstriction involving mitochondrial oxygen sensing. Circ Res 2001;88:1259–66.

82. Wang QS, Zheng YM, Dong L, Ho YS, Guo Z, Wang YX. Role of mitochondrial reactive oxygen species in hypoxia-dependent increase in intracellular calcium in pulmonary artery myocytes. Free Radic Biol Med 2007;42:642–53.

•83. Leach RM, Hill HM, Snetkov VA, Robertson TP, Ward JP. Divergent roles of glycolysis and the mitochondrial electron transport chain in hypoxic pulmonary vasoconstriction of the rat: identity of the hypoxic sensor. J Physiol 2001;536:211–24.

84. Wang Q, Wang YX, Yu M, Kotlikoff MI. Ca^{2+}-activated Cl$^-$ currents are activated by metabolic inhibition in rat pulmonary artery smooth muscle cells. Am J Physiol 1997;273:C520–30.

85. Duchen MR. Contributions of mitochondria to animal physiology: from homeostatic sensor to calcium signaling and cell death. J Physiol 1999;516:1–17.

86. Kang TM, Park MK, Uhm DY. Effects of hypoxia and mitochondrial inhibition on the capacitative calcium entry in rabbit pulmonary arterial smooth muscle cells. Life Sci 2003;72:1467–79.

♦87. Ward JP, Robertson TP, Aaronson PI. Capacitative calcium entry: a central role in hypoxic pulmonary vasoconstriction? Am J Physiol Lung Cell Mol Physiol 2005;289:L2–4.

88. Post JM, Hume JR, Archer SL, Weir EK. Direct role for potassium channel inhibition in hypoxic pulmonary vasoconstriction. Am J Physiol 1992;262:C882–90.

89. Yuan XJ. Voltage-gated K^+ currents regulate resting membrane potential and $[Ca^{2+}]_i$ in pulmonary arterial myocytes. Circ Res 1995;77:370–8.

90. Archer SL, Huang JM, Reeve HL et al. Differential distribution of electrophysiologically distinct myocytes in conduit and resistance arteries determines their response to nitric oxide and hypoxia. Circ Res 1996;78:431–42.

91. Osipenko ON, Evans AM, Gurney AM. Regulation of the resting potential of rabbit pulmonary artery myocytes by a low threshold, O_2-sensing potassium current. Br J Pharmacol 1997;120:1461–70.

92. Vadula MS, Kleinman JG, Madden JA. Effect of hypoxia and norepinephrine on cytoplasmic free Ca^{2+} in pulmonary and cerebral arterial myocytes. Am J Physiol 1993;265:L591–7.

93. Post JM, Gelband CH, Hume JR. $[Ca^{2+}]_i$ inhibition of K^+ channels in canine pulmonary artery. Novel mechanism for hypoxia-induced membrane depolarization. Circ Res 1995;77:131–9.

94. Franco-Obregon A, Lopez-Barneo J. Differential oxygen sensitivity of calcium channels in rabbit smooth muscle cells of conduit and resistance pulmonary arteries. J Physiol 1996;491:511–8.

95. Urena J, Franco-Obregon A, Lopez-Barneo J. Contrasting effects of hypoxia on cytosolic Ca^{2+} spikes in conduit and resistance myocytes of the rabbit pulmonary artery. J Physiol 1996;496:103–9.

96. Bakhramov A, Evans AM, Kozlowski RZ. Differential effects of hypoxia on the intracellular Ca^{2+} concentration of myocytes isolated from different regions of the rat pulmonary arterial tree. Exp Physiol 1998;83:337–47.

●97. Weissmann N, Dietrich A, Fuchs B et al. Classical transient receptor potential channel 6 (TRPC6) is essential for hypoxic pulmonary vasoconstriction and alveolar gas exchange. Proc Natl Acad Sci USA 2006;103:19093–8.

98. Evans AM, Osipenko ON, Gurney AM. Properties of a novel K^+ current that is active at resting potential in rabbit pulmonary artery smooth muscle cells. J Physiol 1996;496:407–20.

99. Albarwani S, Robertson BE, Nye PC, Kozlowski RZ. Biophysical properties of Ca^{2+}- and Mg-ATP-activated K^+ channels in pulmonary arterial smooth muscle cells isolated from the rat. Pflügers Arch 1994;428:446–54.

100. Peng W, Hoidal JR, Farrukh IS. Role of a novel KCa opener in regulating K^+ channels of hypoxic human pulmonary vascular cells. Am J Respir Cell Mol Biol 1999;20:737–45.

101. Nelson MT, Quayle JM. Physiological roles and properties of potassium channels in arterial smooth muscle. Am J Physiol 1995;268:C799–822.

●102. Wyatt CN, Wright C, Bee D, Peers C. O_2-sensitive K^+ currents in carotid body chemoreceptor cells from normoxic and chronically hypoxic rats and their roles in hypoxic chemotransduction. Proc Natl Acad Sci USA 1995;92:295–9.

♦103. Aaronson PI, Robertson TP, Knock GA et al. Hypoxic pulmonary vasoconstriction: mechanisms and controversies. J Physiol 2006;570:53–8.

104. Archer SL, Souil E, Dinh-Xuan AT et al. Molecular identification of the role of voltage-gated K^+ channels, Kv1.5 and Kv2.1, in hypoxic pulmonary vasoconstriction and control of resting membrane potential in rat pulmonary artery myocytes. J Clin Invest 1998;101:2319–30.

105. Hille B. Potassium channels and chloride channels. Ion channels of excitable membranes, 3rd ed. Sunderland: Sinauer Associates, Inc; 2001. pp. 131–67.

106. Pongs O. Molecular biology of voltage-dependent potassium channels. Physiol Rev 1992;72:S69–88.

107. Wang J, Juhaszova M, Rubin LJ, Yuan XJ. Hypoxia inhibits gene expression of voltage-gated K^+ channel α subunits in pulmonary artery smooth muscle cells. J Clin Invest 1997;100:2347–53.

108. Hulme JT, Coppock EA, Felipe A, Martens JR, Tamkun MM. Oxygen sensitivity of cloned voltage-gated K^+ channels expressed in the pulmonary vasculature. Circ Res 1999; 85:489–97.

109. Patel AJ, Lazdunski M, Honore E. Kv2.1/Kv9.3, a novel ATP-dependent delayed-rectifier K^+ channel in oxygen-sensitive pulmonary artery myocytes. EMBO J 1997;16:6615–25.

110. Archer SL, London B, Hampl V et al. Impairment of hypoxic pulmonary vasoconstriction in mice lacking the voltage-gated potassium channel Kv1.5. FASEB J 2001;15:1801–3.

111. Platoshyn O, Brevnova EE, Burg ED, Yu Y, Remillard CV, Yuan JX. Acute hypoxia selectively inhibits KCNA5 channels in pulmonary artery smooth muscle cells. Am J Physiol Cell Physiol 2006;290:C907–16.

112. Conforti L, Bodi I, Nisbet JW, Millhorn DE. O_2-sensitive K^+ channels: role of the Kv1.2 -subunit in mediating the hypoxic response. J Physiol 2000;524:783–93.

113. McMurtry IF, Davidson AB, Reeves JT, Grover RF. Inhibition of hypoxic pulmonary vasoconstriction by calcium antagonists in isolated rat lungs. Circ Res 1976;38:99–104.

114. McMurtry IF. BAYK8644 potentiates and A23187 inhibits hypoxic vasoconstriction in rat lungs. Am J Physiol 1985; 249:H741–6.

115. Tolins M, Weir EK, Chesler E, Nelson DP, From AH. Pulmonary vascular tone is increased by a voltage-dependent calcium channel potentiator. J Appl Physiol 1986;60:942–8.

116. Salvaterra CG, Goldman WF. Acute hypoxia increases cytosolic calcium in cultured pulmonary arterial myocytes. Am J Physiol 1993;264:L323–8.

117. Olschewski A, Hong Z, Nelson DP, Weir EK. Graded response of K^+ current, membrane potential, and $[Ca^{2+}]_i$ to hypoxia in pulmonary arterial smooth muscle. Am J Physiol Lung Cell Mol Physiol 2002;283:L1143–50.

118. Robertson TP, Hague D, Aaronson PI, Ward JP. Voltage-independent calcium entry in hypoxic pulmonary

vasoconstriction of intrapulmonary arteries of the rat. J Physiol 2000;525:669–80.

119. Yuan XJ, Goldman WF, Tod ML, Rubin LJ, Blaustein MP. Hypoxia reduces potassium currents in cultured rat pulmonary but not mesenteric arterial myocytes. Am J Physiol 1993;264:L116–23.

120. Gelband CH, Gelband H. Ca^{2+} release from intracellular stores is an initial step in hypoxic pulmonary vasoconstriction of rat pulmonary artery resistance vessels. Circulation 1997;96:3647–54.

121. Dipp M, Nye PC, Evans AM. Hypoxic release of calcium from the sarcoplasmic reticulum of pulmonary artery smooth muscle. Am J Physiol Lung Cell Mol Physiol 2001;281:L318–25.

•122. Wilson HL, Dipp M, Thomas JM, Lad C, Galione A, Evans AM. ADP-ribosyl cyclase and cyclic ADP-ribose hydrolase act as a redox sensor. A primary role for cyclic ADP-ribose in hypoxic pulmonary vasoconstriction. J Biol Chem 2001;276:11180–8.

◆123. Evans AM, Dipp M. Hypoxic pulmonary vasoconstriction: cyclic adenosine diphosphate-ribose, smooth muscle Ca(2+) stores and the endothelium. Respir Physiol Neurobiol 2002;132:3–15.

◆124. Haworth SG, Hislop AA. Lung development – the effects of chronic hypoxia. Semin Neonatol 2003;8:1–8.

125. Rabinovitch M, Gamble WJ, Miettinen OS, Reid L. Age and sex influence on pulmonary hypertension of chronic hypoxia and on recovery. Am J Physiol 1981;240:H62–72.

126. Meyrick B, Reid L. Hypoxia and incorporation of 3H-thymidine by cells of the rat pulmonary arteries and alveolar wall. Am J Pathol 1979;96:51–70.

◆127. Rabinovitch M. Pathobiology of pulmonary hypertension. Extracellular matrix. Clin Chest Med 2001;22:433–49.

128. Ten VS, Pinsky DJ. Endothelial response to hypoxia: physiologic adaptation and pathologic dysfunction. Curr Opin Crit Care 2002;8:242–50.

129. Ali MH, Schlidt SA, Chandel NS, Hynes KL, Schumacker PT, Gewertz BL. Endothelial permeability and IL-6 production during hypoxia: role of ROS in signal transduction. Am J Physiol 1999;277:L1057–65.

130. Yoon CH, Hur J, Oh IY et al. Intercellular adhesion molecule-1 is upregulated in ischemic muscle, which mediates trafficking of endothelial progenitor cells. Arterioscler Thromb Vasc Biol 2006;26:1066–72.

131. Stewart DJ, Levy RD, Cernacek P, Langleben D. Increased plasma endothelin-1 in pulmonary hypertension: marker or mediator of disease? Ann Intern Med 1991;114: 464–9.

132. Giaid A, Yanagisawa M, Langleben D et al. Expression of endothelin-1 in the lungs of patients with pulmonary hypertension. N Engl J Med 1993;328:1732–9.

133. Rubin LJ, Badesch DB, Barst RJ et al. Bosentan therapy for pulmonary arterial hypertension. N Engl J Med 2002;346: 896–903.

134. Olschewski H, Olschewski A, Rose F et al. Physiologic basis for the treatment of pulmonary hypertension. J Lab Clin Med 2001;138:287–97.

135. Fagan KA, McMurtry IF, Rodman DM. Role of endothelin-1 in lung disease. Respir Res 2001;2:90–101.

136. Li H, Chen SJ, Chen YF et al. Enhanced endothelin-1 and endothelin receptor gene expression in chronic hypoxia. J Appl Physiol 1994;77:1451–9.

137. Li H, Elton TS, Chen YF, Oparil S. Increased endothelin receptor gene expression in hypoxic rat lung. Am J Physiol 1994;266:L553–60.

138. Stelzner TJ, O'Brien RF, Yanagisawa M et al. Increased lung endothelin-1 production in rats with idiopathic pulmonary hypertension. Am J Physiol 1992;262:L614–20.

139. Frasch HF, Marshall C, Marshall BE. Endothelin-1 is elevated in monocrotaline pulmonary hypertension. Am J Physiol 1999;276:L304–10.

140. Aguirre JI, Morrel NW, Long L et al. Vascular remodeling and ET-1 expression in rat strains with different responses to chronic hypoxia. Am J Physiol 2000;278:L981–7.

141. Hocher B, Schwarz A, Fagan KA et al. Pulmonary fibrosis and chronic lung inflammation in ET-1 transgenic mice. Am J Respir Cell Mol Biol 2000;23:19–26.

142. Jeffery TK, Bryan-Lluka LJ, Wanstall JC. Specific uptake of 5-hydroxytryptamine is reduced in lungs from hypoxic pulmonary hypertensive rats. Eur J Pharmacol 2000; 396:137–40.

143. MacLean MR, Herve P, Eddahibi S, Adnot S. 5-hydroxytriptamine and the pulmonary circulation: receptors, transporters and relevance to pulmonary arterial hypertension. Br J Pharmacol 2000;131: 161–8.

144. Lee SL, Wang WW, Moore BJ, Fanburg BL. Dual effect of serotonin in growth of bovine pulmonary artery smooth muscle cells in culture. Circulation 1991;68:1362–8.

145. Pitt BR, Weng W, Steve AR, Blakely RD, Reynolds I, Davies P. Serotonin increase DNA synthesis in rat proximal and distal pulmonary vascular smooth muscle cells in culture. Am J Physiol 1994;266:L178–86.

•146. MacLean MR, Deuchar GA, Hicks MN et al. Overexpression of the 5-hydroxytryptamine transporter gene: effect on pulmonary hemodynamics and hypoxia-induced pulmonary hypertension. Circulation 2004;109:2150–5.

147. Keegan A, Morecroft I, Smillie D, Hicks MN, MacLean MR. Contribution of the 5-HT(1B) receptor to hypoxia-induced pulmonary hypertension: converging evidence using 5-HT(1B)-receptor knockout mice and the 5-HT(1B/1D)- receptor antagonist GR127935. Circ Res 2001;89: 1231–9.

•148. Eddahibi S, Hanoun N, Lanfumey L et al. Attenuated hypoxic pulmonary hypertension in mice lacking the 5-hydroxytriptamine transporter gene. J Clin Invest 2000;105:1555–62.

149. Badesch DB, Orton EC, Zapp LM et al. Decreased arterial wall prostaglandin production in neonatal calves with severe chronic pulmonary hypertension. Am J Respir Cell Mol Biol 1989;1:489–98.

150. Le Cras TD, McMurtry IF. Nitric oxide production in the hypoxic lung. Am J Physiol Lung Cell Mol Physiol 2001;280:L575–82.

◆151. Aaronson PI, Robertson TP, Ward JP. Endothelium-derived mediators and hypoxic pulmonary vasoconstriction. Respir Physiol Neurobiol 2002;132:107–20.

•152. Smirnov SV, Robertson TP, Ward JP, Aaronson PI. Chronic hypoxia is associated with reduced delayed rectifier K^+ current in rat pulmonary artery muscle cells. Am J Physiol 1994;266:H365–70.

•153. Osipenko ON, Alexander D, MacLean MR, Gurney AM. Influence of chronic hypoxia on the contributions of non-inactivating and delayed rectifier K currents to the resting potential and tone of rat pulmonary artery smooth muscle. Br J Pharmacol 1998;124:1335–7.

154. Sweeney M, Yuan JX. Hypoxic pulmonary vasoconstriction: role of voltage-gated potassium channels. Respir Res 2000;1:40–8.

155. Platoshyn O, Yu Y, Golovina VA et al. Chronic hypoxia decreases K(v) channel expression and function in pulmonary artery myocytes. Am J Physiol 2001;280:L801–12.

156. Reeve HL, Michelakis E, Nelson D, Weir EK, Archer SL. Alterations in a redox oxygen sensing mechanism in chronic hypoxia. J Appl Physiol 2001;90:2249–56.

157. Hong Z, Weir EK, Nelson DP, Olschewski A. Sub-acute hypoxia decreases K_v channel expression and function in pulmonary artery myocytes. Am J Respir Cell Mol Biol 2004;31:337–43.

•158. Pozeg ZI, Michelakis ED, McMurtry MS et al. In vivo gene transfer of the O_2-sensitive potassium channel Kv1.5 reduces pulmonary hypertension and restores hypoxic pulmonary vasoconstriction in chronically hypoxic rats. Circulation 2003;107:2037–44.

159. Yu AY, Shimoda LA, Iyer NV et al. Impaired physiological response to chronic hypoxia in mice partially deficient for hypoxia-inducible factor 1α. J Clin Invest 1999;103:691–6.

160. Shimoda LA, Manalo DJ, Sham JS, Semenza GL, Sylvester JT. Partial HIF-1α deficiency impairs pulmonary arterial myocyte electrophysiological responses to hypoxia. Am J Physiol Lung Cell Mol Physiol 2001;281:L202–8.

161. Yu Y, Platoshyn O, Zhang J et al. c-Jun decreases voltage-gated K^+ channel activity in pulmonary artery smooth muscle cells. Circulation 2001;104:1557–63.

162. Webster KA, Discher DJ, Bishopric NH. Induction and nuclear accumulation of Fos and Jun proto-oncogenes in hypoxic cardiac myocytes. J Biol Chem 1993;268:16852–8.

163. Munell F, Burke RE, Bandele A, Gubits RM. Localization of c-fos, c-jun, and hsp70 mRNA expression in brain after neonatal hypoxia-ischemia. Dev Brain Res 1994;77:111–21.

164. Bunn HF, Poyton RO. Oxygen sensing and molecular adaptation to hypoxia. Physiol Rev 1996;76:839–85.

165. Krick S, Platoshyn O, McDaniel SS, Rubin LJ, Yuan JX. Augmented K^+ currents and mitochondrial membrane depolarization in pulmonary artery myocyte apoptosis. Am J Physiol Lung Cell Mol Physiol 2001;281:L887–94.

166. Krick S, Platoshyn O, Sweeney M et al. Nitric oxide induces apoptosis by activating K^+ channels in pulmonary vascular smooth muscle cells. Am J Physiol Heart Circ Physiol 2002;282:H184–93.

167. Brevnova EE, Platoshyn O, Zhang S, Yuan JX. Overexpression of human KCNA5 increases IK V and enhances apoptosis. Am J Physiol Cell Physiol 2004;287:C715–22.

168. Hong ZG, Klein JJ, Nelson DP, Hong FX, Varghese A, Weir EK. Capacitative calcium entry in pulmonary arteries increases in chronic hypoxia. Am J Respir Crit Care Med 2004;169:A401.

169. Wang J, Weigand L, Sylvester JT, Shimoda LA. Enhanced capacitative Ca^{2+} entry (CCE) contributes to elevated resting Ca^{2+} and tension in pulmonary arterial smooth muscle from rats exposed to chronic hypoxia (CH). Am J Respir Crit Care Med 2004;169:A400.

•170. Lin MJ, Leung GP, Zhang WM et al. Chronic hypoxia-induced upregulation of store-operated and receptor-operated Ca^{2+} channels in pulmonary arterial smooth muscle cells: a novel mechanism of hypoxic pulmonary hypertension. Circ Res 2004;95:496–505.

171. Golovina VA, Platoshyn O, Bailey CL et al. Upregulated TRP and enhanced capacitative Ca^{2+} entry in human pulmonary artery myocytes during proliferation. Am J Physiol Heart Circ Physiol 2001;280:H746–55.

172. Yu Y, Sweeney M, Zhang S et al. PDGF stimulates pulmonary vascular smooth muscle cell proliferation by upregulating TRPC6 expression. Am J Physiol Cell Physiol 2003;284:C316–30.

173. Yu Y, Fantozzi I, Remillard CV et al. Enhanced expression of transient receptor potential channels in idiopathic pulmonary arterial hypertension. Proc Natl Acad Sci USA 2004;101:13861–6.

174. Fantozzi I, Zhang S, Platoshyn O, Remillard CV, Cowling RT, Yuan JX. Hypoxia increases AP-1 binding activity by enhancing capacitative Ca^{2+} entry in human pulmonary artery endothelial cells. Am J Physiol Lung Cell Mol Physiol 2003;285:L1233–45.

◆175. McMurtry IF, Bauer NR, Fagan KA, Nagaoka T, Gebb SA, Oka M. Hypoxia and Rho/Rho-kinase signaling. Lung development versus hypoxic pulmonary hypertension. Adv Exp Med Biol 2003;543:127–37.

•176. Robertson TP, Dipp M, Ward JP, Aaronson PI, Evans AM. Inhibition of sustained hypoxic vasoconstriction by Y-27632 in isolated intrapulmonary arteries and perfused lung of the rat. Br J Pharmacol 2000;131:5–9.

177. Fagan KA, Oka M, Bauer NR et al. Attenuation of acute hypoxic pulmonary vasoconstriction and hypoxic pulmonary hypertension in mice by inhibition of Rho-kinase. Am J Physiol Lung Cell Mol Physiol 2004;287:L656–64.

•178. Mehta JP, Campian JL, Guardiola J, Cabrera JA, Weir EK, Eaton JW. Generation of oxidants by hypoxic human pulmonary and coronary smooth-muscle cells. Chest 2008;133:1410–4.

179. Michelakis ED, Hampl V, Nsair A et al. Diversity in mitochondrial function explains differences in vascular oxygen sensing. Circ Res 2002;90:1307–15.

•180. Bonnet S, Michelakis ED, Porter CJ et al. An abnormal mitochondrial-hypoxia inducible factor-1alpha-Kv channel pathway disrupts oxygen sensing and triggers pulmonary arterial hypertension in fawn hooded rats: similarities to human pulmonary arterial hypertension. Circulation 2006;113:2630–41.

181. Archer SL, Nelson DP, Weir EK. Simultaneous measurement of O_2 radicals and pulmonary vascular reactivity in rat lung. J Appl Physiol 1989;67:1903–11.

182. Paky A, Michael JR, Burke-Wolin TM, Wolin MS, Gurtner GH. Endogenous production of superoxide by rabbit lungs: effects of hypoxia or metabolic inhibitors. J Appl Physiol 1993;74:2868–74.

183. Weissmann N, Vogels H, Schermuly RT et al. Measurement of exhaled hydrogen peroxide from rabbit lungs. Biol Chem 2004;385:259–64.

184. Weissmann N, Kuzkaya N, Fuchs B et al. Detection of reactive oxygen species in isolated, perfused lungs by electron spin resonance spectroscopy. Respir Res 2005;6:86.

185. Killilea DW, Hester R, Balczon R, Babal P, Gillespie MN. Free radical production in hypoxic pulmonary artery smooth muscle cells. Am J Physiol Lung Cell Mol Physiol 2000;279:L408–12.

186. Liu JQ, Sham JS, Shimoda LA, Kuppusamy P, Sylvester JT. Hypoxic constriction and reactive oxygen species in porcine distal pulmonary arteries. Am J Physiol Lung Cell Mol Physiol 2003;285:L322–33.

187. Waypa GB, Guzy R, Mungai PT et al. Increases in mitochondrial reactive oxygen species trigger hypoxia-induced calcium responses in pulmonary artery smooth muscle cells. Circ Res 2006;99:970–8.

188. Paddenberg R, Ishaq B, Goldenberg A et al. Essential role of complex II of the respiratory chain in hypoxia-induced ROS generation in the pulmonary vasculature. Am J Physiol Lung Cell Mol Physiol 2003;284:L710–9.

5

Pulmonary vascular remodeling and pathobiology of pulmonary hypertension

NICHOLAS W MORRELL

PULMONARY VASCULAR REMODELING

Pulmonary vascular remodeling involves structural and functional changes to the normal architecture of the walls of pulmonary arteries. The process of vascular remodeling can occur as a primary response to injury, or stimulus such as hypoxia, within the resistance vessels of the lung. Alternatively, the changes seen in more proximal vessels are probably the result of a sustained rise in intravascular pressure. In order to withstand the chronic increase in intraluminal pressure, the vessel wall becomes thickened and stronger. This arises from Laplaces law, i.e. $P = T/r$, where T = tangential tension, P = pressure difference across the wall of the vessel and r = radius. Thus tension within the vessel wall rises as a consequence of increased pressure. This "armoring" of the vessel wall with extra smooth muscle, fibroblasts and extracellular matrix decreases lumen diameter and reduces the capacity for vasodilatation. This maladaptive response results in increased pulmonary vascular resistance and consequently, sustained pulmonary hypertension.

PHYSIOLOGICAL CONSEQUENCES OF PULMONARY VASCULAR REMODELING

The normal adult pulmonary circulation is a high flow, low resistance vascular bed with little or no resting tone. The capacity for recruitment and vasodilatation in the normal pulmonary circulation is such that large increases in cardiac output cause little elevation of pulmonary arterial pressure (Figure 5.1). Thus, pulmonary vascular resistance decreases as pulmonary blood flow increases. However, when the pulmonary circulation is remodeled there is a reduced capacity

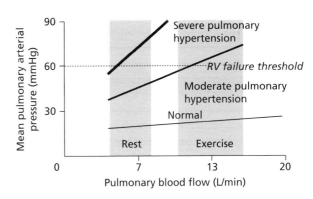

Figure 5.1 Diagramatic representation of pressure/flow curves, at rest and on exercise, in the normal pulmonary circulation and in pulmonary hypertension, in the face of increasing remodeling. The slope of the lines is equivalent to the pulmonary vascular resistance (PVR). Thus, an increase in remodeling leads to increases in PVR and thus pressure. Note that an increase in resting PVR is accompanied by truncation of the pressure/flow curve on exercise and a marked increase in exercise PVR in pulmonary hypertension. RV, right ventricle.

for vasodilatation and a decrease in the cross sectional area of the pulmonary vascular bed. Therefore, pulmonary arterial pressure may be elevated at rest and rises markedly on exercise. The greater the degree of remodeling, the greater the rise in pressure for a given cardiac output. So for example, in patients with idiopathic pulmonary hypertension in whom florid vascular remodeling is observed, severe pulmonary hypertension can lead to right ventricular failure at rest. At a mean right ventricular pressure of > 60 mmHg, right ventricular overload occurs and the capacity to further increase cardiac output is compromised.

MORPHOLOGICAL FEATURES

Normal pulmonary arteries

The anatomy of pulmonary arteries alters in a systematic way from the central "conduit" arteries to the peripheral "resistance" vessels. Proximal arteries are thin walled relative to their luminal diameter. The media is composed of many elastic laminae separated by layers of smooth muscle. These large arteries serve an important role as capacitance vessels and contribute to reducing ventricular afterload. This useful function may be lost as the proximal pulmonary arteries stiffen. In advanced pulmonary hypertension atheromatous change with calcification can be seen in proximal pulmonary arteries. As the diameter of the arterial lumen decreases down the arterial tree, the elastic laminae become less prominent and are replaced by smooth muscle. Beyond the terminal bronchioles, within the respiratory acinus, the arteries become only partially muscularized as the smooth muscle layer tails off in a spiral, with no smooth muscle found within the smaller intra-acinar arteries (reviewed in refs 1, 2). This precapillary segment of the pulmonary vascular bed is the site of the greatest pressure drop along the pulmonary circulation. As this site contributes to the majority of pulmonary vascular resistance, it follows that small changes in tone or wall structure at this level can lead to large elevations of pulmonary arterial pressure. For example, from Poiseuille's law for steady flow:

$$\text{PVR} \propto \frac{8\mu L}{\pi D^4}$$

where L is vascular length, μ is the viscosity of blood, and D is vessel diameter, it can be seen that at constant length, the resistance in a tube doubles if D is decreased by 16 percent. The most distal segments of the precapillary arterioles contain an endothelial layer underlined by a single elastic lamina. Additional smooth muscle-like cell types have been described in the more distal segments, (1) intermediate cells which, unlike smooth muscle cells, lie inside the internal elastic lamina; and (2) pericytes which lie beneath the endothelium in small precapillary vessels that do not possess an elastic lamina.

Distal muscularization of normally non-muscular arteries

A feature common to all forms of pulmonary hypertensive remodeling is the appearance of a layer of smooth muscle in small peripheral, normally non-muscular, pulmonary arteries within the respiratory acinus. The cellular processes underlying muscularization of this distal segment of the pulmonary arterial tree are incompletely understood. In precapillary vessels intermediate cells, inside the internal elastic lamina, may proliferate and differentiate into smooth muscle cells (3). In the most distal vessels, which lack an elastic lamina (20–30 μm diameter), differentiation of pericytes and recruitment of interstitial fibroblasts from the surrounding lung parenchyma contribute to the process of muscularization (4). These cells subsequently take on a smooth muscle-like phenotype.

It has been emphasized that when pulmonary hypertension occurs associated with alveolar hypoxia, such as hypoxic lung disease or from residence at high altitude, the remodeling observed in small pulmonary arteries is rather different from that seen in other forms of pulmonary hypertension. Although distal neomuscularization still occurs, laying down of a longitudinally orientated layer of smooth muscle within the intima of small (80–500 μm) pulmonary arteries, and formation of "inner muscular tubes" is characteristic of hypoxia-induced pulmonary hypertension in man (5).

Increased muscularization of muscular pulmonary arteries

In the more proximal muscular arteries, subjected to a higher intraluminal pressure secondary to vasoconstriction and remodeling in the small peripheral arteries, proliferation and hypertrophy of medial smooth muscle occurs, leading to a "fixed" reduction in the diameter of the vessel lumen (6,7). New elastic laminae are deposited between the muscle layers, and increased type 1 collagen deposition serves to stiffen the vessel wall (7). In addition to the changes in the media, there is proliferation of fibroblasts in the adventitial layer along with collagen deposition. In pulmonary hypertension due to raised left atrial pressure, similar though less marked changes may be observed in the pulmonary veins (8). The mechanism leading to excess vascular muscularization in the proximal pulmonary arteries includes endothelial damage/activation leading to increased permeability to factors in the serum (see below). For example, activation of elastases disrupts the elastic laminae of the vessel and promotes proliferation and hypertrophy of activated smooth muscle cells and deposition of extracellular matrix (9,10).

Neointima formation

A hallmark of severe pulmonary hypertension (e.g. primary pulmonary hypertension, or congenital heart disease) is the formation of a layer of cells and extracellular matrix between the endothelium and the internal elastic lamina, termed the neointima (11,12). This important lesion occurs in small and large arteries and contributes significantly to the increased vascular resistance. Neointima formation appears to be a frequent non-specific response to vascular injury and is also found in restenosis following angioplasty, and the atherosclerosis of coronary arteries in transplant hearts. The commonly used animal models of pulmonary hypertension (e.g. chronically hypoxic rat, or monocrotaline) do not recapitulate this important feature. However, when vascular injury (monocrotaline) is combined with high flow (induced by pneumonectomy) the rat pulmonary artery also develops a neointima (13,14). These observations suggest that increased blood flow, such as that seen in congenital left to right shunts, is an important stimulus to neointima formation and disease progression.

The cells comprising the neointima are myofibroblasts. These cells express smooth muscle markers such as α-smooth muscle actin (α-SM actin), and vimentin, but are distinguished from mature smooth muscle cells by their lack of expression of markers characteristic of highly differentiated smooth muscle cells, such as smooth muscle myosin. Neointimal cells do not express endothelial cell markers such as CD31, CD34 or Factor VIII (12). *In vitro*, myofibroblasts derived from the neointima, exhibit different responses to growth factors than cells derived from the media.

The origin of neointimal cells in severe pulmonary hypertension remains unclear, though diverse origins seem likely. Cells may arise by transdifferentiation of endothelial cells, by migration of "smooth muscle cell-like cells" from the media, or by migration of adventitial fibroblasts. In the systemic circulation, using pulse-labeling of dividing cells with bromodeoxyuridine, the available evidence suggests that proliferating cells arising in the media and adventitia of injured arteries migrate to the subendothelial space (15,16). Furthermore, labeled adventitial fibroblasts stably transfected with a lacZ retrovirus were found capable of migrating from the adventitia to the media and neointima (17). Study of the relative contribution from adventitial fibroblasts and poorly differentiated medial smooth muscle cells to neointima formation is hampered by the lack of specific markers to differentiate between these cells. Labeling of bone marrow derived cells with fluorescent markers has implicated a major role for these cells in the formation of a neointima following arterial injury.

Formation of plexiform lesions

A further important form of vascular remodeling in severe pulmonary hypertension is the disorganized proliferation of endothelial cells leading to formation of the so-called plexiform lesion. This disorganized growth of new vessels is seen in approximately 80 percent of cases of idiopathic

PAH and in severe cases of PAH associated with other conditions. They are typically seen arising from arteries of diameter 200–400 μm. Lesions tend to occur in association with smaller arteries in idiopathic PAH compared with PAH associated with congenital heart disease (12). The cells comprising these lesions are endothelial channels supported by a stroma containing matrix proteins and α-SM actin expressing myofibroblasts. The endothelial cells within these lesions express markers of angiogenesis, such as VEGF and its receptors (18,19). Studies have shown that the cells comprising plexiform lesions in cases of IPAH are monoclonal in origin, whereas cells in cases of associated PAH are polyclonal in origin (20). Therefore, although the lesions themselves may be hemodynamically irrelevant, they may represent more than simply the result of severe elevation of intravascular pressures. Rather, the endothelial proliferation seen in these lesions may be a marker of a fundamental endothelial abnormality in IPAH, possibly playing a key role in the pathogenesis of the condition (21).

CELLULAR CHANGES IN PULMONARY VASCULAR REMODELING

Endothelium

The endothelium is the interface between hemodynamics and the underlying vascular wall. In addition, the endothelium provides the antithrombogenic, semi-permeable barrier between the vascular and extravascular fluid compartments. The endothelium fulfils a variety of metabolic functions as well as exerting profound effects on vascular tone, growth and differentiation, and the response to injury. The initiating injury in the context of pulmonary hypertension may be hypoxia, increased flow (shear stress), inflammation, or the response to drugs (e.g. dexfenfluramine) or toxins (e.g. adulterated rape seed oil, monocrotaline) on a background of genetic susceptibility. The endothelial cell may respond to specific forms of injury in various ways that can affect the process of vascular remodeling. The term endothelial dysfunction is used to describe these changes. As well as influencing cell growth and differentiation, injury or dysfunction may directly damage the normal homeostatic functions of the endothelium, by altering endothelial permeability, metabolism, production of growth factors, and coagulation pathways. For further discussion on this subject, see refs 3, 22–31.

One of the major functions of the pulmonary endothelium under normal conditions is to prevent the formation of thrombus. In addition, small thrombi from the systemic veins will be continuously filtered by the lungs and presumably undergo fibrinolysis in the small pulmonary vessels. Alterations in endothelial coagulation and fibrinolytic factors may therefore contribute to the pathogenesis of idiopathic and thromboembolic pulmonary hypertension. *In situ* thrombosis in small pulmonary arteries is a feature of patients with idiopathic pulmonary hypertension (32).

In addition, anticoagulant therapy with warfarin improves the survival of these patients. Thrombin disrupts the endothelial barrier, causing leak of proteins and interstitial edema, and promotes growth of fibroblasts and stimulates deposition of collagen in the interstitium. Thrombin also promotes neutrophil adherence to the endothelium. Fibrin degradation products (FDPs), formed during fibrinolysis, also contribute to microvascular injury and can stimulate proliferation of lung interstitial fibroblasts (33). Recent studies have shown that there are marked elevations of circulating plasminogen activator inhibitor and von Willebrand factor in severe idiopathic PAH, as well as reduced soluble thrombomodulin, indicating impaired local fibrinolysis (34). The RhoA/ROCK and Rac/PAK signaling pathways have been implicated in thrombin- and TXA_2-induced platelet activation, aggregation, and secretion (35). Whether these changes are involved in the pathogenesis of this condition or are secondary to endothelial injury are not yet known. For example, alterations in blood flow and shear stress can alter the expression of regulators of the coagulation and fibrinolytic pathways (reviewed in ref 36). In addition to changes in shear stress, hypoxia itself exerts profound effects on endothelial cell function leading to increased endothelial permeability, expression of procoagulant factors (e.g. thrombomodulin), and induction of inflammatory molecules (e.g. IL-1, ICAM-1).

In response to these stimuli (hypoxia, increased shear stress, injury), endothelial cells in the hypertensive pulmonary circulation produce more vasoconstricting, proproliferative factors (ET-1, ANG II, thromboxane A_2), and less vasodilating, antiproliferative mediators (NO, PGI_2), which may serve to maintain the vessel wall in the remodeled hypertensive state.

Smooth muscle

During the development of pulmonary hypertension, smooth muscle cells undergo hypertrophy and proliferation, migration and changes in matrix deposition. Hypertrophy of smooth muscle cells makes a greater contribution than hyperplasia in the larger, more proximal arteries, whereas hyperplasia is more prevalent in the smaller resistance arteries (7,22,24). In large hilar arteries, cells take on a more "synthetic" as opposed to the usual "contractile" smooth muscle cell phenotype. They show prominent rough endoplasmic reticulum and Golgi apparatus (7). Cells from hypertensive arteries produce more collagen (types I and IV) and elastin in culture (37).

Under normal conditions, the smooth muscle cells comprising the adult pulmonary arterial media display minimal basal cell division. In contrast, during the development of pulmonary hypertension this suppression of cell proliferation is perturbed by the upregulation of stimulatory pathways (changes in ion channel activity, altered balance of vasoactive mediators, and growth factor expression). Similar to the manner in which endothelial cells respond to changes in shear stress, smooth muscle cells are affected by mechanical stimuli, such as increased transmural pressures

imposing circumferential stretch to the vessel wall. For example, mechanical stretch increases DNA synthesis in pulmonary artery smooth muscle cells, and increases collagen expression in pulmonary artery fibroblasts exposed to cyclical mechanical loading (38,39).

The process of extension of smooth muscle into normally non-muscular arteries is probably brought about by differentiation and hypertrophy of intermediate cells and pericytes, already present in the wall. Indeed pericytes have been shown to exhibit great plasticity in culture, being capable of differentiation into phagocytes, osteoblasts and adipocytes (40). In addition, in hyperoxia-induced pulmonary hypertension, recruitment of interstitial fibroblasts from alveolar walls contributes to the formation of muscularized microvessels in the rat lung (4).

It has become apparent that heterogeneity of pulmonary artery smooth muscle cells exists within the medial layer. This has been most elegantly demonstrated in the media of the bovine main pulmonary artery, where differently oriented cell populations, which differentially express mRNA for procollagen and tropoelastin (41), are visible by light microscopy. By utilizing a panel of antibodies to contractile and cytoskeletal proteins at least four cell phenotypes can be discerned, which arise early during development of the arterial media (42). These subpopulations are distinct with regard to their state of differentiation, expression of smooth muscle markers, proliferative response to growth factors, and to hypoxia (43). When isolated in tissue culture, these subpopulations display markedly different rates of proliferation, and matrix protein expression. Thus, at any given level of the vessel wall there may be distinct smooth muscle cell subpopulations that may play diverse roles in vascular homeostatis and can respond in an injury-specific manner during the development of pulmonary hypertension (44–47). Although the media of the human pulmonary artery appears homogeneous by conventional histochemical staining techniques and light microscopy, heterogeneity is apparent using antibodies directed against contractile proteins. In addition, heterogeneity in medial cell function is apparent *in vitro*, for example the release of adrenomedullin (48) and expression of binding sites for angiotensin II (49). Furthermore, heterogeneity in smooth muscle cells is also observed in cells isolated from different anatomical locations in the lung, i.e. proximal versus peripheral arteries. For example, human pulmonary artery smooth muscle cells from the peripheral pulmonary circulation (arteries 1–2 mm diameter) proliferate more rapidly and are more sensitive to the antiproliferative effects of prostacyclin analogues than cells isolated from the main pulmonary artery (50).

Fibroblasts

Early studies demonstrated that in rats exposed to hypoxia there is an early peak (2–3 days) in fibroblast proliferation and hypertrophy in the adventitia of hilar arteries (7,24). This coincides with increased deposition of type I collagen and elastin. In small peripheral muscular arteries fibroblast hyperplasia and increased production of extracellular matrix protein is also prominent (51). Type 1 collagen deposition and elastin synthesis in the adventitia contribute to the narrowing of the vascular lumen and probably to the reduced capacity for vasodilatation in advanced pulmonary hypertension (52,53).

Recent evidence supports an active role for the adventitial fibroblast in the remodeling of the pulmonary circulation during the development of pulmonary hypertension. Adventitial fibroblasts undergo a transition in phenotype during the development of pulmonary hypertension, as evidenced by the expression of smooth muscle contractile proteins such as α-smooth muscle actin (α-SM actin) (54). These α-SM actin-expressing fibroblasts are often referred to as myofibroblasts, and are thought to represent a response to injury. As such they are found in the adventitial layer of systemic arteries following balloon injury and in the injured dermis contribute to wound healing and scar contraction (55).

Although adventitial remodeling occurs in idiopathic PAH (56), it occurs most dramatically in neonatal forms of pulmonary hypertension (57). The heightened proliferative response of the neonatal fibroblast may be due to developmental differences in PKC signaling (58,59).

Similar to smooth muscle cells, phenotypically distinct subpopulations of fibroblasts exist within the adventitia (60). In addition, fibroblasts are also heterogeneous in their responses to hypertensive stimuli. For example, in response to hypoxia some pulmonary artery fibroblasts proliferate, with increased activity of mitogen activated protein (MAP) kinases (61) whereas in others no response is observed (60). It has been proposed in pulmonary hypertension there is selective expansion of a subpopulation of fibroblasts within the adventitia (61). In fetal cells, the hypoxia-induced proliferation is related to the activity of specific isoforms of protein kinase C (62).

In arterial remodeling, the adventitial layer is now seen as an important modulator of remodeling through its interactions with other layers of the vessel wall. Much of what is known originates from observations in the systemic circulation in the context of vascular injury following balloon angioplasty. The activated adventitial fibroblast may contribute to remodeling by transition of fibroblasts to myofibroblasts (expressing contractile proteins e.g. alpha smooth muscle actin), myofibroblast migration into the intima, adventitial fibrosis and expression of matrix metalloproteinases (see below).

THE EXTRACELLULAR MATRIX

The extracellular matrix (ECM) represents a substrate for tissue morphogenesis. In addition, it instructs many forms of cell behavior at the biophysical and biochemical levels through interactions with multiple receptors, including the heterodimeric integrins composed of α and β sub-units (63). The connections between integrins, ECM ligands and actin-based microfilaments inside the cell are indirect, and are linked via scaffolding proteins, such as talin, paxillin and α-actinin (63). These scaffolds activate or recruit numerous signaling molecules, including focal adhesion kinase and Src kinase family members that then phosphorylate downstream substrates (64).

Although the deposition of collagen is often thought of as an irreversible process, the fractional synthesis rate of collagen is about 3 percent per day in the rabbit pulmonary artery (65). Small changes in the rate of collagen synthesis and metabolism therefore cause a marked alteration in collagen content. Elastin and collagen deposition is increased during the development of pulmonary hypertension (24). Endothelial cells in the microvasculature secrete type IV collagen and elastin. In larger arteries, smooth muscle cells and fibroblasts produce collagen and elastin within the media and adventitia, respectively. This appears to be in response to increased wall tension, since isolated stretched vessels also do this (66). In the hypoxic model, the increased connective tissue maintains its normal relationship to muscle mass. In other models (e.g. neonatal hypoxic calves) there is greatly increased collagen deposition in the adventitia (52,57). Connective tissue turnover is regulated in the vessel wall by the production of collagen and elastin on the one hand and its breakdown on the other. The degradation of matrix proteins is in large part due to the activity of matrix metalloproteinases (collagenases and elastases), the activity of which is in turn regulated by tissue inhibitors of matrix metalloproteinases (TIMPs) (see below).

ROLE OF ENDOGENOUS VASCULAR ELASTASES AND PROTEASES

One of the earliest features of pulmonary vascular remodeling is fragmentation of the internal elastic lamina, implying that elastases are activated in the vessel wall (67). Inhibition of serine elastase activity with serine protease inhibitors (e.g. α1-antitrypsin) during the early stages of monocrotaline or hypoxia-induced pulmonary hypertension prevents disruption of the internal elastic lamina and reduces vascular remodeling (9,68). The mechanism of elastase activation is due to serum factors leaking into the arterial wall because of damage to the endothelium. Within the media, elastase also degrades proteoglycans that serve as storage sites for growth factors, releasing biologically active forms of basic fibroblast growth factors (bFGF) and transforming growth factor-β (TGF-β) (69). In addition, elastase and the matrix metalloproteinases, as well as FGF-2, can induce production of the matrix glycoprotein tenascin-C (70). For more details, see refs 71–77.

APOPTOSIS

Tissue remodeling also involves apoptosis, or programmed cell death. Either excessive or limited apoptosis can lead to the development of a variety of diseases including pulmonary hypertension. In contrast to cell necrosis, apoptosis is a tightly regulated process that requires energy from ATP, gene transcription and protein synthesis. In the monocrotaline model, apoptosis is seen in the endothelial cells of the pulmonary artery, suggesting a mechanism for access of serum factors to the subendothelial space (78). In patients with idiopathic PAH, cells within plexiform lesions exhibit somatic mutations in genes regulating apoptosis (Bax) as well as cell proliferation (MutS Homolog 2 gene and TGF-β type II receptor) (79). It is hypothesized that acquisition of somatic mutations in these genes allows clonal expansion of endothelial cells in idiopathic PAH. These somatic mutations are not found in lesions from patients with familial PAH (80). Bcl-2 is a key anti-apoptotic membrane protein. Expression of Bcl-2 mRNA has been shown to be upregulated in lung tissues from patients with idiopathic and familial PAH (81). Survivin (16.5 kDa) is the smallest member of the mammalian inhibitor of apoptosis family. Survivin is overexpressed in pulmonary arteries from PAH patients and in rats with MCT-induced PAH (82). Wild type survivin delivered via an inhaled adenovirus to normal rats causes PH. Conversely, gene therapy with an adenovirus carrying a phosphorylation-deficient survivin mutant reverses established pulmonary hypertension in monocrotaline exposed rats (82).

Interestingly, hypoxia is a powerful promoter of apoptosis in many cell systems, and resistance to hypoxia-induced apoptosis allows clonal expansion of cells in some tumors. Little or no increase in the number of apoptotic cells is observed within the media of the chronically hypoxic rat. However, on return to room air apoptosis is maximal after 3 days and is likely to be involved in the involution of vascular remodeling during recovery from chronic hypoxic exposure (83). The potential importance of targeting apoptosis in the therapeutic reversal of established pulmonary vascular remodeling was shown in monocrotaline-induced pulmonary hypertensive rats. Treatment of rats with serine elastase inhibitors led to myocyte apoptosis and loss of ECM, and normalized pulmonary artery structure and pressure (68).

THE ROLE OF INFLAMMATION IN PAH PATHOBIOLOGY

Inflammatory processes are prominent in various types of human and experimental pulmonary hypertension (PH) and are increasingly recognized as major pathogenic components of pulmonary vascular remodeling. Macrophages, T and B lymphocytes, and dendritic cells are present in the vascular lesions of PH, whether in idiopathic pulmonary arterial hypertension (PAH), or PAH related to more classical forms of inflammatory syndromes such as connective tissue diseases, HIV or other viral etiologies. Similarly, the presence of circulating chemokines and cytokines, viral protein components (e.g. HIV-1 *Nef*), and increased

expression of growth (such as VEGF and PDGF) and transcriptional (e.g. Nuclear Factor of Activated T cells or NFAT) factors in these patients are thought to contribute directly to further recruitment of inflammatory cells, and proliferation of smooth muscle and endothelial cells.

A role for inflammation in PAH is based on the finding of inflammatory cells, including macrophages and T and B lymphocytes, and dendritic cells around the plexiform lesions of PAH (84). Levels of macrophage inflammatory protein-1 alpha, interleukin-1β and interleukin-6 (85,86), and P-selectin (87) are increased in severe IPAH. Involvement of leukocytes, macrophages, and lymphocytes in the complex vascular lesions of IPAH was initially described by Tuder and colleagues (88) and confirmed in more recent studies by Dorfmuller and coworkers (89). Cytokine and chemokine-dependent mechanisms leading to inflammatory cell recruitment are also prominent in PAH.

Cytokines and chemokines in PAH

Fractalkine (CX3CL1), a unique chemokine which promotes the chemokine (C-X3-C motif) receptor 1 (CX3CR1)-expressing leukocyte recruitment, is upregulated in circulating CD4$^+$ and CD8$^+$ T lymphocytes from PAH patients as compared with controls. These patients also have elevated soluble CX3CL1 plasma concentrations; their lung tissue samples demonstrate increased CX3CL1 mRNA expression as compared with controls, and pulmonary artery endothelial cells (EC) from these lungs express CX3CL1 protein (90). For more details see refs 91–95.

GROWTH FACTORS AND OTHER MEDIATORS INVOLVED IN VASCULAR REMODELING

Numerous cell-derived growth factors, vasoactive peptides and cytokines are involved in modulation of the vascular remodeling process. In addition, small molecules such as nitric oxide and reactive oxygen species play important roles.

The cell surface receptors for many growth factors are transmembrane tyrosine specific protein kinases, also known as receptor tyrosine kinases. These include receptors for platelet-derived growth factor (PDGF), fibroblast growth factors (FGFs), insulin-like growth factor-1 (IGF-1), epidermal growth factor (EGF) and vascular endothelial growth factor (VEGF). Ligand binding leads to phosphorylation of the intracellular part of the receptor and initiation of intracellular signaling cascades. The TGF-β and bone morphogenetic protein family of growth factors signal via receptor serine/threonine kinases. The intracellular signaling pathways downstream of these receptors are complex and depend upon the tissue and cell type under investigation, which lends specificity to the responses. However, many of the factors involved in vascular remodeling converge on common key signaling pathways within the cell.

For example, a number of antiproliferative signaling pathways in vascular smooth muscle stimulate production of the important intracellular second messengers, cyclic nucleotides (cyclic AMP and cyclic GMP). Vasoconstrictors and growth factors tend to converge to stimulate phosphorylation of MAP kinases. Different growth factors operate at different stages of the cell cycle (the process of cell division), underlining the importance of multiple signals operating in concert *in vivo*.

MECHANISMS OF VASCULAR REMODELING IN PAH

Although many factors act in concert to orchestrate pulmonary vascular remodeling, recent advances in our understanding of the pathogenesis of pulmonary arterial hypertension have demonstrated that alterations in certain key pathways may play a central role in initiating disease, or causing disease progression (Figure 5.2).

Nitric oxide and prostacyclin

Endothelial dysfunction in PAH is reflected by reduced production of the vasodilators/growth inhibitors nitric oxide (NO) and prostacyclin (PGI_2). NO signaling is mainly mediated by the guanylate cyclase/cyclic guanosine monophosphate (cGMP) pathway. Degradation of the second messenger of NO, cGMP, by phosphodiesterases (PDEs) is predominantly accomplished by PDE5, which is preferentially expressed in the lung and corpus cavernosum.

Reduced NO bioavailability in PAH can be due to decreased expression of eNOS, inhibition of eNOS enzymatic activity, and inactivation of NO by superoxide anion. Activation of endothelial RhoA/ROCK signaling can be involved in at least the first two processes (96). The activity of arginase II, which reduces NO synthesis by competing with eNOS for the substrate L-arginine, is increased in endothelial cells from PAH patients (97). Patients with IPAH have increased plasma levels of the endogenous inhibitor of eNOS, asymmetric dimethylarginine (ADMA) (98), and the levels of ADMA and the enzyme that degrades it, dimethylarginine dimethyaminohydrolase (DDAH2), are, respectively, increased and decreased in the pulmonary artery endothelium of IPAH patients (98).

Prostacyclin (PGI_2) stimulates the formation of the second messenger cyclic adenosine monophosphate (cAMP). cAMP also inhibits the proliferation of SMCs and decreases platelet aggregation. Christman *et al.* (99) and Tuder *et al.* (100) have shown a deficiency of PGI_2 and PGI_2 synthase and an excess of thromboxane in PAH. Moreover, PGI_2-receptor knockout mice develop more severe hypoxia-induced pulmonary hypertension (101). Conversely, PGI_2

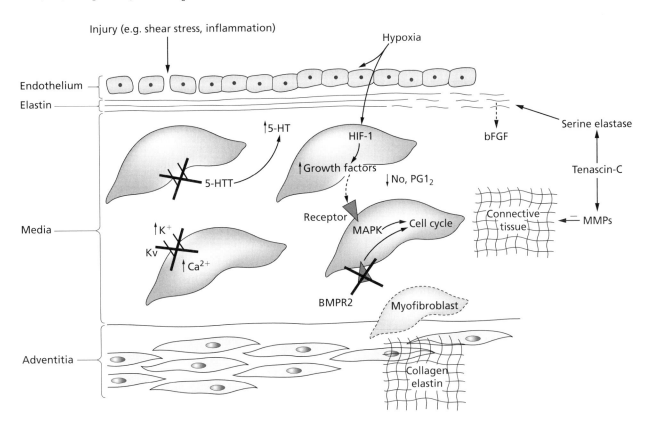

Figure 5.2 Diagramatic representation of the various mechanisms involved in pulmonary vascular remodeling. 5HT, 5-hydroxytryptamine (serotonin); 5HTT, 5-HT transporter; bFGF, basic fibroblast growth factor; BMPR2, bone morphogenetic protein receptor 2; HIF-1, hypoxia inducible factor-1; Kv, voltage-gated K^+ channels; MMP, matrix metalloprotein; PGI_2, prostacyclin.

overexpressing mice are protected against hypoxia-induced pulmonary hypertension (102).

TGF-β/bone morphogenetic proteins

Heterozygous germline mutations in the gene encoding the bone morphogenetic protein type II receptor gene, *BMPR2*, have been found in approximately 80 percent of families with PAH (103,104). In addition, up to 25 percent of patients with apparently sporadic idiopathic PAH have been found to harbor mutations (105). At least a proportion of these are examples of familial PAH, in which the condition has not manifested in relatives due to low penetrance (106), whereas others are examples of *de novo* mutation. To date some 144 distinct mutations have been identified in 210 independent patients with familial PAH (103). See also refs 107–117.

THE CONSEQUENCES OF BMPR2 MUTATION FOR BMP/TGF-β SIGNALING

Studies have shown that the mechanism by which BMPR-II mutants disrupt BMP/Smad signaling is heterogeneous and mutation specific (118,119). See also refs 112, 120, 121.

STUDIES OF BMP SIGNALING CELLS AND TISSUES FROM PAH PATIENTS

BMPR-II is widely expressed in normal tissues and cells (110). See also Figures 5.3, 5.4, and refs 122–128.

BMP SIGNALING IN RODENT MODELS OF PAH

Studies in knockout mice reveal the critical role of the BMP pathway in early embryogenesis and vascular development (129). See also refs 130–136.

Serotonin

The effects of serotonin (5-hydroxytryptamine, 5-HT) on the pulmonary circulation have been of major interest since reports of increased risk of IPAH in patients who used appetite suppressants that interact with 5-HT (137). An association between the anorexigen, aminorex, and idiopathic PAH was first described in the 1960s. In the 1980s, fenfluramine use was shown to be associated with an epidemic of IPAH in France and Belgium (138). In patients with PAH, platelet and plasma 5-HT levels are increased (139,140), and in addition, Fawn Hooded rats, which have a deficiency in the storage of 5-HT by platelets, have a genetic predisposition to the development of PH (141,142).

5-HT induces hyperplasia and hypertrophy of human PASMCs (143,144) although no mitogenic effect has been observed in endothelial cells or fibroblasts (145,146). 5-HT also acts as a co-mitogen since in combination with other growth factors, including PDGF, EGF and FGF, the proliferative response is greater in magnitude than either mitogen alone. Pulmonary artery smooth muscle cells from

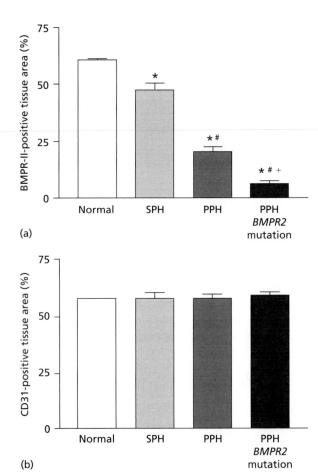

(a)

(b)

Figure 5.3 (a) Pulmonary endothelial expression of *BMPRII* in lung tissue from normal, secondary (SPH) and primary pulmonary hypertensive (PPH) patients (with or without mutations in *BMPR2*). (b) The amount of endothelial positive tissue was determined by staining with the endothelial marker CD31. Image analysis confirmed that expression of *BMPRII* was markedly reduced in the peripheral lung of primary pulmonary hypertensive patients especially in those harboring *BMPR2* mutations.
*, significantly different from control, $P < 0.05$; #, significantly different from SPH, $P < 0.05$; +, significantly different from PPH, $P < 0.05$.

arteries of patients with idiopathic PAH display a greater proliferative response to 5-HT compared with normal cells (147). In contrast to the constricting action of 5-HT on smooth muscle cells, which is mainly mediated by 5-HT receptors (5-HT 1B/D, 2A, and 2B) (138), the mitogenic and co-mitogenic effects of 5-HT require internalization via the 5-HT transporter (5-HTT) (145,148). In patients with idiopathic PAH, 5-HT uptake and binding of the 5-HTT inhibitor, citalopram, is increased in the lungs due to increased expression of 5-HTT (147). Accordingly, drugs that competitively inhibit 5-HTT also block the mitogenic effects of 5-HT on smooth muscle cells (149). The appetite suppressants fenfluramine, D-fenfluramine, and aminorex differ from selective serotonin transporter inhibitors in that they not only inhibit serotonin reuptake but also trigger indoleamine release and interact with 5-HTT and 5-HT

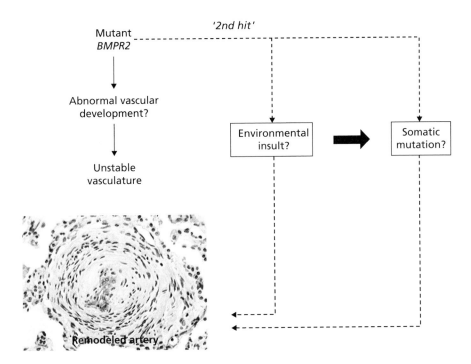

Figure 5.4 Hypothetical mechanisms underlying the pathogenesis of primary pulmonary hypertension associated with *BMPR2* mutation.

receptors in a specific manner (149,150). The importance of 5-HTT in vascular remodeling is further illustrated by the fact that when 5-HTT knockout mice are exposed to hypoxia medial thickening and neo-muscularization is significantly less than in wild type mice (151). Conversely, increased 5-HTT expression was associated with increased severity of hypoxic PH (152,153). Indeed specific overexpression of 5-HTT in PASMCs under the control of the SM22 promoter is sufficient to produce spontaneous PAH (154).

SEROTONIN RECEPTORS IN PULMONARY HYPERTENSION

On release from platelets or from nerve endings, serotonin can activate up to 14 structurally distinct 5HT receptors. These are divided up into seven families ($5HT_{1-7}$). Of these, the $5HT_{2A}$, $5HT_{2B}$ and $5HT_{1B}$ receptors are particularly relevant to PAH. In most non-human mammals, the $5HT_{2A}$ receptor mediates vasoconstriction in both the systemic and pulmonary circulations (155,156). See also refs 157–162.

SEROTONIN SYNTHESIS

The rate-limiting step in 5-HT biosynthesis is catalyzed by the enzyme tryptophan hydroxylase (Tph). Tph exists as two isoforms, Tph1 and Tph2, encoded by separate genes. 5-HT synthesis is thought to be controlled chiefly by Tph2 in the central nervous system and Tph1 in peripheral organs (163). Although peripherally produced 5-HT is synthesized chiefly by the enterochromaffin cells in the gut, human PAECs produce 5-HT and express Tph1. Both 5-HT synthesis and Tph1 expression are increased in cells from patients with IPAH compared with controls (164). Mice lacking Tph1 are resistant to hypoxia- and dexfenfluramine-induced pulmonary hypertension (165,166).

Angiopoietin and TIE-2

Angiopoietin-1 (Ang-1) is an oligomeric secreted glycoprotein, first described by Davis *et al.* in 1996 (167), which along with angiopoietin-2 and angiopoietin-3/4 comprise the angiopoietin family of growth factors. The angiopoietin ligands exert their effects through the endothelial-specific tyrosine kinase TIE2 (168). In lung vascular development, both Ang-1 and TIE2 are expressed in growing blood vessels: Ang-1 is made and secreted by vascular smooth muscle cells and precursor pericytes, whereas TIE2 is a transmembrane receptor expressed in the surface of endothelial cells (169).

Ang-1 is required for correct organization and maturation of newly formed vessels and promotes quiescence, smooth muscle cell encasement, and structural integrity of adult blood vessels (170). The prostabilizing effects of Ang-1 are clearly demonstrated in studies in which Ang-1 is directly administered or overexpressed leading to marked improvement in vascular integrity and smooth muscle cell investment in both growing and adult mice (171). These results suggest that Ang-1/TIE2 signaling plays an essential role in arterial vascular formation and remodeling.

Several lines of evidence have suggested that Ang-1 regulates pathologic smooth muscle cell hyperplasia around vessels in pulmonary hypertension. Ang-1 has been shown to be overexpressed in the lungs of patients with most forms of non-familial PAH compared to the lungs of control patients, at both the mRNA and protein levels (169,172). Ang-1 causes constitutive activation of the TIE2 receptor, by tyrosine autophosphorylation, in the pulmonary vascular endothelium in PAH (172,173). Enhanced TIE2 levels and a 4-fold increase in TIE2 phosphorylation are found in human PAH lung tissue compared to control subjects without pulmonary hypertension (172,174).

In support of a causative role for Ang-1 in pulmonary arterial hypertension, virally mediated overexpression of Ang-1 in the rat lung results in the development of pulmonary hypertension (173,175,176). Ang-1 transgenic animals show augmented levels of pulmonary vascular endothelial TIE2 phosphorylation and manifest severe smooth muscle cell hyperplasia in small and mid-sized pulmonary arterioles. Further, overexpression of a soluble TIE2 ectodomain which sequesters Ang-1, suppresses the pulmonary hypertensive phenotype in monocrotaline and Ang-1-induced models of this disease (176).

There is controversy in this field. In contrast to a causative role, Ang-1 has also been reported to protect against the development of pulmonary hypertension in the rat monocrotoline and hypoxia models of disease. In these studies, Ang-1 expression in the rat lung was achieved by transfection of smooth muscle cells or fibroblasts harboring a vector containing the human Ang-1 gene via an internal jugular route (177). Ang-1 may then protect against endothelial apoptosis (177).

K⁺ and Ca⁺ channels in PAH

In PASMCs the free Ca^{2+} concentration in the cytosol ($[Ca^{2+}]_{cyt}$) is an important determinant of contraction, migration and proliferation. As cytosolic Ca^{2+} increases, so it is bound by calmodulin, which activates myosin light chain kinase (MLCK) that, in turn, phosphorylates the myosin light chain (MLC). The phosphorylated MLC initiates cycling of the myosin crossbridges with the actin filament and causes PASMC contraction and vasoconstriction. In addition, elevated nuclear Ca^{2+} propels quiescent cells into the cell cycle and through mitosis, promoting cellular proliferation. The sarcoplasmic reticulum (SR) is the most prominent intracellular Ca^{2+} store within vascular smooth muscle cells. Depletion of Ca^{2+} from the inositol-1,4,5-trisphosphate (IP_3)-sensitive Ca^{2+} stores with SR Ca^{2+}-Mg^{2+} ATPase inhibitors has been shown to arrest cell growth, while its repletion allows continued sarcoplasmic/endoplasmic reticular function (such as lipid synthesis and protein sorting and processing) and the resumption of the S phase of cell cycle, leading to mitosis and cellular proliferation.

It is also noted that: (1) regulation of $[Ca^{2+}]_{cyt}$ is regulated in pulmonary artery smooth muscle cells; (2) inhibition of K⁺ channel activity causes membrane depolarization; (3) receptor-operated and store-operated Ca^{2+} channels have a role in regulating $[Ca^{2+}]_{cyt}$ (178,179); (4) K⁺ channels are inhibited by Bcl-2 (124); and (5) downregulated Kv channels have a pathogenetic role (124,180).

Circulating progenitor cells in pulmonary vascular remodeling

Damaged organs, especially those characterized by chronic inflammation and fibrosis, appear able to recruit myofibroblast precursors from several sources. Resident fibroblasts as well as SMC seem to be important sources for these highly metabolically active myofibroblast or myofibroblast-like cells. However, studies in many organs, including the lung, suggest that bone marrow derived circulating cells, known as fibrocytes, represent an alternative source for myofibroblast accumulation during reparative processes in the lung as well as in other organs (181–184).

Fibrocytes are bone marrow derived mesenchymal progenitors that co-express hematopoetic stem cell antigens, markers of the monocyte lineage, and fibroblast gene products. They constitutively produce ECM components as well as ECM-modifying enzymes and can further differentiate into myofibroblasts both *in vitro* and *in vivo* under certain conditions. These cells can contribute to the new population of fibroblasts and myofibroblasts that emerge at tissue sites during normal or aberrant wound healing, in ischemic or inflammatory fibrotic processes and as part of the stromal reaction to tumor development (185,186).

The fibrocyte, which appears to arrive at sites of tissue injury through mechanisms similar to those of other monocytes, may differentiate into mature mesenchymal cells *in vivo*. Differentiation of fibrocytes into myofibroblast-like cells occurs in situations where there is increased production of TGFβ-1 and/or endothelin in the wounded tissues. In these settings, fibrocytes or fibrocyte precursor cells demonstrate a progressive downregulation of the expression of leukocytic markers (e.g. CD34 and CD45) with a concomitant upregulation of mesenchymal markers (including α-SM-actin and Type-1 collagen).

Evidence of a causal link between accumulation of fibrocytes at injured sites and ongoing vascular remodeling has been provided in animal models. In the chronically hypoxic rat, monocyte/fibrocyte depletion leads to a marked attenuation of pulmonary vascular remodeling (187). It must be emphasized, however, that fibrocytes themselves produce a number of cytokines and growth factors that induce fibroblast hyperplasia, promote the release of ECM molecules from resident tissues fibroblasts and promote angiogenesis.

The transition of any cell type including endothelial cells, progenitor cells, fibroblasts or even SMC into a myofibroblast becomes relevant to a better understanding of pulmonary hypertension in view of recent work indicating that during fibrotic situations, myofibroblasts developed a capacity of producing a long lasting tension centrally regulated at the level of Rho/Rho-kinase-mediated inhibition of myosin-light chain phosphatase (188). It is thus possible that cells that have transitioned into fibroblast- and myofibroblast-like cells play a role in the contracture and inability of the vessel wall to dilate in response to traditional vasodilating stimuli.

Endothelial progenitor cells are bone marrow derived cells, found in the monocyte pool, which express the stem cell marker CD133, the hematopoietic marker CD34 and the endothelial marker VEGFR2 (189). The role of endothelial progenitor cells in pulmonary vascular remodeling remains controversial. Studies have reported both increased (190) and decreased (191) numbers of circulating EPCs in patients with PAH. The number of circulating EPCs is very small (< 1 percent of the monocyte fraction) and different techniques and antibodies used to identify cells may lead to variation in quantification. Monocytes when cultured under appropriate conditions *in vitro* can be induced to express endothelial markers. Such monocyte derived EPCs have been used therapeutically and have been shown to prevent and reverse monocrotaline-induced pulmonary hypertension when delivered intravenously (192).

THERAPEUTIC REVERSAL OF PULMONARY VASCULAR REMODELING

Most of the current therapies available for the treatment of severe pulmonary hypertension were designed to target the process of vasoconstriction, rather than the remodeling process. The relationship between vasoconstriction and remodeling has not been clearly established. It is probably not true to assume that all vasodilators will inhibit or reverse the process of remodeling, though the mechanisms of action of many vasodilators (e.g. calcium channel blockers, activation of cyclic nucleotides) impact on known growth pathways. Nevertheless, since vessel remodeling is critical in the pathogenesis of pulmonary hypertension it would seem advantageous to design treatments that specifically target this process.

Prostacyclin therapy (i.v., inhaled or oral administration) has been a significant advance in the treatment of PAH. Many trials have found prostacyclin or its analogues to not only reduce pulmonary artery pressure but more importantly improve long-term survival. Although primarily used for its vasodilator properties there is the suggestion that prostacyclin has anti-proliferative effects (50). Indirect evidence for this comes from the observation that patients who do not show an initial acute vasodilator response to prostacyclin still demonstrate a reduction in pulmonary vascular resistance during long-term administration (193,194), though some of these effects are due to an improvement in cardiac function. Direct evidence for the anti-proliferative effects of PGI_2 is derived from both *in vitro* cell culture studies (195) and from animal models of the disease (196).

Endothelin, a potent smooth muscle mitogen, is thought to play an important role in pulmonary hypertension since there are various alterations in the endothelin pathway in PH (197). A number of controlled clinical trials have shown the efficacy of these agents in PAH. Although there are theoretical advantages in selective ET_A blockade, leaving the ETB receptor on the endothelium to undertake the role of ET-1 clearance, clinical trials have not demonstrated any superiority of selective versus dual blockade. The mechanism of action of endothelin receptor antagonists may relate to its vasodilatory properties although anti-mitogenic effects cannot be ruled out since numerous studies in animal models of the disease have found that endothelin antagonists can not only prevent the development of, but also reverse, remodeling.

Enhancement of the NO/cGMP pathway by phosphodiesterase inhibitors such as sildenafil is a further widely used approach in clinical PAH (198). Combinations of agents designed to target different pathways has also been shown to be beneficial in PAH patients (199).

The importance of elastase in the development of vascular remodeling in pulmonary hypertension has already been discussed (see above). Serine elastase inhibitors and even gene therapy, targeting serine elastase, may in the future prove to be beneficial in treating pulmonary vascular remodeling associated with pulmonary hypertension. In animal models of pulmonary hypertension various serine elastase inhibitors have been demonstrated to inhibit, and for some even completely reverse, existing remodeling. Targeted overexpression of the serine elastase inhibitor, elafin, in mice has been found to not only suppress the up-regulation of MMP9 seen in non-transgenic mice exposed to hypoxia but to reduce remodeling (200).

Further experimental approaches under investigation include the inhibition of Rho kinase (201) and the direct targeting of apoptosis pathways. Statins exert pleiotropic effects which are beneficial in animal models of PH (202). The targeting of growth factor pathways mediated by receptor tyrosine kinases is under intense investigation, and one of these, imatinib, which inhibits the PDGF receptors and other kinases, has been shown to be effective in severe PAH (203). Cell based therapies involving the delivery of EPCs are also underway and have shown promise in preliminary studies (204). Future developments are likely to include targeting the serotonin system and the BMP/TGF-β signaling pathways.

KEY POINTS

- The structure of the pulmonary arterial wall varies systematically from the large (proximal) vessels to the small (distal) pre-acinar vessels.
- Vascular remodeling involves thickening of the vessel wall to withstand and increase in intravascular pressure or flow, but also lumen narrowing and reduced capacity for vasodilatation.
- Smooth muscle cells, fibroblasts and endothelial cells contribute to remodeling by a combination of migration, hypertrophy and proliferation.
- Increased synthesis of collagen and elastin serves to reduce vascular wall compliance.
- Animal models mimic some, but not all of the features of human pulmonary vascular remodeling.
- Vascular wall elastases and matrix metalloproteinases (and their inhibitors – TIMPs) regulate matrix protein deposition and smooth muscle during remodeling.

- Disruption of the elastic lamina is an early feature of remodeling, resulting from leak of serum proteins through a damaged endothelium and activation of endogenous vascular elastases.
- Receptor tyrosine kinase growth factors (e.g. EGF, PDGF, IGF, FGF, VEGF) and receptor serine/threonine kinases (BMPs/TGF-β) are involved in cell differentiation and proliferation.
- Activation of mitogen activated protein kinases is a common feature of growth signals acting via G-protein coupled receptors and receptor tyrosine kinases.
- Specific targeting of the pathways regulating pulmonary vascular remodeling may lead to new treatments aimed at preventing or reversing pulmonary hypertension.

REFERENCES

1. deMello DE, Sawyer D, Galvin N, Reid LM. Early fetal development of lung vasculature. Am J Respir Cell Mol Biol 1997;16:568–71.
2. Davies P, Maddalo F, Reid L. Effects of chronic hypoxia on structure and reactivity of rat lung microvessels. J Appl Physiol 1985;58(3):795–801.
3. Meyrick B, Reid L. The effect of continued hypoxia on rat pulmonary arterial circulation. An ultrastructural study. Lab Invest 1978;38(2):188–200.
4. Jones R, Jacobson M, Steudel W. α-smooth muscle actin and microvascular precursor smooth muscle cells in pulmonary hypertension. Am J Respir Cell Mol Biol 1999;20:582–94.
5. Heath D. Pulmonary vascular disease. In: Hasleton PS, editor. Spencer's pathology of the lung. London: McGraw-Hill, 1996:649–93.
6. Hislop A, Reid L. New findings in pulmonary arteries of rats with hypoxia-induced pulmonary hypertension. Br J Exp Pathol 1976;57(5):542–54.
7. Meyrick B, Reid L. Hypoxia-induced structural changes in the media and adventitia of the rat hilar pulmonary artery and their regression. Am J Pathol 1980;100(1):151–78.
8. Wagenvoort C, Wagenvoort N. Primary pulmonary hypertension: a pathological study of vessels in 156 clinically diagnosed cases. Circulation 1970;42:1163–84.
9. Ilkiw R, Todorovich-Hunter L, Maruyama K, Shin J, Rabinovitch M. SC-39026, a serine elastase inhibitor, prevents muscularization of peripheral arteries, suggesting a mechanism of monocrotaline-induced pulmonary hypertension in rats. Circ Res 1989;64(4):814–25.
10. Maruyama K, Ye CL, Woo M, Venkatacharya H, Lines LD, Silver MM et al. Chronic hypoxic pulmonary hypertension in rats and increased elastolytic activity. Am J Physiol 1991;261(6 Pt 2):H1716–26.
11. Botney MD, Kaiser LR, Cooper JD, Mecham RP, Parghi D, Roby J et al. Extracellular matrix protein gene expression in atherosclerotic hypertensive pulmonary arteries. Am J Pathol 1992;140(2):357–64.
12. Yi ES, Kim H, Ahn H, Strother J, Morris T, Masliah E et al. Distribution of obstructive intimal lesions and their cellular phenotypes in chronic pulmonary hypertension. A morphometric and immunohistochemical study. Am J Respir Crit Care Med 2000;162(4 Pt 1):1577–86.
13. Botney MD. Role of hemodynamics in pulmonary vascular remodeling: implications for primary pulmonary hypertension. Am J Respir Crit Care Med 1999;159:361–4.
14. Okada K, Tanaka Y, Bernstein M, Zhang W, Patterson GA, Botney MD. Pulmonary hemodynamics modify the rat pulmonary artery response to injury. A neointimal model of pulmonary hypertension. Am J Pathol 1997;151(4):1019–25.
15. Shi Y, O'Brien JE, Fard A, Mannion JD, Wang D, Zalewski A. Adventitial myofibroblasts contribute to neointimal formation in injured porcine coronary arteries. Circulation 1996;94(7):1655–64.
16. Scott NA, Cipolla GD, Ross CE, Dunn B, Martin FH, Simonet L et al. Identification of a potential role for the adventitia in vascular lesion formation after balloon overstretch injury of porcine coronary arteries. Circulation 1996;93(12):2178–87.
17. Li G, Chen S-J, Oparil S, Chen YF, Thompson AT. Direct in vivo evidence demonstrating neointimal migration of adventitial fibroplasts after balloon injury of rat carotid arteries. Circulation 2000;101:1362–5.
18. Hirose S, Hosoda Y, Furuya S, Otsuki T, Ikeda E. Expression of vascular endothelial growth factor and its receptors correlates closely with formation of the plexiform lesion in human pulmonary hypertension. Pathol Int 2000;50(6):472–9.
19. Tuder RM, Chacon M, Alger L, Wang J, Taraseviciene-Stewart L, Kasahara Y et al. Expression of angiogenesis-related molecules in plexiform lesions in severe pulmonary hypertension: evidence for a process of disordered angiogenesis. J Pathol 2001;195(3):367–74.
20. Cool CD, Stewart JS, Werahera P, Miller GJ, Williams RL, Voelkel NF et al. Three-dimensional reconstruction of pulmonary arteries in plexiform pulmonary hypertension using cell-specific markers. Evidence for a dynamic and heterogeneous process of pulmonary endothelial cell growth. Am J Pathol 1999;155(2):411–9.
21. Tuder RM, Cool CD, Yeager M, Taraseviciene-Stewart L, Bull TM, Voelkel NF. The pathobiology of pulmonary hypertension. Endothelium. Clin Chest Med 2001;22(3):405–18.
22. Meyrick B, Reid L. Hypoxia and incorporation of 3H-thymidine by cells of the rat pulmonary arteries and alveolar wall. Am J Pathol 1979;96(1):51–70.
23. Stiebellehner L, Belknap JK, Ensley B, Tucker A, Orton EC, Reeves JT et al. Lung endothelial cell proliferation in normal and pulmonary hypertensive neonatal calves. Am J Physiol 1998;275:L593–600.

24. McKenzie JC, Clancy J, Jr., Klein RM. Autoradiographic analysis of cell proliferation and protein synthesis in the pulmonary trunk of rats during the early development of hypoxia-induced pulmonary hypertension. Blood Vessels 1984;21(2):80–9.

25. Meyrick B, Reid L. Endothelial and subintimal changes in rat hilar pulmonary artery during recovery from hypoxia. A quantitative ultrastructural study. Lab Invest 1980; 42(6):603–15.

26. Vyas-Somani AC, Aziz SM, Arcot SA, Gillespie MN, Olson JW, Lipke DW. Temporal alterations in basement membrane components in the pulmonary vasculature of the chronically hypoxic rat: impact of hypoxia and recovery. Am J Med Sci 1996;312(2):54–67.

27. Fisher AB, Chien S, Barakat AI, Nerem RM. Endothelial cellular response to altered shear stress. Am J Physiol Lung Cell Mol Physiol 2001;281(3):L529–33.

28. Rabinovitch M, Bothwell T, Hayakawa BN, Williams WG, Trusler GA, Rowe RD et al. Pulmonary artery endothelial abnormalities in patients with congenital heart defects and pulmonary hypertension. A correlation of light with scanning electron microscopy and transmission electron microscopy. Lab Invest 1986;55(6):632–53.

29. Todorovich-Hunter L, Johnson DJ, Ranger P, Keeley FW, Rabinovitch M. Altered elastin and collagen synthesis associated with progressive pulmonary hypertension induced by monocrotaline. A biochemical and ultrastructural study. Lab Invest 1988;58(2):184–95.

30. Csortos C, Kolosova I, Verin AD. Regulation of vascular endothelial cell barrier function and cytoskeleton structure by protein phosphatases of the PPP family. Am J Physiol Lung Cell Mol Physiol 2007;293(4):L843–54.

31. Wojciak-Stothard B, Tsang LY, Paleolog E, Hall SM, Haworth SG. Rac1 and RhoA as regulators of endothelial phenotype and barrier function in hypoxia-induced neonatal pulmonary hypertension. Am J Physiol Lung Cell Mol Physiol 2006;290(6):L1173–82.

32. Hassell KL. Altered hemostasis in pulmonary hypertension. Blood Coagul Fibrinolysis 1998;9(2):107–17.

33. Gray AJ, Bishop JE, Reeves JT, Mecham RP, Laurent GJ. Partially degraded fibrin(ogen) stimulates fibroblast proliferation in vitro. Am J Respir Cell Mol Biol 1995;12(6):684–90.

34. Welsh CH, Hassell KL, Badesch DB, Kressin DC, Marlar RA. Coagulation and fibrinolytic profiles in patients with severe pulmonary hypertension. Chest 1996;110:710–7.

35. Akbar H, Kim J, Funk K, Cancelas JA, Shang X, Chen L et al. Genetic and pharmacologic evidence that Rac1 GTPase is involved in regulation of platelet secretion and aggregation. J Thromb Haemost 2007;5(8):1747–55.

36. Turitto VT, Hall CL. Mechanical factors affecting hemostasis and thrombosis. Thromb Res 1998;92(6 Suppl 2):S25–31.

37. Crouch EC, Parks WC, Rosenbaum JL, Chang D, Whitehouse L, Wu LJ et al. Regulation of collagen production by medial smooth muscle cells in hypoxic pulmonary hypertension. Am Rev Respir Dis 1989;140(4):1045–51.

38. Weiser MC, Majack RA, Tucker A, Orton EC. Static tension is associated with increased smooth muscle cell DNA synthesis in rat pulmonary arteries. Am J Physiol 1995;268(3 Pt 2):H1133–8.

39. Bishop JE, Butt R, Dawes K, Laurent G. Mechanical load enhances the stimulatory effect of PDGF on pulmonary artery fibroblast procollagen synthesis. Chest 1998; 114(1 Suppl):25S.

40. Hirschi KK, D'Amore PA. Pericytes in the microvasculature. Cardiovasc Res 1996;32(4):687–98.

41. Prosser IW, Stenmark KR, Suthar M, Crouch EC, Mecham RP, Parks WC. Regional heterogeneity of elastin and collagen gene expression in intralobar arteries in response to hypoxic pulmonary hypertension as demonstrated by in situ hybridization. Am J Pathol 1989;135(6):1073–88.

42. Frid MG, Moiseeva EP, Stenmark KR. Multiple phenotypically distinct smooth muscle cell populations exist in the adult and developing bovine pulmonary arterial wall. Circ Res 1994;75:669–81.

43. Frid MG, Aldashev AA, Dempsey EC, Stenmark KR. Smooth muscle cells isolated from discrete compartments of the mature vascular media exhibit unique phenotypes and distinct growth capabilities. Circ Res 1997;81(6):940–52.

44. Frid MG, Aldashev A, Dempsey EC, Stenmark KR. Smooth muscle cells isolated from discrete compartments of the mature vascular media exhibit unique phenotypes and distinct growth capabilities. Circ Res 1997;81:940–52.

45. Dempsey EC, Frid MG, Aldashev AA, Das M, Stenmark KR. Heterogeneity in the proliferative response to bovine pulmonary artery smooth muscle cells to mitogens and hypoxia: importance of protein kinase C. Can J Physiol Pharmacol 1997;75:936–44.

46. Wohrley JD, Frid MG, Moiseeva EP, Orton EC, Belknap JK, Stenmark KR. Hypoxia selectively induces proliferation in a specific subpopulation of smooth muscle cells in the bovine neonatal pulmonary arterial media. J Clin Invest 1995;96:273–81.

47. Morrell NW, Yang X, Upton PD, Jourdan KB, Morgan N, Sheares KK et al. Altered growth responses of pulmonary artery smooth muscle cells from patients with primary pulmonary hypertension to transforming growth factor-β1 and bone morphogenetic proteins. Circulation 2001; 104(7):790–5.

48. Upton PD, Wharton J, Davie N, Ghatei MA, Smith DM, Morrell NW. Differential adrenomedullin release and endothelin receptor expression in distinct subpopulations of human airway smooth-muscle cells. Am J Respir Cell Mol Biol 2001;25(3):316–25.

49. Morrell NW, Upton PD, Kotecha S, Huntley A, Yacoub MH, Polak JM et al. Angiotensin II activates MAPK and stimulates growth of human pulmonary artery smooth muscle via AT_1 receptors. Am J Physiol 1999;277:L440–8.

50. Wharton J, Davie N, Upton PD, Yacoub MH, Polak JM, Morrell NW. Prostacyclin analogues differentially inhibit growth of distal and proximal human pulmonary artery smooth muscle cells. Circulation 2000;102:3130–6.

51. Riley DJ, Poiani GJ, Tozzi CA, Rosenbloom J, Pierce RA, Deak SB. Collagen and elastin gene expression in the hypertensive pulmonary artery of the rat. Trans Assoc Am Physicians 1986;99:180–8.

52. Mecham RP, Whitehouse LA, Wrenn DS, Parks WC, Griffin GL, Senior RM et al. Smooth muscle-mediated connective tissue remodeling in pulmonary hypertension. Science 1987;237(4813):423–6.

53. Tozzi CA, Christiansen DL, Poiani GJ, Riley DJ. Excess collagen in hypertensive pulmonary arteries decreases vascular distensibility. Am J Respir Crit Care Med 1994;149(5):1317–26.

54. Stenmark KR, Mecham RP. Cellular and molecular mechanisms of pulmonary vascular remodeling. Annu Rev Physiol 1997;59:89–144.

55. Strauss BH, Rabinovitch M. Adventitial fibroblasts: defining a role in vessel wall remodeling. Am J Respir Cell Mol Biol 2000;22:1–3.

56. Chazova I, Loyd JE, Zhdanov VS, Newman JH, Belenkov Y, Meyrick B. Pulmonary artery adventitial changes and venous involvement in primary pulmonary hypertension. Am J Pathol 1995;146:389–97.

57. Stenmark KR, Fasules J, Hyde DM, Voelkel NF, Henson J, Tucker A et al. Severe pulmonary hypertension and arterial adventitial changes in newborn calves at 4,300 m. J Appl Physiol 1987;62(2):821–30.

58. Das M, Stenmark KR, Ruff LJ, Dempsey EC. Selected isozymes of PKC contribute to augmented growth of fetal and neonatal bovine PA adventitial fibroblasts. Am J Physiol 1997;273:L1276–84.

59. Das M, Stenmark KR, Dempsey EC. Enhanced growth of fetal and neonatal pulmonary artery adventitial fibroblasts is dependent on protein kinase C. Am J Physiol 1995; 269:L660–7.

60. Das M, Dempsey EC, Reeves JT, Stenmark KR. Selective expansion of fibroblast subpopulations from pulmonary artery adventitia in response to hypoxia. Am J Physiol Lung Cell Mol Physiol 2002;282(5):L976–86.

61. Das M, Bouchey DM, Moore MJ, Hopkins DC, Nemenoff RA, Stenmark KR. Hypoxia-induced proliferative response of vascular adventitial fibroblasts is dependent on G protein-mediated activation of mitogen-activated protein kinases. J Biol Chem 2001;276(19):15631–40.

62. Das M, Dempsey EC, Bouchey D, Reyland ME, Stenmark KR. Chronic hypoxia induces exaggerated growth responses in pulmonary artery adventitial fibroblasts. Am J Respir Cell Mol Biol 2000;22:15–25.

63. Boudreau NJ, Jones PL. Extracellular matrix and integrin signalling: the shape of things to come. Biochem J 1999;339(Pt 3):481–8.

64. Miyamoto S, Katz BZ, Lafrenie RM, Yamada KM. Fibronectin and integrins in cell adhesion, signaling, and morphogenesis. Ann N Y Acad Sci 1998;857:119–29.

65. Reeves JT, Bishop JE, Laurent GJ. Functional basis for the structure of the pulmonary arterial tree. In: Bishop JE, Reeves JT, Laurent GJ, editors. Pulmonary vascular remodelling. London: Portland Press, 1995:1–19.

66. Tozzi CA, Poiani GJ, Harangozo AM, Boyd CD, Riley DJ. Pressure-induced connective tissue synthesis in pulmonary artery segments is dependent on intact endothelium. J Clin Invest 1989;84(3):1005–12.

67. Todorovich-Hunter L, Dodo H, Ye C, McCready L, Keeley FW, Rabinovitch M. Increased pulmonary artery elastolytic activity in adult rats with monocrotaline-induced progressive hypertensive pulmonary vascular disease compared with infant rats with nonprogressive disease. Am Rev Respir Dis 1992;146(1):213–23.

68. Cowan KN, Heilbut A, Humpl T, Lam C, Ito S, Rabinovitch M. Complete reversal of fatal pulmonary hypertension in rats by a serine elastase inhibitor. Nature Med 2000:6.

69. Thompson K, Rabinovitch M. Exogenous leukocyte and endogenous elastases can mediate mitogenic activity in pulmonary artery smooth muscle cells by release of extracellular-matrix bound basic fibroblast growth factor. J Cell Physiol 1996;166(3):495–505.

70. Jones PL, Cowan KN, Rabinovitch M. Tenascin-C, proliferation and subendothelial fibronectin in progressive pulmonary vascular disease. Am J Pathol 1997;150(4):1349–60.

71. Jones PL, Crack J, Rabinovitch M. Regulation of tenascin-C, a vascular smooth muscle cell survival factor that interacts with the alpha v beta 3 integrin to promote epidermal growth factor receptor phosphorylation and growth. J Cell Biol 1997;139(1):279–93.

72. Cowan KN, Jones PL, Rabinovitch M. Regression of hypertrophied rat pulmonary arteries in organ culture is associated with suppression of proteolytic activity, inhibition of tenascin-C, and smooth muscle cell apoptosis. Circ Res 1999;84(10):1223–33.

73. Yamamoto K, Onoda K, Sawada Y, Fujinaga K, Imanaka-Yoshida K, Shimpo H et al. Tenascin-C is an essential factor for neointimal hyperplasia after aortotomy in mice. Cardiovasc Res 2005;65(3):737–42.

74. Thakker-Varia S, Tozzi CA, Poiani GJ, Babiarz JP, Tatem L, Wilson FJ et al. Expression of matrix-degrading enzymes in pulmonary vascular remodeling in the rat. Am J Physiol 1998;275:L398–406.

75. Vieillard-Baron A, Frisdal E, Eddahibi S, Deprez I, Baker AH, Newby AC et al. Inhibition of matrix metalloproteinases by lung TIMP-1 gene transfer or doxycycline aggravates pulmonary hypertension in rats. Circ Res 2000;87(5): 418–25.

76. Cowan KN, Jones PL, Rabinovitch M. Regression of hypertrophied rat pulmonary arteries in organ culture is associated with suppression of proteolytic activity, inhibition of tenascin-C, and smooth muscle cell apoptosis. Circ Res 1999;84:1223–33.

77. Cowan KN, Jones PL, Rabinovitch M. Elastase and matrix metalloproteinase inhibitors induce regression, and tenascin-C antisense prevents progression, of vascular disease. J Clin Invest 2000;105(1):21–34.

78. Thomas HC, Lame MW, Dunston SK, Segall HJ, Wilson DW. Monocrotaline pyrrole induces apoptosis in pulmonary artery endothelial cells. Toxicol Appl Pharmacol 1998;151(2):236–44.

79. Yeager ME, Halley GR, Golpon HA, Voelkel NF, Tuder RM. Microsatellite instability of endothelial cell growth and apoptosis genes within plexiform lesions in primary pulmonary hypertension. Circ Res 2001;88:e2–11.

80. Machado RD, James V, Southwood M, Harrison RE, Atkinson C, Stewart S et al. Investigation of second genetic hits at the BMPR2 locus as a modulator of disease progression in familial pulmonary arterial hypertension. Circulation 2005;111(5):607–13.

81. Yeager ME, Halley GR, Golpon HA, Voelkel NF, Tuder RM. Microsatellite instability of endothelial cell growth and apoptosis genes within plexiform lesions in primary pulmonary hypertension. Circ Res 2001;88(1):E2–11.

82. McMurtry MS, Archer SL, Altieri DC, Bonnet S, Haromy A, Harry G et al. Gene therapy targeting survivin selectively induces pulmonary vascular apoptosis and reverses pulmonary arterial hypertension. J Clin Invest 2005; 115(6):1479–91.

83. Riley DJ, Thakker-Varia S, Wilson FJ, Poiani GJ, Tozzi CA. Role of proteolysis and apoptosis in regression of pulmonary vascular remodeling. Physiol Res 2000;49(5):577–85.

84. Dorfmuller P, Perros F, Balabanian K, Humbert M. Inflammation in pulmonary arterial hypertension. Eur Respir J 2003;22(2):358–63.

85. Humbert M, Monti G, Brenot F, Sitbon O, Portier A, Grangeot-Keros L et al. Increased interleukin-1 and interleukin-6 serum concentrations in severe primary pulmonary hypertension. Am J Respir Crit Care Med 1995;151:1628–31.

86. Kasahara Y, Kimura H, Kurosu K, Sugito K, Mukaida N, Matsushima K et al. MCAF/MCP-1 protein expression in a rat model for pulmonary hypertension induced by monocrotaline. Chest 1998;114(1 Suppl):67S.

87. Sakamaki F, Kyotani S, Nagaya N, Sato N, Oya H, Satoh T et al. Increased plasma P-selectin and decreased thrombomodulin in pulmonary arterial hypertension were improved by continuous prostacyclin therapy. Circulation 2000;102(22):2720–5.

88. Tuder RM, Groves B, Badesch DB, Voelkel NF. Exuberant endothelial cell growth and elements of inflammation are present in plexiform lesions of pulmonary hypertension. Am J Pathol 1994;144:275–85.

89. Dorfmuller P, Humbert M, Perros F, Sanchez O, Simonneau G, Muller KM et al. Fibrous remodeling of the pulmonary venous system in pulmonary arterial hypertension associated with connective tissue diseases. Hum Pathol 2007;38(6):893–902.

90. Balabanian K, Foussat A, Dorfmuller P, Durand-Gasselin I, Capel F, Bouchet-Delbos L et al. CX3C chemokine fractalkine in pulmonary arterial hypertension. Am J Respir Crit Care Med 2002;165(10):1419–25.

91. Dorfmuller P, Zarka V, Durand-Gasselin I, Monti G, Balabanian K, Garcia G et al. Chemokine RANTES in severe pulmonary arterial hypertension. Am J Respir Crit Care Med 2002;165(4):534–9.

92. Perros F, Dorfmuller P, Souza R, Durand-Gasselin I, Godot V, Capel F et al. Fractalkine-induced smooth muscle cell proliferation in pulmonary hypertension. Eur Respir J 2007;29(5):937–43.

93. Sanchez O, Marcos E, Perros F, Fadel E, Tu L, Humbert M et al. Role of endothelium-derived CC chemokine ligand 2 in idiopathic pulmonary arterial hypertension. Am J Respir Crit Care Med 2007;176(10):1041–7.

94. Peinado VI, Barbera JA, Abate P, Ramirez J, Roca J, Santos S et al. Inflammatory reaction in pulmonary muscular arteries of patients with mild chronic obstructive pulmonary disease. Am J Respir Crit Care Med 1999;159: 1605–11.

95. Santos S, Peinado VI, Ramirez J, Melgosa T, Roca J, Rodriguez-Roisin R et al. Characterization of pulmonary vascular remodelling in smokers and patients with mild COPD. Eur Respir J 2002;19:632–8.

96. Takemoto M, Sun J, Hiroki J, Shimokawa H, Liao JK. Rho-kinase mediates hypoxia-induced downregulation of endothelial nitric oxide synthase. Circulation 2002; 106(1):57–62.

97. Xu W, Kaneko FT, Zheng S, Comhair SA, Janocha AJ, Goggans T et al. Increased arginase II and decreased NO synthesis in endothelial cells of patients with pulmonary arterial hypertension. FASEB J 2004;18(14):1746–8.

98. Pullamsetti S, Kiss L, Ghofrani HA, Voswinckel R, Haredza P, Klepetko W et al. Increased levels and reduced catabolism of asymmetric and symmetric dimethylarginines in pulmonary hypertension. FASEB J 2005;19(9):1175–7.

99. Christman BW, McPherson CD, Newman JH, King GA, Bernard GR, Groves BM et al. An imbalance between the excretion of thromboxane and prostacyclin metabolites in pulmonary hypertension. N Engl J Med 1992;327(2):70–5.

100. Tuder RM, Cool CD, Geraci MW, Wang J, Abman SH, Wright L et al. Prostacyclin synthase expression is decreased in lungs from patients with severe pulmonary hypertension. Am J Respir Crit Care Med 1999;159(6):1925–32.

101. Hoshikawa Y, Voelkel NF, Gesell TL, Moore MD, Morris KG, Alger LA et al. Prostacyclin receptor-dependent modulation of pulmonary vascular remodeling. Am J Respir Crit Care Med 2001;164(2):314–8.

102. Geraci MW, Gao B, Shepherd DC, Moore MD, Westcott JY, Fagan KA et al. Pulmonary prostacyclin synthase overexpression in transgenic mice protects against development of hypoxic pulmonary hypertension. J Clin Invest 1999;103(11):1509–15.

103. Machado RD, Aldred MA, James V, Harrison RE, Patel B, Schwalbe EC et al. Mutations of the TGF-beta type II receptor BMPR2 in pulmonary arterial hypertension. Hum Mutat 2006;27(2):121–32.

104. Lane KB, Machado RD, Pauciulo MW, Thomson JR, Phillips JA, III, Loyd JE et al. Heterozygous germline mutations in BMPR2, encoding a TGF-beta receptor, cause familial primary pulmonary hypertension. The International PPH Consortium. Nat Genet 2000;26(1):81–4.

105. Thomson JR, Machado RD, Pauciulo MW, Morgan NV, Humbert M, Elliott GC et al. Sporadic primary pulmonary hypertension is associated with germline mutations of the

gene encoding BMPR-II, a receptor member of the TGF-beta family. J Med Genet 2000;37(10):741–5.

106. Newman JH, Wheeler L, Lane KB, Loyd E, Gaddipati R, Phillips JA, III et al. Mutation in the gene for bone morphogenetic protein receptor II as a cause of primary pulmonary hypertension in a large kindred. N Engl J Med 2001;345(5):319–24.

107. Miyazono K, Kusanagi K, Inoue H. Divergence and convergence of TGF-beta/BMP signaling. J Cell Physiol 2001;187(3):265–76.

108. Miyazono K, Maeda S, Imamura T. BMP receptor signaling: transcriptional targets, regulation of signals, and signaling cross-talk. Cytokine Growth Factor Rev 2005;16(3):251–63.

109. Shi Y, Massague J. Mechanisms of TGF-beta signaling from cell membrane to the nucleus. Cell 2003;113(6):685–700.

110. Rosenzweig BL, Imamura T, Okadome T, Cox GN, Yamashita H, ten Dijke P et al. Cloning and characterization of a human type II receptor for bone morphogenetic proteins. Proc Natl Acad Sci USA 1995;92(17):7632–6.

111. Nickel J, Kotzsch A, Sebald W, Mueller TD. A single residue of GDF-5 defines binding specificity to BMP receptor IB. J Mol Biol 2005;349(5):933–47.

112. Upton PD, Long L, Trembath RC, Morrell NW. Functional characterization of bone morphogenetic protein binding sites and Smad1/5 activation in human vascular cells. Mol Pharmacol 2008;73(2):539–52.

113. David L, Mallet C, Mazerbourg S, Feige JJ, Bailly S. Identification of BMP9 and BMP10 as functional activators of the orphan activin receptor-like kinase 1 (ALK1) in endothelial cells. Blood 2007;109(5):1953–61.

114. Trembath RC, Thomson JR, Machado RD, Morgan NV, Atkinson C, Winship I et al. Clinical and molecular genetic features of pulmonary hypertension in patients with hereditary hemorrhagic telangiectasia. N Engl J Med 2001;345(5):325–34.

115. Massague J, Seoane J, Wotton D. Smad transcription factors. Genes Dev 2005;19(23):2783–810.

116. Shi W, Chen H, Sun J, Chen C, Zhao J, Wang YL et al. Overexpression of Smurf1 negatively regulates mouse embryonic lung branching morphogenesis by specifically reducing Smad1 and Smad5 proteins. Am J Physiol Lung Cell Mol Physiol 2004;286(2):L293–300.

117. Chen HB, Shen J, Ip YT, Xu L. Identification of phosphatases for Smad in the BMP/DPP pathway. Genes Dev 2006;20(6):648–53.

118. Rudarakanchana N, Flanagan JA, Chen H, Upton PD, Machado R, Patel D et al. Functional analysis of bone morphogenetic protein type II receptor mutations underlying primary pulmonary hypertension. Hum Mol Genet 2002;11(13):1517–25.

119. Nishihara A, Watabe T, Imamura T, Miyazono K. Functional heterogeneity of bone morphogenetic protein receptor-II mutants found in patients with primary pulmonary hypertension. Mol Biol Cell 2002;13(9):3055–63.

120. Yu PB, Beppu H, Kawai N, Li E, Bloch KD. Bone morphogenetic protein (BMP) type II receptor deletion reveals BMP ligand-specific gain of signaling in pulmonary artery smooth muscle cells. J Biol Chem 2005;280(26):24443–50.

121. Yu PB, Deng DY, Beppu H, Hong CC, Lai C, Hoyng SA et al. Bone morphogenetic protein (BMP) type II receptor is required for BMP-mediated growth arrest and differentiation in pulmonary artery smooth muscle cells. J Biol Chem 2008;283(7):3877–88.

122. Atkinson C, Stewart S, Upton PD, Machado R, Thomson JR, Trembath RC et al. Primary pulmonary hypertension is associated with reduced pulmonary vascular expression of type II bone morphogenetic protein receptor. Circulation 2002;105(14):1672–8.

123. Yang X, Long L, Southwood M, Rudarakanchana N, Upton PD, Jeffery TK et al. Dysfunctional Smad signaling contributes to abnormal smooth muscle cell proliferation in familial pulmonary arterial hypertension. Circ Res 2005;96(10):1053–63.

124. Zhang S, Fantozzi I, Tigno DD, Yi ES, Platoshyn O, Thistlethwaite PA et al. Bone morphogenetic proteins induce apoptosis in human pulmonary vascular smooth muscle cells. Am J Physiol Lung Cell Mol Physiol 2003;285(3):L740–54.

125. Yang J, Davies RJ, Southwood M, Long L, Yang X, Sobolewski A et al. Mutations in bone morphogenetic protein type II receptor cause dysregulation of Id gene expression in pulmonary artery smooth muscle cells: implications for familial pulmonary arterial hypertension. Circ Res 2008;102(10):1212–21.

126. Valdimarsdottir G, Goumans MJ, Rosendahl A, Brugman M, Itoh S, Lebrin F et al. Stimulation of Id1 expression by bone morphogenetic protein is sufficient and necessary for bone morphogenetic protein-induced activation of endothelial cells. Circulation 2002;106(17):2263–70.

127. Teichert-Kuliszewska K, Kutryk MJ, Kuliszewski MA, Karoubi G, Courtman DW, Zucco L et al. Bone morphogenetic protein receptor-2 signaling promotes pulmonary arterial endothelial cell survival: implications for loss-of-function mutations in the pathogenesis of pulmonary hypertension. Circ Res 2006;98(2):209–17.

128. Sakao S, Taraseviciene-Stewart L, Wood K, Cool CD, Voelkel NF. Apoptosis of pulmonary microvascular endothelial cells stimulates vascular smooth muscle cell growth. Am J Physiol Lung Cell Mol Physiol 2006; 291(3):L362–8.

129. Beppu H, Kawabata M, Hamamoto T, Chytil A, Minowa O, Noda T et al. BMP type II receptor is required for gastrulation and early development of mouse embryos. Dev Biol 2000;221(1):249–58.

130. Long L, MacLean MR, Jeffery TK, Morecroft I, Yang X, Rudarakanchana N et al. Serotonin increases susceptibility to pulmonary hypertension in BMPR2-deficient mice. Circ Res 2006;98(6):818–27.

131. Song Y, Jones JE, Beppu H, Keaney JF, Jr., Loscalzo J, Zhang YY. Increased susceptibility to pulmonary hypertension in heterozygous BMPR2-mutant mice. Circulation 2005;112(4):553–62.

132. Long L, MacLean MR, Jeffery TK, Morecroft I, Yang X, Rudarakanchana N et al. Serotonin increases susceptibility to pulmonary hypertension in BMPR2-deficient mice. Circ Res 2006;98(6):818–27.

133. Botney MD, Bahadori L, Gold LI. Vascular remodeling in primary pulmonary hypertension: potential role for transforming growth factor-β. Am J Pathol 1994;144:286–95.

134. Long L, Crosby A, Yang X, Southwood M, Upton PD, Kim DK et al. Altered bone morphogenetic protein and transforming growth factor-β signaling in rat models of pulmonary hypertension: potential for activin receptor-like kinase-5 inhibition in prevention and progression of disease. Circulation 2009;119(4):566–76.

135. Richter A, Yeager ME, Zaiman A, Cool CD, Voelkel NF, Tuder RM. Impaired transforming growth factor-β signaling in idiopathic pulmonary arterial hypertension. Am J Respir Crit Care Med 2004;170(12):1340–8.

136. Chen YF, Feng JA, Li P, Xing D, Zhang Y, Serra R et al. Dominant negative mutation of the TGF-beta receptor blocks hypoxia-induced pulmonary vascular remodeling. J Appl Physiol 2006;100(2):564–71.

137. Abenhaim L, Moride Y, Brenot F, Rich S, Benichou J, Kurz X et al. Appetite-suppressant drugs and the risk of primary pulmonary hypertension. International Primary Pulmonary Hypertension Study Group. N Engl J Med 1996;335(9):609–16.

138. MacLean MR, Herve P, Eddahibi S, Adnot S. 5-hydroxytryptamine and the pulmonary circulation: receptors, transporters and relevance to pulmonary arterial hypertension. Br J Pharmacol 2000;131(2):161–8.

139. Herve P, Drouet L, Dosquet C, Launay JM, Rain B, Simonneau G et al. Primary pulmonary hypertension in a patient with a familial platelet storage pool disease: role of serotonin. Am J Med 1990;89(1):117–20.

140. Herve P, Launay JM, Scrobohaci ML, Brenot F, Simonneau G, Petitpretz P et al. Increased plasma serotonin in primary pulmonary hypertension. Am J Med 1995;99(3):249–54.

141. Gonzalez AM, Smith AP, Emery CJ, Higenbottam TW. The pulmonary hypertensive fawn-hooded rat has a normal serotonin transporter coding sequence. Am J Respir Cell Mol Biol 1998;19(2):245–9.

142. Sato K, Webb S, Tucker A, Rabinovitch M, O'Brien RF, McMurtry IF et al. Factors influencing the idiopathic development of pulmonary hypertension in the fawn hooded rat. Am Rev Respir Dis 1992;145(4 Pt 1):793–7.

143. Fanburg BL, Lee SL. A new role for an old molecule: serotonin as a mitogen. Am J Physiol 1997;272(5 Pt 1):L795–806.

144. Eddahibi S, Fabre V, Boni C, Martres MP, Raffestin B, Hamon M et al. Induction of serotonin transporter by hypoxia in pulmonary vascular smooth muscle cells: relationship with the mitogenic action of serotonin. Circ Res 1999;84(3):329–36.

145. Lee SL, Wang WW, Moore BJ, Fanburg BL. Dual effect of serotonin on growth of bovine pulmonary artery smooth muscle cells in culture. Circ Res 1991;68(5):1362–8.

146. Pitt BR, Weng WL, Steve AR, Blakely RD, Reynolds I, Davies P. Serotonin increases DNA-synthesis in rat proximal and distal pulmonary vascular smooth-muscle cells in culture. Am J Physiol 1994;266(2):L178–86.

147. Eddahibi S, Humbert M, Fadel E, Raffestin B, Darmon M, Capron F et al. Serotonin transporter overexpression is responsible for pulmonary artery smooth muscle hyperplasia in primary pulmonary hypertension. J Clin Invest 2001;108(8):1141–50.

148. Eddahibi S, Fabre V, Boni C, Martres MP, Raffestin B, Hamon M et al. Induction of serotonin transporter by hypoxia in pulmonary vascular smooth muscle cells. Relationship with the mitogenic action of serotonin. Circ Res 1999;84(3):329–36.

149. Eddahibi S, Adnot S. Anorexigen-induced pulmonary hypertension and the serotonin (5-HT) hypothesis: lessons for the future in pathogenesis. Respir Res 2002;3:9.

150. Rothman RB, Ayestas MA, Dersch CM, Baumann MH. Aminorex, fenfluramine, and chlorphentermine are serotonin transporter substrates. Implications for primary pulmonary hypertension. Circulation 1999;100(8):869–75.

151. Eddahibi S, Hanoun N, Lanfumey L, Lesch KP, Raffestin B, Hamon M et al. Attenuated hypoxic pulmonary hypertension in mice lacking the 5-hydroxytryptamine transporter gene. J Clin Invest 2000;105(11):1555–62.

152. MacLean MR, Deuchar GA, Hicks MN, Morecroft I, Shen S, Sheward J et al. Overexpression of the 5-hydroxytryptamine transporter gene: effect on pulmonary hemodynamics and hypoxia-induced pulmonary hypertension. Circulation 2004;109(17):2150–5.

153. Guignabert C, Izikki M, Tu LI, Li Z, Zadigue P, Barlier-Mur AM et al. Transgenic mice overexpressing the 5-hydroxytryptamine transporter gene in smooth muscle develop pulmonary hypertension. Circ Res 2006;98(10):1323–30.

154. Guignabert C, Raffestin B, Benferhat R, Raoul W, Zadigue P, Rideau D et al. Serotonin transporter inhibition prevents and reverses monocrotaline-induced pulmonary hypertension in rats. Circulation 2005;111(21):2812–9.

155. Keegan A, Morecroft I, Smillie D, Hicks MN, MacLean MR. Contribution of the 5-HT(1B) receptor to hypoxia-induced pulmonary hypertension: converging evidence using 5-HT(1B)-receptor knockout mice and the 5-HT(1B/1D)-receptor antagonist GR127935. Circ Res 2001;89(12):1231–9.

156. MacLean MR, Clayton RA, Templeton AG, Morecroft I. Evidence for 5-HT1-like receptor-mediated vasoconstriction in human pulmonary artery. Br J Pharmacol 1996;119(2):277–82.

157. Frishman WH, Huberfeld S, Okin S, Wang YH, Kumar A, Shareef B. Serotonin and serotonin antagonism in cardiovascular and non-cardiovascular disease. J Clin Pharmacol 1995;35(6):541–72.

158. Launay JM, Herve P, Peoc'h K, Tournois C, Callebert J, Nebigil CG et al. Function of the serotonin 5-hydroxytryptamine 2B receptor in pulmonary hypertension. Nat Med 2002;8(10):1129–35.

159. Callebert J, Esteve JM, Herve P, Peoc'h K, Tournois C, Drouet L et al. Evidence for a control of plasma serotonin levels by 5-hydroxytryptamine(2B) receptors in mice. J Pharmacol Exp Ther 2006;317(2):724–31.

160. Blanpain C, Le Poul E, Parma J, Knoop C, Detheux M, Parmentier M et al. Serotonin 5-HT(2B) receptor loss of function mutation in a patient with fenfluramine-associated

primary pulmonary hypertension. Cardiovasc Res 2003; 60(3):518–28.

161. Morecroft I, Heeley RP, Prentice HM, Kirk A, MacLean MR. 5-hydroxytryptamine receptors mediating contraction in human small muscular pulmonary arteries: importance of the 5–HT1B receptor. Br J Pharmacol 1999;128(3):730–4.

162. MacLean MR, Sweeney G, Baird M, McCulloch KM, Houslay M, Morecroft I. 5-Hydroxytryptamine receptors mediating vasoconstriction in pulmonary arteries from control and pulmonary hypertensive rats. Br J Pharmacol 1996;119(5): 917–30.

163. Darmon MC, Guibert B, Leviel V, Ehret M, Maitre M, Mallet J. Sequence of two mRNAs encoding active rat tryptophan hydroxylase. J Neurochem 1988;51(1):312–6.

164. Eddahibi S, Guignabert C, Barlier-Mur AM, Dewachter L, Fadel E, Dartevelle P et al. Cross talk between endothelial and smooth muscle cells in pulmonary hypertension: critical role for serotonin-induced smooth muscle hyperplasia. Circulation 2006;113(15):1857–64.

165. Morecroft I, Dempsie Y, Bader M, Walther DJ, Kotnik K, Loughlin L et al. Effect of tryptophan hydroxylase 1 deficiency on the development of hypoxia-induced pulmonary hypertension. Hypertension 2007;49(1):232–6.

166. Dempsie Y, Morecroft I, Welsh DJ, MacRitchie NA, Herold N, Loughlin L et al. Converging evidence in support of the serotonin hypothesis of dexfenfluramine-induced pulmonary hypertension with novel transgenic mice. Circulation 2008;117(22):2928–37.

167. Davis S, Aldrich TH, Jones PF, Acheson A, Compton DL, Jain V et al. Isolation of angiopoietin-1, a ligand for the TIE2 receptor, by secretion-trap expression cloning. Cell 1996;87(7):1161–9.

168. Kim KT, Choi HH, Steinmetz MO, Maco B, Kammerer RA, Ahn SY et al. Oligomerization and multimerization are critical for angiopoietin-1 to bind and phosphorylate Tie2. J Biol Chem 2005;280(20):20126–31.

169. Thistlethwaite PA, Lee SH, Du LL, Wolf PL, Sullivan C, Pradhan S et al. Human angiopoietin gene expression is a marker for severity of pulmonary hypertension in patients undergoing pulmonary thromboendarterectomy. J Thorac Cardiovasc Surg 2001;122(1):65–73.

170. Brindle NP, Saharinen P, Alitalo K. Signaling and functions of angiopoietin-1 in vascular protection. Circ Res 2006;98(8):1014–23.

171. Thurston G, Rudge JS, Ioffe E, Zhou H, Ross L, Croll SD et al. Angiopoietin-1 protects the adult vasculature against plasma leakage. Nat Med 2000;6(4):460–3.

172. Du L, Sullivan CC, Chu D, Cho AJ, Kido M, Wolf PL et al. Signaling molecules in nonfamilial pulmonary hypertension. N Engl J Med 2003;348(6):500–9.

173. Sullivan CC, Du L, Chu D, Cho AJ, Kido M, Wolf PL et al. Induction of pulmonary hypertension by an angiopoietin 1/TIE2/serotonin pathway. Proc Natl Acad Sci USA 2003;100(21):12331–6.

174. Dewachter L, Adnot S, Fadel E, Humbert M, Maitre B, Barlier-Mur AM et al. Angiopoietin/Tie2 pathway influences smooth muscle hyperplasia in idiopathic

pulmonary hypertension. Am J Respir Crit Care Med 2006;174(9):1025–33.

175. Chu D, Sullivan CC, Du L, Cho AJ, Kido M, Wolf PL et al. A new animal model for pulmonary hypertension based on the overexpression of a single gene, angiopoietin-1. Ann Thorac Surg 2004;77(2):449–56.

176. Kido M, Du L, Sullivan CC, Deutsch R, Jamieson SW, Thistlethwaite PA. Gene transfer of a TIE2 receptor antagonist prevents pulmonary hypertension in rodents. J Thorac Cardiovasc Surg 2005;129(2):268–76.

177. Zhao YD, Campbell AI, Robb M, Ng D, Stewart DJ. Protective role of angiopoietin-1 in experimental pulmonary hypertension. Circ Res 2003;92(9):984–91.

178. Golovina VA, Platoshyn O, Bailey CL, Wang J, Limsuwan A, Sweeney M et al. Upregulated TRP and enhanced capacitative Ca(2+) entry in human pulmonary artery myocytes during proliferation. Am J Physiol Heart Circ Physiol 2001;280(2):H746–55.

179. Yu Y, Fantozzi I, Remillard CV, Landsberg JW, Kunichika N, Platoshyn O et al. Enhanced expression of transient receptor potential channels in idiopathic pulmonary arterial hypertension. Proc Natl Acad Sci USA 2004;101(38):13861–6.

180. Yuan JX, Aldinger AM, Juhaszova M, Wang J, Conte JV, Jr., Gaine SP et al. Dysfunctional voltage-gated K+ channels in pulmonary artery smooth muscle cells of patients with primary pulmonary hypertension. Circulation 1998; 98(14):1400–6.

181. Abe R, Donnelly SC, Peng T, Bucala R, Metz CN. Peripheral blood fibrocytes: differentiation pathway and migration to wound sites. J Immunol 2001;166(12):7556–62.

182. Direkze NC, Forbes SJ, Brittan M, Hunt T, Jeffery R, Preston SL et al. Multiple organ engraftment by bone-marrow-derived myofibroblasts and fibroblasts in bone-marrow-transplanted mice. Stem Cells 2003;21(5):514–20.

183. Forbes SJ, Russo FP, Rey V, Burra P, Rugge M, Wright NA et al. A significant proportion of myofibroblasts are of bone marrow origin in human liver fibrosis. Gastroenterology 2004;126(4):955–63.

184. Hinz B, Phan SH, Thannickal VJ, Galli A, Bochaton-Piallat ML, Gabbiani G. The myofibroblast: one function, multiple origins. Am J Pathol 2007;170(6):1807–16.

185. Quan TE, Cowper SE, Bucala R. The role of circulating fibrocytes in fibrosis. Curr Rheumatol Rep 2006;8(2):145–50.

186. Strieter RM, Gomperts BN, Keane MP. The role of CXC chemokines in pulmonary fibrosis. J Clin Invest 2007; 117(3):549–56.

187. Frid MG, Brunetti JA, Burke DL, Carpenter TC, Davie NJ, Reeves JT et al. Hypoxia-induced pulmonary vascular remodeling requires recruitment of circulating mesenchymal precursors of a monocyte/macrophage lineage. Am J Pathol 2006;168(2):659–69.

188. Tomasek JJ, Vaughan MB, Kropp BP, Gabbiani G, Martin MD, Haaksma CJ et al. Contraction of myofibroblasts in granulation tissue is dependent on Rho/Rho kinase/myosin light chain phosphatase activity. Wound Repair Regen 2006;14(3):313–20.

189. Khakoo AY, Finkel T. Endothelial progenitor cells. Ann Rev Med 2005;56(1):79–101.

190. Asosingh K, Aldred MA, Vasanji A, Drazba J, Sharp J, Farver C et al. Circulating angiogenic precursors in idiopathic pulmonary arterial hypertension. Am J Pathol 2008;172(3):615–27.

191. Junhui Z, Xingxiang W, Guosheng F, Yunpeng S, Furong Z, Junzhu C. Reduced number and activity of circulating endothelial progenitor cells in patients with idiopathic pulmonary arterial hypertension. Respir Med 2008; 102(7):1073–9.

192. Zhao YD, Courtman DW, Deng Y, Kugathasan L, Zhang Q, Stewart DJ. Rescue of monocrotaline-induced pulmonary arterial hypertension using bone marrow-derived endothelial-like progenitor cells: efficacy of combined cell and enos gene therapy in established disease. Circ Res 2005;96(4):442–50.

193. McLaughlin VV, Genthner DE, Panella MM, Rich S. Reduction in pulmonary vascular resistance with long-term epoprostenol (prostacyclin) therapy in primary pulmonary hypertension. N Engl J Med 1998;338(5):273–7.

194. McLaughlin VV, Shillington A, Rich S. Survival in primary pulmonary hypertension: the impact of epoprostenol therapy. Circulation 2002;106:1477–82.

195. Clapp LH, Finney P, Turcato S, Tran S, Rubin LJ, Tinker A. Differential effects of stable prostacyclin analogs on smooth muscle proliferation and cyclic AMP generation in human pulmonary artery. Am J Respir Cell Mol Biol 2002;26(2):194–201.

196. Nagaya N, Yokoyama C, Kyotani S, Shimonishi M, Morishita R, Uematsu M et al. Gene transfer of human prostacyclin synthase ameliorates monocrotaline-induced pulmonary hypertension in rats. Circulation 2000;102(16):2005–10.

197. Dupuis J, Hoeper MM. Endothelin receptor antagonists in pulmonary arterial hypertension. Eur Respir J 2008;31(2): 407–15.

198. Galie N, Ghofrani HA, Torbicki A, Barst RJ, Rubin LJ, Badesch D et al. Sildenafil Citrate Therapy for Pulmonary Arterial Hypertension. N Engl J Med 2005;353(20):2148–57.

199. Clozel M, Hess P, Rey M, Iglarz M, Binkert C, Qiu C. Bosentan, sildenafil, and their combination in the monocrotaline model of pulmonary hypertension in rats. Exp Biol Med (Maywood) 2006;231(6):967–73.

200. Zaidi SH, You XM, Ciura S, Husain M, Rabinovitch M. Overexpression of the serine elastase inhibitor elafin protects transgenic mice from hypoxic pulmonary hypertension. Circulation 2002;105(4):516–21.

201. Hu E, Lee D. Rho kinase as potential therapeutic target for cardiovascular diseases: opportunities and challenges. Expert Opin Ther Targets 2005;9(4):715–36.

202. Nishimura T, Vaszar LT, Faul JL, Zhao G, Berry GJ, Shi L et al. Simvastatin rescues rats from fatal pulmonary hypertension by inducing apoptosis of neointimal smooth muscle cells. Circulation 2003;108(13):1640–5.

203. Schermuly RT, Dony E, Ghofrani HA, Pullamsetti S, Savai R, Roth M et al. Reversal of experimental pulmonary hypertension by PDGF inhibition. J Clin Invest 2005; 115(10):2811–21.

204. Wang XX, Zhang FR, Shang YP, Zhu JH, Xie XD, Tao QM et al. Transplantation of autologous endothelial progenitor cells may be beneficial in patients with idiopathic pulmonary arterial hypertension: a pilot randomized controlled trial. J Am Coll Cardiol 2007;49(14):1566–71.

CLINICAL ASSESSMENT OF PULMONARY HYPERTENSION: DIAGNOSIS & MANAGEMENT

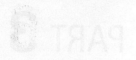

6

Clinical features*

ANDREW J PEACOCK AND COLIN CHURCH

INTRODUCTION

Pulmonary hypertension is not a disease, but a syndrome in which the pressure in the pulmonary circulation is raised. The clinical features of this syndrome are mostly related to the degree of pulmonary artery pressure elevation and its effect on the right ventricle. Although idiopathic pulmonary arterial hypertension (IPAH) is a very rare disease, pulmonary hypertension is remarkably common and is estimated to be the third most common cardiovascular syndrome after coronary artery disease and systemic hypertension. Pulmonary hypertension is common because raised blood pressure in the pulmonary circulation can accompany nearly all cardiac and pulmonary disease. Previous classifications of the causes of pulmonary hypertension distinguished between primary pulmonary hypertension, where there appears to be a primary histological vasculopathy but the cause is unknown, and secondary pulmonary hypertension, where pulmonary hypertension occurs in the response to a known stimulus. This classification outlived its usefulness when it became clear that several types of "secondary pulmonary hypertension" had similar histology to primary unexplained pulmonary hypertension, suggesting common biological pathways. Furthermore, with the advent of successful treatment for pulmonary hypertension it became clear that primary pulmonary hypertension and secondary pulmonary hypertension due to connective tissue disease, HIV and porto-pulmonary syndromes responded in a similar fashion to intravenous therapies such as epoprostenol. This prompted the Evian Symposium

in 1998 and subsequent world symposia in Venice 2003 and Dana Point in 2008 where physicians and scientists gathered from all over the world and spent time developing, amongst other things, new classifications for pulmonary arterial hypertension (PAH) (see Chapter 14).

In the current (Dana Point) classification, pulmonary hypertension is divided into pulmonary hypertension directly affecting the pulmonary vasculature, i.e. idiopathic pulmonary arterial hypertension (PAH), heritable PAH, CTD associated PAH, HIV-PAH, portopulmonary PAH (or associated pulmonary arterial hypertension), pulmonary hypertension associated with disorders of the respiratory system, pulmonary hypertension due to thrombotic or embolic disease and pulmonary venous hypertension. Within the general category of pulmonary arterial hypertension, pathology and response treatment may be similar suggesting a common final pathobiological pathway (see Chapter 5). The cellular processes may be a primary process but may also be a response to the deranged hemodynamics (1) suggesting that the histological change may be, in some way, coupled to the vasomotor response (2). Interestingly, despite similarities in histology there may be marked differences in the rate of onset of the disease, its progression and its response to treatment. For example, congenital heart disease with left-to-right shunt causes a gradual increase in pulmonary vascular remodeling and hence pulmonary artery pressure, which can reach systemic levels. Idiopathic pulmonary arterial hypertension is more rapidly progressive than congenital heart disease associated pulmonary hypertension, but the most rapidly progressive form of PAH is pulmonary hypertension associated with CREST syndrome, which also tends to be resistant to

*Sitaxsentan was withdrawn in December 2010.

vasodilator therapy. The differences in progression and in etiology, whether familial, related to infection, related to autoimmune disease or related to anorexigen use have suggested the "single, dual or multiple hit" hypothesis: a genetic susceptibility is present which only results in clinical signs of disease when an additional factor exists, such as anorexigen use, exposure to high altitude, or pregnancy.

The main problem for clinicians interested in the pulmonary circulation has been the long delays between the onset of disease and its diagnosis.

This delay may be because:

- Pulmonary hypertension is difficult to diagnose because the symptoms and signs are vague and basic investigations are unhelpful.
- Until the new era of treatment for pulmonary hypertension there was little urgency to establish the diagnosis, since the prognosis was bleak and the physicians were unable to offer much in the way of disease modifying therapy.
- Pulmonary hypertension was considered to be a very rare condition and therefore did not prompt a high index of suspicion for the diagnostician.
- There is no sphygmomanometer for the pulmonary circulation. Measurements of pressure and flow could only be made invasively by right heart catheterization. This obvious hurdle in the diagnosis pathway has meant that the average delay between onset of symptoms of pulmonary hypertension and diagnosis was two years in most studies (3).

This delay is now being overcome and the reasons for improved diagnosis are as follows:

- The discovery of the gene for pulmonary hypertension. The discovery of mutations in the bone morphogenetic protein type 2 receptor (*BMPR2*) has given a firm genetic basis for this disease. This is present in up to 80 percent of cases of familial idiopathic pulmonary arterial hypertension and approximately 25 percent of cases of sporadic idiopathic pulmonary arterial hypertension. Its discovery will most likely lead to genetic screening and has also prompted new avenues of pathobiological research (see Chapters 5 and 15.2).
- Non-invasive screening in the form of echocardiography is now widely available (see Chapter 7).
- The availability of non-invasive testing and the new classification of pulmonary hypertension allow us to screen more effectively for the presence of pulmonary hypertension even in the asymptomatic stage.
- The availability of effective treatment. The last decade has seen an explosion of effective treatments for pulmonary hypertension. The first was continuous intravenous epoprostenol (prostacyclin), followed by the prostacyclin analogs iloprost, beroprost, and treprostinil. More recently orally available treatments such as the endothelin receptor antagonists (bosentan, sitaxsentan,

ambrisentan) and phosphodiesterase type 5 inhibitors (sildenafil, tadalafil) have been shown to be of clinical benefit (4,5). At the time of writing, further trials are underway using strategies against novel targets many of which have been identified through a greater understanding of the molecular and cellular pathobiology of the disease process (see Chapters 5 and 16.8).

- There is increased awareness of the condition and physicians are now considering PAH as a potential diagnosis earlier on than before.
- We now have better techniques for evaluating the effectiveness of treatment, in particular sophisticated studies of hemodynamics by cardiac catheter, echocardiography, magnetic resonance imaging or cardiopulmonary exercise testing.

In this chapter, we shall examine the features of pulmonary hypertension, which enhance our clinical understanding of the various conditions whose common feature is an increase in pulmonary artery pressure. We shall discuss the clinical symptoms and signs associated with pulmonary hypertension and right heart dysfunction. We shall discuss symptoms and signs that might lead to the diagnosis of the diseases associated with pulmonary hypertension. Lastly we will discuss those investigations that have improved our understanding of the clinical features of the pulmonary hypertension, both in terms of understanding the effects of a raised pulmonary vascular resistance per se and also our understanding of the various conditions that lead to a change in pulmonary vascular resistance.

EPIDEMIOLOGICAL FEATURES ASSISTING THE CLINICAL DIAGNOSIS OF PULMONARY HYPERTENSION

The syndrome of pulmonary hypertension has many causes, risk factors and associations. A thorough knowledge of these factors may help both in improving clinical diagnosis of pulmonary hypertension and in allowing a better understanding of its clinical and pathobiological course.

Pulmonary arterial hypertension

GENETIC ASPECTS

A germ-line mutation in the bone morphogenetic protein receptor 2 (*BMPR2*) has been found in a number of families with pulmonary arterial hypertension (6–8). This mutation occurs in most cases of familial pulmonary arterial hypertension but also occurs in up to 25 percent of patients with "sporadic" idiopathic pulmonary arterial hypertension (9). Furthermore it is apparent that patients with "sporadic" idiopathic pulmonary arterial hypertension can transmit the disease. *BMPR2* may not, however, be the only important genetic polymorphism. Mutation of the *ALK-1* gene, another member of the TGF-β superfamily (like *BMPR2*) is found in the rare condition of IPAH associated with hereditary hemorrhagic telangectasia (10). The deletion homozygote of the *ACE* gene may be important in patients who have chronic hypoxic lung disease (11) and is also associated with an inability to ascend to extreme altitude, possibly because of the excessive hypoxic pulmonary vasoconstriction limiting exercise. Finally, abnormalities of the serotonin transport gene promoter seems to be more common in patients with IPAH, possibly because the increased transcription of serotonin transporter results in an increased take-up of serotonin into the cell where it can act as a growth promoter (12). At present there is no large scale program of screening of the population for these genetic defects or indeed other genetic defects which may be important (e.g. NO synthase, endothelin receptors, etc.) but the evidence is good enough at present that family members of those with pulmonary hypertension should be screened for the presence of pulmonary hypertension. Progress has been made in this area, e.g. it has been shown that asymptomatic carriers of the gene have abnormal pulmonary artery pressure responses to exercise and hypoxia (13). This, of course, raises three issues:

1. First, should patients with abnormal gene mutations and polymorphisms be subjected to tests to indicate the presence of early pulmonary vascular disease?
2. Second, if early disease is found, should they be treated before symptoms develop?
3. Third, should they receive genetic counseling to try and ensure that the gene is not transmitted?

These are important ethical questions which are discussed later in the chapter.

DEMOGRAPHICS

Idiopathic pulmonary arterial hypertension is more common in women. This has been thought to be due to the fact that males with the condition died *in utero* but, interestingly, in children the female to male ratio is 1:1 and then it becomes 1.7:1 in adults (14). There appears to be no relationship between pulmonary hypertension and race. The mean age for developing the condition is 40, but 8 percent of patients are aged over 60 (14). There is evidence that elderly people have diastolic dysfunction of the heart and decreased compliance of both systemic and pulmonary vessels. It may be these features act as triggers when there is an underlying tendency to pulmonary hypertension. Certainly, in these authors' experience it is common for patients to have a history of systemic hypertension. The association between the two is not yet understood and arteriosclerosis is extremely rare in the pulmonary circulation.

ENVIRONMENTAL FACTORS

The best-known external trigger to pulmonary hypertension is the anorectic drugs. It is ironic that the second WHO symposium was held at the time of the second epidemic of pulmonary hypertension associated with appetite suppressant usage. The first WHO symposium was held after the 1960s epidemic when the appetite suppressant Aminorex was responsible for a 1000-fold increased risk of pulmonary hypertension. This lesson was not learned, however, and new anorectic drugs appeared; subsequently over 5 000 000 prescriptions were written for the fenfluramine anorectics before they were withdrawn from the marketplace (15). Luckily, the association was discovered early and a case-controlled study showed that there was an overall increase in risk using these drugs of 6.3-fold, or 23-fold if they were used for more than 3 months (16). Subsequently, a study of 579 patients in the United States (17) showed that the risk of idiopathic pulmonary arterial hypertension was increased by 7.5 times if anorectics were used for more than 6 months. Not surprisingly, there is an increased female to male ratio of pulmonary hypertension secondary to anorectic drugs, and this is particularly true in Belgium and France where the greatest number of prescriptions per capita were written (18). The exact mechanism by which the anorexigens cause pulmonary hypertension is not understood (see Chapter 15.4). A front-runner is likely to be the change in 5-HT transport that occurs in response to the anorexigens (19).

CONNECTIVE TISSUE DISEASE

The fact that up to 10 percent of patients with idiopathic pulmonary arterial hypertension have Raynaud's phenomenon has prompted exhaustive investigation into the association between autoimmune disease and pulmonary hypertension. Interestingly, the rates of pulmonary hypertension in these diseases seem to vary from one study to another. For example, in France approximately 10 percent of patients with pulmonary arterial hypertension have connective tissue disease (14). However, in the recent treatment trials for pulmonary arterial hypertension approximately 50 percent of the patients had connective tissue disease associated pulmonary hypertension. In order to decide whether or not to screen patients with connective tissue disease for the presence of pulmonary hypertension, it is necessary to look at the figures the other way round. This subject has been reviewed by Hoeper (20) who found that approximately 5–10 percent of patients with systemic lupus erythematosis had pulmonary arterial disease. This is higher in patients with the CREST variant of systemic sclerosis (now known as limited cutaneous scleroderma), where figures range between 10 and 30 percent; post mortem studies suggest that up to 50 percent of patients with CREST have pulmonary arterial disease.

Figures from Japan suggest that 6 percent of patients with SLE (21) have pulmonary vascular disease and that it improves with treatment of the SLE using cyclophosphamide. This is also seen in mixed connective tissue disease (MCTD) (22). The discrepancies between the clinical and the post mortem studies underscore the deficiency of our current methods for the diagnosis and assessment of patients with pulmonary arterial disease. Clearly, pulmonary vascular disease is more common than we have previously thought, but only becomes manifest in those in whom the pulmonary vascular disease progresses faster and further.

HIV INFECTION

The association of pulmonary hypertension with HIV infection has been known for a number of years (see Chapter 15.6) but the mechanism remains unknown. The histologic characteristics are similar to idiopathic pulmonary arterial hypertension, i.e. a plexogenic arteriopathy. The syndrome appears to be particularly prevalent in IV drug abusers (14), suggesting that intravenous injection is an additional risk factor. The incidence of pulmonary hypertension in HIV infection in France is 0.6 percent. Survival of HIV pulmonary hypertension is poor, averaging 6 months in one study (23) although, similarly to SLE, case reports have suggested that anti-retroviral treatment may improve the pulmonary hypertension (24). Furthermore treatment with disease targeted therapy especially epoprostenol has shown improvement in survival (25).

PORTAL HYPERTENSION

The incidence of pulmonary hypertension occurring in the setting of cirrhosis and portal hypertension varies from 0.7 percent to 3.1 percent (14,26). In the NIH Registry (3) 8 percent of the patients with pulmonary arterial hypertension also had portal hypertension. Patients with cirrhosis but without portal hypertension do not develop pulmonary hypertension, suggesting that the development of pulmonary hypertension must be related to changes in the portal circulation (for review see Chapter 15.5). The role of emerging therapies in this condition is as yet undecided although case reports have suggested patients respond to treatment (27).

OTHERS

There are a number of other seemingly unrelated diseases and syndromes associated with pulmonary arterial hypertension and it is to be hoped that these associations will lead us to a clearer understanding of the pathobiology of the disease. For example, pulmonary arterial hypertension is associated with thyroid disease (in one study 22 percent of patients with idiopathic pulmonary arterial hypertension were hypothyroid) (28); with amyloid (29); with hemoglobinopathies (14); with splenectomy (30) and with the ingestion of toxic oil, the infamous outbreak in Spain (31)).

Importantly, some of these syndromes are reversible. For example, approximately 8 percent of those with toxic oil syndrome developed pulmonary arterial hypertension, but this regressed in 74 percent suggesting that once the cause was removed the process was reversed. Also of interest was the high male to female ratio in the toxic oil syndrome. The

cause of pulmonary arterial hypertension in the hemaglobinopathies is unknown. In patients with splenectomy it is possible that the abnormal red cells that would normally be cleared by the spleen result in platelet activation in the pulmonary vascular bed causing *in situ* thrombosis that is often difficult to distinguish from plexogenic pulmonary arteriopathy (32).

Exercise-induced PH

Prior to the most recent WHO world symposium (Dana Point 2008) the definition of PAH took into account the existence of pulmonary hypertension which is absent at rest but develops on exercise. However the clinical relevance of exercise-induced pulmonary hypertension is unclear. Indeed studies have shown that subjects with a PA pressure of greater than 30 mmHg on exercise can be either completely asymptomatic or in contrast have reduced exertional capacity. This fact has led to a change in the definition of pulmonary hypertension at the Dana Point world symposium (see Chapter 14). Exercise has been used in familial PAH cases to try and identify those subjects who may be at risk of developing PAH because of a genetic trait. Yet the natural history of exercise-induced PAH remains unclear, as does whether this condition leads inexorably to the development of PAH at rest.

Tolle *et al.* have recently presented evidence that exercise-induced PAH is indeed an early, mild and clinically important stage in the development of PAH (33). This group found that patients with exercise-induced PAH had mPAP and PVR values (as determined by right heart catheterization) in between those of normal and PAH at rest. Although not as robust, similar findings have been suggested by a study in patients with systemic sclerosis (34).

The importance of determining this finding has been highlighted by the recent EARLY study which showed benefit in treating patients with disease targeted therapy at a very early stage of their disease process (35). Thus exercise-induced PAH, if it was confirmed to be a preclinical stage of the disease process, would be an excellent opportunity to commence therapy. At the very least those who are identified to have this should be closely followed up.

Hypoxic lung disease

It has been known since 1946 that alveolar hypoxia induces pulmonary hypertension. Interestingly, hypoxemia without alveolar hypoxia (such as in cyanotic heart disease) does not cause pulmonary hypertension to the same extent, suggesting that the oxygen sensor is indeed on the alveolar side of the small pulmonary arteries. Because hypoxia is a potent pulmonary vasoconstrictor, hypoxia induced pulmonary hypertension can be found at altitude. It occurs in 5 percent of those residing at altitude between 3000 and 5000 meters and 27 percent of those living between 4500 and 5000 meters (14).

The most common cause of secondary pulmonary hypertension is chronic obstructive pulmonary disease, where it appears that a minimum daily level of hypoxia is necessary (36). There are several mechanisms by which hypoxia could cause pulmonary hypertension: (1) hypoxia causes contraction of the entire pulmonary vascular bed, of isolated pulmonary arteries and even isolated pulmonary artery smooth muscle cells; (2) hypoxia stimulates both the production of hypoxia inducible factor α (HIF-α) and the signaling pathways associated with the stress kinase. This raises the possibility that hypoxia may be an additional element in the development of the pulmonary arterial hypertension even when it is not its primary cause. To this end, it has been noted that patients with idiopathic pulmonary arterial hypertension tend to desaturate particularly at night, possibly related to reduced ventilation. It is also known that up to one-fourth of patients with obstructive sleep apnea develop pulmonary hypertension (37) (for review see Chapter 20.2).

The degree of PH in patients with stable COPD is often mild–moderate with mean pulmonary artery pressures in the range of 20–35 mmHg with preserved cardiac output. These patients may also have a co-morbid condition which may also contribute to their PH such as sleep apnea or left heart disease.

However, there is emerging evidence to suggest the existence of a subgroup of COPD population (maybe as many as 5 percent) who have severe PH as defined by mean PAP > 40 mmHg. These patients have COPD and have pulmonary vascular disease more akin to idiopathic PAH rather than the hypoxic induced group. It is possible that this group may respond to PAH targeted treatment (38,39).

Pulmonary venous hypertension

Another large group of patients with pulmonary hypertension are those that have PH resulting from left heart dysfunction. The most common causes are mitral valve disease or left ventricular diastolic dysfunction. The latter condition is increasing in incidence possibly reflecting the rise in diabetes, although other risk factors are important including systemic hypertension, obesity, coronary artery disease and insulin resistance (40).

Patients can present with similar findings to PAH except orthopnea and PND often occur as a predominant feature; ECG may show left axis deviation and left ventricular hypertrophy; chest x-ray may show pulmonary venous congestion and echo can demonstrate impaired relaxation of the left ventricle. Right heart catheterization is necessary to differentiate between pulmonary venous hypertension and PAH and classically shows an elevated pulmonary wedge pressure and pulmonary artery diastolic pressure. Indeed if the difference between the PA diastolic and PA wedge pressure is less than 10 mmHg, then this favors the diagnosis of PVH. Obviously the accuracy of the wedge measurement is critical. Exercise or fluid challenge to increase the cardiac output can be used to help differentiate between pulmonary venous and arterial disease by measuring the response of the cardiac output and wedge pressure (41).

Treatment of these patients is uncertain. There have been some studies looking at treatment of LV *systolic* failure. Addition of sildenafil suggested a trend to improved hemodynamics; bosentan had no effect and epoprostenol may actually increase mortality. No studies have been completed in LV *diastolic* dysfunction. The definitive treatment for mitral valve disease remains valvular replacement (42).

Thromboembolic pulmonary hypertension

This is defined as obstruction of the pulmonary arteries by a clot causing pulmonary hypertension. Since removal of the clot at surgery does not always cure the pulmonary hypertension, intrinsic abnormalities in the pulmonary vessel, in addition to the mechanical obstruction from the clot, may also be responsible (for review, see Lang Chapter 22.3). Furthermore, controversy exists about whether the clot really migrated from peripheral veins or develops *in situ* (43). To add to this debate it has been found that although thrombotic risk factors are not usually present in idiopathic pulmonary arterial hypertension, antiphospholipid antibodies are present in both idiopathic pulmonary arterial hypertension (10 percent) and thromboembolic pulmonary hypertension (20 percent) (14). The pathological variant of pulmonary hypertension known as thrombotic pulmonary hypertension likely results from thrombosis *in situ* due to low flow in the pulmonary circulation, causing endothelial damage, abnormal circulating platelets, or other elements. Since anticoagulants alone improve survival in idiopathic pulmonary arterial hypertension, thromboembolic pulmonary hypertension and idiopathic pulmonary arterial hypertension might have more in common than previously suggested.

Exercise capacity and pulmonary vascular resistance have been shown to predict outcome and also perioperative survival in pulmonary thromboendarterectomy (44,45).

Congenital heart disease

Approximately 5 percent of patients with congenital heart disease will develop pulmonary hypertension. It is thought that, in the setting of interatrial or interventricular septal defects, left-to-right shunting results in high flow and higher pressure in the low-pressure right circulation causing sheer stress and endothelial damage, and leads to pulmonary vascular remodeling and pulmonary hypertension. However, in some cases the pulmonary hypertension is out of proportion to the degree of shunt (46), suggesting that these pulmonary vessels have a propensity to develop histological changes in the presence of shunt-induced higher flow. Evidence has now shown that patients with Eisenmenger's syndrome could benefit from being on bosentan therapy (47).

SYMPTOMS

The classical, albeit nonspecific, symptom of pulmonary arterial hypertension is exertional breathlessness, which is said to be present in up to 60 percent of cases (3). The fact that breathlessness may not be associated with any additional symptoms of cardiopulmonary disease has led in the past to delays in diagnosis of up to 2 years (3) a problem which persists (16). A typical case was a young woman presenting to another hospital in her 20s with breathlessness. Initially this had been put down to lack of physical fitness. Later it was put down to hyperventilation syndrome and the diagnosis only became apparent when additional factors developed such as chest pain, syncope or ankle swelling (3). The pathophysiology of exertional breathlessness in PAH is multifactorial. The potential mechanisms include (i) the inability of the right heart to raise cardiac out-put on exercise thereby reducing oxygen delivery to tissues; (ii) a lactic acidosis which occurs earlier compared to normal, leading to increased CO_2 production; and (iii) reduced perfusion of ventilated lung. It is now becoming clear that cardiac index is the most useful prognostic factor in patients with pulmonary arterial hypertension. It is said that symptoms do not develop until the pulmonary artery pressure has doubled, but breathlessness can vary depending on the etiology and severity of the pulmonary hypertension. For example Delcroix (18) showed that anorexigen-induced pulmonary hypertension is commonly associated with shortness of breath, but the severity is generally less than that seen in patients from the National Institute of Health Registry for the same degree of pulmonary arterial pressure. An interesting observation is that the duration of breathlessness appears, at least in one study, to be inversely related to survival (48). This might suggest that the breathlessness is not simply related to the pulmonary vascular changes, but has other causes; it is possible that an increased sensation of breathlessness might protect the patient from high exertion which, in turn, induces worsening vascular changes. While breathlessness is the most common symptom the other two symptoms that usually lead to the diagnosis are syncope and chest pain.

Chest pain is thought to be due to relative ischemia of the right ventricular myocardium. The expression "relative ischemia" is used because coronary artery anatomy is usually normal but, because of the grossly thickened right ventricle, there is inadequate coronary supply. Furthermore, the reduced cardiac output and reduced intraortic pressure also reduce the coronary artery perfusion pressure.

Syncope, which usually occurs on exercise, is thought to be due to right ventricular encroachment on the left ventricle, decreasing left ventricular stroke volume particularly on exercise and thus reducing forward systemic cardiac flow. It may however also result from a reduction in the left ventricular end diastolic volume secondary to a lower stroke volume from the failing right ventricle. Whatever the mechanism syncope is usually thought of as an ominous sign because it indicates severe pulmonary arterial changes and dilating right ventricle.

Fatigue is another nonspecific symptom often encountered and is believed to reflect the poor cardiac output. A more unusual presentation is that of Ortner's syndrome in which the patient suffers from hoarseness as a direct result of compression of the left recurrent laryngeal nerve by an enlarged pulmonary artery (49).

Shortness of breath, chest pain and syncope are the classic symptoms of pulmonary hypertension, but other symptoms related to right ventricular dysfunction may also be present, such as ankle swelling, ascites (which appears to occur in patients on prostacyclin even where there is very little ankle swelling suggesting a local hepatic dysfunction) and anorexia presumably due to gastric mucosal edema. Finally, there may be other symptomatic clues which are helpful, for example the syndrome may have been brought on by triggers such as pregnancy (especially in ASD), high altitude (particularly in pulmonary artery vascular abnormalities such as pulmonary artery atresia) and the use of anorexigens. There may also be symptoms of other underlying diseases that are known to be associated with pulmonary hypertension such as HIV infection, thyroid disease, connective tissue disease, venous thrombotic disease or primary cardiac disease (see Table 6.1).

SIGNS

The clinical signs in pulmonary vascular disease should be considered in the same way as the clinical symptoms, i.e. the signs associated with pulmonary hypertension, the signs associated with right ventricular dysfunction and signs associated with primary disorders that cause pulmonary hypertension. Typically the signs of pulmonary

Table 6.1 Symptoms of pulmonary hypertension

Shortness of breath
Syncope
Chest pain

Table 6.2 Symptoms of right heart dysfunction

Breathlessness
Ascites
Ankle swelling
Poor appetite

Table 6.3 Symptoms of disease associated with pulmonary hypertension

Hypoxic lung disease
Congenital heart disease
Left heart disease
Thromboembolic disease
Thyroid disease
HIV
Cirrhosis of the liver

Table 6.4   Signs associated with pulmonary hypertension

Loud split P2
Right ventricular hypertrophy
Increased "a" waves
Increased "v" waves
Diastolic murmur (pulmonary valvular reflux)
Pansystolic murmur (tricuspid reflux)

Table 6.5   Signs of right heart failure

Poor peripheral perfusion
Raised RAP
Right ventricular third and fourth heart sounds
Tricuspid regurgitation
Ejection systolic murmur across the pulmonary valve

Table 6.6   Signs of associated conditions

Connective tissue disease especially scleroderma

Hypoxic lung disease especially:
   COPD
   Interstitial lung disease
   Kyphoscholiosis

Signs of left heart disease

hypertension are difficult to discern even when the examiner already knows that the pulmonary artery pressure is high. Cyanosis can have two causes: (1) the decrease in mixed venous oxygen tension that is characteristic of the low cardiac output in pulmonary hypertension; and (2) the right-to-left shunt that may occur, particularly on exercise, when a patent foramen ovale opens (50). The jugular venous pressure may reveal enlarged "a" waves thought to be secondary to poor compliance of the right ventricle and "v" waves due to tricuspid regurgitation. The tricuspid valve is a naturally leaky valve and the presence of the murmur of tricuspid reflux and the presence of "v" waves does not necessarily indicate right ventricular failure. Right ventricular hypertrophy can be determined from left parasternal or sub-xiphisternal pulsation although this may be absent when there is a relatively hyperinflated chest. Pulmonary hypertension produces a loud pulmonary component of the second heart sound (3) often associated with "normal" splitting of the second sound, i.e. the split widens on inspiration as blood is sucked into the chest and right ventricular preload increases. This is said to be present in up to 93 percent of cases (3). A shunt such as an ASD should be considered when the splitting of the second sound is fixed and wide.

The pansystolic murmur of tricuspid regurgitation or the early diastolic murmur of pulmonary regurgitation can also be appreciated in the failing ventricle as the valve annulus starts to stretch and become dysfunctional. There may also be signs of right ventricular dysfunction including raised jugular venous pressure with prominent "v" waves, ascites, hepatomegaly and swollen ankles. All these features are due to backpressure on the right atrium from

the dilated right ventricle. Interestingly, sometimes the signs are dissociated, for example in patients on prostacyclin it is not uncommon to find ascites, which raises the possibility of primary liver disease: it may simply be that hepatic hemodynamics are changed by the prostacyclin. Hypotension and cool peripheries reflect the development of a severe reduction in cardiac output and is a poor prognostic indicator.

Other physical signs can suggest the underlying cause of the PAH: the skin manifestations of scleroderma and basal crackles on auscultation of the chest suggesting interstitial lung disease are just a few. Digital clubbing can be seen rarely, but may indicate underlying congenital heart disease or pulmonary veno-occlusive disease.

There are a number of important points that can be made about the clinical signs:

- Where there is evidence of an intracardiac shunt it is important to consider whether the shunt is the cause of the pulmonary hypertension or simply coincidental.
- Where there are signs of connective tissue disease one should determine whether the breathlessness and poor exercise tolerance is a consequence of the pulmonary arterial hypertension or associated interstitial lung disease.
- Where there is evidence of peripheral edema, it is important to consider whether this is due to raised right atrial pressure, hypoalbuminemia or vasodilators such as calcium antagonists or the endothelin receptor antagonists, which are used to treat pulmonary hypertension.
- There is great confusion about the term cor pulmonale. The WHO definition is right ventricular hypertrophy as a consequence of pulmonary disease, but it has come to mean the presence of fluid retention in hypoxic lung disease. In hypoxic lung disease fluid retention is likely to be due to renal causes (51) because cardiac output in these patients is usually normal. However, when peripheral edema is seen in the context of idiopathic pulmonary arterial hypertension, it is likely that right ventricular failure is the cause and this will be associated with a low cardiac index.

INVESTIGATION OF PULMONARY HYPERTENSION

When faced with a breathless patient the cardiologist or respiratory physician will normally undertake a number of investigations including electrocardiogram, chest x-ray, pulmonary function tests, V/Q scan, CT scan and echocardiography as well as routine blood tests and arterial blood gases. We have therefore taken these investigations as the starting point. We have divided them into (1) those investigations that suggest the *presence* of pulmonary hypertension; (2) those investigations that suggest the *cause* of pulmonary hypertension; and (3) those investigations that give us some idea of the *severity* of pulmonary hypertension.

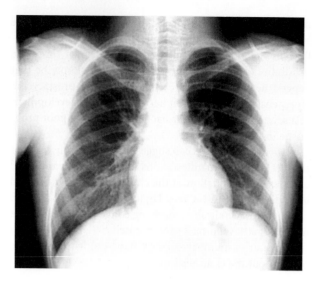

Figure 6.1   Chest x-ray of a young man fatally ill with thromboembolic pulmonary hypertension. There is little evidence of pulmonary hypertension on this x-ray.

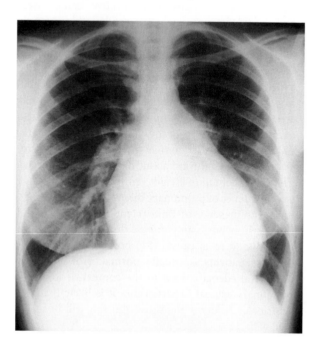

Figure 6.2   Chest x-ray of a young woman with primary pulmonary hypertension who remains symptomatically well on continuous intravenous prostacyclin 7 years after the original diagnosis.

Investigations suggesting the presence of pulmonary hypertension

CHEST X-RAY

Classically the chest x-ray would show enlargement of the right side of the heart, enlargement of the main pulmonary artery and enlargement of both hila due to enlarged pulmonary arteries. There may also be loss of vascularity in the peripheral lung due to diminished blood flow as a consequence of the high peripheral resistance (often referred to as "pruning of the vessels"). The lateral chest x-ray may show loss of the retrosternal space due to enlargement of the right ventricle. The chest x-ray is not, however, wholly reliable; although these features are common when there is severe pulmonary hypertension, the chest x-ray may be entirely normal (Figures 6.1 and 6.2). For review of Radiology see Chapter 8.

ELECTROCARDIOGRAM

The electrocardiogram classically shows features of right atrial and right ventricular hypertension, i.e. large p-wave especially in II, right axis deviation, tall R waves and ST depression in the right-sided chest leads. Once again these features may be absent (Figure 6.3) and a normal ECG does not exclude significant PH. Indeed the lack of sensitivity and specificity has rendered it unsuitable as a screening tool for PH (52). Patients are usually in sinus rhythm, possibly because arrhythmias are often fatal.

PULMONARY FUNCTION TESTS

These are most useful to exclude COPD and interstitial lung disease. In the NIH Registry Study (3) patients with idiopathic pulmonary arterial hypertension had mild restriction, but diminished gas transfer. Similar results were seen in the Israeli study (53). It has always been assumed that the loss of gas transfer is due to diminished pulmonary capillary blood volume, as a consequence of constriction of small peripheral pulmonary arteries, but studies where pulmonary capillary blood volume has been separated from gaseous diffusion have suggested that most of the loss of DLCO in idiopathic pulmonary arterial hypertension and chronic thromboembolic pulmonary hypertension is due to a decrease in the diffusion at the membrane level (54). The mild restriction to ventilation is not really understood but could be due to the thickening of peripheral vessels, which diminishes lung compliance. Other studies have also shown mild airflow obstruction in idiopathic pulmonary arterial hypertension, particularly at the level of peripheral airways, with changes in the flow independent section of the flow volume loop (55). The reason for this peripheral airflow obstruction is not understood.

VENTILATION/PERFUSION SCAN

The ventilation/perfusion scan is classically used as a means for distinguishing pulmonary thromboembolism from other causes of breathlessness. The situation in pulmonary arterial hypertension is, however, more complicated because there may be *in situ* thrombosis in IPAH which can closely mimic pulmonary embolism (56–59). Generally, however, the loss of perfusion is segmental fashion and asymmetric in thromboembolic pulmonary hypertension whereas it is more generalized in IPAH (Figures 6.5 and 6.6). For a review of V/Q see Chapter 8.

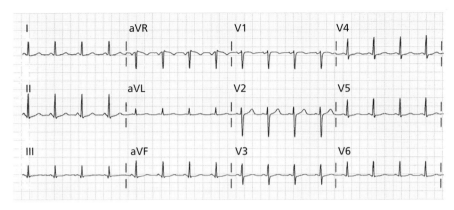

Figure 6.3 Electrocardiogram of a young man dying from thromboembolic pulmonary hypertension: there is little evidence of a right ventricular response to his high pulmonary artery pressures.

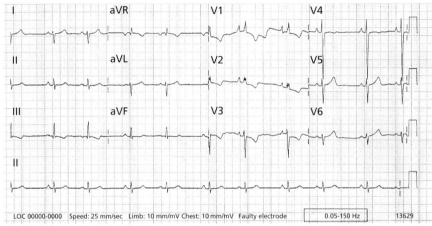

Figure 6.4 Electrocardiogram of a young woman in Figure 6.2 showing right ventricular hypertrophy with right axis deviation.

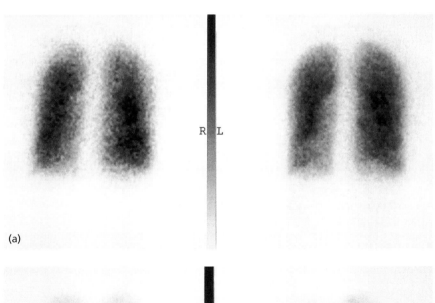

Figure 6.5 Ventilation (a) and perfusion (b) scans from a patient with primary pulmonary hypertension showing patchy ("motheaten") appearances to the perfusion images. These changes are thought to represent pulmonary artery thrombosis.

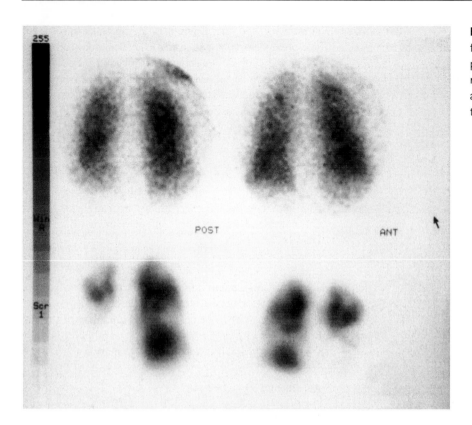

Figure 6.6 Ventilation perfusion scan from a patient with thromboembolic pulmonary hypertension showing normal ventilation (upper panels) but abnormal perfusion (lower panels) due to vascular obstruction by clot.

CT SCAN

The main purpose of the CT scan is to distinguish pulmonary hypertension from other causes of progressive breathlessness, particularly emphysema and interstitial lung disease (60,61). In "pure" idiopathic pulmonary arterial hypertension the CT scan will demonstrate enlarged pulmonary arteries with diminished peripheral vascularity. For a review of CT radiology, see Chapter 8.

BLOOD TESTS

Typically arterial PO_2 is low and there is an accompanying decrease in arterial PCO_2 due to increased ventilation. The low PO_2 is a consequence of low mixed venous O_2, in turn a consequence of the poor cardiac index. There is probably no significant defect in gaseous diffusion despite abnormalities in DLCO as described above.

ECHOCARDIOGRAM

This is the definitive screening test for the presence of pulmonary hypertension and is dealt with elsewhere (Chapter 7). Echocardiogram will demonstrate right ventricular dilation; an estimate of pulmonary artery systolic pressure can be obtained from a measurement of tricuspid regurgitant jet wave velocity. However, recently data have suggested that echo may underestimate the pulmonary artery pressure and cardiac output in up to 50 percent of cases (62).

Investigations suggesting the cause of pulmonary arterial hypertension

From the classification of pulmonary hypertension (see Chapter 14) it is clear that there are many causes, some of which can be determined by basic investigation. Since pulmonary hypertension is difficult to treat it is very important to establish a diagnosis if there is a causative disease which can be independently treated with benefit to the pulmonary circulation (particularly in SLE, HIV, COPD and left heart dysfunction).

CHEST X-RAY

The chest x-ray may show evidence of COPD, interstitial lung disease or abnormalities of the chest wall causing hypoventilation. Focal areas of oligemia may suggest underlying CTEPH.

ELECTROCARDIOGRAM

The electrocardiogram may demonstrate ischemic heart disease or systemic hypertension.

PULMONARY FUNCTION TESTS

These may show the presence of COPD, restriction due to chest wall disease or restriction due to interstitial lung disease. The patients with "pure" idiopathic pulmonary arterial hypertension will also have restriction and low gas transfer. Clearly it can be difficult to determine whether or not there is significant interstitial lung disease from the pulmonary function tests and whether this is contributing to the restriction and loss of gas transfer. Careful evaluation of the pulmonary function tests in conjunction with high resolution CT scan of the chest and clinical examination is necessary.

Screening overnight pulse oximetry can be a simple and very useful test in detecting the presence of underlying sleep disordered breathing, especially obesity hypoventilation which may be the cause of the PH.

VENTILATION/PERFUSION SCAN

This will show patchy loss of ventilation in primary lung disease (56,58) and the presence of asymmetric perfusion defects in thromboembolic pulmonary hypertension, but there can be confusion because of a similar appearance that occurs in the thrombotic variant of idiopathic pulmonary arterial hypertension. The main differentiating factor between the conditions is the localization of the perfusion defects. In IPAH the defects are patchy and nonsegmental and said to be of low probability which contrasts with the multiple segmental and sharply demarcated defects in CTEPH (63,64). In addition while it is true that normal V/Q scans effectively rule out the diagnosis of chronic thromboembolic disease, it is important to state that segmental defects do not always represent CTEPH and other conditions such as mediastinal fibrosis and pulmonary artery vasculitis, and tumors can also give rise to similar appearances. For review of V/Q see Chapter 8.

The perfusion scan may also give some clue about the presence of pulmonary veno-occlusive disease. This variant was thought to be rare, but is now believed to be more common. It is very important to make the diagnosis because treatment with standard vasodilators may be fatal (65).

Recently the role of V/Q scanning has been questioned with the advent of routine CT-pulmonary angiography. However, evidence exists which suggests that V/Q scanning is much more sensitive and specific for picking up CTEPH when compared to CTPA (66). Thus V/Q scanning should remain an integral part of the investigation of PH.

ECHOCARDIOGRAM

The echocardiogram may show evidence of left ventricular disease – either hypertrophy or dysfunction, the presence of proximal thromboembolism or the presence of left-to-right cardiac shunt. For further evaluation of possible shunts a transesophageal echo can be used. If a right-to-left shunt is suspected then "bubble" contrast echocardiography should be performed.

CT SCAN

It is our practice to perform a high resolution CT (HRCT) scan to look for evidence of interstitial lung disease or

pulmonary veno-occlusive disease (PVOD) (61,67–69). The presence of lymphadenopathy, nodular opacities, septal lines and small pleural effusions are typical of PVOD which is difficult to diagnose otherwise, even on cardiac catheterization. We also perform CT pulmonary angiography to look for proximal, surgically removable clot (68,69). For review of Radiology see Chapter 8.

BLOOD TESTS

Arterial blood gases do not help to find the cause of pulmonary hypertension, but other blood tests can be helpful. In particular serology to test for include antinuclear and anti-DNA (systemic lupus erythematosus), anti-Scl-70 and antinuclear (scleroderma), anticentromere (limited scleroderma or CREST syndrome), rheumatoid factor (rheumatoid arthritis), anti-Ro and anti-La (Sjögren's syndrome), anti-Jo-1 (dermatomyositis/polymyositis) and anti-U1 RNP (mixed connective tissue disease). There may also be thrombocytopenia and raised ANCA in CTD, and HIV serology will be positive in HIV associated pulmonary hypertension.

ABDOMINAL ULTRASOUND

Should be performed in all patients with PAH and abnormal liver function to exclude cirrhosis of the liver with or without portal hypertension.

Investigations indicating the severity of pulmonary arterial hypertension (including clinical end points)

The principle complaint of patients with pulmonary hypertension is breathlessness on exertion thus some form of functional test performed on exertion is going to give the most useful information about the severity of pulmonary hypertension. This should be compared with assessments of quality of life in order to determine the functional severity of disease and to determine the impact of therapy. After the 1998 Evian Symposium a classification of breathlessness was formed based on the New York Heart Association Criteria and this is given in Chapter 14.

Basic static investigations that give some idea of severity are as follows:

QUALITY OF LIFE ASSESSMENT

All recent treatment trials in pulmonary hypertension used some measure of quality of life; while none is perfect, these have included: the medical outcomes trust short form 12 (SF12) and 36 (SF36); the EQ-5D and, for most of the trials, a modification of the Minnesota living with heart failure questionnaire. None of these quality of life tests were developed specifically for pulmonary hypertension. However, there is now a quality of life questionnaire which has been specifically developed for assessment of PH patients;

the Cambridge Pulmonary Hypertension Outcome Review (CAMPHOR) (70). This has now been validated in the UK, USA and Canada as an effective tool. In future when we consider the end points for trials with vasodilators in pulmonary hypertension we should now include this as a measure of quality of life.

CHEST X-RAY

An enlarging heart indicates that it is failing in response to the high outflow impedance.

ELECTROCARDIOGRAM

There is some evidence that size of p-wave amplitude and the development of features of right ventricular hypertrophy relate to prognosis in idiopathic pulmonary arterial hypertension (71). Furthermore a linear relationship between the p-wave amplitude in lead II and pulmonary vascular resistance has been demonstrated and this group has also suggested that a treatment response can be determined by follow-up analysis of the p-wave amplitude, QRS axis and T-wave axis as compared to a baseline ECG (72).

This same group have also shown an inverse relationship between a QRS ventricular gradient and RV mass as assessed by cardiac MRI (73). This new evidence may suggest a role for the ECG as a non-invasive test for assessing patient response to treatment.

PULMONARY FUNCTION TESTS

The only pulmonary function variable related to severity is the gas transfer, which has been found to be proportional to the VO_2 max, the oxygen pulse and the ventilation/VCO_2 slope at anaerobic threshold (74). In addition recent evidence has confirmed previous findings that in these patients there is no association between lung function and hemodynamic parameters (75).

BLOOD TESTS

The presence of hyponatremia (sodium $<$ 136 mEq/L) has been shown to indicate a greater degree of right heart failure and be associated with a worse prognosis (76).

Biomarkers such as plasma brain naturetic peptide (BNP) have been found to have prognostic importance in the management of PAH (77). BNP is secreted by ventricular myocytes and the plasma levels correlate with the degree of stretch on the cardiomyocytes. More recently the N-terminal pro-BNP which is the cleaved section of the pro-peptide has been suggested as a better biomarker as it has a longer half life.

V/Q SCAN

This is also essentially a description of the anatomic derangement of the pulmonary circulation but one study reported a perfusion index from the perfusion scans that was proportional to mean pulmonary artery pressure and right ventricular ejection fraction in patients with idiopathic pulmonary arterial hypertension (78).

ECHOCARDIOGRAPHY

This investigation would appear to be the non-invasive investigation of choice for looking at the severity of pulmonary hypertension. It is possible using echocardiography to measure right ventricular size (rather inaccurate) and pulmonary artery systolic pressure (more accurate). Since severity of pulmonary hypertension is only partly related to these two variables there have been attempts to get more information from echocardiography (see Chapter 7). Two studies are worth mentioning here: the Derived Right Ventricular Index was the only independent predictor of mortality in 53 patients with pulmonary hypertension (79). Additionally, a poor outcome could be predicted by the presence of pericardial effusion and increased right atrial size (80). More recently, use of the tricuspid annular planar systolic excursion (TAPSE) has been shown to be a prognostic factor (81). In an attempt to improve the morphological description given by echocardiography, Menzel *et al.* (82) used three-dimensional echo to develop measurements of right ventricular size and systolic function that improved after surgery for thromboembolic disease.

MAGNETIC RESONANCE IMAGING (MRI)

MRI has much greater potential than echocardiography to measure right ventricular mass, right ventricular morphology, pulmonary artery morphology and pulmonary artery physiology in the form of velocity profiles. For review of MR in PH see Chapter 9. At present these investigations are still in their infancy but it is known that right ventricular mass is proportional to mean pulmonary artery pressure (83). In the future we may be able to measure the benefit of therapy by improvements in the right ventricular mass or other variables. At present, physiological variables derived from MRI appear to have poor correlation with invasive hemodynamics (84) but increasingly sophisticated measures of pulse wave profile, reflective waves and other variables may improve this non-invasive assessment. An ongoing multicenter international study is seeking to address the clinical question of whether cardiac MR can be used as a non-invasive investigation to monitor patient response to treatment (Pulmotension: Framework 6).

EXERCISE TESTING

Six-minute walk test

The 6-minute walk test has been widely used in all the trials of the effectiveness of vasodilators in pulmonary hypertension. This test has the advantages of being low tech, easy to administer, and relatively reproducible (85–87). Despite its widespread use there have been remarkably few publications of its value in the assessment of pulmonary hypertension. During the 6-minute walk, measurements are made of SaO_2, heart rate, and the distance walked. It is the distance walked that has been used to evaluate the effectiveness of therapy and the prognosis of patients with these diseases. There appears to be no linear correlation between distance walked and mortality from pulmonary hypertension (86) but there does appear to be a threshold, i.e. if patients can walk more than a certain distance (332 m) (87), their survival is a great deal better. This fits very well with the data from invasive cardiac index studies, which have shown that the resting cardiac index is the best predictor of exercise tolerance and prognosis. Indeed, it has been suggested that the 6-minute walk distance is determined by the cardiac output response to exercise (88).

Cardiopulmonary exercise testing

It would seem obvious that cardiopulmonary exercise testing would be the most useful way of looking at exercise tolerance in pulmonary hypertension. For review see Chapter 10. Measurements are normally made of ventilation, CO_2 production, oxygen consumption, respiratory rate and tidal volume. From these variables oxygen pulse, ventilatory equivalents for O_2 and CO_2 and maximum oxygen uptake are calculated.

Not surprisingly exercise tolerance is dictated by VO_{2max}, which is always diminished in these patients. VO_{2max} may also be a very good way of looking at the response to therapy: for example, it has been shown that by increasing the dose of intravenous prostacyclin it is possible to further increase the cardiac output without improving VO_{2max}. This suggests that the drug is opening up shunts in the skin and visceral organs without further improvement in oxygen delivery.

Since pulmonary hypertension is associated with loss of vascularity in the periphery, there is V/Q mismatching with a high physiological deadspace and hence wasted ventilation. This is reflected in changes in slope of the VE/VCO_2 and VE/O_2 curves. It has recently been shown that the slope of these curves relates directly to the pulmonary artery pressure measured by high fidelity micromanometer tipped catheter during exercise (89). Cardiopulmonary exercise testing will also show an increase in right-to-left shunt when a patent foramen ovale opens due to the high pressures in the pulmonary circulation developed on exercise. This is detected by changes in VO_2 and VCO_2 (74). At present it seems we will get the most information from VO_{2max}, heart rate, VO_2 curves (74) and the slopes of the VE/VCO_2 and VE/VO_2 (89).

All the investigations described above are of course invasive and ultimately we would hope that the investigation and management of these patients can be conducted in a non-invasive faction. At present right heart catheterization is mandatory for all these patients to make the diagnosis of pulmonary hypertension, to allow a measure of the severity of pulmonary hypertension and to look for possible other causes of pulmonary hypertension. Furthermore it can be used to detect serial changes in patients' hemodynamics on treatment, especially during clinical trials (90).

RIGHT HEART CATHETERIZATION

This is normally performed using a triple lumen, fluid-filled Swan–Ganz thermodilution catheter. For methodology see Chapter 12. Measurements are made of right atrial and ventricular pressures, pulmonary artery pressure and cardiac output at baseline and after a vasodilator (91,92). Fluid-filled catheters are notorious for the poor frequency-to-noise ratio and because of the external transducer, poor reliability if there is any patient movement. These problems have been overcome by the development of the micromanometer tipped high fidelity catheter where the transducer is on the tip of the catheter and hence movement of the patient makes no difference to the pressure obtained. Also, because there is no fluid in the catheter, the results are much more accurate. These catheters have been exploited to make measurements in the pulmonary circulation under conditions of changes in posture, changes in exercise, changes in inhaled gases (93) resulting in the demonstration of a fixed relationship between systolic pulmonary artery pressure (sPAP) and mean pulmonary artery pressure (mPAP) which allows calculation of mPAP from the sPAP (94). They have also been used to generate pressure-flow lines which are far more useful than single measurements of pressure or flow. For example, it has been shown that whereas the pressure and flow measured at rest on the catheter table may be identical for a patient before and after prolonged treatment with prostacyclin even though the patient has noted considerable clinical benefit, the slope of the pressure–flow curve is improved by the drug (95).

It is likely that solid state catheters will prove to be more useful in the assessment of patients with pulmonary hypertension particularly since they can be inserted for up to 48 hours with recordings downloaded to a small computer carried on a waistband. Ultimately, however, these invasive tests must be used to correlate with non-invasive measurements that can be performed routinely to follow up patients with pulmonary vascular disease.

One of the advantages of catheterization is being able to obtain accurate measurements of cardiac index. It has been shown that cardiac index in response to exercise correlates with the 6-minute walk and a study of our patients has shown that cardiac index is the most important predictor of survival in patients with pulmonary hypertension regardless of cause (48).

PROGNOSIS AND SURVIVAL

There have been several studies of the prognosis in pulmonary arterial hypertension, some of which were performed in the "pre-prostacyclin" era and some performed subsequently. The NIH Registry in the United States included 194 patients collected between 1981 and 1985. The median survival of these patients was 2.8 years and appeared to relate to cardiac index, right atrial pressure and pulmonary artery pressure (96). A small study in the UK of 34 patients showed a mean survival of 7.3 years (97) but these patients are unusual. In Mexico the median survival in 61 patients diagnosed between 1977 and 1991 was 4 years (98). In Japan the median survival of 223 patients diagnosed between 1980 and 1990 was 32 months (99). It appears that the expected median survival for idiopathic pulmonary arterial hypertension is between 2.5 and 4 years. However, when the pulmonary hypertension is due to other conditions the prognosis may be quite different. For example, the prognosis is worse in anorexigen-induced pulmonary hypertension: in a US study the 3-year survival was only 17 percent, vs. 60 percent for sporadic IPAH (100). Survival of HIV-associated pulmonary hypertension is also poor, but in a study of 82 patients in France a combination of anti-retroviral therapy and prostacyclin could diminish that mortality (101). In connective tissue disease the prognosis also appears to be poor. Although disability from the disease and exercise tolerance can be improved by intravenous prostacyclin (see Chapter 15.3), mortality is not improved by therapy and remains worse than idiopathic pulmonary arterial hypertension. However, newer studies have suggested that there is an improvement in the outcome with the more modern therapies although those patients who have scleroderma related PAH and interstitial lung disease still have a poor outcome (102).

Prognosis in pulmonary arterial hypertension in the original NIH study was related to cardiac index, right atrial pressure and mean pulmonary artery pressure (96). In the Swiss Registry Study of 106 patients survival was related to 6-minute walk distance, NYHA criteria and mixed venous oxygen tension. In a recent French study prognosis of patients receiving prostacyclin related to a history of right heart failure, the presence of NYHA grade 4 breathlessness, a 6-minute walk distance of less than 250 m and a right atrial pressure of more than 12 mmHg (103). A study from our own group of approximately 90 patients suggested that cardiac index is the most important predictor of survival and interestingly this is true no matter what the cause of the pulmonary hypertension (48).

While the bulk of evidence suggests that factors related to hemodynamics and cardiac responses dictate survival, a study in 90 patients with pulmonary hypertension showed that serum uric acid levels are proportional to pulmonary vascular resistance and mortality and inversely proportional to cardiac output. Possibly the poor oxygen delivery from the diminished cardiac output causes a rise in uric acid level (104). Furthermore, plasma BNP is also an independent predictor of survival (77). While we presently need an invasive measurement of cardiac output and pulmonary hemodynamics, preferably on exercise, to predict prognosis, in the future we may be able to obtain similar information from measurements of circulating levels of hormones or other biomarkers of disease severity.

SCREENING FOR PULMONARY HYPERTENSION

From the above it is evident that we now understand the natural history of severe pulmonary arterial hypertension quite well. Since the symptoms and signs of pulmonary arterial hypertension are so vague and the basic investigations are often unhelpful it would be useful if we had screening tests (particularly non-invasive screening tests) to allow us to make an earlier diagnosis before hemodynamics are changed and therapy becomes difficult. The question is who should we screen and how should we screen them?

Furthermore, as new therapies become available for the management of PAH and the prognosis improves, the question of screening asymptomatic individuals who are deemed at risk is becoming more of an issue. Screening includes both genetic testing and non-invasively investigating subjects for evidence of raised pulmonary artery pressure.

Genetic screening

Up to 10 percent of cases of PAH are due to familial or heritable PAH. This condition seems to be inherited as an autosomal dominant pattern, with incomplete penetrance and genetic anticipation (105). In as many as 70 percent of those cases a mutation in the member of the TGF-β receptor family, *BMPRII*, has been found. These mutations have also been identified in IPAH although to a much lesser degree (10 percent) (9). These factors mean that genetic counseling can prove complex. For example possession of the genetic mutation in the *BMPRII* gene does not necessarily indicate development of the disease due to the incomplete penetrance of only 20 percent. This obviously implies the need for a so-called second hit to make the disease clinically expressed and important interactions between serotonin and BMPRII have been reported (106).

Furthermore the mutations are distinct between families and so an individual can only really be tested if the mutation in an affected individual in that family has already been characterized. This is further complicated by the fact that in only about 50 percent of affected families can an exonic mutation be found. The technical side of testing for the mutations can also be troublesome as the *BMPRII* gene is some 13 exons long.

For the individual taking the test there are a few important facts which they must understand (107). There can be significant psychological stress in knowing that you have a genetic predisposition to developing an incurable disease and moreover that there currently is no preventative therapy which could help in reducing the risk of developing the disease. There may also be discrimination from employers and insurance companies. Despite these considerations many individuals wish to be tested and one of the major reasons cited is the concern that they can pass on this mutation to their offspring who will then develop the disease. With the development of preimplantation screening of embryos, this becomes an important and emotive area to consider (108). Perhaps one of the most important advances in the management of familial cases is the need for physicians to liaise with geneticists and allow patients access to genetic counseling (108).

One of the advantages of genetic screening is that it allows the identification of those individuals who do not have the mutation and are therefore at no higher risk of developing the disease than the general population. In those asymptomatic individuals in whom a mutation is located then it would be very helpful if there was a way of identifying those that would be at risk of developing the disease. Currently this does not exist in PAH although screening with Doppler echocardiography or right heart catheterization has been proposed. Indeed the guidelines in 2004 suggested first degree relatives of an affected individual with a known genetic mutation be screened every 3–5 years (105). The exact timescale and frequency of monitoring has not been fully elucidated. Furthermore there are emerging data which suggest that asymptomatic individuals with a *BMPRII* mutation who develop an increase in their mean pulmonary artery pressure to above 40 mmHg during exercise might represent a preclinical stage of the disease, which has already been discussed in this chapter (33). Clearly though this would only be useful if treatment initiated at this early stage could alter the natural course of the disease. The EARLY trial may prove this to be the case (35) since it has shown a benefit in treating patients who are in functional class II as compared to the traditional time to treat in functional class 3 or 4.

Currently, because of the heterogeneity in the *BMPRII* mutations, genetic screening in IPAH is not recommended although patients should be informed of the availability of genetic testing and that it can be performed if clinical need dictates (109,110). They should also be informed of the low risk of recurrence (estimated at 5 percent).

Screening of at-risk populations

Those who have a familial tendency to PAH are at risk and should be tested as above. However, it has been recognized for a number of years that certain patients are at a higher risk of developing PAH than others by virtue of having other underlying conditions – for example connective tissue disease, sickle cell, portal hypertension and HIV infection.

CONNECTIVE TISSUE DISEASES

Guidelines have suggested that patients with systemic sclerosis and mixed connective tissue disease should undergo annual clinical and echocardiographic assessment to detect early signs of PAH whether they are breathless or not. As the development of PAH in this group is associated with such a poor outcome it is hoped that by detecting and treating patients earlier the prognosis would be improved.

Recognition of those patients who should be referred for right heart catheterization include a Doppler peak velocity of >2.8 m/s and a reduction in lung diffusion measurement (TLCO) of >50 percent (105).

Other connective tissue disease groups should be screened if they develop symptoms of PAH. A recent study has suggested that right heart catheterization is still essential for establishing the diagnosis in this population, but that echocardiography was the best non-invasive screening test compared to cardiac MR and lung function tests (111).

PORTAL HYPERTENSION

Patients with portal hypertension are at increased risk of developing porto-pulmonary hypertension. This condition can make liver transplantation more risky and so patients who are being considered for transplant should be screened with echo.

OTHER GROUPS

There is an increased recognition of association of PAH with sickle cell and HIV infection but as yet no routine screening is proposed. However, in a patient with dyspnea and one of these conditions, PAH should be actively excluded.

In summary, as tests for PAH become less invasive and earlier treatment becomes more effective, screening should become routine in many predisposing diseases.

KEY POINTS

Causative factors

- Since the histology in pulmonary arterial hypertension from various causes such as IPAH, HIV associated PAH, CTD associated PAH, portal hypertension PAH is similar, it is likely that these conditions share a final path of, consistent with the "double hit" hypothesis, i.e. an initial propensity and a subsequent secondary trigger.
- Since in some cases the pulmonary arterial hypertension will regress with treatment of the underlying disease as is seen particularly in SLE or HIV, it is possible that the histological lesions seen in pulmonary hypertension can regress provided the causative stimulus is removed.
- There is clearly an interaction within the pulmonary circulation between vasospasm, histological changes and the presence of intravascular thrombosis. Understanding the link between these will be critical if we are to unravel the pathobiological pathways for pulmonary hypertension and develop treatments that will reverse these pathways.

Symptoms and signs

- Symptoms and signs of pulmonary arterial hypertension are vague and are often missed.
- The symptom of excessive exertional breathlessness in association with "normal" physical examination should alert the physician to the possibility of pulmonary arterial disease.
- Resting pulmonary artery pressure has already risen considerably by the time symptoms due to pulmonary hypertension develop – methods for earlier screening are necessary.
- The clue to the presence of pulmonary hypertension is often given by the associated condition such as connective tissue disorder, congenital heart disease or hypoxic lung disease. Patients with any of these syndromes should be examined with a view to determining the functional status of the pulmonary circulation.

Investigations

- Basic investigations may be unhelpful.
- Pulmonary function tests showing normal lung volumes and spirometry but diminished gas transfer should arouse suspicion.
- Exercise tolerance and survival in pulmonary hypertension appears to relate to cardiac output.
- Echocardiography remains the screening investigation of choice for those at risk from pulmonary hypertension.

REFERENCES

1. Botney MD. Role of hemodynamics in pulmonary vascular remodeling: implications for primary pulmonary hypertension. Am J Resp Crit Care Med 1999;159(2):361–4.
2. Scott PH, Peacock AJ. Cell signalling in pulmonary vascular cells: do not shoot the messenger! Thorax 1996;51(8):864–6.
●3. Rich S, Dantzker DR, Ayres SM, Bergofsky EH, Brundage BH, Detre KM et al. Primary pulmonary hypertension. A national prospective study. Ann Intern Med 1987; 107(2):216–23.
4. Galie N, Ghofrani HA, Torbicki A, Barst RJ, Rubin LJ, Badesch D et al. Sildenafil citrate therapy for pulmonary arterial hypertension. N Engl J Med 2005;353(20):2148–57.
5. Rubin LJ, Badesch DB, Barst RJ, Galie N, Black CM, Keogh A et al. Bosentan therapy for pulmonary arterial hypertension. N Engl J Med 2002;346(12):896–903.
●6. Lane KB, Machado RD, Pauciulo MW, Thomson JR, Phillips JA, 3rd, Loyd JE et al. Heterozygous germline mutations in BMPR2, encoding a TGF-beta receptor, cause familial primary pulmonary hypertension. The International PPH Consortium. Nat Genet 2000;26(1):81–4.
●7. Deng Z, Morse JH, Slager SL, Cuervo N, Moore KJ, Venetos G et al. Familial primary pulmonary hypertension (gene PPH1) is caused by mutations in the bone morphogenetic protein receptor-II gene. Am J Hum Genet 2000;67(3):737–44.
8. Newman JH, Wheeler L, Lane KB, Loyd E, Gaddipati R, Phillips JA, 3rd et al. Mutation in the gene for bone morphogenetic protein receptor II as a cause of primary pulmonary hypertension in a large kindred. N Engl J Med 2001;345(5):319–24.
●9. Thomson JR, Machado RD, Pauciulo MW, Morgan NV, Humbert M, Elliott GC et al. Sporadic primary pulmonary hypertension is associated with germline mutations of the gene encoding BMPR-II, a receptor member of the TGF-beta family. J Med Genet 2000;37(10):741–5.
10. Trembath RC, Thomson JR, Machado RD, Morgan NV, Atkinson C, Winship I et al. Clinical and molecular genetic features of pulmonary hypertension in patients with hereditary hemorrhagic telangiectasia. N Engl J Med 2001;345(5):325–34.
11. Montgomery HE, Shall R, Hemingway H, Myerson S, Clarkson P, Dollery C et al. Human gene for physical performance. Nature 1998;393(6682):221–2.
12. Eddahibi S, Humbert M, Fadel E, Raffestin B, Darmon M, Capron F et al. Serotonin transporter overexpression is responsible for pulmonary artery smooth muscle hyperplasia in primary pulmonary hypertension. J Clin Invest 2001;108(8):1141–50.
13. Grunig E, Janssen B, Mereles D, Barth U, Borst MM, Vogt IR et al. Abnormal pulmonary artery pressure response in asymptomatic carriers of primary pulmonary hypertension gene. Circulation 2000;102(10):1145–50.
◆14. Humbert M, Nunes H, Sitbon O, Parent F, Herve P, Simonneau G. Risk factors for pulmonary arterial hypertension. Clin Chest Med 2001;22(3):459–75.
15. Voelkel NF, Clarke WR, Higenbottam T. Obesity, dexfenfluramine, and pulmonary hypertension. A lesson not learned? Am J Respir Crit Care Med 1997;155(3):786–8.
●16. Abenhaim L, Moride Y, Brenot F, Rich S, Benichou J, Kurz X et al. Appetite-suppressant drugs and the risk of primary pulmonary hypertension. International Primary Pulmonary Hypertension Study Group. N Engl J Med 1996; 335(9):609–16.
●17. Rich S, Rubin L, Walker AM, Schneeweiss S, Abenhaim L. Anorexigens and pulmonary hypertension in the United States: results from the surveillance of North American pulmonary hypertension. Chest 2000;117(3):870–4.
18. Delcroix M, Kurz X, Walckiers D, Demedts M, Naeije R. High incidence of primary pulmonary hypertension associated with appetite suppressants in Belgium. Eur Respir J 1998;12(2):271–6.
19. Eddahibi S, Adnot S. Anorexigen-induced pulmonary hypertension and the serotonin (5-HT) hypothesis: lessons for the future in pathogenesis. Resp Res 2002;3:9.
20. Hoeper MM. Pulmonary hypertension in collagen vascular disease. Eur Respir J 2002;19(3):571–6.
21. Tanaka E, Harigai M, Tanaka M, Kawaguchi Y, Hara M, Kamatani N. Pulmonary hypertension in systemic lupus erythematosus: evaluation of clinical characteristics and

response to immunosuppressive treatment. J Rheumatol 2002;29(2):282–7.

22. Sanchez O, Sitbon O, Jais X, Simonneau G, Humbert M. Immunosuppressive therapy in connective tissue diseases – associated pulmonary arterial hypertension. Chest 2006;130(1):182–9.

23. Mehta NJ, Khan IA, Mehta RN, Kowitz DA. HIV-related pulmonary hypertension: analytic review of 131 cases. Chest 2000;118(4):1133–41.

24. Speich R, Jenni R, Opravil M, Jaccard R. Regression of HIV-associated pulmonary arterial hypertension and long-term survival during antiretroviral therapy. Swiss Med Wkly 2001;131(45–46):663–5.

25. Sitbon O. HIV-related pulmonary arterial hypertension: clinical presentation and management. AIDS (London) 2008;22 Suppl 3:S55–62.

26. Yang YY, Lin HC, Lee WC, Hou MC, Lee FY, Chang FY et al. Portopulmonary hypertension: distinctive hemodynamic and clinical manifestations. J Gastroenterol 2001;36(3):181–6.

27. Porres-Aguilar M, Zuckerman MJ, Figueroa-Casas JB, Krowka MJ. Portopulmonary hypertension: state of the art. Ann Hepatol 2008;7(4):321–30.

28. Curnock AL, Dweik RA, Higgins BH, Saadi HF, Arroliga AC. High prevalence of hypothyroidism in patients with primary pulmonary hypertension. Am J Med Sci 1999;318(5):289–92.

29. Dingli D, Utz JP, Gertz MA. Pulmonary hypertension in patients with amyloidosis. Chest 2001;120(5):1735–8.

30. Hoeper MM, Niedermeyer J, Hoffmeyer F, Flemming P, Fabel H. Pulmonary hypertension after splenectomy? Ann Intern Med 1999;130(6):506–9.

31. James TN. The toxic oil syndrome. Clinical Cardiol 1994;17(9):463–70.

32. Peacock AJ. Pulmonary hypertension after splenectomy: a consequence of loss of the splenic filter or is there something more? Thorax 2005;60(12):983–4.

33. Tolle JJ, Waxman AB, Van Horn TL, Pappagianopoulos PP, Systrom DM. Exercise-induced pulmonary arterial hypertension. Circulation 2008;118(21):2183–9.

34. Callejas-Rubio JL, Moreno-Escobar E, de la Fuente PM, Perez LL, Fernandez RR, Sanchez-Cano D et al. Prevalence of exercise pulmonary arterial hypertension in scleroderma. J Rheumatol 2008;35(9):1812–6.

35. Galie N, Rubin L, Hoeper M, Jansa P, Al-Hiti H, Meyer G et al. Treatment of patients with mildly symptomatic pulmonary arterial hypertension with bosentan (EARLY study): a double-blind, randomised controlled trial. Lancet 2008;371(9630):2093–100.

36. Weitzenblum E, Chaouat A. Hypoxic pulmonary hypertension in man: what minimum daily duration of hypoxaemia is required? Eur Respir J 2001;18(2):251–3.

37. Yamakawa H, Shiomi T, Sasanabe R, Hasegawa R, Ootake K, Banno K et al. Pulmonary hypertension in patients with severe obstructive sleep apnea. Psychiatr Clin Neurosci 2002;56(3):311–2.

38. Chaouat A, Bugnet AS, Kadaoui N, Schott R, Enache I, Ducolone A et al. Severe pulmonary hypertension and chronic obstructive pulmonary disease. Am J Respir Crit Care Med 2005;172(2):189–94.

39. Chaouat A, Naeije R, Weitzenblum E. Pulmonary hypertension in COPD. Eur Respir J 2008;32(5):1371–85.

40. Angeja BG, Grossman W. Evaluation and management of diastolic heart failure. Circulation 2003;107(5):659–63.

41. Nootens M, Wolfkiel CJ, Chomka EV, Rich S. Understanding right and left ventricular systolic function and interactions at rest and with exercise in primary pulmonary hypertension. Am J Cardiol 1995;75(5):374–7.

42. Rich S, Rabinovitch M. Diagnosis and treatment of secondary (non-category 1) pulmonary hypertension. Circulation 2008;118(21):2190–9.

43. Fedullo PF, Rubin LJ, Kerr KM, Auger WR, Channick RN. The natural history of acute and chronic thromboembolic disease: the search for the missing link. Eur Respir J 2000; 15(3):435–7.

44. Condliffe R, Kiely DG, Gibbs JS, Corris PA, Peacock AJ, Jenkins DP et al. Improved outcomes in medically and surgically treated chronic thromboembolic pulmonary hypertension. Am J Respir Crit Care Med 2008;177(10): 1122–7.

45. Condliffe R, Kiely DG, Gibbs JS, Corris PA, Peacock AJ, Jenkins DP et al. Prognostic and aetiological factors in chronic thromboembolic pulmonary hypertension. Eur Respir J 2009;33(2):332–8.

46. Rich S, Abenheim L. Executive summary from the World Symposium on Primary Pulmonary Hypertension. World Health Organization. http://www.who.int/ncd/cvd/pph.html.

47. Galie N, Beghetti M, Gatzoulis MA, Granton J, Berger RM, Lauer A et al. Bosentan therapy in patients with Eisenmenger syndrome: a multicenter, double-blind, randomized, placebo-controlled study. Circulation 2006;114(1):48–54.

48. Impey VCA, Hamilton G, Peacock AJ. Cardiac index is the most important predictor of survival in patients with all types of pulmonary hypertension. Am J Respir Crit Care Med 2002;165:A97.

49. Hegewald MJ, Kewitz B, Elliott CG. Pulmonary hypertension: clinical manifestations, classification and diagnosis. Internat J Clin Pract 2007;156:5–14.

50. Sun XG, Hansen JE, Oudiz RJ, Wasserman K. Gas exchange detection of exercise-induced right-to-left shunt in patients with primary pulmonary hypertension. Circulation 2002;105(1):54–60.

51. MacNee W. Pathophysiology of cor pulmonale in chronic obstructive pulmonary disease. Part two. Am J Respir Crit Care Med 1994;150(4):1158–68.

52. Ahearn GS, Tapson VF, Rebeiz A, Greenfield JC, Jr. Electrocardiography to define clinical status in primary pulmonary hypertension and pulmonary arterial hypertension secondary to collagen vascular disease. Chest 2002;122(2):524–7.

53. Appelbaum L, Yigla M, Bendayan D, Reichart N, Fink G, Priel I et al. Primary pulmonary hypertension in Israel: a national survey. Chest 2001;119(6):1801–6.

54. Steenhuis LH, Groen HJ, Koeter GH, van derk TW. Diffusion capacity and hemodynamics in primary and chronic

thromboembolic pulmonary hypertension. Eur Respir J 2000;16(2):276–81.

55. Meyer FJ, Ewert R, Hoeper MM, Olschewski H, Behr J, Winkler J et al. Peripheral airway obstruction in primary pulmonary hypertension. Thorax 2002;57(6):473–6.

56. D'Alonzo GE, Bower JS, Dantzker DR. Differentiation of patients with primary and thromboembolic pulmonary hypertension. Chest 1984;85(4):457–61.

57. Azarian R, Brenot F, Sitbon O, Parent F, Petitpretz P, Musset D et al. Pulmonary arterial hypertension of chronic thromboembolic origin; therapeutic indications. Arch Malad Coeur Vaisseaux 1994;87(12):1709–13.

58. Moser KM,er WR, Fedullo PF, Jamieson SW. Chronic thromboembolic pulmonary hypertension: clinical picture and surgical treatment. Eur Respir J 1992;5(3):334–42.

59. Lang IM, Klepetko W. Chronic thromboembolic pulmonary hypertension: an updated review. Curr Opin Cardiol 2008;23(6):555–9.

60. Pauwels RA, Buist AS, Calverley PM, Jenkins CR, Hurd SS. Global strategy for the diagnosis, management, and prevention of chronic obstructive pulmonary disease. NHLBI/WHO Global Initiative for Chronic Obstructive Lung Disease (GOLD) Workshop summary. Am J Respir Crit Care Med 2001;163(5):1256–76.

61. Kazerooni EA, Martinez FJ, Flint A, Jamadar DA, Gross BH, Spizarny DL et al. Thin-section CT obtained at 10-mm increments versus limited three-level thin-section CT for idiopathic pulmonary fibrosis: correlation with pathologic scoring. AJR 1997;169(4):977–83.

62. Fisher MR, Forfia PR, Chamera E, Housten-Harris T, Champion HC, Girgis RE et al. Accuracy of Doppler echocardiography in the hemodynamic assessment of pulmonary hypertension. Am J Respir Crit Care Med 2009;179(7):615–21.

63. Lisbona R, Kreisman H, Novales-Diaz J, Derbekyan V. Perfusion lung scanning: differentiation of primary from thromboembolic pulmonary hypertension. AJR 1985; 144(1):27–30.

64. Worsley DF, Palevsky HI, Alavi A. Ventilation–perfusion lung scanning in the evaluation of pulmonary hypertension. J Nucl Med 1994;35(5):793–6.

65. Bailey CL, Channick RN, Auger WR, Fedullo PF, Kerr KM, Yung GL et al. "High probability" perfusion lung scans in pulmonary venoocclusive disease. Am J Respir Crit Care Med 2000;162(5):1974–8.

66. Tunariu N, Gibbs SJ, Win Z, Gin-Sing W, Graham A, Gishen P et al. Ventilation–perfusion scintigraphy is more sensitive than multidetector CTPA in detecting chronic thromboembolic pulmonary disease as a treatable cause of pulmonary hypertension. J Nucl Med 2007;48(5):680–4.

67. Resten A, Maitre S, Humbert M, Sitbon O, Capron F, Simoneau G et al. Pulmonary arterial hypertension: thin-section CT predictors of epoprostenol therapy failure. Radiology 2002;222(3):782–8.

68. Swensen SJ, Tashjian JH, Myers JL, Engeler CE, Patz EF, Edwards WD et al. Pulmonary venoocclusive disease: CT findings in eight patients. AJR 1996;167(4):937–40.

69. Remy-Jardin M, Remy J, Deschildre F, Artaud D, Beregi JP, Hossein-Foucher C et al. Diagnosis of pulmonary embolism with spiral CT: comparison with pulmonary angiography and scintigraphy. Radiology 1996;200(3):699–706.

70. McKenna SP, Doughty N, Meads DM, Doward LC, Pepke-Zaba J. The Cambridge Pulmonary Hypertension Outcome Review (CAMPHOR): a measure of health-related quality of life and quality of life for patients with pulmonary hypertension. Qual Life Res 2006;15(1):103–15.

71. Bossone E, Paciocco G, Iarussi D, Agretto A, Iacono A, Gillespie BW et al. The prognostic role of the ECG in primary pulmonary hypertension. Chest 2002;121(2):513–8.

72. Henkens IR, Gan CT, van Wolferen SA, Hew M, Boonstra A, Twisk JW et al. ECG monitoring of treatment response in pulmonary arterial hypertension patients. Chest 2008; 134(6):1250–7.

73. Henkens IR, Mouchaers KT, Vonk-Noordegraaf A, Boonstra A, Swenne CA, Maan AC et al. Improved ECG detection of presence and severity of right ventricular pressure load validated with cardiac magnetic resonance imaging. Am J Physiol Heart Circ Physiol 2008;294(5):H2150–7.

74. Sun X-G HJ, Oudiz R, Wasserman K. Heart rate–oxygen uptake (VO_2) hysteresis during incremental exercise and recovery in primary pulmonary hypertension (PPH). Am J Respir Crit Care Med 2002;165:A573.

75. Escribano PM, Sanchez MA, de Atauri MJ, Frade JP, Garcia IM. Lung function testing in patients with pulmonary arterial hypertension. Arch Bronchoneumol 2005;41(7):380–4.

76. Forfia PR, Mathai SC, Fisher MR, Housten-Harris T, Hemnes AR, Champion HC et al. Hyponatremia predicts right heart failure and poor survival in pulmonary arterial hypertension. Am J Respir Crit Care Med 2008;177(12): 1364–9.

77. Nagaya N, Nishikimi T, Uematsu M, Satoh T, Kyotani S, Sakamaki F et al. Plasma brain natriuretic peptide as a prognostic indicator in patients with primary pulmonary hypertension. Circulation 2000;102(8):865–70.

78. Fukuchi K, Hayashida K, Nakanishi N, Inubushi M, Kyotani S, Nagaya N et al. Quantitative analysis of lung perfusion in patients with primary pulmonary hypertension. J Nucl Med 2002;43(6):757–61.

79. Yeo TC, Dujardin KS, Tei C, Mahoney DW, McGoon MD, Seward JB. Value of a Doppler-derived index combining systolic and diastolic time intervals in predicting outcome in primary pulmonary hypertension. Am J Cardiol 1998; 81(9):1157–61.

80. Raymond RJ, Hinderliter AL, Willis PW, Ralph D, Caldwell EJ, Williams W et al. Echocardiographic predictors of adverse outcomes in primary pulmonary hypertension. J Am Coll Cardiol 2002;39(7):1214–9.

81. Forfia PR, Fisher MR, Mathai SC, Housten-Harris T, Hemnes AR, Borlaug BA et al. Tricuspid annular displacement predicts survival in pulmonary hypertension. Am J Respir Crit Care Med 2006;174(9):1034–41.

82. Menzel T, Wagner S, Kramm T, Mohr-Kahaly S, Mayer E, Braeuninger S et al. Pathophysiology of impaired right and left ventricular function in chronic embolic pulmonary

hypertension: changes after pulmonary thromboendarterectomy. Chest 2000;118(4):897–903.

83. Saba TS, Foster J, Cockburn M, Cowan M, Peacock AJ. Ventricular mass index using magnetic resonance imaging accurately estimates pulmonary artery pressure. Eur Respir J 2002;20(6):1519–24.

84. Tardivon AA, Mousseaux E, Brenot F, Bittoun J, Jolivet O, Bourroul E et al. Quantification of hemodynamics in primary pulmonary hypertension with magnetic resonance imaging. Am J Respir Crit Care Med 1994;150(4):1075–80.

85. Kadikar A, Maurer J, Kesten S. The six-minute walk test: a guide to assessment for lung transplantation. J Heart Lung Transplant 1997;16(3):313–9.

86. Paciocco G, Martinez FJ, Bossone E, Pielsticker E, Gillespie B, Rubenfire M. Oxygen desaturation on the six-minute walk test and mortality in untreated primary pulmonary hypertension. Eur Respir J 2001;17(4):647–52.

87. Miyamoto S, Nagaya N, Satoh T, Kyotani S, Sakamaki F, Fujita M et al. Clinical correlates and prognostic significance of six-minute walk test in patients with primary pulmonary hypertension. Comparison with cardiopulmonary exercise testing. Am J Respir Crit Care Med 2000;161(2 Pt 1):487–92.

88. Chabot F SF, Borgna M, Malvestio P, Polu JM. Six minute walking test is related to pulmonary hemodynamic data on exercise in patients with primary pulmonary hypertension. Am J Respir Crit Care Med 2002;2002(165):A37.

89. Raeside DA, Smith A, Brown A, Patel KR, Madhok R, Cleland J et al. Pulmonary artery pressure measurement during exercise testing in patients with suspected pulmonary hypertension. Eur Respir J 2000;16(2):282–7.

90. Chatterjee K. The Swan–Ganz catheters: past, present, and future. A viewpoint. Circulation 2009 6;119(1):147–52.

91. Galie N, Ussia G, Passarelli P, Parlangeli R, Branzi A, Magnani B. Role of pharmacologic tests in the treatment of primary pulmonary hypertension. Am J Cardiol 1995;75(3):55A–62A.

92. Sitbon O, Humbert M, Jagot JL, Taravella O, Fartoukh M, Parent F et al. Inhaled nitric oxide as a screening agent for safely identifying responders to oral calcium-channel blockers in primary pulmonary hypertension. Eur Respir J 1998;12(2):265–70.

93. Raeside DA, Chalmers G, Clelland J, Madhok R, Peacock AJ. Pulmonary artery pressure variation in patients with connective tissue disease: 24 hour ambulatory pulmonary artery pressure monitoring. Thorax 1998;53(10):857–62.

94. Syyed R, Reeves JT, Welsh D, Raeside D, Johnson MK, Peacock AJ. The relationship between the components of pulmonary artery pressure remains constant under all conditions in both health and disease. Chest 2008;133(3):633–9.

95. Castelain V, Chemla D, Humbert M, Sitbon O, Simonneau G, Lecarpentier Y et al. Pulmonary artery pressure–flow relations after prostacyclin in primary pulmonary hypertension. Am J Respir Crit Care Med 2002;165(3):338–40.

96. D'Alonzo GE, Barst RJ, Ayres SM, Bergofsky EH, Brundage BH, Detre KM et al. Survival in patients with primary pulmonary hypertension. Results from a national prospective registry. Ann Intern Med 1991;115(5):343–9.

97. Rozkovec A, Montanes P, Oakley CM. Factors that influence the outcome of primary pulmonary hypertension. Br Heart J 1986;55(5):449–58.

98. Sandoval J, Bauerle O, Palomar A, Gomez A, Martinez-Guerra ML, Beltran M et al. Survival in primary pulmonary hypertension. Validation of a prognostic equation. Circulation 1994;89(4):1733–44.

99. Okada O, Tanabe N, Yasuda J, Yoshida Y, Katoh K, Yamamoto T et al. Prediction of life expectancy in patients with primary pulmonary hypertension. A retrospective nationwide survey from 1980–1990. Intern Med (Tokyo) 1999;38(1):12–6.

100. McLaughlin VV, Shillington A, Rich S. Survival in primary pulmonary hypertension: the impact of epoprostenol therapy. Circulation 2002;106(12):1477–82.

101. Nunes H, Humbert M, Sitbon O, Morse JH, Deng Z, Knowles JA et al. Prognostic factors for survival in human immunodeficiency virus-associated pulmonary arterial hypertension. Am J Respir Crit Care Med 2003;167(10):1433–9.

102. Condliffe R, Kiely DG, Peacock AJ, Corris PA, Gibbs JS, Vrapi F et al. Connective tissue disease-associated pulmonary arterial hypertension in the modern treatment era. Am J Respir Crit Care Med 2009;179(2):151–7.

103. Sitbon O, Humbert M, Nunes H, Parent F, Garcia G, Herve P et al. Long-term intravenous epoprostenol infusion in primary pulmonary hypertension: prognostic factors and survival. J Am Coll Cardiol 2002;40(4):780–8.

104. Nagaya N, Uematsu M, Satoh T, Kyotani S, Sakamaki F, Nakanishi N et al. Serum uric acid levels correlate with the severity and the mortality of primary pulmonary hypertension. Am J Respir Crit Care Med 1999;160(2):487–92.

105. McGoon M, Gutterman D, Steen V, Barst R, McCrory DC, Fortin TA et al. Screening, early detection, and diagnosis of pulmonary arterial hypertension: ACCP evidence-based clinical practice guidelines. Chest 2004;126(1 Suppl): 14S–34S.

106. Long L, MacLean MR, Jeffery TK, Morecroft I, Yang X, Rudarakanchana N et al. Serotonin increases susceptibility to pulmonary hypertension in BMPR2-deficient mice. Circulation Res 2006;98(6):818–27.

107. Jones DL, Sandberg JC, Rosenthal MJ, Saunders RC, Hannig VL, Clayton EW. What patients and their relatives think about testing for BMPR2. J Genet Counsel 2008; 17(5):452–8.

108. Sztrymf B, Yaici A, Girerd B, Humbert M. Genes and pulmonary arterial hypertension. Respir Internat Rev Thorac Dis 2007;74(2):123–32.

109. Durrington HJ, Morrell NW. What we know and what we would like to know about genetics and pulmonary arterial hypertension. Internat J Clin Pract 2009;161:11–6.

110. Robin NH, Tabereaux PB, Benza R, Korf BR. Genetic testing in cardiovascular disease. J Am Coll Cardiol 2007;50(8):727–37.

111. Hsu VM, Moreyra AE, Wilson AC, Shinnar M, Shindler DM, Wilson JE et al. Assessment of pulmonary arterial hypertension in patients with systemic sclerosis: comparison of non-invasive tests with results of right-heart catheterization. J Rheumatol 2008;35(3):458–65.

7

Imaging: Echocardiography

MARCIN KURZYNA AND ADAM TORBICKI

INTRODUCTION

Under normal conditions pulmonary circulation is a low-resistance vascular bed. Remodeling of the right ventricle (RV) which occurs soon after birth transforms this heart chamber into a "low-pressure high-volume" pump. Any pathological increase in pulmonary arterial input impedance, which represents RV afterload, significantly affects the morphology and function of the right heart. Therefore it is imperative that evaluation of pulmonary circulation includes a comprehensive dynamic assessment of the right heart.

Echocardiography has proved to be highly useful in assessment of the morphology and function of the heart. Moreover, it enables the recording and measurement of flow velocities using pulsed and continuous wave Doppler in pre-specified sites within the cardiovascular system. While cardiac magnetic resonance offers more reliable measurements and less operator dependency, echocardiography is more versatile, less expensive, and is also widely available as a bedside "point-of-care" test. All this makes echocardiography useful for non-invasive evaluation of right heart chambers and pulmonary hemodynamics in everyday practice.

This chapter will describe echocardiography of the right heart and discuss the role of echocardiography in:

- assessment of morphology of the right heart structures
- assessment of pulmonary hemodynamics
- screening, diagnosis and differential diagnosis of pulmonary hypertension

- prognostic staging and follow-up of patients with pulmonary hypertension.

ECHOCARDIOGRAPHIC WINDOWS TO THE RIGHT HEART

Modern echocardiographic imaging permits high resolution dynamic visualization of the heart, including right heart structures. Several echocardiographic windows and planes can be used for this purpose.

Transthoracic echocardiography

Apical view allows simultaneous assessment of all four cardiac chambers, including RV and right atrium (RA). RV maximal transverse dimensions as well as its areas can be measured in diastole and systole (1,2) (Figure 7.1). See also refs 3–7.

Parasternal view of the left ventricle, left atrium and the aorta enables the measurement of the RV outflow tract diameter. Despite some limitations, this continues to be one of the most frequently used and best validated measures of RV size. By tilting the transducer, a parasternal long axis view of the right heart can also be obtained.

Rotation and then tilting of the transducer permits cross-sectional visualization of both ventricles at various levels from apex to base, as well as visualization of the large vessels at the base of the heart. The former view is particularly useful for assessment of the shape of the RV in the

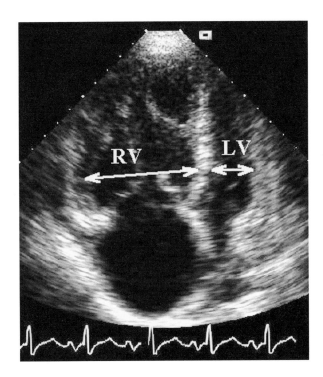

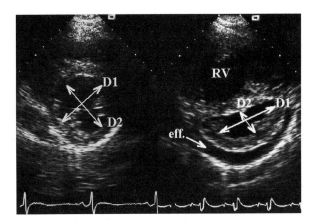

Figure 7.2 Parasternal short axis view. Left panel: normal morphology of both ventricles. Right panel: flattening of interventricular septum and compression of the left ventricle by severely enlarged right ventricle (RV). Diastolic dimensions of left ventricle measured perpendicularly (D2) and in parallel (D1) to the septum for assessment of its eccentricity index (LVEI = D1/D2); eff., pericardial effusion.

Figure 7.1 Apical four-chamber view. Enlarged right ventricle (RV) and compressed left ventricle (LV) in a patient with severe primary pulmonary hypertension. Right ventricle is usually measured in end-diastole at the place of its maximum widths, with left ventricle measured along the same line.

plane perpendicular to its long axis and of the diastolic and systolic position of the septum (8) (Figure 7.2). Tilting the transducer towards the base of the heart offers a useful view of the RA, tricuspid valve, RV outflow tract, pulmonary valve and proximal pulmonary artery up to its bifurcation into right and left main branches.

Subcostal view is used mostly to assess inferior vena cava diameter. It is also particularly helpful in patients with lung hyperinflation (9–11), in whom transthoracic windows are limited by the dispersion of ultrasound beam due to the air in the lungs covering the heart.

Supracostal view may offer some insight into superior vena cava and right pulmonary artery where it passes below the aortic arch.

Three dimensional real-time (3DRT) imaging is based on ultra-fast integration of data derived from several adjacent planes reflecting ultrasound beams. It has become a standard element of software provided by echocardiographic machines allowing also analysis of strain rates within the RV wall, but its suggested role in clinical assessment of the right heart awaits confirmation (12).

Transesophageal echocardiography (TEE)

This semi-invasive procedure requires positioning of the echocardiographic probe in the esophagus, behind the heart. While TEE provides almost unrestricted access to the left heart it usually does not add much to the transthoracic morphological assessment of the RV and tricuspid valve.

However, it may be useful for assessing superior vena cava at the entrance to the RA as well as intracardiac structures such as the Chiari network, vegetations and thrombi. Differentiation between intracardiac thrombi and extension of tumors from inferior and superior vena cava is one of the reasons for performing TEE of the right heart in our laboratory. It is also of great importance in diagnosing or excluding congenital heart disease in patients with unexplained pulmonary hypertension (PH). Sinus venosus type of ASD, abnormal pulmonary venous drainage, patent ductus arteriosus as well as patent foramen ovale missed by transthoracic echocardiography, can be easily detected by TEE (13).

Intracardiac echocardiography

Intracardiac echocardiography is an invasive method, which requires the Seldinger technique for percutaneous introduction of an echocardiograpic micro-probe fixed at the top of an 8F steerable catheter. When introduced via the internal jugular vein, it may be advanced through superior vena cava to the RA. This allows excellent visualization of adjacent structures, particularly the proximal right pulmonary artery and interatrial septum. The latter is very useful for guiding interatrial septum puncture and stepwise balloon inflations during atrial septostomy (14): a palliative intervention used in severe pulmonary arterial hypertension (PAH) to increase systemic cardiac output.

In summary: echocardiography offers several windows of access to the right heart. As in the case of the left-heart examination, it is imperative to consider various complementary echocardiographic approaches and always try to confirm the presence of any suspected, clinically relevant anomalies by at least one additional independent echocardiographic window.

Morphological examination with two-dimensional and M-mode echocardiography should be followed by two-dimensional (color-coded) pulsed and continuous wave Doppler assessment.

CLINICAL IMPLICATIONS OF MORPHOLOGICAL ASSESSMENT OF THE RIGHT HEART

The detailed two-dimensional echocardiographic analysis of the morphology of the RV validated using casts of human ventricles as well as the range of normal values derived from healthy adults were described three decades ago (1,2,15). The most widely used measurement is the maximum short axis diameter assessed in apical or subcostal 4-chamber view (Figure 7.1). Right ventricular end-diastolic dimension either alone or indexed for body surface area was reported to correlate with mean PAP in patients with chronic PH (9–11). However, RV dilation may be also caused by its primary failure and/or increased preload.

Increased thickness of the RV free wall might support suspicion of its chronic pressure overload. Unfortunately, trabeculations of the RV endocardial surface affects reproducibility of the measurements (16). Calculations of the RV mass is even less practical due to complex RV shape (15). Differential diagnosis of RV dilatation may include the analysis of systolic and diastolic position of the interventricular septum. In pure RV pressure overload, intraventricular septal (IVS) flattening was reported to be most marked in end-systole, while increased RV preload resulted in predominantly diastolic leftward IVS displacement (8). Even among patients with primary RV volume overload due to ASD, those with significant PH could be identified on the basis of leftward displacement of interventricular septum persisting until end-systole (17). The degree of this displacement can be expressed by left ventricular eccentricity index (EI). To assess EI, the left ventricle should be imaged in short axis and measured perpendicularly (D2) and in parallel (D1) to interventricular septum (Figure 7.2). In healthy adults, systolic and diastolic LV EI calculated as D1/D2 was 1.00 ± 0.06 and 1.01 ± 0.04, respectively. Patients with RV volume overload had normal systolic but elevated diastolic LVEI (1.02 ± 0.04 and 1.26 ± 0.12, respectively) while patients with RV pressure overload presented with more markedly increased systolic than diastolic LVEI (1.44 ± 0.16 and 1.26 ± 0.11, respectively) (8).

In summary: dilated RV and/or eccentrically distorted left ventricle found at transthoracic echocardiography should always prompt a more specific diagnostic process including a search for congenital heart disease and an attempt of non-invasive estimation of PAP.

ASSESSMENT OF PULMONARY HEMODYNAMICS

Modern echocardiographic equipment may be considered a "non-invasive hemodynamic laboratory." Evaluation of heart chambers and main vessels combined with Doppler measurements of instantaneous blood flow velocities in sites of interest provide data which can be used to quantify most hemodynamic variables measured at right heart catheterization (RHC). This includes systolic and diastolic PAP, stroke volume, pulmonary and systemic cardiac output. A rough estimate of RA pressure can be made from inferior vena cava diameter. Though based on solid theoretical background, hemodynamic calculations derived from echocardiographic measurements suffer from their high intra- and inter-operator variability. This limits clinical implications of calculating mean pulmonary artery pressure (PAP), cardiac output (CO) and particularly pulmonary vascular resistance (PVR) from raw echocardiographic measurements in individual patients, despite correlations reported in clinical trials (18,19). However, when comparing echocardiographic and catheter measurements one should remember that routine RHC also suffers from its own problems, related to zero leveling, intrathoracic pressure shifts and signal damping if fluid-filled catheters are used (20).

On the other hand, echocardiographic signs of PH may be modified by the duration and character of underlying changes within the pulmonary vascular bed, as well as by the right ventricular preload, contractility and dynamic coupling to the arterial system. Therefore, non-invasive assessment of PAP with echocardiography should always take into account coexisting clinical and pathophysiological context.

Pulmonary arterial pressure

The most widely used and straightforward methods of assessment of intracardiac and intravascular pressures are based on continuous wave Doppler measurements of peak velocities of blood traversing narrow orifices within the cardiovascular system. The pressure gradient driving blood through an orifice can be calculated according to the simplified Bernoulli equation as $PG = 4V^2$ (mmHg). While the jet of pulmonary insufficiency (21) as well as peak flow velocities across ventricular septal defect (22,23) and patent ductus arteriosus (24) allow for calculations of pulmonary artery pressures, tricuspid valve regurgitant jets (25) are by far most widely used for this purpose.

Estimation of systolic PAP

Even trivial tricuspid valve regurgitation permits the calculation of systolic pressure gradient between the contracting RV and the RA (tricuspid insufficiency pressure gradient, TIPG). Even beat-to-beat changes in directly measured pressures can be reflected by respective TIPG changes (26). For calculation of systolic PAP, stenosis of RV outflow must be excluded, and an estimate of the right atrial pressure (RAP) should be added to the pressure gradient: systolic PAP = TIPG + estimated RAP (Figure 7.3).

Most of the data regarding the reliability of echocardiographic assessment of systolic PAP date back two decades (Table 7.1). Reported correlations were excellent ($r = 0.89-0.97$). This was partly due to the broad range of directly measured pressures – from normal to suprasystemic levels – in the studied groups. Nevertheless,

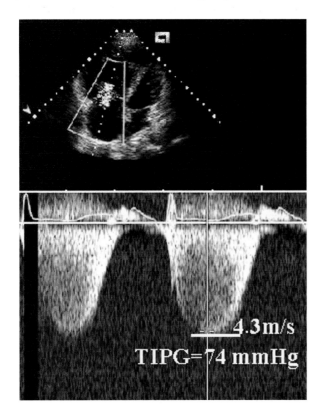

Figure 7.3 Top panel: continuous-wave Doppler beam guided by 'color-coded' Doppler visualization of the jet of tricuspid insufficiency. Bottom panel: Doppler measurement of the peak velocity of the jet. According to the Bernoulli equation, a velocity of 4.3 m/s indicates a maximum systolic pressure gradient between the right ventricle and atrium of 74 mmHg.

the standard error of estimation was relatively high (4.9–8.0 mmHg), making precise estimation of PAP in an individual patient less reliable (27). Part of the discrepancies could be attributed to non-simultaneous invasive and Doppler-derived measurements (25,28,29) and to errors of velocity measurements. While the interobserver and intraobserver variability reported in an early landmark trial were low, with mean ± SD discrepancy of -1.8 ± 4.9 mmHg and -0.2 ± 3.4 mmHg, respectively (25) this is clearly in contrast to everyday clinical experience. See refs 30–38 for more details.

Estimation of diastolic PAP

End-diastolic velocity of the pulmonary regurgitant jet correlates with diastolic pulmonary arterial pressure (PADP). In a study of 32 patients the end-diastolic pulmonary to right ventricular pressure gradients derived from the Doppler flow profiles correlated well with the catheter measurements ($r = 0.95$) (39). A correlation was observed between pulmonary arterial diastolic pressure and Doppler-derived end-diastolic pressure gradient ($r = 0.91$) (39). However, when directly compared in the same patients, Doppler-derived pressure calculations based on diastolic velocities across the pulmonary valve were less accurate than those based on tricuspid jet velocity measurements ($r = 0.83$ vs. 0.98 respectively) (40). The reported prevalence of pulmonary regurgitation on Doppler echocardiography ranged from 22 percent in healthy women to 86 percent in patients with PH.

Estimation of mean PAP

If both tricuspid and pulmonary regurgitant jets are clearly recorded, the complete PA pressure curve can be reconstructed, and mean PAP can be calculated. However, despite reported excellent correlations with catheterization

Table 7.1 Correlations of directly measured pressures with non-invasive pressure estimate based on measurement of peak velocity of tricuspid jet and Bernoulli equation

Author (year)	n	% patients with measurable peak jet velocity	r	versus	SEE	Comments
Yock Popp (1984)	62	87	0.93	RVSP	8 mmHg	
Berger (1985)	69	59	0.97	PASP	4.9 mmHg	
Skjaerpe (1986)	70	?	0.96	RVSP	7.1 mmHg	
Currie (1985)	127	75	0.89	PASP	8 mmHg	
Laaban (1986)	34	65	0.65	PASP	-	COPD
Torbicki (1989)	70	25	0.92	PASP	7.7 mmHg	Lung diseases
Himelman (1989)	36	56%		PASP	-	COPD
		92*	0.98*			Contrast*

COPD, chronic obstructive pulmonary disease; PASP, pulmonary artery systolic pressure; RVSP, right ventricular systolic pressure; SEE, standard error of estimate.
*After saline contrast enhancement of Doppler spectrum.

data (r = 0.97) this approach was probably too cumbersome to gain popularity (40). A simplified strategy based on measurement of the peak (early) diastolic pulmonary to right ventricular pressure gradient derived from the Doppler flow profiles was also suggested (39). See also refs 40–45.

Estimation of intracardiac pressure gradients in congenital shunts

Other jets have been used for assessment of right ventricular and pulmonary arterial systolic pressure, mostly in infants and newborns with congenital heart disease. Peak flow velocity through ventricular septal defect reflected the systolic pressure gradient between contracting ventricles while peak flow velocity across ductus arteriosus in newborns correlated with the pressure gradients between the aorta and pulmonary artery (23,46). In both cases systemic arterial pressure had to be accounted for to calculate PAP. Right and left ventricular outflow must be checked for the presence of additional gradients. If present, these gradients should be appropriately considered in the calculations.

Estimation of right atrial pressure

Several approaches to account for RA pressure, required for estimation of systolic and diastolic PAP from tricuspid and pulmonary regurgitation jets, respectively, have been reported. See refs 25, 38, 47–50. Estimation of RA pressure based on echocardiographic inferior vena cava collapsibility index (IVCCI) has been suggested. This index is calculated by subtracting inspiratory from expiratory IVC diameter, and dividing the result by expiratory IVC diameter (Figure 7.4).

In summary: echocardiographic methods estimating right ventricular and pulmonary arterial pressure based on peak velocity of jets within the heart and proximal arteries are firmly established in clinical practice. In studies directly comparing various echocardiographic methods, the tricuspid jet method was the most valuable in predicting pulmonary arterial pressures both in patients with cardiovascular and respiratory pathology (Tables 7.2 and 7.3) (34,51). However, results obtained with this method should also be considered as an approximation and used for clinical decision making bearing in mind its limitations.

Based on the authors' experience, several specific issues should be considered when using tricuspid jet velocity for estimation of systolic PAP in clinical practice:

- Sub-optimal spectral tracings should be discarded. Even a small inaccuracy in jet velocity measurement (e.g. 5.0 instead of 4.5 m/sec) translates into a substantial error in calculated pressure gradient (100 mmHg instead of 80 mmHg, respectively).

- Angle correction based on the difference between the direction of Doppler beam and regurgitant jet, as visualized by two-dimensional Doppler echocardiography, should be discouraged. Angles below 10 deg do not affect the calculations (25). Those exceeding 20 deg in most cases result in sub-optimal spectral envelope and should be discarded, anyway.

- After inspiration the Doppler spectrum may be more clearly recorded, but the peak velocity of the jet might be slightly higher due to increased RV preload and enhanced RV contractility (25). Therefore, TV jet recordings for velocity measurements should be made either during relaxed expiration or averaged over 5–10 consecutive cycles during quiet respiration. Methodological

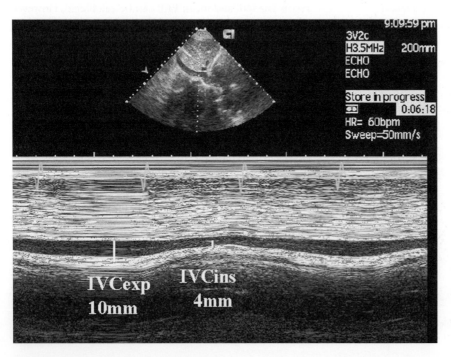

Figure 7.4 Inferior vena cava measured at expiration (IVCexp) and inspiration (IVCins) to calculate its collapsibility index: IVCCI = (IVCexp − IVCins)/IVCexp = 60%.

Table 7.2 Comparison of Doppler methods used for assessment of pulmonary arterial pressure: patients with cardiovascular diseases (Currie *et al.*, 1987; n = 50)

Method used	Success rate (%)	Correlation		SEE (mmHg)
		Coefficient (r)	With	
TVR jet velocity	72	0.89	PASP	7.4
AcT	88	−0.66	PAMP	10
AcT*	52	−0.85		7
RVIRT	64	–		
RVIRT**	22		PASP	11

AcT, acceleration time of right ventricular ejection; PAMP, mean pulmonary arterial pressure; PASP, systolic pulmonary arterial pressure; RVIRT, right ventricular isovolumic relaxation time; SEE, standard error of estimate; TVR, tricuspid valve regurgitation.
*Patients with heart rate between 60 and 100/min.
**Patients in sinus rhythm.

Table 7.3 Comparison of Doppler methods used for assessment of pulmonary arterial pressure: patients with respiratory diseases (Torbicki *et al.*, 1989; n = 70)

Method used	Success rate (%)	Correlation		SEE (mmHg)
		Coefficient (r)	With	
TVR jet velocity	25	0.91	PASP	7.9
AcT	97	−0.72	PAMP	8.3
RVIRT*	84	0.66	PASP	11.6

AcT, acceleration time of right ventricular ejection; PAMP, mean pulmonary arterial pressure; PASP, systolic pulmonary arterial pressure; RVIRT, right ventricular isovolumic relaxation time; SEE, standard error of estimate; TVR, tricuspid valve regurgitation.
*Patients in sinus rhythm.

consistency makes follow-up of individual patients more reliable.

- While TIPG is a straightforward measurement, calculation of systolic PAP requires assumption of RA pressure which may introduce additional error. Therefore, if an estimated systolic PAP is given in the echocardiographic report, the method which was used to account for RA pressure should be clearly stated. This is essential for reproducibility of results.
- For unclear reasons, the Doppler TIPG method may underestimate systolic PAP, particularly in patients with very high PH. During a simultaneous study TIPG underestimated systolic pressure gradient assessed with high fidelity tip-transducers by up to 20–30 mmHg (29). Such significant overestimation of systolic PAP in cases with good quality tricuspid jet velocity tracing is less likely, but still possible (37).

RV stroke volume and output

Echo-Doppler assessment of RV stroke volume may be calculated from flow velocity integral assessed by pulsed

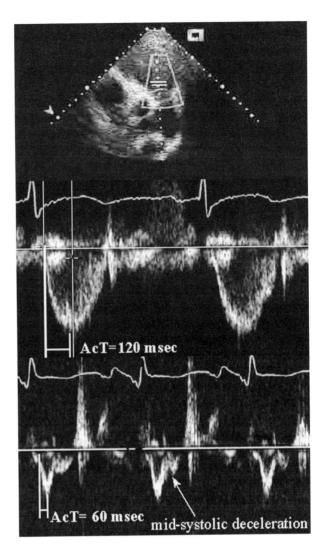

Figure 7.5 Assessment of the pattern of the flow velocity curve in the right ventricular outflow tract just below the level of the pulmonary valve. Tracing from a healthy individual (upper panel) with normal acceleration time (AcT) compared with severely disturbed pattern characterized by short AcT and the presence of mid-systolic deceleration of flow recorded in a patient with PH.

wave Doppler (Figure 7.5) and the area of the RV outflow tract measured by two-dimensional echocardiography. Stroke volume multiplied by heart rate gives a non-invasive estimate of RV output, usually equal to pulmonary flow. While absolute values suffer from error introduced mostly by measurement of RV outflow tract area, the changes in stroke volume and RV output induced by exercise, vasodilators, oxygen or passive leg lifting in individual patients correlated with respective changes simultaneously assessed by thermodilution (52).

Pulsatile pulmonary hemodynamics

Pulsed wave Doppler analysis of time intervals derived from flow velocity curve in the RV outflow tract or proximal PA received some attention as potentially related to elements of pulsatile pulmonary hemodynamics. With increasing PAP the interval between the onset and peak velocity of RV ejection (acceleration time, AcT) was reported to decrease (53). Also, in severe PH midsystolic deceleration of RV ejection to the pulmonary artery was often noted, and occurred earlier with higher PAP (54) (Figure 7.5). Reports suggesting excellent correlations of AcT and PAP followed, offering regression equations which permitted non-invasive pressure calculations. However, significant differences in suggested equations precluded their universal application (55). While heart rate (56) and the presence of tricuspid regurgitation apparently did not affect AcT (57), several other factors did. For the same level of PAP, acceleration time tended to be longer in patients with low cardiac index (58) and with increased pulmonary flow due to pretricuspid shunts (57). Conversely, AcT tended to be shorter with more distal Doppler sample volume positions (59,60), in individuals with body surface area $> 2.0\,m^2$ and in adults > 30 years old (61). Also, proximal pulmonary emboli, especially when acute, profoundly disturbed the flow velocity curve resulting in particularly short AcT and prominent mid- or even early systolic deceleration, regardless of the level of pulmonary arterial pressure (62). A clinically useful Doppler sign suggesting acute pulmonary embolism and indicating patients with chronic thrombo-embolic PH who were most suitable for pulmonary endarterectomy was reported, based on those findings (63,64).

While correlation of simultaneous AcT and PAP measurements were reported (65), acutely induced changes in PAP were not accurately reflected by AcT changes in a simultaneous Doppler-catheter study (66).

In summary: available data from clinical and experimental studies indicate that the characteristics of flow velocity curve of the RV ejection, including AcT, are not directly related to PAP. Differences in dynamic coupling between the ejecting RV and pulmonary arterial bed with its characteristic impedance and reflected pressure waves probably account for much of the observed variability of flow velocity pattern. Therefore, information contained in the dynamics of RV ejection into the pulmonary artery may be even more closely related to the true RV afterload, than variables measured during standard RHC (20).

DIAGNOSIS, SCREENING, AND DIFFERENTIAL DIAGNOSIS OF PULMONARY HYPERTENSION

Echocardiographic definitions of pulmonary hypertension

Pulmonary hypertension is defined as mean PAP exceeding 25 mmHg at rest as measured during RHC. While rise of mean PAP above 30 mmHg during exercise was included in the definition as an independent, alternative criterion it has been recently criticized as not adequately standardized in terms of type and intensity of the exercise which should be

implemented. The definition of PH based on systolic PAP is lacking.

For practical purposes search for non-invasive diagnostic criteria of PH was attempted. In contrast to arbitrary values, e.g. TIPG ≥ 30 mmHg used by some authors (67), others (68) tried first to define the upper limits of tricuspid jet velocity at rest.

In 53 healthy non-smokers aged 14 to 55 years TIPG ranged from 12.6 to 29.3 mmHg (mean 19.3 ± 4.0) (69). Another study of 134 subjects, including older persons, reported correlation between systolic PAP and age ($r = 0.47$, $p = 0.0001$). Systolic PAP increased progressively, from 13 ± 5 mmHg in subject 20 to 29 years old to 22 ± 6 mmHg in those ≥ 80 years old (70). A recent multicenter echocardiographic study, which collected results from 191 healthy control subjects, reported systolic PAP of 20.4 ± 5.3 mmHg and failed to confirm its correlation with age, but the studied population was predominantly young (32 ± 10 years old) (71). The Massachusetts General Hospital echocardiographic database was analyzed for tricuspid jet velocities in patients with otherwise normal transthoracic examination and no clinically suspected diseases potentially leading to elevated PAP (30). Among 3212 such patients mean peak tricuspid jet velocity was 2.6 m/s and TIPG 18.0 ± 4.7 mmHg, with 95 percent CI 8.8–27.2 mmHg. Multiple linear regressions revealed that age, BMI, sex, left ventricular ejection fraction and clinical referral category independently influenced tricuspid velocity. In subjects aged over 60 years and/or presenting with BMI $> 30\,kg/m^2$ the 95 percent confidence intervals for TIPG measurement slightly exceeded 30 mmHg (Table 7.4).

An alternative approach to echocardiographic definition of PH might be based on correlation reported between mean and systolic PAP. Chemla *et al.* found that regardless of the diseases potentially leading to PH there is a universal equation allowing estimation of mean PAP from systolic PAP with negligible error (41). Those data were derived from a high-fidelity tip pressure transducer. Though not validated for echocardiographic measurements, the Chemla equation offers a way to translate Doppler-derived systolic

Table 7.4 Reference ranges for normal systolic pressure gradients assessed with Doppler between right ventricle and right atrium (TIPG) according to McQuillan *et al.* (2001)

Age (years)	n	95% CI for TIPG (mmHg)	
		Women (n = 2065)	Men (n = 1147)
< 20	856	8.6–24.2	8.2–26.2
20–29	669	9.2–24.4	9.9–26.3
30–39	650	9.3–25.7	8.7–27.5
40–49	494	9.9–27.5	9.1–28.3
50–59	344	10.2–29.4	11.0–30.6
> 60	19	10.5–32.1	11.2–33.6

PAP into mean PAP, making it more clinically understandable. According to Chemla *et al.* mean PAP = 0.61 systolic PAP + 2 mmHg. Following this idea, a tricuspid jet velocity of 2.8 m/sec (i.e. TIPG of 31.36 mmHg and a systolic PAP of 36.36 mmHg) would mean PAP of 24.18 mmHg.

Thus, based on existing population and pathophysiological data it appears justified to consider tricuspid jet velocities exceeding in resting conditions 2.8 m/s, and corresponding to TIPG greater than 31 mmHg, as elevated, except for elderly and/or very obese patients.

In an executive summary from the PPH Symposium held in Evian in 1998, mild PH was indeed defined, as tricuspid jet velocity between 2.8 and 3.4 m/sec, which corresponds to TIPG 31–46 mmHg and to systolic PAP 36–51 mmHg (assuming fixed RA pressure of 5 mmHg for its calculation) (72). However, because of intrinsic and operator-dependent limitations of echocardiographic pressure estimations there is a suggestion to limit the conclusions based on tricuspid jet velocity measurements to statements addressing "likelihood" of PH rather than attempting its formal diagnosis or exclusion. According to these suggestions TVI < 2.8 m/sec should be reported as "PH unlikely", 2.8–3.4 m/sec as "PH probable" and > 3.4 m/sec as "PH likely".

Despite multiple factors influencing the relationship between PAP and AcT, several authors assessed clinical value of this variable for diagnosing PH both in cardiovascular and lung diseases (Table 7.5). Reported results indicate, that if interpreted with caution, short AcT may be a reliable supporting sign of PH, especially useful when tricuspid jet cannot be clearly recorded and measured. Conversely, a long AcT suggests normal PAP, particularly if no significant systemic to pulmonary shunt is present (57).

In summary: tricuspid jet velocities, but also other echocardiographic, clinical and laboratory signs should be considered before deciding whether and when to proceed to RHC in order to formally exclude or confirm PH, and assess its severity.

Echocardiographic tests for latent pulmonary hypertension

Similarly to catheter evaluation, Doppler echocardiography may also be performed during exercise to estimate

PAP. Though technically difficult, tricuspid jets were recorded and its velocity could be measured during supine exercise, especially after tilting the patient to the left during pedaling or enhancing the jet signal with peripheral saline contrast injection (73). The correlation with simultaneously performed catheter measurements of pulmonary artery systolic pressure seemed excellent (r = 0.98) (73). Exercise echo was used to assess systolic PAP in several specific groups of patients: with chronic lung diseases (73), after heart transplantation (74), with ASD (75) as well as in individuals susceptible to high altitude lung edema (76) and in asymptomatic carriers of a PPH gene mutation (77). In all these studied groups systolic pulmonary arterial pressure significantly increased on exercise when compared to controls. Prolonged hypoxia (FiO_2 12.5 percent) was also used to induce PH which could be quantified with Doppler echocardiography (76).

In healthy controls systolic pulmonary arterial pressure, as assessed with the Doppler tricuspid jet method remained low despite exercise and averaged: 31 ± 7 mm, 20.5 ± 3.8 mmHg, 19 ± 8 mmHg, 36 ± 3 mmHg and 37 ± 3 mmHg, for the five studies listed above, respectively. One of the groups arbitrarily defined systolic PAP ≤ 40 mmHg, calculated after assuming fixed RA pressure of 5 mmHg, as a normal hemodynamic reaction during stress echocardiography. Interestingly, athletes were reported to generate higher PAP when exercising under the same workload as non-athletes when assessed with tricuspid jet method (78) (Table 7.6). Recently a term "hypertensive response" was suggested to describe exaggerated rise of systolic PAP during exercise echo at workload ≤ 125 Watt or during prolonged breathing air with reduced oxygen content (FiO_2 12 percent). Tricuspid jet velocity > 3.08 m/sec was chosen as a cut-off value, as in 90 percent of normal subjects it fell below this value (71). Hypertensive response was more frequent in family members of patients with PH, and particularly in carriers of BMPRII mutation. However, no upper limit of normal could be identified, as significant increases of Doppler derived systolic PAP were observed during exercise also in healthy controls (71).

Another approach to latent PH was attempted with the pulsed wave Doppler method assessing flow velocity curve in the RV outflow tract during various interventions. Acceleration time (AcT) showed divergent trends during RV preload challenge induced by passive legs rising in patients with normal and even slightly elevated PAP (78–80).

Table 7.5 Sensitivity and specificity of diagnosis of pulmonary hypertension (PH) with acceleration time (AcT) and related time intervals

Author (year)	Definition of PH; mean PAP =	Cut-off value	Sensitivity (%)	Specificity (%)	Comments
Matsuda (1986)	> 25; 'prominent PH'	AcT ≤ 90 ms	–	100	
Isobe (1986)	≥ 20 mmHg	PEP/AcT > 1.1	93	97	
Torbicki (1989)	≥ 20 mmHg	AcT < 90 ms	79	78	COPD
		PEP/AcT > 1.0	93	69	

COPD, chronic obstructive pulmonary disease; PAP, pulmonary arterial pressure; PEP, right ventricular pre-ejection time.

Table 7.6 Reference ranges for systolic pressure gradients assessed at rest and during exercise in athletes and healthy non-athletes with Doppler between right ventricle and right atrium (TIPG) according to Bossone *et al.*

Workload (watts)	5% CI for TIPG (mmHg)	
	Athletes (n = 26)	Non-athletes (n = 14)
Rest	17.5–23.2	9.0–12.1
40	21.7–29.4	9.9–26.3
120	26.6–36.0	17.8–29.4
240	38.4–55.4	12.3–26.6

In summary: exercise Doppler studies were expected to improve the sensitivity of echocardiographic diagnosis of latent or mild PH. This became questionable in view of removing exercise PAP from the definition of PH, because it did not account for the differences related to age, sex, type and intensity of applied exercise tests. While "hypertensive response" during exercise was found in echo more often in family members of patients with idiopathic PAH, and in carriers of the BMPRII gene mutations, the clinical significance of those findings for prediction of development of symptomatic PAH are unknown. Also the significance of echocardiographic changes induced by other interventions, such as hypoxia or preload challenge is not clear.

Screening for pulmonary hypertension

Echocardiography is a natural candidate method for screening of asymptomatic or mildly symptomatic patients at increased risk for PH, and particularly for PAH. Textbook and even guideline recommendations suggested periodic screening of family members of patients with hereditary PAH, patients with scleroderma and patients with portal hypertension considered for liver transplantation. Few trials assessed the feasibility and practical yield of such an approach. A landmark retrospective trial by Mukerjee *et al.* focused on patients with scleroderma with or without lung fibrosis and comprised 137 patients (81). The authors tried to find the echocardiographically measured TIPG which would provide best positive and negative predictive value (PPV and NPV, respectively) for the diagnosis of PH, defined as resting mean PAP > 25 mmHg or exercise PAP exceeding 30 mmHg at RHC. The TIPG cut-of-value of 30 mmHg (corresponding to systolic PAP of 35 mmHg and TR jet velocity of about 2.75 m/sec) had 88 percent sensitivity, but only 42 percent specificity and aNPV of 57 percent. Tricuspid gradients of ≥ 45 mmHg (corresponding to systolic PAP ≥ 50 mmHg and to tricuspid jet velocity ≥ 3.35 m/sec) had 97 percent specificity but only 47 percent sensitivity and 41 percent NPV. Moreover, the authors concluded that no tricuspid jet cut-off value permitted reliable exclusion of PH among patients with scleroderma.

Another trial also addressing patients with scleroderma utilized cut-off value for TIPG > 40 mmHg. Such Doppler "diagnosis" of PH was confirmed in all 32 such patients who were studied with RHC (82). The design of the trial did not allow assessing the rate of false negative results for this cut-off value.

Two important prospective attempts to use echocardiography as a screening test were recently reported from France. Hachulla *et al.* studied 599 patients with scleroderma using Doppler echocardiography. All patients with TR jet velocity > 3.0 m/sec and all those with > 2.5 m/sec and exertional dyspnea were catheterized (83). Only 18 out of 33 such patients had PH at RHC. In most cases PH was mild and in four it was only detectable during exercise, defined as mean PAP > 30 mmHg. According to current definition of PH, applied criteria resulted in 19/33 (58 percent) "unnecessary" RHC. The other trial assessed the prevalence of PAH in 247 patients with HIV and exertional dyspnea, without a previous diagnosis of PAH (84). Among 18 patients with TV peak velocity > 2.5 m/sec and dyspnea only five were found to have PAH at RHC. Retrospectively, the cut-off value of TI peak velocity was moved to > 2.8 m/sec (which would correspond to the mean PAP of > 24.2 mmHg according to the Chemla equation). This reduced the number of positive echo results from 18 to 7 and only in two patients was PH not confirmed at RHC (false positive 29 percent). Still, the number of patients with HIV who needed to be tested (NNT) with echo in order to detect a PAH patient was 50.

In summary: prospective echocardiographic screening of mildly symptomatic patients at risk for PAH, based solely on TIPG is feasible, but the rate of false positive results leading to "unnecessary" RHC, and the number of subjects needed to test with echo to detect a single PAH patients, are both high.

Differential diagnosis of pulmonary hypertension

Echocardiography may reveal the cause of PH such as left ventricular dysfunction, mitral valve disease, or intracardiac shunt, if present. However, some congenital defects potentially leading to PH may be missed during transthoracic examination. These include atypically located ASD, especially of sinus venosus type, anomalous pulmonary venous drainage, patent ductus arteriosus and atypical interventricular septal defects (85). Additional data which significantly altered surgical therapy were found at TEE in 25 percent (12 out of 48) of patients awaiting lung transplantation for severe PH (86). Therefore, complete echocardiographic work-up of unexplained PH should probably include either transesophageal echocardiographic evaluation or cardiac magnetic resonance imaging. In some patients TEE may disclose centrally located PA thrombi. Such a finding usually suggests chronic thromboembolic PH, suitable for surgical treatment (87). However, in cases of severe PH with RV dysfunction and stagnant flow in

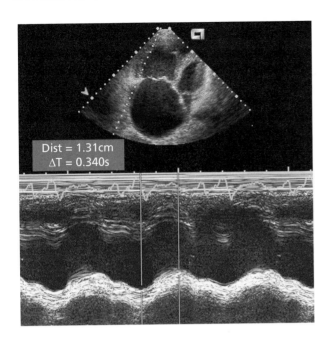

Figure 7.6 Assessment of tricuspid annular plane systolic excursion (TAPSE): under two-dimensional echocardiographic guidance in four-chamber apical view, the cursor is directed towards the lateral part of tricuspid valve (TV) annulus. The displacement of this part of the TV during systole can be easily measured from M-mode tracing. In this case TAPSE = 1.31 cm suggests significantly reduced systolic RV function.

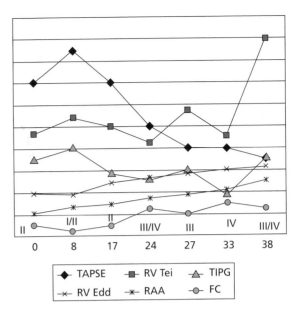

Figure 7.7 Trends of the selected echocardiographic variables and WHO functional class in a patient with progressive PAH followed for up to 3 years. Note improvements in FC at months 8, 27, and 38 related to escalation of treatment. TAPSE reflected the initial improvement at month 8, and thereafter followed progressive remodeling of the right heart, evidenced by continuously increasing RV and RA dimensions. Neither Tei index nor tricuspid jet gradient (TIPG) reflected the clinical course of the disease.

dilated proximal pulmonary arteries, secondary *in situ* thrombi have been described (88).

Right ventricular dilatation can be also due to causes other than chronic PH. Primary RV dysfunction such as in advanced right ventricular arrhythmogenic dysplasia or right ventricular infarction can be suspected in case tricuspid jet velocity is low. If TIPG is only moderately elevated (<60 mmHg) but flow velocity curve in the RV outflow tract shows short acceleration time (<60 msec) and/or marked midsystolic deceleration, acute pulmonary embolism rather than chronic PH should be suspected (63). Acute pulmonary embolism may also cause a particular RV regional contraction pattern known as "McConnell sign." It consists of isolated hyperkinesis of apical part of the RV contrasting with otherwise hypokinetic RV free wall (89).

PROGNOSTIC STAGING AND FOLLOW-UP OF PATIENTS WITH PULMONARY HYPERTENSION

Prognostic stratification in PH is predominantly based on its consequences on the RV function. In acute PH, such as caused by an episode of pulmonary embolism, signs of RV dysfunction found at echocardiography are related to worse short term prognosis. However, the criteria defining RV dysfunction varied between the trials, and were often limited to arbitrarily diagnosed RV "hypokinesis" [90–94]. Nevertheless, echocardiographic signs of RV overload are

considered by recent guidelines as an important marker of risk of early death, helping in stratification of patients into intermediate and low risk category, with different suggested management strategies [95].

In chronic PH echocardiography could theoretically provide estimates of RA pressure, pulmonary arterial pressure and even total pulmonary resistance [19]. All those hemodynamic variables were found by the NH registry to be of prognostic value in patients with "primary" PAH. Evidence accumulated in chronic PH found some new variables, specific for echocardiography, to be prognostically relevant. Leftward shifting of the interventricular septum, supramedian RA area and the presence of pericardial effusion, were all reported to independently increase the risk of death or transplantation among 81 PPH patients followed-up for a mean of 36.9 ± 15.4 months [96]. The presence of pericardial effusion on echocardiography was most consistently reported to indicate poor prognosis in patients with "primary" subtraction of RV ejection time (ET) from total RV systolic time (the latter measured as the interval between cessation and re-appearance of tricuspid diastolic flow). In such a way combined duration of systolic and diastolic isovolumetric time intervals of RV (ICT and IRT, respectively) can be assessed. In a retrospective study involving 55 PPH patients this index of myocardial dysfunction, calculated as (ICT + IRT)/ET was independent from heart rate, RV pressure, dilation, or tricuspid regurgitation but correlated with symptoms and survival [99,100]. In an even smaller group of 26 PPH patients multivariate analysis identified two Doppler-derived indices related to left and right ventricular filling suggesting diastolic dysfunction as independent predictors of survival [98].

More recently tricuspid annular plane systolic excursion (TAPSE) was suggested as useful for staging of patients with PAH (Figure 6.). Forfia et al. [5] reported that TAPSE below a cut-off value of 18 mm, as defined by receiver-operator-curve analysis, indicated worse prognosis in patients with PAH, with survival estimates at 2 years of 50%, compared to 88%, in subjects with a TAPSE above 18 mm. Recently pulmonary vascular capacitance, accounting for pulmonary pulse pressure and RV stroke volume assessed by echo and Doppler was reported as of prognostic significance in idiopathic pulmonary arterial hypertension. Peak systolic tricuspid regurgitation velocity and the end-diastolic pulmonary regurgitation velocity were used to calculate the systolic and diastolic PAP pressures, respectively, while stroke volume was obtained using the volumetric flow through the left ventricular outflow tract. Patients with pulmonary vascular capacitance in the lowest quartile had a 4-year mortality of 39% vs. 7% of those in highest quartile [101].

In summary: multiple echocardiographic variables, most of them reflecting RV systolic or diastolic dysfunction, correlate with survival when assessed at baseline. Their relative value has not been adequately compared.

Follow-up

In view of its non-invasive character, serial echocardiographic evaluations of patients with PH are often attempted.

Spectacular echocardiographic regression of signs of RV overload was observed after thrombolytic treatment of acute PE, lung transplantation, pulmonary thrombendarterectomy or even during acute vasoreactivity tests [102–105]. However, pharmacological treatment of primary PH usually results in changes in PAP, which are too small to be followed in individual patients by Doppler echocardiography [27]. Therefore, echocardiographic indices related to RV systolic and left ventricular diastolic function are more useful to follow effects of treatment than echocardiographic estimates of PAP.

A landmark trial followed trends of about 20 echocardiographic and Doppler variables of potential pathophysiological and/or clinical interest in patients with PAH who received bosentan or placebo for 16 weeks in the frame of a RCT [106]. Particular attention was paid to methodology. Echocardiographic tapes were evaluated blindly by readers not aware of treatment assignment and time sequence of the recordings.

All evaluated parameters showed trend towards improvement in the actively treated vs. placebo group. Treatment effect of the Doppler-derived cardiac index was +0.4 l/min/m (p = 0.007). The difference in the ratio of RV to LV diastolic area (p = 0.007), RV ejection time (p = 0.007), Doppler "Tei" RV index of dysfunction (p = 0.03), and percentage

of patients with an improvement in pericardial effusion score (p = 0.05) were among those most significant, TAPSE was not evaluated in this study. Significant differences were also found in the left heart echo-Doppler variables with improvement in LV early diastolic filling velocity (p = 0.003), LV end-diastolic area (p = 0.003), and LV systolic eccentricity index (p = 0.047) seen in the actively treated when compared to placebo group. The design of the trial did not allow verifying prognostic implication of the observed echocardiographic changes for individual patients.

In summary: while useful for comparison between the groups in a setting of a clinical trial, echocardiographic follow-up might be less reliable in the follow-up of individual patients with PAH. Only integrated assessment of multiple echocardiographic parameters and several sequential observations may provide clinically relevant insight into progression of the disease and effects of treatment (Figure 7.7). Echocardiographic trends should always be interpreted in the context of changes in functional class, exercise capacity and biomarkers.

KEY POINTS

- Enlarged or dominating right ventricle on echocardiography may indicate acute or chronic PH, as well as congenital heart disease, and requires comprehensive differential diagnosis.
- Continuous wave Doppler measurement of peak velocity of the jet of tricuspid regurgitation is the most reliable non-invasive method of assessing systolic PAP.
- Normal ranges of tricuspid jet velocity at rest and on exercise are becoming better defined by recent trials. However, echocardiography can be only used to provide likelihood of PH, while its formal diagnosis or exclusion always requires right heart catheterization.
- Prospective echocardiographic screening of mildly symptomatic patients at risk for PAH, based solely on tricuspid jet velocity is feasible, but the rate of false positive results leading to "unnecessary" right heart catheterization, and the number of subjects needed to test with echo to detect a single PAH patients, are both high.
- Other Doppler and echocardiographic variables have only a supporting role in the assessment of PAP, but may contain relevant pathophysiological information regarding pulmonary circulation.
- Doppler echocardiography is useful for prognostic stratification in acute and chronic PH.
- Follow-up of individual patients with PH should focus on the serial assessment of multiple echocardiographic indices of RV function and left ventricular filling, rather than on attempts at estimation of changes in PAP.

REFERENCES

1. Bommer W, Weinert L, Neumann A, Neef J, Mason DT, DeMaria A. Determination of right atrial and right ventricular size by two-dimensional echocardiography. Circulation 1979;60:91–100.

2. Levine RA, Gibson TC, Aretz T et al. Echocardiographic measurement of right ventricular volume. Circulation 1984;69:497–505.

3. Lebeau R, Di LM, Sauve C et al. Two-dimensional echocardiography estimation of right ventricular ejection fraction by wall motion score index. Can J Cardiol 2004;20:169–76.

4. Zornoff LA, Skali H, Pfeffer MA et al. Right ventricular dysfunction and risk of heart failure and mortality after myocardial infarction. J Am Coll Cardiol 2002;39:1450–5.

5. Forfia PR, Fisher MR, Mathai SC et al. Tricuspid annular displacement predicts survival in pulmonary hypertension. Am J Respir Crit Care Med 2006;174:1034–41.

6. Kalogeropoulos AP, Georgiopoulou VV, Howell S et al. Evaluation of right intraventricular dyssynchrony by two-dimensional strain echocardiography in patients with pulmonary arterial hypertension. J Am Soc Echocardiogr 2008;21:1028–34.

7. Pirat B, McCulloch ML, Zoghbi WA. Evaluation of global and regional right ventricular systolic function in patients with pulmonary hypertension using a novel speckle tracking method. Am J Cardiol 2006;98:699–704.

8. Ryan T, Petrovic O, Dillon JC, Feigenbaum H, Conley MJ, Armstrong WF. An echocardiographic index for separation of right ventricular volume and pressure overload. J Am Coll Cardiol 1985;5:918–27.

9. Zenker G, Forche G, Harnoncourt K. Two-dimensional echocardiography using a subcostal approach in patients with COPD. Chest 1985;88:722–5.

10. Danchin N, Cornette A, Henriquez A et al. Two-dimensional echocardiographic assessment of the right ventricle in patients with chronic obstructive lung disease. Chest 1987;92:229–33.

11. Oswald-Mammosser M, Oswald T, Nyankiye E, Dickele MC, Grange D, Weitzenblum E. Non-invasive diagnosis of pulmonary hypertension in chronic obstructive pulmonary disease. Comparison of ECG, radiological measurements, echocardiography and myocardial scintigraphy. Eur J Respir Dis 1987;71:419–29.

12. Jenkins C, Chan J, Bricknell K, Strudwick M, Marwick TH. Reproducibility of right ventricular volumes and ejection fraction using real-time three-dimensional echocardiography: comparison with cardiac MRI. Chest 2007;131:1844–51.

13. Ayres NA, Miller-Hance W, Fyfe DA et al. Indications and guidelines for performance of transesophageal echocardiography in the patient with pediatric acquired or congenital heart disease: report from the task force of the Pediatric Council of the American Society of Echocardiography. J Am Soc Echocardiogr 2005;18:91–8.

14. Kurzyna M, Dabrowski M, Bielecki D et al. Atrial septostomy in treatment of end-stage right heart failure in patients with pulmonary hypertension. Chest 2007;131:977–83.

15. Foale R, Nihoyannopoulos P, McKenna W et al. Echocardiographic measurement of the normal adult right ventricle. Br Heart J 1986;56:33–44.

16. Prakash R, Matsukubo H. Usefulness of echocardiographic right ventricular measurements in estimating right ventricular hypertrophy and right ventricular systolic pressure. Am J Cardiol 1983;51:1036–40.

17. Shimada R, Takeshita A, Nakamura M. Noninvasive assessment of right ventricular systolic pressure in atrial septal defect: analysis of the end-systolic configuration of the ventricular septum by two-dimensional echocardiography. Am J Cardiol 1984;53:1117–23.

18. Abbas AE, Fortuin FD, Schiller NB, Appleton CP, Moreno CA, Lester SJ. A simple method for noninvasive estimation of pulmonary vascular resistance. J Am Coll Cardiol 2003;41:1021–7.

19. Kouzu H, Nakatani S, Kyotani S, Kanzaki H, Nakanishi N, Kitakaze M. Noninvasive estimation of pulmonary vascular resistance by Doppler echocardiography in patients with pulmonary arterial hypertension. Am J Cardiol 2009;103:872–6.

20. Naeije R, Torbicki A. More on the noninvasive diagnosis of pulmonary hypertension: Doppler echocardiography revisited (editorial). Eur Respir J 1995;8:1445–9.

21. Masuyama T, Kodama K, Kitabatake A, Sato H, Nanto S, Inoue M. Continuous-wave Doppler echocardiographic detection of pulmonary regurgitation and its application to noninvasive estimation of pulmonary artery pressure. Circulation 1986;74:484–92.

22. Matsuoka Y, Hayakawa K. Noninvasive estimation of right ventricular systolic pressure in ventricular septal defect by a continuous wave Doppler technique. Jpn Circ J 1986;50:1062–70.

23. Marx GR, Allen HD, Goldberg SJ. Doppler echocardiographic estimation of systolic pulmonary artery pressure in pediatric patients with interventricular communications. J Am Coll Cardiol 1985;6:1132–7.

24. Musewe NN, Poppe D, Smallhorn JF et al. Doppler echocardiographic measurement of pulmonary artery pressure from ductal Doppler velocities in the newborn (see comments). J Am Coll Cardiol 1990;15:446–56.

25. Yock PG, Popp RL. Noninvasive estimation of right ventricular systolic pressure by Doppler ultrasound in patients with tricuspid regurgitation. Circulation 1984;70:657–62.

26. Currie PJ, Seward JB, Chan KL et al. Continuous wave Doppler determination of right ventricular pressure: a simultaneous Doppler-catheterization study in 127 patients. J Am Coll Cardiol 1985;6:750–6.

27. Hinderliter AL, Willis PW, Barst RJ et al. Effects of long-term infusion of prostacyclin (epoprostenol) on echocardiographic measures of right ventricular structure and function in primary pulmonary hypertension.

Primary Pulmonary Hypertension Study Group (see comments). Circulation 1997;95:1479–86.

28. Richards AM, Ikram H, Crozier IG, Nicholls MG, Jans S. Ambulatory pulmonary arterial pressure in primary pulmonary hypertension: variability, relation to systemic arterial pressure, and plasma catecholamines. Br Heart J 1990;63:103–8.

29. Brecker SJ, Gibbs JS, Fox KM, Yacoub MH, Gibson DG. Comparison of Doppler derived haemodynamic variables and simultaneous high fidelity pressure measurements in severe pulmonary hypertension. Br Heart J 1994; 72:384–9.

30. McQuillan BM, Picard MH, Leavitt M, Weyman AE. Clinical correlates and reference intervals for pulmonary artery systolic pressure among echocardiographically normal subjects. Circulation 2001;104:2797–802.

31. Higham MA, Dawson D, Joshi J, Nihoyannopoulos P, Morrell NW. Utility of echocardiography in assessment of pulmonary hypertension secondary to COPD. Eur Respir J 2001;17:350–5.

32. Laaban JP, Diebold B, Zelinski R, Lafay M, Raffoul H, Rochemaure J. Noninvasive estimation of systolic pulmonary artery pressure using Doppler echocardiography in patients with chronic obstructive pulmonary disease. Chest 1989;96:1258–62.

33. Tramarin R, Torbicki A, Marchandise B, Laaban JP, Morpurgo M. Doppler echocardiographic evaluation of pulmonary artery pressure in chronic obstructive pulmonary disease. A European multicentre study. Working Group on Noninvasive Evaluation of Pulmonary Artery Pressure. European Office of the World Health Organization, Copenhagen. Eur Heart J 1991;12:103–11.

34. Torbicki A, Skwarski K, Hawrylkiewicz I, Pasierski T, Miskiewicz Z, Zielinski J. Attempts at measuring pulmonary arterial pressure by means of Doppler echocardiography in patients with chronic lung disease. Eur Respir J 1989;2:856–60.

35. Beard JT, Byrd BF III. Saline contrast enhancement of trivial Doppler tricuspid regurgitation signals for estimating pulmonary artery pressure. Am J Cardiol 1988;62:486–8.

36. Himelman RB, Struve SN, Brown JK, Namnum P, Schiller NB. Improved recognition of cor pulmonale in patients with severe chronic obstructive pulmonary disease. Am J Med 1988;84:891–8.

37. Fisher MR, Forfia PR, Chamera E et al. Accuracy of Doppler echocardiography in the hemodynamic assessment of pulmonary hypertension. Am J Respir Crit Care Med 2009;179:615–21.

38. Skjaerpe T, Hatle L. Noninvasive estimation of systolic pressure in the right ventricle in patients with tricuspid regurgitation. Eur Heart J 1986;7:704–10.

39. Lei MH, Chen JJ, Ko YL, Cheng JJ, Kuan P, Lien WP. Reappraisal of quantitative evaluation of pulmonary regurgitation and estimation of pulmonary artery pressure by continuous wave Doppler echocardiography. Cardiology 1995;86:249–56.

40. Ensing G, Seward J, Darragh R, Caldwell R. Feasibility of generating hemodynamic pressure curves from noninvasive Doppler echocardiographic signals. J Am Coll Cardiol 1994;23:434–42.

41. Chemla D, Castelain V, Humbert M et al. New formula for predicting mean pulmonary artery pressure using systolic pulmonary artery pressure. Chest 2004;126: 1313–7.

42. Chemla D, Castelain V, Provencher S, Humbert M, Simonneau G, Herve P. Evaluation of various empirical formulas for estimating mean pulmonary artery pressure by using systolic pulmonary artery pressure in adults. Chest 2009;135:760–8.

43. Boyd MJ, Williams IP, Turton CW, Brooks N, Leech G, Millard FJ. Echocardiographic method for the estimation of pulmonary artery pressure in chronic lung disease. Thorax 1980;35:914–9.

44. Stevenson JG, Kawabori I, Guntheroth WG. Noninvasive detection of pulmonary hypertension in patent ductus arteriosus by pulsed Doppler echocardiography. Circulation 1979;60:355–9.

45. Torbicki A, Hawrylkiewicz I, Zielinski J. Value of M-mode echocardiography in assessing pulmonary arterial pressure in patients with chronic lung disease. Bull Eur Physiopathol Respir 1987;23:233–9.

46. Musewe NN, Poppe D, Smallhorn JF et al. Doppler echocardiographic measurement of pulmonary artery pressure from ductal Doppler velocities in the newborn (see comments). J Am Coll Cardiol 1990;15:446–56.

47. Kircher BJ, Himelman RB, Schiller NB. Noninvasive estimation of right atrial pressure from the inspiratory collapse of the inferior vena cava. Am J Cardiol 1990;66:493–6.

48. Pepi M, Tamborini G, Galli C et al. A new formula for echo-Doppler estimation of right ventricular systolic pressure. J Am Soc Echocardiogr 1994;7:20–6.

49. Simonson JS, Schiller NB. Sonospirometry: a new method for noninvasive estimation of mean right atrial pressure based on two-dimensional echographic measurements of the inferior vena cava during measured inspiration. J Am Coll Cardiol 1988;11:557–64.

50. Nakao S, Come PC, McKay RG, Ransil BJ. Effects of positional changes on inferior vena caval size and dynamics and correlations with right-sided cardiac pressure. Am J Cardiol 1987;59:125–32.

51. Chan KL, Currie PJ, Seward JB, Hagler DJ, Mair DD, Tajik AJ. Comparison of three Doppler ultrasound methods in the prediction of pulmonary artery pressure. J Am Coll Cardiol 1987;9:549–54.

52. Torbicki A, Tramarin R, Fracchia C et al. Simultaneous Doppler and thermodilution assessment of pulmonary artery flow during acute interventions in patients with chronic obstructive pulmonary disease. Cor Vasa 1990;32:197–205.

53. Kitabatake A, Inoue M, Asao M et al. Noninvasive evaluation of pulmonary hypertension by a pulsed Doppler technique. Circulation 1983;68:302–9.

54. Turkevich D, Groves BM, Micco A, Trapp JA, Reeves JT. Early partial systolic closure of the pulmonic valve relates to severity of pulmonary hypertension. Am Heart J 1988;115:409–18.

55. Robinson PJ, Macartney FJ, Wyse RK. Non-invasive diagnosis of pulmonary hypertension. Int J Cardiol 1986;11:253–9.

56. Mallery JA, Gardin JM, King SW, Ey S, Henry WL. Effects of heart rate and pulmonary artery pressure on Doppler pulmonary artery acceleration time in experimental acute pulmonary hypertension. Chest 1991;100:470–3.

57. Matsuda M, Sekiguchi T, Sugishita Y, Kuwako K, Iida K, Ito I. Reliability of non-invasive estimates of pulmonary hypertension by pulsed Doppler echocardiography. Br Heart J 1986;56:158–64.

58. Isobe M, Yazaki Y, Takaku F et al. Prediction of pulmonary arterial pressure in adults by pulsed Doppler echocardiography. Am J Cardiol 1986;57:316–21.

59. Okamoto M, Miyatake K, Kinoshita N, Sakakibara H, Nimura Y. Analysis of blood flow in pulmonary hypertension with the pulsed Doppler flowmeter combined with cross sectional echocardiography. Br Heart J 1984;51:407–15.

60. Panidis IP, Ross J, Mintz GS. Effect of sampling site on assessment of pulmonary artery blood flow by Doppler echocardiography. Am J Cardiol 1986;58:1145–7.

61. Gardin JM, Davidson DM, Rohan MK et al. Relationship between age, body size, gender, and blood pressure and Doppler flow measurements in the aorta and pulmonary artery. Am Heart J 1987;113:101–9.

62. Torbicki A, Kurzyna M, Ciurzynski M et al. Proximal pulmonary emboli modify right ventricular ejection pattern. Eur Respir J 1999;13:616–21.

63. Kurzyna M, Torbicki A, Pruszczyk P et al. Disturbed right ventricular ejection pattern as a new Doppler echocardiographic sign of acute pulmonary embolism. Am J Cardiol 2002;90:507–11.

64. Hardziyenka M, Reesink HJ, Bouma BJ et al. A novel echocardiographic predictor of in-hospital mortality and mid-term haemodynamic improvement after pulmonary endarterectomy for chronic thrombo-embolic pulmonary hypertension. Eur Heart J 2007;28:842–9.

65. Marangoni S, Quadri A, Dotti A et al. Noninvasive assessment of pulmonary hypertension: a simultaneous echo-Doppler hemodynamic study. Cardiology 1988;75:401–8.

66. Torbicki A, Tramarin R, Fracchia F et al. Reliability of pulsed wave Doppler monitoring of acute changes in pulmonary artery pressure in patients with chronic obstructive pulmonary disease. Progr Respir Res 1990;26:133–41.

67. Murata I, Takenaka K, Yoshinoya S et al. Clinical evaluation of pulmonary hypertension in systemic sclerosis and related disorders. A Doppler echocardiographic study of 135 Japanese patients. Chest 1997;111:36–43.

68. Elstein D, Klutstein MW, Lahad A, Abrahamov A, Hadas-Halpern I, Zimran A. Echocardiographic assessment of pulmonary hypertension in Gaucher's disease (see comments). Lancet 1998;351:1544–6.

69. Aessopos A, Farmakis D, Taktikou H, Loukopoulos D. Doppler-determined peak systolic tricuspid pressure gradient in persons with normal pulmonary function and tricuspid regurgitation. J Am Soc Echocardiogr 2000; 13:645–9.

70. Dib JC, Abergel E, Rovani C, Raffoul H, Diebold B. The age of the patient should be taken into account when interpreting Doppler assessed pulmonary artery pressures. J Am Soc Echocardiogr 1997;10:72–3.

71. Grunig E, Weissmann S, Ehlken N et al. Stress Doppler echocardiography in relatives of patients with idiopathic and familial pulmonary arterial hypertension: results of a multicenter European analysis of pulmonary artery pressure response to exercise and hypoxia. Circulation 2009;119:1747–57.

72. McGoon MD. The assessment of pulmonary hypertension. Clin Chest Med 2001;22:493–508, ix.

73. Himelman RB, Stulbarg M, Kircher B et al. Noninvasive evaluation of pulmonary artery pressure during exercise by saline-enhanced Doppler echocardiography in chronic pulmonary disease. Circulation 1989;79:863–71.

74. Barbant SD, Redberg RF, Tucker KJ et al. Abnormal pulmonary artery pressure profile after cardiac transplantation: an exercise Doppler echocardiographic study. Am Heart J 1995;129:1185–92.

75. Oelberg DA, Marcotte F, Kreisman H, Wolkove N, Langleben D, Small D. Evaluation of right ventricular systolic pressure during incremental exercise by Doppler echocardiography in adults with atrial septal defect. Chest 1998;113: 1459–65.

76. Grunig E, Mereles D, Hildebrandt W et al. Stress Doppler echocardiography for identification of susceptibility to high altitude pulmonary edema. J Am Coll Cardiol 2000;35:980–7.

77. Grunig E, Janssen B, Mereles D et al. Abnormal pulmonary artery pressure response in asymptomatic carriers of primary pulmonary hypertension gene. Circulation 2000;102:1145–50.

78. Bossone E, Avelar E, Bach DS, Gillespie B, Rubenfire M, Armstrong WF. Diagnostic value of resting tricuspid regurgitation velocity and right ventricular ejection flow parameters for the detection of exercise induced pulmonary arterial hypertension. Int J Card Imaging 2000;16:429–36.

79. Torbicki A, Tramarin R, Fracchia F et al. Effect of increased right ventricular preload on pulmonary artery flow velocity in patients with normal or increased pulmonary artery pressure. Am J Noninvas Cardiol 1994;8:151–5.

80. Ohashi M, Sato K, Suzuki S et al. Doppler echocardiographic evaluation of latent pulmonary hypertension by passive leg raising. Coron Artery Dis 1997;8:651–5.

81. Mukerjee D, St GD, Knight C et al. Echocardiography and pulmonary function as screening tests for pulmonary arterial hypertension in systemic sclerosis. Rheumatology (Oxford) 2004;43:461–6.

82. Launay D, Mouthon L, Hachulla E et al. Prevalence and characteristics of moderate to severe pulmonary hypertension in systemic sclerosis with and without interstitial lung disease. J Rheumatol 2007;34:1005–11.

83. Hachulla E, Gressin V, Guillevin L et al. Early detection of pulmonary arterial hypertension in systemic sclerosis: a French nationwide prospective multicenter study. Arthritis Rheum 2005;52:3792–800.

84. Sitbon O, Lascoux-Combe C, Delfraissy JF et al. Prevalence of HIV-related pulmonary arterial hypertension in the current antiretroviral therapy era. Am J Respir Crit Care Med 2008;177:108–13.

85. Chen WJ, Chen JJ, Lin SC, Hwang JJ, Lien WP. Detection of cardiovascular shunts by transesophageal echocardiography in patients with pulmonary hypertension of unexplained cause. Chest 1995;107:8–13.

86. Gorcsan J III, Edwards TD, Ziady GM, Katz WE, Griffith BP. Transesophageal echocardiography to evaluate patients with severe pulmonary hypertension for lung transplantation. Ann Thorac Surg 1995;59:717–22.

87. Pruszczyk P, Torbicki A, Pacho R et al. Noninvasive diagnosis of suspected severe pulmonary embolism: transesophageal echocardiography vs spiral CT (see comments). Chest 1997;112:722–8.

88. Moser KM, Fedullo PF, Finkbeiner WE, Golden J. Do patients with primary pulmonary hypertension develop extensive central thrombi? Circulation 1995;91:741–5.

89. McConnell MV, Solomon SD, Rayan ME, Come PC, Goldhaber SZ, Lee RT. Regional right ventricular dysfunction detected by echocardiography in acute pulmonary embolism. Am J Cardiol 1996;78:469–73.

90. Goldhaber SZ. Echocardiography in the management of pulmonary embolism. Ann Intern Med 2002;136:691–700.

91. Grifoni S, Olivotto I, Cecchini P et al. Short-term clinical outcome of patients with acute pulmonary embolism, normal blood pressure, and echocardiographic right ventricular dysfunction. Circulation 2000;101:2817–22.

92. Kasper W, Konstantinides S, Geibel A, Tiede N, Krause T, Just H. Prognostic significance of right ventricular afterload stress detected by echocardiography in patients with clinically suspected pulmonary embolism. Heart 1997;77:346–9.

93. Ribeiro A, Lindmarker P, Juhlin-Dannfelt A, Johnsson H, Jorfeldt L. Echocardiography Doppler in pulmonary embolism: right ventricular dysfunction as a predictor of mortality rate. Am Heart J 1997;134:479–87.

94. Ribeiro A, Lindmarker P, Johnsson H, Juhlin-Dannfelt A, Jorfeldt L. Pulmonary embolism: one-year follow-up with echocardiography Doppler and five-year survival analysis. Circulation 1999;99:1325–30.

95. Torbicki A, Perrier A, Konstantinides S et al. Guidelines on the diagnosis and management of acute pulmonary embolism: the Task Force for the Diagnosis and Management of Acute Pulmonary Embolism of the European Society of Cardiology (ESC). Eur Heart J 2008;29:2276–315.

96. Raymond RJ, Hinderliter AL, Willis PW et al. Echocardiographic predictors of adverse outcomes in primary pulmonary hypertension. J Am Coll Cardiol 2002;39:1214–9.

97. Hinderliter AL, Willis PW, Long W et al. Frequency and prognostic significance of pericardial effusion in primary pulmonary hypertension. PPH Study Group. Primary pulmonary hypertension. Am J Cardiol 1999;84:481–4, A10.

98. Eysmann SB, Palevsky HI, Reichek N, Hackney K, Douglas PS. Two-dimensional and Doppler-echocardiographic and cardiac catheterization correlates of survival in primary pulmonary hypertension. Circulation 1989;80:353–60.

99. Tei C, Dujardin KS, Hodge DO et al. Doppler echocardiographic index for assessment of global right ventricular function (see comments). J Am Soc Echocardiogr 1996;9:838–47.

100. Yeo TC, Dujardin KS, Tei C, Mahoney DW, McGoon MD, Seward JB. Value of a Doppler-derived index combining systolic and diastolic time intervals in predicting outcome in primary pulmonary hypertension. Am J Cardiol 1998;81:1157–61.

101. Mahapatra S, Nishimura RA, Oh JK, McGoon MD. The prognostic value of pulmonary vascular capacitance determined by Doppler echocardiography in patients with pulmonary arterial hypertension. J Am Soc Echocardiogr 2006;19:1045–50.

102. Katz WE, Gasior TA, Quinlan JJ et al. Immediate effects of lung transplantation on right ventricular morphology and function in patients with variable degrees of pulmonary hypertension. J Am Coll Cardiol 1996;27:384–91.

103. Dittrich HC, Nicod PH, Chow LC, Chappuis FP, Moser KM, Peterson KL. Early changes of right heart geometry after pulmonary thromboendarterectomy. J Am Coll Cardiol 1988;11:937–43.

104. Menzel T, Wagner S, Mohr-Kahaly S et al. (Reversibility of changes in left and right ventricular geometry and hemodynamics in pulmonary hypertension. Echocardiographic characteristics before and after pulmonary thromboendarterectomy). Z Kardiol 1997;86:928–35.

105. Ritchie M, Waggoner AD, Davila-Roman VG, Barzilai B, Trulock EP, Eisenberg PR. Echocardiographic characterization of the improvement in right ventricular function in patients with severe pulmonary hypertension after single-lung transplantation. J Am Coll Cardiol 1993;22:1170–4.

106. Galie N, Hinderliter AL, Torbicki A et al. Effects of the oral endothelin-receptor antagonist bosentan on echocardiographic and Doppler measures in patients with pulmonary arterial hypertension. J Am Coll Cardiol 2003;41:1380–6.

8

Imaging: Chest radiography, ventilation/perfusion scintigraphy and computed tomography

MICHAEL SPROULE

INTRODUCTION

There is no cure for pulmonary arterial hypertension. However, in recent years, several different therapies have been developed which have led to improvements in symptoms, exercise tolerance and, in some cases, survival (1,2). This is true for both idiopathic pulmonary arterial hypertension (IPAH) and pulmonary hypertension secondary to various cardiac and respiratory disorders, and has emphasized the importance of early and accurate detection of raised pulmonary artery pressure and its underlying etiology. Right heart catheterization remains the most accurate method of measuring pulmonary artery (PA) pressure (3) but is an invasive and relatively expensive test. There are, of course, non-invasive tests which may not only indicate raised PA pressure but also suggest an underlying etiology. Echocardiography and magnetic resonance imaging are discussed elsewhere (Chapters 7 and 9); in this chapter, the role of the chest radiograph (CXR), ventilation/perfusion scintigraphy (V/Q) and computed tomography (CT) will be reviewed. A large number of radiographic signs may be seen in patients with pulmonary hypertension. The value and the limitations of these signs, and their pitfalls will be assessed. Taken individually, the radiographic signs can be of limited worth due to lack of sensitivity and specificity. However, taken together in the appropriate clinical context, it is often possible to make a confident diagnosis, not just of raised PA pressure but also of the underlying etiology.

In routine clinical practice, pulmonary hypertension has become an increasingly important condition for the radiologist to recognize. With effective treatment now available, awareness of the possibility of pulmonary hypertension has risen and consequently referrals for imaging for patients with possible pulmonary hypertension have multiplied. In this context, the role of the imaging is to confirm the diagnosis of pulmonary hypertension, assess its severity and, if possible, suggest the underlying etiology. In the case of chronic thromboembolic pulmonary hypertension (CTEPH), it is also important to determine if it is amenable to surgical correction and whether a good outcome can be anticipated. Alternatively, pulmonary hypertension may not be suspected by the referrer, which is hardly surprising given the entirely nonspecific presenting symptoms of the condition (4). However, because so many of these patients with nonspecific respiratory and cardiac symptoms now routinely undergo imaging, especially thoracic CT, the radiologist may be in a position to be the first to suggest a diagnosis of pulmonary hypertension.

CHEST RADIOGRAPHY

The CXR is inexpensive, widely available and non-invasive. It may give the first clue to the presence of pulmonary hypertension, providing invaluable information about the pulmonary vasculature, the heart size and the lung parenchyma.

The characteristic radiographic features of pulmonary arterial hypertension consist of enlargement of the central PAs and rapid tapering of the vessels as they extend to the

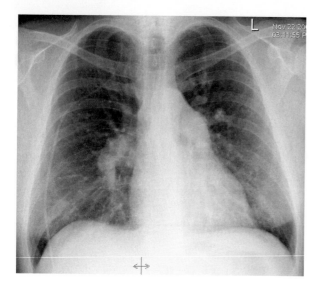

Figure 8.1 IPAH: enlarged central pulmonary arteries and "peripheral pruning." Central line *in situ* for prostacyclin treatment.

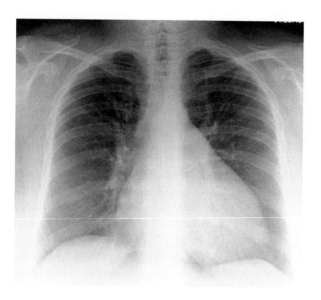

Figure 8.2 Calcification in the right interlobar artery.

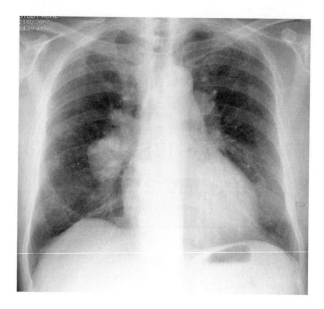

Figure 8.3 CTEPH: bulging and asymmetrical hilar vessels.

Enlargement of the hilar PAs can be assessed by measuring the diameter of the interlobar arteries at the hilar point; the upper limit of normal being 16 mm in men and 15 mm in women (8).

The characteristic findings in chronic thromboembolic pulmonary hypertension (CTEPH) are, like idiopathic pulmonary arterial hypertension (IPAH), enlargement of the right ventricle, prominence of the central PAs and rapid tapering of the distal pulmonary arteries giving the appearance of peripheral oligemia. When thrombosis or embolism occurs in the central PAs, then bulging and/or asymmetrical hilar vessels is characteristic (9,10) (Figure 8.3). Another feature of CTEPH, is decreased vascularity (mosaic oligemia) (10). The areas of decreased vascularity visible on plain radiographs can be confirmed by pulmonary angiography to be associated with chronic emboli (Figure 8.4).

The chest radiograph may, in addition, usefully suggest an underlying cause of pulmonary hypertension by showing parenchymal lung disease (Figure 8.5).

Although it is clear that the presence of pulmonary hypertension can be recognized from the chest radiograph, the sensitivity and degree of accuracy with which severity can be estimated is controversial (11,12). Measurement of the interlobar PAs are affected by variable magnification related to the size of the patient and distance between the x-ray tube and film. Measurements may also be difficult, or impossible, in the presence of severe parenchymal lung disease. Assessment of vascular pruning is subjective, and the degree of pruning does not correlate well with the level of pulmonary hypertension (13). Although it is not known precisely at what stage in the development of pulmonary hypertension that the characteristic chest radiographic features become visible, it is likely that they become conspicuous only in more severe disease. Clearly, this limits the role of the chest radiograph in the diagnosis of early or mild pulmonary hypertension.

periphery of the lungs, giving rise to peripheral oligemia (Figure 8.1). "Peripheral pruning," or discordance in caliber between central and peripheral pulmonary arteries, is a distinct feature of pulmonary arterial hypertension (5,6) regardless of etiology (with the caveat of large left to right shunts when pulmonary plethora is expected). The heart, particularly the right sided chambers, is usually enlarged but may be of normal size. An unusual manifestation of severe chronic pulmonary hypertension is the presence of vascular calcification, usually in the main pulmonary artery (MPA) or its hilar branches (Figure 8.2). Such calcification is regarded as evidence of high pulmonary vascular resistance (PVR) and irreversible vascular disease; most often in association with Eisenmenger's syndrome (7).

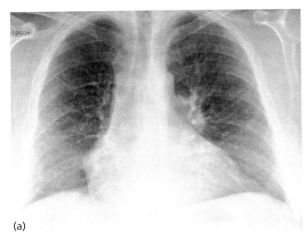

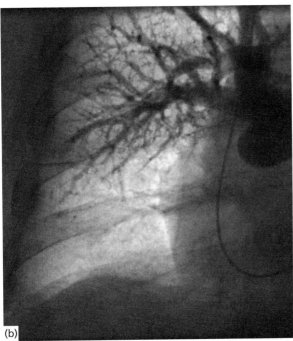

Figure 8.4 (a) CTEPH: CXR showing decreased vascularity in the right lower zone. (b) CTEPH: pulmonary angiogram from the same patient confirming absent flow in the right lower lobe.

VENTILATION/PERFUSION SCINTIGRAPHY

The role of ventilation perfusion (V/Q) scintigraphy is mainly in distinguishing IPAH from hypertension associated with chronic thromboembolic disease. With CTEPH, the V/Q scan is invariably high probability showing multiple mismatched segmental or larger perfusion defects. A normal or low probability scan virtually excludes CTEPH. In contrast, with IPAH, the V/Q scan is usually normal or shows heterogeneous perfusion (14–16) (Figure 8.6). Rarely, larger mismatched perfusion defects may be seen in IPAH, presumably due to thrombosis *in situ*. Where patients have intermediate or high probability scans, the diagnosis of CTEPH can usually be confirmed by CT pulmonary angiography (CTPA). However, it is worth noting that some

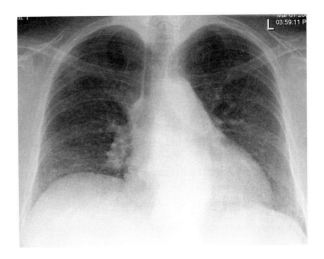

Figure 8.5 Pulmonary hypertension in a patient with severe pulmonary fibrosis.

investigators have found that a significant minority of patients with CTEPH have evidence of thromboembolic disease on V/Q scintigraphy but not on CTPA (17).

Although V/Q scintigraphy is a safe and highly sensitive test for suspected CTEPH, large mismatched perfusion defects may arise in other processes that result in obliteration of the central arteries and veins. For example, large vessel vasculitis, pulmonary artery sarcoma, extrinsic compression due to cancer, lymphadenopathy, fibrosing mediastinitis and pulmonary veno-occlusive disease (PVOD) (18–21) (Figure 8.7).

COMPUTED TOMOGRAPHY

Given the dramatic technological advances over the last 10–15 years, computed tomography (CT) now has a central role in the diagnosis of pulmonary hypertension. With multidetector CT (MDCT), it is possible to cover the chest in submillimeter thick slices in 3–4 seconds, which even the most breathless patients can manage in a single breath-hold. With optimal contrast enhancement, submillimeter thick slices, and improved post processing power, the images can be reviewed in any plane without loss of detail (isotropic spatial resolution). Unlike other modalities, with CT it is possible to image the main and peripheral pulmonary arteries, the heart and the lung parenchyma.

The main pulmonary artery

Because the main PA is intrapericardial, it cannot be measured on conventional chest radiography. It can, however, readily be identified and measured on CT: best measured at a right angle to the long axis of the main PA, lateral to the ascending aorta, and near the left of the bifurcation (22,23) (Figure 8.8). There have been several studies over the last 30 years or so that have examined the reliability of CT in detecting pulmonary hypertension (22–27). These

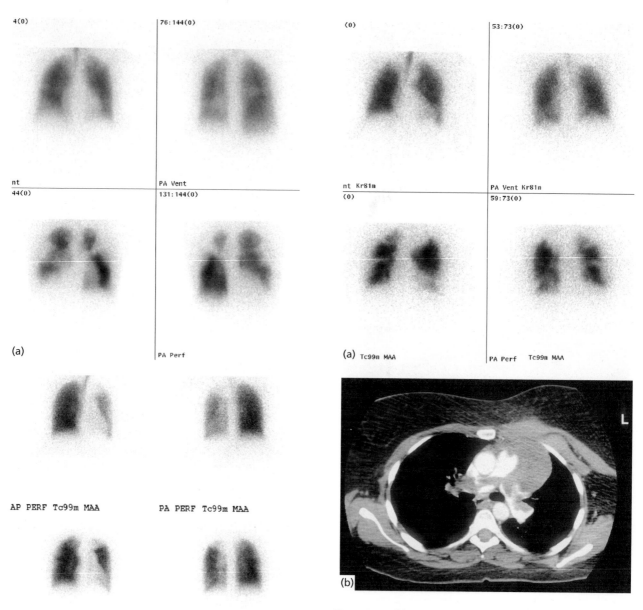

Figure 8.6 (a) CTEPH: high probability V/Q scan showing multiple large mismatched perfusion defects. (b) IPAH: V/Q scan showing relatively subtle heterogeneous perfusion.

Figure 8.7 (a) High probability V/Q scan in a patient with pulmonary hypertension which turned out to be due to pulmonary artery sarcoma. (b) CT of same patient showing pulmonary artery sarcoma (biopsy proven via CT guidance).

studies were conducted using different methodologies; in particular, different definitions of mean pulmonary artery pressure (mPAP). It is hardly surprising, therefore, that the results are inconsistent. Nonetheless, despite great variation in the size of the PA in normal subjects, up to 36 mm (23), there is linkage between PA size and pulmonary arterial hypertension. In one study of 36 patients who had pulmonary arterial hypertension, the main PA measurements on CT were correlated with right heart hemodynamic data (24). A main PA diameter on CT of ≥ 29 mm had a sensitivity of 87 percent, a specificity of 89 percent and a positive predictive value of 97 percent for pulmonary arterial hypertension. Based on the results of this and various other studies, it is

reasonable to conclude that a main PA diameter of ≥ 29 mm on CT is suggestive of, but not diagnostic, for the presence of pulmonary hypertension (or increased blood flow due a left-to-right shunt). Some studies have failed to show a linear correlation between the degree of pulmonary hypertension and the main PA diameter (24). Other studies have shown that the strength of the relationship between the main PA size and the mPAP is greater in patients with more severe pulmonary hypertension than in patients with mild pulmonary hypertension (23).

The large variation in the reported diameter of the main PA suggests that its size is dependent on factors other than the mPAP; for example, patient body surface area. Factors such as this would be expected to affect the morphology of the ascending aorta to the same extent as the mean PA,

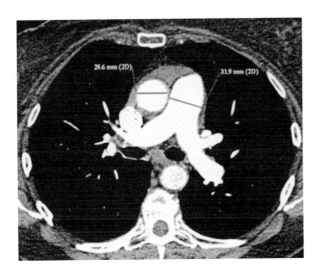

Figure 8.8 CT showing enlargement of the main pulmonary artery near the level of the bifurcation, and a PA:AA ratio of >1.

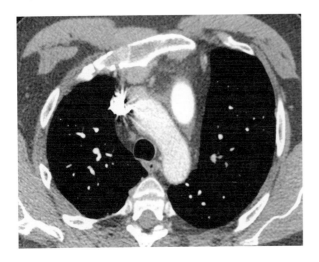

Figure 8.9 IPAH: "Egg and banana" sign. The top of the dilated main PA (white arrow) appears on the same axial section as the arch of the aorta (black arrow).

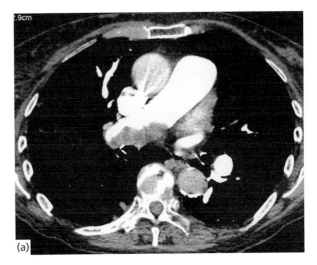

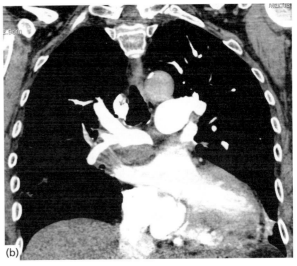

Figure 8.10 (a) CTPA axial section showing eccentric thrombus in the main PA. (b) CTPA coronal reformatted section from the same patient showing eccentric thrombus in the main PA.

which has lead to the concept of the ratio between the PA and ascending aorta (AA). In a study by Ng *et al.* (27) a PA:AA ratio of >1 was highly specific for pulmonary hypertension (92 percent specificity) and correlated strongly with mPAP. However, it must be emphasized that it was no more specific and does not correlate any more strongly than PA size alone. Nonetheless, along with an absolute PA diameter of >29 mm, the PA:AA ratio has become a widely accepted, quick and easy sign which is useful in supporting the diagnosis of pulmonary hypertension.

As noted above, when assessing the main PA for dilatation, it is usually measured in the axial plane, near the bifurcation. This may be somewhat arbitrary, given the complex shape and position of the main PA, especially as it elongates in pulmonary arterial hypertension. Nevertheless, a simple and specific sign for severe pulmonary arterial hypertension, on axial CT, occurs when the main PA is visible at the same level as aortic arch (the "egg and banana" sign) (28) (Figure 8.9).

Abnormalities in the main PA may be highly suggestive of pulmonary hypertension due to chronic thromboembolic disease. The most common finding is an eccentric location of thrombus, resulting in a crescentic filling defect adjacent to the vessel wall (29,30) (Figure 8.10). It is worth noting that this peripheral laminated filling defect in the central PAs is not specific for CTEPH. There are a number of conditions which may give rise to a similar appearance on CT, thus mimicking CTEPH. In Eisenmenger's syndrome, due to very slow flow and giant pulmonary arteries, laminated thrombus may develop *in situ* in the proximal pulmonary arteries (31) (Figure 8.11). Other mimics of CTEPH include large vessel vasculitis (20) (Figure 8.12) and pulmonary artery sarcoma (21) (Figure 8.7).

Pulmonary arteries and bronchial arteries

Measuring the caliber of the right and left PAs and the right interlobar artery does not appear to offer any advantage

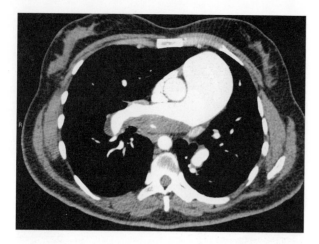

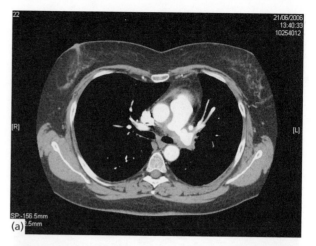

Figure 8.11   CTPA showing grossly dilated central pulmonary arteries and thrombosis *in situ* (black arrow) in a patient with Eisenmenger's syndrome.

over the main PA (22,23,25). Within the lung, the diameter of the pulmonary arteries should be approximately the same as the accompanying bronchi. In patients with pulmonary hypertension or increased blood flow due to left to right shunts, there may be significant dilatation of intrapulmonary arteries relative to their accompanying bronchi (Figure 8.13). It has been suggested that pulmonary hypertension can be confidently predicted if the ratio of the segmental artery-to-bronchus diameter is >1 in three or more lobes (32). Increased segmental artery-to-bronchus ratios in one or two lobes would be unreliable as this may be seen in normal individuals or in patients with regional pulmonary abnormalities; for example, emphysema and pulmonary fibrosis.

The bronchial arterial anatomy is notoriously variable; though they most commonly arise from the proximal descending aorta (33). They supply blood to the walls of the bronchial tree and proximal pulmonary arteries. Bronchial artery hypertrophy occurs most commonly in chronic inflammatory diseases of the airways, for example, cystic fibrosis, and in chronic pulmonary hypoperfusion, when the bronchial arteries act as a collateral blood supply to the pulmonary parenchyma. Hypertrophy of the bronchial arteries has been defined as curvilinear mediastinal vessels >1.5 mm in diameter, seen along the course of the proximal bronchial tree (34). In practice, given that the bronchial arteries are inconspicuous on CT in normal individuals, hypertrophied arteries are usually easily identified, especially on coronal reformatted projections (Figure 8.14). Bronchial artery hypertrophy occurs in approximately half the patients with CTEPH and only rarely in IPAH (35–37). The explanation for this seems to be due to the primary site of pulmonary vascular disease. In chronic thromboembolic disease, the distal circulation may be morphologically normal and therefore able to accommodate an increased collateral supply, whilst in IPAH the pathological process (plexogenic arteriopathy) is centered at arteriolar level. However, bronchial artery hypertrophy does occur with sufficient frequency in

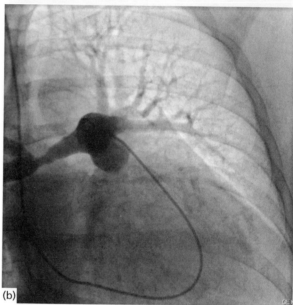

Figure 8.12   (a) CTPA of a patient with pulmonary hypertension due to large vessel vasculitis mimicking eccentric thrombus of CTEPH. (b) Pulmonary angiogram from the same patient showing narrowing and irregularity of central pulmonary arteries, thus mimicking CTEPH.

other causes of pulmonary hypertension, such as IPAH and Eisenmenger's syndrome, as to make it an unreliable sign on its own for the diagnosis of CTEPH (31).

Other vascular signs of CTEPH, visible on CT, are recanalization within intraluminal filling defects and arterial webs and stenoses (38) (Figures 8.15 and 8.16). These abnormalities often lie in the transaxial plane and, as such, are best demonstrated in multiplanar reformatted projections.

Cardiac signs

Cardiac abnormalities are readily appreciated with MDCT. Enlargement and hypertrophy of the right ventricle and atrium are common in patients with pulmonary hypertension, along with flattening or reversal of intraventricular septum (39,40) (Figure 8.17). However, it must be stressed,

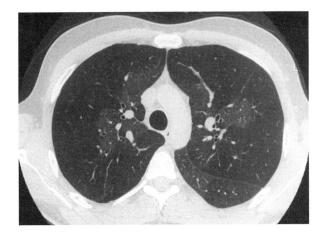

Figure 8.13 HRCT in a patient with CTEPH showing enlargement of segmental pulmonary arteries relative to their accompanying bronchi.

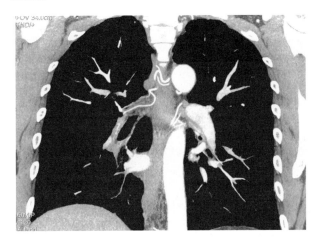

Figure 8.14 Coronal reformatted CT in a patient with CTEPH showing hypertrophied bronchial arteries in the mediastinum.

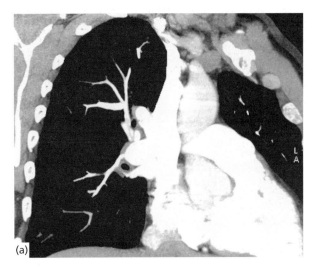

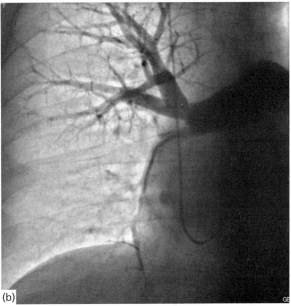

Figure 8.15 (a) Oblique coronal reformatted CT in a patient with CTEPH showing recanalization of the right interlobar artery. (b) Pulmonary angiogram from the same patient showing recanalization of the right interlobar artery.

the reliability of this CT sign in determining PA pressures in patients with mild or moderate pulmonary hypertension is unknown. The left ventricle is usually compressed and displaced posteriorly unless the pulmonary hypertension has developed secondary to left sided cardiac dysfunction; in which case, left atrial and ventricle dilatation may be present.

Reflux of contrast from the right atrium into the IVC during its first pass is another useful sign of pulmonary hypertension on CT (Figure 8.18). It occurs because of secondary tricuspid regurgitation in patients with pulmonary hypertension and the degree of reflux correlates with mPAP at RHC (41,42). Caution is required when interpreting this sign as IVC reflux may be seen in normal individuals when contrast injection rates exceed 3 mL/second (43). However, in routine practice, it is unusual to see reflux into the hepatic veins in patients without significant right heart dysfunction or tricuspid regurgitation.

Pericardial effusions are not an infrequent finding in pulmonary hypertension (44) (Figure 8.19). Their pathogenesis is unclear but they are usually refractory to diuretics and larger effusions are associated with evidence of heart failure, impaired exercise tolerance and poor prognosis. Smaller amounts of fluid (but still at least 10–15 mm in depth) within the anterior pericardial recess, have been reported to occur more frequently in patients with pulmonary hypertension than in normal individuals (45). This creates an infilling of the space between the main PA and the AA, resembling a "bikini bottom" (Figure 8.20). Again, it is important to remember that this sign is not specific for pulmonary hypertension.

Lung parenchyma

Mosaic pattern refers to regional differences in density of lung parenchyma. It is usually caused by patchy involvement of the lungs by infiltrative lung disease, small airways

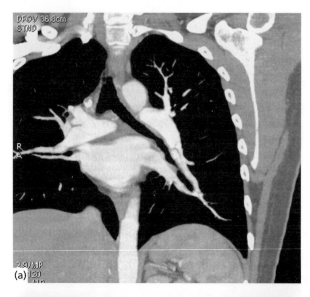

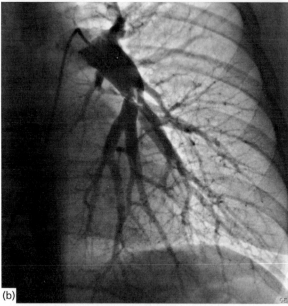

Figure 8.16   (a) Coronal reformatted CT in a patient with CTEPH showing a vascular web in the left interlobar artery. (b) Pulmonary angiogram from the same patient confirming the constriction/web at the branch point of the left interlobar artery.

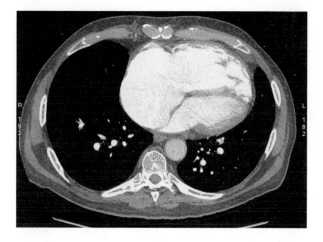

Figure 8.17   CT in a patient with IPAH showing dilated right atrium and ventricle (white arrows), flattening of the interventricular septum (black arrow) and posterior displacement and compression of left ventricle (broad white arrow).

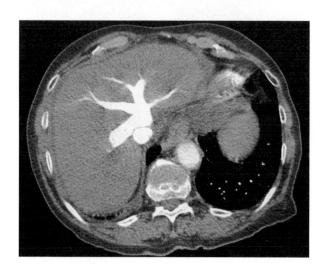

Figure 8.18   CT from a patient with IPAH showing reflux of contrast into the IVC and hepatic veins.

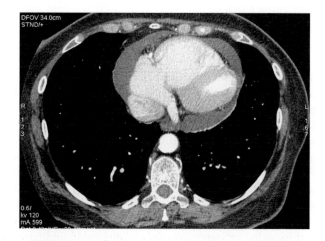

Figure 8.19   CT from a patient with IPAH (note large RV and displaced and compressed LV) showing a moderately large pericardial effusion (white arrows).

disease or CTEPH. In CTEPH, the mosaic pattern is caused by obliteration of parts of the vascular bed. This results in hypoperfusion with arteries of diminished size in some areas, and normal or increased perfusion with enlarged arteries in others; "mosaic oligemia" (Figure 8.21). In the context of pulmonary hypertension, this finding used to be considered virtually pathogneumonic of CTEPH (46). However, some studies have been published, albeit with small population sizes, which suggest that a mosaic pattern is not as uncommon in other causes of pulmonary hypertension as was previously thought (47–49).

In small airways disease (obliterative or constrictive bronchiolitis), focal hypoventilation and reflex vasoconstriction also give rise to mosaic oligemia. On expiratory

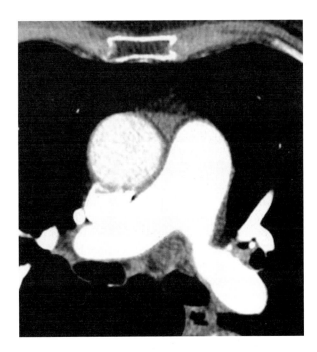

Figure 8.20 CT showing small amount of fluid in the anterior pericardial recess resembling a "bikini bottom".

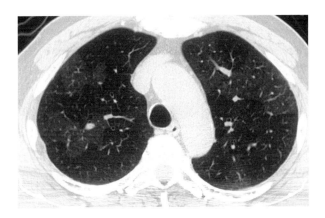

Figure 8.21 HRCT from a patient with CTEPH showing a mosaic pattern with a paucity of vascular markings in the "lucent" lung.

high resolution CT (HRCT) studies, these patients demonstrate air trapping, causing an increase in the conspicuity of the mosaic pattern (50). It used to be thought that a confident distinction between small airways disease and CTEPH could be made on the basis of expiratory HRCT studies. However, once again, this CT sign has to be interpreted with some caution as air trapping has also been reported in CTEPH (51,52). The mechanism is unclear, but it may be due to increased levels of the potent vasoconstrictor endothelin-1 in patients with pulmonary hypertension (51). In addition to air trapping, it is also recognized that bronchial dilatation, possibly related to ischemia, may also occur in areas of hypoperfusion in patients with CTEPH (52). Therefore, the presence of both small and large airway abnormalities (air trapping and bronchial dilatation), does

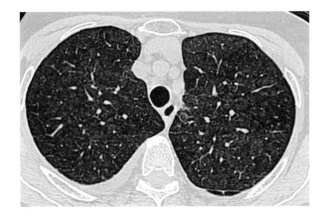

Figure 8.22 HRCT from a patient with PVOD showing multiple, small, ill-defined ground glass nodules scattered diffusely throughout both lungs. Note the small right pleural effusion (black arrow).

not allow reliable distinction to be made between CTEPH and primary airways disease. Nonetheless, most patients with CTEPH and mosaicism do not have air trapping and therefore expiratory HRCT studies are frequently helpful.

Small centrilobular ground-glass nodules are sometimes seen in patients with pulmonary arterial hypertension (Figure 8.22). There is no consensus as to their cause but possible explanations include cholesterol granulomas, hemorrhage and vascular proliferation (that is, direct visualization of large plexogenic arterial lesions) (49,53,54). Centrilobular ground-glass nodules and patching ground-glass opacity are a common finding in pulmonary veno-occlusive disease (PVOD) and capillary hemangiomatosis. However, unlike patients with pulmonary arterial hypertension, smooth interlobular septal thickening, pleural effusions and mediastinal lymphadenopathy are also characteristic features of PVOD (55,56) (Figure 8.23). Normal left sided cardiac chambers, and normal precapillary wedge pressure (PCWP) on right heart catheterization, allows distinction from other causes of pulmonary venous hypertension.

Peripheral lung parenchymal opacities are a common finding in CTEPH (57,58) (Figure 8.24). They represent pulmonary infarcts due to occlusion of segmental and smaller pulmonary arteries and therefore occur more commonly in "peripheral type" CTEPH than "central type."

Chronic thromboembolic pulmonary hypertension: CT findings and prediction of surgical outcome

The morbidity and mortality from pulmonary thromboendarterectomy has fallen steadily over the last 10–15 years. However, the procedure is still associated with significant mortality (approximately 10 percent) and fails to reduce pulmonary vascular resistance (PVR) in 10–15 percent of patients (57). A reliable method of predicting surgical success would clearly be of great value. The location and

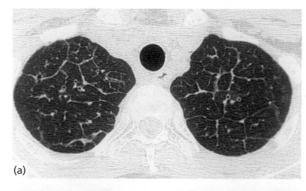

(a)

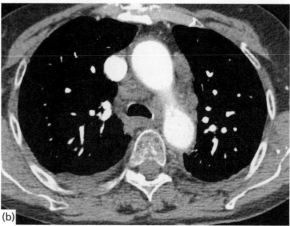

(b)

Figure 8.23 (a) HRCT from a patient with PVOD showing smooth interlobular septal thickening. (b) CT from a patient with PVOD showing mediastinal lymphadenopathy (white arrows) and small right pleural effusion (black arrow).

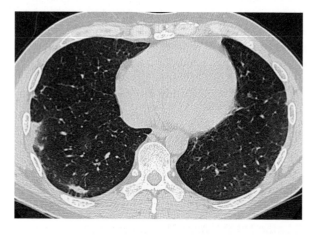

Figure 8.24 CT from a patient with CTEPH showing peripheral lung parenchymal opacities representing pulmonary infarcts.

extent of thromboembolic obstruction are the most critical determinants of operability. Occluding thrombus must involve the main, lobar or proximal segmental arteries. Persistent pulmonary hypertension and right ventricular failure occur when a substantial component of the hemodynamic impairment arises from thromboembolic obstruction that is beyond

the limits of surgical accessibility. In other words, an acceptable hemodynamic outcome requires that the preoperative hemodynamic impairment is due, in large part, to surgically accessible thromboembolic material.

CT is an excellent non-invasive method of directly visualizing thrombus in the central pulmonary arteries (Figure 8.10). However, the hemodynamic impairment in CTEPH is primarily caused by scar tissue in the pulmonary arteries which develops through organization of the original fresh thrombi. This may or may not be associated with overlying laminated thrombus. It is removal of the scar tissue, rather than removal of the chronic thrombus, which determines the hemodynamic improvement. Therefore, the absence of morphologically demonstrable central thrombus on CT scanning does not predict a poor hemodynamic outcome. However, when there is visible central thrombus, there is likely to be a good outcome (58,59).

Bronchial artery dilatation (Figure 8.14) is seen in approximately 50 percent of patients with CTEPH and only rarely in IPAH (35,36,37). There is no difference in the preoperative hemodynamics between patients with and without bronchial artery dilatation, indicating that elevated pulmonary artery pressure *per se* is not the stimulus for the development of bronchial artery dilatation. Postoperatively, it has been reported that patients with dilated bronchia arteries have a greater fall in pulmonary vascular resistance, suggesting that those patients without dilated bronchial arteries have a higher proportion of distal vascular disease (either distal thromboembolism or secondary small vessel arteriopathy) (7,36).

Peripheral subpleural densities (Figure 8.24) are a well known finding in patients with pulmonary emboli, which are thought to reflect previous episodes of infarction (57). A significant correlation between multiple peripheral densities and high postoperative pulmonary vascular resistance has been reported (independent of preoperative correlation). It has also been observed that pulmonary infarction is uncommon when central arteries are obstructed but frequent when peripheral arteries are occluded. It would therefore appear that patients with multiple peripheral densities have a greater proportion of distal artery occlusion which is surgically inaccessible.

As discussed above, dilatation of the main PA and a main PA to AA ratio of >1 are common findings in pulmonary hypertension which correlate with PA pressure (Figure 8.8). They do not, however, correlate with pulmonary vascular resistance. The measurements can therefore be used to support the diagnosis of pulmonary hypertension but cannot be used to predict postoperative hemodynamics (57–59).

It would therefore appear that the presence of bronchial artery dilatation and the absence of peripheral densities on preoperative CT are predictors of a good hemodynamic outcome post pulmonary artery thromboendarterectomy. When there is visible central thrombus, there is likely to be a good outcome but the absence of central thrombus does not predict an adverse result.

IMAGING PATHWAY

There is no perfect algorithm for imaging patients with suspected pulmonary hypertension. It is clear from the above discussion that there is no single radiographic sign, on any modality, which allows one to make a reliable diagnosis of raised PA pressure, never mind the underlying etiology. In any given patient, it is the *combination* of findings that is critical in increasing the confidence of the reporting radiologist. For example, one would hesitate to make a confident diagnosis of PH if the only abnormality was an enlarged main PA. However, the combination of an enlarged main PA with dilated right sided cardiac chambers, reflux of contrast into the IVC and fluid in the anterior pericardial recess, would be highly suggestive of PH. In routine clinical practice it is therefore usual to perform more rather than less imaging.

In our institution, patients with suspected pulmonary hypertension have a CXR and echocardiogram performed. If these examinations are abnormal, or even if they are normal but the clinical index of suspicion is high, then further imaging is indicated. Intravenous contrast enhanced MDCT examinations of the thorax are acquired in both the pulmonary arterial and systemic arterial phases of contrast enhancement. This allows optimal visualization of the pulmonary arterial tree as well as the heart and bronchial arteries. Depending on the findings in the lung parenchyma, in particular any suggestion of mosaicism, HRCT examinations are obtained in both inspiration and expiration. We find V/Q scintigraphy useful. A normal examination virtually excludes CTEPH, and in some patients with chronic thromboembolic disease the V/Q study may be high probability despite a normal CTPA (17). Conventional pulmonary angiography is the modality with the greatest spatial resolution and therefore gives the most information about the pulmonary vascular tree. It is performed whenever there is doubt regarding the possibility of CTEPH. In practice this is usually in differentiating "peripheral type" CTEPH and IPAH. Conventional pulmonary angiography is also performed whenever there is a confident diagnosis of CTEPH, as part of the pre-surgical work-up.

Cases of pulmonary hypertension are frequently complex and the imaging findings nonspecific. Therefore, when interpreting the imaging studies, the confidence one has in the significance of the various radiographic signs is influenced by the clinical context and physiological data. It is therefore of great benefit if the radiology is reviewed in a clinical-radiological meeting.

CONCLUSION

In recent years, several different therapies have been developed which are of proven benefit in both IPAH and pulmonary hypertension secondary to a range of cardiac and respiratory disorders. This has raised awareness of the possibility of pulmonary hypertension in patients presenting with nonspecific respiratory and cardiac symptoms and has highlighted the need for early and accurate diagnosis. The role of imaging is to confirm the diagnosis of pulmonary hypertension, assess the severity and determine the underlying etiology. In the case of CTEPH, it is important to assess surgical resectability and predict outcome. Patients with pulmonary hypertension may have a wide range of radiographic signs on CXR, V/Q scanning and CT; especially CT. Taken individually, these signs are frequently of limited value due to lack of sensitivity and specificity. This is especially true in milder forms of the disease when there may be considerable overlap between normal individuals and patients with pulmonary hypertension. However, when these signs are taken collectively, in the appropriate clinical context, it is usually possible to make a confident diagnosis.

KEY POINTS

- The role of imaging is to confirm the diagnosis of PH, assess the severity and suggest the underlying etiology.
- Patients with pulmonary hypertension may have a large number of radiographic signs. In isolation these signs are of limited value due to lack of sensitivity and specificity. It is the *combination* of findings that allow a confident diagnosis to be made.
- Due to the complexity of the cases, and the nonspecific nature of the imaging findings, it is of great value if the radiology is reviewed in a clinical–radiological meeting.

REFERENCES

1. Humbert M, Sitbon O, Simonneau G. Treatment of pulmonary arterial hypertension. N Engl J Med 2004;351:1425–36.
2. Barst RJ, Gibbs JSR, Ghofrani HA *et al.* Evidence based treatment algorithm in pulmonary arterial hypertension. J Am Coll Cardiol 2009;54:78–84.
3. Badesch DB, Champion HC, Sanchez MAG *et al.* Diagnosis and assessment of pulmonary arterial hypertension. J Am Coll Cardiol 2009;54:55–66.
4. Humbert M, Sitbon O, Chaouat A *et al.* Pulmonary arterial hypertension in France: results from a national registry. Am J Respir Crit Care Med 2006;173:1023–30.
5. Revin CE. Pulmonary vascularity: radiographic considerations. J Thorac Imaging 1988;3:1–14.
6. Randall PA, Heitzman ER, Bull NJ *et al.* Pulmonary hypertension: a contemporary review. RadioGraphics 1989;9:905–27.
7. Mallamo GT, Baum RS, Simon AL. Diffuse pulmonary artery calcifications in a case of Eisenmenger's syndrome. Radiology 1971;99:549–50.

8. Chang CH. The normal roentgenographic measurement of the right descending pulmonary artery in 1,085 cases. AJR Am J Roentgenol 1962;87:927–35.

9. Woodruff WW, Hoeck BE, Chitwood WR et al. Radiographic findings in pulmonary hypertension from unresolved embolism. AJR Am J Roentgenol 1985;144:681–6.

10. Chitwood WR, Sabiston DC, Wechsler AS. Surgical treatment of chronic unresolved pulmonary embolism. Clin Chest Med 1984;5:507–36.

11. Turner AF, Lau FYK, Jacobson G. A method for the estimation of pulmonary venous and arterial pressures from the routine chest roentgenogram. AJR Am J Roentgenol 1972;116:97–106.

12. Anderson G, Reid L, Simon G. The radiographic appearances in primary and thromboembolic pulmonary hypertension. Clin Radiol 1973;24:113–20.

13. Ormond RS, Drake EH, Hildner FJ. Pulmonary hypertension: an angiographic study. Radiology 1967;88:680–5.

14. Worsley DF, Palevsky HI, Alavi A. Ventilation–perfusion lung scanning in the evaluation of pulmonary hypertension. J Nucl Med 1994;35:793–6.

15. Fishman AJ, Moser KM, Fedullo PF. Perfusion lung scan versus pulmonary angiography in evaluation of suspected pulmonary hypertension. Chest 1983;84:679–83.

16. Bow JE, Palevsky HI, McCarthy KE et al. Pulmonary arterial hypertension: value of perfusion scintigraphy. Radiology 1987;164:727–30.

17. Tunariu N, Gibbs SJ, Win Z et al. Ventilation–perfusion scintigraphy is more sensitive than multidetector CTPA in detecting chronic thromboembolic pulmonary disease as a treatable cause of pulmonary hypertension. J Nucl Med 2007;48:680–4.

18. Berry DF, Buccigrossi D, Peabody J et al. Pulmonary vascular occlusion and fibrosing mediastinitis. Chest 1986;89:296–301.

19. Weisser K, Wyler F, Gloor F. Pulmonary veno-occlusive disease. Arch Dis Child 1967;42:322–7.

20. Martin K, Schnyder P, Schirg E et al. Pattern-based differential diagnosis in pulmonary vasculitis using volumetric CT. AJR Am J Roentgenol 2005;184:720–33.

21. Widera E. Pulmonary artery sarcoma misdiagnosed as chronic thromboembolic pulmonary hypertension. Mt Sinai J Med 2005;72:360–4.

22. Kuriyama K, Gamsu G, Stern RG et al. CT-determined pulmonary artery diameters in predicting pulmonary hypertension. Invest Radiol 1984;19:16–22.

23. Haimovici JB, Trotman-Dickenson B, Halpern EF et al. Relationship between pulmonary artery diameter at computed tomography and pulmonary artery pressures at right heart catheterization. Acad Radiol 1997;4:327–34.

24. Tan RT, Kuzo R, Goodman LR et al. Utility of CT scan evaluation for predicting pulmonary hypertension in patients with parenchymal lung disease. Chest 1998;113:1250–6.

25. Schmidt HC, Kauczor HU, Schild HH et al. Pulmonary hypertension in patients with chronic pulmonary thromboembolism: chest radiograph and CT evaluation before and after surgery. Eur Radiol 1996;6:817–25.

26. Edwards PD, Bull RK, Coulden R. CT measurement of main pulmonary artery diameter. Br J Radiol 1998;71:1018–20.

27. Ng CS, Wells AU, Padley SP. A CT sign of chronic pulmonary arterial hypertension: the ratio of main pulmonary artery to aortic diameter. J Thorac Imaging 1999;14:270–8.

28. Devaraj A, Hansell D. Computed tomography signs of pulmonary hypertension: old and new observations. Clin Radiol 2009;64:751–60.

29. Teigen CL, Maus TP, Sheedy PF et al. Pulmonary embolism: diagnosis with electron-beam CT. Radiology 1993;188:839–45.

30. Roberts HC, Kauczor HU, Schweden F et al. Spiral CT of pulmonary hypertension and chronic thromboembolism. J Thorac Imaging 1997;12:118–27.

31. Perloff K, Hart EM, Greaves SM et al. Proximal pulmonary arterial and intrapulmonary radiologic features of Eisenmenger syndrome and primary pulmonary hypertension. Am J Cardiol 2003;92:182–7.

32. Tan RT, Kuzo R, Goodman LR et al. Utility of CT scan evaluation for predicting pulmonary hypertension in patients with parenchymal lung disease. Medical College of Winsconsin Lung Transplant Group. Chest 1998;113:1250–6.

33. Riquet M. Bronchial arteries and lymphatics of the lung. Thorac Surg Clin 2007;17:619–38.

34. Remy-Jardin M, Duhamel A, Deken V et al. Systematic collateral supply in patients with chronic thromboembolic and primary pulmonary hypertension: assessment with multidetector row helical CT angiography. Radiology 2005;235:274–81.

35. Endrys J, Hayat N, Cherian G. Comparison of broncho-pulmonary collaterals and collateral blood flow in patients with chronic thromboembolic and primary hypertension. Heart 1997;78:171–6.

36. Shimizu H, Tanabe N, Terada J et al. Dilatation of bronchial arteries correlates with extent of central disease in patients with chronic thromboembolic pulmonary hypertension. Circ J 2008;72:1136–41.

37. Kauczor HU, Schwickert HC, Mayer E et al. Spiral CT of bronchial arteries in chronic thromboembolism. J Comput Assis Tomogr 1994;6:855–60.

38. Schwickert HC, Schweden F, Schild HH et al. Pulmonary arteries and pulmonary parenchyma in chronic pulmonary embolism: preoperative and post operative CT findings. Radiology 1994;191:351–7.

39. Bossone E, Duong-Wagner H, Paciocco G et al. Echocardiographic features of primary pulmonary hypertension. J Am Soc Echocardiogr 1999;12:655–62.

40. Reid JH, Murchison JT. Acute right ventricular dilatation: a new helical CT sign of massive pulmonary embolism. Clin Radiol 1998;53:694–8.

41. Daniels LV, Krummen BE, Blanchard DG. Echocardiography in pulmonary vascular disease. Cardiol Clin 2004;22:383–99.

42. Groves AM, Win T, Charman SC et al. Semi-quantitative assessment of tricuspid regurgitation on contrast-enhanced multidetector CT. Clin Radiol 2004;59:715–9.

43. Yeh BM, Kurzman P, Foster E, *et al.* Clinical relevance of retrograde inferior vena cava or hepatic vein opacification during contrast-enhanced CT. AJR Am J Roentgenol 204;183:1227–32.

44. Hinderliter AL, Willis PW, Long W *et al.* Frequency and prognostic significance of pericardial effusion in primary pulmonary hypertension. Am J Cardiol 1999;84:481–4.

45. Baque-Juston MC, Wells AU, Hansell DM. Pericardial thickening or effusion in patients with pulmonary artery hypertension: a CT study. AJR Am J Roentgenol 1999;172: 361–4.

46. Bergin CL, Rios G, King MA *et al.* Accuracy of high-resolution CT in identifying chronic pulmonary thromboembolic disease. AJR Am J Roentgenol 1996;166:1371–7.

47. Griffin N, Allen D, Wort J *et al.* Eisenmenger syndrome and idiopathic pulmonary arterial hypertension: do parenchymal lung changes reflect etiology? Clin Radiol 2007;62:587–95.

48. Sherrick AD, Swensen SJ, Hartman TE. Mosaic pattern of lung attenuation on CT scans: frequency among patients with pulmonary artery hypertension of different causes. AJR Am J Roentgenol 1997;169:79–82.

49. Chaudry G, MacDonald C, Aditia I *et al.* CT of the chest in the evaluation of idiopathic pulmonary arterial hypertension in children. Pediatr Radiol 2007;37:345–50.

50. Chen D, Webb WR, Storto ML *et al.* Assessment of air trapping using post-expiratory high resolution computed tomography. J Thorac Imaging 1998;13:135–43.

51. Arakawa H, Stern EJ, Nakamoto WT *et al.* Chronic pulmonary thromboembolism. Air trapping on computed tomography and correlation with pulmonary function tests. J Comput Assist Tomogr 2003;27:735–42.

52. Remy–Jardin M, Remy J, Louvegny *et al.* Airway changes in chronic pulmonary embolism: CT findings in 33 patients. Radiology 1997;203:355–60.

53. Nolan HP, McAdams, Sporn TA *et al.* Pulmonary cholesterol granulomas in patients with pulmonary artery hypertension: chest radiographic and CT findings. AJR Am J Roentgenol 1999;172:1317–9.

54. Horton MR, Tuder RM. Primary pulmonary arterial hypertension presenting as diffuse micronodules on CT. Crit Rev Comput Tomogr 2004;45:335–41.

55. Swensen SJ, Tashjian JH, Myers JL *et al.* Pulmonary veno-occlusive disease: CT findings in 8 patients. AJR Am J Roentgenol 1996;167:937–40.

56. Resten A, Maitre S, Humbert *et al.* Pulmonary hypertension: CT of the chest in pulmonary veno-occlusive disease. AJR Am J Roentgenol 2004;183:65–70.

57. Heinrich M, Uder M, Tscholl D *et al.* CT findings in chronic thromboembolic pulmonary hypertension: predictors of hemodynamic improvement after pulmonary thromboendarterectomy. Chest 2005; 127:1606–13.

58. Jamieson SW, Kapelanski DP, Sakakibara N *et al.* Pulmonary endarterectomy: experience and lessons learned in 1500 cases. Ann Thorac Surg 2003;76:1457–62.

59. Bergin CJ, Sirlin C, Deutsch R *et al.* Predictors of patient response to pulmonary thromboendarterectomy. AJR Am J Roentgenol 2000;174:509–15.

9

Imaging: Emerging modalities (MR, PET and others)

ANTON VONK-NOORDEGRAAF

INTRODUCTION

Accurate assessment of right ventricular (RV) and arterial structure and function in pulmonary hypertension (PH) is essential for several reasons:

1. First, since direct visualization of the effects of the disease on the vessel wall is not possible, the assessment of disease severity and monitoring of therapeutic effects is only possible by studying RV and pulmonary arterial function. Since the effects of treatment on right ventricular and pulmonary arterial function are small, a prerequisite for such measurements is that they are accurate, reproducible, observer independent, and do not require geometric assumptions.
2. Second, the primary cause of death in most types of PH is RV failure. The diagnosis of early RV failure is thus of great clinical importance. In addition, the mechanisms of RV failure are currently poorly understood and can only be unravelled if the complex interaction between altered RV structure and function and the pivotal role of myocardial perfusion and metabolism on these parameters can be elucidated.
3. Third, since it is known that most medications used in the field of pulmonary arterial hypertension, not only act on the pulmonary vasculature, but also have an effect on the myocardium, discrimination of the effects of PH medication on both the right ventricle and the pulmonary vasculature are important.

Magnetic resonance imaging (MRI) and nuclear techniques are both emerging techniques in the field of PH and offer novel possibilities to study the role of the RV in PH and the effects of treatment thereon. In addition, these techniques allow us to determine the role of the different factors involved in RV failure, and subsequently to develop new therapeutic strategies. This chapter provides an overview of the application of MRI and nuclear imaging techniques in the field of PH and discusses future possibilities.

MAGNETIC RESONANCE IMAGING

Quantification of right ventricular geometry and mass

In the early years of MRI, it was already recognized that this technique allows accurate measurement of the RV volume (1–3). Initially, the accuracy of global RV volume and function measurements was verified by using water-filled latex balloons and ventricular casts of excised bovine hearts (3).

In recent years, temporal and spatial resolution has been further improved, allowing more accurate quantification of global function of both the left and right ventricle and the complex interaction between both ventricles in PH (4,5). Short-axis images are used to reconstruct a 3D image of the right and left ventricle, allowing the measurements of ventricular volumes and wall mass at all moments in the cardiac cycle. Figure 9.1 shows short axis images covering the complete cardiac cycle made at the mid-ventricular level. Endocardial contours are drawn during post-processing on end-diastolic and end-systolic frames, and total LV and

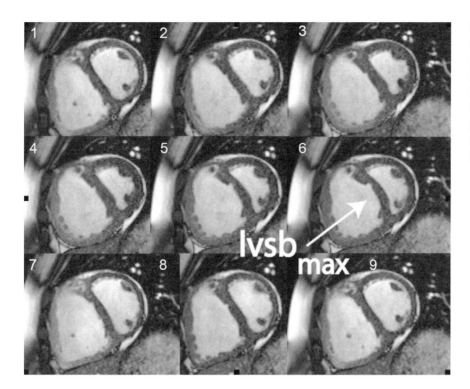

Figure 9.1 Short axis images covering the complete cardiac cycle made at the mid-ventricular level. The first image represents the end-diastolic phase. Leftward ventricular septal bowing (LVSB) is observed in the early diastolic phase of the left ventricle, while the right ventricle is still contracting (left-to-right ventricular asynchrony).

RV volumes are calculated using the so called "Simpson's rule," which takes into account the sum of individual slice volumes and the interslice gap. Left and right ventricular end-systolic volumes are subtracted from the end-diastolic volumes yielding stroke volumes. From the contours of epicardial and endocardial tracings ventricular wall volume is derived and wall mass is the product of myocardial volume and muscle density (1.05 g/cm^3). From the volume changes of the right ventricle over time, parameters of systolic and diastolic function can be derived (5–7). Previously the post-processing was time consuming since all the contours were drawn manually, but new software solutions make a semiautomatic analysis possible.

The accuracy and inter-study reproducibility of volume measurements using semi-automatic analysis has been validated in several reports (4,9–12) and appears to be superior to echocardiography (13). Another advantage of MRI-based ventricular measurements is that this technique does not require geometric assumptions and can also be assessed in a subset of patients difficult to study by means of echocardiography, such as is the case in COPD (14). Bottini *et al.* showed that estimates of RV mass measured by MR acquired pre-mortem in COPD patients corresponds closely with RV mass measured at autopsy (15).

The clinical value of the different MR parameters in PH has been assessed in several studies. Earlier studies by MRI revealed that in PH RV volumes at end-diastole and end-systole are increased together with an increase in RV mass, whereas left ventricular end-diastolic volume and stroke volume are decreased (2,3,16). As a consequence, RV ejection fraction is decreased, whereas left ventricular

ejection fraction is preserved or even increased (6,7,17). Figure 9.2 shows a long axis image of a healthy control and a patient with severe PH. Several studies showed that single MRI parameters of the RV are related to hemodynamic parameters and disease severity. For instance, two independent studies showed that MRI-measured right ventricular ejection fraction is inversely related to NT-proBNP (6,7) and that RV mass is related to pulmonary arterial pressure (18,19). In a group of 64 idiopathic PAH patients, van Wolferen showed that RV end-diastolic volume, stroke volume and left ventricular end-diastolic volume all measured at baseline conditions were strong predictors for first year mortality (19). Several studies have demonstrated the possibilities of MRI to monitor the effects of PAH therapy on the RV over time (20–23). In these studies, an increased RV stroke volume and a decrease in wall mass were associated with improvement of symptoms and 6-minute walking distance. In addition it was shown that a progressive dilation of the RV during therapy accompanied with a decrease in stroke volume is associated with a poor outcome (20).

The potential of MRI-derived parameters to be used as a primary end-point to compare different treatment strategies was demonstrated in the Seraph study; a randomized prospective study aimed to measure the different effects of bosentan and sildenafil on RV mass (24). This study demonstrated that sildenafil, in contrast to bosentan, reduces RV mass. This finding is of interest; since it underlines that MR provides additional insights in comparison to the functional parameters currently used to evaluate the efficacy of medication.

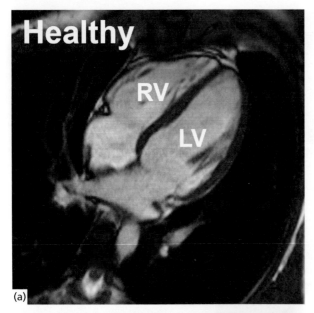

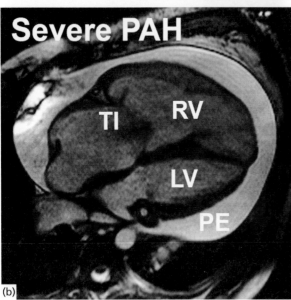

Figure 9.2   Long axis view of a healthy subject (a) and a patient with severe pulmonary arterial hypertension (b). RV, right ventricle; LV, left ventricle; PE, pleural effusion; TI, tricuspid regurgitation.

Advanced techniques to characterize the right ventricle

The MRI protocol can be extended with more advanced techniques that recently have been used in the study of the RV in PH. These techniques include delayed contrast enhancement to measure the presence of scar tissue in the RV wall, myocardial tagging to analyze regional myocardial shortening and measurement of coronary artery flow to the right ventricle.

- Delayed contrast enhancement (DCE) can be used to visualize and quantify the deposition of collagen in the

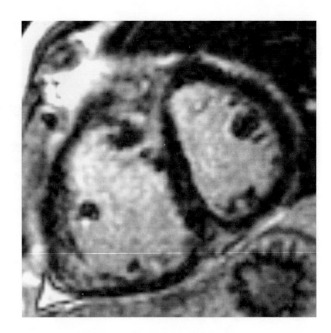

Figure 9.3   Delayed contrast enhancement in a scleroderma patient with pulmonary hypertension. This figure shows extensive delayed contrast enhancement at the insertion points.

RV myocardium. Delayed contrast enhancement imaging is performed about ten minutes after injection of MRI contrast agent. In healthy myocardium, the contrast agent then has been washed out, but in non-viable, damaged and fibrotic myocardium the contrast agent is still present. Thus, "bright is dead" with this technique. In two studies it was shown that abnormal DCE is present in the right ventricle and confined to the insertion points of the right ventricle and interventricular septum (25–27). Interestingly, these findings may suggest that mechanical factors contribute to the occurrence of fibrosis. The extent of contrast enhancement correlated in both studies associated positively with mean PAP, and pulmonary vascular resistance and was inversely related with RV ejection fraction. Figure 9.3 shows a typical example of delayed contrast enhancement in PAH.

- A method to study regional myocardial contraction patterns is myocardial tagging, allowing for the measurement of segmental myocardial strains. This method labels the myocardial tissue with parallel lines or a grid (typical distance 7 mm) of magnetic pre-saturation at the beginning of the cardiac cycle (R-wave of ECG). These lines remain visible as "dark" lines in MRI cine images, and thereby display the regional myocardial strains over the cardiac cycle by changes in the line- or grid-pattern. In PH, the RV myocardial wall is thick enough to explore RV contraction patterns by this technique, but in the non-hypertrophied RV wall spatial resolution of the technique is insufficient. This technique has been successfully used in the study of the mechanisms of ventricular interdependency (28–29). Results of these studies show that there is a left-to-right asynchrony in the peak of circumferential shortening,

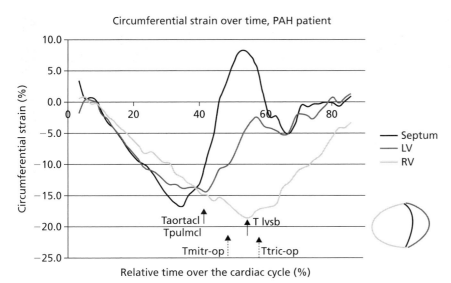

Circumferential strain over time, PAH patient

Figure 9.4 Circumferential strain curves after the electrocardiographic R-wave for the septum, right and left ventricle in a patient with severe pulmonary hypertension. MRI myocardial tagging is used to calculate the circumferential strain. From this image it is clear that time to right ventricular peak shortening is delayed in comparison to the left ventricle. As a consequence leftward septal bowing occurs. Note that right ventricular contraction continues after pulmonary valve closure leading to the so called end-systolic right ventricular isovolumetric shortening (adapted from Marcus JT *et al.* J Am Coll Cardiol 2008;51:750–7).

which is caused by RV overload and plays a role in the leftward septal bowing thereby impairing LV filling (Figure 9.4).

- Finally, advances in MR make it possible to visualize and measure coronary artery flow. From animal studies it is known that RV coronary perfusion is not or little impeded in systole. By using MR-based coronary flow assessment it was shown that in patients with right ventricular hypertrophy coronary arterial flow in systole is impeded, and in severe right ventricular hypertrophy even total mean flow to the right ventricle is reduced (30). Whether this reduction of coronary blood flow per gram might contribute to right ventricular failure is unknown.

Although the direct clinical value of these techniques is presently still uncertain, their application has advanced our understanding of RV function and failure and offers tools to increase our understanding in the near future.

Assessment of pulmonary artery flow and distensibility

Velocity encoded cine MRI provides an accurate and reproducible tool for quantification of pulmonary artery flow (31–33). Kondo *et al.* described in 1992 for the first time the application of this technique in PAH patients (34). It was found that in comparison to controls, flow acceleration time and distensibility of the pulmonary artery were decreased in patients with primary PAH, a finding similar to that observed in studies using Doppler echocardiography for measuring velocity flow. Several attempts have been made to estimate pulmonary artery pressure from the flow signal (35–37). However, a validation study performed by Roeleveld *et al.* showed that all these approaches fail to estimate pulmonary

arterial pressure sufficiently accurately (22). This can be explained by the fact that acceleration time is not only a parameter of the pulmonary vascular bed, but is also influenced by the pump function characteristics of the right ventricle.

The major advantage of flow measurements, however, is not the estimation of pulmonary artery pressure but the accurate assessment of effective stroke volume of the right ventricle from MRI flow measurement in the pulmonary artery (31–34). Stroke volume can be considered as one of the most important hemodynamic parameters in PAH, since it is a direct reflection of right ventricular function in relation to its increased afterload. Earlier studies showed that stroke volume is decreased in pulmonary hypertension and that exercise does not lead to an increase in stroke volume (38). In addition, it was shown that baseline stroke volume accurately predicts 6-minute walking distance in PAH and that improvements in stroke volume in patients under treatment are directly related to an improvement in the 6-minute walking distance (22,39). In addition it was shown that stroke volume derived from the pulmonary artery flow measured by MRI is a strong predictor of mortality in PAH (19).

Since the aorta flow can be measured in the same plane as the pulmonary artery flow, the ratio of right-to-left flow and vice versa can be used in the assessment of intracardiac shunts. Beerbaum *et al.* validated this MRI based shunt measurement approach, showing that right-to-left and left-to-right intracardiac shunts in children with congenital heart disease can be measured accurately in less than 60 seconds (33,40). A limitation of this technique is that in dilated pulmonary arteries turbulent flow can occur, causing an inaccuracy of the pulmonary blood flow estimates by MRI (40).

Another parameter that can be assessed from the flow measurements is the distensibility of the pulmonary artery. From invasive studies it is known that elasticity of the pulmonary vascular bed is decreased in advanced disease, and that this decrease is related to a poor outcome (41,42). Since compliance is quantitative measure of the elasticity of the large pulmonary vessels, this gives an important functional characterization of the vascular tree. Indeed, it was shown that loss of compliance of the large pulmonary vessels measured by MRI is related to a poor outcome (43).

Combining MRI flow measurements with invasive measurements

Measurement of the pulmonary vascular resistance requires an accurate assessment of pulmonary blood flow and pressure. Certain conditions, such as congenital heart disease might preclude a reliable invasive estimation of pulmonary blood flow. In these cases, combined MR measured flow with invasive measured pulmonary artery pressure, provides accurate estimations of pulmonary vascular resistance. In a group of 24 children with either suspected PAH or congenital heart disease it was shown that this approach provides more reliable data than invasive measurements (45).

Another application of the combined measurements of pressure and flow is the assessment of arterial input impedance (46,47), as a comprehensive representation of right ventricular load. Input impedance takes into account the pulsatile nature of blood flow and pressure and not only consists of pulmonary vascular resistance but also of compliance and characteristic impedance. The assessment of input impedance can only be obtained from spectral analysis of pressure and flow curves. Although the relevance of such measurements has been acknowledged for a long period of time, clinical application has been hampered by the requirement of simultaneous and instantaneous pulmonary pressure and flow, and sophisticated analysis techniques. With the advent of MR scanners in the catheterization laboratory (48–51), pressure and flow can be measured simultaneously; enabling advanced hemodynamic characterization of individual patients in clinical practice (52).

A limitation of the combined measurement of pressure and MR flow is that a right sided heart catheterization is still required and that for simultaneous measurements an interventional (X-)MRI suite together with a special catheterization set must be used. Thus although this approach can be of use in conditions where accurate invasive stroke volume measurement is not possible, or in experimental settings, it is unlikely that this type of measurement will be performed routinely in the near future.

MRI pulmonary angiography and perfusion measurements

Although digital subtraction angiography of the pulmonary artery is still regarded as the reference technique

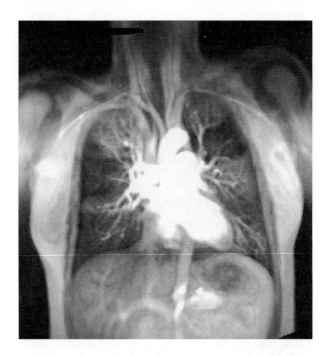

Figure 9.5 MR perfusion image of a patient with chronic thromboembolic pulmonary hypertension.

for the diagnosis of chronic thromboembolic pulmonary hypertension, recent studies showed that MR angiography is a sensitive non-invasive alternative for the depiction of central thromboembolic material (53). Typically, one static 3D image acquisition is performed, tailored for spatial resolution and signal to noise ratio during a breath-hold period of about 15 s. The advantage of MRI is not only that it provides high quality 3D images of the pulmonary vasculature, but also that these measurements can be combined with the assessment of right ventricular function and perfusion measurements (54) (Figure 9.5). MRI based dynamic pulmonary perfusion imaging is a technique visualizing the passage of a contrast bolus of an MRI-contrast agent through the lungs in a 3-dimensional way, enabling the visualization of sub-segmental perfusion defects in chronic thromboembolic PAH (54,55). In addition, post-processing of the perfusion images makes it possible to derive quantitative data from the dynamic perfusion scan such as pulmonary blood volume, flow and transit time defined as the time required for the contrast to transit through the lungs (56). Although it has been shown that all of these MRI derived parameters are directly related to hemodynamic parameters such as pulmonary artery pressure and cardiac output, accurate calculation of the main determinant of the pulmonary vascular bed, pulmonary vascular resistance, is not yet possible (57).

NUCLEAR TECHNIQUES

Nuclear techniques can be used for imaging the lung and the heart. The application of lung perfusion scintigraphy

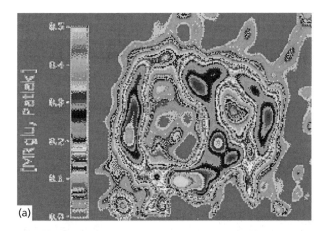

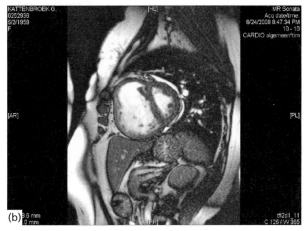

Figure 9.6   (a) Glucose consumption in the right and left ventricle as indicated as MRglu (metabolic rate of glucose (μmol/ml/min) measured by ¹⁸FDG-PET. (b) Corresponding short axis view measured by MRI.

in the diagnosis of chronic thromboembolic PH is well established, and its role is further discussed in Chapter 13. A refinement of perfusion scintigraphy is single photon emission computed tomography (SPECT). This technique enables the reconstruction of perfusion images in a way similar to the reconstruction of CT images, further improving the diagnostic accuracy of perfusion scintigraphy (58).

The role of nuclear techniques in the diagnosis of right ventricular failure is less well established despite the fact that these techniques play a pivotal role in the diagnosis of left heart disease. In the past ventricular angiography was frequently used to assess right ventricular volumes and function. Several approaches have been described to measure right ventricular volumes, including SPECT equilibrium radionuclide angiography (59,60). Despite the fact that these approaches provide reliable data on right ventricular volume, their role is limited and they have been replaced by echocardiography, MRI and computed tomography. Recent insights obtained by nuclear techniques are that the metabolic function of the right ventricle is altered in PAH. Several studies showed that in PH the uptake of

free fatty acids is decreased whereas the uptake of glucose is increased (61,62). In normal persons, glucose uptake in the right ventricle can barely be seen using positron emission tomography (PET) and fluoro-18-deoxyglucose (¹⁸FDG). Figure 9.6 shows an example of glucose consumption measured by ¹⁸FDG-PET in the right ventricle in a patient with severe PAH. This image shows that glucose uptake of the right ventricle exceeds glucose uptake of the left ventricle. Kluge *et al.* found that glucose uptake in the right ventricle is closely related to right ventricular function as measured by echocardiography indicating that a failing right ventricle switches from free fatty acids metabolism to glucose metabolism (63). In a study by Oikawa *et al.* it was shown that glucose uptake in the right ventricle can be reversed by epoprostenol therapy (64). Although the mechanisms responsible for this metabolic switch remain to be elucidated, one possibility is that RV ischemia might induce such changes. Gomez *et al.* showed by using stress myocardial scintigraphy that 9 of the 23 PAH patients examined had images consistent with RV ischemia (65). In addition, they found a significant correlation between RV ischemia obtained through myocardial perfusion scintigraphy and hemodynamic measures of RV failure, underpinning the possible contribution of ischemia to RV failure.

A future application of nuclear techniques in the field of PH is the use of radioligands to image the site of action of drugs and by that guide treatment decisions and monitoring. An example of such a ligand is [¹¹C]RAL-01PDE, a potential phosphodieseterase 5 ligand (66). In the study by Jacobsen *et al.* it was shown that this ligand binds to the binding site of PDE5 on the myocardium and lung. The results of this study showed that this ligand has the potential to quantify PDE5 expression in the lung of PAH patients and by that guide therapeutic decisions.

CONCLUDING REMARKS

Both MRI and nuclear techniques are promising emerging techniques in the field of pulmonary hypertension. MRI offers not only the possibility to measure accurately RV structure and function and its relation with changes in the pulmonary vasculature, but also provides information on morphological changes of the RV wall and coronary flow. In addition, although the role of MR is not defined yet, the advantage of MR to monitor PAH patients is presently well recognized by many clinicians. Table 9.1 summarizes the strength and weakness of MRI in comparison to echocardiography and right heart catheterization (67). Although nuclear techniques have not been frequently used in the study of RV failure, lessons learned from the left ventricle, especially with respect to perfusion and metabolism show that this modality can play an important role in the near future.

Table 9.1   A comparison of the usefulness of the different imaging modalities and RHC for characterizing different parameters

Parameter	Modality		
	Cardiac MRI	Echocardiography (Including 3-dimensional echocardiography)	RHC (Including right-sided angiocardiography)
RV assessment			
Volumes	+++	++	+
Ejection fraction	+++	++	+
Strain	+++	++	−
RV pressure	−/+	++	+++
Stroke volume	+++	+	+++
Mass	++	−/+	−
RV remodeling including septal curvature	+++	++	−
Tricuspid regurgitation	++	+++	+
Miscellaneous (pericardial effusion, pulmonary embolism, and other incidental findings)	++	+	+
RA assessment	++	+	−
RA pressure	−	−	+++
PA dimensions	+++	+	+
PA distensibility	+++	+	−/+
PA hemodynamics	−/+	+	+++
Quantitative lung flow	+++	−	−

−, not useful; +, may be useful; ++, useful; +++, extremely useful. MRI, magnetic resonance imaging; PA, pulmonary artery; RA, right atria; RHC, right heart catheterization; RV, right ventricle (adapted from: Benza R *et al.* J Am Coll Cardiol 2008;52:1683–92).

KEY POINTS

- MRI offers precise measures of right and left ventricular volume and mass.
- Stroke volume and right ventricular end-diastolic volume are key prognostic parameters in PAH. MRI can measure both parameters accurately.
- MR angiography and perfusion imaging of the lung can be combined.
- MR tagging is a technique to study right-to-left ventricular interaction in PAH.
- Delayed contrast imaging of the wall shows abnormal enhancement at the insertion points of the ventricular septum in PAH.
- Right ventricular perfusion can be measured by means of MRI and nuclear techniques.
- Increased FDG uptake and decreased RV perfusion of the right ventricle are indicators of right ventricular failure.
- The use of novel radioligands might be helpful to study the pathobiology of PAH in patients.

REFERENCES

1. Bouchard A, Higgins CB, Byrd BF 3rd, Amparo EG, Osaki L, Axelrod R. Magnetic resonance imaging in pulmonary arterial hypertension. Am J Cardiol 1985;56:938–42.

2. Katz J, Whang J, Boxt LM, Barst RJ. Estimation of right ventricular mass in normal subjects and in patients with primary pulmonary hypertension by nuclear magnetic resonance imaging. J Am Coll Cardiol 1993;21: 1475–81.

3. Boxt LM, Katz J, Kolb T, Czegledy FP, Barst RJ. Direct quantitation of right and left ventricular volumes with nuclear magnetic resonance imaging in patients with primary pulmonary hypertension. J Am Coll Cardiol 1992;19:1508–15.

4. Roeleveld RJ, Marcus JT, Fes TJ, Gan TJ, Boonstra A, Postmus PE, Vonk-Noordegraaf A. Interventricular septal configuration at MR imaging and pulmonary arterial pressure in pulmonary hypertension. Radiology 2005;234:710–7.

5. Gan CT, Lankhaar JW, Marcus JT, Westerhof N, Marques KM, Bronzwer JG, Boonstra A, Postmus PE, Vonk-Noordegraaf A. Impaired left ventricular filling due to right-to-left ventricular interaction in patients with pulmonary arterial hypertension. Am J Physiol Heart Circ Physiol 2006;290:H1528–33.

6. Gan CT, McCann GP, Marcus JT, van Wolferen SA, Twisk JW, Boonstra A, Postmus PE, Vonk-Noordegraaf A. NT-proBNP reflects right ventricular structure and function in pulmonary hypertension. Eur Respir J 2006;28:1190–4.

7. Blyth KG, Groenning BA, Mark PB, Martin TN, Foster JE, Steedman T, Morton JJ, Dargie HJ, Peacock AJ. NT-proBNP can be used to detect right ventricular systolic dysfunction in pulmonary hypertension. Eur Respir J 2007;29:737–44.

8. Gan TC, Holverda B, Marcus JT, Paulus WJ, Westerhof N, Marques KM, Bronzwer JGF, Boonstra A, Postmus PE, Vonk-Noordegraaf A. Right ventricular diastolic dysfunction in pulmonary arterial hypertension. Chest 2007;132:11–7.

9. Suzuki J, Caputo GR, Masui T, Chang JM, O'Sullivan M, Higgins CB. Assessment of right ventricular diastolic and systolic function in patients with dilated cardiomyopathy using cine magnetic resonance imaging. Am Heart J 1991;122:1035–40.

10. Doherty NE 3rd, Fujita N, Caputo GR, Higgins CB. Measurement of right ventricular mass in normal and dilated cardiomyopathic ventricles using cine magnetic resonance imaging. Am J Cardiol 1992;69:1223–28.

11. Semelka RC, Tomei E, Wagner S, Mayo J, Kondo C, Suzuki J, et al. Normal left ventricular dimensions and function: interstudy reproducibility of measurements with cine MR imaging. Radiology 1990;174:763–8.

12. Grothues F, Moon JC, Bellenger NG, Smith GS, Klein HU, Pennell DJ. Interstudy reproducibility of right ventricular volumes, function, and mass with cardiovascular magnetic resonance. Am Heart J 2004;147:218–23.

13. Grothues F, Smith GC, Moon JC, Bellenger NG, Collins P, Klein HU, Pennell DJ. Comparison of interstudy reproducibility of cardiovascular magnetic resonance with two-dimensional echocardiography in normal subjects and in patients with heart failure or left ventricular hypertrophy. Am J Cardiol 2002;90:29–34.

14. Vonk Noordegraaf A, Marcus JT, Holverda S, Roseboom B, Postmus PE. Early changes of cardiac structure and function in COPD patients with mild hypoxemia. Chest 2005;127:1898–903.

15. Bottini PB, Carr AA, Prisant, Calverley PM, Howatson R, Flenley DC, Lamb D. Clinicopathological correlations in cor pulmonale. Thorax 1992;47:494–8.

16. Pattynama PM, Willems LN, Smit AH, van der Wall EE, de Roos A. Early diagnosis of cor pulmonale with MR imaging of the right ventricle. Radiology 1992;182:375–9.

17. Marcus JT, Vonk Noordegraaf A, Roeleveld RJ, Postmus PE, Heethaar RM, Van Rossum AC, Boonstra A. Impaired left ventricular filling due to right ventricular pressure overload in primary pulmonary hypertension: noninvasive monitoring using MRI. Chest 2001;119:1761–5.

18. Saba TS, Foster J, Cockburn M, Cowan M, Peacock AJ. Ventricular mass index using magnetic resonance imaging accurately estimates pulmonary artery pressure. Eur Respir J 2002;20:1519–24.

19. Roeleveld RJ, Marcus JT, Boonstra A, Postmus PE, Marques KM, Bronzwer JG, Vonk-Noordegraaf A. A comparison of noninvasive MRI-based methods of estimating pulmonary artery pressure in pulmonary hypertension. J Magn Reson Imaging 2005;22:67–72.

20. Van Wolferen SA, Marcus JT, Boonstra A, Marques KM, Bronzwer JG, Spreeuwenberg MD, Postmus PE, Vonk-Noordegraaf A. Prognostic value of right ventricular mass, volume, and function in idiopathic pulmonary arterial hypertension. Eur Heart J 2007;28:1250–7.

21. Michelakis ED, Tymchak W, Noga M, Webster L, Wu XC, Lien D, Wang SH, Modry D, Archer SL. Long-term treatment with oral sildenafil is safe and improves functional capacity and hemodynamics in patients with pulmonary arterial hypertension. Circulation 2003;108:2066–9.

22. Roeleveld RJ, Vonk-Noordegraaf A, Marcus JT, Bronzwer JG, Marques KM, Postmus PE, Boonstra A. Effects of epoprostenol on right ventricular hypertrophy and dilatation in pulmonary hypertension. Chest 2004;125:572–9.

23. Van Wolferen SA, Boonstra A, Marcus JT, Marques KM, Bronzwer JG, Postmus PE, Vonk-Noordegraaf A. Right ventricular reverse remodelling after sildenafil in pulmonary arterial hypertension. Heart 2006;92:1860–1.

24. Wilkins MR, Paul GA, Strange JW, Tunariu N, Gin-Sing W, Banya WA, Westwood MA, Stefanidis A, Ng LL, Pennell DJ, Mohiaddin RH, Nihoyannopoulos P, Gibbs JS. Sildenafil versus Endothelin Receptor Antagonist for Pulmonary Hypertension (SERAPH) study. Am J Respir Crit Care Med 2005;171:1292–7.

25. Blyth KG, Groenning BA, Martin TN, Foster JE, Mark PB, Dargie HJ, Peacock AJ. Contrast enhanced-cardiovascular magnetic resonance imaging in patients with pulmonary hypertension. Eur Heart J 2005;26:1993–9.

26. McCann GP, Beek AM, Vonk-Noordegraaf A, van Rossum AC. Delayed contrast-enhanced magnetic resonance imaging in pulmonary arterial hypertension. Circulation 2005;112:e268.

27. McCann GP, Gan CT, Beek AM, Niessen HW, Vonk-Noordegraaf A, van Rossum AC. Extent of MRI delayed enhancement of myocardial mass is related to right ventricular dysfunction in pulmonary artery hypertension. Am J Roentgenol 2007;188:349–55.

28. Vonk-Noordegraaf A, Marcus JT, Gan CT, Boonstra A, Postmus PE. Interventricular mechanical asynchrony due to right ventricular pressure overload in pulmonary hypertension plays an important role in impaired left ventricular filling. Chest 2005;128(6 Suppl):628S–30S.

29. Marcus JT, Gan CT, Zwanenburg JJ, Boonstra A, Allaart CP, Götte MJ, Vonk-Noordegraaf A. Interventricular mechanical asynchrony in pulmonary arterial hypertension: left-to-right delay in peak shortening is related to right ventricular overload and left ventricular underfilling. J Am Coll Cardiol 2008;51:750–7.

30. Van Wolferen SA, Marcus JT, Westerhof N, Spreeuwenberg MD, Marques KM, Bronzwer JG, Henkens IR, Gan CT, Boonstra A, Postmus PE, Vonk-Noordegraaf A. Right coronary artery flow impairment in patients with pulmonary hypertension. Eur Heart J 2008;29:120–7.

31. Rebergen SA, van der Wall EE, Doornbos J, de Roos A. Magnetic resonance measurement of velocity and flow: technique, validation, and cardiovascular applications. Am Heart J 1993;126:1439–56.

32. Fratz S, Hess J, Schwaiger M, Martinoff S, Stern HC. More accurate quantification of pulmonary blood flow by magnetic resonance imaging than by lung perfusion scintigraphy in patients with Fontan circulation. Circulation 2002;106:1510–3.

33. Beerbaum P, Korperich H, Barth P, Esdorn H, Gieseke J, Meyer H. Noninvasive quantification of left-to-right shunt in pediatric patients: phase-contrast cine magnetic resonance imaging compared with invasive oximetry. Circulation 2001;103:2476–82.

34. Kondo C, Caputo GR, Masui T, Foster E, O'Sullivan M, Stulbarg MS, Golden J, Catterjee K, Higgins CB. Pulmonary hypertension: pulmonary flow quantification and flow profile analysis with velocity-encoded cine MR imaging. Radiology 1992;183:751–8.

35. Muthurangu V, Taylor A, Andriantsimiavona R, Hegde S, Miquel ME, Tulloh R, Baker E, Hill DLG, Razavi RS. Novel method of quantifying pulmonary vascular resistance by use of simultaneous invasive pressure monitoring and phase-contrast magnetic resonance flow. Circulation 2004;110:826–34.

36. Bogren HG, Klipstein RH, Mohiaddin RH, Firmin DN, Underwood SR, Rees RS, Longmore DB. Pulmonary artery distensibility and blood flow patterns: a magnetic resonance study of normal subjects and of patients with pulmonary arterial hypertension. Am Heart J 1989;118:990–99.

37. Laffon E, Vallet C, Bernard V, Montaudon M, Ducassou D, Laurent F, Marthan R. A computed method for noninvasive MRI assessment of pulmonary arterial hypertension. J Appl Physiol 2004;96:463–8.

38. Holverda S, Gan CT-J, Marcus JT, Postmus PE, Boonstra A, Vonk-Noordegraaf A. Impaired stroke volume response to exercise in pulmonary arterial hypertension. J Am Coll Cardiol 2006;47:1732–3.

39. Provencher S, Chemla D, Hervé P, Sitbon O, Humbert M, Simonneau G. Heart rate responses during the 6-minute walk test in pulmonary arterial hypertension. Eur Respir J 2006;27:114–20.

40. Beerbaum P, Korperich H, Gieseke J, Barth P, Peuster M, Meyer H. Rapid left-to-right shunt quantification in children by phase-contrast magnetic resonance imaging. combined with sensitivity encoding (SENSE). Circulation 2003;108:1355–61.

41. Mauritz GJ, Marcus JT, Boonstra A, Postmus PE, Westerhof N, Vonk-Noordegraaf A. Non-invasive stroke volume assessment in patients with pulmonary arterial hypertension: left-sided data mandatory. J Cardiovasc Magn Reson 2008;10:51.

42. Mahapatra S, Nishimura RA, Sorajja P, Cha S, McGoon MD. Relationship of pulmonary arterial capacitance and mortality in idiopathic pulmonary arterial hypertension. J Am Coll Cardiol 2006;47:799–803.

43. Lankhaar JW, Westerhof N, Fes TJ, Gan CT, Marques KM, Boonstra A, van den Berg FG, Postmus PE, Vonk-Noordegraaf A. Pulmonary vascular resistance and compliance stay inversely related during treatment of pulmonary hypertension. Eur Heart J 2008;29:1688–95.

44. Gan CT, Lankhaar JW, Westerhof N, Marcus JT, Becker A, Twisk JW, Boonstra A, Postmus PE, Vonk-Noordegraaf A. Noninvasively assessed pulmonary artery stiffness predicts mortality in pulmonary arterial hypertension. Chest 2007;132:1906–12.

45. Razavi R, Hill DL, Keevil SF, Miquel ME, Muthurangu V, Hegde S, Rhode K, Barnett M, van Vaals J, Hawkes PD, Baker E. Cardiac catheterisation guided by MRI in children and adults with congenital heart disease. Lancet 2003;362:1877–82.

46. Murgo JP, Westerhof N. Input impedance of the pulmonary arterial system in normal man. Effects of respiration and comparison to systemic impedance. Circ Res 1984;54:666–73.

47. Grant BJ, Paradowski LJ. Characterization of pulmonary arterial input impedance with lumped parameter models. Am J Physiol 1987;252:H585–93.

48. Kuehne T, Yilmaz S, Schulze-Neick I, Wellnhofer E, Ewert P, Nagel E, Lange P. Magnetic resonance imaging guided catheterisation for assessment of pulmonary vascular resistance: in vivo validation and clinical application in patients with pulmonary hypertension. Heart 2005;91:1064–9.

49. Bock M, Muller S, Zuehlsdorff S, Speier P, Fink C, Hallscheidt P, Umathum R, Semmler W. Active catheter tracking using parallel MRI and real-time image reconstruction. Magn Reson Med 2006;55:1454–9.

50. Muthurangu V, Atkinson D, Sermesant M et al. Measurement of total pulmonary arterial compliance using invasive pressure monitoring and MR flow quantification during MR guided cardiac catheterization. Am J Physiol Heart Circ Physiol 2005;289:H1301–6.

51. Gaynor SL, Maniar HS, Bloch JB, Steendijk P, Moon MR. Right atrial and ventricular adaptation to chronic right ventricular pressure overload. Circulation 2005;112:1212–8.

52. Lankhaar JW, Westerhof N, Fes TJC, Marques KM, Marcus JT, Postmus PE, Vonk-Noordegraaf A. Quantification of right ventricular afterload in patients with and without pulmonary hypertension. Am J Physiol Heart Circ Physiol 2006;291:H1731–7.

53. Kreitner KF, Ley S, Kauczor HU, Mayer E, Kramm T, Pitton MB, Krummenauer F, Thelen M. Chronic thromboembolic pulmonary hypertension: pre- and postoperative assessment with breath-hold MR imaging techniques. Radiology 2004;232:535–43.

54. Nikolaou K, Schoenberg SO, Attenberger U et al. Pulmonary arterial hypertension: diagnosis with fast perfusion MR imaging and high-spatial-resolution MR angiography – preliminary experience. Radiology 2005;236(2):694–703.

55. Ley S, Fink C, Zaporozhan J, Borst MM et al. Value of high spatial and high temporal resolution magnetic resonance angiography for differentiation between idiopathic and thromboembolic pulmonary hypertension: initial results. Eur Radiol 2005;15(11):2256–63.

56. Ohno Y, Hatabu H, Murase K et al. Quantitative assessment of regional pulmonary perfusion in the entire lung using three-dimensional ultrafast dynamic contrast-enhanced magnetic resonance imaging: preliminary experience in 40 subjects. J Magn Reson Imaging 2004;20:353–65.

57. Ohno Y, Koyama H, Nogami M et al. Dynamic perfusion MRI: capability for evaluation of disease severity and

progression of pulmonary arterial hypertension in patients with connective tissue disease. J Magn Reson Imaging 2008;28:887–99.

58. Harris B, Bailey D, Miles S *et al.* Objective analysis of tomographic ventilation–perfusion scintigraphy in pulmonary embolism. Am J Respir Crit Care Med 2007;175:1173–80.

59. Schulman DS. Assessment of the right ventricle with radionuclide techniques. J Nucl Cardiol 1996;3:253–64.

60. Nichols K, Saouaf R, Ababneh AA *et al.* Validation of SPECT equilibrium radionuclide angiographic right ventricular parameters by cardiac magnetic resonance imaging. J Nucl Cardiol 2002;9:153–60.

61. Matsushita T, Ikeda S, Miyahara Y *et al.* Use of [123I]-BMIPP myocardial scintigraphy for the clinical evaluation of a fatty-acid metabolism disorder of the right ventricle in chronic respiratory and pulmonary vascular disease. J Int Med Res 2000;28:111–23.

62. Nagaya N, Goto Y, Satoh T *et al.* Impaired regional fatty acid uptake and systolic dysfunction in hypertrophied right ventricle. J Nucl Med 1998;39:1676–80.

63. Kluge R, Barthel H, Pankau H *et al.* Different mechanisms for changes in glucose uptake of the right and left ventricular myocardium in pulmonary hypertension. J Nucl Med 2005;46:25–31.

64. Oikawa M, Kagaya Y, Otani H *et al.* Increased [18F] fluorodeoxyglucose accumulation in right ventricular free wall in patients with pulmonary hypertension and the effect of epoprostenol. J Am Coll Cardiol 2005;45: 1849–55.

65. Gomez A, Bialostozky D, Zajarias A, Santos E, Palomar A, Martinez ML, Sandoval J. Right ventricular ischemia in patients with primary pulmonary hypertension. J Am Coll Cardiol 2001;38:1137–42.

66. Jakobsen S, Kodahl GM, Olsen AK, Cumming P. Synthesis, radiolabeling and in vivo evaluation of [11C]RAL-01, a potential phosphodiesterase 5 radioligand. Nucl Med Biol 2006;33:593–7.

67. Benza R, Biederman R, Murali S, Gupta H. Role of cardiac magnetic resonance imaging in the management of patients with pulmonary arterial hypertension. J Am Coll Cardiol 2008;52:1683–92.

10

Exercise testing and pulmonary hypertension: Six-minute walk testing and cardiopulmonary exercise testing*

DANIEL DUMITRESCU AND RONALD J OUDIZ

PULMONARY HYPERTENSION: IMPORTANCE OF DIAGNOSTIC ASSESSMENT DURING EXERCISE

Pulmonary hypertension is not only a disease whose pathology is limited to the pulmonary vasculature. The consequences of increased pressure in the pulmonary circulation affect right ventricular function, cardiopulmonary gas exchange, oxygen (O_2) transport and peripheral muscle metabolism. Indeed, at rest, there are reserves in cardiac function, pulmonary vascular capacity and energy stores for ATP regeneration in the peripheral muscles, so that impairments in one or more of these systems may not be recognized at rest. Only during exercise can cardiopulmonary reserve be challenged, so that even slight limitations in O_2 uptake, transport or metabolism can be revealed at this stage.

SUBMAXIMAL AND MAXIMAL EXERCISE TESTING

Metabolic adaptations to exercise vary with the work intensity, or from a physiologic point of view, with the availability of O_2 in the exercising muscles. During moderate exercise, the generation of high-energy phosphate (ATP) for muscle contraction is O_2 flow-independent. Arterial capillary O_2 content is higher than the O_2 demand in the muscles, so that nutritional substrates (carbohydrates, fatty acids, proteins) can be aerobically metabolized. With higher work intensity, exceeding this range, O_2 demand exceeds the available arterial O_2 content, so that even maximal O_2 extraction up to the critical capillary partial pressure of O_2 (about 14–22 mmHg) will lead to an O_2 deficit (28). Substrates will be anaerobically metabolized, meaning that ATP will be generated faster, but with less than 20 percent efficiency relative to aerobic metabolism. During anaerobic metabolism, lactate is produced, lowering blood pH, increasing ventilatory drive, and further stressing metabolism. While aerobic metabolism can be sustained for long periods of time, anaerobic metabolism is not sustainable.

The range in which aerobic metabolism is sufficient to sustain the required exercise level can be variable, so that the terms "moderate" and "heavy" exercise are relative for each individual. Sedentary subjects have a lower anaerobic threshold (*AT*) than physically active subjects, because ATP regeneration is not as effective in the untrained vs. the

---

*Abbreviations: $\dot{V}E$, minute ventilation (L); HR, heart rate (1/min) = oxygen uptake (L/min); $\dot{V}CO_2$, carbon dioxide output (L/min); O_2 pulse, oxygen pulse, equals $\dot{V}O_2 \div$ HR (mL O_2/min); $\dot{V}E/\dot{V}O_2$, ventilatory equivalent for oxygen (no unit); $\dot{V}E/\dot{V}CO_2$, ventilatory equivalent for carbon dioxide (no unit); VC, vital capacity (L); IC, inspiratory capacity (L); MVV, maximum voluntary ventilation (L/min); RER, respiratory exchange ratio, equals $\dot{V}CO_2 \div \dot{V}O_2$; $P_{ET}O_2$, end-expiratory oxygen partial pressure (mmHg); $P_{ET}CO_2$, end-expiratory carbon dioxide partial pressure (mmHg).

trained muscle. Patients with significant cardiac, pulmonary or pulmonary vascular impairment also have a significantly reduced AT, as O_2 uptake and/or O_2 transport are impaired, further exacerbated by physical inactivity as a consequence of their disease.

During maximum exercise, the ability to increase cardiac output (cardiac reserve) reaches a minimum whereby additional pulmonary vascular bed cannot be recruited, and ventilation is optimized to perfusion in the lungs. When one of these functions is impaired, maximal exercise is reached earlier because compensatory cardiac, ventilatory, and pulmonary vascular mechanisms are only operational at submaximal exercise levels, when significant reserves are still present.

Submaximal exercise testing is easier to perform than maximal exercise testing. Submaximal exercise requires less time and is safer in patients with cardiopulmonary disease than maximal exercise. Submaximal exercise can provide a good estimate of disease severity, and can be an objective method for differentiating between mild and more severe stages of pulmonary hypertension. Maximal exercise testing is a more complex procedure, in technical terms as well as in terms of duration and interpretation of results.

In patients with pulmonary hypertension, the most common tests used in clinical practice as well as in clinical trials are the six-minute walk (6MW) test, as a submaximal testing procedure, and cardiopulmonary exercise testing (CPET), as a submaximal or maximal test of exercise capacity, depending on the exercise protocol.

SIX-MINUTE WALK TESTING

Performing the test

The 6MW test is an unencouraged, self-paced test to determine submaximal exercise capacity, and has been used as a surrogate for peak VO_2 (27). Patients are asked to walk on a flat surface for six minutes, covering as much distance as possible at their own pace without running or jogging. Typically, dyspnea at the completion of the test is rated by the patients as a score on the Borg scale, ranging from 0 (no breathlessness at all) to 10 (maximal breathlessness) (1). The test can be performed by physicians or technicians with training on the methodology, and does not require equipment other than a marked hallway of at least 100 ft in length and a chronometer. It is recommended that a mobile chair and an oxygen source as well as an emergency cart be made available in the immediate proximity to the test site. The 6MW test can be performed with supplemental O_2; however if supplemental O_2 is needed and serial measurements are planned, it is important to perform all tests with the same equipment and at the same O_2 flow rate where possible, so that fair comparisons between tests can be made. Pulse oximetry can be measured during the 6MW test; however the pulse oximeter should be lightweight and held

in place so that the patient is not required to focus on handling the device during the test. The technician should not follow the patient to obtain oximetry measurements, so as not to interfere with the patient's test performance. Patients should be given adequate time for resting before starting the test. The use of a treadmill instead of a hallway to administer the 6MW test is not recommended according to recent guidelines (1).

Normal 6MW values

Age, sex, height and weight may influence 6MW distance, thus these factors should be taken into consideration when interpreting a 6MW test. However, there are no published recommendations for correcting the 6MW distance for these factors in healthy subjects or in patients. In addition, there are no reference values defining a normal 6MW distance. In one study, the lowest reported median value for a healthy population was 580 m for men and 500 m for women (2). Other smaller studies have reported distances of 630 m in a healthy elderly population (3), and 698 m in a population ranging in age between 20 and 80 years old, however in this latter study, subjects were tested four times in one day (4).

The short-term reproducibility of the 6MW test under standardized conditions is excellent (5); however a learning effect has been described, whereby test results improve in consecutive tests, with the greatest difference between tests occurring between the first and the third test (6).

Value of the 6MW for clinical practice

The 6MW test is a simple, reliable and cost-effective test which correlates with severity of the disease in patients with pulmonary hypertension (2). However, there are little data on how to best document improvement in walking distance. It is common practice to document change in 6MW distance as an absolute change rather than as a relative change.

6MW results must be carefully interpreted, as the 6MW test is nonspecific and does not provide physiologic information. The 6MW distance thus must be interpreted in the context of the patient's clinical status, and with other diagnostic findings, such as hemodynamics, echocardiography, pulmonary function tests, cardiopulmonary exercise testing, and/or or biomarker measurements. Further, a reduced 6MW distance must be thoroughly evaluated since there are many causes of reduced exercise capacity, such as musculoskeletal abnormalities which may impair walking.

Slight changes in 6MW distance correlate better with clinical status in patients with severe pulmonary hypertension, rather than in cases of milder disease (26). This may be attributed to the fact that the 6MW test becomes an almost maximal exercise test in these patients, and that they reproducibly exhaust their pulmonary vascular and cardiac reserves while walking, so that these patients are not able to vary their walking speed as much as patients with mild disease.

The distance walked during a 6MW test has prognostic value in patients with PAH. It has been shown that a walking distance < 330 m is associated with higher mortality (2). Another trial demonstrated worse outcome for patients with a 6MWD of 380 m or less after initiation of epoprostenol therapy (7).

Value of 6MW testing for clinical trials

The 6MW test has been widely used as an outcome measure in clinical trials for chronic lung and heart diseases. In most trials done for regulatory approval of drugs to treat pulmonary arterial hypertension, the primary endpoint has been improvement in 6MW distance (8–11). Despite the nonspecific nature of the test, general improvements in functional capacity appear to be reliably detectable with the test, although statistically significant differences in walking distance are generally of smaller magnitude than what may be considered clinically relevant differences for individual patients. Finally, the short time required to administer the 6MW test and its small cost have contributed to the popularity of the test.

Limitations of six-minute walk testing

The major disadvantage of 6MW testing is the fact that it evaluates exercise capacity generically; it does not yield any specific information regarding a patient's underlying disease process. Improvement or worsening can be attributed to a variety of factors such as patient motivation, learning effect, and other etiologies of impaired ability to walk. This is especially important in pulmonary hypertension patients with concomitant diseases such as scleroderma. The utility of the absolute walking distance may be hampered by factors such as Raynaud's-related pain and/ or joint pain affecting the ability to walk in these patients. Serial measurements over time may be more reliable, however they always have to be evaluated in the clinical context together with other findings and must be critically interpreted.

CARDIOPULMONARY EXERCISE TESTING

Methodological aspects

CPET is a non-invasive assessment of cardiopulmonary and metabolic adaptations to exercise. At rest, and at defined workloads on a cycle ergometer or a treadmill, parameters of cardiac, ventilatory and pulmonary vascular function are continuously recorded and analyzed. In addition to classical stress ergometry measurements such as ECG, blood pressure and peripheral O_2 saturation recordings,

gas exchange is measured on a breath-by-breath basis. This integrative test can therefore be used for performance diagnostics as well as for detection and evaluation of heart and lung diseases (12).

Gas exchange measurement systems primarily measure air flow and minute ventilation ($\dot{V}E$), O_2 uptake ($\dot{V}CO_2$), carbon dioxide output ($\dot{V}O_2$), and the end expiratory partial pressures for O_2 ($P_{ET}O_2$) and for carbon dioxide ($P_{ET}CO_2$).

CPET is widely used for performance diagnostics in athletes, however it is also useful for a variety of clinical applications and serves in determining the cause for exercise intolerance, as well as for quantifying the extent of cardiopulmonary limitation in exercise performance (13–15).

Therefore, CPET serves several important functions in pulmonary hypertension. For the initial evaluation of patients who are suspected to have pulmonary hypertension, and for the evaluation of patient groups at high risk of developing pulmonary hypertension, CPET is an important tool for early detection of the disease, and for differential diagnosis. In patients with known pulmonary hypertension, CPET can provide important information on the effectiveness of treatment and on the pathophysiological mechanisms of treatment effects (29). Furthermore, CPET allows risk stratification for pulmonary hypertension patients and is able to generate prognostic information (19).

Performing the test

Cardiopulmonary exercise testing should require physical examination of the patient, both for safety considerations, for evaluating contraindications to exercise, and for obtaining a focused medical history and medication list, which complement the interpretation of the results. CPET can be performed on a cycle ergometer or a treadmill. For patients with pulmonary hypertension, a cycle ergometer may be safer than treadmill exercise for patients that may not be able to keep up with the incremental speed increases of the treadmill and for those at risk of falling. For diagnostic purposes, a ramp test, in which the work rate (WR) is incremental, is preferable to a constant WR test, as a ramp test helps describe adaptation to low, moderate and high work intensities. Additionally, the determination of the anaerobic threshold (*AT*) during constant WR test may be more difficult to determine the *AT* than with a ramp test.

The slope of the WR incrementation (ramp) should be chosen with the aim of achieving an exercise time of about 6–10 minutes (16), and should be maintained at the same rate for each follow-up test, if clinically possible. This ensures the ability to make comparison between tests in a simple way. There is no consensus on whether or not patients should be encouraged during the test, however a very cautious approach is highly suggested, since patients with pulmonary hypertension might exceed their right ventricular output reserves with encouragement, and may acutely decompensate clinically. Unfortunately, submaximal tests may be a major source of result misinterpretation. Therefore, it is important to document the reason for stopping in any test, and to determine whether a maximal test was reached or not. In particular, patients with concomitant medical problems may stop exercising before reaching their maximum exercise capacity, so that proper documentation of peak exercise is essential.

Pathophysiological mechanisms and patterns in CPET

Pulmonary hypertension is a heterogenous disease – the consequence of a pathologic increase in pulmonary vascular resistance (PVR) in the precapillary pulmonary vasculature. It is the result of a process with several possible pathophysiological mechanisms that may be due to a structural change of pulmonary arteries in the precapillary vasculature itself, a chronic lung disease, or a postcapillary process as a consequence of left-sided heart disease.

Pulmonary arterial hypertension (PAH) is thought to be the result of structural damage to the precapillary pulmonary circulation, often termed a pulmonary vasculopathy. The earliest changes of PAH consist of a loss of elasticity in these vessels, which affects maximal pulmonary blood flow. While in the systemic circulation an increase in cardiac output during exercise is accompanied by an elevation in systemic blood pressure, the pulmonary circulation is designed to respond to an increase in cardiac output by vasodilation. The cross-sectional area of the pulmonary vascular bed increases, so that pulmonary arterial pressure does not significantly rise in response to the increase in cardiac output in healthy subjects, even at peak exercise levels.

It is thought that at early stages, the pulmonary vasculopathy of PAH limits recruitment of the pulmonary vascular bed, only during exercise. At later stages, the limitation in pulmonary vascular bed recruitment is manifested more overtly at rest. An increase in cardiac output during exercise is accompanied by an elevation in PVR. As a consequence, the right ventricle must hypertrophy in order to overcome the elevated PVR. Depending on extent and rate of progress of the vasculopathy, the right ventricle may not be able to maintain adequate pulmonary blood flow, and this may be manifest by clinical decompensation with right ventricular failure.

There are two pathophysiological mechanisms which cause impaired exercise tolerance in PAH patients, and can be measured with CPET:

- an impaired O_2 transport.
- ventilation/perfusion mismatching.

Impaired O_2 transport during exercise leads to arterial hypoxemia and an early onset of lactic acidosis from anaerobic metabolism, therefore stimulating ventilatory drive by excess production of CO_2 and H^+ as acid stimuli. Additionally, well-ventilated lung areas are not adequately perfused because of the structural damage to the pulmonary arteries. Physiological dead space/tidal volume ratio (V_D/V_T) is therefore elevated during exercise, so that gas exchange becomes less efficient than normal, leading to lowered arterial O_2 content and early lactate production further increasing ventilatory drive and adding to dyspnea early during exercise (17).

The structural changes in the pulmonary vasculature and the resulting consequences in O_2 transport as well as the impaired matching of ventilation to perfusion can be detected and quantitated with gas exchange measurements obtained during exercise (Table 10.1). While parameters of O_2 transport, such as peak O_2 uptake ($\dot{V}O_2$), anaerobic threshold (AT), peak O_2 pulse ($\dot{V}O_2$/HR) and the relationship between increase in workload and increase in O_2 consumption ($\Delta\dot{V}O_2/\Delta WR$) are not specific for pulmonary vascular disease, abnormalities of ventilation/perfusion mismatching ($\dot{V}E/\dot{V}CO_2$ @ AT, PETCO$_2$ @ AT) seen with CPET are more specific for pulmonary arterial hypertension and may even assist in differentiating between precapillary and postcapillary reasons for pulmonary hypertension (30).

Figure 10.1 shows the typical CPET findings in a patient with PAH. Reduced peak $\dot{V}O_2$ (panel 3) and reduced anaerobic threshold (panel 5) may be seen in a variety of cardiac

---

Table 10.1   Gas exchange parameters reflecting pathophysiology of pulmonary arterial hypertension (PAH)

Parameter	Change in PAH	Interpretation
Peak $\dot{V}O_2$	(↓)	Maximum achievable O_2 transport
Maximum peak O_2 pulse ($\dot{V}O_2$/HR)	(↓)	Cardiovascular function, indicator for ability to increase cardiac output
Anaerobic threshold (AT)	(↓)	Maximal ability to sustain aerobic metabolism
$\Delta VO_2/\Delta WR$	(↓)	Indicator of adequate O_2 delivery with increasing workload
$\dot{V}E/\dot{V}CO_2$ at the AT	(↑)	Indicator of ventilatory efficiency
$P_{ET}CO_2$ at the AT	(↓)	Dead space ventilation, ventilatory drive

and pulmonary diseases. The inability to adequately increase cardiac output with exercise can be seen in panels 3 and 5. The slope of $\Delta \dot{V}O_2/\Delta WR$ (panel 3) is blunted below and above the anaerobic threshold (normal 10 mL/min/watt). Panel 5 shows a higher heart rate response than expected with rising O_2 consumption, indicating an impaired ability to increase stroke volume during exercise. More specific for PAH, panel 6 demonstrates that ventilation does not become more efficient after start of exercise, reflected by an increased relationship between minute ventilation and CO_2 output. The patient has to breathe more during exercise in order to eliminate 1 liter of CO_2, contrary to what would be physiologically expected. In terms of gas exchange, $\dot{V}E/\dot{V}CO_2$ rises during exercise.

The partial pressure of end-tidal carbon dioxide ($P_{ET}CO_2$) is low (normal 32–40 mmHg) during the entire test, and continuously falls during exercise (panel 9), reflecting an increased ventilatory drive with early lactic acidosis as well as

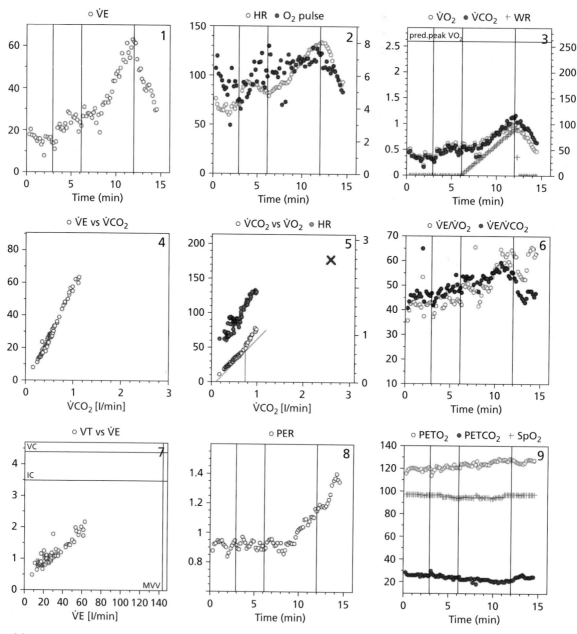

Abbreviations:

$\dot{V}E$ = minute ventilation (L)   HR = heart rate (1/min) = oxygen uptake (L/min) $\dot{V}CO_2$ = carbon dioxide output (L/min)
O_2 pulse = oxygen pulse, equals $\dot{V}O_2 \div$ HR (mL O_2/min) $\dot{V}E/\dot{V}O_2$ = ventilatory equivalent for oxygen (no unit)

Figure 10.1 Standardized 9-panel plot (12) of a cardiopulmonary exercise test in a 42-year-old male (170 cm, 74 kg) at initial diagnosis of idiopathic pulmonary arterial hypertension (IPAH).

an impaired ability to eliminate CO_2. Low $P_{ET}CO_2$ is also commonly seen with voluntary hyperventilation; however in this case respiratory exchange ratio (RER, panel 8) is elevated, with values > 1. In the example illustrated in Figure 10.1 RER values are normal, confirming that hyperventilation is due to an involuntary increase in ventilatory drive.

Initial patient evaluation with CPET

The symptoms of pulmonary hypertension are nonspecific. Patients mainly present with dyspnea, early fatigue, dizziness and other symptoms that might be caused by other cardiac or pulmonary diseases. It is helpful to include CPET in the initial diagnostic work-up of patients presenting with unexplained dyspnea which could be caused by PH:

- Peak $\dot{V}O_2$ and AT values measured with CPET are reproducible (22). Baseline assessment of maximal exercise capacity with CPET is therefore also valuable for follow-up evaluations, independent of the cause of exercise limitation.
- CPET can demonstrate findings characteristic for pulmonary arterial hypertension, and it can aid in the differential diagnosis of unexplained dyspnea, uncovering other causes of cardiac and/or pulmonary disease.
- CPET is a non-invasive test which provides comprehensive information on cardiopulmonary status at rest and during exercise.

Early detection of pulmonary vascular disease

The earliest structural changes in the pulmonary vasculature are difficult to detect, because they are not present at rest. A considerable amount of pulmonary vascular bed has to be affected before the mismatching of ventilation to perfusion becomes obvious. However during exercise, when pulmonary vascular reserve is impaired, these changes may be seen with earlier disease; this may be seen as abnormal $\dot{V}E/\dot{V}CO_2$ and $P_{ET}CO_2$, and these measures may correlate with disease severity (17,18,25), although in a recent study, $\dot{V}E/\dot{V}CO_2$ was not sufficiently sensitive to distinguish exercise-induced PAH from normal (31).

Patient follow-up

CPET, when correctly performed, is highly reproducible at rest and during all phases of exercise. Although in many cases only slight differences may be seen in the key gas exchange parameters, even these slight changes in gas exchange may be clinically relevant (29). In most cases, improvement in O_2 transport (peak $\dot{V}O_2$, AT) will be more prominent than improvement of V/Q mismatching ($\dot{V}E/\dot{V}CO_2$, $P_{ET}CO_2$) due to the fact that the latter phenomenon reflects the structural damage to the pulmonary vasculature, which is not reversible at present, while O_2 transport can very well be improved by medication or with rehabilitation. Furthermore, O_2 transport and ventilation/perfusion mismatching can change independently, even in opposite directions. CPET allows monitoring each of these mechanisms. As a result, changes in disease state can be seen early, and be attributed to a mechanism, which is clinically relevant for therapeutic decisions.

Prognostic considerations

CPET allows prognostication in patients with PAH. Measures of O_2 transport and V/Q mismatching have been shown to be prognostic. Wensel et al. showed that the strongest CPET predictors of poor outcome were a peak $\dot{V}O_2$ below 10.4 mL/min/kg, and peak systolic blood pressure below 120 mmHg, both measures of O_2 transport (19). More recent data showed a peak VO_2 of 13.2 mL/min/kg as a threshold value for poorer outcome; an elevated $VE/\dot{V}CO_2$ slope > 48 as well as a blunting of O_2 pulse (change start to peak exercise less than 3.3 mL O_2/beat) were additional predictors of mortality in patients with PAH (20).

Limitations of cardiopulmonary exercise testing

The performance and interpretation of CPET requires technical expertise. Improvements in software and testing equipment have made tremendous progress in user-friendliness and sensor accuracy; however calibration of the equipment may be a persistent source or error in a CPET laboratory with a poorly trained technician. Therefore, technical prowess in the CPET laboratory is still necessary to ensure that the technical procedures, including equipment calibration, are adequately followed. Strict quality control is essential for acquiring reliable and reproducible data.

Quality control in the CPET laboratory consists of calibration and validation of the equipment, as well as proper documentation of these processes. While calibration should be done before each test, validation should be performed at regular time periods with a mechanical validator (21), or with a healthy reference person performing a test with a standardized protocol.

Standardization of CPET interpretation is highly desirable. During each test, a large amount of data is generated, which should be interpreted in a systematic fashion. Plotting the results in a standardized 9-panel plot, as set forth by Wasserman et al. (12) has been a major advance in standardization for comparing different tests. Unfortunately, the formatting of these plots still differs in layout and scaling among the different CPET equipment manufacturers, which can make data comparison and data exchange more difficult.

A high inter-observer variability in the interpretation of CPET results has been criticized, in particular in the context of the use of CPET as an endpoint in clinical trials; this is likely due to the lack of standardization in the determination of key CPET parameters. Results differ with different forms of data averaging and with the number and selection of data points that are taken into calculation for each CPET measure. It has been shown that adherence to strict and specific criteria minimizes variability (22). In clinical practice as well as in clinical trials, standardization for determining key CPET is strongly advised.

Finally, as with the 6MW test, CPET may be limited in its diagnostic power in patients who have other causes of impaired limb mobility such as joint pain or stiff legs, not permitting adequate levels of exercise for interpretation of the response to exercise.

CORRELATION BETWEEN SUBMAXIMAL AND MAXIMAL TESTING

Physiologically, measures of submaximal and maximal exercise testing are expected to show a correlation. The 6MWD was originally developed as a surrogate for peak $\dot{V}O_2$, because of its ease of administration and reproducibility (23). It has been shown that a correlation between peak $\dot{V}O_2$ and 6MWD exists, and that the best results are achieved when using weight-adapted 6MWD results instead of the absolute values (24). Unexpectedly, a learning effect was seen in this multi-center study, showing correlation improvement over time in less experienced centers.

REFERENCES

1. Brooks D, Solway S, Gibbons WJ. ATS statement on six-minute walk test. Am J Respir Crit Care Med 2002; 166(1):111–17.
2. Miyamoto S, Nagaya N, Satoh T, Kyotani S, Sakamaki F, Fujita M, Nakanishi N, Miyatake K. Clinical correlates and prognostic significance of six-minute walk test in patients with primary pulmonary hypertension. Am J Respir Crit Care Med 2000;161:487–92.
3. Stevens D, Elpern E, Sharma K, Szidon P, Ankin M, Kesten S. Comparison of hallway and treadmill six-minute walk tests. Am J Respir Crit Care Med 1999;160:1540–43.
4. Gibbons WJ, Fruchter N, Sloan S, Levy RD. Reference values for a multiple repetition 6-minute walk test in healthy adults older than 20 years. J Cardiopulm Rehabil 2001; 21(2):87–93.
5. Guyatt GH, Thompson PJ, Berman LB, Sullivan MJ, Townsend M, Jones NL, Pugsley SO. How should we measure function in patients with chronic heart and lung disease? J Chronic Dis 1985;38:517–24.
6. Wu G, Sanderson B, Bittner V. The 6-minute walk test: how important is the learning effect? Am Heart J 2003;146(1):129–33.
7. Sitbon O, Humbert M, Nunes H et al. Long-term intravenous epoprostenol infusion in primary pulmonary

8. hypertension: prognostic factors and survival. J Am Coll Cardiol 2002;40:780–8.
8. Rubin LJ, Badesch DB, Barst RJ et al. Bosentan therapy for pulmonary arterial hypertension. N Engl J Med 2002;346(12):896–903.
9. Olschewski H, Simonneau G, Galie N et al. Inhaled iloprost for severe pulmonary arterial hypertension. N Engl J Med 2002;347(5):322–9.
10. Galie N, Ghofrani A, Torbicki A et al. Sildenafil citrate therapy for pulmonary arterial hypertension. N Engl J Med 2005;353:2148–57.
11. Galie N, Olschewski H, Oudiz RJ et al. Ambrisentan for the treatment of pulmonary arterial hypertension. Results of the Ambrisentan in Pulmonary Arterial Hypertension, Randomized, Double-Blind, Placebo-Controlled, Multicenter Efficacy (ARIES) Study 1 and 2. Circulation 2008;117:3010–9.
12. Wasserman K, Hansen JE, Sue DY, Stringer WW, Whipp BJ (eds). Principles of Exercise Testing and Interpretation, 4th edn. Philadelphia: Lippincott Williams & Wilkins, 2005.
13. Sun XG, Oudiz RJ, Hansen JE, Wasserman K. Exercise pathophysiology in primary pulmonary vascular hypertension. Circulation 2001;104:429–35.
14. Riley MS, Porszasz J, Engelen MPKJ, Brundage B, Wasserman K. Gas exchange responses to continuous incremental cycle ergometry exercise in primary pulmonary hypertension in humans. Eur J Appl Physiol 2000;83:63–70.
15. Hansen JE, Ulubay G, Fai Chow B, Sun XG, Wasserman K. Mixed-expired and end-tidal CO_2 distinguish between ventilation and perfusion defects during exercise testing in lung and heart diseases. Chest 2007;132:977–83.
16. Wasserman K, Hansen JE, Sue DY, Casaburi R, Whipp BJ (eds). Principles of Exercise Testing and Interpretation, 4th edn, Chapter 6. Philadelphia: Lippincott Williams & Wilkins, 1994.
17. Yasunobu Y, Oudiz RJ, Sun XG, Hansen JE, Wasserman K. End-tidal PCO_2 abnormality and exercise limitation in patients with primary pulmonary hypertension. Chest 2005;127:1637–46.
18. Markowitz DH, Systrom DM. Diagnosis of pulmonary vascular limit to exercise by cardiopulmonary exercise testing. J Heart Lung Transplant 2004;23:88–95.
19. Wensel R, Opitz CF, Anker SD et al. Assessment of survival in patients with primary pulmonary hypertension: importance of cardiopulmonary exercise testing. Circulation 2002;106:319–24.
20. Groepenhoff H, Vonk-Noordegraaf A, Boonstra A, Spreeuwenberg MD, Postmus PE, Bogaard HJ. Exercise testing to estimate survival in pulmonary hypertension. Med Sci Sports Exerc 2008;40(10):1725–32.
21. Huszczuk A, Whipp BJ, Wasserman K. A respiratory gas exchange simulator for routine calibration in metabolic studies. Eur Respir J 1990;3(4):465–8.
22. Hansen JE, Sun XG, Yasunobu Y, Garafano RP, Gates G, Barst RJ, Wasserman K. Reproducibility of cardiopulmonary

exercise measurements in patients with pulmonary arterial hypertension. Chest 2004;126:816–24.

23. Guyatt GH, Sullivan MJ, Thompson PJ, Fallen EL, Pugsley SO, Taylor DW, Berman LB. The 6-minute walk: a new measure of exercise capacity in patients with chronic heart failure. Can Med Assoc J 1985;132:919–23.

24. Oudiz RJ, Barst RJ, Hansen JE *et al.* Cardiopulmonary exercise testing and six-minute walk correlations in pulmonary arterial hypertension. Am J Cardiol 2006; 97(1):123–6.

25. Sun XG, Hansen JE, Garatchea N, Storer TW, Wasserman K. Ventilatory efficiency during exercise in healthy subjects. Am J Respir Crit Care Med 2002;166:1443–8.

26. Frost AE, Langleben D, Oudiz R *et al.* The 6-min walk test (6MW) as an efficacy endpoint in pulmonary arterial hypertension clinical trials: demonstration of a ceiling effect. Vascul Pharmacol 2005;43:36–9.

27. Guyatt GH, Sullivan MJ, Thompson PJ, Fallen EL, Pugsley SO, Taylor DW, Berman LB. The 6-minute walk: a new measure of exercise capacity in patients with chronic heart failure. Can Med Assoc J 1985;132:919–23.

28. Wasserman K. Critical capillary pO_2 and the role of lactate production in oxyhemoglobin dissociation during exercise. Adv Exp Med Biol 1999;471:321–33.

29. Oudiz RJ, Roveran G, Hansen JE, Sun XG, Wasserman K. Effect of sildenafil on ventilatory efficiency and exercise tolerance in pulmonary hypertension. Eur J Heart Fail 2007; 9:917–21.

30. Deboeck G, Niset G, Lamotte M, Vachiéry JL, Naeije R. Exercise testing in pulmonary arterial hypertension and in chronic heart failure. Eur Respir J 2004;23:747–51.

31. Tolle JJ, Waxman AB, Van Horn TL, Pappagianopoulos PP, Systrom DM. Exercise-induced pulmonary arterial hypertension. Circulation 2008;118:2183–9.

11

Blood biomarkers

CHRISTOPHER RHODES, VAHITHA ABDUL-SALAM, JOHN WHARTON AND MARTIN R WILKINS

INTRODUCTION

A "biomarker" can be defined as follows: "Any characteristic that is objectively measured and evaluated as an indicator of normal biological processes, pathogenic processes, or pharmacologic responses to a therapeutic intervention" (1).

Any signal that informs about the state of health of a biological system may hold some value as a biomarker and this includes biochemical and physical measurements (2), as well as more qualitative measurements such as questionnaires (3). The focus of this chapter is soluble or biochemical blood biomarkers which hold potential value in pulmonary hypertension (PH), specifically pulmonary arterial hypertension (PAH) and chronic thromboembolic pulmonary hypertension (CTEPH).

BIOMARKERS: AN OVERVIEW

Soluble (or biochemical) biomarkers have a number of advantages. Among these are that they use samples, blood and urine, that can be obtained relatively easily, and are therefore easy to deploy at the bedside and can be repeated serially at follow-up. They can also be quantified objectively and should be relatively low cost.

For any biomarker to be useful, however, it has to be qualified as fit for purpose. The evidence needed to qualify a biomarker depends upon the nature of the decisions that will be made based on the information it provides. Clearly the supporting evidence will be less where the biomarker is reporting on a proposed mechanism of drug effect (for example, to aid an in-house decision on whether to proceed with the development of that drug), than where it is used as a surrogate endpoint in a clinical trial and used as a basis on which to licence a drug for a clinical indication. In the latter case, the biomarker needs approval from the regulatory authorities.

The general conditions that need to be satisfied when considering the utility of a biomarker include:

- **Biological plausibility:** There should be a reasonable scientific argument that links the biomarker with the disease process.
- **Strength of association:** There should be a strong statistical correlation between changes in the biomarker and the event it is reporting.
- **Consistency:** The association should hold irrespective of the intervention.
- **Specificity:** The biomarker should be associated with the disease of interest and not confounded by co-existing disease or other factors. This is measured practically as the percentage of individuals without the corresponding disease state correctly identified.
- **Sensitivity:** The biomarker should be able to clearly distinguish between those with or without the disease of interest. This is measured practically as the percentage of individuals with the corresponding disease state correctly identified.
- **Temporality:** Changes in the biomarker should reflect changes in the disease in a suitable timeframe.

- **Biological gradient:** The biomarker should have a reasonable dynamic range that enables grading of the disease or its response to interventions.
- **Experimental evidence:** The clinical utility of a biomarker needs to be supported by data from clinical scenarios. This is most robust when gathered in the context of a clinical trial and is an iterative process, refined by the findings from the latest study.
- **Robustness of the assay:** The biomarker assay should be accurate and reliable and reproducible in other laboratories.

There are a variety of potential uses of biomarkers, as outlined in Table 11.1. In all cases these remain unmet clinical needs in PH. Our current understanding of the natural history of idiopathic PAH (IPAH) suggests individual variation in susceptibility to the condition, with a genetic basis in some cases, and a sub-clinical phase before presentation. There are therefore opportunities for screening for the disease and for its detection at an early stage. The diagnosis of PH is often delayed as other diagnoses are considered, and it is dependent upon an invasive procedure, cardiac catheterization. While at present the latter remains essential for a definitive diagnosis, it has been replaced in some centres in the regular follow-up of patients by skilled imaging techniques. This is an important development but cannot match the potential of a suitable blood or urine test for ease of deployment and cost. The clinical classification of PH into subtypes assists with treatment choice but there is considerable room for refinement through a better understanding of the disease processes at the molecular level. The translation of that molecular understanding into biomarkers could provide a classification or algorithm that enables more personalised prescribing. Studies to evaluate the efficacy of new treatments for PH are highly dependent upon surrogate clinical endpoints to filter out ineffective and unsafe interventions and enable resource to be given to more promising approaches. Soluble biomarkers have great appeal in this regard and once accepted, can be incorporated into goal-oriented treatment programmes for PH patients based upon repetitive monitoring during follow-up (4).

Arguably, at the present time, *BMPR2* genotype is the only biomarker of PAH universally recognized (5–14), although brain natriuretic peptide-32 (BNP-32) and N-terminal (NT) pro-BNP have been studied extensively and have utility in clinical trials, if not day-to-day patient management (15–28). Other potential biomarkers which have been and are actively under investigation which will be discussed include troponin, growth and differentiation factor (GDF)-15, uric acid, endothelin, creatinine and apelin.

GENETIC BIOMARKERS

Alterations in the bone morphogenetic protein (BMP) signaling pathway are well described in PAH (5–12,29) and the use of screening for mutations in the *BMPR2* gene, which encodes the BMP type-2 receptor, in patients with family histories of PAH, has value in predicting the susceptibility of patients to PAH. *ALK1* has also been identified as a susceptibility gene for PAH (30,31).

Bone morphogenetic protein biology

BMPR2 is a member of the TGF-β superfamily of kinase receptors and is activated upon ligand binding to extracellular ligand-binding domains on both type 1 and type 2 receptors. Ligand-binding causes receptor dimerization and activation of BMPR1 by BMPR2. Receptor-regulated or R-Smads (Smad-1, -5 and -8) and the common Smad-4 are responsibile for intracellular signal transduction (32). R-Smads, along with Smad-4 can translocate to the nucleus, and with other cofactors, regulate gene expression (33); in smooth muscles cells this can lead to inhibition of cell proliferation and apoptosis induction (Figure 11.1). Non-Smad-regulated pathways including the mitogen activated protein (MAP) kinase pathway (34) may also be important in BMPR2 signaling and recently an apparent BMP/apolipoprotein E/peroxisome proliferator-associated receptor-γ axis has been identified (35), by which BMPR2 might mediate further effects. The anti-proliferative and

Table 11.1 Uses of soluble/biochemical biomarkers in pulmonary hypertension

Biomarker use	Example	Notes
Susceptibility	BMPR2, ALK1 genotype	In patients with a family history
Screening	BNP-32 and NT-proBNP	Not sensitive enough to detect subclinical disease
Diagnostic	BNP-32 and NT-proBNP	Helpful in the context of a consistent medical exam
Risk stratification	NT-proBNP, BNP-32, ANP, serum troponin, serum creatinine, uric acid, GDF-15	Natriuretic peptides useful. GDF-15 and creatinine need independent confirmation. Troponin raised in end stage disease. Uric acid affected by diuretics/renal disease
Therapeutic monitoring	BNP-32 or NT-proBNP	Need to interpret in context of all patient information

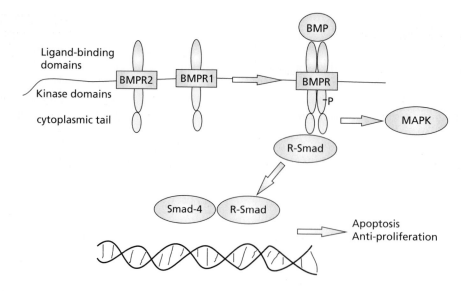

Figure 11.1   A schematic representation of the bone morphogenetic protein type-2 (BMPR2) receptor pathway. BMP, bone morphogenetic protein; MAPK, mitogen activated protein kinase.

pro-apoptotic effects of BMPR2 signaling are important in PAH, where excessive proliferation in the pulmonary vasculature contributes to the disease progression.

Bone morphogenetic protein in PAH

BMPR2 mutations are found in around 60 percent (50–80 percent) of familial PAH (5,7,10,11,29), 25 percent of IPAH patients (36) and rarely in PAH associated with anorexic drugs or congenital heart disease (6,8). Mutations vary but all predict a reduction in BMPR2 function (37). Penetrance of PAH in carriers of a *BMPR2* mutation is relatively low (~20%) but may vary from 33 percent to 80 percent dependent on single nucleotide polymorphisms of TGF-β which can alter gene expression (12). Patients with *BMPR2* mutations are less likely to respond to vasodilator therapy (14) and present on average 10 years before those without a defined *BMPR2* mutation (13). Their hemodynamic measurements also indicate more severe PAH (e.g. mean pulmonary artery pressure (mPAP) 64 ± 13 versus 56 ± 13 mmHg, $p < 0.0001$), and life expectancy is significantly reduced ($p = 0.002$) (13).

Whilst the link between *BMPR2* mutations and PAH is clear, the relatively low frequency of mutations in non-familial PAH and low penetrance of the disease in carriers without further TGF-β dysfunction means that screening for mutations should be restricted to relatives of patients with an identified *BMPR2* mutation.

ALK1 in PAH

Activin receptor-like kinase-1 (ALK1) is another member of the TGF-β superfamily which may signal through the same Smad proteins described above (10,30). Mutation to *ALK1* has been identified as the main cause of PAH in patients with hereditary hemorrhagic telangiectasia (31).

Transcript profiling in peripheral blood monocytes

A microarray transcriptomics approach using peripheral blood monocytes (PBMCs) in PAH patients and healthy controls identified a large signature set of 106 genes which could distinguish between patients with PAH ($p < 0.002$) (38). Quantitative polymerase chain reaction confirmed the differential expression of two of these genes (adrenomedullin and endothelial cell growth factor-1) in PAH PBMCs. Furthermore, the herpesvirus entry mediator gene was differentially expressed in PBMCs from IPAH patients compared with those from patients with secondary PAH. Further characterization of genetic "fingerprints" for PAH disease states in these accessible PBMCs could hold diagnostic or even prognostic value (39).

NATRIURETIC PEPTIDES

Natriuretic peptide biology

There are three members of the natriuretic protein family: atrial (ANP), brain (BNP) and C-type (CNP) natriuretic peptides (28). ANP and BNP are synthesized in the myocardium and circulate in plasma, regulating natriuresis, diuresis (40) and vasomotor tone (41). Both are synthesized in the cardiac atria but with pressure and volume overload, the hypertrophied ventricle becomes the major

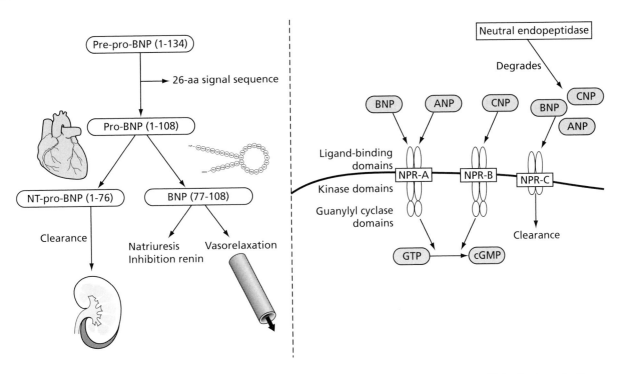

Figure 11.2   Left: A schematic diagram of the processing of BNP pro-peptides and downstream functions. Right: A schematic diagram of the mechanism of action and clearance of natriuretic peptides (NP) types A, B and C. NPR, natriuretic peptide receptor; GTP, guanosine triphosphate; cGMP, cyclic guanosine monophosphate.

source of circulating BNP (42). CNP is expressed in endothelial cells and has a paracrine role regulating vascular tone but it may possess some protective properties post-myocardial infarction (43).

While cytokines can influence natriuretic peptide synthesis, the most important stimulus to release is wall stress. ANP is stored in granules and readily secreted in response to rises in atrial pressure, such as may occur with exercise, atrial tachycardias and even postural change. Relatively low amounts of BNP are stored in myocardium but wall stress increases both synthesis and release (44). Both ANP and BNP are produced as pro-hormones, with biological activity residing in the C-terminus. BNP is synthesized as pre-proBNP, which is cleaved to form a 108-amino acid pro-peptide, proBNP and subsequently BNP-32 and a 76 amino acid peptide, N-terminal-proBNP (NT-proBNP).

ANP has a plasma half-life of around 4 minutes, while for BNP-32 and NT-proBNP, the half-life is 20 minutes and 1 hour, respectively (45,46). There are two recognized active clearance pathways for circulating ANP and BNP-32. Both are substrates for neutral endopeptidase and both bind to the natriuretic peptide clearance receptor (NPR-C, Figure 11.2). All natriuretic peptides are filtered by the kidney, but renal clearance is likely to be the main route for removing NT-proBNP from plasma. Circulating NT-proBNP levels are higher than those of BNP-32, and more dependent upon renal function (26). Both BNP-32 and NT-proBNP levels are higher in women, rise with age and are inversely related to body mass index.

Collectively, ANP and BNP act to reduce the workload of the heart. That PH is frequently a progressive disease despite high circulating levels likely reflects resistance to the biological actions of these peptides in PH, perhaps mediated in part by high levels of hormones with opposing actions. There is considerable interest in the extent to which circulating ANP and BNP levels can be used as biomarkers in a number of cardiovascular diseases, particularly left (LV) (47) and right ventricular (RV) (15–28) dysfunction. This reduces their specificity as a diagnostic tool and stresses the need to interpret values in context, rather than in isolation.

BNP and ANP in PAH

Circulating levels of ANP and BNP-32 levels have been found to correlate significantly with resting mean pulmonary artery pressure (mPAP), pulmonary vascular resistance (PVR), right atrial pressure (RAP), cardiac output (CO), right ventricular hypertrophy and right ventricular ejection fraction (15,22). The data support the thesis that circulating levels report on RV function in PH. Moreover a reduction in BNP levels with long-term vasodilator therapy which correlated strongly ($p < 0.001$) with reductions in PVR suggests that changes in BNP-32 levels may be useful as a measure of treatment efficacy (15). Changes in BNP-32 levels have also been reported to correlate with changes in 6-minute walk distance (6MWD) (22), but this has not been the experience of all investigators (unpublished data). This may reflect the utility of 6MWD as a measure of therapeutic response, which has its detractors.

Resting ANP and BNP-32 levels correlate with New York Health Association (NYHA) functional class, although there is overlap between the groups (16,18). In a multivariable analysis, only BNP-32 proved an independent predictor of mortality. A baseline BNP-32 level > 150 pg/mL was associated with significantly higher mortality (log rank test, $p < 0.05$) and a fall in BNP-32 levels to < 180 pg/mL or > 180 pg/mL after 3 months treatment with prostacyclin distinguished survivors and non-survivors ($p < 0.0001$) (16). It should be noted, however, that the response was not uniform in either group; BNP-32 levels increased in some survivors while some non-survivors showed a reduction.

NT–proBNP in PAH

Baseline NT-proBNP levels have also been reported to correlate with hemodynamic measurements, such as PVR, cardiac index (CI), RAP (20,24,25), and mPAP (20,25), as well as functional class (25) and prognosis (24,26). In a study of 55 patients with a mean follow-up of 36 months (24), a cut-off level of 1400 pg/mL predicted fatal outcome with 88 percent sensitivity and 53 percent specificity (log rank test, $p = 0.0089$). The influence of renal insufficiency on BNP-32 and NT-proBNP levels was examined in a study of 118 patients (26). In a multivariable analysis with a mean follow-up of 10 months, only NT-proBNP levels and creatinine clearance were independent predictors of mortality. It is likely that NT-proBNP, like BNP-32, informs about right ventricular function in PH. In one small study of 25 patients, a baseline NT-proBNP level of 1685 pg/mL was associated with RV systolic dysfunction (RVSD), defined as a RV ejection fraction (RVEF) > 2 standard deviations below controls as measured by cardiac magnetic resonance, with 100 percent sensitivity and 94 percent specificity (27). There are no published data on serial NT-proBNP measurements and response to treatment.

BNP assays

Several commercial immunoassays are available for BNP. Some (Shionogi & Co. Ltd., Japan) require 20 hours. Others are more rapid [Shionoria-IRMA (Shionogi and Co. Ltd., Osaka, Japan), Triage BNP (Biosite Inc., San Diego, CA), ADVIA Centaur BNP (Bayer Diagnostics, Tarrytown, NY), Access BNP (Beckman Coulter Inc., Fullerton, CA), and AxSYM BNP (Abbott Laboratories, Abbott Park, IL)] and allow analysis at room temperature within 4 hours of collection. The dynamic range on a drop of blood is between 5 pg/mL and 5000 pg/mL (48). For NT-proBNP, available systems include Elecsys (Roche Diagnostics, Indianapolis, IN, USA); Dimension (Siemens Healthcare Diagnostics, Deerfield, IL, USA); RAMP (Response Biomedical Corporation, Vancouver, British Colombia, Canada); VIDAS (BioMerieur Canada Inc., St. Laurent, Quebec, Canada) and VITROS (Orthoclinical Diagnostics, Rochester, NY, USA). EDTA heparinized plasma samples collected in glass or plastic tubes can be used, and samples are stable at room temperature or 4°C for up to 3 days (49). The integration of BNP measurements have been reported to improve the management and reduce cost in some presentations of cardiovascular disease (50,51). The absolute values vary between assays, as each assay is based on a different antibody and there is evidence of alternative forms of BNP, which might influence measurements to an extent that may vary between assays (52). Clinicians must be aware of this when interpreting the results of BNP tests and should use the same assay for serial measurements in patients.

Natriuretic peptides in diagnosis, prognosis, clinical trials and individual patient management

Circulating natriuretic peptide levels inform about cardiac workload. The measurement of natriuretic peptide levels has been advocated in screening and diagnostic programmes for a range of heart diseases. In this regard, the strength of data favours BNP-32 and NT-proBNP over ANP. Moreover, the stability of NT-proBNP in blood samples *ex-vivo* gives this peptide an advantage over BNP-32.

The utility of the result depends upon the clinical context. A normal value in an asymptomatic person has a high negative predictive value for heart disease. A raised level merits further investigation. In a dyspneic patient, a raised level suggests a cardiac problem but does not provide the diagnosis.

Once the diagnosis of PH is made, BNP levels predict prognosis and can be used to risk stratify patients. But there are too few data on the day-to-day variability of natriuretic peptide levels in PH to recommend their use to tailor treatment in individual patients. Serial measurements give more information than isolated values but there are no objective data on how to interpret a change in levels. Does, say, a 40 percent fall represent a significant response to treatment or is it commensurate with the variability seen in the disease? Should therapy be adjusted until values fall to normal or below a threshold value? Using BNP measurements as part of a management algorithm (4) may be useful but this needs full evaluation in a clinical trial setting.

BNP measurements have established a key role in clinical trials evaluating new treatments. Although individual responses may vary, an effective treatment would be expected to reduce cardiac workload in a group of patients and so their circulating BNP levels. While new imaging technologies might provide more detailed information about RV function in PH, serial BNP measurements are more practical for large scale trials and are likely to remain a useful informative tool.

URIC ACID

Uric acid biology

Uric acid (UA) is the final degradation product of purines. Tissue ischemia and hypoxia are known to deplete adenosine triphosphate and promote degradation of adenine nucleotides, producing uric acid (53). Circulating UA levels may therefore reflect oxidative stress. High levels have been detected in hypoxic pathologies including chronic obstructive pulmonary disease (54), chronic heart failure (55) and cyanotic congenital heart disease (56).

Uric acid in PAH

Hyperuricemia has been documented in PAH (57–62); in one study average UA in 90 IPAH patients was 7.5 ± 2.5 mg/dL (average UA in control subjects 4.9 ± 1.2 mg/dL, $p < 0.001$) (58). UA levels correlated with CO ($r = -0.52$, $p < 0.001$) and total pulmonary resistance ($r = 0.57$, $p < 0.001$) and fell from 7.1 ± 1.9 to 5.9 ± 1.6 mg/dL after chronic vasodilator therapy. Serum UA levels above control values predicted mortality (log rank test, $p < 0.01$). UA levels could also distinguish significantly between functional classes II, III and IV. Serum creatinine levels were also raised in the high-UA group and it is important to note that patients with severe renal dysfunction were excluded from the study (due to a large confounding effect on circulating UA levels). Diuretic therapy is also known to affect UA levels (63) and these confounding factors detract from the value of measuring UA in PAH. However, as with NT-proBNP (see above) and in chronic heart failure, where UA levels have been suggested to reflect circulating xanthine oxidase levels (64), the reflection of renal function in UA levels may add to its value (58,65).

GDF-15

GDF-15 biology

Growth and differentiation factor-15 (GDF-15) was originally identified as a factor secreted by macrophages activated by cytokines such as interleukins 1β and 2, or tumor necrosis factor-alpha, but not by interferon-γ or lipopolysaccharide, suggesting it was involved in the limitation of the later phases of macrophage activation, but not primary activation (66). It was identified as a member of the TGF-β cytokine family, with closest homology (15–29 percent) to the bone morphogenetic proteins. Since then it has been identified as a member of the GDF subgroup, which have been shown to be important in growth, differentiation, wound healing and tissue repair (67). Only minimal GDF-15 expression occurs in tissues under normal conditions (68) but under pathologic conditions, such as tissue hypoxia, inflammation and oxidative stress, it can be upregulated

(69,70) and has been shown to have a protective and anti-hypertrophic role associated with Smad activation (71).

Recent studies have demonstrated increased circulating levels of GDF-15 in acute coronary syndrome (72) and left-sided heart failure (73), and it appears to have prognostic value in patients with pulmonary embolism (74). Its release from cardiomyocytes can be triggered by mechanical stretch (75).

GDF-15 in PAH

Fifty-five percent of 76 treatment-naïve PAH patients had circulating GDF-15 levels above the pre-determined threshold of 1200 ng/L (upper limit of normal range in elderly healthy individuals) (62). The risk of death or transplantation at 1 and 3 years were significantly higher in patients with GDF-15 levels above than below 1200 ng/L ($p = 0.035$ and 0.006, respectively). A value of 2097 ng/L predicted adverse outcomes at 3 years with 74 percent sensitivity, 82 percent specificity. Increased GDF-15 levels were associated with increased RAP and pulmonary capillary wedge pressures, and decreased mixed venous oxygen saturations (SvO_2), along with increased UA and NT-proBNP. After adjustments for hemodynamic and biochemical variables, GDF-15 still independently predicted adverse outcomes ($p = 0.002$). GDF-15 did not correlate with mPAP, CO, CI or PVR and therefore does not hold diagnostic value in PH, but may represent a quantitative measure of pathological processes that are not reflected in other biomarkers. In a second cohort of 22 patients, GDF-15 levels correlated again with NT-proBNP measurements and SvO_2 ($r = -0.74$, $p < 0.001$). The subgroup of patients with raised NT-proBNP and GDF-15 levels had a significantly worse prognosis than either elevated NT-proBNP or GDF-15 levels alone.

GDF-15 appears to have prognostic value in PH, which may be more powerful in combination with NT-proBNP measurements, but independent prospective studies are required to further qualify this molecule as a true biomarker in PH.

CREATININE

Renal dysfunction is a potent and independent predictor of cardiovascular morbidity and mortality (76–78) and has been linked to prognosis in PH (26). In a comprehensive study involving 500 PAH patients (79), serum creatinine (SCr) levels, used as a crude but highly practical measurement of renal function, were correlated with prognosis, hemodynamics, exercise capacity and functional class in PH, although there was no correlation with mPAP or CI. With a median follow-up of 3.5 years, 279 deaths occurred and SCr intervals of < 1.0 mg/dL (low), 1.0–1.4 mg/dL (normal) and > 1.4 mg/dL (slightly raised) predicted mortality ($p < 0.0001$ for normal and slightly raised SCr versus low SCr). In a multivariable analysis, SCr correlated with

RAP with high significance (p < 0.0001) and best predicted mortality in those patients with RAP < 10 mmHg, probably due to the confounding power of RAP as a predictor of mortality in PH. Other possible confounding factors include age, gender, systemic hypertension, diabetes mellitus and diuretic use. Most patients in this study were added retrospectively and independent prospective data is required to confirm creatinine as a biomarker in PH.

OTHER CARDIAC MARKERS

Cardiac troponin T

Cardiac troponin T (cTnT) is a specific marker of myocyte injury, and detectable levels have been associated with in-hospital mortality in acute precapillary PH (80–82). Detectable levels in PH have been associated with significantly lower survival (29 percent versus 81 percent in PH without detectable cTnT, log rank test p = 0.001) and increased heart rate and NT-proBNP (4528 ± 3170 versus 2054 ± 2168 pg/mL, p = 0.03); also decreased SvO_2 (p = 0.04) and 6MWD (298 ± 132 versus 396 ± 101 m, p = 0.02) (83). It has not been directly demonstrated that the source of cTnT in these patients is the failing RV. cTnT was only detectable in 14 percent of the patients studied (83), which indicates that it may be a marker of late stage disease.

Fatty acid binding protein

Another marker of myocardial injury, heart-type fatty acid binding protein (H-FABP) has been identified as a negative prognostic marker in CTEPH in a study of 93 patients with a median follow-up of 1260 days. H-FABP is a cytosolic protein and is not found outside the cell under normal conditions (84). Baseline H-FABP levels of above 2.7 ng/mL indicated a significantly lower probability of event-free survival after pulmonary endarterectomy (85). It has also been validated for use in risk stratification in pulmonary embolism (86). Further studies will be required to characterize the use of H-FABP in PH.

OTHER HORMONES

Endothelin

Endothelin-1(ET-1), a potent vasoconstrictor expressed in the lungs (87), was identified as upregulated in PH shortly after its discovery (88,89). ET-1 acts on both ET_A and ET_B receptors and the effects are related to the site of the receptor. Vascular smooth muscle cells express both ET_A and ET_B receptors and ligand binding to either receptor causes vasoconstriction and cell proliferation. Endothelial cells express only ET_B receptors and the activation of this receptor causes vasodilatation and ET-1 clearance. Circulating ET-1 levels correlate with RAP, pulmonary artery oxygen saturation and PVR (90–92).

Big ET-1, an ET-1 precursor, was found elevated in 16 IPAH patients with significant positive correlation with PVR and RAP, and a negative correlation with CO, cardiac index and disease severity (93). Big ET-1 has been proposed as a more reliable indicator of activation of the ET-1 system as it has a longer half life than ET-1 (94). Iloprost inhalation reduces the ratio of big ET-1 in the radial artery to the PA (95). One study has shown ET-1 levels inversely correlate with survival in PAH (96). Data in this area are sparse and interpretation will be confounded by endothelin B receptor antagonists, which increase levels of ET-1.

Apelin

Apelin, the endogenous ligand for the angiotensin receptor-like 1 APJ receptor (97), is a recently characterized inotropic hormone, which can also stimulate vasodilatation (98,99). It is primarily expressed in lung and mammary tissue in normal rats (100) and plasma levels were 4-fold lower in 10 IPAH patients versus 26 control subjects (p < 0.001) (101). Levels are decreased in patients with chronic parenchymal lung disease or chronic heart failure (101). This study proposed that apelin levels could be of use in distinguishing pulmonary and systemic disease in patients who present with dyspnea. Further studies are required to establish if measuring this novel hormone is of any value in PH.

Serotonin

Plasma levels of the vasoconstrictor serotonin are raised in PAH and correlate with PVR, but do not respond to therapeutic chronic vasodilator treatment (102).

Nitric oxide (NO)

NO is an important vasodilator and reduced activity has long been proposed as a factor in the pathogenesis of PH. Exhaled NO levels and urine NO metabolites have been reported to be reduced in IPAH in one small study, and reversed by bosentan treatment (103). NO measurement is technically demanding, has a small dynamic range in PH and requires patients to adhere to a strict diet. Measurements of circulating NO and NO metabolites may be useful in assessing the response to treatments targeted at this pathway in both experimental and clinical trials. Due to the short half-life of NO, measurements of circulating nitrite and nitrate metabolites may provide more consistent and informative data (104).

Asymmetric dimethyl arginine

Asymmetric dimethyl arginine (ADMA) is an endogenous inhibitor of nitric oxide synthase (NOS) and a potential marker of endothelial dysfunction in PAH (105). ADMA levels are upregulated and correlate with hemodynamics in IPAH (106), CTEPH (107) and PAH associated with congenital heart disease (108). In two of these studies, raised ADMA was linked to increased mortality (106,107), with a sensitivity of 81.1 percent and a specificity of 79.3 percent. Following pulmonary endarterectomy in CTEPH patients, ADMA levels fell to levels comparable with controls (107).

OTHER CIRCULATING BIOMARKERS

Circulating endothelial and endothelial progenitor cells

Circulating endothelial cells and endothelial cell microparticles have been proposed as markers of vascular endothelial damage and disease progression in a variety of cardiovascular disorders (109,110), including PH (111). Attention has focussed on circulating endothelial progenitor cells (EPCs) as biomarkers and possible therapeutic targets (112–114). These cells arise from mesodermal stem cells or hemangioblasts in the bone marrow, but also occur in other tissues, and are generally considered to have a regenerative role in vascular homeostasis and neovascularization (112–114). Indeed, the number and function of EPCs has been shown to correlate with cardiovascular risk factors and impaired endothelial function (115,116) and predict clinical outcome (117). Interest is therefore growing in the possible diagnostic and therapeutic applications of EPCs in PAH, where they have been found to promote pulmonary reperfusion in monocrotaline-induced PH (118). Recent studies have also observed a reduction of circulating EPCs in patients with IPAH or PAH associated with Eisenmenger's syndrome (104,119,120) whereas others have described a higher level of angiogenic precursors in IPAH, compared with healthy controls, and suggested that they may contribute to vascular remodeling (121). This uncertainty reflects the current lack of consensus concerning the identification of EPCs, the term having been widely applied to describe a heterogeneous population of cells that probably serve a variety of functions. These issues will need to be resolved in order to determine whether EPCs have prognostic value as biomarkers in PAH.

Cyclic guanosine monophosphate

NO stimulates soluble guanylyl cyclase to produce cyclic guanosine monophosphate (cGMP). Plasma cGMP levels are increased in patients with PH and are decreased by iloprost inhalation (122). cGMP correlates with PVR ($r = 0.62$, $p < 0.001$) (123) but the increases in cGMP seen in response to an acute pulmonary vasodilator challenge with NO inhalation do not discriminate between responders and non-responders. Urinary cGMP levels have also been found to be significantly higher in IPAH patients, compared to respiratory disease patients without PH or normal healthy controls, and correlated with disease severity (124).

Von Willebrand factor

Plasma von Willebrand factor (vWF) is the carrier of coagulation factor VIII and has been used as a marker for endothelial cell injury, along with its antigen vWF:Ag. Levels of vWF were elevated and responded to prostacyclin therapy in 10 patients with severe PAH (125) and circulating vWF:Ag is raised in PH (126,127), a cut-off of >240 percent predicting death at 1 year (53 percent sensitivity, 93 percent specificity, $p = 0.003$) (127).

D-dimer

D-dimer is a degradation product of fibrin and may reflect microvascular thrombosis, which is seen in PAH. In two small studies, D-dimer levels were elevated in IPAH patients, correlating with NYHA class, PAP and 1-year survival (128,129), but further studies have yet to be undertaken.

Complement 4a des Arg

In a proteomic study of differentially expressed proteins in 27 IPAH plasma samples versus 26 controls, complement component 4a des Arg was discovered to be elevated in IPAH (130). This was confirmed in a second cohort of 30 IPAH and 19 controls and enzyme-linked immunoassays confirmed that the levels were significantly higher ($p < 0.0001$) in IPAH patients (2.12 ± 0.27 mg/mL) compared with normal controls (0.53 ± 0.05 mg/mL). A cut-off level of 0.6 mg/mL correctly classified 92 percent of IPAH patients and 80 percent of controls. Clinical utility of this factor is currently compromised until we better understand its biological origins.

Osteoprotegerin

Osteoprotegerin, a member of the TNF-α receptor superfamily, has increased expression in human PAH vascular lesions and was significantly elevated in serum by more than threefold (1530 ± 191.3 pg/mL, $n = 33$ control patients versus 4710 ± 369.2 pg/mL, $n = 38$ IPAH patients; $p < 0.0001$) compared with healthy control subjects (131). BMP-R2 RNA interference increased osteoprotegerin levels *in vitro* but no evidence of a link to *BMPR2* mutations or hemodynamics was shown in the patient set.

BIOMARKER DISCOVERY AND QUALIFICATION

The availability of new high-throughput technologies in genomics, proteomics, transcriptomics and metabolomics has opened up approaches for novel biomarker discovery.

Screening blood samples, circulating cells and tissue from well-phenotyped patient groups is an active area of research in a number of centres (38,39,132–134). In principle, the pulmonary vascular bed should be a rich source of new biomarkers. The techniques for identifying markers that discriminate between disease and health are well established and the prospects for innovation exciting, but the effort required to qualify a biomarker for a particular purpose should not be underestimated. By way of example, BNP-32 has been proposed as a biomarker of value in the management of heart disease almost since its isolation in 1989 but its acceptance by regulatory authorities for specific indications is very recent.

CONCLUDING REMARKS

The gold standard for the diagnosis of PH, right heart catheterization, is invasive and very expensive. Echocardiography and magnetic resonance are less invasive but are skilled techniques and not easily deployed. A simple, cheap and non-invasive blood biomarker could be very useful in a number of clinical scenarios in PH, including identifying susceptible individuals, screening, diagnosis, risk stratification and therapeutic monitoring. Despite the clear value of easily measurable biomarkers, only two have entered clinical practice at present and both have limited utility. *BMPR2* and *ALK1* gene profiling is valuable in identifying at risk relatives of patients with established mutations. BNP-32/NT-proBNP measurements are markers of right heart dysfunction in PH and have value in assessing group responses to interventions in clinical trials. BNP-32/NT-proBNP measurements carry information on prognosis and can be useful in individual patient management when integrated into the complete package of clinical information gathered about that patient. The possibility that BNP measurements might be more useful in patient management in combination with other blood biomarkers, for example, GDF-15, merits prospective study. New high-throughput technologies and the vast surface area of the pulmonary vasculature offer the potential for new discoveries and the identification of a biomarker that reflects vascular damage rather than cardiac stress. The qualification of new biomarkers in PH is no small feat and requires access to large well-phenotyped patient populations, with serial sampling.

KEY POINTS

- Biomarkers include any accessible, quantifiable signal that informs about the state of health of a biological system.
- A simple, cheap and non-invasive blood biomarker could be useful in a number of clinical scenarios in PH, including identifying susceptible individuals, screening, diagnosis, risk stratification and therapeutic monitoring, where current methods including right heart catheterization and magnetic resonance imaging are invasive and/or very expensive.
- Mutations in *BMPR2* and *ALK1* can be used in context (i.e. patients with a family history) to identify susceptible individuals.
- Brain natriuretic peptide (BNP-32) and N-terminal proBNP (NT-proBNP) have some clinical utility in PH, in particular for risk stratification and for measuring responses to novel therapeutics in clinical trials.
- Other potential novel biomarkers in PH include growth and differentiation factor-15 (GDF-15), uric acid and creatinine.
- Other markers of cardiomyocyte stress may help identify late stage disease, indicating an increase in therapy or more invasive treatments.
- New high-throughput technologies and the vast surface area of the pulmonary vasculature offer the potential for new discoveries and the identification of a biomarker that reflects vascular damage rather than cardiac stress.
- The road from biomarker discovery to biomarker qualification is a long one and requires access to large well-phenotyped patient populations in order to gain confidence in any signal and acceptance by the research and regulatory communities.

REFERENCES

1. The Biomarker Definitions Working Group. Biomarkers and surrogate endpoints: preferred definitions and conceptual framework. Clin Pharmacol Ther 2001;69:89–95.
2. Ventetuolo CE, Benza RL, Peacock AJ *et al.* Surrogate and combined end points in pulmonary arterial hypertension. Proc Am Thorac Soc 2008;5:617–22.
3. Chen H, Taichman DB, Doyle RL. Health-related quality of life and patient-reported outcomes in pulmonary arterial hypertension. Proc Am Thorac Soc 2008;5:623–30.
4. Hoeper MM, Markevych I, Spiekerkoetter E *et al.* Goal-oriented treatment and combination therapy for pulmonary arterial hypertension. Eur Respir J 2005;26:858–63.
5. Lane KB, Machado RD, Pauciulo MW *et al.* Heterozygous germline mutations in BMPR2, encoding a TGF-beta receptor, cause familial primary pulmonary hypertension. The International PPH Consortium. Nat Genet 2000;26:81–4.
6. Humbert M, Deng Z, Simonneau G *et al.* BMPR2 germline mutations in pulmonary hypertension associated with fenfluramine derivatives. Eur Respir J 2002;20:518–23.
7. Morisaki H, Nakanishi N, Kyotani S *et al.* BMPR2 mutations found in Japanese patients with familial and sporadic primary pulmonary hypertension. Hum Mutat 2004;23:632.

8. Roberts KE, McElroy JJ, Wong WP *et al.* BMPR2 mutations in pulmonary arterial hypertension with congenital heart disease. Eur Respir J 2004;24:371–4.

9. Aldred MA, Vijayakrishnan J, James V *et al.* BMPR2 gene rearrangements account for a significant proportion of mutations in familial and idiopathic pulmonary arterial hypertension. Hum Mutat 2006;27:212–3.

10. Machado RD, Aldred MA, James V *et al.* Mutations of the TGF-beta type II receptor BMPR2 in pulmonary arterial hypertension. Hum Mutat 2006;27:121–32.

11. Cogan JD, Pauciulo MW, Batchman AP *et al.* High frequency of BMPR2 exonic deletions/duplications in familial pulmonary arterial hypertension. Am J Respir Crit Care Med 2006;174:590–8.

12. Phillips JA, III, Poling JS, Phillips CA *et al.* Synergistic heterozygosity for TGFbeta1 SNPs and BMPR2 mutations modulates the age at diagnosis and penetrance of familial pulmonary arterial hypertension. Genet Med 2008;10:359–65.

13. Sztrymf B, Coulet F, Girerd B *et al.* Clinical outcomes of pulmonary arterial hypertension in carriers of BMPR2 mutation. Am J Respir Crit Care Med 2008;177:1377–83.

14. Rosenzweig EB, Morse JH, Knowles JA *et al.* Clinical implications of determining BMPR2 mutation status in a large cohort of children and adults with pulmonary arterial hypertension. J Heart Lung Transplant 2008;27:668–74.

15. Nagaya N, Nishikimi T, Okano Y *et al.* Plasma brain natriuretic peptide levels increase in proportion to the extent of right ventricular dysfunction in pulmonary hypertension. J Am Coll Cardiol 1998;31:202–8.

16. Nagaya N, Nishikimi T, Uematsu M *et al.* Plasma brain natriuretic peptide as a prognostic indicator in patients with primary pulmonary hypertension. Circulation 2000;102:865–70.

17. Yamaguchi H, Yoshida J, Yamamoto K *et al.* Elevation of plasma brain natriuretic peptide is a hallmark of diastolic heart failure independent of ventricular hypertrophy. J Am Coll Cardiol 2004;43:55–60.

18. Leuchte HH, Holzapfel M, Baumgartner RA *et al.* Clinical significance of brain natriuretic peptide in primary pulmonary hypertension. J Am Coll Cardiol 2004;43:764–70.

19. Leuchte HH, Neurohr C, Baumgartner R *et al.* Brain natriuretic peptide and exercise capacity in lung fibrosis and pulmonary hypertension. Am J Respir Crit Care Med 2004;170:360–5.

20. Souza R, Bogossian HB, Humbert M *et al.* N-terminal-pro-brain natriuretic peptide as a haemodynamic marker in idiopathic pulmonary arterial hypertension. Eur Respir J 2005;25:509–13.

21. Wilkins MR, Paul GA, Strange JW *et al.* Sildenafil versus Endothelin Receptor Antagonist for Pulmonary Hypertension (SERAPH) study. Am J Respir Crit Care Med 2005;171:1292–7.

22. Leuchte HH, Holzapfel M, Baumgartner RA *et al.* Characterization of brain natriuretic peptide in long-term follow-up of pulmonary arterial hypertension. Chest 2005;128:2368–74.

23. Leuchte HH, Baumgartner RA, Nounou ME *et al.* Brain natriuretic peptide is a prognostic parameter in chronic lung disease. Am J Respir Crit Care Med 2006;173:744–50.

24. Fijalkowska A, Kurzyna M, Torbicki A *et al.* Serum N-terminal brain natriuretic peptide as a prognostic parameter in patients with pulmonary hypertension. Chest 2006;129:1313–21.

25. Souza R, Jardim C, Julio Cesar FC *et al.* NT-proBNP as a tool to stratify disease severity in pulmonary arterial hypertension. Respir Med 2007;101:69–75.

26. Leuchte HH, El NM, Tuerpe JC *et al.* N-terminal pro-brain natriuretic peptide and renal insufficiency as predictors of mortality in pulmonary hypertension. Chest 2007;131:402–9.

27. Blyth KG, Groenning BA, Mark PB *et al.* NT-proBNP can be used to detect right ventricular systolic dysfunction in pulmonary hypertension. Eur Respir J 2007;29:737–44.

28. Daniels LB, Maisel AS. Natriuretic peptides. J Am Coll Cardiol 2007;50:2357–68.

29. Deng Z, Morse JH, Slager SL *et al.* Familial primary pulmonary hypertension (gene PPH1) is caused by mutations in the bone morphogenetic protein receptor-II gene. Am J Hum Genet 2000;67:737–44.

30. Trembath RC. Mutations in the TGF-beta type 1 receptor, ALK1, in combined primary pulmonary hypertension and hereditary haemorrhagic telangiectasia, implies pathway specificity. J Heart Lung Transplant 2001;20:175.

31. Harrison RE, Flanagan JA, Sankelo M *et al.* Molecular and functional analysis identifies ALK-1 as the predominant cause of pulmonary hypertension related to hereditary haemorrhagic telangiectasia. J Med Genet 2003; 40:865–71.

32. Kawabata M, Chytil A, Moses HL. Cloning of a novel type II serine/threonine kinase receptor through interaction with the type I transforming growth factor-beta receptor. J Biol Chem 1995;270:5625–30.

33. Massague J. TGF-beta signal transduction. Annu Rev Biochem 1998;67:753–91.

34. Adachi-Yamada T, Nakamura M, Irie K *et al.* p38 mitogen-activated protein kinase can be involved in transforming growth factor beta superfamily signal transduction in Drosophila wing morphogenesis. Mol Cell Biol 1999;19:2322–9.

35. Hansmann G, de Jesus Perez, V, Alastalo TP *et al.* An antiproliferative BMP-2/PPARgamma/apoE axis in human and murine SMCs and its role in pulmonary hypertension. J Clin Invest 2008;118:1846–57.

36. Newman JH, Phillips JA, III, Loyd JE. Narrative review: the enigma of pulmonary arterial hypertension: new insights from genetic studies. Ann Intern Med 2008;148:278–83.

37. Atkinson C, Stewart S, Upton PD *et al.* Primary pulmonary hypertension is associated with reduced pulmonary vascular expression of type II bone morphogenetic protein receptor. Circulation 2002;105:1672–8.

38. Bull TM, Coldren CD, Moore M *et al.* Gene microarray analysis of peripheral blood cells in pulmonary arterial hypertension. Am J Respir Crit Care Med 2004; 170:911–9.

39. Bull TM, Coldren CD, Geraci MW, Voelkel NF. Gene expression profiling in pulmonary hypertension. Proc Am Thorac Soc 2007;4:117–20.

40. Yoshimura M, Yasue H, Morita E et al. Hemodynamic, renal, and hormonal responses to brain natriuretic peptide infusion in patients with congestive heart failure. Circulation 1991;84:1581–8.

41. Nakao K, Ogawa Y, Suga S, Imura H. Molecular biology and biochemistry of the natriuretic peptide system. II: Natriuretic peptide receptors. J Hypertens 1992;10:1111–4.

42. Yasue H, Yoshimura M, Sumida H et al. Localization and mechanism of secretion of B-type natriuretic peptide in comparison with those of A-type natriuretic peptide in normal subjects and patients with heart failure. Circulation 1994;90:195–203.

43. Soeki T, Kishimoto I, Okumura H et al. C-type natriuretic peptide, a novel antifibrotic and antihypertrophic agent, prevents cardiac remodeling after myocardial infarction. J Am Coll Cardiol 2005;45:608–16.

44. Yoshimura M, Yasue H, Okumura K et al. Different secretion patterns of atrial natriuretic peptide and brain natriuretic peptide in patients with congestive heart failure. Circulation 1993;87:464–9.

45. Yandle TG, Richards AM, Nicholls MG et al. Metabolic clearance rate and plasma half life of alpha-human atrial natriuretic peptide in man. Life Sci 1986;38:1827–33.

46. Holmes SJ, Espiner EA, Richards AM et al. Renal, endocrine, and hemodynamic effects of human brain natriuretic peptide in normal man. J Clin Endocrinol Metab 1993;76:91–6.

47. Chen HH. Heart failure: a state of brain natriuretic peptide deficiency or resistance or both! J Am Coll Cardiol 2007;49:1089–91.

48. Vogeser M, Jacob K. B-type natriuretic peptide (BNP) – validation of an immediate response assay. Clin Lab 2001;47:29–33.

49. Yeo KT, Wu AH, Apple FS et al. Multicenter evaluation of the Roche NT-proBNP assay and comparison to the Biosite Triage BNP assay. Clin Chim Acta 2003;338:107–15.

50. Mueller C, Scholer A, Laule-Kilian K et al. Use of B-type natriuretic peptide in the evaluation and management of acute dyspnea. N Engl J Med 2004;350:647–54.

51. Moe GW, Howlett J, Januzzi JL, Zowall H. N-terminal pro-B-type natriuretic peptide testing improves the management of patients with suspected acute heart failure: primary results of the Canadian prospective randomized multicenter IMPROVE-CHF study. Circulation 2007;115:3103–10.

52. Friedewald VE, Jr., Burnett JC, Jr., Januzzi JL, Jr. et al. The editor's roundtable: B-type natriuretic peptide. Am J Cardiol 2008;101:1733–40.

53. Mentzer RM, Jr., Rubio R, Berne RM. Release of adenosine by hypoxic canine lung tissue and its possible role in pulmonary circulation. Am J Physiol 1975;229:1625–31.

54. Braghiroli A, Sacco C, Erbetta M et al. Overnight urinary uric acid: creatinine ratio for detection of sleep hypoxemia. Validation study in chronic obstructive pulmonary disease

55. Leyva F, Chua TP, Anker SD, Coats AJ. Uric acid in chronic heart failure: a measure of the anaerobic threshold. Metabolism 1998;47:1156–9.

56. Hayabuchi Y, Matsuoka S, Akita H, Kuroda Y. Hyperuricaemia in cyanotic congenital heart disease. Eur J Pediatr 1993;152:873–6.

57. Hoeper MM, Hohlfeld JM, Fabel H. Hyperuricaemia in patients with right or left heart failure. Eur Respir J 1999;13:682–5.

58. Nagaya N, Uematsu M, Satoh T et al. Serum uric acid levels correlate with the severity and the mortality of primary pulmonary hypertension. Am J Respir Crit Care Med 1999;160:487–92.

59. Voelkel MA, Wynne KM, Badesch DB et al. Hyperuricemia in severe pulmonary hypertension. Chest 2000;117: 19–24.

60. Bendayan D, Shitrit D, Ygla M et al. Hyperuricemia as a prognostic factor in pulmonary arterial hypertension. Respir Med 2003;97:130–3.

61. Njaman W, Iesaki T, Iwama Y et al. Serum uric acid as a prognostic predictor in pulmonary arterial hypertension with connective tissue disease. Int Heart J 2007;48:523–32.

62. Nickel N, Kempf T, Tapken H et al. Growth differentiation factor-15 in idiopathic pulmonary arterial hypertension. Am J Respir Crit Care Med 2008;178:534–41.

63. Darlington LG. Study to compare the relative hyperuricaemic effects of frusemide and bumetanide. Adv Exp Med Biol 1986;195(Pt A):333–9.

64. Bakhtiiarov ZA. [Changes in xanthine oxidase activity in patients with circulatory failure]. Ter Arkh 1989;61:68–9.

65. Anker SD, Doehner W, Rauchhaus M et al. Uric acid and survival in chronic heart failure: validation and application in metabolic, functional, and hemodynamic staging. Circulation 2003;107:1991–7.

66. Bootcov MR, Bauskin AR, Valenzuela SM et al. MIC-1, a novel macrophage inhibitory cytokine, is a divergent member of the TGF-beta superfamily. Proc Natl Acad Sci USA 1997;94:11514–9.

67. Roberts AB, Sporn MB. Physiological actions and clinical applications of transforming growth factor-beta (TGF-beta). Growth Factors 1993;8:1–9.

68. Su AI, Wiltshire T, Batalov S et al. A gene atlas of the mouse and human protein-encoding transcriptomes. Proc Natl Acad Sci USA 2004;101:6062–7.

69. Schlittenhardt D, Schober A, Strelau J et al. Involvement of growth differentiation factor-15/macrophage inhibitory cytokine-1 (GDF-15/MIC-1) in oxLDL-induced apoptosis of human macrophages in vitro and in arteriosclerotic lesions. Cell Tissue Res 2004;318:325–33.

70. Kempf T, Eden M, Strelau J et al. The transforming growth factor-beta superfamily member growth-differentiation factor-15 protects the heart from ischemia/reperfusion injury. Circ Res 2006;98:351–60.

and obstructive sleep apnea before and after treatment with nasal continuous positive airway pressure. Am Rev Respir Dis 1993;148:173–8.

71. Xu J, Kimball TR, Lorenz JN *et al.* GDF15/MIC-1 functions as a protective and antihypertrophic factor released from the myocardium in association with SMAD protein activation. Circ Res 2006;98:342–50.

72. Wollert KC, Kempf T, Peter T *et al.* Prognostic value of growth-differentiation factor-15 in patients with non-ST-elevation acute coronary syndrome. Circulation 2007; 115:962–71.

73. Kempf T, von HS, Peter T *et al.* Prognostic utility of growth differentiation factor-15 in patients with chronic heart failure. J Am Coll Cardiol 2007;50:1054–60.

74. Lankeit M, Kempf T, Dellas C *et al.* Growth differentiation factor-15 for prognostic assessment of patients with acute pulmonary embolism. Am J Respir Crit Care Med 2008;177:1018–25.

75. Frank D, Kuhn C, Brors B *et al.* Gene expression pattern in biomechanically stretched cardiomyocytes: evidence for a stretch-specific gene program. Hypertension 2008;51:309–18.

76. Sarnak MJ, Levey AS, Schoolwerth AC *et al.* Kidney disease as a risk factor for development of cardiovascular disease: a statement from the American Heart Association Councils on Kidney in Cardiovascular Disease, High Blood Pressure Research, Clinical Cardiology, and Epidemiology and Prevention. Circulation 2003;108:2154–69.

77. Go AS, Chertow GM, Fan D *et al.* Chronic kidney disease and the risks of death, cardiovascular events, and hospitalization. N Engl J Med 2004;351:1296–305.

78. Smith GL, Lichtman JH, Bracken MB *et al.* Renal impairment and outcomes in heart failure: systematic review and meta-analysis. J Am Coll Cardiol 2006;47: 1987–96.

79. Shah SJ, Thenappan T, Rich S *et al.* Association of serum creatinine with abnormal hemodynamics and mortality in pulmonary arterial hypertension. Circulation 2008;117:2475–83.

80. Giannitsis E, Muller-Bardorff M, Kurowski V *et al.* Independent prognostic value of cardiac troponin T in patients with confirmed pulmonary embolism. Circulation 2000;102:211–7.

81. Meyer T, Binder L, Hruska N *et al.* Cardiac troponin I elevation in acute pulmonary embolism is associated with right ventricular dysfunction. J Am Coll Cardiol 2000;36:1632–6.

82. Douketis JD, Crowther MA, Stanton EB, Ginsberg JS. Elevated cardiac troponin levels in patients with submassive pulmonary embolism. Arch Intern Med 2002;162:79–81.

83. Torbicki A, Kurzyna M, Kuca P *et al.* Detectable serum cardiac troponin T as a marker of poor prognosis among patients with chronic precapillary pulmonary hypertension. Circulation 2003;108:844–8.

84. Alhadi HA, Fox KA. Do we need additional markers of myocyte necrosis: the potential value of heart fatty–acid–binding protein. QJM 2004;97:187–98.

85. Lankeit M, Dellas C, Panzenbock A *et al.* Heart-type fatty acid-binding protein for risk assessment of chronic

86. Puls M, Dellas C, Lankeit M *et al.* Heart-type fatty acid-binding protein permits early risk stratification of pulmonary embolism. Eur Heart J 2007;28:224–9.

87. Galie N, Manes A, Branzi A. The endothelin system in pulmonary arterial hypertension. Cardiovasc Res 2004;61:227–37.

88. Stewart DJ, Levy RD, Cernacek P, Langleben D. Increased plasma endothelin-1 in pulmonary hypertension: marker or mediator of disease? Ann Intern Med 1991;114:464–9.

89. Giaid A, Yanagisawa M, Langleben D *et al.* Expression of endothelin-1 in the lungs of patients with pulmonary hypertension. N Engl J Med 1993;328:1732–9.

90. Cacoub P, Dorent R, Maistre G *et al.* Endothelin-1 in primary pulmonary hypertension and the Eisenmenger syndrome. Am J Cardiol 1993;71:448–50.

91. Nootens M, Kaufmann E, Rector T *et al.* Neurohormonal activation in patients with right ventricular failure from pulmonary hypertension: relation to hemodynamic variables and endothelin levels. J Am Coll Cardiol 1995;26:1581–5.

92. Cacoub P, Dorent R, Nataf P *et al.* Endothelin-1 in the lungs of patients with pulmonary hypertension. Cardiovasc Res 1997;33:196–200.

93. Rubens C, Ewert R, Halank M *et al.* Big endothelin-1 and endothelin-1 plasma levels are correlated with the severity of primary pulmonary hypertension. Chest 2001;120:1562–9.

94. Hemsen A, Ahlborg G, Ottosson-Seeberger A, Lundberg JM. Metabolism of Big endothelin-1 (1–38) and (22–38) in the human circulation in relation to production of endothelin-1 (1–21). Regul Pept 1995;55:287–97.

95. Wilkens H, Bauer M, Forestier N *et al.* Influence of inhaled iloprost on transpulmonary gradient of big endothelin in patients with pulmonary hypertension. Circulation 2003;107:1509–13.

96. Galie N, Grigioni F, Bacchi-Reggiani L *et al.* Relation of endothelin-1 to survival in patients with primary pulmonary hypertension. Eur J Clin Invest 1996;26(Suppl. 1):273.

97. Tatemoto K, Hosoya M, Habata Y *et al.* Isolation and characterization of a novel endogenous peptide ligand for the human APJ receptor. Biochem Biophys Res Commun 1998;251:471–6.

98. Szokodi I, Tavi P, Foldes G *et al.* Apelin, the novel endogenous ligand of the orphan receptor APJ, regulates cardiac contractility. Circ Res 2002;91:434–40.

99. Berry MF, Pirolli TJ, Jayasankar V *et al.* Apelin has in vivo inotropic effects on normal and failing hearts. Circulation 2004;110:II187–93.

100. Kawamata Y, Habata Y, Fukusumi S *et al.* Molecular properties of apelin: tissue distribution and receptor binding. Biochim Biophys Acta 2001;1538:162–71.

101. Goetze JP, Rehfeld JF, Carlsen J *et al.* Apelin: a new plasma marker of cardiopulmonary disease. Regul Pept 2006;133:134–8.

102. Kereveur A, Callebert J, Humbert M *et al.* High plasma serotonin levels in primary pulmonary hypertension. Effect

thromboembolic pulmonary hypertension. Eur Respir J 2008;31:1024–9.

of long-term epoprostenol (prostacyclin) therapy. Arterioscler Thromb Vasc Biol 2000;20:2233–9.

103. Girgis RE, Champion HC, Diette GB *et al.* Decreased exhaled nitric oxide in pulmonary arterial hypertension: response to bosentan therapy. Am J Respir Crit Care Med 2005;172:352–7.

104. Diller GP, van ES, Okonko DO *et al.* Circulating endothelial progenitor cells in patients with Eisenmenger syndrome and idiopathic pulmonary arterial hypertension. Circulation 2008;117:3020–30.

105. Cooke JP. A novel mechanism for pulmonary arterial hypertension? Circulation 2003;108:1420–1.

106. Kielstein JT, Bode-Boger SM, Hesse G *et al.* Asymmetrical dimethylarginine in idiopathic pulmonary arterial hypertension. Arterioscler Thromb Vasc Biol 2005;25: 1414–8.

107. Skoro-Sajer N, Mittermayer F, Panzenboeck A *et al.* Asymmetric dimethylarginine is increased in chronic thromboembolic pulmonary hypertension. Am J Respir Crit Care Med 2007;176:1154–60.

108. Gorenflo M, Zheng C, Werle E *et al.* Plasma levels of asymmetrical dimethyl-L-arginine in patients with congenital heart disease and pulmonary hypertension. J Cardiovasc Pharmacol 2001;37:489–92.

109. Boos CJ, Lip GY, Blann AD. Circulating endothelial cells in cardiovascular disease. J Am Coll Cardiol 2006;48: 1538–47.

110. Erdbruegger U, Haubitz M, Woywodt A. Circulating endothelial cells: a novel marker of endothelial damage. Clin Chim Acta 2006;373:17–26.

111. Bull TM, Golpon H, Hebbel RP *et al.* Circulating endothelial cells in pulmonary hypertension. Thromb Haemost 2003;90:698–703.

112. Hristov M, Weber C. Endothelial progenitor cells: characterization, pathophysiology, and possible clinical relevance. J Cell Mol Med 2004;8:498–508.

113. Khakoo AY, Finkel T. Endothelial progenitor cells. Annu Rev Med 2005;56:79–101.

114. Liew A, Barry F, O'Brien T. Endothelial progenitor cells: diagnostic and therapeutic considerations. Bioessays 2006;28:261–70.

115. Vasa M, Fichtlscherer S, Aicher A *et al.* Number and migratory activity of circulating endothelial progenitor cells inversely correlate with risk factors for coronary artery disease. Circ Res 2001;89:E1–7.

116. Hill JM, Zalos G, Halcox JP *et al.* Circulating endothelial progenitor cells, vascular function, and cardiovascular risk. N Engl J Med 2003;348:593–600.

117. Werner N, Kosiol S, Schiegl T *et al.* Circulating endothelial progenitor cells and cardiovascular outcomes. N Engl J Med 2005;353:999–1007.

118. Zhao YD, Courtman DW, Deng Y *et al.* Rescue of monocrotaline-induced pulmonary arterial hypertension using bone marrow-derived endothelial-like progenitor cells: efficacy of combined cell and eNOS gene therapy in established disease. Circ Res 2005;96:442–50.

119. Fadini GP, Schiavon M, Rea F *et al.* Depletion of endothelial progenitor cells may link pulmonary fibrosis and pulmonary hypertension. Am J Respir Crit Care Med 2007;176:724–5.

120. Junhui Z, Xingxiang W, Guosheng F *et al.* Reduced number and activity of circulating endothelial progenitor cells in patients with idiopathic pulmonary arterial hypertension. Respir Med 2008;102:1073–9.

121. Asosingh K, Aldred MA, Vasanji A *et al.* Circulating angiogenic precursors in idiopathic pulmonary arterial hypertension. Am J Pathol 2008;172:615–27.

122. Wiedemann R, Ghofrani HA, Weissmann N *et al.* Atrial natriuretic peptide in severe primary and nonprimary pulmonary hypertension: response to iloprost inhalation. J Am Coll Cardiol 2001;38:1130–6.

123. Ghofrani HA, Wiedemann R, Rose F *et al.* Lung cGMP release subsequent to NO inhalation in pulmonary hypertension: responders versus nonresponders. Eur Respir J 2002;19:664–71.

124. Bogdan M, Humbert M, Francoual J *et al.* Urinary cGMP concentrations in severe primary pulmonary hypertension. Thorax 1998;53:1059–62.

125. Veyradier A, Nishikubo T, Humbert M *et al.* Improvement of von Willebrand factor proteolysis after prostacyclin infusion in severe pulmonary arterial hypertension. Circulation 2000;102:2460–2.

126. Friedman R, Mears JG, Barst RJ. Continuous infusion of prostacyclin normalizes plasma markers of endothelial cell injury and platelet aggregation in primary pulmonary hypertension. Circulation 1997;96:2782–4.

127. Lopes AA, Maeda NY. Circulating von Willebrand factor antigen as a predictor of short-term prognosis in pulmonary hypertension. Chest 1998;114:1276–82.

128. Shitrit D, Bendayan D, Rudensky B *et al.* Elevation of ELISA d-dimer levels in patients with primary pulmonary hypertension. Respiration 2002;69:327–9.

129. Shitrit D, Bendayan D, Bar-Gil-Shitrit A *et al.* Significance of a plasma D-dimer test in patients with primary pulmonary hypertension. Chest 2002;122:1674–8.

130. Abdul-Salam VB, Paul GA, Ali JO *et al.* Identification of plasma protein biomarkers associated with idiopathic pulmonary arterial hypertension. Proteomics 2006; 6:2286–94.

131. Lawrie A, Waterman E, Southwood M *et al.* Evidence of a role for osteoprotegerin in the pathogenesis of pulmonary arterial hypertension. Am J Pathol 2008;172:256–64.

132. Yu M, Wang XX, Zhang FR *et al.* Proteomic analysis of the serum in patients with idiopathic pulmonary arterial hypertension. J Zhejiang Univ Sci B 2007;8:221–7.

133. Moreno-Vinasco L, Gomberg-Maitland M, Maitland ML *et al.* Genomic assessment of a multikinase inhibitor, sorafenib, in a rodent model of pulmonary hypertension. Physiol Genomics 2008;33:278–91.

134. Terrier B, Tamby MC, Camoin L *et al.* Identification of target antigens of antifibroblast antibodies in pulmonary arterial hypertension. Am J Respir Crit Care Med 2008;177:1128–34.

12

Cardiac catheterization of patients with pulmonary hypertension

TODD M BULL, BERTRON M GROVES AND DAVID B BADESCH

INTRODUCTION

An essential part of the evaluation of patients with pulmonary hypertension (PH) includes an invasive measurement of the patient's cardiopulmonary hemodynamics, or right heart catheterization (RHC). The RHC confirms accuracy of the diagnosis of PH, allows appropriate classification of the disease, provides accurate assessment of the severity of the condition and allows selection of appropriate therapy. In addition to characterizing the patient's pulmonary hemodynamics, the catheterization procedure should be designed to safely answer the following questions:

1. Is the PH in part or predominantly due to pulmonary venous hypertension as indicated by elevation of the pulmonary arterial wedge pressure/pulmonary artery occlusion pressure (PCWP/PAOP), or is the PH "precapillary" due to pulmonary arterial/arteriolar obstructive disease?
2. Does the patient have an intracardiac communication or "shunt" which might cause or contribute to the development of PH as a result of increased pulmonary vascular flow? Such shunts include atrial septal defects (ASD), ventricular septal defects (VSD), anomalous pulmonary venous return and patent ductus arteriosus (PDA). Increased flow to the pulmonary vasculature from a left-to-right shunt can result in remodeling of the pulmonary arterial bed, elevation in pulmonary arterial pressure and eventually reversal of flow with

development of Eisenmenger's syndrome. Is isolated surgical or transcatheter correction of the congenital heart defect possible or will the patient also require medical therapy and consideration of simultaneous lung or heart/lung transplantation?
3. Does the patient have an intracardiac right-to-left shunt via a patent foramen ovale or atrial septal defect which markedly increases the challenge of accurately measuring pulmonary/systemic blood flow (QP/QS)?
4. Does the patient have sufficient acute pulmonary vasoreactivity to warrant a long-term trial of oral calcium channel blocker treatment, or does such a trial subject the patient to significant risk with minimal benefit?
5. In patients with PH secondary to left ventricular cardiomyopathy who are undergoing evaluation as potential candidates for heart transplantation, is there enough reversibility of the elevated pulmonary vascular resistance for the patient to be accepted as a heart transplant recipient?

PRECATHETERIZATION EVALUATION

To address all issues of importance for a pulmonary hypertensive patient's hemodynamic assessment, a thorough precatheterization evaluation should be performed (see Chapters 7–9). Depending on the patient's clinical evaluation, appropriate modification in the details of the right heart catheterization should be planned ahead. For example, if chronic thromboembolic disease is strongly suspected, digital subtraction angiography of the pulmonary vasculature may be added to the evaluation. Suspicion of congenital heart disease should prompt a careful and detailed oximetry series. If portal PH is being considered, assessment of portal pressures and measurement of a portal gradient can be performed by measuring the hepatic vein wedge pressure.

CARDIAC CATHETERIZATION PROCEDURE: TECHNIQUES AND MEASUREMENTS

For the initial cardiac catheterization procedure, a standardized approach to cardiac catheterization is recommended. This approach can help to minimize intrapatient variability related to technical factors and allows members of the catheterization team to perform the RHC more efficiently. Our approach is outlined below.

Sedation

We do not routinely use conscious sedation prior to or during the cardiac catheterization procedure, as pulmonary hypertensive patients can react adversely to sedatives and systemic vasodilatation may alter the baseline hemodynamics. However, when local anesthesia is insufficient for an anxious patient, we use low-dose intravenous midazolam and fentanyl.

Percutaneous placement of venous sheath for right heart catheterization

Our preferred approach for RHC in patients being assessed for PH is the right internal jugular (IJ) vein. The right IJ vein is the most direct route and thus easiest position from which to manipulate the PA catheter into the pulmonary vasculature. This approach facilitates catheterization of patients with severe elevation of their pulmonary artery pressures and dilatation of the right ventricle and pulmonary arteries with moderate to severe pulmonary and or tricuspid valvular insufficiency. Another benefit of this approach is the patient's rapid recovery time. Frequently, patients are discharged directly from the cath lab following a few minutes of manual compression to close the IJ venotomy site. Since catheter manipulation into the pulmonary artery is much easier from the neck, an 8.0 Fr sheath with a self-sealing hemostatic valve and side arm port is satisfactory for the IJ vein approach in most pulmonary hypertensive patients when a 7.5 Fr standard or "guidewire" Swan–Ganz thermodilution catheter is used. If an 8.0 Fr oximetric balloon-tipped pulmonary artery catheter (Opticath, #P7110-EP8-H, Abbott Laboratories, Chicago, IL) is used, a 9.0 Fr sheath is needed to accommodate the larger catheter size.

The other frequently used approach to the RHC is the right femoral vein. This approach is desirable if the patient also requires left heart catheterization or if the right IJ approach is not possible, for example due to altered anatomy or the presence of other catheters. We also prefer the femoral vein approach if measurement of IVC oxygen saturation is needed for an oximetry series to quantitate an intracardiac shunt or if measurement of the intrahepatic venous wedge pressure is needed. Due to the increased technical difficulty that is frequently encountered secondary to marked enlargement of the RA and RV in association with severe tricuspid and/or pulmonary valvular regurgitation, we have found it is helpful to use an 8.0 Fr sheath without a side arm port and hemostatic valve that limits the freedom of catheter manipulation. To provide hemostasis and optimal freedom of catheter manipulation through this type of femoral venous sheath, an adjustable Luer lock adapter (#PMLLA-UCC-L, Cook Cardiology, Bloomington, IN) is used.

Following RIJ venous catheterization, patients who are hemodynamically stable are discharged directly from the cardiac catheterization laboratory without the need for further observation. When femoral venous catheterization is performed, patients are observed in the supine position in a recovery unit for one hour following removal of the sheath to ensure adequate venous hemostasis prior to ambulation and discharge.

"Guidewire" Swan–Ganz thermodilution catheter

Hemodynamic evaluation of patients with severe PH is frequently difficult due to marked enlargement of the right atrium and right ventricle associated with severe tricuspid valvular regurgitation + /– severe pulmonary valvular regurgitation. Because of the significant back pressure associated with the increased RV afterload, there is a tendency to prolapse a standard balloon tipped Swan–Ganz catheter from the right ventricle back into the right atrium. To overcome these difficulties that are magnified when the femoral venous approach is used, Dr Groves developed a "guidewire" Swan–Ganz balloon-tipped thermodilution catheter (#93A-821H, Baxter Healthcare, Irvine, CA) in collaboration with the American Edwards Co. in 1983 (1). The catheter has a "blind-end" lumen which allows the insertion of an indwelling guidewire. The guidewire serves to stiffen the catheter facilitating its advancement into the pulmonary artery and in helping to maintain its position within the pulmonary artery for prolonged periods. The "guidewire" lumen of this catheter ends proximal to the location of the thermistor near the end of the thermodilution balloon-tipped catheter (Figure 12.1). The blind lumen accommodates a 0.025–0.028 inch guidewire and does not allow exit of the guidewire outside the catheter which could initiate arrhythmias or cause cardiac perforation.

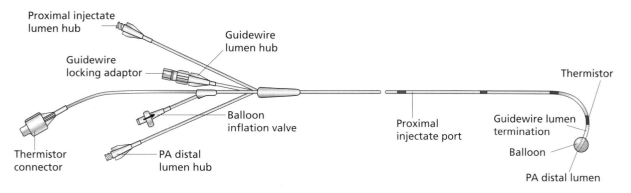

Figure 12.1 "Guidewire" Swan–Ganz catheter design. The anatomy of this catheter is identical to the venous infusion port (VIP) Swan–Ganz balloon-tipped thermodilution catheter with the exception that the VIP port is used as the guidewire lumen which is a blind-end lumen that terminates near the thermistor. The guidewire lumen is preloaded with a 0.028 inch guidewire before the catheter is inserted into the venous access sheath to stiffen the shaft of the catheter for navigation through an enlarged, hypertensive right ventricle that is usually associated with moderate to severe tricuspid valvular regurgitation. Once the tip of the catheter is positioned appropriately in the right or left pulmonary artery, the guidewire is retracted approximately 10 cm from the tip of the catheter so that it still traverses the pulmonary valve, but softens the catheter tip enough to prevent inadvertent wedging that could cause a life-threatening pulmonary infarction in patients with severe pulmonary hypertension. The guidewire locking adaptor is then tightened to secure the desired guidewire position within the catheter.

Once the catheter is properly positioned within the right or left pulmonary artery, the balloon tip can readily be inflated to allow recording of a wedge pressure, which can be difficult in many patients with severe PH. After optimal positioning of this catheter, we recommend that the guidewire be retracted approximately 10 cm from the tip of the catheter to soften its distal segment and minimize the likelihood of prolonged entrapment in the wedge position that could produce pulmonary infarction or rupture of the pulmonary artery. The distal lumen is still available for blood sampling and pressure measurement, while the guidewire is positioned in the "guidewire" lumen.

In the rare patient in whom the pulmonary arterial wedge pressure cannot be successfully obtained using either a standard Swan–Ganz balloon tipped PA catheter or a "guidewire" catheter, the left ventricular end diastolic pressure (LVEDP) can be measured directly. The right or left femoral artery is accessed and a 5 Fr pigtail catheter is inserted retrograde across the aortic valve into the left ventricle. A normal LVEDP associated with echocardiographic evidence of a normal left atrium/mitral valve excludes "left-sided" etiologies of pulmonary hypertension.

Percutaneous systemic arterial catheterization

We perform most of our hemodynamic studies without using percutaneous insertion of an intra-arterial catheter in patients only being assessed for PH. The systemic arterial pressure and oxygen saturation are monitored non-invasively using a combined automated brachial arterial blood pressure cuff and finger pulse oximeter (Propaq 104,

Protocol Systems, Beaverton, OR). However, in hemodynamically unstable patients, we recommend placement of a 20 gauge percutaneous radial or brachial arterial cannula which has a flexible guidewire stylet (#RA-04120, Arrow International, Reading, PA) for continuous systemic arterial pressure monitoring. In such patients, the systemic arterial oxygen saturation is continuously monitored using a finger pulse oximeter to ensure adequate oxygenation. This combination also optimizes patient comfort and mobility and provides painless monitoring of arterial blood gases if subsequent hemodynamic monitoring in the ICU is required.

Echo/Doppler detection of intracardiac shunting

Prior to cardiac catheterization, transthoracic echocardiography with Doppler color flow and intravenous injection of agitated saline (shunt "bubble study") to detect intracardiac shunting is performed routinely in all patients with PH (see Chapter 8).

Methods used to detect and quantify intracardiac shunts during cardiac catheterization

OXIMETRY "SERIES"

If the precatheterization echo/Doppler study suggests the presence of an intracardiac shunt, it is our preference to perform the right heart catheterization using the femoral vein approach. This approach facilitates inter-atrial trans-septal catheterization using an endhole multipurpose catheter loaded with a 0.035 inch J guidewire. Small samples (0.5–1.0 mL) of whole blood are withdrawn for measurement of O_2 saturation and O_2 content (Hemoximeter #OSM 3, Radiometer, Copenhagen) from multiple sites including: high SVC, low SVC, high RA, mid RA, low RA, high IVC, low IVC, LA (if trans-septal catheter passage is possible through a patent foramen ovale or ASD), pulmonary vein (usually technically accessible from the LA via retrograde catheterization when a patent foramen ovale or ASD is present), RV, main PA and right or left PA, and AO (by finger pulse oximetry). If there is a physiologically significant left-to-right shunt, there will be a > 5–7 percent "step-up" in O_2 saturation in the chamber into which the shunt flows compared to the "mixed venous" or average O_2 saturation proximal to that chamber.

Because of the relative imprecision of this technique secondary to streaming and inadequate mixing in the RA and RV, especially in the presence of severe tricuspid regurgitation, a small left-to-right shunt may be undetected or falsely identified as being present by analysis of oximetry data. To detect and quantify left-to-right shunting from an atrial septal defect, we recommend compensating for the known higher oxygen saturation of "high" IVC blood (due to the contribution of renal vein blood, which normally contains a higher oxygen saturation in comparison to systemic venous blood sampled from the SVC or "low" IVC) when computing the "mixed venous" O_2 saturation by using the Flamm equation (4):

$$\text{Mixed venous O}_2 \text{ saturation} = \frac{(\text{SVC O}_2 \text{ sat} \times 3) + (\text{IVC O}_2 \text{ sat} \times 1)}{4}$$

The standard Fick equation is used to calculate the pulmonary (QP) and systemic (QS) blood flows from the measured (or estimated) oxygen consumption and oxygen contents obtained from the oximetry series (2). A physiologically significant left-to-right shunt will have a QP/QS ratio of $\geq 1.5/1.0$. Patients with the Eisenmenger syndrome resulting from an intracardiac communication such as an ASD or VSD usually have a QP/QS < 1.0 demonstrating right-to-left flow.

ANGIOGRAPHY

Contrast injection with angiographic imaging of antegrade flow can also be used to localize and semi-quantitate left-to-right shunts. An injection into the aortic arch will opacify a PDA, a left ventricular injection in the LAO projection with cranial angulation (parallel to the interventricular septum) will localize a VSD with contrast streaming through the defect into the RV and/or PA, and injection of contrast into the left atrium or pulmonary artery with levophase angiography will demonstrate contrast flowing from the left atrium into the right atrium through an ASD.

Catheterization methods used to detect and quantify right–to–left shunts

OXIMETRY SERIES

Using oximetry data from the sites sampled above for detection of a left-to-right shunt, one can also detect and quantify the size of a right-to-left shunt which is reflected by a "step-down" in oxygen saturation between the pulmonary vein and the left sided chamber which receives the right-to-left shunt: (1) left atrium (LA) if an ASD or patent foramen ovale is present; (2) left ventricle if there is a VSD; or (3) descending thoracic aorta when a PDA is present. Most commonly, right-to-left shunts in pulmonary hypertensive adults occur at the atrial level via an ASD or patent foramen ovale that has been stretched open resulting in a drop in O_2 saturation from ≥ 95 percent in the pulmonary veins to a lower level in the LA depending upon the size of the right-to-left shunt. If a pulmonary vein cannot be sampled through the ASD, the room air pulmonary vein saturation can be estimated as 95–98 percent for the purpose of shunt calculation. The LV and AO will have approximately the same saturation as the LA; however, LA sampling is susceptible to "streaming" or incomplete mixing artifacts. In the presence of significant right-to-left intracardiac shunting, the thermodilution cardiac output method overestimates the cardiac output. Therefore, we recommend that the Fick method be used to measure pulmonary and systemic flow and vascular resistances in these patients.

HYPEROXIA

If the oximetry series is suggestive of a right-to-left shunt, we have found it useful to administer 100 percent oxygen for 10 minutes and repeat the arterial blood gases and hemodynamics. If the PaO_2 exceeds 300 mmHg in our laboratory (5280 feet above sea level), a physiologically significant right-to-left shunt is unlikely. Conversely, if the PaO_2 is < 300 mmHg, a right-to-left shunt remains a consideration and further investigation may be warranted. At sea level the PaO_2 should exceed 400 mmHg in the absence of a right-to-left shunt.

ANGIOGRAPHY

Injection of contrast into the involved right sided chamber will visualize the right-to-left shunt in patients with Eisenmenger's syndrome. An ASD or patent foramen ovale with right-to-left shunting causes contrast injected into the RA to opacify the LA directly, a VSD opacifies the LV directly if the RV is injected, and a PDA causes the descending thoracic AO to be visualized early if contrast injection into the main pulmonary artery is performed.

INTRACARDIAC ECHOCARDIOGRAPHY (ICE)

The development of miniaturized ultrasound tipped catheters has allowed the application of intracardiac echocardiography (ICE) to aid in a number of interventional procedures (3). ICE permits detailed identification of normal and abnormal cardiac anatomy facilitating assessment of intracardiac communications. When there is consideration of closure of an ASD or PFO, the use of ICE can provide assistance with devise implantation, reduce procedural and fluoroscopy time and decease procedural risk by allowing visualization of the specific anatomic relationship between the occluder device and surrounding structures (4).

MEASURED VARIABLES

Baseline invasive pressures (RA, RV, PA, and pulmonary arterial "wedge") and the brachial arterial cuff pressure are recorded in a computerized physiologic recorder (Prucka Mac-Lab 7000 Cath Lab Physiological Monitoring System; General Electric Medical Systems, Milwaukee, Wisconsin, US). Cardiac output is measured by the thermodilution technique using a computer (Edwards #COM-2, Baxter, Irvine, CA). In a previous study of RHC in the assessment of pulmonary hypertensive patients we found the thermodilution cardiac output to be an over-estimate when compared to simultaneously measured Fick cardiac output if the thermodilution value was < 3.5 L/min (5). However, we observed that the thermodilution cardiac outputs which were > 3.5 L/min compared favorably to measured Fick cardiac outputs even in the presence of significant tricuspid regurgitation. Therefore, for multiple repeat cardiac output measurements during the titration of vasodilator drugs, we use serial thermodilution cardiac output measurements to avoid excessive blood loss and logistical difficulties which are inherent in the measured Fick technique. For comparison with the thermodilution cardiac output, we calculate an "estimated" baseline Fick cardiac output by estimating the oxygen consumption and measuring the A–V O_2 difference using the classic Fick equation:

$$\text{Fick cardiac output} = \frac{\text{oxygen consumption (estimated or measured)}}{\text{arterial } O_2 \text{ content} - \text{mixed venous } O_2 \text{ content}}$$

where cardiac output is in liters/minute; oxygen consumption is in mL/min; O_2 content is in volumes percent; mixed venous is pulmonary artery in the absence of a left-to-right shunt.

In the presence of a left-to-right shunt, the thermodilution cardiac output reflects pulmonary flow (QP) and not systemic flow (QS). A right-to-left shunt invalidates the thermodilution method for measurement of pulmonary flow since some of the indicator (cold saline) is shunted from the RA to LA if an ASD or patent foramen ovale is present or RV to LV if a VSD is present. Therefore, the area beneath the curve is reduced and the calculated thermodilution pulmonary flow is erroneously increased.

Pulmonary capillary wedge pressure (PCWP)

One of the important measurements obtained during the assessment of cardiopulmonary hemodynamics in patients with suspected PH is the pulmonary capillary wedge pressure (PCWP), also referred to as the pulmonary artery occlusion pressure (PAOP). It is essential this assessment of left sided filling pressures is accurate to appropriately classify the etiology of the patient's elevated pulmonary artery pressure and to help select appropriate therapy. However, accurate measurement of the PCWP can be difficult to obtain in this patient population requiring experience in the manipulation of the catheter and interpretation of the wave forms to confirm the validity of the measurement. The assumption that the PCWP reflects the left atrial pressure is true only if the catheter tip is in the appropriate zone of the lung (West Zone 3). At this position pulmonary arterial pressure is greater then pulmonary venous pressure which is greater then pulmonary alveolar pressure (Ppa > Pv > Palv), therefore blood flow is not interrupted and a direct fluid column connects the catheter tip to the let atrium. Fortunately, in the supine patient the majority of the lung is effectively in West Zone 3 facilitating this measurement. Visualization of the appropriate components of the left atrial wave form (a wave, v wave, x descent, y descent) timed against the electrocardiogram (ECG) also indicate appropriate placement of the catheter tip. Finally, respiratory variation of the wave form should be noted. In patients with severe elevation of pulmonary arterial pressures or in those with occlusion of segments or sub-segments of the pulmonary vasculature such as occurs in thromboembolic disease confirmation of all these parameters can be challenging and requires persistence on part of the operator. Techniques which may assist in obtaining an accurate PCWP include decreasing the amount of air used to fill the catheter tip balloon and repositioning the catheter into different segments of the pulmonary vasculature. As discussed previously, in some cases it is not possible to obtain an acceptable PCWP. In these situations the LVEDP can be measured directly with a retrograde pigtail catheter via the percutaneous femoral arterial approach.

DERIVED VARIABLES

Pulmonary vascular resistance

Vascular resistance calculations are based on the principles of Ohm's law hydraulic fluid flow. Resistance is defined as the ratio of the decrease in pressure between two points in a vascular segment and the blood flow through the segment. Though it is true this calculation represents an oversimplification of the complex behavior of pulsatile flow of blood in a dynamic vascular bed, measurement of resistance based on these principles has been demonstrated of clinical use.

Pulmonary vascular resistance (PVR) is calculated according to the following equation:

$$\text{PVR} = \frac{(\text{PAM} - \text{PAWM})}{\text{CO}}$$

where PVR is pulmonary vascular resistance in Wood units; PAM is pulmonary artery mean pressure (mmHg); PAWM is pulmonary artery wedge mean pressure (mmHg);

CO is cardiac output (L/min). PVR can be expressed as dyne sec/cm^{-5} by multiplying Wood units by 80.

The normal resting pulmonary vascular resistance ranges between 0.3 and 1.6 Wood units or 20–130 dyne sec/cm^{-5}.

SYSTEMIC OXYGEN TRANSPORT

Systemic oxygen transport (SO_2T) is an important measurement for monitoring oxygen delivery to the tissues and organs of the body which is calculated by the following equation:

$$SO_2T = aO_2 \text{ content} \times CO$$

where SO_2T is systemic oxygen transport (oxygen delivery in mL/min); aO_2 content is arterial oxygen content (mL/L); CO is cardiac output (L/min).

When measurement of the cardiac output is not readily available, the dynamic physiologic status of the pulmonary hypertensive patient can be inferred from following the A–V O_2 content differences (arterial-mixed venous oxygen contents in volumes percent). If an oximetric balloon tipped catheter (Opticath #P7110-EP8-H, Abbott Laboratories, Chicago, IL) and optical module (Oximetric 3 SO_2/CO computer, Abbott Laboratories, Chicago, IL) are used to monitor the pulmonary arterial pressure, oxygen saturation, and thermodilution cardiac output, and a pulse oximeter is used for monitoring systemic arterial oxygen saturation, the A–V O_2 content difference can be calculated and monitored as a meaningful parameter to assess a pulmonary hypertensive patient's hemodynamic response to vasodilator treatment in the acute setting. This approach also eliminates the necessity for repetitive withdrawal of blood.

$$\text{Oxygen content (vol\%)} = Hb (g\%) \times 1.36 \times O_2 \text{ sat} \times 100$$

where $1.36 = O_2$ carrying capacity/g Hb and A–V O_2 content difference (vol%) is systemic arterial – mixed venous O_2 content.

As the cardiac output decreases, the pulmonary arterial O_2 content falls and the A–V O_2 content difference widens. Conversely, when a pulmonary hypertensive patient responds favorably to a pulmonary vasodilator, the pulmonary arterial pressure decreases, cardiac output increases, A–V O_2 content difference narrows as systemic oxygen transport is increased.

TRANSPULMONARY GRADIENT

Measurement of the transpulmonary gradient (TPG) is another means of assessing the function of the pulmonary vascular bed. Because the pulmonary vasculature is a high capacitance low resistance system, left sided filling pressures should approximate right sided pressures. A significant difference in this gradient is indicative of pulmonary vascular bed pathology. The transpulmonary gradient is calculated by the following equation:

$$TPG = PAM - PAWM$$

where TPG is transpulmonary gradient; PAM is mean pulmonary artery pressure (mmHg); PAWM is pulmonary artery wedge mean pressure (mmHg).

A normal TPG is < 12 mmHg. Values greater then 12 mmHg imply dysfunction of the pulmonary vascular bed.

Assessing pulmonary vasoreactivity

VARYING THE FRACTION OF INSPIRED OXYGEN (FIO_2)

If the pulmonary hypertensive patient being evaluated for the first time in our cardiac catheterization laboratory does not have significant resting hypoxemia, we prefer to perform all resting hemodynamic measurements with the patient breathing room air. If the patient is being treated with chronic supplemental oxygen therapy at home, the initial hemodynamics are measured while the patient receives his or her baseline supplemental oxygen dosage. If the history indicates chronic residency at high altitude (above 6000 feet) or suggests the possibility of hypoxic pulmonary vasoconstriction, we may repeat all hemodynamics including measurement of the cardiac output with the patient breathing a hypoxic gas mixture containing 16 percent oxygen for 10 minutes using a noseclip and mouth-piece with a one-way valve. At our altitude of 5280 feet, this simulates an altitude exposure of approximately 11 000 feet. At sea level, to achieve a similar level of hypoxic challenge, 14 percent oxygen may be used. Once a full set of hemodynamic and blood gas measurements have been collected, we replace the hypoxic mixture with 100 percent oxygen for 10 minutes and repeat the hemodynamic and blood gas measurements. Patients with pulmonary arterial hypertension secondary to pulmonary thromboembolic disease, alveolar hypoventilation or chronic obstructive lung disease, may demonstrate marked improvement in pulmonary hemodynamics (including a reduction in the mean PAP without a concomitant fall in cardiac output) in response to acute hyperoxia. Cardiac output in these patients may increase in response to 100 percent oxygen. It is also important to reassess such patients after prolonged home oxygen therapy, since the improvement in pulmonary hemodynamics may require weeks or months to achieve the maximal benefit which is not always predicted by the response to acute hyperoxia.

EXERCISE DURING CARDIAC CATHETERIZATION

The use of exercise during RHC to assess for abnormalities in the pulmonary vasculature (exercised induced pulmonary hypertension) is an area of burgeoning interest. It is hypothesized that an abnormal physiologic response to exercise resulting in significant increases in pulmonary artery pressure and pulmonary vascular resistance *may* identify patients at risk for developing progressive pulmonary vascular disease (6). Exercise studies may also help identify the cause of dyspnea in patients with limited exercise tolerance, but normal hemodynamic parameters at rest. However the use of exercise studies during cardiac catheterization is currently limited by the lack of data regarding utility and lack of standardization of approach among catheterization laboratories. Here we discuss our approach to exercise cardiac catheterization.

A high exercise workload can be achieved during supine clinical cardiac catheterization by using leg exercise via a supine cycle ergometer attached to the catheterization table. Optimally, when employing this approach the catheterization is performed through the IJ approach to lessen the dislodgement of the sheath during vigorous movement of the lower extremities. The patient's feet are positioned in the stirrups of the ergometer and the catheter and manifolds are positioned to be readily available and undisturbed during exercise. The patient is instructed that a variable degree of workload will occur during the procedure, with the first minute starting at a minimal workload and then gradual advancement over the ensuing 4–10 minutes, depending on the individual's exercise capacity. The patient is asked to alert the catheterization team when they believe they can exercise for a total of 2 minutes more so that appropriate measurements can be obtained prior to cessation of exercise. During this 2-minute window, we repeat the hemodynamic measurements obtained at baseline including RA pressure, PA pressure, PCWP, CO, systemic blood pressure and pulmonary arterial saturation measurement. The patient's systemic saturation is monitored continuously via pulse oximetry as is the patient's ECG during the procedure. The workload can be adjusted based on the patient's severity of disease, leg strength and ability to exercise.

We have also used supine straight-arm-raising exercise using small weighted barbells in each hand as an alternative form of exercise. In pulmonary hypertensive patients, we have been able to achieve satisfactory exercise workloads by having the supine patient hold a small 1, 2, or 3 pound barbell (secured with Velcro straps around the back of the hand) in each hand while rapidly raising the extended arms to a position of apposition directly above the chest and lowering the extended arms to a position level with the mid axillary line. We apply an appropriate sized blood pressure cuff to the thigh for recording the popliteal arterial pressure while monitoring arterial saturation with a pulse oximeter attached to a toenail on the opposite foot. Again, the patient is instructed to signal us approximately 2 minutes before he/she anticipates having to stop from exhaustion so that we can rapidly record the RA, PA, wedge, and popliteal arterial (cuff) pressures, thermodilution cardiac output, and sample PA (mixed venous) and arterial oxygen saturation (using the toe pulse oximeter) during peak exercise. Other laboratories have applied different techniques to measure exercise catheterization including upright bicycle ergometry and straight-leg-raising exercise reporting satisfactory results.

During strenuous exercise, the PAP can increase in response to marked elevation of the cardiac output without a concomitant increase in pulmonary vascular resistance. In a sea level study of eight normal, conditioned, male athletes who had a resting mean pulmonary artery pressure of $15.0 + 0.9$ mmHg, mean cardiac output of 6.7 L/min, and pulmonary vascular resistance of 1.2 Wood units, we observed an increase in cardiac output during extreme upright cycle ergometric exercise to a mean value of $27.2 + 2.0$ L/min (range 19.1–35.9) which was associated with an increase in the mean pulmonary artery pressure to $33 + 1$ mmHg (range 25–45) (7). The mean pulmonary arterial wedge pressure in these subjects also increased to 21 mmHg during extreme exercise and contributed to the elevation of the pulmonary artery pressure. Therefore, despite having a significant increase in pulmonary arterial pressure during extreme exercise, the pulmonary vascular resistance was decreased to 0.4 Wood units in these conditioned athletes. In pulmonary hypertensive patients, we have observed that symptom limited exercise is usually not associated with more than a twofold increase in cardiac output and we have never observed an increase in the mean wedge pressure above the normal range unless there was associated left ventricular disease.

ASSESSMENT OF ACUTE PULMONARY VASOREACTIVITY

An important part of the assessment of cardiopulmonary hemodynamics during right heart catheterization in patients with pulmonary arterial hypertension is the assessment of acute vasoreactivity. The degree to which the pulmonary vascular bed acutely dilates in response to pharmacologic therapy provides information essential to the selection of long-term treatment. Currently, the main question to be answered when performing an acute vasodilator challenge is whether the patient should receive a trial of oral calcium channel blockers as chronic therapy for pulmonary arterial hypertension. Patients that meet specific criteria for acute vasoreactivity (discussed below) can receive such a trial. However the criteria defining acute vasoreactivity have changed over the years. Early reports defined vasoreactivity as percentage decreases in mean pulmonary arterial pressure and pulmonary vascular resistance. For example, in a landmark study, Rich et al. defined a positive acute vasoreactivity study as a decrease in both mean PA pressure and PVR by 20 percent following exposure to a pulmonary vasodilator. Patients meeting these criteria were reported to have an excellent long-term response to orally administered calcium channel blockers with a significantly improved survival compared to non-responders (8). A more recent study published by Sitbon et al. has since further refined the definition of acute vasoreactivity (9). Their retrospective analysis of patients initially defined as acutely vasoreactive by a decrease in mean PA pressure and PVR of > 20 percent (the definition proposed by Rich et al.) demonstrated that only a subset of these patients in fact had long-term improvement while taking calcium channel blockers. Sitbon defined long-term improvement as patients who clinically remained in NYHA functional class I or II, one year after initiating therapy with calcium channel blockers and who did not require the addition of other PAH specific therapy during this interval. Their review indicated these patients had a more pronounced initial reduction in PA pressures during the acute vasoreactivity study then the previously accepted > 20 percent decrease in mean PA pressure and PVR. The definition of acute vasoreactivity suggested by Sitbon and accepted by the American College of Chest Physicians (ACCP) now requires that the mean PA pressure decrease by a least 10 mmHg to an absolute value of ≤ 40 mmHg and that CO increases or remains the same (no decrease in CO) (10). However, it is important to note that in this same manuscript by Sitbon, there were patients who did not meet these strict criteria and yet were still noted to be "long-term" responders (9). It is therefore important to consider these patients on a case-by-case basis when deciding on the use of calcium channel blockade as therapy for PAH.

A vasodilator challenge should not be performed if there is elevation of PCWP or LVEDP noted at baseline for fear of inducing acute pulmonary edema. We use a PCWP cut-off value of 18 mmHg as the upper limit for performing an acute vasodilator challenge in patients with PAH. It is controversial as to whether acute vasoreactivity studies should be performed on all patients with WHO group I forms of PAH or rather limited to only patients suspected to have IPAH. Most studies which have examined the utility of acute vasodilator testing have limited their patient populations to those with IPAH only and it is generally recognized that acute vasoreactivity is unusual in some subsets of patients with PAH such as those with limited stage scleroderma. It is also unclear what the efficacy of long-term calcium channel blockade is in these other patient populations. It has been our approach to perform acute vasoreactivity challenges as part of our standard RHC evaluation on all patients with PAH with normal left sided filling pressures (PCWP or LVEDP) barring any other contraindication, and we have indeed noted positive responses in patient populations other then IPAH. It remains unclear at this time as to whether these patients should receive a trial of calcium channel blockers.

CHOICE OF PULMONARY VASCULAR VASODILATORS: A HISTORICAL PERSPECTIVE

Intravenous vasodilators with short duration of action

BACKGROUND

Daoud reported in 1978 that acutely administered IV isoproterenol could be used to assess pulmonary vasoreactivity in patients with PPH (IPAH) (11). We also found that IV isoproterenol produced pulmonary vasodilation in some PPH (IPAH) patients; however, its potent inotropic and chronotropic effects frequently produced marked sinus tachycardia, increased cardiac output, and higher PAP. Thus, patients were prone to experience ischemic-like chest pain (presumed to be secondary to right ventricular ischemia reflecting an imbalance in myocardial oxygen supply and demand) despite having a significant decrease in pulmonary vascular resistance. Rubin reported a beneficial acute vasodilatory effect of IV hydralazine in PPH (IPAH) patients in 1980 (12).

Prostaglandins

PROSTACYCLIN

In 1982 Rubin reported that intravenous prostacyclin (PGI_2) produced acute pulmonary vasodilation in patients with PPH (IPAH) (13). The hemodynamic effects of prostacyclin were subsequently reported to be similar to, but more potent than, intravenous hydralazine (14). Between 1981 and 1988 we studied 44 PPH (IPAH) patients in whom we compared the acute IV response to PGI_2 with oral diltiazem or nifedipine (15). Prostacyclin was titrated from 1.0 to a maximum of 12.0 ng/kg/min with the mean tolerated dosage being 8.0 ng/kg/min. The mean hemodynamic effects of PGI_2 included a 14 percent increase in heart rate, 5 percent decrease in mean PA pressure, 47 percent increase in cardiac output, and a 32 percent decrease in pulmonary vascular resistance. We defined a favorable individual patient response to PGI_2 to be a > 30 percent decrease in pulmonary vascular resistance *and* a > 10 percent decrease in mean pulmonary artery pressure that was observed in 30 percent of the untreated PPH (IPAH) patients. Side effects including cutaneous flushing, headache, nausea, systemic hypotension and vomiting were observed, but remitted within 10–15 minutes after stopping the prostacyclin. The response to IV PGI_2 was predictive of the subsequent response to oral calcium blocker treatment (8).

ILOPROST

We have used IV iloprost, a more stable analogue of prostacyclin, in a similar protocol for assessing acute pulmonary vasoreactivity in 26 untreated patients with PPH (IPAH) (16). Intravenous iloprost was titrated from 1.0 to a maximum of 8.0 ng/kg/min with the mean tolerated dosage being 4.0 ng/kg/min. The mean hemodynamic responses to IV iloprost included an 11 percent increase in heart rate, 9 percent decrease in mean PA pressure, 40 percent increase in cardiac output, and a 31 percent decrease in pulmonary resistance. A favorable vasodilatory response to intravenous iloprost (using the same arbitrary definition of > 30 percent decrease in pulmonary resistance *and* a > 10 percent decrease in mean pulmonary artery pressure) was observed in 42 percent of the PPH (IPAH) patients. Side effects were similar to those noted above for IV prostacyclin and cleared within 15–30 minutes after stopping iloprost. Thus, we consider IV PGI_2 and iloprost to be effective and safe vasodilators in acutely assessing pulmonary vasoreactivity in IPAH patients. We have observed similar hemodynamic results when administering IV PGI_2 or IV iloprost to patients with PAH associated with other disease states.

ADENOSINE

Other reports have indicated that adenosine injected into the pulmonary artery or intravenously (17) is another pulmonary vasodilator which is attractive because of its potency on the pulmonary circulation and short duration of action (18–20). Since adenosine is rapidly metabolized by adenosine deaminase in endothelial cells and erythrocytes, it has a limited effect on the systemic circulation. Thus, intravenous adenosine titrated from 50 to 500 micrograms/kg/min is an alternative agent for acutely assessing pulmonary vasoreactivity that is predictive of subsequent responsiveness to oral calcium blocker treatment in pulmonary hypertensive patients (21).

Nitrates

NITROGLYCERIN

Intravenous nitroglycerin has also been used in assessing pulmonary vasoreactivity in pulmonary hypertensive patients but is generally considered to be a less potent pulmonary vasodilator in comparison with intravenous prostacyclin, iloprost, or adenosine (22).

NITROPRUSSIDE

Intravenous nitroprusside has been established as being useful in evaluating the reversibility of pulmonary arterial hypertension in patients with left ventricular decompensation from ischemic or idiopathic cardiomyopathy who are undergoing precardiac transplantation evaluation (23). We administer IV nitroprusside to all patients being considered for cardiac transplantation who have pulmonary hypertension with a pulmonary vascular resistance above 2.5 Wood units. We begin the IV nitroprusside infusion at 0.1 mcg/kg/min and increase the dosage by 0.2 mcg/kg/min every 3 minutes until either the PVR falls below 2.5 Wood units based upon serial thermodilution cardiac output measurements, or the mean systemic arterial pressure falls below 65 mmHg. Arterial saturation is monitored continuously by finger pulse oximetry and the A–V O_2 content difference is measured at the peak nitroprusside dosage. Occasionally, patients with refractory congestive heart failure and systemic hypotension require concurrent intravenous dobutamine to maintain an adequate systemic pressure to allow this study of the pulmonary vascular bed. Patients whose PVR can be decreased to $\leq$ 2.5 Wood units during this challenge are further considered for cardiac transplantation.

Inhaled vasodilators

NITRIC OXIDE

Inhaled nitric oxide (iNO) is another agent with proven efficacy in the assessment of acute pulmonary vasoreactivity.

Because iNO is rapidly inactivated by hemoglobin, it has minimal effects on the systemic vascular resistance. The dose of iNO used in reported vasoreactivity studies has ranged from 10 to 80 ppm (24–26). In our laboratory, we have adopted an acute vasoreactivity protocol using iNO at 40 ppm + 50% FIO_2 for 10 minutes. If the patient appears to meet criteria for an acute response prior to 10 minutes that allows selection of appropriate therapy, the study can be terminated after pulmonary hemodynamics have been re-measured. The delivery of iNO is regulated using an INOvent delivery system (Daytex–Ohmeda, Inc; Madison, WI USA) which can deliver 1 to 80 ppm NO via an air tight mask with the patient breathing room air or supplemental oxygen from 21 to 100 percent. The acute response to inhaled NO in patients with pulmonary hypertension has been reported to be predictive of their responsiveness to oral calcium blocker treatment (21). Persistent pulmonary hypertension of the newborn formerly requiring extra corporeal membrane oxygenation (ECMO) may also be responsive to NO inhalation therapy (27). Due to its safety profile and ease of use, many catheterization laboratories including ours now use iNO as the favored pulmonary vasodilator for assessing acute pulmonary vasoreactivity.

ILOPROST

Inhaled iloprost has also been reported to be a safe and effective agent for acutely assessing pulmonary vasoreactivity in pulmonary hypertensive patients (28).

Recommended agents for acute vasodilator challenge

Based on the above mentioned studies, their relative safety profiles and expert opinion the four mediations currently favored for assessment of acute vasoreactivity are intravenous adenosine, intravenous epoprostenol, inhaled nitric oxide and inhaled iloprost (29).

It is important to again note that the acute pulmonary effect of short-acting vasodilators is believed to predict the long-term efficacy of oral calcium channel blockers in some patients with PAH. However, there are no studies which predict the chronic impact of other classes of mediations (endothelin receptor blockers, phosphodiesterase-5 inhibitors, prostanoids) on patients who demonstrate acute pulmonary vasoreactivity.

COMPLICATIONS OF RIGHT HEART CARDIAC CATHETERIZATION

Complications which are particularly important in patients with severe pulmonary hypertension and relatively "fixed" low cardiac outputs include the following:

1. Vasovagal reactions with bradycardia and systemic hypotension are life-threatening and must be treated

immediately with intravenous atropine and volume expansion.

2. Supraventricular tachycardias including paroxysmal atrial tachycardia and atrial fibrillation which can be induced by guidewire and/or catheter manipulation through the right heart. The rapid rate during SVT with inadequate ventricular filling or loss of atrial contraction during atrial fibrillation with a rapid ventricular response can quickly cause right ventricular decompensation requiring immediate electrical cardioversion to sustain an adequate systemic blood pressure.

3. A large hematoma at an arterial catheter entry site with significant blood loss can produce systemic hypotension requiring immediate hemostasis and intravenous fluid administration to maintain systemic pressures.

4. With the exception of inhaled nitric oxide and inhaled iloprost, pulmonary vasodilators are also systemic vasodilators. Therefore, if the pulmonary vascular resistance is relatively "fixed" and the systemic vascular resistance is responsive to the acute administration of a vasodilator, systemic hypotension is a potential side effect of any IV or oral vasodilator treatment trial. For this reason, vasodilators with a short duration of action are favored for acutely assessing pulmonary vasoreactivity.

FOLLOW-UP OUTPATIENT CARDIAC CATHETERIZATION PROCEDURES

A follow-up or repeat RHC can be useful in assessing progression of disease and response to therapy. The hemodynamic information can help guide addition of other medications or prompt a more aggressive approach towards evaluation for transplantation. Some centers advocate annual RHCs of their patients to closely monitor for disease progression and for assessment of medical therapeutic efficacy. Our approach has evolved to the point that we normally repeat invasive RHC only when a careful history, physical exam and echocardiography provide inadequate data to guide therapy. Prior to a repeat cardiac catheterization we obtain a repeat ECG and echocardiogram so these studies can be correlated directly with the invasive hemodynamic measurements and used as future noninvasive reference points. The patient is instructed to continue his/her usual dosage of PH specific therapy prior to reporting to the catheterization laboratory to ensure the hemodynamic data obtained reflects steady-state efficacy of the current therapeutic regimen. The hemodynamic measurements are the same as the initial catheterization procedure. We generally do not repeat an acute vasodilator study during the repeat RHC assuming the vasoreactivity was accurately assessed during the initial procedure. If there are questions regarding the initial assessment of the acute

vasoreactivity study, it may be repeated to clarify the patient's current hemodynamic status. During the repeat hemodynamic evaluation we also consider including an assessment of the added physiologic effect of exercise if the initial catheterization demonstrated significant abnormalities which may have been improved by vasodilator treatment.

Unfortunately, 80–90 percent of patients with pulmonary arterial hypertension do not demonstrate significant pulmonary vasoreactivity acutely and thus will not respond favorably to the chronic administration of oral calcium channel antagonists. However, the chronic treatment of such patients has advanced dramatically in the past decade, and potential therapies are covered in detail in other chapters. Briefly, these patients will often respond hemodynamically and clinically to chronic therapy with continuous intravenous and subcutaneous prostacyclin analogs as well as inhaled formulations of prostacyclin, oral endothelin receptor antagonists and phosphodiesterase inhibitors. Repeat RHC with direct measurement of the pulmonary arterial pressure and cardiac output may be helpful for the objective assessment of the efficacy of all these treatment modalities of pulmonary hypertension, depending on the clinical scenario.

KEY POINTS

- Right heart cardiac catheterization is an essential part of the evaluation of patients with suspected PH.
- When performed correctly, RHC ensures accuracy of the diagnosis, appropriate classification and assessment of disease severity and facilitates selection of appropriate therapy.
- Catheterization also provides the opportunity to detect and quantify intracardiac shunts.
- Patients with severe PH present unique technical challenges due to elevation of right-sided pressures, dilation of the right ventricle and atrium, and coexistent severe tricuspid and/or pulmonary valvular regurgitation.
- Accurate hemodynamic measurements can be safely obtained despite these obstacles; however, proper RHC technique requires experience, patience and persistence of the cath lab team.
- Invasive procedures in pulmonary hypertensive patients are associated with increased morbidity due to hemodynamic intolerance to significant bradycardia and/or hypovolemia.
- Proper team and patient preparation for the catheterization procedure minimizes the risk taken and maximizes the information obtained.

REFERENCES

1. Groves BM, Ditchey RV, Reeves JT. Multicenter trial of a new guidewire thermodilution catheter. J Am Coll Cardiol 2008;3(599). [abstract]

2. Grossman W. Shunt detection and quantification. In: Baim DS, Grossman W, eds. Grossman's Cardiac Catheterization, Angiography and Intervention, 6th edn. Philadelphia: Lippincott Williams and Wilkins, 2000:179–91.

3. Ren JF, Schwartzman D, Callans DJ, Brode SE, Gottlieb CD, Marchlinski FE. Intracardiac echocardiography (9 MHz) in humans: methods, imaging views and clinical utility. Ultrasound Med Biol 1999;25:1077–86.

4. Hijazi Z, Wang Z, Cao Q, Koenig P, Waight D, Lang R. Transcatheter closure of atrial septal defects and patent foramen ovale under intracardiac echocardiographic guidance: feasibility and comparison with transesophageal echocardiography. Catheter Cardiovasc Interv 2001; 52:194–9.

5. van Grondelle A, Ditchey RV, Groves BM, Wagner WW Jr., Reeves JT. Thermodilution method overestimates low cardiac output in humans. Am J Physiol 1983;245:H690–2.

6. Tolle JJ, Waxman AB, Van Horn TL, Pappagianopoulos PP, Systrom DM. Exercise-induced pulmonary arterial hypertension. Circulation 2008;118:2183–89.

7. Groves BM, Reeves JT, Sutton JR, Wagner PD, Cymerman A, Malconian MK et al. Operation Everest II: elevated high-altitude pulmonary resistance unresponsive to oxygen. J Appl Physiol 1987;63:521–30.

8. Rich S, Kaufmann E, Levy PS. The effect of high doses of calcium-channel blockers on survival in primary pulmonary hypertension. N Engl J Med 1992;327:76–81.

9. Sitbon O, Humbert M, Jais X, Ioos V, Hamid AM, Provencher S et al. Long-term response to calcium channel blockers in idiopathic pulmonary arterial hypertension. Circulation 2005;111:3105–11.

10. Badesch DB, Abman SH, Simonneau G, Rubin LJ, McLaughlin VV. Medical therapy for pulmonary arterial hypertension: updated ACCP evidence-based clinical practice guidelines. Chest 2007;131:1917–28.

11. Daoud FS, Reeves JT, Kelly DB. Isoproterenol as a potential pulmonary vasodilator in primary pulmonary hypertension. Am J Cardiol 1978;42:817–22.

12. Rubin LJ, Peter RH. Oral hydralazine therapy for primary pulmonary hypertension. N Engl J Med 1980;302:69–73.

13. Rubin LJ, Groves BM, Reeves JT, Frosolono M, Handel F, Cato AE. Prostacyclin-induced acute pulmonary vasodilation in primary pulmonary hypertension. Circulation 1982;66:334–8.

14. Groves BM, Rubin LJ, Frosolono MF, Cato AE, Reeves JT. A comparison of the acute hemodynamic effects of prostacyclin and hydralazine in primary pulmonary hypertension. Am Heart J 1985;110:1200–4.

15. Groves BM, Badesch DB, Turkevich D. Ion Flux in Pulmonary Vascular Disease. Weir EK, Hume JR, Reeves JT, eds. New York: Plenum Publishing Corporation, 1993:317–30.

16. Groves B, Badesch D, Donnellan K. Acute hemodynamic effects of iloprost in primary (unexplained) pulmonary hypertension. Semin Respir Crit Care Med 1994;15: 230–37.

17. Schrader BJ, Inbar S, Kaufmann L, Vestal RE, Rich S. Comparison of the effects of adenosine and nifedipine in pulmonary hypertension. J Am Coll Cardiol 1992;19: 1060–4.

18. Morgan JM, McCormack DG, Griffiths MJ, Morgan CJ, Barnes PJ, Evans TW. Adenosine as a vasodilator in primary pulmonary hypertension. Circulation 1991;84:1145–9.

19. Reeves JT, Groves BM, Weir EK. Adenosine and selective reduction of pulmonary vascular resistance in primary pulmonary hypertension. Circulation 1991;84:1437–9.

20. Schrader BJ, Inbar S, Kaufmann L, Vestal RE, Rich S. Comparison of the effects of adenosine and nifedipine in pulmonary hypertension. J Am Coll Cardiol 1992;19: 1060–4.

21. Schrader BJ, Inbar S, Kaufmann L, Vestal RE, Rich S. Comparison of the effects of adenosine and nifedipine in pulmonary hypertension. J Am Coll Cardiol 1992;19: 1060–4.

22. Pearl RG, Rosenthal MH, Schroeder JS, Ashton JP. Acute hemodynamic effects of nitroglycerin in pulmonary hypertension. Ann Intern Med 1983;99:9–13.

23. Costard-Jackle A, Fowler MB. Influence of preoperative pulmonary artery pressure on mortality after heart transplantation: testing of potential reversibility of pulmonary hypertension with nitroprusside is useful in defining a high risk group. J Am Coll Cardiol 1992;19: 48–54.

24. Pepke-Zaba J, Higenbottam TW, Dinh-Xuan AT, Stone D, Wallwork J. Inhaled nitric oxide as a cause of selective pulmonary vasodilatation in pulmonary hypertension. Lancet 1991;338:1173–4.

25. Ricciardi MJ, Knight BP, Martinez FJ, Rubenfire M. Inhaled nitric oxide in primary pulmonary hypertension: a safe and effective agent for predicting response to nifedipine. J Am Coll Cardiol 1998;32:1068–73.

26. Hoeper MM, Olschewski H, Ghofrani HA, Wilkens H, Winkler J, Borst MM et al. A comparison of the acute hemodynamic effects of inhaled nitric oxide and aerosolized iloprost in primary pulmonary hypertension. German PPH study group. J Am Coll Cardiol 2000;35: 176–82.

27. Kinsella JP, Neish SR, Shaffer E, Abman SH. Low-dose inhalation nitric oxide in persistent pulmonary hypertension of the newborn. Lancet 1992;340:819–20.

28. Olschewski H, Walmrath D, Schermuly R, Ghofrani A, Grimminger F, Seeger W. Aerosolized prostacyclin and iloprost in severe pulmonary hypertension. Ann Intern Med 1996;124:820–4.

29. Barst RJ, McGoon M, Torbicki A, Sitbon O, Krowka MJ, Olschewski H et al. Diagnosis and differential assessment of pulmonary arterial hypertension. J Am Coll Cardiol 2004;43:40S–7S.

13

An integrated approach to the diagnosis of pulmonary hypertension

ROBERT P FRANTZ AND MICHAEL D McGOON

INTRODUCTION

The term "pulmonary hypertension (PH)" refers to the presence of a mean resting pulmonary arterial pressure ≥ 25 mmHg independent of cause. Disorders having PH as a component are classified based on a combination of the underlying mechanism, presentation, clinical context, histopathology and response to treatment. "Pulmonary arterial hypertension (PAH)" pertains to PH caused by elevated pre-capillary pulmonary resistance, and is considered to be present when pulmonary venous pressure is ≤ 15 mmHg. PAH is also the term attached to WHO Group I types of PH.

The diagnostic process for PH entails two conceptual stages: detection and characterization. "Detection" is the process of establishing the presence of PH. The purpose of this phase of diagnosis is to determine a cause of a patient's symptoms or to detect the presence of PH in a high-risk patient (screening). PH can also be discovered incidentally during the course of general evaluation. Detection requires awareness of the clinical presentation and maintenance of a high level of suspicion when circumstances warrant. "Characterization" is the process of determining the specific clinical context of the PH, including causal factors, associated diseases or substrates, hemodynamic perturbations and their localization, and sequelae. The purpose of this stage of diagnosis is to identify optimal treatment strategies and estimate prognosis. Characterization demands understanding the appropriate utilization and capabilities of a broad range of diagnostic modalities.

The tools for the assessment of PH range from the history and physical examination and basic laboratory assessment to a multiplicity of imaging procedures and careful hemodynamic analyses. These modalities are examined in more detail in Chapters 6–12. Figure 13.1 is a diagnostic flowchart that provides a general strategy for integrating these tools into the overall evaluation of a patient with PH, or with a presentation potentially attributable to PH. In this schema, tests which are required for an adequate evaluation are pivotal tests; contingent tests are those which may or may not be required to complete the evaluation depending on the results of prior tests.

DETECTION

The initial consideration of PH as a potential diagnosis in an individual patient may arise from one of three general scenarios: (1) evaluation of symptoms for which PH is in the differential diagnosis; (2) screening for the presence of PH in a high risk individual without suggestive symptoms; or (3) the incidental discovery of PH as a consequence of a general evaluation for unrelated issues. The context of the discovery of PH may have an impact on the further strategy of diagnosis and treatment.

Symptom evaluation

Since PH is less prevalent than many types of cardiovascular diseases which are associated with the same nonspecific

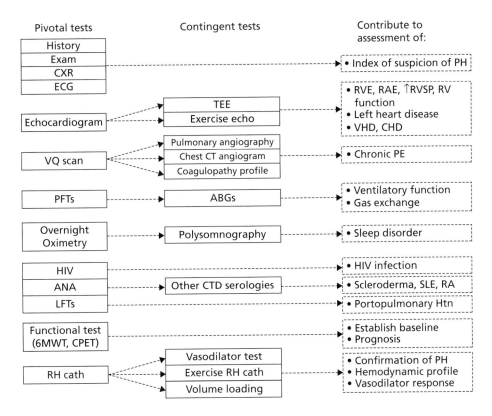

Figure 13.1 General guidelines for the evaluation of pulmonary hypertension. Since the suspicion of PH may arise in various ways, the sequence of tests may vary. However, the diagnosis of PAH requires that certain data support a specific diagnosis. In addition, the diagnosis of idiopathic pulmonary arterial hypertension is one of excluding all other reasonable possibilities. **Pivotal tests** are those that are essential to establishing a diagnosis of any type of PAH either by identification of criteria of associated disease or exclusion of diagnoses other than IPAH. All pivotal tests are required for a definitive diagnosis and baseline characterization. An abnormality of one assessment (such as obstructive pulmonary disease on PFTs), does not preclude that another abnormality (chronic thromboembolic disease on VQ scan and pulmonary angiogram) is contributing or predominant. **Contingent tests** are recommended to elucidate or confirm results of the pivotal tests, and need only be performed in the appropriate clinical context. The **combination** of pivotal and appropriate contingent tests contributes to assessment of the differential diagnoses in the right-hand column. It should be recognized that definitive diagnosis may require additional specific evaluations not necessarily included in this general guideline. 6MWT = six-minute walk test; ABGs = arterial blood gases; ANA = antinuclear antibody serology; CHD = congenital heart disease; CPET = cardiopulmonary exercise test; CT = computerized tomography; CTD = connective tissue disease; CXR = chest X-ray; ECG = electrocardiogram; HIV = human immunodeficiency virus screening; Htn = hypertension; LFTs = liver function tests; PE = pulmonary embolism; PFTs = pulmonary function tests; PH = pulmonary hypertension; RA = rheumatoid arthritis; RAE = right atrial enlargement; RH Cath = right heart cath; RVE = right ventricular enlargement; RVSP = right ventricular systolic pressure; SLE = systemic lupus erythematosus; TEE = transesophageal echocardiography; VHD = valvular heart disease; VQ Scan = lung ventilation-perfusion scintigram. From ref 271.

symptoms, the clinician needs a high index of suspicion to direct further evaluation. Among the symptoms which should raise the possibility of PH, exertional dyspnea is the presenting symptom in 60 percent of symptomatic patients and ultimately develops during the course of the disease in 98 percent. (1) Exercise intolerance may also be expressed as fatigue or weakness. Angina occurs in about one-third of patients with PH. The cause may due to any of the following factors: (1) decreased myocardial oxygen supply due to decreased systolic coronary flow to the right ventricle caused by reduction in the systolic pressure gradient across the right ventricular myocardium (2); (2) increased myocardial oxygen demand due to elevated right ventricular wall stress and increased right ventricular muscle mass; (3) compression of the left main coronary artery by the dilated central pulmonary artery (3–8); or atherosclerotic coronary artery disease. Syncope may occur in approximately one-third of patients for multiple reasons, including atrial or ventricular arrhythmias, and systemic vasodilatation producing hypotension due to inability to increase cardiac output through the high resistance pulmonary vasculature (9). Peripheral edema and abdominal distension from ascites suggest right ventricular failure with associated tricuspid regurgitation.

A clear quantification of subjective activity tolerance should be determined and documented in order to provide a baseline for serial follow-up of disease progression, response to treatment and prognostication. NYHA or WHO functional classification is most commonly utilized and correlates with survival (10–14).

Screening

Recognized risk factors for PH include history of appetite suppressant use, liver disease with portal hypertension, deep vein thrombosis or symptoms suggestive of past pulmonary thromboembolism, residence at high altitude, connective tissue disease, congenital heart disease or human immunodeficiency virus infection, chronic hypoxic restrictive or obstructive lung disease, sleep apnea, or a family history of pulmonary arterial hypertension. Periodic assessment of patients with an underlying predisposition may be warranted in order to introduce therapy at an early stage, or to initiate more aggressive surveillance to detect progression (15).

Incidental discovery

Discovery of unsuspected PH, especially of milder degrees, has become more frequent with the widespread use of Doppler echocardiographic techniques. The clinical significance and natural history of asymptomatic or mild PH is unclear, so the implications for further assessment and treatment remain uncertain. In general, the observation of PH should prompt an attempt to define or exclude possible causes, since it may be the first evidence of a modifiable substrate. However, the severity of the PH and the reliability of the measurement should temper the aggressiveness of the evaluation. An echocardiographic RVSP of 44 mmHg in a patient without attributable symptoms and without supportive evidence by other screening procedures (physical examination, electrocardiogram, chest x-ray or other echocardiographic features) may merit only re-examination in 6–12 months, whereas the same observation in a patient with a history of deep vein thrombosis would justify evaluation for possible chronic pulmonary thromboembolism. Even under those circumstances, however, confirmation (and more detailed characterization) of abnormal pulmonary hemodynamics by right heart catheterization may be appropriate before embarking on extensive evaluation.

Possible explanations for mildly elevated PA systolic pressure detected by echocardiography (or right heart catheterization) include (1) overestimation of the RVSP in a patient with true normal pulmonary pressure; (2) serendipitous observation of a rare transient pressure elevation in an otherwise healthy individual; (3) discovery of stable mild PH, possibly of long duration; or (4) discovery of early progressive PH in an individual with intrinsic pulmonary vascular disease. In addition, PA pressure differences may be observed in different populations and conditions, including age and weight (16), level of conditioning, and exercise or stress. Quantification of hemodynamics, either invasively or by echocardiography, must be tempered by the recognition that there is spontaneous variation which may result in measurement at one time that may change over time (17). No clear guidelines are available which delineate normal from pathologic in all circumstances.

Physical examination

The importance of the physical examination cannot be overstated, as it is the first step in narrowing the extensive differential diagnosis raised by presenting symptoms and in assessing the severity and consequences of the disease. The physical findings in PH, and their implications, are provided in Tables 13.1–13.3.

Chest x-ray

The chest x-ray in PH classically shows central pulmonary and right ventricular enlargement (1,18). Findings specific to advanced PH include a prominent pulmonary trunk and hilar pulmonary arteries and peripheral attenuation of pulmonary arteries producing a hypovascular appearance of the lung fields. The retrosternal space, which normally shows a wedge of radiolucent pulmonary tissue, is encroached upon by the more radiodense tissue of the enlarged anteriorly displaced right ventricle (Figure 13.2). Additional clues to possible associated diseases should be carefully considered, such as pulmonary venous hypertension, septal lines and pleural effusions (pulmonary venous hypertension due to left heart filling abnormality, pulmonary veno-occlusive disease (19)); hyperinflation (chronic obstructive pulmonary disease), or kyphosis (restrictive pulmonary disease). Marked asymmetry of the enlarged central pulmonary arteries (20), the presence of an avascular area and right pulmonary artery diameter over 20 mm together with pleural changes (21) may be clues to chronic thromboembolic disease.

Table 13.1 Physical signs the indicate presence of pulmonary hypertension (272)

Sign	Implication
Accentuated pulmonary component of S2 (pulmonic component audible at apex)	High pulmonary pressure and reflected pressure wave increases force of pulmonary valve closure
Early systolic click	Sudden interruption of opening of pulmonary valve into high pressure artery; reflected pressure wave from high resistance pulmonary vessels
Midsystolic ejection murmur	Turbulent transvalvular pulmonary outflow
Left parasternal lift	High right ventricular pressure and hypertrophy present
Increased jugular "a" waves	High right ventricular filling pressure

Table 13.2 Physical signs that indicate severity of pulmonary hypertension (272)

Sign	Implication
Moderate to severe pulmonary hypertension	
Diastolic murmur	Pulmonary regurgitation
Holosystolic murmur that increases with inspiration	Tricuspid regurgitation
Increased jugular "v" waves	Tricuspid regurgitation
Hepatojugular reflux	Tricuspid regurgitation
Pulsatile liver	Tricuspid regurgitation; right ventricular failure
Advanced pulmonary hypertension with right ventricular failure	
Right ventricular S3	Right ventricular dysfunction
Marked distention of jugular veins	Right ventricular dysfunction or tricuspid regurgitation or both
Hepatomegaly	Right ventricular dysfunction or tricuspid regurgitation or both
Peripheral edema	Right ventricular dysfunction or tricuspid regurgitation or both
Ascites	Right ventricular dysfunction or tricuspid regurgitation or both
Low blood pressure, diminished pulse pressure, cool extremities	Right ventricular dysfunction or tricuspid regurgitation or both

Table 13.3 Physical signs that detect possible underlying cause or associations of pulmonary hypertension. Adapted from ref 272

Sign	Implication
Central cyanosis	Hypoxemia, right-to-left shunt
Clubbing	Congenital heart disease, interstitial lung disease, hypoxia, pulmonary veno-occlusive disease (19)
Cardiac auscultatory findings, including systolic murmurs, diastolic murmurs, opening snap, and gallop	Congenital or acquired heart or valvular disease
Rales, dullness, or decreased breath sounds	Pulmonary congestion or effusion or both
Fine rales, accessory muscle use, wheezing, protracted expiration, productive cough	Pulmonary parenchymal disease
Obesity, kyphoscoliosis, enlarged tonsils	Possible substrate for disordered ventilation
Sclerodactyly, arthritis, rash, telangiectasia, calcinosis	Connective tissue disorder
Peripheral venous insufficiency or obstruction	Possible venous thrombosis

Electrocardiography

Electrocardiographic examination in patients with advance symptomatic PH characteristically shows evidence of right ventricular hypertrophy and right atrial enlargement (Figure 13.3) (22). In the NIH Registry of Primary Pulmonary Hypertension, 87 percent of patients had electrocardiographic criteria right ventricular hypertrophy and 79 percent had right axis deviation (1). The electrocardiogram alone, however, is not sufficiently sensitive to exclude the presence of PH even in high risk populations such as patients with connective tissue disease (23). In patients with known idiopathic pulmonary arterial hypertension (IPAH), increased P-wave amplitude or presence of qR in lead V1 are predictors of decreased survival (24).

Transthoracic echocardiography

If screening or preliminary evaluation of symptoms supports the possibility of PH, validation and initial exploration of severity and underlying cause is most easily pursued by Doppler echocardiographic techniques. Echocardiography is useful for the evaluation of the right heart and pulmonary hemodynamics because of its ability to assess reliably and noninvasively the morphology of cardiac and vascular structures and to record flow velocities in precisely selected sites (25,26). For more details see also Figure 13.4 and refs 27–43.

CHARACTERIZATION

Once PH is suspected or confirmed, evaluation to define the nature and severity of the disease is warranted.

Transthoracic echocardiography

The Doppler echocardiographic examination conceptually consists of the detection aspect (above) which discovers or confirms the probability of PH, and the aspect which initiates the process of characterizing the severity and possible causes of the hemodynamic abnormality.

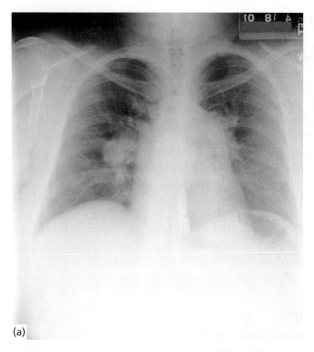

(a)

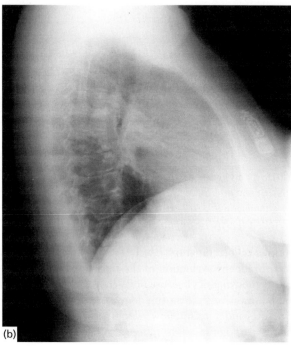

(b)

Figure 13.2   The posteroanterior (a) and lateral (b) chest X-ray findings specific to advanced pulmonary hypertension.

ASSESSMENT OF SEVERITY OF PH

Estimation of RVSP (above) is the most direct and commonly used method to detect and quantitate severity of PH. Other parameters have been employed to further hemodynamically characterize PH. These are:

- Pulmonary artery diastolic pressure (Figure 13.5 A and B) (44,45).
- Pulmonary artery mean pressure (46–49).

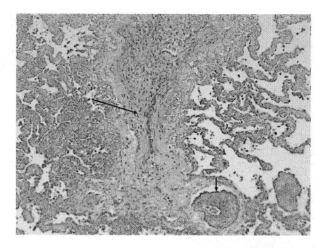

Figure 13.3   Electrocardiogram of patient with primary PH, demonstrating right atrial enlargement, right axis deviation and right ventricular hypertrophy.

- Continuous pulmonary artery pressure (50).
- Pulmonary vascular resistance (Figure 13.6) (51–56).

DIFFERENTIAL DIAGNOSIS OF PH

Two-dimensional transthoracic echocardiography may elucidate causes underlying PH such as left ventricular dysfunction, mitral valve disease, and intracardiac shunt. Some congenital defects may be missed if transesophageal echocardiographic techniques are not used. These include atypically situated atrial septal defects, especially of sinus venosus type with abnormal pulmonary venous drainage. The amplitude of pulmonary artery "pulse pressure" as assessed with Doppler in patients with significant PH has been found to reliably distinguish between patients with IPAH and proximal chronic pulmonary thromboembolism (57).

ASSESSMENT OF RIGHT VENTRICULAR FUNCTION AND RIGHT VENTRICULAR TO PULMONARY ARTERIAL COUPLING

The right ventricle, as the "end organ" most directly affected by PH, is important to assess during the evaluation of PH. Techniques for measuring right ventricular volume and function have been described, but are limited due to the complexity of derived formulas and difficult imaging imposed by the crescentic shape of the right ventricle. Simple measurements, such as right ventricular outflow tract fractional shortening correlate with other measurements of right ventricular function (58). A relatively simple method derived from *in-vitro* measurements (59) has been subsequently applied in children with PH (60). Ejection fraction is (EDV-ESV)/EDV in which EDV is right ventricular end-diastolic volume and ESV is right ventricular end-systolic volume. Volumes are estimated by either or both of two calculations: (1) volume = 2/3 area in the apical four-chamber view times length in the subcostal short

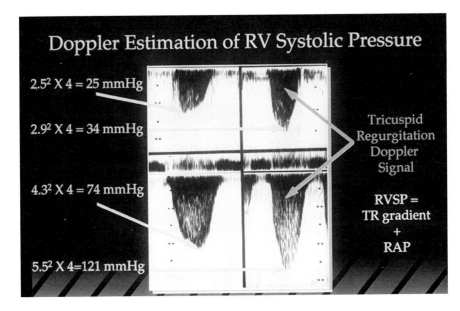

Figure 13.4 Doppler-echocardiographic signals of tricuspid regurgitant velocity illustrating incorporation into the modified Bernoulli equation to estimate the ventricular-to-atrial pressure gradient across the tricuspid valve.

axis view; or (2) 2/3 area in the subcostal short axis view times length in the apical four-chamber view. Using these techniques, ejection fraction correlated with measures obtained by magnetic resonance imaging (r = 0.9) in 21 patients (60). Three-dimensional echocardiographic techniques may provide greater accuracy and consistency of measurement of right ventricular volumes and ejection fractions than two-dimensional imaging (61,62).

Since complex right ventricular geometry generally precludes reliable echocardiographic assessment of ejection fraction and related indices, quantitative assessment of right ventricular function using other Doppler echocardiographic techniques has been explored. Continuous wave Doppler measurement of tricuspid valve jet velocity was suggested as a means of non-invasive evaluation of dP/dt of the right ventricle. However, right ventricular dP/dt varies with the level of PH and thus is not an independent marker of right ventricular function (63).

An alternative index of right ventricular dysfunction is the right ventricular index of myocardial performance (RIMP; Figure 13.7) (64). For more details, see refs 65–88.

EVALUATION OF PROGNOSIS AND RESPONSE TO TREATMENTS

Echocardiographic data have prognostic relevance. Parameters including elevated pulmonary artery pressure, right atrial pressure and decreased cardiac output were found to identify patients with PH and poor survival (11). In addition, pericardial effusions (which occur frequently in primary PH (89)) and short acceleration time correlate with poor prognosis (76), as do right atrial enlargement and septal displacement (90). Pulmonary artery systolic pressure, whether estimated echocardiographically or measured directly, correlates poorly with survival. Echocardiographic and Doppler indices of right ventricular pressure overload and dysfunction improve after successful treatment of chronic severe PH either by thromboendarterectomy (91)

or continuous intravenous infusion of prostacyclin (92). In patients with chronic pulmonary disease, right ventricular end-diastolic filling and velocity of late diastolic fillings tend to portend worse survival (93).

FOLLOW-UP

Patients with high quality echocardiographic studies and good correlation of noninvasively measured pulmonary hemodynamics with catheterization data can be followed with serial echocardiograms to assess progression of disease or response to treatment. Despite high correlation with catheter measured pulmonary artery pressures in populations with PH, however, operator technique and interpretation may introduce errors in measurement. Consequently, comparison of measurements over time in a single individual should be considered in light of corroborative data (including newer indices noted above) and experience of the echocardiographic laboratory.

Transesophageal echocardiography (TEE)

Transesophageal echocardiography can be performed safely in patients with severe PH, and provides additional clinically important data that may alter treatment in up 25 percent of patients (94). TEE is useful in the detection of otherwise occult intracardiac shunts, especially atrial septal defects.

TEE can detect central pulmonary emboli (Figure 13.8), including chronic thromboemboli causing pulmonary hypertension, with a reported sensitivity of 80 percent (95), and up to 96 percent, with a specificity of 88 percent, in patients with documented severe central acute or chronic thromboembolism (96).

Intravascular ultrasound (IVUS)

IVUS techniques have recently disclosed increased pulmonary arterial wall thickness in patients with PH, particularly

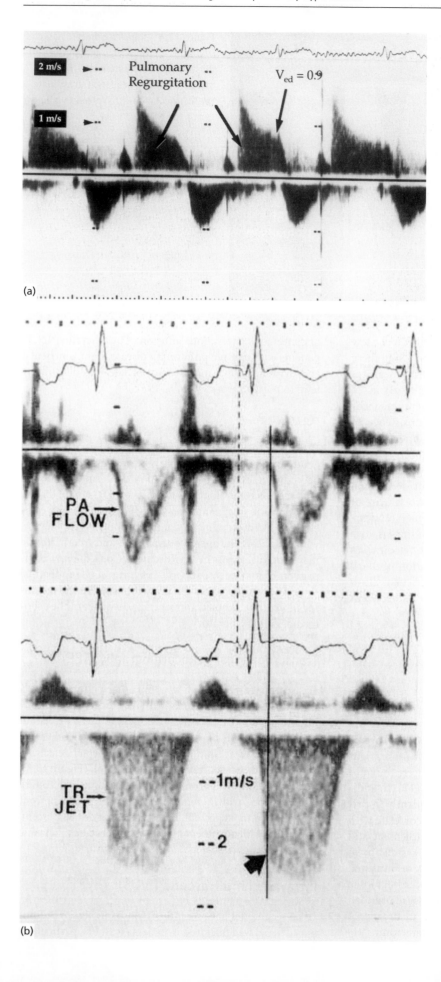

Figure 13.5 (a) Continuous-wave Doppler echocardiographic recording of pulmonary flow velocity illustrating measurement of the velocity at end-diastole. Estimated diastolic pulmonary artery pressure is 4 (0.9)^2 + right atrial pressure. (b) Top: pulsed-wave Doppler echocardiographic recording of the pulmonary artery. Bottom: a continuous-wave Doppler echocardiographic recording of the tricuspid regurgitant jet. ECG is used as a reference point to determine the tricuspid regurgitant velocity at the time of pulmonary valve opening. This is indicated by the point at which the solid line intersects with the outer border of the tricuspid regurgitant envelope (dark arrow). PA = pulmonary artery; TR = tricuspid regurgitation. From ref 45.

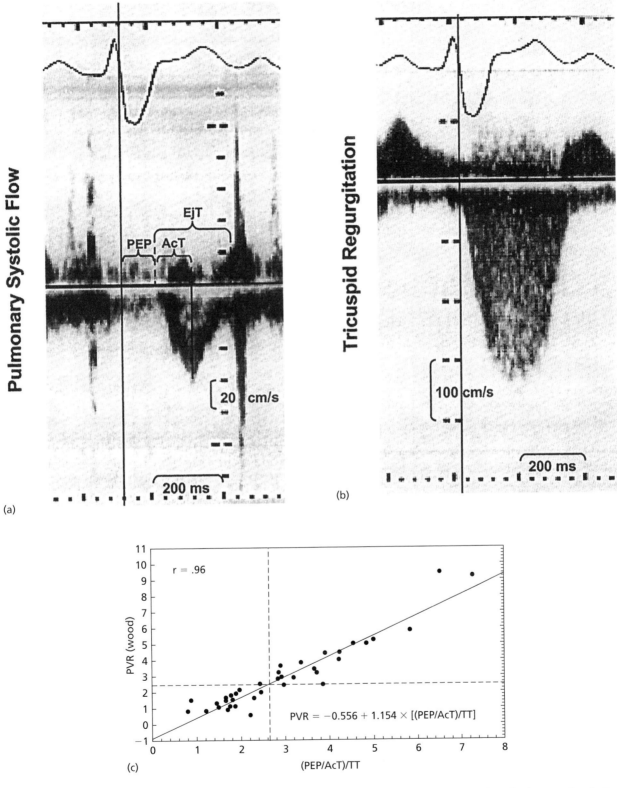

Figure 13.6 (a) Continuous-wave Doppler recording of tricuspid regurgitant flow. (b) Pulsed-wave recording of pulmonary flow in the same patient. (c) Scatterplot of linear correlation between measured and Doppler-determined pulmonary vascular resistance (PVR). Vertical dashed line marks the value of 2.6 in Doppler-determined PVR that predicts a value of 2.5 Wood units in measured PVR (horizontal dashed line). AcT = acceleration time; EjT = ejection time; PEP = pre-ejection period; TT = total systolic time. From ref 51.

in the lower lobes, which correlate with the degree of endothelin abnormalities (97). Reports about correlation of wall thickness and hemodynamic abnormalities vary from a direct correlation (97) to no correlation whatsoever (98).

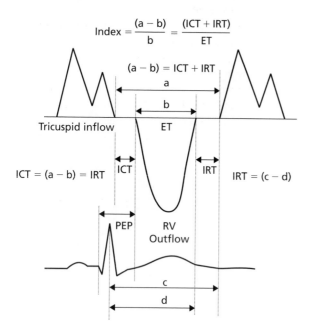

Figure 13.7   Schema of Doppler intervals. The index ([a−b]/b) is calculated by measuring two intervals: (1) a is the interval between cessation and onset of tricuspid inflow and (2) b is the ejection time (ET) of right ventricular (RV) outflow. Other available intervals include isovolumetric relaxation time (IRT) measure (c−d) by subtracting the interval (d) between the R wave and cessation of RV outflow from interval (c) between the R wave and onset of tricuspid flow; isovolumetric contraction time (ICT) obtained by subtracting IRT from (a−b); and pre-ejection period (PEP) measured from onset of QRS wave to onset of RV ejection flow. From ref 64.

Whether such modalities will have a clinical role remains to be determined.

Specific blood tests for evaluation of PH

The search for an etiology of PH requires evaluation with some blood tests which should be routinely obtained under most circumstances, followed by more directed evaluation if necessary. Antinuclear antibody (ANA) titer to screen for connective tissue disease and human immunodeficiency virus (HIV) serologies should be obtained in all cases of undifferentiated PH. Among patients with idiopathic PAH, 40 percent have positive but low antinuclear antibody titers ($\geq$ 1:80 dilutions) (99). Patients with a substantially elevated ANA or suspicious clinical features may require further serologic assessment, which may be guided by Table 13.4. For more details see refs 100–153.

Ventilation–perfusion (V/Q) scintigraphy

V/Q scanning is a widely available and highly sensitive screening modality to detect chronic pulmonary thromboemboli in patients with suspected or proven PH (154). Lung scans of patients with chronic pulmonary embolism show at least one segmental-sized or larger perfusion defect. Most have several segmental or lobar defects bilaterally (Figure 13.9A), which are typically mismatched and larger than ventilation abnormalities (111). Large perfusion defects which are not segmental or lobar in distribution should not be considered indicative of pulmonary embolism, especially when in the lower lung distribution, but may be due to diversion of flow to upper lung zones in patients with high left sided filling pressures and secondary lower zone vasoconstriction (155).

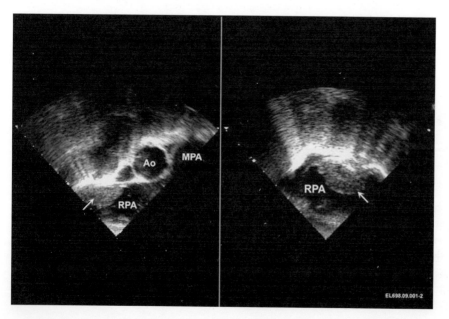

Figure 13.8   Multiplane transesophageal echocardiogram showing central chronic pulmonary embolus in a 73-year-old woman with chronic severe pulmonary hypertension. Left: horizontal view at the level of the great vessels. Right: oblique cross-sectional view of the right pulmonary artery. Additional thrombi (not shown) were visible in the left pulmonary artery. The white arrow indicates the chronic thrombus. Ao = aortic root; MPA = main pulmonary artery; RPA = right pulmonary artery.

Table 13.4   Summary of autoantibodies in connective tissue disease, from ref 273

Autoantibody	Frequency of occurrence	Comments
ANA	SLE, 95 percent, many other CTD	Sensitive but not specific for CTD
Double-stranded DNA	SLE, 30–70 percent	Specific but not sensitive for SLE; levels correlate with disease activity
Sm	SLE, < 30 percent	Specific but not sensitive for SLE
U_1RNP	MCTD; SLE, 40 percent; other CTD	By definition, present with MCTD
Anti-SS-A/Ro	Sjögren's, 75 percent; SLE, 25 percent; other CTD especially associated with Sjögren's	Evident with skin involvement in SLE, complete heart block in babies of mothers with this antibody
Anti-SS-B/La	Sjögren's, 40 percent; SLE, 10 percent; other CTD	Usually occurs with anti-SS-A/Ro
Anti-histone	Drug-induced SLE, > 90 percent; idiopathic SLE, > 50 percent; RA and Felty's syndrome occasionally	Not specific but sensitive for drug-induced SLE
Anti-centromere	CREST syndrome, > 80 percent	Staining pattern on ANA, relatively specific and sensitive for CREST
Anti-Scl 70	Progressive systemic sclerosis, 26–76 percent	Specific but not sensitive for progressive systemic sclerosis
c-ANCA	Active Wegener's granulomatosis	Titers tend to vary with disease activity
p-ANCA	Wegener's granulomatosis, 10 percent; glomerulonephritis, inflammatory bowel disease	Less specific and sensitive for Wegener's granulomatosis than is c-ANCA
Rheumatoid factor	Rheumatoid arthritis, 80 percent; Sjögren's, 50 percent; other CTD	High levels tend to correlate with severe rheumatoid arthritis

Patients with normal V/Q scans, including those with inhomogeneous flow patterns (Figure 13.9B) are very unlikely to have chronic pulmonary embolism, and more likely to have idiopathic PAH (156–160). Patchy nonsegmental diffuse defects are less specific, but may be associated with thromboembolic disease (161). Perfusion scans consistently tend to underestimate the degree of severity of large vessel obstruction in PH (162).

Computerized tomography (CT)

CT scanning measurements that correlate with severity of PH are the cross-sectional area of the pulmonary artery (163), the diameter of the main pulmonary artery (164), the ratio of the diameter of the artery to the bronchus (165), the ratio of the diameter of the pulmonary artery to the pulmonary vein (166), the ratio of the main pulmonary artery to aortic diameter (164,167), and the presence of pericardial thickening or effusion (168). A mosaic pattern of lung attenuation in a noncontrast CT scan raises the possibility of chronic thromboembolism (169). Although such observations may be useful in noninvasively adding strength to a diagnosis of PH and assessment of severity, they do not take the place of more precise and validated Doppler echocardiographic measurements. Rather, the role of CT is to explore possible etiologic factors.

Spiral (or helical) CT (170) or electron-beam CT (EBCT) (171) can visualize central chronic pulmonary thromboemboli (Figure 13.10), in some cases more accurately than angiography or MRI (as assessed at the time of thromboendarterectomy) (172). Serial spiral CT scans in

patients with acute pulmonary embolism suggest that up to 39 percent of pulmonary emboli do not completely resolve after a mean follow-up of 11 months (173). CT features of chronic thromboembolic disease are complete occlusion of pulmonary arteries, eccentric filling defects consistent with thrombi, recanalization, and stenoses or webs (174). The sensitivity of spiral CT for detecting central pulmonary embolism is higher than 85–90 percent, exceeding 98 percent for 64-detector row CT (175). Though sensitivity for detecting distal emboli generally is felt to be lower, detection rates of up to 97 percent for distal emboli (compared to high probability ventilation-perfusion scans or angiography) have been reported (95,175). The presence of central pulmonary arterial chronic thromboembolism is associated with a better result of thromboendarterectomy (176,177).

CT can provide important clues to the presence of pulmonary venous obstruction, such as the presence of stricture or hypoplasia in children with congenital heart disease (178). Other signs of possible pulmonary vein obstruction, including pulmonary veno-occlusive disease are smooth thickening of interlobular septa, peribronchovascular cuffing and, alveolar ground-glass opacification (19,178,179). See also ref 180.

High resolution CT

See refs 181, 182. High resolution CT can be done with either spiral or electron beam CT. More detailed views of the lung parenchyma during evaluation of PH or hypoxia can help in the diagnosis of pulmonary fibrosis.

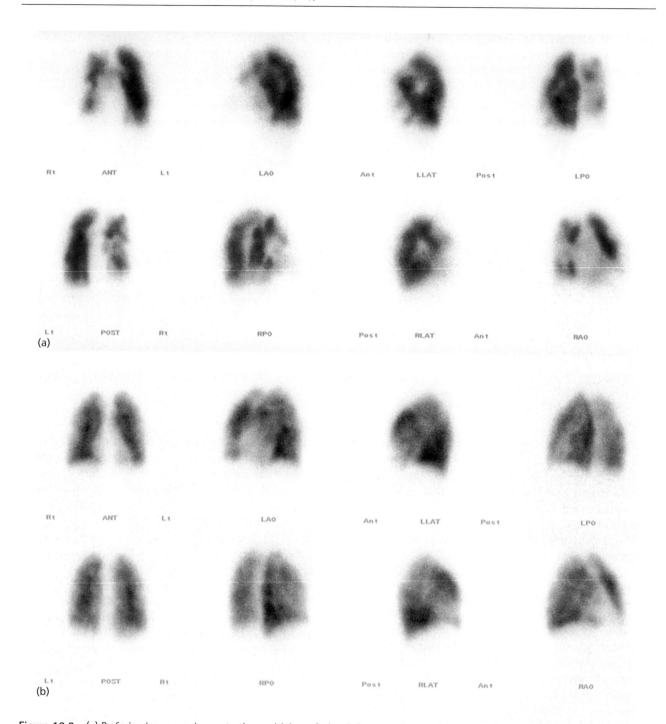

Figure 13.9 (a) Perfusion lung scan demonstrating multiple perfusion defects consistent with chronic thromboemboli in a patient with chronic pulmonary hypertension (5331418). (b) Perfusion lung scan demonstrating inhomogeneous flow pattern in a patient with primary pulmonary hypertension. From ref 272.

A mosaic pattern of the lung parenchyma and variation of segmental vessel size are suggestive of chronic thromboembolic disease (183).

Features of high resolution CT scans may be helpful in suggesting diagnoses that may be difficult to otherwise suspect. Diffuse bilateral thickening of the interlobular septae and the presence of small, centrilobular, poorly circumscribed nodular opacities are suggestive of pulmonary capillary hemangiomatosis. Patients with pulmonary veno-occlusive disease may demonstrate diffuse predominantly central ground-glass opacification and thickening of interlobular septa (184).

Magnetic resonance imaging (MRI)

Several recent reviews have summarized the role of MRI in the assessment of pulmonary vascular disease (185–187). MRI can provide noninvasive clues to the presence and impact of PH by evaluation of right ventricular chamber size, shape and volume; myocardial thickness and mass;

and the presence of fat or edema (188). Compared to normal right ventricular reference values (189), MRI-measured right ventricular systolic and diastolic volumes are significantly increased and left ventricular end-diastolic volume decreased in patients with primary PH. In addition, right and left ventricular ejection fractions are depressed in primary PH, and right ventricular stroke volume index is higher than left stroke volume index due to tricuspid regurgitation (190). Patients with PH exhibit myocardial delayed contrast enhancement specifically at the right ventricular insertion points, proportionately to right ventricular systolic dysfunction (191,192). Finally, right ventricular

myocardial contractility can be accurately derived from pressure-volume loops incorporating MRI volume and invasive pressure measurements (193). For more details, see Figure 13.11 and refs 194–213.

Pulmonary angiography

Pulmonary angiography is important to confirm or exclude the diagnosis of chronic pulmonary embolism, and to define the extent and location of thrombus. It can be performed safely in patients with severe PH and right ventricular failure (1,214), with about a 1 percent chance

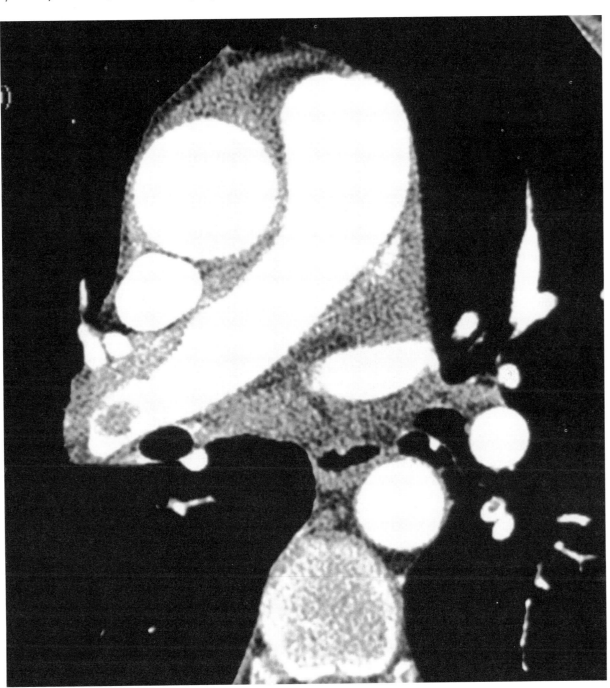

Figure 13.10   Electron beam CT of pulmonary chronic pulmonary embolism.

of adverse events, most of which are mild and reversible, in patients undergoing right heart catheterization with or without angiography (215). Appropriate precautions include using a brachial or jugular approach (to reduce risk of femoral thrombus), continuous monitoring of ECG and arterial saturation, single injections into right (using posterior – anterior projection) and left (using slight left anterior-oblique) main pulmonary arteries, nonionic contrast, and pretreatment with atropine 1 mg iv.

Chronic thrombi appear different than acute thrombi and occur in highly variable locations, often incorporated into and retracting the vessel wall. Obstructions can take the form of bands or webs, sometimes with post stenotic dilation (Figure 13.12). Irregular intimal surface (Figure 13.12), rounded or pouch-like termination of segmental branches, luminal narrowing of the central vessel, odd-shaped pulmonary arteries all may indicate the presence of chronic pulmonary embolism (216).

Pulmonary angioscopy

Fiberoptic angioscopy has been reported to enhance diagnostic accuracy in evaluation of chronic pulmonary thromboembolism (217). Currently this technique is employed at University of California San Diego as a staging procedure prior to thromboendarterectomy (218,219).

Pulmonary function testing (PFT)

Pulmonary function testing is required to exclude or characterize the contribution of underlying airways or parenchymal lung disease. Although obstructive pulmonary disease with hypoxemia may be confirmed by testing, abnormalities may occur in other types of PH. Approximately 20 percent of patients with chronic pulmonary embolism have a restrictive defect (a reduction in lung volumes to <80 percent of normal) (111), and may have near normal diffusing capacity for carbon monoxide (DL_{CO}) (220). Twenty percent of patients with systemic sclerosis have an isolated reduction in DL_{CO} (221), which when severe (<55 percent of predicted) may be associated with future development of PH in the limited cutaneous form (CREST) (222), but only correlates weakly with pulmonary pressure when PH is present (223). Patients with IPAH generally have mild reduction in forced vital capacity (FVC), forced expiratory volume in 1 second (FEV1), and effective alveolar volume; normal FEV1/FVC suggesting the presence of a mild restrictive ventilatory defect; and about 75 percent of patients have a percent predicted DL_{CO} below the lower limit of normal (224).

Arterial blood gas measurement

Arterial oxygen desaturation is both a promoter and consequence of PH, but is in itself nonspecific regarding underlying cause. It may signal abnormal gas exchange,

right-to-left shunting and ventilation/perfusion mismatching, interstitial fibrosis or other parenchymal lung disease, or hypoventilation. Failure to normalize with high FiO_2 oxygen inhalation supports a component of right-to-left shunting.

A search for abnormal oxygenation is warranted even when resting oxygen saturation is unremarkable. Arterial blood gas measurement or oximetry during exercise may disclose desaturation requiring supplemental oxygen treatment to improve exercise capacity and promote pulmonary vasodilation. Overnight oximetry may disclose disordered sleep with frequent desaturations and may be the first clue to sleep apnea sufficient to contribute to PH. Nocturnal hypoxemia occurs in over 75 percent of patients with primary PH independently of the occurrence of apneas or hypopneas, and many also had hypoxemia with walking (225). Since hypoxemia is a potent pulmonary vasoconstrictor, all patients with unexplained PH require assessment of both sleep and exercise oxygen saturation.

Exercise assessment

Formal assessment of exercise capacity is an integral part of the evaluation of PH. The goals of exercise testing vary under different clinical circumstances, and determine the specific testing modality to employ. These objectives include searching for alternative or contributory reasons for symptoms, such as myocardial ischemia; determining maximal exercise tolerance; characterizing comfortable activity level (functional capacity) of the patient; obtaining predictive data; establishing a baseline measure of exercise capacity and following the response to therapy; assessing the interaction of the circulatory and ventilatory systems; or attempting to discover abnormal pulmonary hemodynamic responses to exercise prior to clinically evident PH at rest.

The most commonly used exercise tests specifically for the evaluation of PH are the six-minute walk test, standard treadmill exercise test generally utilizing a low intensity graduated exercise protocol, cardiopulmonary exercise testing with gas exchange measurement, exercise testing in conjunction with noninvasive Doppler echocardiographic assessment of pulmonary artery pressure, and exercise testing in conjunction with right heart catheterization.

The six-minute walk test was developed as an objective measure of exercise capacity in patients with congestive heart failure, and was modified from prior protocols used in patients with obstructive pulmonary disease (226). It proved to be reproducible and correlated with other measures of functional status. The test was consequently applied in the evaluation of patients with primary PH, and has been used as a primary end-point in a number of clinical drug treatment trials. An additional observation derived from these studies was that six-minute walk performance was predictive of survival (227). Subsequent studies confirm a high level of clinical relevance. The distance patients with

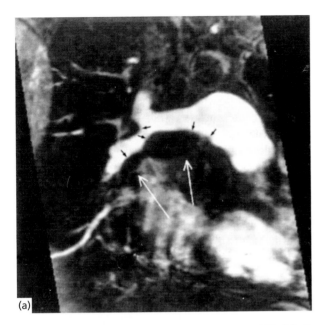

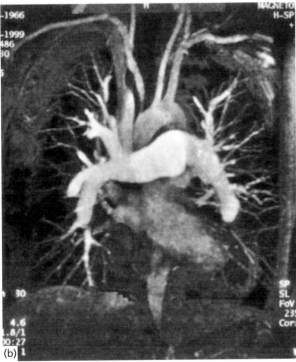

Figure 13.11 Magnetic resonance angiography shows
(a) massive central and irregular wall thickening due to organized
thrombotic material (white and black arrows), and (b) in another
patient dilatation of the central pulmonary arteries, abrupt
changes of vascular caliber, peripheral vascular cut-offs and
abnormal tapering. Both patients had chronic thromboembolic
pulmonary hypertension. From ref 207.

idiopathic PAH walk correlates inversely with New York
Heart Association functional status severity, correlates
moderately with baseline cardiac output and total pulmonary resistance (but not mean pulmonary arterial pressure), and strongly with peak exercise oxygen consumption

(peak VO$_2$), peak oxygen pulse, minute ventilation – carbon dioxide output slope (VE-VCO$_2$ slope) (228). In a
multivariate analysis which included clinical, echocardiographic and neurohumoral factors, six-minute walk was
the only independent predictor of death in a mean follow-
up period of 21+/− 16 months among 43 patients with
idiopathic PAH (228). In addition, a drop in arterial oxygen
saturation of more than 10 percent during six-minute walk
testing predicts an increase in mortality risk of 2.9 times
over a median 26 months of follow-up (229). At the Mayo
Clinic, unencouraged six-minute walk tests are performed
on a 20-meter back-and-forth course during monitoring by
a trained PH nurse specialist. Measured parameters are
distance walked, baseline and peak oxygen saturation by
finger, earlobe or forehead oximetry, supplemental oxygen
rate if present, baseline and peak blood pressure and pulse,
number of breaks, and self-reported Borg dyspnea scale
rating. For more details, see refs 230–247.

Right heart hemodynamic catheterization

Catheter measurement of mean pulmonary artery pressure
(P$_p$ [mmHg]), pulmonary arterial blood flow (Q$_p$ [L/min]),
pulmonary capillary wedge pressure (PCWP [mmHg]),
right atrial pressure (P$_{RA}$), and mixed venous oxygen saturation (MVO$_2$ [percent]) provide the most definitive characterization of pulmonary hemodynamics.

ASSESSMENT OF INTRACARDIAC SHUNT

While significant right-to-left shunting can most often be
excluded by bubble-contrast echocardiography (above),
right heart catheterization with a hydrogen curve, oximetry run, or double sampling indocyanine green dye curve
may be required to exclude left-to-right shunting and
thus the presence of a potentially treatable intracardiac
shunt.

MEASUREMENT OF PULMONARY ARTERY WEDGE (OCCLUSION) PRESSURE

Assessment of pulmonary vein pressure and transpulmonary gradient is needed for calculation of pulmonary arteriolar resistance, and requires knowing pulmonary artery
occlusion pressure. If necessary, left atrial pressure or left
ventricular end-diastolic pressure should be measured. An
elevated pulmonary arterial occlusion pressure supports
the presence of left heart disease or pulmonary vein
obstruction, but is very insensitive for pulmonary veno-
occlusive disease (19).

MEASUREMENT OF PULMONARY RESISTANCE

By analogy to Ohm's law, P$_p$ and Q$_p$ provide the basis
for calculating total pulmonary vascular resistance
(TPR [U] = P$_p$/Q$_p$) and pulmonary arterial resistance

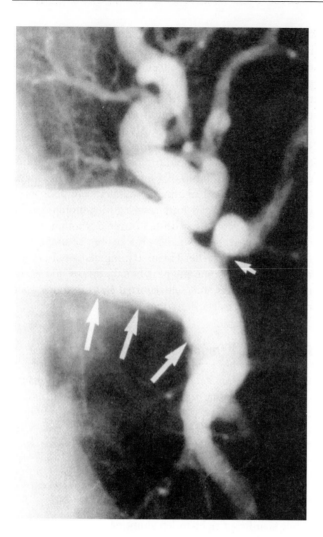

Figure 13.12   Pulmonary angiogram of a patient with chronic thromboembolic pulmonary hypertension showing vessel narrowing due to a band (small arrow) and luminal irregularities due to a large amount of thrombus lining the vessel wall. From ref 216.

$(PAR [U] = (P_p - PCWP)/Q_p)$. Blood flow and resistance can be indexed to body surface area (m^2). Calculation of Q_p by the Fick method and thermodilution correlate reasonably well, including in patients with low cardiac output or tricuspid regurgitation, so that either technique may be used in most cases (248), though the Fick technique is preferable with significant tricuspid regurgitation. In reality, it is recognized that this calculation reflects an artificial situation applicable to steady flow in a system of smooth-walled, regular, nondistensible conduits with laminar flow. In such a system, pressure increases proportionally with flow and the slope of the increase defines the resistance (which is constant) (249).

   A more accurate reflection of physiologic pulmonary vascular resistance has been advocated. The pulmonary vasculature is compliant and recruitable, and flow is pulsatile; thus volume and luminal diameter increase with increasing pressure. Consequently, resistance may decrease

as flow increases, though this may play only a rather minor role in maintaining low resistance during high flow in the normal lung (249). Pulmonary vessels also display a critical pressure (either due to extrinsic compression by lung parenchyma or due to vascular elastic or muscular recoil) (250) at which flow may cease even while the pulmonary pressure is higher than left atrial pressure. In normal individuals, critical pressure is approximately 10 mmHg (249). If the critical pressure is considered the effective "downstream" pressure, then elevated pressure–flow relationships can be a consequence of either an elevated critical pressure, elevated resistance or a combination.

MEASUREMENT OF PULMONARY VASODILATOR RESPONSE

Vasodilator study should be performed whenever PH is discovered or confirmed during right heart catheterization of patients in whom symptoms or severity of hypertension would warrant treatment. All patients in whom vasodilator treatment is to be initiated require hemodynamic monitoring for detection of either beneficial or detrimental effects of acute treatment. A decrease in P_p and PAR of 20–26 percent is required to confidently attribute the effect to an intervention (17,251). To minimize spontaneous fluctuation, the patient should be allowed to stabilize before the initiation of testing (252). Measurements should be obtained at predetermined intervals following drug administration and results should be interpreted cautiously unless decreases of pressure or resistance exceed the criteria above. Ideally, the critical pressure (intercept on the pressure axis of the pressure–flow relation) must be subtracted from the pressure gradient (249,252). Otherwise, an increase in flow (i.e., secondary to sympathetic stimulation due to systemic vasodilatation) may falsely suggest a decrease in pulmonary resistance in the absence of actual vasodilatation (252).

PROGNOSTICATION

Baseline hemodynamic measurements provide information which can be used to estimate the natural history of the disease in an individual patient. The probability of survival P(t) 1, 2, or 3 years after diagnosis can be estimated as $P(t) = (H(t))^{A(x,y,z)}$, where $H(t) = (0.88 - 0.14t + 0.01t^2)$, $A(x,y,z) = e^{(0.007325x + 0.0526y - 0.3275z)}$, t = years, x = mPAP (mmHg), y = mRAP (mmHg), and z = CI (L/min/m^2) (11). However, the predictive value of this equation has been altered by development of more effective therapies so that current survival consistently exceeds that predicted by this baseline assessment. Other logistic regression equations have been reported to predict survival or death within one year (253). Implantable hemodynamic monitors, although still investigational, hold promise as tools that can provide rapid remote provider access to continuous hemodynamics utilizing secure web-based technology (238).

SELECTION OF TREATMENT

The acute pulmonary hemodynamic effect of intravenously administered short-acting vasodilators predicts the hemodynamic response to oral long-acting vasodilators. Thus the efficacy of the short-acting drug can be used to determine optimal treatment (252,254–259). Short-acting vasodilators reportedly used in this capacity are prostacyclin (257,260–263), nitric oxide (264), adenosine, (255,257,265) acetylcholine (257) and L-arginine (266). Patients who respond with a reduction in mean pulmonary artery pressure of 10 mmHg or more, achieving a mean pulmonary artery pressure of less than 40 mmHg, and associated with no change or an increase in cardiac output warrant a trial of calcium channel antagonists. Those who are nonresponders may warrant a trial of endothelin receptor antagonists or phosphodiesterase inhibitors, but chronic continuous prostanoids should be considered early in patients with poor prognostic signs in view of observations that hemodynamic, symptomatic and survival benefit may occur in spite of absence of a significant acute beneficial hemodynamic effect (227,267).

Abrupt development of pulmonary edema during acute vasodilator testing suggests the presence of pulmonary veno-occlusive disease (268).

Lung biopsy

Open or thoracoscopic lung biopsy entails substantial risk of morbidity and mortality (269). Because of the low likelihood of altering the clinical diagnosis, routine biopsy is discouraged. Histopathologic findings in small pulmonary arteries obtained at biopsy may not even reliably distinguish between chronic thromboembolic disease and primary PH (270). Under certain circumstances, histopathologic diagnosis may provide useful information by excluding or establishing a diagnosis of active vasculitis, granulomatous pulmonary disease, pulmonary veno-occlusive disease, interstitial lung disease or bronchiolitis.

KEY POINTS

- Pulmonary hypertension of clinically significant degree is detectable by careful attention to history and examination coupled with appropriate interpretation of chest x-ray and electrocardiogram. Failure to appropriately diagnose pulmonary hypertension or attribute symptoms to it accounts for the largest delay in initiating treatment in these patients.
- Detection of pulmonary hypertension of mild degree generally warrants further evaluation for confirmation, identification of potentially treatable causes, initiation of monitoring progression, and treatment of related symptoms.
- Detection and confirmation of pulmonary hypertension of moderate or severe degree requires full evaluation of underlying causes and identification of an optimal treatment regimen.
- Full Doppler-echocardiographic examination is pivotal in characterizing pulmonary hypertension and screening for a broad range of potential causes, but invasive hemodynamic assessment is required for complete evaluation.
- Left-sided cardiac disease and chronic thromboembolism are the most frequently treatable causes of pulmonary hypertension and must be fully evaluated as potential causes.
- The diagnostic process should ideally occur at referral centers where complex treatment regimens can most effectively be initiated and followed.

REFERENCES

1. Rich S, Dantzker DR, Ayres SM et al. Primary pulmonary hypertension: a national prospective study. Ann Intern Med 1987;107(2):216–23.
2. Wolferen SAv, Marcus TJ, Westerhof N et al. Right coronary artery flow impairment in patients with pulmonary hypertension. Eur Heart J 2007:ehm567.
3. Rich S, McLaughlin VV, O'Neill W. Stenting into reverse left ventricular ischemia due to left main coronary artery compression in primary pulmonary hypertension. Chest 2001;120(4):1412–5.
4. Kawut SM, Silvestry FE, Ferrari VA et al. Extrinsic compression of the left main coronary artery by the pulmonary artery in patients with long-standing pulmonary hypertension. Am J Cardiol 1999;83(6):984–6.
5. Bonderman D, Fleischmann D, Prokop M, Klepetko W, Lang IM. Left main coronary artery compression by the pulmonary trunk in pulmonary hypertension: images in cardiovascular medicine. Circulation 2002;105(2):265.
6. Mesquita S, Castro C, Ikari N, Oliveira S, Lopes A. Likelihood of left main coronary artery compression based on pulmonary trunk diameter in patients with pulmonary hypertension. Am J Med 2004;116(6):369–74.
7. Dodd JD, Maree A, Palacios I et al. Left main coronary artery compression syndrome: evaluation with 64-slice cardiac multidetector computed tomography. Circulation 2007;115(1):e7–8.
8. Lindsey JB, Brilakis ES, Banerjee S. Acute coronary syndrome due to extrinsic compression of the left main coronary artery in a patient with severe pulmonary hypertension: successful treatment with percutaneous coronary intervention. Cardiovasc Revasc Med 2008;9(1):47–51.
9. Mikhail GW, Gibbs JSR, Yacoub MH. Pulmonary and systemic arterial pressure changes during syncope in primary pulmonary hypertension. Circulation 2001; 104(11):1326–7.

10. Appelbaum L, Yigla M, Bendayan D et al. Primary pulmonary hypertension in Israel: a national survey. Chest 2001;119:1801–6.

11. D'Alonzo GE, Barst RJ, Ayres SM et al. Survival in patients with primary pulmonary hypertension: results from a national prospective registry. Ann Intern Med 1991;115:343–9.

12. Higenbottam T, Wheeldon D, Wells F, Wallwork J. Long-term treatment of primary pulmonary hypertension with continuous intravenous epoprostenol (prostacyclin). Lancet 1984:1046–7.

13. Kuhn KP, Byrne DW, Arbogast PG, Doyle TP, Loyd JE, Robbins IM. Outcome in 91 consecutive patients with pulmonary arterial hypertension receiving epoprostenol. Am J Respir Crit Care Med 2003;167(4):580–3.

14. McLaughlin VV, Presberg KW, Doyle RL et al. Prognosis of pulmonary arterial hypertension: ACCP evidence-based clinical practice guidelines. Chest 2004;126(1 Suppl):78S–92S.

15. McLaughlin VV, McGoon MD. Pulmonary arterial hypertension. Circulation 2006;114(13):1417–31.

16. McQuillan BM, Picard MH, Leavitt M, Weymann AE. Clinical correlates and reference intervals for pulmonary artery systolic pressure among echocardiographically normal subjects. Circulation 2001;104(23):2797–802.

17. Rich S, D'Alonzo GE, Dantzker DR, Levy PS. Magnitude and implications of spontaneous hemodynamic variability in primary pulmonary hypertension. Am J Cardiol 1985;55(1):159–63.

18. McGoon MD. Pulmonary hypertension. In: Murphy JG, Lloyd MA, eds. Mayo Clinic Cardiology: Concise Textbook. Rochester, MN: Mayo Clinic Scientific Press and Informa Healthcare USA, 2007:929–50.

19. Holcomb BW Jr., Loyd JE, Ely W, Johnson J, Robbins IM. Pulmonary veno-occlusive disease: a case series and new observations. Chest 2000;118:1671–9.

20. Moser KM, Olson LK, Schlusselberg M, Daily PO, Dembitsky WP. Chronic thromboembolic occlusion in the adult can mimic pulmonary artery agenesis. Chest 1989;95:503–8.

21. Satoh T, Kyotani S, Okano Y, Nakanishi N, Kunieda T. Descriptive patterns of severe chronic pulmonary hypertension by chest radiography. Respir Med 2005;99:329–36.

22. Bossone E, Butera G, Bodini BD, Rubenfire M. The interpretation of the electrocardiogram in patients with pulmonary hypertension: the need for clinical correlation. Italian Heart J 2003;4(12):850–4.

23. Ahearn GS, Tapson VF, Rebeiz A, Greenfield JC. Electrocardiography to define clinical status in primary pulmonary hypertension and pulmonary arterial hypertension secondary to collagen vascular disease. Chest 2002;122:524–7.

24. Bossone E, Paciocco G, Iarussi D et al. The prognostic role of the ECG in primary pulmonary hypertension. Chest 2002;121:513–8.

25. Lee KS, Abbas AE, Khandheria BK, Lester SJ. Echocardiographic assessment of right heart hemodynamic parameters. J Am Soc Echocardiogr 2007;20:773–82.

26. Bossone E, Bodini BD, Mazza A, Allegra L. Pulmonary arterial hypertension – The key role of echocardiography. Chest 2005;127:1836–43.

27. Borgeson DD, Seward JB, Miller Jr. FA, Oh JK, Tajik AJ. Frequency of Doppler measurable pulmonary artery pressures. J Am Soc Echocardiogr 1996;9:832–7.

28. Jeon D, Luo H, Iwami T et al. The usefulness of a 10 percent air–10 percent blood–80 percent saline mixture for contrast echocardiography: Doppler measurement of pulmonary artery systolic pressure. J Am Coll Cardiol 2002;39:124–9.

29. Brecker SJ, Gibbs JS, Fox KM, Yacoub MH, Gibson DG. Comparison of Doppler derived haemodynamic variables and simultaneous high fidelity pressure measurements in severe pulmonary hypertension. Br Heart J 1994;72:384–9.

30. Chan KL, Currie PJ, Seward JB. Comparison of three Doppler ultrasound methods in the prediction of pulmonary artery pressure. J Am Coll Cardiol 1987;9:549–54.

31. Chapatou L, Metz D, Jolly D et al. Diagnostic, prognostic and therapeutic value of Doppler echocardiography in pulmonary embolism. Ann Cardiol Angiol 1989;38:523–9.

32. Currie PJ, Seward JB, Chan KL et al. Continuous wave Doppler determination of right ventricular pressure: a simultaneous Doppler-catheterization study in 127 patients. J Am Coll Cardiol 1985;6(4):750–6.

33. Isobe M, Yazaki Y, Takaku K et al. Prediction of pulmonary artery pressure in adults by pulsed Doppler echocardiography. Am J Cardiol 1986;56:316–21.

34. Kosturakis D, Goldberg SJ, Allen HD, Loeber C. Doppler echocardiographic prediction of pulmonary hypertension in congenital heart disease. Am J Cardiol 1984;53:1110–5.

35. Laaban JP, Diebold B, Zielinski R, Lafay M, Raffoul H, Rochemaure J. Noninvasive estimation of systolic pulmonary artery pressure using Doppler echocardiography in patients with chronic obstructive pulmonary disease. Chest 1989;96:1258–62.

36. Marangoni S, Quadri A, Dotti A et al. Noninvasive assessment of pulmonary hypertension: a simultaneous echo-Doppler study. Cardiology 1988;75:401–8.

37. Marchandise B, De Bruyne B, Delaunis L, Kremer R. Noninvasive prediction of pulmonary hypertension in chronic obstructive pulmonary disease by Doppler echocardiography. Chest 1987;91:361–5.

38. Torbicki A, Skwarski K, Hawrylkiewicz I, Pasierski T, Miskiewicz Z, Zielinski J. Attempts at measuring pulmonary arterial pressure by means of Doppler echocardiography in patients with chronic lung disease. Eur Respir J 1989;2:856–60.

39. Kim W, Krowka M, Plevak D et al. Accuracy of Doppler echocardiography in the assessment of pulmonary hypertension in liver transplant candidates. Liver Transplant 2000;6(4):453–8.

40. Arcasoy SM, Christie JD, Ferrari VA et al. Echocardiographic assessment of pulmonary hypertension in patients with advanced lung disease. Am J Respir Crit Care Med 2003;167(5):735–40.

41. Homma A, Anzueto A, Peters JI *et al.* Pulmonary artery systolic pressures estimated by echocardiogram vs. cardiac catheterization in patients awaiting lung transplantation. J Heart Lung Transplant 2001;20:833–9.

42. Ommen SR, Nishimura RA, Hurrell DG, Klarich KW. Assessment of right atrial pressure with 2-dimensional and Doppler echocardiography: a simultaneous catheterization and echocardiographic study. Mayo Clin Proc 2000;75:24–9.

43. Bossone E, Duong-Wagner T, Paciocco G *et al.* Echocardiographic features of primary pulmonary hypertension. J Am Soc Echocardiogr 1999:655–62.

44. Hatle L, Angelsen B. Doppler Ultasound in Cardiology: Physical Principles and Clinical Applications. 2nd ed. Philadelphia: Lean & Febiger, 1985.

45. Stephen B, Dalal P, Berger M, Schweitzer P, Hecht S. Noninvasive estimation of pulmonary artery diastolic pressure in patients with tricuspid regurgitation by Doppler echocardiography. Chest 1999;116:73–7.

46. Kitabatake A, Inoue M, Asao M *et al.* Noninvasive evaluation of pulmonary hypertension by a pulsed Doppler technique. Circulation 1983;68(2):302–9.

47. Dabestani A, Mahan G, Gardin JM. Evaluation of pulmonary artery pressure and resistance by pulsed Doppler echocardiography. Am J Cardiol 1987;59:661–8.

48. Masuyama T, Kodama K, Kitabatake A, Sato H, Nanto S, Inoue M. Continuous-wave Doppler echocardiographic detection of pulmonary regurgitation and its application to noninvasive estimation of pulmonary artery pressure. Circulation 1986;74:784–92.

49. Abbas AE, Fortuin FD, Schiller NB, Appleton CP, Moreno CA, Lester SJ. Echocardiographic determination of mean pulmonary artery pressure. Am J Cardiol 2003;92:1373–6.

50. Ensing G, Seward JB, Darragh R, Caldwell R. Feasibility of generating hemodynamic pressure curves from noninvasive Doppler echocardiographic signals. J Am Coll Cardiol 1994;23:434–42.

51. Scapellato F, Temporelli PL, Eleuteri E, Corra U, Imparato A, Giannuzzi P. Accurate noninvasive estimation of pulmonary vascular resistance by Doppler echocardiography in patients with chronic heart failure. J Am Coll Cardiol 2001;37:1813–9.

52. Abbas AE, Fortuin FD, Schiller NB, Appleton CP, Moreno CA, Lester SJ. A simple method for noninvasive estimation of pulmonary vascular resistance. J Am Coll Cardiol 2003; 41(6):1021–6.

53. Vlahos AP, Feinstein JA, Schiller NB, Silverman NH. Extension of Doppler-derived echocardiographic measures of pulmonary vascular resistance to patients with moderate or severe pulmonary vascular disease. J Am Soc Echocardiogr 2008;21(6):711–4.

54. Ulett KB, Marwick TH. Incorporation of pulmonary vascular resistance measurement into standard echocardiography: implications for assessment of pulmonary hypertension. Echocardiography 2007;24(10):1020–2.

55. Shandas R, Weinberg CE, Ivy D *et al.* Development of a noninvasive ultrasound color M-mode means of estimating pulmonary vascular resistance in pediatric pulmonary hypertension: mathematical analysis, in vitro validation, and preliminary clinical studies. Circulation 2001;104: 908–13.

56. Nagaya N, Satoh T, Uematsu M *et al.* Shortening of Doppler-derived deceleration time of early diastolic transmitral flow in the presence of pulmonary hypertension through ventricular interaction. Am J Cardiol 1997; 79:1502–6.

57. Nakayama Y, Sugimachi M, Nakanishi N *et al.* Noninvasive differential diagnosis between chronic pulmonary thromboembolism and primary pulmonary hypertension by means of Doppler ultrasound measurement. J Am Coll Cardiol 1998;31:1367–71.

58. Lindqvist P, Henein M, Kazzam E. Right ventricular outflow-tract fractional shortening: an applicable measure of right ventricular systolic function. Eur J Echocardiogr 2003;4(1):29–35.

59. Levine RA, Gibson TC, Aretz T. Echocardiographic measurement of right ventricular volume. Circulation 1984;69:497–505.

60. Apfel HD, Solowiejczyk DE, Printz BF *et al.* Feasibility of a two-dimensional echocardiographic method for the clinical assessment of right ventricular volume and function in children. J Am Soc Echocardiogr 1996;9: 637–45.

61. Jenkins C, Chan J, Bricknell K, Strudwick M, Marwick TH. Reproducibility of right ventricular volumes and ejection fraction using real-time three-dimensional echocardio-graphy: comparison with cardiac MRI. Chest 2007; 131(6):1844–51.

62. Menzel T, Kramm T, Bruckner A, Mohr-Kahaly S, Mayer E, Meyer J. Quantitative assessment of right ventricular volumes in severe chronic thromboembolic pulmonary hypertension using transthoracic three-dimensional echocardiography: changes due to pulmonary thrombo-endarterectomy. Eur J Echocardiogr 2002;3(1):67–72.

63. Pai RG, Bansal RC, Shah PM. Determinants of the rate of right ventricular pressure rise by Doppler echocardiography: potential value in the assessment of right ventricular function. J Heart Valve Dis 1994;3:179–84.

64. Tei C, Dujardin KS, Hodge DO *et al.* Doppler echocardiographic index for assessment of global right ventricular function. J Am Soc Echocardiogr 1996;9:838–47.

65. Seyfarth HJ, Pankau H, Winkler J, Wirtz H. Correlation of TEI index and invasive parameters of right heart function in PAH. Pneumologie 2004;58(4):206–7.

66. Yeo TC, Dujardin KS, Tei C, Mahoney DW, McGoon MD, Seward JB. Value of a Doppler-derived index combining systolic and diastolic time intervals in predicting outcome in primary pulmonary hypertension. Am J Cardiol 1998; 81:1157–61.

67. Vonk MC, Sander MH, van den Hoogen FHJ, van Riel PLCM, Verheugt FWA, van Dijk APJ. Right ventricle Tei-index: a tool to increase the accuracy of non-invasive detection of pulmonary arterial hypertension in connective tissue diseases. Eur J Echocardiogr 2007;8(5):317–21.

68. Sebbag I, Rudski LG, Therrien J, Hirsch A, Langleben D. Effect of chronic infusion of epoprostenol on echocardiographic right ventricular myocardial performance index and its relation to clinical outcome in patients with primary pulmonary hypertension. Am J Cardiol 2001; 88(9):1060–3.

69. Dyer KL, Pauliks LB, Das B et al. Use of myocardial performance index in pediatric patients with idiopathic pulmonary arterial hypertension. J Am Soc Echocardiogr 2006;19:21–7.

70. Torbicki A, Hawrylkiewicz I, Zielinski J. Value of M-mode echocardiography in assessing pulmonary arterial pressure in patients with chronic lung disease. Bull Eur Pathophysiol Respir 1987;23:233–9.

71. Kussmaul WG, Noordegraaf A, Laskey WK. Right ventricular-pulmonary arterial interactions. Ann Biomed Eng 1992; 20:63–80.

72. Furuno Y, Nagamoto Y, Fujita M, Kaku T, Sakurai S, Kuroiea A. Reflection as a cause of midsystolic deceleration of pulmonary flow wave in dogs with acute pulmonary hypertension: comparison of pulmonary artery constriction with embolization. Circulat Res 1991;25:118–24.

73. Milnor WR, Conti CR, Lewis KB, O'Rourke MF. Pulmonary arterial pulse wave velocity and impedance in man. Circulat Res 1969;25:637–49.

74. Turkevich D, Groves BM, Micco A, Trapp JA, Reeves JT. Early partial closure of the pulmonic valve relates to severity of pulmonary hypertension. Am Heart J 1988; 115:409–18.

75. Torbicki A, Kurzyna M, Ciurzynski M et al. Proximal pulmonary emboli modify right ventricular ejection pattern. Eur Respir J 1999;13:616–21.

76. Eysmann SB, Palevsky HI, Reichek N, Hackney K, Douglas PS. Two-dimensional and Doppler echocardiography and cardiac catheterisation correlates of survival in primary pulmonary hypertension. Circulation 1989;80:353–60.

77. Mahapatra S, Nishimura RA, Oh JK, McGoon MD. The prognostic value of pulmonary vascular capacitance determined by Doppler echocardiography in patients with pulmonary arterial hypertension. J Am Soc Echocardiogr 2006;19(8):1045–50.

78. Mahapatra S, Nishimura RA, Sorajja P, Cha S, McGoon MD. Relationship of pulmonary arterial capacitance and mortality in idiopathic pulmonary arterial hypertension. J Am Coll Cardiol 2006;47(4):799–803.

79. Schwartz DJ, Kop WJ, Park MH et al. Evidence for early right ventricular and septal mechanical activation (interventricular dyssynchrony) in pulmonary hypertension. Am J Cardiol 2008;102(9):1273–7.

80. Ruan Q, Nagueh SF. Clinical application of tissue Doppler imaging in patients with idiopathic pulmonary hypertension. Chest 2007;131(2):395–401.

81. Borges AC, Knebel F, Eddicks S et al. Right ventricular function assessed by two-dimensional strain and tissue Doppler echocardiography in patients with pulmonary arterial hypertension and effect of vasodilator therapy. Am J Cardiol 2006;98(4):530–4.

82. Urheim S, Cauduro S, Frantz R et al. Relation of tissue displacement and strain to invasively determined right ventricular stroke volume. Am J Cardiol 2005;96:1173–8.

83. Kittipovanonth M, Bellavia D, Chandrasekaran K, Villarraga HR, Abraham TP, Pellikka PA. Doppler myocardial imaging for early detection of right ventricular dysfunction in patients with pulmonary hypertension. J Am Soc Echocardiogr 2008;21(9):1035–41.

84. Rajdev S, Nanda NC, Pate V et al. Tissue Doppler assessment of longitudinal right and left ventricular strain and strain rate in pulmonary artery hypertension. Echocardiography 2006;23(10):872–9.

85. Pirat B, McCulloch ML, Zoghbi WA. Evaluation of global and regional right ventricular systolic function in patients with pulmonary hypertension using a novel speckle tracking method. Am J Cardiol 2006;98(5):699–704.

86. Forfia PR, Fisher MR, Mathai SC et al. Tricuspid annular displacement predicts survival in pulmonary hypertension. Am J Respir Crit Care Med 2006;174:1034–41.

87. Saxena N, Rajagopalan N, Edelman K, Lopez-Candales A. Tricuspid annular systolic velocity: a useful measurement in determining right ventricular systolic function regardless of pulmonary artery pressures. Echocardiography 2006;23(9):750–5.

88. De Castro S, Cavarretta E, Milan A et al. Usefulness of tricuspid annular velocity in identifying global RV dysfunction in patients with primary pulmonary hypertension: a comparison with 3D echo-derived right ventricular ejection fraction. Echocardiography 2008; 25(3):289–93.

89. Hinderliter AL, Willis PW, Long WA et al. Frequency and prognostic significance of pericardial effusion in primary pulmonary hypertension. Am J Cardiol 1999; 84:481–4.

90. Raymond RJ, Hinderliter AL, Willis PW et al. Echocardiographic predictors of adverse outcomes in primary pulmonary hypertension. J Am Coll Cardiol 2002;39:1214–9.

91. Menzel T, Wagner S, Mohr-Kahaly S et al. Reversibility of changes in left and right ventricular geometry and hemodynamics in pulmonary hypertension: echocardiographic characteristics before and after pulmonary thromboendarterectomy. Z Kardiol 1997;86:928–35.

92. Hinderliter AL, Willis IV PW, Barst RJ et al. Effects of long-term infusion of prostacyclin (epoprostenol) on echocardiographic measures of right ventricular structure and function in primary pulmonary hypertension. Circulation 1997;95:1479–86.

93. Burgess MI, Mogulkoc N, Bright-Thomas RJ, Bishop P, Egan JJ, Ray SG. Comparison of echocardiographic markers of right ventricular function in determining prognosis in chronic pulmonary disease. J Am Soc Echocardiogr 2002;15:633–9.

94. Gorcsan J, Edwards TD, Ziady GM, Katz WE, Griffith BP. Transesophageal echocardiography to evaluate patients with severe pulmonary hypertension for lung transplantation. Ann Thorac Surg 1995;59:717–22.

95. Pruszczyk P, Torbicki A, Pacho R *et al.* Noninvasive diagnosis of suspected severe pulmonary embolism: transesophageal echocardiography vs spiral CT. Chest 1997;112(3):722–8.

96. Wittlich N, Erbel R, Eichler A *et al.* Detection of central pulmonary artery thromboemboli by transesophageal echocardiography in patients with severe pulmonary embolism. J Am Soc Echocardiogr 1992;5(5):515–24.

97. Bressollette E, Dupuis J, Bonan R, Doucet S, Cernacek T, Tardif JC. Intravascular ultrasound assessment of pulmonary vascular disease in patients with pulmonary hypertension. Chest 2001;120:809–15.

98. Rodes-Cabau J, Domingo E, Roman A *et al.* Intravascular ultrasound of the elastic pulmonary arteries: a new approach for the evaluation of primary pulmonary hypertension. Heart 2003;89(3):311–5.

99. Rich S, Kieras K, Hart K, Groves BM, Stobo JD, Brundage BH. Antinuclear antibodies in primary pulmonary hypertension. J Am Coll Cardiol 1986;8:1307–11.

100. Petitpretz P, Brenot F, Azarian R *et al.* Pulmonary hypertension in patients with human immunodeficiency virus infection: comparison with primary pulmonary hypertension. Circulation 1994;89:2722–7.

101. Sitbon O, Lascoux-Combe C, Delfraissy J-F *et al.* Prevalence of HIV-related pulmonary arterial hypertension in the current antiretroviral therapy era 10.1164/rccm.200704-541OC. Am J Respir Crit Care Med 2008;177(1):108–13.

102. Barnett CF, Hsue PY, Machado RF. Pulmonary hypertension: an increasingly recognized complication of hereditary hemolytic anemias and HIV infection. JAMA 2008; 299(3):324–31.

103. de Chadarevian JP, Lischner HW, Karmazin N, Pawel BR, Schultz TE. Pulmonary hypertension and HIV infection: new observations and review of the syndrome. Mod Pathol 1994;7:685–9.

104. Mani S, Smith GW. HIV and pulmonary hypertension: a review. Southern Med J 1994;87:357–62.

105. Mette SA, Palevsky HI, Pietra GG *et al.* Primary pulmonary hypertension in association with human immunodeficiency virus infection: a possible viral etiology for some forms of hypertensive pulmonary arteriopathy. Rev Respir Dis 1992;145:1196–200.

106. Polos PG, Wolfe D, Harley RA, Strange C, Sahn SA. Pulmonary hypertension and human inmunodeficiency virus infection: two reports and a review of the literature. Chest 1992;101:474–8.

107. Speich R, Jenni R, Opravil M, Pfab M, Russi EW. Primary pulmonary hypertension in HIV infection. Chest 1991; 100:1268–71.

108. Heron E, Laaban JP, Capron F, Quieffin J, Brechot JM, Rochemaure J. Thrombotic primary pulmonary hypertension in HIV+ patient. Eur Heart J 1994;15:394–6.

109. Maliakkal R, Friedman SA, Sridhar S. Progressive pulmonary thromboembolism in association with HIV disease. NY State J Med 1992;92:403–4.

110. Nunes H, Humbert M, Sitbon O *et al.* Prognostic factors for survival in human immunodeficiency virus-associated pulmonary arterial hypertension. Am J Respir Crit Care Med 2003;167(10):1433–9.

111. Viner SM, Bagg BR, Auger WR, Ford GT. The management of pulmonary hypertension secondary to chronic thromboembolic disease. Prog Cardiovasc Dis 1994;37(2):79–92.

112. Wolf M, Boyer-Neumann C, Parent F *et al.* Thrombotic risk factors in pulmonary hypertension. Eur Respir J 2000; 15(2):395–9.

113. Petri M. Diagnosis of antiphospholipid antibodies. Rheumat Dis Clin North Am 1994;20:443–69.

114. Bonderman D, Skoro-Sajer N, Jakowitsch J *et al.* Predictors of outcome in chronic thromboembolic pulmonary hypertension. Circulation 2007.

115. Ridker PM, Miletich JP, Stampfer MJ *et al.* Factor V Leiden and risks of recurrent idiopathic venous thromboembolism. Circulation 1995;92(10):2800–2.

116. Manten B, Westendorp RG, Koster T, Reitsma PH, Rosendaal FR. Risk factor profiles in patients with different clinical manifestations of venous thromboembolism: a focus on the factor V Leiden mutation. Thromb Haemostas 1997; 76(4):510–3.

117. Lang IM, Klepetko W, Pabinger I. No increased prevalence of the factor V Leiden mutation in chronic major vessel thromboembolic pulmonary hypertension (CTEPH) [letter]. Thromb Haemostas 1996;76(3):476–7.

118. Lang I, Kerr K. Risk factors for chronic thromboembolic pulmonary hypertension. Proc Am Thorac Soc 2006; 3(7):568–70.

119. Cody RJ, Haas GJ, Binkley PF, Capers Q, Kelley RT. Plasma endothelin correlates with the extent of pulmonary hypertension in patients with chronic congestive heart failure. Circulation 1992;85:504–9.

120. Nootens M, Kaufman E, Rector T *et al.* Neurohormonal activation in patients with right ventricular failure from pulmonary hypertension: relation to hemodynamic variables and endothelin levels. J Am Coll Cardiol 1995; 26:1581–5.

121. Rubens C, Ewert R, Halank M *et al.* Big endothelin-1 and endothelin-1 plasma levels are correlated with the severity of primary pulmonary hypertension. Chest 2001;120:1562–9.

122. Stewart DJ, Levy RD, Cernacek P, Langleben D. Increased plasma endothelin-1 in pulmonary hypertension: marker or mediator of disease? Ann Intern Med 1991;114:464.

123. Andreassen AK, Wergeland R, Simonsen S, Geiran O, Guevara C, Ueland T. N-terminal pro-B-type natriuretic peptide as an indicator of disease severity in a heterogeneous group of patients with chronic precapillary pulmonary hypertension. The Am J Cardiol 2006;98(4):525–9.

124. Souza R, Sitbon O, Parent F, Simonneau G, Humbert M. Long term imatinib treatment in pulmonary arterial hypertension. Thorax 2006;61(8):736.

125. Souza R, Jardim C, Fernandes CJC, Lapa MS, Rabelo R, Humbert M. NT-proBNP as a tool to stratify disease severity in pulmonary arterial hypertension. Respir Med 2007;101(1):69–75.

126. Nagaya N, Nishikimi T, Uematsu M *et al.* Plasma brain natriuretic peptide as a prognostic indicator in patients

with primary pulmonary hypertension. Circulation 2000; 102(8):865–70.

127. Park MH, Scott RL, Uber PA, Ventura HO, Mehra MR. Usefulness of B-type natriuretic peptide as a predictor of treatment outcome in pulmonary arterial hypertension. Congest Heart Fail 2004;10(5):221–5.

128. Leuchte HH, Holzapfel M, Baumgartner RA, Neurohr C, Vogeser M, Behr J. Characterization of brain natriuretic peptide in long-term follow-up of pulmonary arterial hypertension. Chest 2005;128:2368–74.

129. Fijalkowska A, Kurzyna M, Torbicki A et al. Serum N-terminal brain natriuretic peptide as a prognostic parameter in patients with pulmonary hypertension. Chest 2006; 129(5):1313–21.

130. Allanore Y, Borderie D, Avouac J et al. High N-terminal pro-brain natriuretic peptide levels and low diffusing capacity for carbon monoxide as independent predictors of the occurrence of precapillary pulmonary arterial hypertension in patients with systemic sclerosis. Arthrit Rheumat 2008;58(1):284–91.

131. Dimitroulas T, Giannakoulas G, Karvounis H et al. N-terminal probrain natriuretic peptide as a biochemical marker in the evaluation of bosentan treatment in systemic-sclerosis-related pulmonary arterial hypertension. Clin Rheumatol 2008;27(5):655–8.

132. Galie N, Olschewski H, Oudiz RJ et al. Ambrisentan for the treatment of pulmonary arterial hypertension: results of the ambrisentan in pulmonary arterial hypertension, randomized, double-blind, placebo-controlled, multicenter, efficacy (ARIES) Study 1 and 2. Circulation 2008;117(23):3010–9.

133. O'Byrne ML, Rosenzweig ES, Barst RJ. The effect of atrial septostomy on the concentration of brain-type natriuretic peptide in patients with idiopathic pulmonary arterial hypertension. Cardiol Young 2007;17(5):557–9.

134. Simeoni S, Lippi G, Puccetti A et al. N-terminal pro-BNP in sclerodermic patients on bosentan therapy for PAH. Rheumatol Internat 2008;28(7):657–60.

135. Wilkins MR, Paul GA, Strange JW et al. Sildenafil versus endothelin receptor antagonist for pulmonary hypertension (SERAPH) study. Am J Respir Crit Care Med 2005;171:1292–7.

136. Machado RF, Anthi A, Steinberg MH et al. N-terminal pro-brain natriuretic peptide levels and risk of death in sickle cell disease. JAMA 2006;296(3):310–8.

137. Suntharalingam J, Goldsmith K, Toshner M et al. Role of NT-proBNP and 6MWD in chronic thromboembolic pulmonary hypertension. Respir Med 2007;101(11): 2254–62.

138. Diller G-P, van Eijl S, Okonko DO et al. Circulating endothelial progenitor cells in patients with Eisenmenger syndrome and idiopathic pulmonary arterial hypertension. Circulation 2008;117(23):3020–30.

139. Arroliga AC, Dweik RA, Rafanan AL. Primary pulmonary hypertension and thyroid disease (letter). Chest 2000; 118:1224.

140. Ferris A, Jacobs T, Widlitz A, Barst RJ, Morse JH. Pulmonary arterial hypertension and thyroid disease (letter). Chest 2001;119:1980–1.

141. Nakchbandi IA, Wirth JA, Inzucchi SE. Pulmonary hypertension caused by Graves' thyrotoxicosis: normal pulmonary hemodynamics restored by 131 I treatment. Chest 1999;116:1483–5.

142. Badesch DB, Wynne KM, Bonvallet S, Voelkel NF, Ridgway C, Groves BM. Hypothyroidism and primary pulmonary hypertension: an autoimmune pathogenetic link? Ann Intern Med 1993;119(1):44–6.

143. Curnock AL, Dweik RA, Higgins BH, H.F. S, Arroliga AC. High prevalence of hypothyroidism in patients with primary pulmonary hypertension. Am J Med Sci 1999; 318:289–92.

144. Ghamra ZW, Dweik RA, Arroliga AC. Hypothyroidism and pulmonary arterial hypertension (letter). Am J Med 2004; 116(5):354–5.

145. Chu JW, Kao PN, Faul JL, Doyle RL. High prevalence of autoimmune thyroid disease in pulmonary arterial hypertension. Chest 2002;122(5):1668–73.

146. Li JH, Safford RE, Aduen JF, Heckman MG, Crook JE, Burger CD. Pulmonary hypertension and thyroid disease. Chest 2007;132(3):793–7.

147. Marvisi M, Zambrelli P, Brianti M, Civardi G, Lampugnani R, Delsignore R. Pulmonary hypertension is frequent in hyperthyroidism and normalizes after therapy. Eur J Intern Med 2006;17:267–71.

148. Merce J, Ferras S, Oltra C et al. Cardiovascular abnormalities in hyperthyroidism: a prospective Doppler echocardiographic study. Am J Med 2005;118:126–31.

149. Lozano H, Sharma C. Reversible pulmonary hypertension, tricuspid regurgitation, and right-sided heart failure associated with hyperthyroidism; case report and review of the literature. Cardiol Rev 2004;12:299–305.

150. Virani SS, Mendoza CE, Ferreira AC, de Marchena E. Graves' disease and pulmonary hypertension. Texas Heart Inst J 2003;30(4):314–5.

151. Abboud B, Badaoui G, Aoun Z, Tabet G, Jebara V. Substernal goitre: a rare cause of pulmonary hypertension and heart failure. J Laryngol Otol 2000;114:719–20.

152. Voelkel MA, Wynne KM, Badesch DB, Groves BM, Voelkel NF. Hyperuricemia in severe pulmonary hypertension. Chest 2000;117:19–24.

153. Nagaya N, Uematsu M, Satoh T et al. Serum uric acid levels correlate with the severity and mortality of primary pulmonary hypertension. Am J Respir Crit Care Med 1999;160:487–92.

154. Tunariu N, Gibbs SJR, Win Z et al. Ventilation-perfusion scintigraphy is more sensitive than multidetector CTPA in detecting chronic thromboembolic pulmonary disease as a treatable cause of pulmonary hypertension. J Nucl Med 2007;48(5):680–4.

155. Au V, Jones D, Slavotinek J. Pulmonary hypertension secondary to left-sided heart disease: a cause for ventilation-perfusion mismatch mimicking pulmonary embolism. Br J Radiol 2001;74:86–8.

156. Chapman PJ, Bateman ED, Benatar SR. Primary pulmonary hypertension and thromboembolic pulmonary hypertension – similarities and differences. Respir Med 1990;84:485–8.

157. D'Alonzo GE, Bower JS, Dantzker DR. Differentiation of patients with primary and thromboembolic pulmonary hypertension. Chest 1984;85(4):457–61.

158. Fishman AJ, Moser KM, Fedullo PF. Perfusion lung scans versus pulmonary angiography in evaluation of suspected primary pulmonary hypertension. Chest 1983;84:679–83.

159. Hull RD, Hirsch J, Carter CJ. Pulmonary angiography, ventilation lung scanning, and venography for clinically suspected pulmonary embolism with abnormal perfusion lung scan. Ann Intern Med 1983;98:891–9.

160. Worsley DF, Palevsky HI, Alavi A. Ventilation-perfusion lung scanning in the evaluation of pulmonary hypertension. J Nucl Med 1994;35:793–6.

161. Rich S, Pietra GG, Kieras K, Hart K, Brundage BH. Primary pulmonary hypertension: radiographic and scintigraphic patterns of histologic subtypes. Ann Intern Med 1986; 105:499–502.

162. Ryan KL, Fedullo PF, Davis GB, Vasquez TE, Moser KM. Perfusion scan findings understate the severity of angiographic and hemodynamic compromise in chronic thromboembolic pulmonary hypertension. Chest 1988; 93:1180–5.

163. Kuriyama K, Gamsu G, Stern RG, Cann CE, Herfkens RJ, Brundage BH. CT-determined pulmonary artery diameters in predicting pulmonary hypertension. Invest Radiol 1984;19:16–22.

164. Heinrich M, Uder M, Tscholl D, Grgic A, Kramann B, Schafers HJ. CT scan findings in chronic thromboembolic pulmonary hypertension. Chest 2005;127:1606–13.

165. Tan RT, Kuzo R, Goodman LR, Siegel R, Haasler GB, Presberg KW. Utility of CT scan evaluation for predicting pulmonary hypertension in patients with parenchymal lung disease. Chest 1998;113:1250–6.

166. Choe KO, Hong YK, Kim HJ et al. The use of high-resolution computed tomography in the evaluation of pulmonary hemodynamics in patients with congenital heart disease: in pulmonary vessels larger than 1 mm in diameter. Pediatr Cardiol 2000;21:202–10.

167. Ng CS, Wells AU, Padley SG. A CT sign of chronic pulmonary arterial hypertension: the ratio of main pulmonary artery to aortic diameter. J Thorac Imag 1999;14:270–8.

168. Baque-Juston MC, Wells AU, Hansell DM. Pericardial thickening or effusion in patients with pulmonary artery hypertension: a CT study. Am J Roentgenol 1999;172: 361–4.

169. King MA, Bergin CJ, Yeung DW et al. Chronic pulmonary thromboembolism: detection of regional hypoperfusion with CT. Radiology 1994;191(2):359–63.

170. Remy-Jardin M, Remy J, Wattinne L, Giraud F. Central pulmonary thromboembolism: diagnosis with spiral volumetric CT with the single breath-hold technique: comparison with pulmonary angiography. Radiology 1992;185:381–7.

171. Teigen CL, Maus TP, Sheedy PF, Johnson CM, Stanson AW, Welch TJ. Pulmonary embolism: diagnosis with electron-beam CT. Radiology 1993;188:839–45.

172. Bergin CJ, Sirlin CB, Hauschildt JP et al. Chronic thromboembolism: diagnosis with helical CT and MR imaging with angiographic and surgical correlation. Radiology 1997;204(3):695–702.

173. Remy-Jardin M, Louvegny S, Remy J et al. Acute central thromboembolic disease: post-therapeutic follow-up with sprial CT angiography. Radiology 1997;203:173–80.

174. Remy-Jardin M, Ramy J. Spiral CT angiography of the pulmonary circulation. Radiology 1999;212:615–36.

175. Reichelt A, Hoeper MM, Galanski M, Keberle M. Chronic thromboembolic pulmonary hypertension: evaluation with 64-detector row CT versus digital substraction angiography. Eur J Radiol 2008;doi:10.1016/j.ejrad.2008.03.016.

176. Bergin C, Sirlin CB, Deutsch R et al. Predictors of patient response to pulmonary thromboendarterectomy. Am J Roentgenol 2000;174:509–15.

177. Oikonomou A, Dennie CJ, Muller NL, Seely JM, Matzinger FR, Ruben FD. Chronic thromboembolic pulmonary arterial hypertension: correlation of postoperative results of thromboendarterectomy with preoperative helical contrast-enhanced computed tomography. J Thorac Imag 2004;19(2):67–73.

178. Chen SJ, Wang JK, Li YW, Chiu IS, Su C, Lue HC. Validation of pulmonary venous obstruction by electron beam computed tomography in children with congenital heart disease. Am J Cardiol 2001;87:589–93.

179. Resten A, Maitre S, Humbert M et al. Pulmonary hypertension: CT of the chest in pulmonary veno-occlusive disease. Am J Roentgenol 2004;183:65–70.

180. Jones AT, Hansell DM, Evans TW. Quantifying pulmonary perfusion in primary pulmonary hypertension using electron-beam computed tomography. Eur Respir J 2004; 23(2):202–7.

181. Zisman DA, Karlamangla AS, Ross DJ et al. High-resolution chest CT findings do not predict the presence of pulmonary hypertension in advanced idiopathic pulmonary fibrosis. Chest 2007;132(3):773–9.

182. Filipek MS, Gosselin MV. Multidetector pulmonary CT angiography: advances in the evaluation of pulmonary arterial diseases. Semin Ultrasound CT, MRI 2004;25: 83–98.

183. Bergin CJ, Rios G, King MA, Belezzuoli E, Luna J, Auger WR. Accuracy of high-resolution CT in identifying chronic pulmonary thromboembolic disease. AJR Am J Roentgenol 1996;166(6):1371–7.

184. Dufour B, Maitre S, Humbert M, Capron F, Simonneau G, Musset D. High-resolution CT of the chest in four patients with pulmonary capillary hemangiomatosis or pulmonary veno-occlusive disease. Am J Radiol 1998;171:1321–4.

185. Ley S, Kauczor H-U. MR Imaging/magnetic resonance angiography of the pulmonary arteries and pulmonary thromboembolic disease. Magnet Resonan Imag Clin North Am 2008;16(2):263–73.

186. Ley S, Kreitner KF, Fink C, Heussel C, Borst M, Kauczor H. Assessment of pulmonary hypertension by CT and MR imaging. Eur Radiol 2004;14(3):359–68.

187. Pedersen MR, Fisher MT, Beek EJRv. MR imaging of the pulmonary vasculature: an update. Eur Radiol 2006; V16(6):1374–86.

188. Boxt LM. MR imaging of pulmonary hypertension and right ventricular dysfunction. Magnet Reson Imag Clin North Am 1996;4(2):307–25.

189. Tandri H, Daya SK, Nasir K et al. Normal reference values for the adult right ventricle by magnetic resonance imaging. The Am J Cardiol 2006;98(12):1660–4.

190. Boxt LM, Katz J, Kolb T, Czegledy FP, Barst RJ. Direct quantitation of right and left ventricular volumes with nuclear magnetic resonance imaging in patients with primary pulmonary hypertension. J Am Coll Cardiol 1992;19(7):1508–15.

191. Blyth KG, Groenning BA, Martin TN et al. Contrast enhanced-cardiovascular magnetic resonance imaging in patients with pulmonary hypertension. Eur Heart J 2005;26(19):1993–9.

192. McCann GP, Gan CT, Beek AM, Niessen HWM, Noordegraaf AV, van Rossum AC. Extent of MRI delayed enhancement of myocardial mass is related to right ventricular dysfunction in pulmonary artery hypertension. Am J Roentgenol 2007; 188(2):349–55.

193. Kuehne T, Yilmaz S, Steendijk P et al. Magnetic resonance imaging analysis of right ventricular pressure–volume loops. Circulation 2004;110:2010–6.

194. Frank H, Globits S, Glogar D, Neuhold A, Kneussl M, Mlczoch J. Detection and quantification of pulmonary artery hypertension with MR imaging: results in 23 patients. Am J Roentgenol 1993;161(1):27–31.

195. Katz J, Whang J, Boxt LM, Barst RJ. Estimation of right ventricular mass in normal subjects and in patients with primary pulmonary hypertension by nuclear magnetic resonance imaging. J Am Coll Cardiol 1993;21:1475–81.

196. Murray TI, Boxt LM, Katz J, Reagan K, Barst RJ. Estimation of pulmonary artery pressure in patients with primary pulmonary hypertension by quantitative analysis of magnetic resonance images. J Thorac Imag 1994;9:198–204.

197. Laffon E, Laurent F, Bernard V, De Boucaud L, Ducassou D, Marthan R. Noninvasive assessment of pulmonary arterial hypertension by MR phase-mapping method. J Appl Physiol 2001;90:2197–202.

198. Ohno Y, Hatabu H, Murase K et al. Primary pulmonary hypertension: 3D dynamic perfusion MRI for quantitative analysis of regional pulmonary perfusion. Am J Roentgenol 2007;188(1):48–56.

199. Roeleveld R, Marcus J, Boonstra A et al. A comparison of noninvasive MRI-based methods of estimating pulmonary artery pressure in pulmonary hypertension. J Magnet Reson Imag 2005;22:67–22.

200. Mousseaux E, Tasu JP, Jolivet O, Simonneau G, Bittoun J, Gaux JC. Pulmonary arterial resistance: noninvasive measurement with indexes of pulmonary flow estimated at velocity-encoded MR imaging: preliminary experience. Radiology 1999;212:896–902.

201. Muthurangu V, Taylor A, Andriantsimiavona R et al. Novel method of quantifying pulmonary vascular resistance by use of simultaneous invasive pressure monitoring and phase-contrast magnetic resonance flow. Circulation 2004;110:826–34.

202. Levin DL, Hatabu H. MR evaluation of pulmonary blood flow. J Thorac Imag 2004;19(4):241–9.

203. Gan CT-J, Lankhaar J-W, Westerhof N et al. Noninvasively assessed pulmonary artery stiffness predicts mortality in pulmonary arterial hypertension. Chest 2007;132(6): 1906–12.

204. Nael K, Michaely HJ, Kramer U et al. Pulmonary circulation: contrast-enhanced 3.0-T MR angiography – initial results. Radiology 2006;240(3):858–68.

205. Hatabu H, Gefter WB, Axel L et al. MR imaging with spatial modulation of magnetization in the evaluation of chronic central pulmonary thromboemboli. Radiology 1994; 190(3):791–6.

206. Wielopolski P. Magnetic resonance pulmonary angiography. Coron Art Dis 1999;10:157–75.

207. Kauczor HU, Kreitner KF. Contrast-enhanced MRI of the lung. Eur J Radiol 2000;34:196–207.

208. Kruger S, Haage P, Hoffmann R et al. Diagnosis of pulmonary arterial hypertension and pulmonary embolism with magnetic resonance angiography. Chest 2001;120: 1556–61.

209. Bergin CJ, Hauschildt J, Rios G, Belezzuoli EV, Huynh TV, Channick RN. Accuracy of MR angiography compared with radionuclide scanning in identifying the cause of pulmonary arterial hypertension. Am J Roentgenol 1997;168:1549–55.

210. Frist WH, Lorenz CH, Walker ES et al. MRI complements standard assessment of right ventricular function after lung transplantation. Ann Thorac Surg 1995;60(2):268–71.

211. Globits S, Burghuber OC, Koller J et al. Effect of lung transplantation on right and left ventricular volumes and function measured by magnetic resonance imaging. Am J Respir Crit Care Med 1994;149(4):1000–4.

212. Moulton MJ, Creswell LL, Ungacta FF, Downing SW, Szabo BA, Pasque MK. Magnetic resonance imaging provides evidence for remodeling of the right ventricle after single lung transplantation for pulmonary hypertension. Circulation 1996;94(9 Suppl):II312–9.

213. Silverman JM, Julien PJ, Herfkens RJ, Pelc NJ. Quantitative differential pulmonary perfusion: MR imaging versus radionuclide lung scanning. Radiology 1993;189(3): 699–701.

214. Nicod P, Peterson KL, Levine M. Pulmonary angiography in severe chronic pulmonary hypertension. Ann Int Med 1987;107:565–8.

215. Hoeper MM, Lee SH, Voswinckel R et al. Complications of right heart catheterization procedures in patients with pulmonary hypertension in experienced centers. J Am Coll Cardiol 2006;48(12):2546–52.

216. Auger WR, Fedullo PF, Moser KM. Chronic major-vessel thromboembolic pulmonary artery obstruction: appearance at angiography. Radiology 1992;182:393–8.

217. Shure D, Gregoratos G, Moser KM. Fiberoptic angioscopy: role in the diagnosis of chronic pulmonary arterial obstruction. Ann Intern Med 1985;103(6):844–50.

218. Auger WR, Channick RN, Kerr KM, Fedullo PF. Evaluation of patients with suspected chronic thromboembolic

pulmonary hypertension. Semin Thorac Cardiovasc Surg 1999;11:179–90.

219. Fedullo PF, Auger WR, Kerr KM, Rubin LJ. Chronic thromboembolic pulmonary hypertension. N Engl J Med 2001;345:1465–72.

220. Moser KM, Auger WR, Fedullo PF. Chronic thromboembolic pulmonary hypertension: clinical picture and surgical treatment. Eur Respir J 1992;5:334–42.

221. Owens GR, Fino GJ, Herbert DL et al. Pulmonary function in progressive systemic sclerosis: comparison of CREST syndrome variant with diffuse scleroderma. Chest 1983; 84:546–50.

222. Steen VD, Graham G, Conte C, Owens GR, Medsger TA. Isolated diffusing capacity reduction in systemic sclerosis. Arthrit Rheumat 1992;35:765–70.

223. Mukerjee D, St. George D, Knight C et al. Echocardiography and pulmonary function as screening tests for pulmonary arterial hypertension in systemic sclerosis. Rheumatology (Oxford) 2004;43(4):461–6.

224. Sun XG, Hansen JE, Oudiz R, Wasserman K. Pulmonary function in primary pulmonary hypertension. J Am Coll Cardiol 2003;41(6):1027–35.

225. Rafanan AL, Golish JA, Dinner DS, Hague LK, Arroliga AC. Nocturnal hypoxemia is common in primary pulmonary hypertension. Chest 2001;120:894–9.

226. Guyatt GH, Sullivan MJ, Thompson PJ et al. The 6-minute walk: a new measure of exercise capacity in patients with chronic heart failure. Can Med Ass J 1985; 132:91923.

227. Barst RJ, Rubin LJ, Long WA et al. A comparison of continuous intravenous epoprostenol (prostacyclin) with conventional therapy for primary pulmonary hypertension. New Eng J Med 1996;334(5):296–301.

228. Miyamoto S, Nagaya N, Satoh T et al. Clinical correlates and prognostic significance of six-minute walk test in patients with primary pulmonary hypertension: comparison with cardiopulmonary exercise testing. Am J Respir Crit Care Med 2000;161:487–92.

229. Paciocco G, Martinez F, Bossone E, Pielsticker E, Gillespie B, Rubenfire M. Oxygen desaturation on the six-minute walk test and mortality in untreated primary pulmonary hypertension. Eur Respir J 2001;17:647–52.

230. Riley MS, Porszasz J, Engelen MJ, Shapiro SM, Brundage BH, Wasserman K. Responses to constant work rate bicycle ergometry exercise in primary pulmonary hypertension: the effect of inhaled nitric oxide. J Am Coll Cardiol 2000; 36:547–56.

231. Sun XG, Hansen JE, Oudiz RJ, Wasserman K. Exercise pathophysiology in patients with primary pulmonary hypertension. Circulation 2001;104:429–35.

232. Garofano RP, Barst RJ. Exercise testing in children with primary pulmonary hypertension. Pediatr Cardiol 1999; 20:61–4.

233. Yasunobu Y, Oudiz R, Sun XG, Hansen JE, Wasserman K. End-tidal PCO_2 abnormality and exercise limitation in patients with primary pulmonary hypertension. Chest 2005;127(5):1637–46.

234. Yetman A, Taylor A, Doran A, Ivy D. Utility of cardiopulmonary stress testing in assessing disease severity in children with pulmonary arterial hypertension. Am J Cardiol 2005; 95:697–9.

235. Wensel R, Opitz CF, Anker SD et al. Assessment of survival in patients with primary pulmonary hypertension: importance of cardiopulmonary exercise testing. Circulation 2002;106:319–24.

236. Iwase T, Nagaya N, Ando M et al. Acute and chronic effects of surgical thromboendarterectomy on exercise capacity and ventilatory efficiency in patients with chronic thromboembolic pulmonary hypertension. Heart 2001; 86:188–92.

237. Oudiz R, Barst R, Hansen JE et al. Cardiopulmonary exercise testing and six-minute walk correlations in pulmonary arterial hypertension. Am J Cardiol 2006; 997:123–6.

238. Frantz RP, Benza RL, Kjellstrom B et al. Continuous hemodynamic monitoring in patients with pulmonary arterial hypertension. J Heart Lung Transplant 2008; 27(7):780–8.

239. James KB, Maurer J, Wolski K et al. Exercise hemodynamic findings in patients with exertional dyspnea. Texas Heart Inst J 2000;27:100–5.

240. Raeside DA, Chalmers G, Clelland J, Madhok R, Peacock AJ. Pulmonary artery pressure variation in patients with connective tissue disease: 24 hour ambulatory pulmonary artery pressure monitoring. Thorax 1998;53:857–62.

241. Raeside DA, Smith AL, Brown A et al. Pulmonary artery pressure measurement during exercise testing in patients with suspect pulmonary hypertension. Eur Respir J 2000; 16:282–7.

242. Bach DS. Stress echocardiography for evaluation of hemodynamics: valvular heart disease, prosthetic valve function, and pulmonary hypertension. Prog Cardiovasc Dis 1997;39(6):543–54.

243. Himelman RB, Stulbarg MS, Lee E. Noninvasive evaluation of pulmonary artery systolic pressure during dynamic exercise by saline enhanced Doppler echocardiography: serial studies in a patient with severe pulmonary hypertension. Am Heart J 1990;119:685–8.

244. Kuecherer HF, Will M, da Silva KG. Contrast enhanced Doppler ultrasound for noninvasive assessment of pulmonary artery pressure during exercise in patients with congestive heart failure. Am J Cardiol 1996;78:229–32.

245. Bidart CM, Abbas AE, Parish JM, Chaliki HP, Moreno CA, Lester SJ. The noninvasive evaluation of exercise-induced changes in pulmonary artery pressure and pulmonary vascular resistance. J Am Soc Echocardiogr 2007; 20(3):270–5.

246. Steen V, Chou M, Shanmugam V, Mathias M, Kuru T, Morrissey R. Exercise-induced pulmonary arterial hypertension in patients with systemic sclerosis. Chest 2008;134(1):146–51.

247. Tolle JJ, Waxman AB, Van Horn TL, Pappagianopoulos PP, Systrom DM. Exercise-induced pulmonary arterial hypertension. Circulation 2008;118(21):2183–9.

248. Hoeper MM, Maier R, Tongers J *et al.* Determination of cardiac output by the Fick method, thermodilution, and acetylene rebreathing in pulmonary hypertension. Am J Respir Crit Care Med 1999;160:535–41.

249. McGregor M, Sniderman A. On pulmonary resistance: the need for more precise definition. Am J Cardiol 1985; 55:217–21.

250. Burton AC. On the physical equilibrium of small blood vessels. Am J Physiol 1951;164:319–29.

251. Simonneau G, Herve P, Petitpretz P *et al.* Detection of a reversible component in primary pulmonary hypertension: value of prostacyclin infusion (abstr). Ann Rev Respir Dis 1986;133:223.

252. Galie N, Ussia G, Passarelli P, Parlangeli R, Branzi A, Magnani B. Role of pharmacologic tests in the treatment of primary pulmonary hypertension. Am J Cardiol 1995; 75:55A–62A.

253. Okada O, Tanabe N, Yasuda Y, Katoh K, Yanamoto T, Kuriyama T. Prediction of life expectancy in patients with primary pulmonary hypertension. A retrospective nationwide survey from 1980–1990. Intern Med 1999;38:12–6.

254. Groves BM, Rubin LJ, Frosolono MF, Cato AE, Reeves JT. A comparison of the acute hemodynamic effects of prostacyclin and hydralazine in primary pulmonary hypertension. Am Heart J 1985;110:1200–4.

255. Morgan MJ, McCormack DG, Griffiths MD, Morgan CJ, Barnes PJ, Evans TW. Adenosine as a vasodilator in primary pulmonary hypertension. Circulation 1991;84:1145–9.

256. Nootens M, Schrader BJ, Kaufmann E, Vestal RE, Long WA, Rich S. Comparative acute effects of adenosine and prostacyclin in primary pulmonary hypertension. Chest 1995;107:54–7.

257. Palevsky HI, Long WA, Crow JW, Fishman AP. Prostacyclin and acetylcholine as screening agents for acute pulmonary vasodilator responsiveness in primary pulmonary hypertension. Circulation 1990;82:2018–26.

258. Shapiro SM, Oudiz RJ, Cao T *et al.* Primary pulmonary hypertension: improved long-term effects and survival with continuous intravenous epoprostenol infusion. J Am Coll Cardiol 1997;30:343–9.

259. Sitbon O, Brenot F, Denjean A *et al.* Inhaled nitric oxide as a screening vasodilator agent in primary pulmonary hypertension: a dose–response study and comparison with prostacyclin. Am J Respir Crit Care Med 1995; 151:384–9.

260. Barst RJ. Pharmacologically induced pulmonary vasodilatation in children and young adults with primary pulmonary hypertension. Chest 1986;89(4):497–503.

261. Jones DK, Higenbottam TW, Wallwork J. Treatment of primary pulmonary hypertension with intravenous epoprostenol (prostacyclin). Br Heart J 1987;57:270–8.

262. Rubin LJ, Groves BM, Reeves JT, Frosolono MF, Handel F, Cato AE. Prostacyclin-induced acute pulmonary vasodilation in primary pulmonary hypertension. Circulation 1982;66(2):334–8.

263. Weir EK, Rubin LJ, Ayres SM, *et al.* The acute administration of vasodilators in primary pulmonary hypertension: experience from the National Institutes of Health Registry on Primary Pulmonary Hypertension. Am Rev Respir Dis 1989;140:1623–30.

264. Pepke-Zaba J, Higenbottam TW, Dinh'Xuan AT, Stone D, Wallwork J. Inhaled nitric oxide as a cause of selective pulmonary vasodilation in pulmonary hypertension. Lancet 1991;338:1173–4.

265. Inbar S, Schrader BJ, Kaufmann E, Vestal RE, Rich S. Effects of adenosine in combination with calcium channel blockers in patients with primary pulmonary hypertension. J Am Coll Cardiol 1993;21(2):413–8.

266. Mehta S, Stewart DJ, Langleben D, Levy RD. Short-term pulmonary vasodilation with L-arginine in pulmonary hypertension. Circulation 1995;92:1539–45.

267. McLaughlin VV, Genthner DE, Panella MM, Rich S. Reduction in pulmonary vascular resistance with long-term epoprostenol (prostacyclin) therapy in primary pulmonary hypertension. N Engl J Med 1998; 338:273–7.

268. Palmer SM, Robinson LJ, Wang A, Gossage JR, Bashore TM, Tapson VF. Massive pulmonary edema and death after prostacyclin infusion in a patient with pulmonary veno-occlusive disease. Chest 1998;113:237–40.

269. Nicod P, Moser KM. Primary pulmonary hypertension: risk and benefit of lung biopsy. Circulation 1989;80: 1486–8.

270. Moser KM, Bloor CM. Pulmonary vascular lesions occurring in patients with chronic major vessel thromboembolic pulmonary hypertension. Chest 1993;103:685–92.

271. McLaughlin VV, Archer SL, Badesch DB *et al.* ACCF/AHA Clinical Expert Consensus Document on Pulmonary Hypertension: a Report of the American College of Cardiology Foundation Task Force on Clinical Expert Consensus Documents. J Am Coll Cardiol 2009; In Press.

272. McGoon MD. The assessment of pulmonary hypertension. Clin Chest Med 2001;22:493–508.

273. Moder KG. Use and interpretation of rheumatologic tests: a guide for clinicians. Mayo Clin Proc 1996;71:391–6.

PART 4

DISORDERS ASSOCIATED WITH PULMONARY HYPERTENSION

14

Updated clinical classification of pulmonary hypertension

DAVID MONTANI AND GERALD SIMONNEAU

INTRODUCTION

The classification of pulmonary hypertension (PH) has gone through a series of changes since the first classification proposed in 1973 which designated only two categories, PPH or secondary pulmonary hypertension, depending on the presence or absence of identifiable causes or risk factors (1,2). In 1998, a second World Symposium on Pulmonary Arterial Hypertension was held in Evian (France) and this classification attempted to create categories of PH that shared similar pathogenesis, clinical features and therapeutic options (3). This classification allowed us to define homogenous groups of patients to conduct clinical trials and to obtain approval for specific PAH therapies worldwide. In 2003, the third World Symposium on Pulmonary Arterial Hypertension (Venice, Italy) did not propose major changes, except the introduction of the terms idiopathic PAH, familial PAH, or associated PAH (Table 14.1). In recent years, it has become clear that these three groups share broadly similar physiopathology and response to therapy. The other prominent change was to move pulmonary veno-occlusive disease (PVOD) and pulmonary capillary hemangiomatosis (PCH) from separate categories into a single subcategory of PAH. These two entities have many similarities with idiopathic PAH, including clinical presentation, hemodynamic characteristics and risk factors, that justified placing them together in Group 1 (Table 14.1).

In 2008, the fourth World Symposium on PH held in Dana Point (California, USA) and the consensus of an international group of experts was to revise previous classifications in order to accurately reflect information published over the past 5 years, as well as to clarify some areas that were unclear. The current Dana Point classification is presented in Table 14.2.

GROUP 1: PULMONARY ARTERIAL HYPERTENSION

The nomenclature of the subgroups and associated conditions has evolved since the first classification, and additional modifications were added in this revised classification.

Group 1.1/1.2: Idiopathic and heritable PAH

Idiopathic PAH corresponds to sporadic disease in which there is neither a family history of PAH nor an identified risk factor. When PAH occurs in a familial context, germline mutations in the bone morphogenetic protein receptor 2 (*BMPR2*) gene, a member of the transforming growth factor beta (TGF-β) signaling family, can be detected in about 70 percent of cases (4,5). For more details, see refs 6–13.

Table 14.1 Venice Clinical Classification of Pulmonary Hypertension (2003)

1. Pulmonary arterial hypertension (PAH)
    1.1. Idiopathic (idiopathic PAH)
    1.2. Familial (FPAH)
    1.3. Associated with (APAH):
        1.3.1. Collagen vascular disease
        1.3.2. Congenital systemic-to-pulmonary shunts
        1.3.3. Portal hypertension
        1.3.4. HIV infection
        1.3.5. Drugs and toxins
        1.3.6. Other (thyroid disorders, glycogen storage disease, Gaucher disease, hereditary hemorrhagic telangiectasia, hemoglobinopathies, myeloproliferative disorders, splenectomy)
    1.4. Associated with significant venous or capillary involvement
        1.4.1. Pulmonary veno-occlusive disease (PVOD)
        1.4.2. Pulmonary capillary hemangiomatosis (PCH)
    1.5. Persistent pulmonary hypertension of the newborn
2. Pulmonary hypertension with left heart disease
    2.1. Left-sided atrial or ventricular heart disease
    2.2. Left-sided valvular heart disease
3. Pulmonary hypertension associated with lung diseases and/or hypoxemia
    3.1. Chronic obstructive pulmonary disease
    3.2. Interstitial lung disease
    3.3. Sleep-disordered breathing
    3.4. Alveolar hypoventilation disorders
    3.5. Chronic exposure to high altitude
    3.6. Developmental abnormalities
4. Pulmonary hypertension due to chronic thrombotic and/or embolic disease
    4.1. Thromboembolic obstruction of proximal pulmonary arteries
    4.2. Thromboembolic obstruction of distal pulmonary arteries
    4.3. Nonthrombotic pulmonary embolism (tumor, parasites, foreign material)
5. Miscellaneous
Sarcoidosis, histiocytosis X, lymphangiomatosis, compression of pulmonary vessels (adenopathy, tumor, fibrosing mediastinitis)

Table 14.2 Updated Clinical Classification of Pulmonary Hypertension (Dana Point, 2008)

1. Pulmonary arterial hypertension
    1.1. Idiopathic PAH
    1.2. **Heritable**
        1.2.1. **BMPR2**
        1.2.2. **ALK1, endoglin (with or without hereditary hemorrhagic telangiectasia)**
        1.2.3. **Unknown**
    1.3. Drug- and toxin-induced
    1.4. Associated with
        1.4.1. Connective tissue diseases
        1.4.2. HIV infection
        1.4.3. Portal hypertension
        1.4.4. Congenital heart diseases
        1.4.5. **Schistosomiasis**
        1.4.6. **Chronic hemolytic anemia**
    1.5. Persistent pulmonary hypertension of the newborn
1'. **Pulmonary veno-occlusive disease (PVOD) and/or pulmonary capillary hemangiomatosis (PCH)**
2. Pulmonary hypertension due to left heart disease
    2.1. **Systolic dysfunction**
    2.2. **Diastolic dysfunction**
    2.3. Valvular disease
3. Pulmonary hypertension due to lung diseases and/or hypoxia
    3.1. Chronic obstructive pulmonary disease
    3.2. Interstitial lung disease
    3.3. **Other pulmonary diseases with mixed restrictive and obstructive pattern**
    3.4. Sleep-disordered breathing
    3.5. Alveolar hypoventilation disorders
    3.6. Chronic exposure to high altitude
    3.7. Developmental abnormalities
4. **Chronic thromboembolic pulmonary hypertension (CTEPH)**
5. **PH with unclear multifactorial mechanisms**
    5.1. **Hematologic disorders: myeloproliferative disorders splenectomy**
    5.2. **Systemic disorders, sarcoidosis, pulmonary Langerhans cell histiocytosis,** lymphangioleiomyomatosis, neurofibromatosis, vasculitis
    5.3. **Metabolic disorders: glycogen storage disease, Gaucher disease, thyroid disorders**
    5.4. **Others: tumoral obstruction, fibrosing mediastinitis, chronic renal failure on dialysis.**

Main modifications to the previous Venice classification are set in bold in table body.

Group 1.3: Drug- and toxin-induced PAH

A number of risk factors for the development of PAH have been included in the previous classifications (3,14). In the current classification, the categorization of risk factors and the likelihood of developing PAH have been modified (Table 14.3). For more details, see refs 15–18.

Group 1.4.1: PAH associated with connective tissue diseases

PAH associated with connective tissue diseases represents an important clinical subgroup. The prevalence of PAH has been well established only for systemic sclerosis. Two recent prospective studies using echocardiography as a screening method and right-heart catheterization for confirmation found a prevalence of PAH of between 7 and 12 percent (19,20). For more details, see refs 21–30.

Group 1.4.2: HIV infection

PAH is a rare but well-established complication of HIV infection (31,32). See also refs 33–37.

Table 14.3   Updated risk factors and associated conditions for PAH

Definite	Possible
Aminorex	Cocaine
Fenfluramine	Phenylpropanolamine
Dexfenfluramine	St. John's Wort
Toxic rapeseed oil	Chemotherapeutic agents
	SSRI
Likely	**Unlikely**
Amphetamines	Oral contraceptives
L-tryptophan	Estrogen
Methamphetamines	Cigarette smoking

Group 1.4.3: Portopulmonary hypertension

Portopulmonary hypertension (POPH) is defined by the development of PAH associated with increased pressure in the portal circulation (38,39). See also refs 40–43.

Group 1.4.4: Congenital heart diseases

A significant proportion of patients with congenital heart disease, in particular those with systemic-to-pulmonary shunts, will develop PAH if left untreated. Eisenmenger's syndrome is defined as congenital heart disease with an initial large systemic-to-pulmonary shunt that induces progressive pulmonary vascular disease and PAH, with resultant reversal of the shunt and central cyanosis (44,45). See also Tables 14.4 and 14.5, and refs 46–48.

Group 1.4.5: Schistosomiasis

In the new classification, PH associated with schistosomiasis was included in Group 1, even though it was subcategorized in Group 4 as PH due to chronic embolic disease in the previous classification. For more details, see refs 49–53.

Group 1.4.6: Chronic hemolytic anemia

The chronic hemolytic anemias represent a new subcategory of PAH previously subcategorized under "other condition" associated with PAH. There has been increasing evidence that PAH is a complication of chronic hereditary and acquired hemolytic anemias, including sickle cell disease (54,55), thalassemia (56), hereditary spherocytosis (57), stomatocytosis (58), and microangiopathic hemolytic anemia (59). For more details, see refs 60–64.

GROUP 1′: PULMONARY VENO-OCCLUSIVE DISEASE AND/OR PULMONARY CAPILLARY HEMANGIOMATOSIS

PVOD and PCH are uncommon conditions, but they are increasingly recognized as causes of PH (65). In the Evian

Table 14.4   Anatomic-pathophysiologic classification of congenital systemic-to-pulmonary shunts associated with pulmonary arterial hypertension (Modified from Venice 2003)

1. **Type**
   1.1. **Simple pre-tricuspid shunts**
      1.1.1. Atrial septal defect (ASD)
         1.1.1.1. Ostium secundum
         1.1.1.2. Sinus venosus
         1.1.1.3. Ostium primum
      1.1.2. Total or partial unobstructed anomalous pulmonary venous return
   1.2. **Simple post-tricuspid shunts**
      1.2.1. Ventricular septal defect (VSD)
      1.2.2. Patent ductus arteriosus
   1.3. **Combined shunts**
      Describe combination and define predominant defect
   1.4. **Complex CHD**
      1.4.1. Complete atrioventricular septal defect
      1.4.2. Truncus arteriosus
      1.4.3. Single ventricle physiology with unobstructed pulmonary blood flow
      1.4.4. Transposition of the great arteries with VSD (without pulmonary stenosis) and/or patent ductus arteriosus
      1.4.5. Other
2. **Dimension** (specify for each defect if more than one congenital heart defect)
   2.1. **Hemodynamic (specify Qp/Qs)***
      2.1.1. Restrictive (pressure gradient across the defect)
      2.1.2. Nonrestrictive
   2.2. **Anatomic**
      2.2.1. Small to moderate (ASD $\leq$ 2.0 cm and VSD $\leq$ 1.0 cm)
      2.2.2. Large (ASD $>$ 2.0 cm and VSD $>$ 1.0 cm)
3. **Direction of shunt**
   3.1. Predominantly systemic-to-pulmonary
   3.2. Predominantly pulmonary-to-systemic
   3.3. Bidirectional
4. **Associated cardiac and extracardiac abnormalities**
5. **Repair status**
   5.1. Unoperated
   5.2. Palliated (specify type of operation/s, age at surgery)
   5.3. Repaired (specify type of operation/s, age at surgery)

*Ratio of pulmonary (Qp) to systemic (Qs) blood flow.

classification, these two entities were placed in two different groups, both distinct from PAH (Table 14.1). Similarities in pathologic features and clinical presentation suggest that these disorders may overlap (66); thus, PVOD and PCH were included in the same subgroup of PAH. The decision to leave PVOD and PCH in the same subgroup is supported by a recent clinicopathologic study (66) analyzing specimens from 35 patients diagnosed as having either PVOD (n = 30) or PCH (n = 5). PCH was identified in 24 (73 percent) of cases diagnosed as PVOD. Indeed, venous involvement was present in 4/5 cases initially diagnosed as PCH. These findings suggest that PCH may be an angioproliferative process frequently associated with PVOD.

Table 14.5 Clinical classification of congenital systemic-to-pulmonary shunts associated to pulmonary arterial hypertension (PAH)

(A) Eisenmenger syndrome

Includes all systemic-to-pulmonary shunts resulting from large defects and leading to a severe increase in pulmonary vascular resistance (PVR) and a reversed (pulmonary-to-systemic) or bidirectional shunt. Cyanosis, erythrocytosis, and multiple organ involvement are present.

(B) Pulmonary arterial hypertension associated with systemic-to-pulmonary shunts

Includes moderate to large defects. PVR is mildly to moderately increased, systemic-to-pulmonary shunt is still prevalent, and no cyanosis is present at rest.

(C) Pulmonary arterial hypertension with small defects

Small defects (usually ventricular septal defects < 1 cm and atrial septal defect < 2 cm of effective diameter assessed by echocardiography). The clinical picture is very similar to idiopathic PAH.

(D) Pulmonary arterial hypertension after corrective cardiac surgery

Congenital heart disease has been corrected, but PAH is still present immediately after surgery or recurs several months or years after surgery in the absence of significant postoperative residual lesions.

PVOD and PCH were included in Group 1 because the two entities share a number of characteristics with idiopathic PAH. First, some histologic changes in the small pulmonary arteries (intimal fibrosis and medial hypertrophy) observed in PAH were also found in PVOD/PCH. Second, the clinical presentations and hemodynamics of PVOD/PCH and PAH are often indistinguishable (14,65,67). Third, PVOD/PCH and PAH share similar risk factors, including the scleroderma spectrum of disease (68), HIV infection (69,70), and the use of anorexigens (65). Lastly, familial occurrence has been reported with both PVOD and PCH, and mutations in the *BMPR2* gene have been documented in patients with PVOD (67,71). These findings suggest that PVOD, PCH, and PAH may represent different components of a single spectrum of disease.

Although PVOD and PCH may present similarly to idiopathic PAH, there are a number of important differences. These include the presence of crackles on examination, radiologic abnormalities on high-resolution computed tomography of the chest (ground glass opacities, septal thickening, mediastinal adenopathy) (67,72–74), hemosiderin-laden macrophages on bronchoalveolar lavage (75), and a lower DLCO and PaO_2 in patients with PVOD or PCH (67). In addition, the response to medical therapy and prognosis of PVOD/PCH are quite different from PAH. A recent study compared 24 patients with histologic evidence of PVOD with or without PCH and 24 randomly selected patients with idiopathic, familial, or anorexigen-associated PAH (65). Among the 16 PVOD patients who received

PAH-specific therapy, seven (43.8 percent) developed pulmonary edema. These patients were treated mainly with continuous intravenous epoprostenol, but also with oral therapies, bosentan, and calcium-channel blockers and clinical outcomes were worse in PVOD patients than in idiopathic PAH patients.

PVOD/PCH remains a difficult disorder to categorize, as it shares characteristics with idiopathic PAH, but also has a number of distinct differences. Given the current evidence, it was decided that PVOD/PCH should be a distinct category but not completely separated from PAH and PVOD/PCH are designated as 1′ in the current classification.

GROUP 2: PULMONARY HYPERTENSION DUE TO LEFT HEART DISEASE

Left-sided ventricular or valvular diseases may produce an increase of left atrial pressure, leading to a backward transmission of the pressure and a passive increase of pulmonary arterial pressure. Left heart disease, probably represents the most frequent cause of PH (76). In this situation, PVR is normal or near normal (< 3.0 Wood units) and there is no gradient between mean PAP and pulmonary wedge pressure (transpulmonary gradient < 12 mmHg). In the previous classification, these entities were divided in two subgroups based on the presence or absence of valvular disease. In the recent classification, the increasing recognition of left-sided heart dysfunction with preserved ejection fraction leads to changes in the subcategories of Group 2 and now this group includes three distinct etiologies: left heart systolic dysfunction, left heart diastolic dysfunction, and left heart valvular disease. In some patients with left heart disease, the elevation of pulmonary arterial pressure is out of proportion to that expected from the elevation of left arterial pressure (transpulmonary gradient > 12 mmHg), and PVR is increased to > 3.0 Wood units (19–35 percent of patients) (76). Some patients with left heart valvular disease or even left heart dysfunction can develop severe PH of the same magnitude as that seen in PAH (77–79). The elevation of PAP and PVR may be due to either the increase of pulmonary artery vasomotor tone and/or pulmonary vascular remodeling (80,81). No studies using medications approved for PAH have been performed in this patient population, and the efficacy and safety of PAH medications remain unknown.

GROUP 3: PULMONARY HYPERTENSION DUE TO LUNG DISEASES AND/OR HYPOXIA

In this group, the predominant cause of PH is alveolar hypoxia as a result of either chronic lung disease, impaired control of breathing, or residence at high altitude; however, the precise prevalence of PH in all these conditions remains largely unknown. In the revised classification, the heading has been modified to reinforce the link with the development of PH. A category of lung disease characterized by a mixed obstructive and restrictive pattern was added, including chronic bronchiectasis, cystic fibrosis and the recently described syndrome of combined pulmonary fibrosis and emphysema in which the prevalence of PH is almost 50 percent (82,83). In PAH associated with parenchymal lung disease, the increase of pulmonary arterial pressure is usually modest (mean PAP lower than 35 mmHg) (84). Interestingly, in some patients, increase of pulmonary arterial pressure is out of proportion and can be higher than 35 mmHg (85). In a retrospective study of 998 patients with chronic obstructive pulmonary disease who underwent right-heart catheterization, only 1 percent had severe PH (86). These patients with more severe PH were characterized by mild-to-moderate airway obstruction, severe hypoxemia, hypocapnia, and a very low diffusing capacity for carbon monoxide. Large control randomized studies of specific PAH therapies are not available for PH "out of proportion" associated with parenchyma lung disease.

GROUP 4: CHRONIC THROMBOEMBOLIC PULMONARY HYPERTENSION

In the Venice classification, Group 4 was heterogeneous including obstruction of pulmonary arterial vessels by thromboemboli, tumors or foreign bodies. However, depending on the origin of the obstruction, the clinical and radiologic findings are different, and management is unique to each etiology. Even if the incidence of chronic thromboembolic pulmonary hypertension (CTEPH) is uncertain, CTEPH represents a frequent cause of PH and occurs in up to 4 percent of patients after an acute pulmonary embolism (87,88). In contrast, other etiologies of "obstructive PH" are very rare. Therefore, in the new classification, only CTEPH was included in Group 4. In the previous classification, CTEPH was divided into two subgroups: proximal CTEPH and distal CTEPH, depending on the feasibility of performing pulmonary thromboendarterectomy. Currently, there is no consensus about the definitions of proximal and distal CTEPH and the decision of surgery may vary depending on individual centers (89). Thus, in the new classification, it was decided to maintain in Group 4 only a single category of CTEPH without distinction between proximal and distal forms. However, patients with suspected or confirmed CTEPH need to be referred to a center with expertise in the management of CTEPH, to consider the feasibility of performing surgery, which depends on the location of the obstruction, the correlation between hemodynamic findings and the degree of mechanical obstruction assessed by angiography, comorbidities, the willingness of the patient, and the experience of the surgeon (90,91). Patients who are not candidates for surgery may benefit from PAH-specific medical therapy (27,92); however, further evaluation of these therapies in randomized control trials are needed (93).

GROUP 5: PH WITH UNCLEAR OR MULTIFACTORIAL ETIOLOGIES

Group 5 is divided into:

- **Group 5.1: Hematologic disorders** (95–100).
- **Group 5.2: Systemic disorders** (101–115). The second subgroup includes systemic disorders, including sarcoidosis, pulmonary Langerhans cell histiocytosis, lymphangioleiomyomatosis, neurofibromatosis or vasculitis. See refs 101–115 for more details.
- **Group 5.3: Metabolic disorders** (116–127).
- **Group 5.4: Miscellaneous conditions** (128–137). The last subgroup includes a number of miscellaneous conditions, including tumoral obstruction, fibrosing mediastinitis, chronic renal failure on dialysis.

KEY POINTS

- In this updated classification of PH, recent findings were incorporated to clarify areas of ambiguity.
- The major modifications adopted principally concern Group 1, pulmonary arterial hypertension in order to define a more homogeneous group.
- The subgroup pulmonary arterial hypertension introduces the term of "heritable PAH" for patients with a family history or idiopathic PAH patients with germline mutations (e.g., *BMPR2*, *ACVRL1* or *endoglin*).
- In the new classification, schistosomiasis and chronic hemolytic anemia appear as separate entities in the subgroup of PAH associated with identified conditions.
- It was decided to place pulmonary veno-occlusive disease and pulmonary capillary hemoangiomatosis in a separate group, distinct from but very close to Group 1 (now called Group 1′).

REFERENCES

1. Hatano S, Strasser T. Primary Pulmonary Hypertension. Report on a WHO meeting. October 15–17, 1973, Geneva: WHO, 1975.
2. Wagenvoort CA, Wagenvoort N. Primary pulmonary hypertension: a pathological study of the lung vessels in 156 clinically diagnosed cases. Circulation 1970;42: 1163–84.
3. Fishman AP. Clinical classification of pulmonary hypertension. Clin Chest Med 2001;22:385–91, vii.
4. Cogan JD, Pauciulo MW, Batchman AP, Prince MA, Robbins IM, Hedges LK, Stanton KC, Wheeler LA, Phillips JA, 3rd, Loyd JE, Nichols WC. High frequency of BMPR2 exonic deletions/duplications in familial

pulmonary arterial hypertension. Am J Respir Crit Care Med 2006;174:590–8.

5. Aldred MA, Vijayakrishnan J, James V, Soubrier F, Gomez-Sanchez MA, Martensson G, Galie N, Manes A, Corris P, Simonneau G, Humbert M, Morrell NW, Trembath RC. BMPR2 gene rearrangements account for a significant proportion of mutations in familial and idiopathic pulmonary arterial hypertension. Hum Mutat 2006; 27:212–3.

6. Sztrymf B, Coulet F, Girerd B, Yaici A, Jais X, Sitbon O, Montani D, Souza R, Simonneau G, Soubrier F, Humbert M. Clinical outcomes of pulmonary arterial hypertension in carriers of BMPR2 mutation. Am J Respir Crit Care Med 2008;177:1377–83.

7. Elliott CG, Glissmeyer EW, Havlena GT, Carlquist J, McKinney JT, Rich S, McGoon MD, Scholand MB, Kim M, Jensen RL, Schmidt JW, Ward K. Relationship of BMPR2 mutations to vasoreactivity in pulmonary arterial hypertension. Circulation 2006;113:2509–15.

8. Rosenzweig EB, Morse JH, Knowles JA, Chada KK, Khan AM, Roberts KE, McElroy JJ, Juskiw NK, Mallory NC, Rich S, Diamond B, Barst RJ. Clinical implications of determining BMPR2 mutation status in a large cohort of children and adults with pulmonary arterial hypertension. J Heart Lung Transplant 2008;27:668–74.

9. Machado RD, Aldred MA, James V, Harrison RE, Patel B, Schwalbe EC, Gruenig E, Janssen B, Koehler R, Seeger W, Eickelberg O, Olschewski H, Elliott CG, Glissmeyer E, Carlquist J, Kim M, Torbicki A, Fijalkowska A, Szewczyk G, Parma J, Abramowicz MJ, Galie N, Morisaki H, Kyotani S, Nakanishi N, Morisaki T, Humbert M, Simonneau G, Sitbon O, Soubrier F, Coulet F, Morrell NW, Trembath RC. Mutations of the TGF-beta type II receptor BMPR2 in pulmonary arterial hypertension. Hum Mutat 2006;27: 121–32.

10. Thomson JR, Machado RD, Pauciulo MW, Morgan NV, Humbert M, Elliott GC, Ward K, Yacoub M, Mikhail G, Rogers P, Newman J, Wheeler L, Higenbottam T, Gibbs JSR, Egan J, Crozier A, Peacock A, Allcock R, Corris P, Loyd JE, Trembath RC, Nichols WC. Sporadic primary pulmonary hypertension is associated with germline mutations of the gene encoding BMPR-II, a receptor member of the TGF-ß family. J Med Genet 2000;37:741–5.

11. Chaouat A, Coulet F, Favre C, Simonneau G, Weitzenblum E, Soubrier F, Humbert M. Endoglin germline mutation in a patient with hereditary haemorrhagic telangiectasia and dexfenfluramine associated pulmonary arterial hypertension. Thorax 2004;59:446–8.

12. Trembath RC, Thomson JR, Machado RD, Morgan NV, Atkinson C, Winship I, Simonneau G, Galie N, Loyd JE, Humbert M, Nichols WC, Morrell NW, Berg J, Manes A, McGaughran J, Pauciulo M, Wheeler L. Clinical and molecular genetic features of pulmonary hypertension in patients with hereditary hemorrhagic telangiectasia. N Engl J Med 2001;345:325–34.

13. McGoon M, Gutterman D, Steen V, Barst R, McCrory DC, Fortin TA, Loyd JE. Screening, early detection, and diagnosis

of pulmonary arterial hypertension: ACCP Evidence-Based Clinical Practice Guidelines. Chest 2004;126:14S–34.

14. Simonneau G, Galie N, Rubin LJ, Langleben D, Seeger W, Domenighetti G, Gibbs S, Lebrec D, Speich R, Beghetti M, Rich S, Fishman A. Clinical classification of pulmonary hypertension. J Am Coll Cardiol 2004;43:5S–12S.

15. Souza R, Humbert M, Sztrymf B, Jais X, Yaici A, Le Pavec J, Parent F, Herve P, Soubrier F, Sitbon O, Simonneau G. Pulmonary arterial hypertension associated with fenfluramine exposure: report of 109 cases. Eur Respir J 2008;31:343–8.

16. Walker AM, Langleben D, Korelitz JJ, Rich S, Rubin LJ, Strom BL, Gonin R, Keast S, Badesch D, Barst RJ, Bourge RC, Channick R, Frost A, Gaine S, McGoon M, McLaughlin V, Murali S, Oudiz RJ, Robbins IM, Tapson V, Abenhaim L, Constantine G. Temporal trends and drug exposures in pulmonary hypertension: an American experience. Am Heart J 2006;152:521–6.

17. Chambers CD, Hernandez-Diaz S, Van Marter LJ, Werler MM, Louik C, Jones KL, Mitchell AA. Selective serotonin-reuptake inhibitors and risk of persistent pulmonary hypertension of the newborn. N Engl J Med 2006;354:579–87.

18. Chin KM, Channick RN, Rubin LJ. Is methamphetamine use associated with idiopathic pulmonary arterial hypertension? Chest 2006;130:1657–63.

19. Hachulla E, Gressin V, Guillevin L, Carpentier P, Diot E, Sibilia J, Kahan A, Cabane J, Frances C, Launay D, Mouthon L, Allanore Y, Tiev KP, Clerson P, de Groote P, Humbert M. Early detection of pulmonary arterial hypertension in systemic sclerosis: a French nationwide prospective multicenter study. Arthritis Rheum 2005;52:3792–800.

20. Mukerjee D, St George D, Coleiro B, Knight C, Denton CP, Davar J, Black CM, Coghlan JG. Prevalence and outcome in systemic sclerosis associated pulmonary arterial hypertension: application of a registry approach. Ann Rheum Dis 2003;62: 1088–93.

21. Launay D, Mouthon L, Hachulla E, Pagnoux C, de Groote P, Remy-Jardin M, Matran R, Lambert M, Queyrel V, Morell-Dubois S, Guillevin L, Hatron PY. Prevalence and characteristics of moderate to severe pulmonary hypertension in systemic sclerosis with and without interstitial lung disease. J Rheumatol 2007;34:1005–11.

22. de Groote P, Gressin V, Hachulla E, Carpentier P, Guillevin L, Kahan A, Cabane J, Frances C, Lamblin N, Diot E, Patat F, Sibilia J, Petit H, Cracowski JL, Clerson P, Humbert M. Evaluation of cardiac abnormalities by Doppler echocardiography in a large nationwide multicentric cohort of patients with systemic sclerosis. Ann Rheum Dis 2008;67:31–6.

23. Meune C, Avouac J, Wahbi K, Cabanes L, Wipff J, Mouthon L, Guillevin L, Kahan A, Allanore Y. Cardiac involvement in systemic sclerosis assessed by tissue-Doppler echocardiography during routine care: A controlled study of 100 consecutive patients. Arthritis Rheum 2008;58: 1803–9.

24. Tanaka E, Harigai M, Tanaka M, Kawaguchi Y, Hara M, Kamatani N. Pulmonary hypertension in systemic lupus

erythematosus: evaluation of clinical characteristics and response to immunosuppressive treatment. J Rheumatol 2002;29:282–7.

25. Asherson RA, Higenbottam TW, Dinh Xuan AT, Khamashta MA, Hughes GR. Pulmonary hypertension in a lupus clinic: experience with twenty-four patients. J Rheumatol 1990; 17:1292–8.

26. Burdt MA, Hoffman RW, Deutscher SL, Wang GS, Johnson JC, Sharp GC. Long-term outcome in mixed connective tissue disease: longitudinal clinical and serologic findings. Arthritis Rheum 1999;42:899–909.

27. Jais X, Launay D, Yaici A, Le Pavec J, Tcherakian C, Sitbon O, Simonneau G, Humbert M. Immunosuppressive therapy in lupus- and mixed connective tissue disease-associated pulmonary arterial hypertension: a retrospective analysis of twenty-three cases. Arthritis Rheum 2008;58: 521–31.

28. Launay D, Hachulla E, Hatron PY, Jais X, Simonneau G, Humbert M. Pulmonary arterial hypertension: a rare complication of primary Sjogren syndrome: report of 9 new cases and review of the literature. Medicine (Baltimore) 2007;86:299–315.

29. Bunch TW, Tancredi RG, Lie JT. Pulmonary hypertension in polymyositis. Chest 1981;79:105–7.

30. Dawson JK, Goodson NG, Graham DR, Lynch MP. Raised pulmonary artery pressures measured with Doppler echocardiography in rheumatoid arthritis patients. Rheumatology (Oxford) 2000;39:1320–5.

31. Kim KK, Factor SM. Membranoproliferative glomerulonephritis and plexogenic pulmonary arteriopathy in a homosexual man with acquired immunodeficiency syndrome. Hum Pathol 1987;18:1293–6.

32. Mehta NJ, Khan IA, Mehta RN, Sepkowitz DA. HIV-related pulmonary hypertension: analytic review of 131 cases. Chest 2000;118:1133–41.

33. Opravil M, Pechere M, Speich R, Joller-Jemelka HI, Jenni R, Russi EW, Hirschel B, Luthy R. HIV-associated primary pulmonary hypertension. A case control study. Swiss HIV Cohort Study. Am J Respir Crit Care Med 1997;155:990–5.

34. Sitbon O, Lascoux-Combe C, Delfraissy JF, Yeni PG, Raffi F, De Zuttere D, Gressin V, Clerson P, Sereni D, Simonneau G. Prevalence of HIV-related pulmonary arterial hypertension in the current antiretroviral therapy era. Am J Respir Crit Care Med 2008;177: 108–13.

35. Nunes H, Humbert M, Sitbon O, Morse JH, Deng Z, Knowles JA, Le Gall C, Parent F, Garcia G, Herve P, Barst RJ, Simonneau G. Prognostic factors for survival in human immunodeficiency virus-associated pulmonary arterial hypertension. Am J Respir Crit Care Med 2003;167: 1433–9.

36. Sitbon O, Gressin V, Speich R, Macdonald PS, Opravil M, Cooper DA, Fourme T, Humbert M, Delfraissy JF, Simonneau G. Bosentan for the treatment of human immunodeficiency virus-associated pulmonary arterial hypertension. Am J Respir Crit Care Med 2004;170:1212–7.

37. Degano B, Yaïci A, Le Pavec J, Savale L, Jaïs X, Camara B, Humbert M, Simonneau G, Sitbon O. Long-term effects of bosentan in patients with HIV-associated pulmonary arterial hypertension. Eur Respir J 2008; In Press.

38. Herve P, Lebrec D, Brenot F, Simonneau G, Humbert M, Sitbon O, Duroux P. Pulmonary vascular disorders in portal hypertension. Eur Respir J 1998;11:1153–66.

39. Rodriguez-Roisin R, Krowka MJ, Herve P, Fallon MB. On behalf of the ERS Task Force Pulmonary-Hepatic Vascular Disorders Scientific Committee ERS Task Force PHD Scientific Committee. Pulmonary-Hepatic vascular Disorders (PHD). Eur Respir J 2004;24:861–80.

40. Hadengue A, Benhayoun MK, Lebrec D, Benhamou JP. Pulmonary hypertension complicating portal hypertension: prevalence and relation to splanchnic hemodynamics. Gastroenterology 1991;100:520–8.

41. Krowka MJ, Swanson KL, Frantz RP, McGoon MD, Wiesner RH. Portopulmonary hypertension: results from a 10-year screening algorithm. Hepatology 2006;44:1502–10.

42. Kawut SM, Krowka MJ, Trotter JF, Roberts KE, Benza RL, Badesch DB, Taichman DB, Horn EM, Zacks S, Kaplowitz N, Brown RS, Jr., Fallon MB. Clinical risk factors for portopulmonary hypertension. Hepatology 2008;48:196–203.

43. Le Pavec J, Souza R, Herve P, Lebrec D, Savale L, Tcherakian C, Jais X, Yaici A, Humbert M, Simonneau G, Sitbon O. Portopulmonary hypertension: survival and prognostic factors. Am J Respir Crit Care Med 2008;178:637–43.

44. Eisenmenger V. Die Angeborene Defecte der Kammersheidewand das Herzen. Z Klin Med 1897;132:131.

45. Wood P. The Eisenmenger syndrome or pulmonary hypertension with reversed central shunt. I. Br Med J 1958;2:701–9.

46. Daliento L, Somerville J, Presbitero P, Menti L, Brach-Prever S, Rizzoli G, Stone S. Eisenmenger syndrome. Factors relating to deterioration and death. Eur Heart J 1998;19:1845–55.

47. Besterman E. Atrial septal defect with pulmonary hypertension. Br Heart J 1961;23:587–98.

48. Hoffman JI, Rudolph AM. The natural history of ventricular septal defects in infancy. Am J Cardiol 1965;16:634–53.

49. Shaw AP, Ghareed A. The pathogenesis of pulmonary schistosomiasis in Egypt with special reference to Ayerza's disease. J Pathol Bacteriol 1938;46:401–24.

50. Lapa MS, Ferreira EV, Jardim C, Martins Bdo C, Arakaki JS, Souza R. [Clinical characteristics of pulmonary hypertension patients in two reference centers in the city of Sao Paulo]. Rev Assoc Med Bras 2006;52:139–43.

51. Chaves E. The pathology of the arterial pulmonary vasculature in Manson's schistosomiasis. Dis Chest 1966;50:72–7.

52. de Cleva R, Herman P, Pugliese V, Zilberstein B, Saad WA, Rodrigues JJ, Laudanna AA. Prevalence of pulmonary hypertension in patients with hepatosplenic Mansonic schistosomiasis – prospective study. Hepatogastroenterology 2003;50:2028–30.

53. Lapa M, Dias B, Jardim C, Fernandes CJ, Dourado PM, Figueiredo M, Farias A, Tsutsui J, Terra-Filho M, Humbert M, Souza R. Cardiopulmonary manifestations of hepatosplenic schistosomiasis. Circulation 2009;119:1518–23.

54. Castro O, Hoque M, Brown BD. Pulmonary hypertension in sickle cell disease: cardiac catheterization results and survival. Blood 2003;101:1257–61.

55. Gladwin MT, Sachdev V, Jison ML, Shizukuda Y, Plehn JF, Minter K, Brown B, Coles WA, Nichols JS, Ernst I, Hunter LA, Blackwelder WC, Schechter AN, Rodgers GP, Castro O, Ognibene FP. Pulmonary Hypertension as a risk factor for death in patients with sickle cell disease. N Engl J Med 2004;350:886–95.

56. Aessopos A, Stamatelos G, Skoumas V, Vassilopoulos G, Mantzourani M, Loukopoulos D. Pulmonary hypertension and right-heart failure in patients with beta-thalassemia intermedia. Chest 1995;107:50–3.

57. Smedema JP, Louw VJ. Pulmonary arterial hypertension after splenectomy for hereditary spherocytosis. Cardiovasc J Afr 2007;18:84–9.

58. Jais X, Till SJ, Cynober T, Ioos V, Garcia G, Tchernia G, Dartevelle P, Simonneau G, Delaunay J, Humbert M. An extreme consequence of splenectomy in dehydrated hereditary stomatocytosis: gradual thrombo-embolic pulmonary hypertension and lung–heart transplantation. Hemoglobin 2003;27:139–47.

59. Stuard ID, Heusinkveld RS, Moss AJ. Microangiopathic hemolytic anemia and thrombocytopenia in primary pulmonary hypertension. N Engl J Med 1972;287:869–70.

60. Parent F, Egels S, Stzrymf B, Girot R, Dreiss F, Galacteros F, Simonneau G. Haemodynamic characteristics of patients with sickle cell disease and suspected pulmonary hypertension on the basis of a tricuspid regurgitation jet velocity > 2.5 m/s on Doppler echocardiography. Eur Respir J 2006;28:544s (Abstract).

61. Anthi A, Machado RF, Jison ML, Taveira-Dasilva AM, Rubin LJ, Hunter L, Hunter CJ, Coles W, Nichols J, Avila NA, Sachdev V, Chen CC, Gladwin MT. Hemodynamic and functional assessment of patients with sickle cell disease and pulmonary hypertension. Am J Respir Crit Care Med 2007;175:1272–9.

62. Haque AK, Gokhale S, Rampy BA, Adegboyega P, Duarte A, Saldana MJ. Pulmonary hypertension in sickle cell hemoglobinopathy: a clinicopathologic study of 20 cases. Hum Pathol 2002;33:1037–43.

63. Reiter CD, Wang X, Tanus-Santos JE, Hogg N, Cannon RO, 3rd, Schechter AN, Gladwin MT. Cell-free hemoglobin limits nitric oxide bioavailability in sickle-cell disease. Nat Med 2002;8:1383–9.

64. Gladwin MT, Lancaster JR, Jr., Freeman BA, Schechter AN. Nitric oxide's reactions with hemoglobin: a view through the SNO-storm. Nat Med 2003;9:496–500.

65. Montani D, Achouh L, Dorfmuller P, Le Pavec J, Sztrymf B, Tcherakian C, Rabiller A, Haque R, Sitbon O, Jais X, Dartevelle P, Maitre S, Capron F, Musset D, Simonneau G, Humbert M. Pulmonary veno-occlusive disease: clinical, functional, radiologic, and hemodynamic characteristics and outcome of 24 cases confirmed by histology. Medicine (Baltimore) 2008;87:220–33.

66. Lantuejoul S, Sheppard MN, Corrin B, Burke MM, Nicholson AG. Pulmonary veno-occlusive disease and pulmonary capillary hemangiomatosis: a clinicopathologic study of 35 cases. Am J Surg Pathol 2006;30:850–7.

67. Montani D, Price LC, Dorfmuller P, Achouh L, Jais X, Yaici A, Sitbon O, Musset D, Simonneau G, Humbert M. Pulmonary veno-occlusive disease. Eur Respir J 2009;33:189–200.

68. Dorfmuller P, Humbert M, Perros F, Sanchez O, Simonneau G, Muller KM, Capron F. Fibrous remodeling of the pulmonary venous system in pulmonary arterial hypertension associated with connective tissue diseases. Hum Pathol 2007;38:893–902.

69. Escamilla R, Hermant C, Berjaud J, Mazerolles C, Daussy X. Pulmonary veno-occlusive disease in a HIV-infected intravenous drug abuser. Eur Respir J 1995;8:1982–4.

70. Ruchelli ED, Nojadera G, Rutstein RM, Rudy B. Pulmonary veno-occlusive disease. Another vascular disorder associated with human immunodeficiency virus infection? Arch Pathol Lab Med 1994;118:664–6.

71. Runo JR, Vnencak-Jones CL, Prince M, Loyd JE, Wheeler L, Robbins IM, Lane KB, Newman JH, Johnson J, Nichols WC, Phillips JA, 3rd. Pulmonary veno-occlusive disease caused by an inherited mutation in bone morphogenetic protein receptor II. Am J Respir Crit Care Med 2003;167:889–94.

72. Resten A, Maitre S, Humbert M, Rabiller A, Sitbon O, Capron F, Simonneau G, Musset D. Pulmonary hypertension: CT of the chest in pulmonary venoocclusive disease. AJR Am J Roentgenol 2004;183:65–70.

73. Holcomb BW, Jr., Loyd JE, Ely EW, Johnson J, Robbins IM. Pulmonary veno-occlusive disease: a case series and new observations. Chest 2000;118:1671–9.

74. Dufour B, Maitre S, Humbert M, Capron F, Simonneau G, Musset D. High-resolution CT of the chest in four patients with pulmonary capillary hemangiomatosis or pulmonary venoocclusive disease. AJR Am J Roentgenol 1998;171:1321–4.

75. Rabiller A, Jais X, Hamid A, Resten A, Parent F, Haque R, Capron F, Sitbon O, Simonneau G, Humbert M. Occult alveolar haemorrhage in pulmonary veno-occlusive disease. Eur Respir J 2006;27:108–13.

76. Oudiz RJ. Pulmonary hypertension associated with left-sided heart disease. Clin Chest Med 2007;28:233–41.

77. Abramson SV, Burke JF, Kelly JJ, Jr., Kitchen JG, 3rd, Dougherty MJ, Yih DF, McGeehin FC, 3rd, Shuck JW, Phiambolis TP. Pulmonary hypertension predicts mortality and morbidity in patients with dilated cardiomyopathy. Ann Intern Med 1992;116:888–95.

78. Zener JC, Hancock EW, Shumway NE, Harrison DC. Regression of extreme pulmonary hypertension after mitral valve surgery. Am J Cardiol 1972;30:820–6.

79. Braunwald E, Braunwald NS, Ross J, Jr., Morrow AG. Effects of mitral-valve replacement on the pulmonary vascular dynamics of patients with pulmonary hypertension. N Engl J Med 1965;273:509–14.

80. Delgado JF, Conde E, Sanchez V, Lopez-Rios F, Gomez-Sanchez MA, Escribano P, Sotelo T, Gomez de la Camara A, Cortina J, de la Calzada CS. Pulmonary vascular remodeling in pulmonary hypertension due to chronic heart failure. Eur J Heart Fail 2005;7:1011–6.

81. Moraes DL, Colucci WS, Givertz MM. Secondary pulmonary hypertension in chronic heart failure: the role of the endothelium in pathophysiology and management. Circulation 2000;102:1718–23.

82. Fraser KL, Tullis DE, Sasson Z, Hyland RH, Thornley KS, Hanly PJ. Pulmonary hypertension and cardiac function in adult cystic fibrosis: role of hypoxemia. Chest 1999;115: 1321–8.

83. Cottin V, Nunes H, Brillet PY, Delaval P, Devouassoux G, Tillie-Leblond I, Israel-Biet D, Court-Fortune I, Valeyre D, Cordier JF. Combined pulmonary fibrosis and emphysema: a distinct underrecognised entity. Eur Respir J 2005;26:586–93.

84. Weitzenblum E, Hirth C, Ducolone A, Mirhom R, Rasaholinjanahary J, Ehrhart M. Prognostic value of pulmonary artery pressure in chronic obstructive pulmonary disease. Thorax 1981;36:752–8.

85. Thabut G, Dauriat G, Stern JB, Logeart D, Levy A, Marrash-Chahla R, Mal H. Pulmonary hemodynamics in advanced COPD candidates for lung volume reduction surgery or lung transplantation. Chest 2005;127:1531–6.

86. Chaouat A, Bugnet AS, Kadaoui N, Schott R, Enache I, Ducolone A, Ehrhart M, Kessler R, Weitzenblum E. Severe pulmonary hypertension and chronic obstructive pulmonary disease. Am J Respir Crit Care Med 2005;172:189–94.

87. Tapson VF, Humbert M. Incidence and prevalence of chronic thromboembolic pulmonary hypertension: from acute to chronic pulmonary embolism. Proc Am Thorac Soc 2006;3:564–7.

88. Pengo V, Lensing AW, Prins MH, Marchiori A, Davidson BL, Tiozzo F, Albanese P, Biasiolo A, Pegoraro C, Iliceto S, Prandoni P. Incidence of chronic thromboembolic pulmonary hypertension after pulmonary embolism. N Engl J Med 2004; 350:2257–64.

89. Kim NH. Assessment of operability in chronic thromboembolic pulmonary hypertension. Proc Am Thorac Soc 2006;3:584–8.

90. Dartevelle P, Fadel E, Mussot S, Chapelier A, Herve P, de Perrot M, Cerrina J, Ladurie FL, Lehouerou D, Humbert M, Sitbon O, Simonneau G. Chronic thromboembolic pulmonary hypertension. Eur Respir J 2004;23:637–48.

91. Jamieson SW, Kapelanski DP, Sakakibara N, Manecke GR, Thistlethwaite PA, Kerr KM, Channick RN, Fedullo PF, Auger WR. Pulmonary endarterectomy: experience and lessons learned in 1,500 cases. Ann Thorac Surg 2003;76: 1457–62; discussion 62–4.

92. Suntharalingam J, Treacy CM, Doughty NJ, Goldsmith K, Soon E, Toshner MR, Sheares KK, Hughes R, Morrell NW, Pepke-Zaba J. Long-term use of sildenafil in inoperable chronic thromboembolic pulmonary hypertension. Chest 2008;134:229–36.

93. Rubin LJ, Hoeper MM, Klepetko W, Galie N, Lang IM, Simonneau G. Current and future management of chronic thromboembolic pulmonary hypertension: from diagnosis to treatment responses. Proc Am Thorac Soc 2006;3:601–7.

94. Dingli D, Utz JP, Krowka MJ, Oberg AL, Tefferi A. Unexplained pulmonary hypertension in chronic myeloproliferative disorders. Chest 2001;120:801–8.

95. Guilpain P, Montani D, Damaj G, Achouh L, Lefrère F, Marfaing-Koka A, Dartevelle P, Simonneau G, Humbert M, Hermine O. Pulmonary hypertension associated with myeloproliferative disorders: a retrospective study of ten cases. Respiration 2008;76:295–302.

96. Marvin KS, Spellberg RD. Pulmonary hypertension secondary to thrombocytosis in a patient with myeloid metaplasia. Chest 1993;103:642–4.

97. Nand S, Orfei E. Pulmonary hypertension in polycythemia vera. Am J Hematol 1994;47:242–4.

98. Peacock AJ. Pulmonary hypertension after splenectomy: a consequence of loss of the splenic filter or is there something more? Thorax 2005;60:983–4.

99. Jais X, Ioos V, Jardim C, Sitbon O, Parent F, Hamid A, Fadel E, Dartevelle P, Simonneau G, Humbert M. Splenectomy and chronic thromboembolic pulmonary hypertension. Thorax 2005;60:1031–4.

100. Hoeper MM, Niedermeyer J, Hoffmeyer F, Flemming P, Fabel H. Pulmonary hypertension after splenectomy? Ann Intern Med 1999;130:506–9.

101. Gluskowski J, Hawrylkiewicz I, Zych D, Wojtczak A, Zielinski J. Pulmonary haemodynamics at rest and during exercise in patients with sarcoidosis. Respiration 1984;46:26–32.

102. Handa T, Nagai S, Miki S, Fushimi Y, Ohta K, Mishima M, Izumi T. Incidence of pulmonary hypertension and its clinical relevance in patients with sarcoidosis. Chest 2006;129:1246–52.

103. Shorr AF, Helman DL, Davies DB, Nathan SD. Pulmonary hypertension in advanced sarcoidosis: epidemiology and clinical characteristics. Eur Respir J 2005;25:783–8.

104. Bourbonnais JM, Samavati L. Clinical predictors of pulmonary hypertension in sarcoidosis. Eur Respir J 2008;32:296–302.

105. Nunes H, Humbert M, Capron F, Brauner M, Sitbon O, Battesti JP, Simonneau G, Valeyre D. Pulmonary hypertension associated with sarcoidosis: mechanisms, haemodynamics and prognosis. Thorax 2006;61:68–74.

106. Dauriat G, Mal H, Thabut G, Mornex JF, Bertocchi M, Tronc F, Leroy-Ladurie F, Dartevelle P, Reynaud-Gaubert M, Thomas P, Pison C, Blin D, Stern M, Bonnette P, Dromer C, Velly JF, Brugiere O, Leseche G, Fournier M. Lung transplantation for pulmonary Langerhans' cell histiocytosis: a multicenter analysis. Transplantation 2006;81:746–50.

107. Fartoukh M, Humbert M, Capron F, Maitre S, Parent F, Le Gall C, Sitbon O, Herve P, Duroux P, Simonneau G. Severe pulmonary hypertension in histiocytosis X. Am J Respir Crit Care Med 2000;161:216–23.

108. Taveira-DaSilva AM, Hathaway OM, Sachdev V, Shizukuda Y, Birdsall CW, Moss J. Pulmonary artery pressure in lymphangioleiomyomatosis: an echocardiographic study. Chest 2007;132:1573–8.

109. Harari S, Simonneau G, De Juli E, Brenot F, Cerrina J, Colombo P, Gronda E, Micallef E, Parent F, Dartevelle P. Prognostic value of pulmonary hypertension in patients with chronic interstitial lung disease referred for lung or heart-lung transplantation. J Heart Lung Transplant 1997;16:460–3.

110. Simeoni S, Puccetti A, Chilosi M, Tinazzi E, Prati D, Corrocher R, Lunardi C. Type 1 neurofibromatosis complicated by pulmonary artery hypertension: a case report. J Med Invest 2007;54:354–8.

111. Engel PJ, Baughman RP, Menon SG, Kereiakes DJ, Taylor L, Scott M. Pulmonary hypertension in neurofibromatosis. Am J Cardiol 2007;99:1177–8.

112. Aoki Y, Kodama M, Mezaki T, Ogawa R, Sato M, Okabe M, Aizawa Y. von Recklinghausen disease complicated by pulmonary hypertension. Chest 2001;119:1606–8.

113. Samuels N, Berkman N, Milgalter E, Bar-Ziv J, Amir G, Kramer MR. Pulmonary hypertension secondary to neurofibromatosis: intimal fibrosis versus thromboembolism. Thorax 1999;54:858–9.

114. Stewart DR, Cogan JD, Kramer MR, Miller WT, Jr., Christiansen LE, Pauciulo MW, Messiaen LM, Tu GS, Thompson WH, Pyeritz RE, Ryu JH, Nichols WC, Kodama M, Meyrick BO, Ross DJ. Is pulmonary arterial hypertension in neurofibromatosis type 1 secondary to a plexogenic arteriopathy? Chest 2007;132:798–808.

115. Launay D, Souza R, Guillevin L, Hachulla E, Pouchot J, Simonneau G, Humbert M. Pulmonary arterial hypertension in ANCA-associated vasculitis. Sarcoidosis Vasc Diffuse Lung Dis 2006;23:223–8.

116. Hamaoka K, Nakagawa M, Furukawa N, Sawada T. Pulmonary hypertension in type I glycogen storage disease. Pediatr Cardiol 1990;11:54–6.

117. Inoue S, Nakamura T, Hasegawa K, Tadaoka S, Samukawa M, Nezuo S, Sawayama T, Higashi Y, Shirabe T. [Pulmonary hypertension due to glycogen storage disease type II (Pompe's disease): a case report.] J Cardiol 1989;19:323–32.

118. Humbert M, Labrune P, Sitbon O, Le Gall C, Callebert J, Herve P, Samuel D, Machado R, Trembath R, Drouet L, Launay JM, Simonneau G. Pulmonary arterial hypertension and type-I glycogen-storage disease: the serotonin hypothesis. Eur Respir J 2002;20:59–65.

119. Pizzo CJ. Type I glycogen storage disease with focal nodular hyperplasia of the liver and vasoconstrictive pulmonary hypertension. Pediatrics 1980;65:341–3.

120. Elstein D, Klutstein MW, Lahad A, Abrahamov A, Hadas-Halpern I, Zimran A. Echocardiographic assessment of pulmonary hypertension in Gaucher's disease. Lancet 1998;351:1544–6.

121. Lee R, Yousem S. The frequency and type of lung involvement in patients with Gaucher's disease. Lab Invest 1998;58: 54 A (Abstract).

122. Theise ND, Ursell PC. Pulmonary hypertension and Gaucher's disease: logical association or mere coincidence? Am J Pediatr Hematol Oncol 1990;12:74–6.

123. Li JH, Safford RE, Aduen JF, Heckman MG, Crook JE, Burger CD. Pulmonary hypertension and thyroid disease. Chest 2007;132:793–7.

124. Ferris A, Jacobs T, Widlitz A, Barst RJ, Morse JH. Pulmonary arterial hypertension and thyroid disease. Chest 2001;119: 1980–1.

125. Merce J, Ferras S, Oltra C, Sanz E, Vendrell J, Simon I, Camprubi M, Bardaji A, Ridao C. Cardiovascular abnormalities in hyperthyroidism: a prospective Doppler echocardiographic study. Am J Med 2005; 118:126–31.

126. Kokturk N, Demir N, Demircan S, Memis L, Kurul C, Akyurek N, Turktas H. Pulmonary veno-occlusive disease in a patient with a history of Hashimoto's thyroiditis. Indian J Chest Dis Allied Sci 2005;47:289–92.

127. Chu JW, Kao PN, Faul JL, Doyle RL. High prevalence of autoimmune thyroid disease in pulmonary arterial hypertension. Chest 2002;122:1668–73.

128. Mayer E, Kriegsmann J, Gaumann A, Kauczor HU, Dahm M, Hake U, Schmid FX, Oelert H. Surgical treatment of pulmonary artery sarcoma. J Thorac Cardiovasc Surg 2001;121:77–82.

129. Anderson MB, Kriett JM, Kapelanski DP, Tarazi R, Jamieson SW. Primary pulmonary artery sarcoma: a report of six cases. Ann Thorac Surg 1995;59: 1487–90.

130. Kim HK, Choi YS, Kim K, Shim YM, Sung K, Lee YT, Park PW, Kim J. Surgical treatment for pulmonary artery sarcoma. Eur J Cardiothorac Surg 2008;33:712–6.

131. Ishiguro T, Kasahara K, Matsumoto I, Waseda R, Minato H, Kimura H, Katayama N, Yasui M, Ohta Y, Fujimura M. Primary pulmonary artery sarcoma detected with a pulmonary infarction. Intern Med 2007;46:601–4.

132. Roberts KE, Hamele-Bena D, Saqi A, Stein CA, Cole RP. Pulmonary tumor embolism: a review of the literature. Am J Med 2003;115:228–32.

133. Dot JM, Sztrymf B, Yaici A, Dorfmuller P, Capron F, Parent F, Jais X, Sitbon O, Simonneau G, Humbert M. [Pulmonary arterial hypertension due to tumor emboli.] Rev Mal Respir 2007;24:359–66.

134. Davis AM, Pierson RN, Loyd JE. Mediastinal fibrosis. Semin Respir Infect 2001;16:119–30.

135. Loyd JE, Tillman BF, Atkinson JB, Des Prez RM. Mediastinal fibrosis complicating histoplasmosis. Medicine (Baltimore) 1988;67:295–310.

136. Goodwin RA, Nickell JA, Des Prez RM. Mediastinal fibrosis complicating healed primary histoplasmosis and tuberculosis. Medicine (Baltimore) 1972;51:227–46.

137. Yigla M, Nakhoul F, Sabag A, Tov N, Gorevich B, Abassi Z, Reisner SA. Pulmonary hypertension in patients with end-stage renal disease. Chest 2003;123:1577–82.

138. Nakhoul F, Yigla M, Gilman R, Reisner SA, Abassi Z. The pathogenesis of pulmonary hypertension in haemodialysis patients via arterio-venous access. Nephrol Dial Transplant 2005;20:1686–92.

Idiopathic and heritable pulmonary hypertension: Introduction to pathophysiology and clinical aspects

KELLY CHIN, FERNANDO TORRES AND LEWIS J RUBIN

INTRODUCTION

Idiopathic pulmonary arterial hypertension (IPAH) is a disease of unclear etiology that is characterized by a mean pulmonary arterial pressure > 25 mmHg and a pulmonary capillary wedge pressure of $\leqslant 15$ mmHg, in the absence of other causes. IPAH can be diagnosed only when pulmonary arterial hypertension is present in patients without other defined risk factors. These include congenital heart disease, connective tissue disease, significant parenchymal lung disease, chronic thromboembolic disease or left-sided valvular or myocardial disease, among others (1).

Pulmonary hypertension is suspected when echocardiographic estimates of systolic pulmonary artery pressure exceed 40 mmHg, corresponding to a tricuspid regurgitant velocity on Doppler echocardiography of 3.0 to 3.5 m/sec (2). However, these estimates of pulmonary artery systolic pressure are not reliable enough to make a definitive diagnosis. *Idiopathic* PAH is also rare, with prevalence estimated at between 5 and 25 cases per million population. Because other forms of pulmonary hypertension are more common, they should still be considered, even when overt signs and symptoms are lacking.

The pathophysiology and clinical characteristics of idiopathic pulmonary arterial hypertension will be briefly reviewed here. The treatment and prognosis of this disorder are discussed separately.

ETIOLOGY AND PATHOGENESIS

It is likely that IPAH and related disorders represent a final common response to a number of potential inciting factors, likely in conjunction with a genetically determined susceptibility (see Chapter 6).

Observed abnormalities in endothelial function

Studies suggest that abnormalities in endothelial function may be present in IPAH, including impaired production of prostacyclin and nitric oxide, and excessive synthesis of endothelin (3,4,5,6,7,8). These abnormalities could lead to vasoconstriction and vascular growth and remodeling. However, it is unknown whether these abnormalities cause the disease or are the result of progressive vascular damage as the disease advances (see Chapters 3 and 5).

The inability to normally terminate the proliferative response to injury may explain the observation that endothelial cell proliferation within plexiform lesions of patients with IPAH tends to be monoclonal. Lee *et al.* have demonstrated monoclonal endothelial cell proliferation within 17 of 22 plexiform lesions from four patients with IPAH, in contrast to none of 19 plexiform lesions from four patients with other forms of pulmonary hypertension (9).

It is likely that many of the observed risk factors for IPAH have in common their ability to damage the pulmonary artery endothelium. Such damage could provoke an endothelial proliferative response which, if dysregulated, could progress to clinical IPAH or similar conditions.

Heritable PAH

Germline mutations in the bone morphogenetic protein receptor type II (*BMPR2*) gene, a member of the transforming growth factor β signaling family, are the most commonly identified abnormality in familial PAH. These mutations are found in approximately 70 percent of familial cases, 10–25 percent of sporadic cases and 9 percent of patients with PAH associated with fenfluramine use (10,11,12). The gene is transmitted as an autosomal dominant trait, with incomplete penetrance and in some cases, genetic anticipation.

BMPR2 carriers without pulmonary hypertension may show greater exercise associated increases in estimated pulmonary artery systolic pressure by Doppler echocardiography (13), perhaps signifying the presence of early, subclinical disease. However, only 10–20 percent of all carriers develop overt disease. The relatively low penetrance can lead to under-recognition of heritable PAH, due to immediate family members being unaffected. This was demonstrated in a registry study where five apparently unrelated families were subsequently linked by pedigree analysis to a pair of common ancestors in the 1850s. Identical *BMPR2* mutations were found in 18 individuals with PAH in these families, 12 of whom had initially been classified as sporadic IPAH (14).

Heritable PAH may also occur in the presence of two gene mutations associated with hereditary hemorrhagic telangiectasis (HHT), activin receptor-like kinase (ALK-1) and endoglin (ENG). HHT causes a vascular dysplasia characterized by mucocutaneous telangiectasias, nasal and gastrointestinal bleeding, and arteriovenous malformations (15).

Reduced *BMPR2* function

Reduced *BMPR2 function* may also be important in sporadic PAH: *BMPR2* expression is reduced in the monocrotaline animal model of acquired pulmonary hypertension (16), and reduced expression of a required *BMPR2* co-receptor has been described in patients with idiopathic PAH and other forms of acquired pulmonary hypertension (17).

Diet pill exposure and PAH

There is an increased risk of developing pulmonary arterial hypertension when the fenfluramine appetite-suppressant medications have been taken for the treatment of obesity (18,19), and monoclonal endothelial proliferation has been observed in this setting (20) (see Chapter 15.4). In one retrospective study, 15 of 73 patients (20 percent) with IPAH had used fenfluramine; in 10, there was a close temporal relationship between drug use and the onset of dyspnea (21). The International Primary Pulmonary Hypertension Study (IPPHS), a case–control study of 95 patients, found an adjusted odds ratio for pulmonary hypertension in users of appetite suppressants for more than three months of 23 (22).

These medications were subsequently withdrawn from the market, but occasional cases of diet-pill associated PAH continue to be identified, sometimes many years after the most recent exposure. The absolute risk with fenfluramine

and dexfenfluramine exposure is relatively low, estimated at 28 cases per million person-years of exposure.

Fenfluramine is thought to contribute to pulmonary hypertension through its ability to alter serotonin signaling. The earliest theories were that fenfluramine simply increased circulating 5HT levels, leading to vasoconstriction. However, the increase in free serotonin is fairly modest (from <1 nM to 1–2 nM), and thus other mechanisms likely contribute (23). This may include growth promoting effects of fenfluramine itself, mediated through the serotonin transporter (24), direct serotonin receptor agonist effects of norfenfluramine, a serotonin metabolite (25), and/or greater increases in *tissue* serotonin levels within the lung, relative to serotonin free in circulation (lung serotonin content is very high).

Whether serotonin might also contribute to IPAH without drug exposure is less clear. Animal studies have suggested a potential role for serotonin, as infusion promotes the development of pulmonary hypertension, and serotonin receptor and transporter blockers reduce pulmonary hypertension (26,27), but human studies are so far very limited.

Stimulants

Pulmonary arterial hypertension has also been reported in association with prior use of "stimulants." In one single-center study, 29 percent of patients reported prior exposure to methamphetamine, amphetamine or cocaine, compared with 4 percent of controls (OR 8–10, p < 0.05). Methamphetamine use was most commonly reported, with or without concomitant amphetamine or cocaine use (28). No other case–control studies have been completed *focusing* on stimulant use, but the association had been suggested by earlier case-reports as well as the IPPHS diet-pill study where a non-significant but elevated OR of 2.8 was reported for prior use of cocaine or amphetamines (22,29,30).

Associated conditions

Patients with connective tissue disease, congenital heart disease, portal hypertension and human immunodeficiency virus (HIV), among others, are at increased risk of developing PAH. Prevalence of PAH varies, with the highest overall risk seen among patients with certain forms of congenital heart disease such as a large ventricular septal defect or patent ductus arteriosus (see Chapter 15.7). Scleroderma patients also have very high prevalence rates, reported at 9–27 percent in various studies (31,32,33,34). *How* these conditions increase risk of PAH is not fully understood, but potential contributing factors may include shear stress, autoantibodies, immune cell activation, viral infection, and increased production of or reduced clearance of vasoconstrictors such as endothelin-1, among others (35,36,37,38,39). On a molecular level, numerous signaling pathways have been identified that may contribute to both idiopathic and other forms of PAH, and a growing number of potential targets for therapy have been identified (40,41). However, it still remains difficult to determine which processes are occurring early in the disease process, given the difficulty in identifying early stage patients with IPAH, as well as the lack of optimal animal models of the disease.

CLINICAL PRESENTATION

Most patients with IPAH present with exertional dyspnea, which is indicative of an inability to increase cardiac output with exercise (42). Exertional chest pain, syncope, and edema are indications of more severe pulmonary hypertension and impaired right heart function. Patients of all ages and of both genders may be affected, but more women than men are diagnosed with IPAH, and young to middle-aged women appear to be at highest risk (median age 30s–50s in various studies) (18,43,44). Establishing the diagnosis of IPAH is frequently delayed, due to the subtle findings on physical examination and the nonspecific symptoms experienced by most patients (see Chapters 7 and 11).

DIAGNOSTIC EVALUATION

The diagnosis of IPAH rarely requires histopathologic confirmation because:

- There are no pathologic features that are diagnostic of IPAH.
- Invasive procedures carry an increased risk in this population.
- The diagnosis of IPAH can be made on clinical grounds, based on a comprehensive evaluation that includes pulmonary function testing, connective tissue serology, echocardiography, complete cardiac catheterization, ventilation–perfusion lung scanning, and/or pulmonary angiography (see Chapter 11).

Instead, the following diagnostic tests should be performed:

- Echocardiography is usually the first diagnostic test suggesting the presence of pulmonary vascular disease, typically showing evidence of right heart chamber enlargement, paradoxic motion of the interventricular septum, and tricuspid insufficiency. Trace to moderate pericardial effusions may be visualized and correlates with elevations in right atrial pressure (45).
- The pulmonary artery systolic pressure can be estimated noninvasively using Doppler techniques, although these measurements are not uniformly accurate as compared with invasive measurements, particularly when performed by less experienced individuals.
- Chest radiographs typically demonstrate enlarged central pulmonary arteries and right heart dilation.
- The electrocardiogram shows right axis deviation and right ventricular hypertrophy with a strain pattern.

Electrocardiographic changes are generally not helpful in assessing disease severity or prognosis (46,47).

- Pulmonary function testing is often slightly abnormal, with over half of all patients demonstrating a mild-to-moderate decrease in FEV1 and FVC compared to age- and sex-matched control subjects (48). The diffusing capacity for carbon monoxide (DLCO) is typically reduced; lung volume measurements may reveal an increase in residual volume, consistent with airway obstruction (49).
- Ventilation–perfusion scanning in IPAH may be normal or may show a mottled pattern, but segmental or larger defects should raise the question of chronic thromboembolic pulmonary hypertension (50). Of note, ventilation–perfusion scanning rather than CT angiography should be used to exclude chronic pulmonary emboli, as its sensitivity for *chronic* but not acute pulmonary emboli is higher (51).
- Pulmonary arteriography should be performed when the perfusion lung scan does not exclude unresolved chronic thromboembolic disease, since patients with proximal chronic thromboembolic disease may be a candidate for pulmonary thromboendarterectomy (see Chapter 17).

Right heart catheterization is ultimately necessary to establish the diagnosis by excluding other cardiovascular conditions that can cause pulmonary hypertension. Catheterization is also required to perform acute vasoreactivity testing, and to obtain measurements of important prognostic variables such as right atrial pressure and cardiac output.

Pulmonary veno-occlusive disease, an unusual form of pulmonary hypertension, may be suggested on clinical grounds when severe pulmonary artery hypertension, accompanied by normal pulmonary capillary wedge and left ventricular diastolic pressures, is associated with evidence of venous congestion on chest radiograph and a patchy appearance of tracer activity on a perfusion scan (52). Occasionally, a lung biopsy or findings at postmortem examination are required to confirm the diagnosis (see Chapter 19.2).

KEY POINTS

- Primary pulmonary hypertension is a rare disease that can be diagnosed only when pulmonary artery hypertension is documented in the absence of other demonstrable cause.
- A mutation in the *BMPR2* gene appears to be responsible for most cases of familial IPAH.
- Other conditions, including connective tissue diseases, congenital heart disorders, liver disease and HIV infection may result in pulmonary vascular disease, likely through common pathways of vascular injury and/or proliferative processes.

REFERENCES

1. Simonneau G, Robbins IM, Beghetti M, Channick RN, Delcroix M, Denton CP et al. Updated clinical classification of pulmonary hypertension. J Am Coll Cardiol 2009;54:S43–54.

2. Rich, S (ed). Executive summary from the World Symposium on Primary Pulmonary Hypertension, Evian, France, September 6–10, 1998, co-sponsored by The World Health Organization. (http://www.who.int/ncd/cvd/pph.html).

3. Christman BW, McPherson CD, Newman JH et al. An imbalance between the excretion of thromboxane and prostacyclin metabolites in pulmonary hypertension. N Engl J Med 1992;327:70.

4. Giaid A, Yanagisawa M, Langleben D et al. Expression of endothelin-1 in the lungs of patients with pulmonary hypertension. N Engl J Med 1993;328:173.

5. Giaid A, Saleh D. Reduced expression of endothelial nitric oxide synthase in the lungs of patients with pulmonary hypertension. N Engl J Med 1995;333:214.

6. Archer SL, Djaballah K, Humbert M et al. Nitric oxide deficiency in fenfluramine- and dexfenfluramine-induced pulmonary hypertension. Am J Respir Crit Care Med 1998;158:1061.

7. Tuder RM, Cool CD, Geraci MW et al. Prostacyclin synthase expression is decreased in lungs from patients with severe pulmonary hypertension. Am J Respir Crit Care Med 1999;159:1925.

8. Bauer M, Wilkens H, Langer F et al. Selective upregulation of endothelin B receptor gene expression in severe pulmonary hypertension. Circulation 2002;105:1034.

9. Lee SD, Shroyer KR, Markham NE et al. Monoclonal endothelial cell proliferation is present in primary but not secondary pulmonary hypertension. J Clin Invest 1998;101:927.

10. Aldred MA, Vijayakrishnan J, James V et al. BMPR2 gene rearrangements account for a significant proportion of mutations in familial and idiopathic pulmonary arterial hypertension. Hum Mutat 2006;27:212–3.

11. Machado RD, Eickelberg O, Elliott CG et al. Genetics and genomics of pulmonary arterial hypertension. J Am Coll Cardiol 2009;54:S32–42.

12. Austin ED, Loyd JE, Phillips JA, 3rd. Genetics of pulmonary arterial hypertension. Semin Respir Crit Care Med 2009;30:386–98.

13. Grunig E, Janssen B, Mereles, D et al. Abnormal pulmonary artery pressure response in asymptomatic carriers of primary pulmonary hypertension gene. Circulation 2000;102:1145.

14. Newman JH, Wheeler L, Lane KB et al. Mutation in the gene for bone morphogenetic protein receptor II as a cause of primary pulmonary hypertension in a large kindred. N Engl J Med 2001;345:319.

15. Faughnan ME, Granton JT, Young LH. The pulmonary vascular complications of hereditary haemorrhagic telangiectasia. Eur Respir J 2009;33:1186–94.

16. Morty RE, Nejman B, Kwapiszewska G et al. Dysregulated bone morphogenetic protein signaling in monocrotaline-induced pulmonary arterial hypertension. Arterioscler Thromb Vasc Biol 2007;27:1072–8.

17. Du L, Sullivan CC, Chu D et al. Signaling molecules in nonfamilial pulmonary hypertension. N Engl J Med 2003;348:500–9.

18. Rich S, Rubin L, Walker AM, Schneeweiss S, Abenhaim L. Anorexigens and pulmonary hypertension in the United States: results from the surveillance of North American pulmonary hypertension. Chest 2000;117:870–4.

19. Voelkel NF, Clarke WR, Higenbottam T. Obesity, dexfenfluramine, and pulmonary hypertension. A lesson not learned? Am J Respir Crit Care Med 1997;155:786.

20. Tuder RM, Radisavljevic Z, Shroyer KR et al. Monoclonal endothelial cells in appetite suppressant-associated pulmonary hypertension. Am J Respir Crit Care Med 1998;158:1999.

21. Brenot F, Herve P, Petitpretz P et al. Primary pulmonary hypertension and fenfluramine use. Br Heart J 1993;70:537.

22. Abenhaim L, Moride Y, Brenot F et al. Appetite-suppressant drugs and the risk of primary pulmonary hypertension. International Primary Pulmonary Hypertension Study Group. N Engl J Med 1996;335:609–16.

23. Rothman RB, Ayestas MA, Dersch CM, Baumann MH. Aminorex, fenfluramine, and chlorphentermine are serotonin transporter substrates. Implications for primary pulmonary hypertension. Circulation 1999;100:869–75.

24. Lee SL, Wang WW, Fanburg BL. Dexfenfluramine as a mitogen signal via the formation of superoxide anion. Faseb J 2001;15:1324–5.

25. Ni W, Li MW, Thakali K, Fink GD, Watts SW. The fenfluramine metabolite (+)-norfenfluramine is vasoactive. J Pharmacol Exp Ther 2004;309:845–52.

26. Marcos E, Adnot S, Pham MH, Nosjean A, Raffestin B, Hamon M et al. Serotonin transporter inhibitors protect against hypoxic pulmonary hypertension. Am J Respir Crit Care Med 2003;168:487–93.

27. Guignabert C, Raffestin B, Benferhat R et al. Serotonin transporter inhibition prevents and reverses monocrotaline-induced pulmonary hypertension in rats. Circulation 2005;111:2812–9.

28. Chin KM, Channick RN, Rubin LJ. Is methamphetamine use associated with idiopathic pulmonary arterial hypertension? Chest 2006;130:1657–63.

29. Schaiberger PH. Pulmonary hypertension associated with long-term inhalation of "crack" methamphetamine. Chest 1993;104:614.

30. Albertson TE, Walby WF, Derlet RW. Stimulant-induced pulmonary toxicity. Chest 1995;108:1140.

31. McLaughlin VV, Presberg KW, Doyle RL et al. Prognosis of pulmonary arterial hypertension: ACCP evidence-based clinical practice guidelines. Chest 2004;126(1 Suppl):78S–92S.

32. Wigley FM, Lima JA, Mayes M, McLain D, Chapin JL, Ward-Able C. The prevalence of undiagnosed pulmonary arterial

hypertension in subjects with connective tissue disease at the secondary health care level of community-based rheumatologists (the UNCOVER study). Arthritis Rheum 2005;52(7):2125–32.

33. Matucci-Cerinic M, Steen V, Nash P, Hachulla E. The complexity of managing systemic sclerosis: screening and diagnosis. Rheumatology (Oxford) 2009;48 Suppl 3:iii8–13.

34. Chang B, Schachna L, White B, Wigley FM, Wise RA. Natural history of mild–moderate pulmonary hypertension and the risk factors for severe pulmonary hypertension in scleroderma. J Rheumatol 2006;33:269–74.

35. Beghetti M, Galie N. Eisenmenger syndrome a clinical perspective in a new therapeutic era of pulmonary arterial hypertension. J Am Coll Cardiol 2009;53:733–40.

36. Abraham DJ, Krieg T, Distler J, Distler O. Overview of pathogenesis of systemic sclerosis. Rheumatology (Oxford) 2009;(48 Suppl 3):iii3–7.

37. Kawut SM, Krowka MJ, Trotter JF et al. Clinical risk factors for portopulmonary hypertension. Hepatology 2008;48: 196–203.

38. Benjaminov FS, Prentice M, Sniderman KW, Siu S, Liu P, Wong F. Portopulmonary hypertension in decompensated cirrhosis with refractory ascites. Gut 2003;52:1355–62.

39. Mesa RA, Edell ES, Dunn WF, Edwards WD. Human immunodeficiency virus infection and pulmonary hypertension: Two new cases and a review of 86 reported cases. Mayo Clin Proc 1998;73:37.

40. Archer S, Rich S. Primary pulmonary hypertension: A vascular biology and translational research "work in progress". Circulation 2000;102:2781.

41. Morrell NW, Adnot S, Archer SL et al. Cellular and molecular basis of pulmonary arterial hypertension. J Am Coll Cardiol 2009;54:S20–31.

42. Peacock AJ. Primary pulmonary hypertension. Thorax 1999;54:1107.

43. Rich S, Dantzker DR, Ayres SM et al. Primary pulmonary hypertension: A national prospective study. Ann Intern Med 1987;107:216.

44. Humbert M, Sitbon O, Chaouat A, Bertocchi M, Habib G, Gressin V et al. Pulmonary arterial hypertension in France: results from a national registry. Am J Respir Crit Care Med 2006;173:1023–30.

45. Hinderliter AL, Willis PW 4th, Long W et al. Frequency and prognostic significance of pericardial effusion in primary pulmonary hypertension. PPH Study Group. Primary pulmonary hypertension. Am J Cardiol 1999;84:481.

46. Bossone E, Paciocco G, Iarussi D et al. The prognostic role of the ECG in primary pulmonary hypertension. Chest 2002;121:513.

47. Ahearn GS, Tapson VF, Rebeiz A, Greenfield JC Jr. Electrocardiography to define clinical status in primary pulmonary hypertension and pulmonary arterial hypertension secondary to collagen vascular disease. Chest 2002;122:524.

48. Sun XG, Hansen JE, Audis RJ, Wasserman K. Pulmonary function in primary pulmonary hypertension. J Am Coll Cardiol 2003;41:1028.

49. Meyer FJ, Ewert R, Hoeper MM et al. Peripheral airway obstruction in primary pulmonary hypertension. Thorax 2002;57:473.

50. Fishman AJ, Moser KM, Fedullo PF. Perfusion lung scans vs. pulmonary angiography in evaluation of suspected primary pulmonary hypertension. Chest 1983;84:679–83.

51. Tunariu N, Gibbs SJ, Win Z et al. Ventilation–perfusion scintigraphy is more sensitive than multidetector CTPA in detecting chronic thromboembolic pulmonary disease as a treatable cause of pulmonary hypertension. J Nucl Med 2007;48:680–4.

52. Mandel J, Mark EJ, Hales CA. Pulmonary veno-occlusive disease. Am J Respir Crit Care Med 2000;162:1964.

Genetics of pulmonary arterial hypertension

ERIC D AUSTIN, JAMES E LLOYD AND JOHN H NEWMAN

INTRODUCTION

Pulmonary arterial hypertension (PAH), formerly known as primary pulmonary hypertension (PPH) is a progressive disease characterized by widespread obstruction in the smallest pulmonary arteries. PAH may be heritable (HPAH), idiopathic (IPAH), or associated with other medical conditions or exposures to drugs or toxins. Familial cases have been recognized for the last half century and are usually due to mutations in bone morphogenic protein receptor 2 (*BMPR2*), or rarely to mutations in other members of the TGF-β family, activin-like kinase-type I (*ALK1*) or endoglin (*ENG*), which are associated with hereditary hemorrhagic telangiectasia.

Without treatment, most PAH patients die in less than three years due to right heart failure. Although PPH was originally described in 1951 (1), only in the past decade has real progress in understanding its pathogenesis and effective treatment been developed. Despite substantial progress in treatments, as evidenced by FDA approval of six medications in the US for PAH, the treatment effect for many patients is partial or transient, and long-term prospective studies have not yet been conducted to establish their effects on long-term survival.

DEFINITIONS

Pulmonary arterial hypertension is defined by mean pulmonary artery pressure above 25 mmHg at rest in the absence of elevation of the pulmonary capillary wedge pressure confirmed by catheterization and testing that excludes known causes, including lung disease, heart disease, pulmonary embolism, or various conditions associated with PAH (2). Clinical criteria for diagnosis of PAH are described in Chapters 6 and 14.

The current classification scheme for pulmonary hypertension (see Chapter 14) revises the category of familial PAH (FPAH) to heritable PAH (HPAH), which includes the additional cases thought clinically to be sporadic, before they were found to carry identifiable mutations in *BMPR2* (3). A family history may be absent in PAH with *BMPR2* mutation because the genetic basis may go unrecognized because of transmission through multiple unaffected generations (incomplete penetrance) which limit its recognition, or it may result from *de novo* mutation.

INCIDENCE/EPIDEMIOLOGY

Only a few studies have described the incidence and prevalence of PAH. In the mid-1980s, a US national prospective study of PPH was conducted at 32 centers that defined PAH clinical features and outcome prior to development of specific therapy. This benchmark investigation defined the clinical characteristics (4), and survival data (5) of the 187 patients enrolled. The prevalence of a positive PAH family history was 6 percent.

A recent collaborative network across France prospectively studied PAH incidence at 17 university hospitals (6). Among the 674 adult patients included during the one year enrollment, 121 patients were new and 553 had been previously diagnosed. The low end of the range of estimates for incidence of PAH in France was 2.4 cases per million adult inhabitants per year and the prevalence was 15 cases per million, including 5.9 cases of idiopathic PAH per million. The proportion of different causes were idiopathic 39.2 percent, familial 3.9 percent, anorexigen exposure 9.5 percent, connective tissue diseases 15.3 percent, congenital heart diseases 11.3 percent, portal hypertension 10.4 percent, and HIV-associated PAH 6.2 percent of the cohort. This report described less severe clinical impairment at first presentation in familial PAH patients (better walk testing and none were class IV) as compared with idiopathic PAH, although the hemodynamics were similar between the two groups. However, a comprehensive follow-up study by these investigators examining severity did determine a significantly lower age at diagnosis and death, and worse hemodynamic status in *BMPR2* mutation carriers at diagnosis compared to noncarriers, but no difference in survival (7).

Another prospective study with a much larger cohort is currently being conducted. The Registry to Evaluate Early and Long term PAH Disease Management (REVEAL) was designed to provide current information about patients with pulmonary arterial hypertension (8). REVEAL has the goal to collect clinical data from 3500 consecutively enrolled PAH patients. The primary outcome will be survival, and other outcome data will include functional class, 6-minute walk distance, cardiopulmonary exercise, pulmonary function, hemodynamics, and hospitalization. REVEAL is expected to provide important information about current PAH incidence and prevalence as well as other clinical parameters and outcomes (8).

ETIOLOGY

PAH in families/transmission features

Primary pulmonary hypertension was described by Dresdale in 1951 (1), and in 1954 he reported a family with PPH in a mother, son and her sister (9). In 1984 we reviewed and contacted authors of the 13 families reported in the English literature (10) and found that eight new cases had occurred in the interval since the original reports. We added description of a Tennessee family with six PAH deaths in four sisters and two daughters in that report. This same extended family has now had 28 patients (24 women and four men) with PAH and another 41 unaffected individuals (20 women and 21 men) who have progeny with PAH, which indicates that they also carry the mutation (Figure 15.2.1).

Disease transmission in PAH families is most consistent with autosomal dominant mode with incomplete penetrance (10,11) but has several unusual features of clinical expression that remain poorly understood. Some of these features include female predominance (2.4:1), decreased penetrance (range 20–80 percent) and variable age of onset (ages 1–70). Decreased penetrance suggests participation by susceptibility or modifier genes, but it is unknown whether these might be genes whose action promotes clinical expression of *BMPR2* mutation in those who develop PAH, or

conversely, whether these are protective modifiers that prevent disease in mutation carriers who never develop disease, or both.

Interestingly, fewer males are born than would normally be expected (11). Several studies (11,12) have shown earlier age of onset in subsequent generations, but it remains unknown whether this finding is due to ascertainment artifact or has a biologic basis. In other diseases, two different causes of genetic anticipation have a known molecular basis. Trinucleotide repeat expansion was discovered for fragile X syndrome in the early 1990s, and this mechanism is now known to be the basis for more than 40 different neurologic diseases, most of which exhibit genetic anticipation (13). The other known biologic explanation for genetic anticipation is progressive telomere shortening in dyskeratosis congenita, which is due to mutation in telomerase reverse transcriptase (14). Neither of these molecular explanations has been shown to explain genetic anticipation in FPAH. Because numerous statistical biases possibly contribute, it will remain uncertain whether the earlier age of onset in successive generations in FPAH has a biologic basis or is statistical artifact, until a biologic mechanism is shown.

Currently we follow a cohort of 110 families with FPAH at Vanderbilt, who have experienced 364 PAH patients (256 females and 108 males). Age at FPAH death occurs across the entire age spectrum, with a mean age at diagnosis of approximately 36 years (Figure 15.2.2). These families contain another 4085 bloodline family members, half of whom are predicted to inherit the mutation, are at risk to develop FPAH. A similar size cohort recruited at Columbia University by Drs Robyn Barst and Dr Jane Morse during the past decade, is currently directed by Dr Wendy Chung and includes an additional 106 families with 278 patients (personal communication). These figures suggest that in the US there are at least 216 families who have had 642 patients, along with several thousand family members who have an estimated risk about 1 in 10 to develop disease during their lifetime.

A small percentage of HPAH families (15–20 percent) have multiple affected individuals but do not have mutations identified in *BMPR2* despite comprehensive testing. It seems likely that mutations in other genes, possibly also in the TGF-β family, are responsible.

Linkage of familial PAH and discovery of *BMPR2* in families

Two investigative teams utilized microsatellite markers and linkage analysis to focus the familial PPH gene search in 1996 (15,16). Nichols reported six families who had autosomal dominant pattern of gene transmission, in whom he established linkage to a 30 million base pair region on chromosome 2q33. Morse *et al.* independently identified the locus of a familial PPH gene to chromosome 2q31–32. A few years later, both teams demonstrated that mutation in

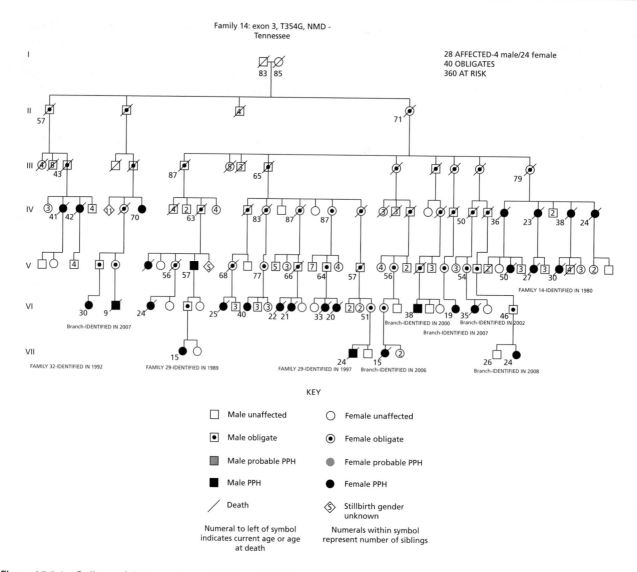

Figure 15.2.1   Pedigree of the largest known family with familial pulmonary arterial hypertension (PAH), with 24 affected females and four affected males over multiple generations, as well as 41 known unaffected mutation heterozygotes. Heritable PAH in this family is due to a mutation in the bone morphogenetic protein receptor type II (*BMPR2*) gene.

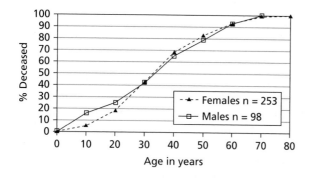

Figure 15.2.2   Cumulative mortality curve for patients (253 females and 98 males) diagnosed with familial pulmonary arterial hypertension, and enrolled in the Vanderbilt University research registry. While more females than males are diagnosed with disease, patient death occurs across the spectrum of ages for both males and females.

the gene encoding bone morphogenetic protein receptor 2 (*BMPR2*) is responsible (17,18).

Various mutation detection methodologies have been employed to screen for mutations, including direct sequencing, melting curve analysis, denaturing high-performance liquid chromatography (DHPLC), Southern blotting and multiplex ligation-dependent probe amplification (MLPA). Nearly 300 different mutations have been described in *BMPR2* (19). Genetic testing for *BMPR2* is available at many different approved sites in the US and Europe.

BMPR2 in IPAH

BMPR2 mutations have been described in IPAH, and have been reported in 11 to 40 percent of cases that clinically appeared to be sporadic (3,20–25). The spectrum of *BMPR2* mutations in hereditary and spontaneous PAH is similar and comprises all of the major classes of mutations.

BMPR2 mutation in other forms of PAH

BMPR2 variations were found in six of 106 children and adults with congenital heart disease due to multiple causes (26). Mutations were not found in 24 patients with PAH and scleroderma. No mutations were found in 19 patients with PAH associated with HIV infection (27). No mutations were found in a series of 103 patients with chronic thromboembolic pulmonary hypertension (28).

Mutations in other genes

Hereditary hemorrhagic telangiectasia (HHT) is characterized by arteriovenous malformation in the lung, brain, intestine, or liver, and is caused by mutations of either the TGF-β type I receptor *ALK-1* or the accessory receptor endoglin (ENG). A small group of HHT patients have PAH, which is clinically and pathologically indistinguishable from other heritable forms of PAH, while others have PAH along with pulmonary arteriovenous fistulas (29), which typically are due to mutation of *ALK-1*. Up to 20 percent (16/83) of all detected mutations in *ALK-1* have been associated with the development of PAH and, of these, 81 percent (13/16) are consistently observed with PAH (30).

CLINICAL PRESENTATION

Common symptoms and signs of PAH include dyspnea during exertion, syncope, and chest pain and are described in Chapter 6. Whether clinical features are changed in the presence of a *BMPR2* mutation is a question of great importance, as it could be useful for diagnosis, prognosis or treatment selection.

A recent study examined the relationship of *BMPR2* mutation to vasoreactivity (31) in 67 consecutive unrelated patients with idiopathic or familial PAH. Nonsynonymous *BMPR2* variations were found in 27 of 67 patients with idiopathic (n = 16 of 52) or familial (n = 11 of 15) PAH. Vasoreactivity was identified in 3.7 percent of 27 patients with nonsynonymous *BMPR2* variations and in 35 percent of 40 patients without nonsynonymous *BMPR2* variations ($P = 0.003$). None of the remaining 22 patients with other *BMPR2* variations demonstrated vasoreactivity. The authors concluded that patients with PAH and nonsynonymous *BMPR2* variations are unlikely to demonstrate vasoreactivity.

Other investigators also examined the role of *BMPR2* mutation on acute vasoreactivity and disease severity in IPAH/FPAH (32). *BMPR2* mutations were sought in 147 patients (69 adults, 78 children; 114 with IPAH, 33 with FPAH) including 124 (84 percent) who were *BMPR2* mutation negative and 23 (16 percent) who were mutation positive. Mutation positive patients were less likely to respond

to acute vasodilator testing than mutation negative patients (4 percent vs. 33 percent; $P < 0.003$; n = 147). Mutation positive patients had lower mixed venous oxygen saturation (57 ± 9 percent vs. 62 ± 10 percent; $P < 0.05$) and cardiac index (CI; 2.0 ± 1.1 vs. 2.4 ± 1.5 L/min; $P < 0.05$) than mutation negative patients. The authors concluded that patients with *BMPR2* mutations are less likely to respond to acute vasodilator testing than mutation negative patients, and thus appear to have more severe disease at diagnosis.

A collaborative study in France compared 68 *BMPR2* mutation positive PAH patients (28 familial and 40 idiopathic) with 155 mutation negative patients (all idiopathic) (7). Mutation positive patients were younger at diagnosis (36.5 ± 14.5 vs. 46.0 ± 16.1 year, $P < 0.0001$), had higher mean pulmonary artery pressure (64 ± 13 vs. 56 ± 13 mmHg, $P < 0.0001$), lower cardiac index (2.13 ± 0.68 vs. 2.50 ± 0.73 L/min/m², $P = 0.0005$), shorter time to death or lung transplantation ($P = 0.044$), and younger age at death ($P = 0.002$), but similar overall survival ($P = 0.51$). The authors concluded that patients with *BMPR2* mutation present approximately 10 years younger than PAH patients without mutation, and have more severe hemodynamic compromise at diagnosis.

In summary, several groups have described that patients with *BMPR2* mutations are less likely to respond to acute vasodilator testing or have worse hemodynamic alterations (31–34). Because these findings would predict worse outcomes, it is surprising that *BMPR2* mutation has not been shown to affect PAH survival.

INVESTIGATIONS

BMPR2 structure and function

The *BMPR2* gene encodes a type 2 receptor for bone morphogenetic proteins (BMP), which belong to the transforming growth factor-β family. The TGF-β family comprises more than 40 protein cytokines and is a strong functional candidate pathway for the stimulus that drives proliferation of the pulmonary arteries in PAH (35). The TGF-β family and their receptors mediate the sequence of cell and tissue growth, stimulate wound healing and inflammatory responses, and induce neoplastic transformation of cells.

Four functional domains of TGF-β type 2 receptors, including *BMPR2*, are highly conserved and include N-terminal ligand binding, transmembrane, serine/threonine kinase and cytoplasmic tail domains. BMPR2 differs from other TGF-β receptors by its very long cytoplasmic tail encoded by exon 12.

Signal transduction in the TGF-β pathway has been investigated extensively for two decades, but BMP signaling remains less well described (19). A hetero-tetrameric complex consisting of type I receptors, including ALK1, BMPR1A or BMPR1B and BMPR2 associate to bind extracellular dimeric ligand. The type I receptors, then bind and phosphorylate members of the Smad family, Smad 1,

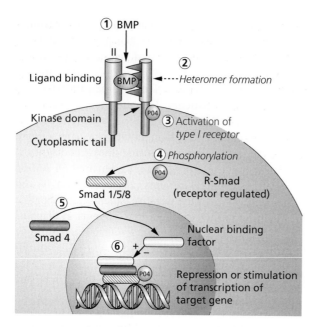

Figure 15.2.3 Signal pathway for the bone morphogenetic proteins (BMPs). BMPs bind to the extracellular domain of BMPRII, resulting in a heteromeric complex with BMPRI. BMPRII then phosphorylates the transmembrane region of BMPRI, activating its kinase domain. The activated BMPRI phosphorylates a receptor Smad (R-Smad), one or more receptor-dependent cytoplasmic Smad proteins (Smad 1 or Smad 5 or Smad 8), which bind with Smad 4 and migrate to the nucleus. This complex interacts with a nuclear binding factor in the nucleus to alter gene transcription.

Smad 5 or Smad 8. Activation increases affinity of the Smads for a nuclear chaperone, Smad 4. These signaling molecules shuttle to the nucleus where, in concert with specific nuclear co-factors and repressors they influence regulation of target genes (Figure 15.2.3) (36). Specificity and flexibility of signaling is tightly maintained, including sequestration of extracellular ligand, competition of type I receptors by decoy receptors, and interactions with other pathways including p38 MAPK, the cytoskeleton associated proteins Tctex-1 and LIMK-1 (36–39) and c-src and RACK-1 (40,41).

Pathogenesis of *BMPR2* mutations

Functional genomic studies and transgenic animal models have investigated BMP-induced effects in the pulmonary vasculature, as well as the cellular effects of *BMPR2* mutations on vascular cell phenotypes (42). While these studies have significantly increased our knowledge about the biologic effects of BMP and TGF-β signaling in the lung vasculature, the molecular mechanisms leading to pulmonary arteriopathy in the context of *BMPR2* mutations in PAH remain largely unknown. Even knowing that *BMPR2*

mutation is the basis for PAH in most families and many IPAH patients, it remains a mystery why vasculature elsewhere in the body is spared, and only the smallest pulmonary arteries are affected.

Several studies addressed expression of TGF-β/BMP system components in human lung (42). BMPR2 is highly expressed in the endothelium and smooth muscle layer of the pulmonary vasculature (43,44). Aberrant vascular remodeling in PAH may not be secondary to global loss of BMP/TGF-β responsiveness but, rather, to changes in the balance of different heteromeric BMP/TGF-β receptor complexes, which shift the balance from a growth inhibitory to a mitogenic response (45).

It appears that BMP/TGF-β signaling plays important but opposite roles in the maintenance and growth of pulmonary artery smooth muscle cells versus pulmonary artery endothelial cells, with important consequences for the onset and development of PAH (42). Investigation of the expression patterns of BMPR2 protein variants in lungs and possibly other tissues from patients with PAH will undoubtedly enrich our understanding of how *BMPR2* mutations lead to the dramatic phenotype of vascular remodeling in IPAH and possibly explain why this disease, in the presence of germline mutations occurring in all cells throughout the body, selectively affects only the pulmonary vasculature (42).

Pathogenesis – nonsense mediated decay (NMD) of RNA transcripts

Some genetic mutations produce stable RNA transcripts, whereas premature termination codons usually generate RNA which is rapidly degraded through the nonsense mediated decay pathway (46,47). Mutations which cause NMD exert their effects via a mechanism of haploinsufficiency rather than dominant negative action (48). We hypothesized that *BMPR2* mutations which cause NMD have a less severe phenotype, because dominant negative mechanisms generally have greater functional impact. We found that NMD of mRNAs encoded by *BMPR2* mutation is active in 24 FPAH families, but does not participate in 21 others. The average age of onset of FPAH with NMD mutations is 36 years, while in those without NMD it is 29 years ($P < 0.002$). We believe that *BMPR2* mutations which are associated with NMD have a milder phenotype manifested as later onset. Mutations which do not cause NMD appear to have more severe phenotype attributable to dominant negative effects (46).

Pathogenesis – decreased expression of normal allele of *BMPR2*

Although all members in FPAH kindreds with *BMPR2* mutations which cause NMD are at risk for disease from haploinsufficiency, only 20 percent ever develop FPAH. We hypothesized that variable expression of the normal wild type (WT) transcripts contribute to the severity of haploinsufficiency, and thereby to penetrance, in individuals carrying NMD causing mutations (49). Individuals who carry a mutation but do not have PAH are clinically normal subjects, thus the cell types of greatest interest (i.e. lung vasculature) are not available from them, so the use of a surrogate cell line is necessary. Transformed lymphoblastoid (LB) cell lines from normal controls and FPAH patients were used to show that WT *BMPR2* transcripts can be quantitatively determined by real-time PCR and that the expression levels vary between individuals (49). Hamid *et al.* compared WT *BMPR2* expression in four kindreds due to NMD causing mutations and found that cells from the affected family members had significantly lower levels of WT *BMPR2* transcripts compared to those from unaffected relatives with the same mutation. This association of transcript levels with penetrance is not limited to a single NMD causing mutation since all four kindreds analyzed have different mutations. These data support the possibility that variation in the amount of WT *BMPR2* transcript acts as a modifier that influences the penetrance of FPAH in individuals who carry NMD causing mutations. The mechanisms underlying variable expression of the WT *BMPR2* allele are not known.

Pathogenesis – modifiers for clinical expression of *BMPR2* mutation

The complex clinical features of PAH, including decreased penetrance, variable age of onset and excess females suggests that additional genetic or environmental features contribute to disease expression. Several studies of the contribution of functional candidate genes, considered to have biological plausibility in PAH, have been conducted. Some among these are serotonin transporter, prostacyclin synthase, angiotensin converting enzyme, endoglin, potassium channels, and carbomyl phosphate synthetase (50–60). All of these studies are constrained by small sample size, so conclusive evidence for contributions by such functional candidates remains modest. It remains possible that an environmental exposure could contribute to clinical expression of *BMPR2*, and is suggested by the appetite suppressant episodes, by excess females affected implicating estrogens, and by the observation that several pairs of monozygotic twins are discordant for PAH (19).

Pathogenesis – TGF-β polymorphisms modify *BMPR2* mutation

Relatively common genetic variants in TGF-β affect its activation in humans (61). The recent finding of a significant association between more severe lung disease in cystic fibrosis and *TGF-β1* rs1982073 CC genotype group (codon 10: odds ratio ~2.2) confirmed an association (62). We examined whether functional *TGFβ1* SNPs increase TGF-β/BMP signaling imbalance in *BMPR2* mutation carriers, and whether these SNPs affect the clinical expression and

SMAD2 expression in lung tissue in FPAH (57). We studied 81 FPAH patients and 39 unaffected *BMPR2* mutation carriers. We found that *BMPR2* mutation carriers without nonsense mediated decay, and who carry the least, intermediate and most active −509 *TGFβ1* SNP genotypes had penetrances of 33, 72 and 80 percent, respectively ($P = 0.003$) while those with 0–1, 2 or 3–4 active SNP alleles had penetrances of 33, 72 and 75 percent ($P = 0.005$). We also showed that relative expression of TGF-β dependent phosphorylated Smad 2, a marker of TGF-β pathway activation, was increased in lung sections of FPAH patients. We conclude that *TGFβ1* SNPs modulate age at diagnosis and penetrance of FPAH in *BMPR2* mutation carriers (57).

Pathogenesis – *BMPR2* mouse models

Many investigations have studied the impact of *BMPR2* deficiency on development of PAH in mice (63). Mice with severe reductions in BMPR2 level, such as *Bmpr2* hypomorphs and *Bmpr2*^{+/−} mice demonstrate embryonic lethal phenotypes (64,65). Mice heterozygous for a *Bmpr2*-null allele (*Bmpr2*^{+/−}) showed modest elevation of mean pulmonary artery pressure and pulmonary vascular resistance (66). However, more recent studies using the same mouse strain, show no significant difference in RV systolic pressure (RVSP) between *Bmpr2*^{+/−} and control mice (67,68).

Specific downregulation of BMPR2 in smooth muscle using a dominant-negative form of BMPR2, Tg(SM22α-dnBmpr2), show elevated RVSP (69). Both *Bmpr2*^{+/−} and Tg (SM22α-dnBMPR2) mice show moderate increase in small pulmonary artery muscle, but they do not fully recapitulate the pathological features of severe PAH (66,69). *Bmpr2*-knockdown by shRNA in mice shows a 90 percent reduction in BMPR2 expression but no significant elevation in pulmonary pressure (70). Investigators using a Cre/loxP system showed that deficiency in BMPR2 signaling in pulmonary endothelial cells can elicit PAH (63).

West *et al.* recently created a smooth muscle-specific doxycycline-inducible *BMPR2* mutation. These SM22-rtTA × TetO(7)-BMPR2(R899X) mice all developed pulmonary vascular pruning, and 33 percent developed elevated right ventricular systolic pressures, muscularization of small pulmonary vessels, and development of large structural pulmonary vascular changes (71). However, a newly developed inducible transgenic mouse model that universally expresses the R899X *BMPR2* mutation fully recapitulates human PAH, with higher penetrance and more rapid disease onset than the smooth muscle specific version. Early manifestations in this mouse include recruitment of circulating cells, alterations in actin organization, and increased TGF-β signaling (West, personal communication). The *BMPR2*-R899X is the most common mutation in our familial cohort, as it is the basis of disease in four different families.

In summary, recently developed *BMPR2* mutation models do recapitulate human PAH, and should form the basis for exciting studies to better understand the pathogenesis and to test novel treatment approaches.

TREATMENT/MANAGEMENT

Treatment of symptomatic PAH is addressed comprehensively in Chapters 13, 16, 17, and 23.

The approach in heritable pulmonary hypertension is the same, except that absence of acute vasoreactivity discussed earlier would predict poor response to calcium channel blockers. It remains unknown and untested whether any treatment recommendations should be offered for the many thousands of individuals who have *BMPR2* mutation in families, but who have no signs or symptoms of PAH. Caring for families with PAH also includes providing education and emotional support as well as genetic testing and counseling and serial screening for signs of disease. Emotional support is often needed for individuals in families regardless of whether they themselves ever have PAH.

Genetic testing and counseling

Siblings or children of heterozygotes for a *BMPR2* mutation have an overall risk of 50 percent to inherit the abnormal gene. Assuming an average gene penetrance of 20 percent, they have an estimated overall risk of 10 percent to express clinical PAH during their lifetime.

CLINICAL SCREENING OF BLOODLINE FAMILY MEMBERS AND MUTATION HETEROZYGOTES

Prospective studies of early detection or clinical evaluation of known carriers of *BMPR2* mutation have not been reported. The 1998 World Pulmonary Hypertension Conference advised first-degree relatives of known FPAH patients to be screened every 3 to 5 years using clinical examination and echocardiography (72).

The pulmonary circulation can tolerate extensive and widespread loss of small pulmonary arteries without provoking any symptoms or clinical signs. It is estimated that the normal human lung has 8 million small arteries of the size which are diseased by PAH. More than half of these vessels can be lost (i.e. 4 million arteries) in PAH, with no clinical signs and no increase in PVR, or any clinical method currently shown to detect disease in a patient in this phase. A test to detect small pulmonary artery occlusive disease, which might be used for presymptomatic detection, is greatly needed for screening the thousands of individuals in families who have *BMPR2* mutation, but who have no symptoms or clinical signs.

TESTING AND COUNSELING

Genetic testing for the *BMPR2* gene is clinically available, so patients with IPAH and FPAH, and members of their families, should be educated about the availability of genetic testing and the potential risk to others in their families. Genetic testing should only be provided after professional genetic counseling (72,73). If the family mutation is known

and the individual tests negative, the risk estimate for an individual family member to express disease falls from 1 in 10 to that of the general population, which is approximately 1 in 1 000 000 (100 000-fold risk reduction). Conversely, if an asymptomatic individual at risk is found to carry the known familial *BMPR2* mutation, risk increases modestly, to 1 in 5 (2-fold risk increase) to express clinical disease throughout their lifetime.

Detection of a *BMPR2* mutation in a patient with IPAH is often received with surprise and disappointment. Finding a mutation in IPAH converts the concept of disease from one of a "sporadic" finding to that of a genetic disease. As such, family members are then recognized to be at increased risk for the first time. They should be offered counseling about their risk and about testing for the known mutation. Using all the mutation detection approaches mentioned earlier, approximately 80 percent of HPAH have mutations in *BMPR2*. In circumstances where no affected family members are available to identify the specific mutation for a family, prior participation by an affected family member in research studies may make it possible to find stored DNA to learn the family mutation.

Clinical genetic testing is available in North America and Europe at a cost ranging from approximately US$1000–3000 to analyze the first member of a family to identify the specific mutation. Testing other family members for a known specific mutation is US$300–500 in 2008. Genetic testing seems most helpful for the half of the individuals who test negative so they are not genetically at risk for PAH, as they can then forgo serial clinical evaluation for detection of PAH. The most common reasons that individuals report that they pursue genetic testing is concern for their progeny, or to inform decisions about family planning (74). In the past, many patients declined genetic testing due to concerns regarding genetic discrimination. Recognition of these concerns led many countries to approve laws to protect individuals who have genetic testing. The Genetic Information Non-Discrimination Act in the US was passed in May 2008, and protects members of both individual and group health insurance plans from discrimination in health insurance coverage on the basis of genetic predisposition and protects against discrimination in employment based upon a genetic predisposition. Genetic testing of children should be performed with caution due to the potentially significant psychological impact on a child.

FUTURE DIRECTIONS OF THERAPY

Better understanding of the central pathogenesis discussed here has been associated with new emphasis on treatments directed against proliferative vascular disease, such as imatinib. All of the formerly approved agents were chosen for testing based on the concepts of PAH pathogenesis as primarily vasoreactive or procoagulant. New agents are greatly needed, and hopefully the new understanding of PAH pathogenesis which is evolving from understanding its central mechanisms discussed here will address proliferative arteriopathy with greater specificity and efficacy. Furthermore, different types of *BMPR2* mutations may respond to different therapeutic interventions.

KEY POINTS

- Familial PAH is a heritable condition, while 10–20 percent of cases of idiopathic PAH are due to heritable mutations.
- Germline mutations in the *BMPR2* gene are associated with the majority of heritable cases of PAH.
- *BMPR2* gene-associated PAH is transmitted in autosomal dominant manner with incomplete penetrance and other features of variable expressivity, including a variable age at diagnosis and marked female predominance.
- Heterozygotes for a *BMPR2* gene mutation have an approximately 20 percent chance of expressing PAH disease in their lifetime, due to the incomplete penetrance of the *BMPR2* gene mutation.
- The variable expressivity of *BMPR2* gene mutations suggest that additional genetic and environmental modifiers of disease exist.
- Identification of a familial mutation can be important for reproductive and disease surveillance planning, but should only be performed in concert with thorough genetic counseling and support.

ACKNOWLEDGMENT

Funding was provided by NIH PO1 HL072058, NIH K12 RR1 7697, and GCRC RR000095.

REFERENCES

• = Key primary paper
◆ = Major review article

•1. Dresdale DT, Schultz M, Michtom RJ. Primary pulmonary hypertension. I. Clinical and hemodynamic study. Am J Med 1951;11(6):686–705.
•2. Simonneau G, Galie N, Rubin LJ, Langleben D, Seeger W, Domenighetti G et al. Clinical classification of pulmonary hypertension. J Am Coll Cardiol 2004;43(12 Suppl S): 5S–12S.
3. Thomson JR, Machado RD, Pauciulo MW, Morgan NV, Humbert M, Elliott GC et al. Sporadic primary pulmonary hypertension is associated with germline mutations of the gene encoding BMPR-II, a receptor member of the TGF-beta family. J Med Genet 2000;37(10):741–5.
◆4. Rich S, Dantzker DR, Ayres SM, Bergofsky EH, Brundage BH, Detre KM et al. Primary pulmonary hypertension. A national prospective study. Ann Intern Med 1987;107(2):216–23.
5. D'Alonzo GE, Barst RJ, Ayres SM, Bergofsky EH, Brundage BH, Detre KM et al. Survival in patients with primary pulmonary hypertension. Results from a national prospective registry. Ann Intern Med 1991;115(5):343–9.
6. Humbert M, Sitbon O, Chaouat A, Bertocchi M, Habib G, Gressin V et al. Pulmonary arterial hypertension in France: results from a national registry. Am J Respir Crit Care Med 2006;173(9):1023–30.
7. Sztrymf B, Coulet F, Girerd B, Yaici A, Jais X, Sitbon O et al. Clinical outcomes of pulmonary arterial hypertension in carriers of BMPR2 mutation. Am J Respir Crit Care Med 2008;20:1300–1.
8. McGoon MD, Krichman A, Farber HW, Barst RJ, Raskob GE, Liou TG et al. Design of the REVEAL registry for US patients with pulmonary arterial hypertension. Clin Proc 2008;83(8): 923–31.
9. Dresdale DT, Michtom RJ, Schultz M. Recent studies in primary pulmonary hypertension, including pharmacodynamic observations on pulmonary vascular resistance. Bull NY Acad Med 1954;30(3):195–207.
•10. Loyd JE, Primm RK, Newman JH. Familial primary pulmonary hypertension: clinical patterns. Am Rev Respir Dis 1984; 129(1):194–7.
11. Loyd JE, Butler MG, Foroud TM, Conneally PM, Phillips JA, 3rd, Newman JH. Genetic anticipation and abnormal gender ratio at birth in familial primary pulmonary hypertension. Am J Respir Crit Care Med 1995;152(1):93–7.
12. Sztrymf B, Yaici A, Jais X, Simonneau G, Sitbon O, Humbert M. [Genetics of pulmonary arterial hypertension: recent data and practical applications.] Rev Mal Respir 2005;22(5 Pt 1):796–805.
13. Pearson CE, Nichol Edamura K, Cleary JD. Repeat instability: mechanisms of dynamic mutations. Nat Rev Genet 2005;6(10):729–42.
14. Armanios M, Chen JL, Chang YP, Brodsky RA, Hawkins A, Griffin CA et al. Haploinsufficiency of telomerase reverse transcriptase leads to anticipation in autosomal dominant dyskeratosis congenita. Proc Natl Acad Sci USA 2005; 102(44):15960–4.
15. Nichols WC, Koller DL, Slovis B, Foroud T, Terry VH, Arnold ND et al. Localization of the gene for familial primary pulmonary hypertension to chromosome 2q31–32. Nat Genet 1997;15(3):277–80.
16. Morse JH, Jones AC, Barst RJ, Hodge SE, Wilhelmsen KC, Nygaard TG. Mapping of familial primary pulmonary hypertension locus (PPH1) to chromosome 2q31–q32. Circulation 1997;95(12):2603–6.
•17. Lane KB, Machado RD, Pauciulo MW, Thomson JR, Phillips JA, 3rd, Loyd JE et al. Heterozygous germline mutations in BMPR2, encoding a TGF-beta receptor, cause familial primary pulmonary hypertension. The International PPH Consortium. Nat Genet 2000;26(1):81–4.

●18. Deng Z, Morse JH, Slager SL, Cuervo N, Moore KJ, Venetos G *et al.* Familial primary pulmonary hypertension (gene PPH1) is caused by mutations in the bone morphogenetic protein receptor-II gene. Am J Hum Genet 2000;67(3): 737–44.

◆19. Machado R, Chung W, Eickelberg O, Elliot G, Hanaoka M, Geraci M *et al.* Genetics and genomics of pulmonary arterial hypertension. J Am Coll Cardiol 2009;54: 532–42.

20. Aldred MA, Vijayakrishnan J, James V, Soubrier F, Gomez-Sanchez MA, tensson G *et al.* BMPR2 gene rearrangements account for a significant proportion of mutations in familial and idiopathic pulmonary arterial hypertension. Human Mutat 2006;27(2):212–3.

21. Kato GJ, McGowan V, Machado RF, Little JA, Taylor JT, Morris CR *et al.* Lactate dehydrogenase as a biomarker of hemolysis-associated nitric oxide resistance, priapism, leg ulceration, pulmonary hypertension, and death in patients with sickle cell disease. Blood 2006;107(6):2279–85.

22. Thomson JR, Machado RD, Pauciulo MW, Morgan NV, Humbert M, Elliott GC *et al.* Sporadic primary pulmonary hypertension is associated with germline mutations of the gene encoding BMPR-II, a receptor member of the TGF-beta family. J Med Genet 2000;37(10):741–5.

23. Humbert M, Deng Z, Simonneau G, Barst RJ, Sitbon O, Wolf M *et al.* BMPR2 germline mutations in pulmonary hypertension associated with fenfluramine derivatives. Eur Respir J 2002;20(3):518–23.

24. Morisaki H, Nakanishi N, Kyotani S, Takashima A, Tomoike H, Morisaki T. BMPR2 mutations found in Japanese patients with familial and sporadic primary pulmonary hypertension. Hum Mutat 2004;23(6):632.

25. Grunig E, Koehler R, Miltenberger-Miltenyi G, Zimmermann R, Gorenflo M, Mereles D *et al.* Primary pulmonary hypertension in children may have a different genetic background than in adults. Pediatr Res 2004;56(4):571–8.

26. Roberts KE, McElroy JJ, Wong WP, Yen E, Widlitz A, Barst RJ *et al.* BMPR2 mutations in pulmonary arterial hypertension with congenital heart disease. Eur Respir J 2004;24(3):371–4.

27. Nunes H, Humbert M, Sitbon O, Morse JH, Deng Z, Knowles JA *et al.* Prognostic factors for survival in human immunodeficiency virus-associated pulmonary arterial hypertension. Am J Respir Crit Care Med 2003;167(10): 1433–9.

28. Suntharalingam J, Machado RD, Sharples LD, Toshner MR, Sheares KK, Hughes RJ *et al.* Demographic features, BMPR2 status and outcomes in distal chronic thromboembolic pulmonary hypertension. Thorax 2007;62(7):617–22.

29. Harrison RE, Flanagan JA, Sankelo M, Abdalla SA, Rowell J, Machado RD *et al.* Molecular and functional analysis identifies ALK-1 as the predominant cause of pulmonary hypertension related to hereditary haemorrhagic telangiectasia. J Med Genet 2003;40(12):865–71.

30. Prigoda NL, Savas S, Abdalla SA, Piovesan B, Rushlow D, Vandezande K *et al.* Hereditary haemorrhagic telangiectasia: mutation detection, test sensitivity and novel mutations. J Med Genet 2006;43(9):722–8.

●31. Elliott CG, Glissmeyer EW, Havlena GT, Carlquist J, McKinney JT, Rich S *et al.* Relationship of BMPR2 mutations to vasoreactivity in pulmonary arterial hypertension. Circulation 2006;113(21):2509–15.

●32. Rosenzweig EB, Morse JH, Knowles JA, Chada KK, Khan AM, Roberts KE *et al.* Clinical implications of determining BMPR2 mutation status in a large cohort of children and adults with pulmonary arterial hypertension. J Heart Lung Transplant 2008;27(6):668–74.

●33. Sztrymf B, Coulet F, Girerd B, Yaici A, Jais X, Sitbon O *et al.* Clinical outcomes of pulmonary arterial hypertension in carriers of BMPR2 mutation. Am J Respir Crit Care Med 2008;177(12):1377–83.

34. Sztrymf B, Yaïci A, Sitbon O, Simonneau G, Humbert M. Clinical presentation, hemodynamical characteristics and survival of patients with pulmonary arterial hypertension carrying or not a BMPR2 mutation Eur Respir J 2005;26(352S).

◆35. Newman JH, Phillips JA, 3rd, Loyd JE. Narrative review: the enigma of pulmonary arterial hypertension: new insights from genetic studies. Ann Intern Med 2008;148(4):278–83.

◆36. Shi Y, Massague J. Mechanisms of TGF-beta signaling from cell membrane to the nucleus. Cell 2003 13;113(6):685–700.

37. Adachi-Yamada T, Nakamura M, Irie K, Tomoyasu Y, Sano Y, Mori E *et al.* p38 mitogen-activated protein kinase can be involved in transforming growth factor beta superfamily signal transduction in Drosophila wing morphogenesis. Mol Cell Biol 1999;19(3):2322–9.

38. Foletta VC, Lim MA, Soosairajah J, Kelly AP, Stanley EG, Shannon M *et al.* Direct signaling by the BMP type II receptor via the cytoskeletal regulator LIMK1. J Cell Biol 2003;162(6):1089–98.

39. Machado RD, Rudarakanchana N, Atkinson C, Flanagan JA, Harrison R, Morrell NW *et al.* Functional interaction between BMPR-II and Tctex-1, a light chain of Dynein, is isoform-specific and disrupted by mutations underlying primary pulmonary hypertension. Hum Mol Genet 2003;12(24):3277–86.

40. Wong WK, Knowles JA, Morse JH. Bone morphogenetic protein receptor type II C-terminus interacts with c-Src: implication for a role in pulmonary arterial hypertension. Am J Respir Cell Mol Biol 2005;33(5):438–46.

41. Zakrzewicz A, Hecker Marsh LM, Kwapiszewska G, Nejman B, Long L *et al.* Receptor for activated C-kinase 1, a novel interaction partner of type II bone morphogenetic protein receptor, regulates smooth muscle cell proliferation in pulmonary arterial hypertension. Circulation 2007; 115(23):2957–68.

42. Eickelberg O, Morty RE. Transforming growth factor beta/ bone morphogenic protein signaling in pulmonary arterial hypertension: remodeling revisited. Trends Cardiovasc Med 2007;17(8):263–9.

43. Atkinson C, Stewart S, Upton PD, Machado R, Thomson JR, Trembath RC *et al.* Primary pulmonary hypertension is

associated with reduced pulmonary vascular expression of type II bone morphogenetic protein receptor. Circulation 2002;105(14):1672–8.

•44. Richter A, Yeager ME, Zaiman A, Cool CD, Voelkel NF, Tuder RM. Impaired transforming growth factor-beta signaling in idiopathic pulmonary arterial hypertension. Am J Respir Crit Care Med 2004;170(12):1340–8.

45. Frank DB, Abtahi A, Yamaguchi DJ, Manning S, Shyr Y, Pozzi A et al. Bone morphogenetic protein 4 promotes pulmonary vascular remodeling in hypoxic pulmonary hypertension. Circ Res 2005;97(5):496–504.

46. Cogan JD, Vnencak-Jones CL, Phillips JA, 3rd, Lane KB, Wheeler LA, Robbins IM et al. Gross BMPR2 gene rearrangements constitute a new cause for primary pulmonary hypertension. Genet Med 2005;7(3): 169–74.

47. Cogan JD, Pauciulo MW, Batchman AP, Prince MA, Robbins IM, Hedges LK et al. High frequency of BMPR2 exonic deletions/duplications in familial pulmonary arterial hypertension. Am J Respir Crit Care Med 2006;174(5):590–8.

48. Khajavi M, Inoue K, Lupski JR. Nonsense-mediated mRNA decay modulates clinical outcome of genetic disease. Eur J Hum Genet 2006;14(10):1074–81.

49. Hamid R, Cogan JD, Hedges LU, Austin E, Phillips JA 3rd, Newman JH et al. Penetrance of pulmonary arterial hypertension is modulated by the expression of normal BMPR2 allele. Hum Mutat 2009;30(4):649–54.

50. Abraham WT, Raynolds MV, Badesch DB, Wynne KM, Groves BM, Roden RL et al. Angiotensin-converting enzyme DD genotype in patients with primary pulmonary hypertension: increased frequency and association with preserved haemodynamics. J Renin Angiotensin Aldosterone Syst 2003;4(1):27–30.

51. Aldashev AA, Sarybaev AS, Sydykov AS, Kalmyrzaev BB, Kim EV, Mamanova LB et al. Characterization of high-altitude pulmonary hypertension in the Kyrgyz: association with angiotensin–converting enzyme genotype. Am J Respir Crit Care Med 2002;166(10):1396–402.

52. Amano S, Tatsumi K, Tanabe N, Kasahara Y, Kurosu K, Takiguchi Y et al. Polymorphism of the promoter region of prostacyclin synthase gene in chronic thromboembolic pulmonary hypertension. Respirology 2004;9(2):184–9.

53. Eddahibi S, Humbert M, Fadel E, Raffestin B, Darmon M, Capron F et al. Serotonin transporter overexpression is responsible for pulmonary artery smooth muscle hyperplasia in primary pulmonary hypertension. J Clin Invest 2001;108(8):1141–50.

54. Hoeper MM, Tacacs A, Stellmacher U, Lichtinghagen R. Lack of association between angiotensin converting enzyme (ACE) genotype, serum ACE activity, and haemodynamics in patients with primary pulmonary hypertension. Heart 2003;89(4):445–6.

55. Koehler R, Olschewski H, Hoeper M, Janssen B, Grunig E. Serotonin transporter gene polymorphism in a cohort of German patients with idiopathic pulmonary arterial hypertension or chronic thromboembolic pulmonary hypertension. Chest 2005;128(6 Suppl):619S.

56. Machado RD, Koehler R, Glissmeyer E, Veal C, Suntharalingam J, Kim M et al. Genetic association of the serotonin transporter in pulmonary arterial hypertension. Am J Respir Crit Care Med 2006;173(7):793–7.

57. Phillips JA, 3rd, Poling JS, Phillips CA, Stanton KC, Austin ED, Cogan JD et al. Synergistic heterozygosity for TGFbeta1 SNPs and BMPR2 mutations modulates the age at diagnosis and penetrance of familial pulmonary arterial hypertension. Genet Med 2008;10(5):359–65.

58. Remillard CV, Tigno DD, Platoshyn O, Burg ED, Brevnova EE, Conger D et al. Function of Kv1.5 channels and genetic variations of KCNA5 in patients with idiopathic pulmonary arterial hypertension. Am J Physiol 2007;292(5):C1837–53.

59. Willers ED, Newman JH, Loyd JE, Robbins IM, Wheeler LA, Prince MA et al. Serotonin transporter polymorphisms in familial and idiopathic pulmonary arterial hypertension. Am J Respir Crit Care Med 2006;173(7):798–802.

60. Wipff J, Kahan A, Hachulla E, Sibilia J, Cabane J, Meyer O et al. Association between an endoglin gene polymorphism and systemic sclerosis-related pulmonary arterial hypertension. Rheumatology 2007;46(4):622–5.

61. Grainger DJ, Heathcote K, Chiano M, Snieder H, Kemp PR, Metcalfe JC et al. Genetic control of the circulating concentration of transforming growth factor type beta1. Hum Mol Genet 1999;8(1):93–7.

62. Drumm ML, Konstan MW, Schluchter MD, Handler A, Pace R, Zou F et al. Genetic modifiers of lung disease in cystic fibrosis. N Engl J Med 2005;353(14):1443–53.

63. Hong KH, Lee YJ, Lee E, Park SO, Han C, Beppu H et al. Genetic ablation of the BMPR2 gene in pulmonary endothelium is sufficient to predispose to pulmonary arterial hypertension. Circulation 2008;118(7):722–30.

64. Delot EC, Bahamonde ME, Zhao M, Lyons KM. BMP signaling is required for septation of the outflow tract of the mammalian heart. Development 2003;130(1): 209–20.

65. Beppu H, Kawabata M, Hamamoto T, Chytil A, Minowa O, Noda T et al. BMP type II receptor is required for gastrulation and early development of mouse embryos. Dev Biol 2000;221(1):249–58.

66. Beppu H, Ichinose F, Kawai N, Jones RC, Yu PB, Zapol WM et al. BMPR-II heterozygous mice have mild pulmonary hypertension and an impaired pulmonary vascular remodeling response to prolonged hypoxia. Am J Physiol Lung Cell Mol Physiol 2004;287(6):L1241–7.

67. Song Y, Jones JE, Beppu H, Keaney JF, Jr., Loscalzo J, Zhang YY. Increased susceptibility to pulmonary hypertension in heterozygous BMPR2-mutant mice. Circulation 2005;112(4):553–62.

68. Long L, MacLean MR, Jeffery TK, Morecroft I, Yang X, Rudarakanchana N et al. Serotonin increases susceptibility to pulmonary hypertension in BMPR2-deficient mice. Circ Res 2006;98(6):818–27.

69. West J, Fagan K, Steudel W, Fouty B, Lane K, Harral J et al. Pulmonary hypertension in transgenic mice expressing a dominant-negative BMPRII gene in smooth muscle. Circ Res 2004;94(8):1109–14.

70. Liu D, Wang J, Kinzel B, Mueller M, Mao X, Valdez R *et al.* Dosage-dependent requirement of BMP type II receptor for maintenance of vascular integrity. Blood 2007; 110(5):1502–10.

71. West J, Harral J, Lane K, Deng Y, Ickes B, Crona D *et al.* Mice expressing BMPR2R899X transgene in smooth muscle develop pulmonary vascular lesions. Am J Physiol Lung Cell Mol Physiol 2008;295(5):L744–55.

♦72. Newman JH, Trembath RC, Morse JA, Grunig E, Loyd JE, Adnot S *et al.* Genetic basis of pulmonary arterial hypertension: current understanding and future directions. J Am Coll Cardiol 2004;43(12 Suppl S):33S–9S.

73. McGoon M, Gutterman D, Steen V, Barst R, McCrory DC, Fortin TA *et al.* Screening, early detection, and diagnosis of pulmonary arterial hypertension: ACCP evidence-based clinical practice guidelines. Chest 2004;126(1 Suppl): 14S–34S.

74. Lientz EA, Clayton EW. Psychosocial implications of primary pulmonary hypertension. Am J Hum Genet 2000;2(59):209–11.

Pulmonary arterial hypertension associated with connective tissue diseases

PAUL M HASSOUN

INTRODUCTION

Pulmonary arterial hypertension (PAH), defined as a mean pulmonary arterial pressure of greater than 25 mmHg in the absence of elevation of the pulmonary capillary wedge pressure, is a cause of significant morbidity and mortality (1–3). PAH includes a heterogeneous group of clinical entities sharing similar pathological changes that have been subcategorized as idiopathic PAH (IPAH, formerly known as "primary pulmonary hypertension" or PPH); familial PAH; pulmonary hypertension associated with other diseases such as connective tissue diseases (CTD, such as systemic sclerosis, systemic lupus erythematosus, and mixed connective tissue disease or MCTD); portopulmonary hypertension; and pulmonary hypertension related to HIV infection, drugs and toxins (4). PAH is characterized by increased pulmonary vascular resistance due to remodeling and occlusion of the small pulmonary arterioles. Left untreated, PAH leads irremediably to right ventricular (RV) hypertrophy, pressure overload and dilation resulting in death within 2–3 years (1).

While the mechanisms involved in the pathogenesis of PAH are vastly unknown, there are several lines of evidence implicating autoimmunity in the development of the pulmonary vascular changes, including the presence of circulating autoantibodies (5), proinflammatory cytokines (e.g., IL-1 and IL-6) (6), and association of PAH with autoimmune diseases such as systemic sclerosis (SSc) and systemic lupus erythematosus (SLE). From a pathologic standpoint, the pulmonary vascular lesions in PAH associated with SSc (SSc-PAH) are indistinguishable from those present in IPAH (with the exception of a higher rate of veno-occlusive disease in SSc-PAH (7)) although the two diseases have quite divergent outcomes and response to therapy. Survival is significantly worse in SSc-PAH compared to IPAH despite the use of modern medical therapy (8,9). While there are serologic and pathologic features suggestive of inflammation in both IPAH and SSc-PAH, it is likely that inflammatory pathways and autoimmunity are more pronounced in SSc-PAH and may explain survival discrepancies between the two syndromes and a differential response to therapy (8,9). As such, SSc-PAH may be considered an ideal prototypic example to study inflammatory processes potentially operative in the pathogenesis of PAH. Other connective tissue diseases such as SLE, MCTD, and to a lesser extent rheumatoid arthritis (RA), dermatomyositis, and Sjögren's syndrome can also be complicated by PAH and will be discussed separately in this chapter.

SCLERODERMA

Systemic sclerosis (SSc) is a heterogeneous disorder characterized by dysfunction of the endothelium, dysregulation of fibroblasts resulting in excessive production of collagen, and abnormalities of the immune system (10). These processes lead to progressive fibrosis of the skin and internal organs resulting in organ failure and death. Although the etiology of SSc is unknown, genetic and environmental factors are thought to contribute to host susceptibility (11) in the context of autoimmune dysregulation. SSc, whether presenting in the limited or diffuse form, is a systemic disease with the potential for multiple organ system involvement including the gastrointestinal, cardiac, renal, and pulmonary systems (12). Pulmonary manifestations include PAH, interstitial fibrosis, and increased susceptibility to lung neoplasms.

Estimates of incidence and prevalence of systemic sclerosis have varied widely by the period of observation, disease definition, and population studied (13). Although the incidence seemed to be increasing over the period from 1940 to 1970, the rate of occurrence has stabilized since the widespread use of a standard classification system (14). However, there continues to be marked geographic variation in the occurrence of the disease, supporting a role for environmental factors in disease pathogenesis. Prevalence of SSc ranges from 30–70 cases per million in Europe and Japan (15–17) to ~240 cases per million in the United States (14). Incidence varies similarly by geographic area, with the highest rates found in the United States (~19 persons per million per year) (13).

SCLERODERMA-ASSOCIATED PAH (SSc-PAH)

Estimates of the prevalence of PAH in patients with SSc have varied widely based on the definition of pulmonary hypertension and the method of obtaining the measurements (i.e., echocardiography or cardiac catheterization). In patients with limited SSc (formerly called CREST syndrome for Calcinosis cutis, Raynaud's phenomenon, Esophageal dysfunction, Sclerodactily and Telangiectasias), the prevalence of elevated RV systolic pressure may be as high as 60 percent (18–21) when based on echocardiographic criteria. However, when using strict cardiac catheterization criteria for diagnosis the prevalence of pulmonary hypertension is 8–12 percent (22,23). However, it is likely that SSc-PAH remains underdiagnosed as suggested by the lower than expected prevalence of the disease in the few registries available (24,25).

Pathophysiology: vascular changes in systemic sclerosis – evidence for autoimmunity as a central component of remodeling

Vascular changes occur at an early state in SSc (26), and include gaps between endothelial cells (27), apoptosis (28), endothelial activation with expression of cell adhesion molecules, inflammatory cell recruitment, procoagulant state (29), and intimal proliferation and adventitial fibrosis leading to vessel obliteration. Prognosis and outcome of patients with SSc depends on the extent and severity of the vascular lesions (30). Endothelial injury is reflected by increased levels of soluble vascular cell adhesion molecule (sVCAM-1) (31), disturbances in angiogenesis as reflected by increased levels

of circulating vascular endothelial growth factor (VEGF) (32,33) and presence of angiostatic factors (32,34). Increased VEGF, a glycoprotein with potent angiogenic and vascular permeability-enhancing properties, may be a consequence of increased angiogenesis or profound disturbances in signaling in SSc. The role of dysregulated angiogenesis in SSc-PAH, whether driven by the inflammatory process or other mechanisms, appears to be a predominant feature of the disease and should be the focus of future studies.

Autoantibodies in scleroderma-related PAH

A role for an autoimmune process has been proposed in the pathogenesis of SSc-PAH. Antifibrillarin antibodies (anti-U3-RNP) are frequently found in SSc-PAH patients (35), and the poorly characterized anti-endothelial antibodies (aECA) correlate with digital infarcts (36). IgG antibodies directed against endothelial cells and obtained from patients with IPAH and SSc-PAH display distinct reactivity profiles against antigens from the micro- and macrovascular beds (37). Antibodies to fibrin-bound tissue plasminogen activator in CREST patients (38) and in IPAH patients with HLA-DQ7 antigen (39), and anti-topoisomerase II-alpha antibodies, particularly in association with HLA-B35 antigen (40), have been reported in SSc-PAH. Nicolls *et al.* suggested that aECA which can activate endothelial cells and induce the expression of adhesion molecules, as well as trigger apoptosis, can potentially play a role in the pathogenesis of APAH (41). *In vitro* experiments using auto-antibodies from patients with connective tissue diseases (anti-U1-RNP and anti-dsDNA) can upregulate adhesion molecules (e.g., endothelial leukocyte adhesion molecule-1) and histocompatibility complex class II molecules on human pulmonary arterial endothelial cells (42), suggesting that such an inflammatory process could lead to proliferative and inflammatory pulmonary vasculopathy.

Fibroblasts are essential components of the pulmonary vascular wall remodeling in PAH and can be found in the remodeled neointimal layer in both SSc-PAH and IPAH. The detection of anti-fibroblast antibodies in the serum of SSc and IPAH patients (37,43) has significant pathogenic importance since these antibodies can activate fibroblasts and induce collagen synthesis, thus contributing potentially directly to the remodeling process. Antibodies from sera of patients with SSc have been shown to induce a proadhesive and proinflammatory response in normal fibroblasts (43). IgG antifibroblast antibodies are present in sera of patients with IPAH and SSc-PAH and have distinct reactivity profiles in these two conditions, as assessed by one-dimension immunoblotting (44). By using a two-dimension immunoblotting technique, several fibroblast antigens recognized by serum IgG from IPAH and SSc-PAH patients were identified, including proteins involved in regulation of cytoskeletal function, cell contraction, oxidative stress, cell energy metabolism and in different key cellular pathways (45). Although the specific membrane antigens targeted by these auto-antibodies remain to be determined, it is likely that they react to membrane components since they typically bind to unpermeabilized fibroblasts, and may mediate the release of cytokines and growth factors which in turn might contribute to the pathogenesis of vascular remodeling in PAH (44).

Taken together, particularly in light of the positive response to immunosuppressive therapy for some patients with PAH associated with SLE and MCTD (46), these studies suggest that inflammation and autoimmunity could play a major role in the pathogenesis of PAH. Therefore, a search for specific biomarkers of inflammation should be a focus of future studies in IPAH, SSc-PAH and other autoimmune conditions associated with PAH.

Genetic factors in systemic sclerosis and scleroderma–related PAH

Recent advances in molecular genetics have contributed to the understanding that there is indeed a genetic contribution to the development of PAH. To date, linkage studies have been limited to the subphenotype IPAH and have mostly been performed with modest datasets of multiplex families, i.e. those with two or more affected individuals (47). Polymorphisms involving the bone morphogenetic protein receptor-2 (BMPRII) are present in about 80 percent of familial IPAH (48,49) and up to 20 percent of sporadic (50,51) cases of IPAH. Additional candidate genes have been proposed to influence the pathogenesis of PAH (52). Polymorphisms of the activin-receptor-like kinase 1 (ALK1) gene, which encodes a type 1 TGF-β receptor, have been reported in patients with hereditary hemorrhagic telangiectasia (HHT) and PAH (53).

Although case studies to date suffer from limited statistical power, an increasing number of candidate genes have been reported to be associated with SSc in different populations. A limited list from the burgeoning literature includes the following: a variant in the promoter of monocyte chemotactic protein-1 (MCP-1) (54); two variants in CD19 (−499G > T and a GT repeat polymorphism in the 3′-UTR region) (55); a promoter and coding polymorphism in TNFA (TNFA −238A > G, TNFA 489A > G) (56); a variant in the promoter of the IL-1 alpha gene (IL1A −889T) (57,58); and a 3-SNP haplotype in IL10 (59). In one of the few genetic studies including ethnic minorities, an association was observed for a variant in the first exon of the gene encoding cytotoxic T lymphocyte associated antigen 4 CTLA4 (+49A > G) (60). A genome-wide association analysis provided evidence for association to multiple loci in a Native American population (61). Thus, there are compelling data supporting a genetic basis for SSc. Despite these recent advances in genetics, little is known about genetic involvement in SSc-PAH (62). BMPR2 mutations have not been identified in two small cohorts of SSc-PAH patients (62,63).

Recently, an association between an endoglin gene (ENG) polymorphism and SSc-related PAH was identified. Wipff

and colleagues demonstrated a significant lower frequency of the 6bINS allele in SSc-PAH patients as compared to controls or patients with SSc but no PAH (64). Endoglin, a homodimeric membrane glycoprotein primarily present on human vascular endothelium, is part of the TGF-β receptor complex. The functional significance of the ENG polymorphism in SSc patients remains to be determined.

Aside from the few examples cited above, the genes relevant to the pathogenesis and generally poor outcome associated with SSc-PAH have not been identified, and their definition will require robust, well-characterized patient populations to provide adequate power for analysis.

Clinical features

Risk factors for the development of PAH in SSc patients include late-onset disease (65), an isolated reduction in DLCO, an FVC%/DLCO% ratio greater than 1.6 (66,67), or a combined decreased DLCO/alveolar volume with elevation of serum N-terminal pro-brain natriuretic peptide levels (68) (Table 15.3.1). Typically, patients with SSc-PAH are predominantly women, have limited sclerosis, are older and have seemingly less severe hemodynamic impairment compared to IPAH patients (9). Like in IPAH, clinical symptoms are non-specific, including dyspnea, functional limitation which may be more severe than in IPAH due not only to older age but also to frequent involvement of the musculoskeletal system in these patients. SSc-PAH patients also tend to have other organ involvement such as renal dysfunction and intrinsic heart disease. Indeed patients with SSc (even in the absence of PAH) tend to have depressed RV function (69,70) and left ventricular systolic as well as diastolic dysfunction (71). Like IPAH patients, SSc-PAH patients have severe RV dysfunction at time of presentation but have more severely depressed RV contractility compared to IPAH patients (72). In addition, SSc-PAH patients tend to have more commonly LV diastolic dysfunction and a higher prevalence of pericardial effusion (34 percent compared to 13 percent for IPAH) (9). In both groups, pericardial effusion portends a particularly poor prognosis (9). SSc-PAH patients also tend to have more severe hormonal and metabolic dysfunction such as high levels of N-terminal

Table 15.1 Risk factors for development of pulmonary arterial hypertension in systemic sclerosis

	Reference
Limited systemic sclerosis	67
Late age of onset	65
Raynaud's phenomenon	67
↓ DLCO	66
FVC%/DLCO% > 1.6	67
↑ NT-pro BNP serum level	68
Antibodies (e.g., anti-U3 RNP)	35

brain natriuretic peptide (N-TproBNP) (73) and hypo-natremia (74). Both N-TproBNP and hyponatremia have been shown, at baseline and with serial changes (for N-TproBNP (73)), to correlate with survival in PAH (73,74).

Detection of the disease

An algorithm for detection of PAH in patients with SSc may be helpful if based on a combination of symptoms and screening echocardiography (Figure 15.3.1). In a large French registry, patients with SSc with tricuspid regurgita-tion velocity (TRV) jet by transthoracic echocardiography greater than 3 m/sec or between 2.5 and 3 m/sec if accom-panied by unexplained dyspnea, were systematically referred for right heart catheterization (22). This approach allowed to detect incident cases of SSc-PAH with less severe disease (as judged on hemodynamic data) compared to patients with known disease. Therefore, unexplained dyspnea should prompt a search for PAH in these patients, in particular in the setting of a low single breath DLCO or declining DLCO over time (67), echocardiographic findings suggestive of the disease (elevated TRV jet or dilated RV or right atrium), or elevated levels of N-TproBNP which can reflect cardiac dysfunction and have been found to predict the presence of SSc-PAH (73). Systematic screening should allow for detection of early disease and prompt therapy which, according to some experts, may be beneficial from a prog-nostic standpoint (75).

Prognosis

In general, patients with SSc-PAH tend to have a worse prog-nosis compared to patients with other forms of PAH such as IPAH (Figure 15.3.2). Indeed, one-year survival rates for SSc-PAH patients range from 50 to 81 percent (8,21,23,76), considerably lower than the estimated 88 percent one year survival for IPAH patients (77). In all patients with SSc, PAH significantly worsens survival and is one of the leading causes of mortality in these patients (14,76,78).

PAH ASSOCIATED WITH OTHER CONNECTIVE TISSUE DISEASES

PAH can complicate any connective tissue disease, most frequently systemic sclerosis as discussed above, but also SLE, MCTD, RA, or other diseases such as Sjögren's syn-drome and dermatomyositis.

Systemic lupus erythematosus

There are many reasons for a pulmonary vascular involve-ment in SLE. Like in SSc, there is evidence of endothelial dysfunction in SLE with a potential consequent imbalance between vasodilators and vasoconstrictors. Endothelin lev-els are high in patients with SLE and particularly in those patients with pulmonary hypertension. Release of ET-1

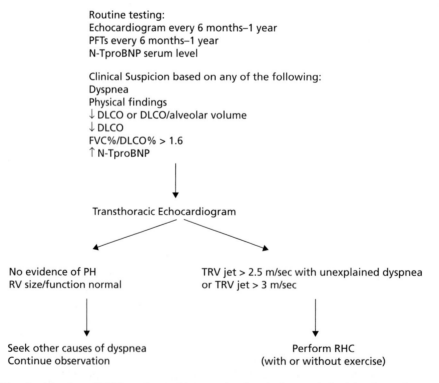

Routine testing:
Echocardiogram every 6 months–1 year
PFTs every 6 months–1 year
N-TproBNP serum level

Clinical Suspicion based on any of the following:
Dyspnea
Physical findings
↓ DLCO or DLCO/alveolar volume
↓ DLCO
FVC%/DLCO% > 1.6
↑ N-TproBNP

Transthoracic Echocardiogram

No evidence of PH
RV size/function normal

TRV jet > 2.5 m/sec with unexplained dyspnea
or TRV jet > 3 m/sec

Seek other causes of dyspnea
Continue observation

Perform RHC
(with or without exercise)

Figure 15.3.1 Algorithm for detection of PAH in patients with systemic sclerosis. Proposed algorithm for performance of routine clinical tests in patients with systemic sclerosis which may allow early detection of pulmonary arterial hypertension or other causes of cardiac dysfunction (e.g., left ventricular dysfunction). PFTs, pulmonary function tests; DLCO, single breath diffusing capacity to carbon monoxide; FVC, forced vital capacity; RV, right ventricle; TRV, tricuspid regurgitation jet; RHC, right heart catheterization.

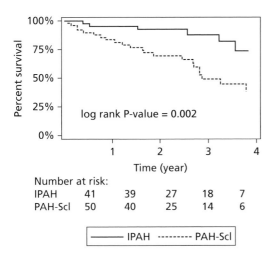

Figure 15.2.2 Survival differences between SSc-PAH and IPAH patients treated with modern therapy: a single-center experience. One- and three-year survival rates are around 87 percent and 48 percent, respectively, in patients with SSc-PAH and 95 percent and 83 percent, respectively, in IPAH patients. SSc-PAH patients are three times more likely to die than IPAH patients despite similar treatment (endothelin receptor antoagonists, prostaglandins or phosphodiesterase inhibitors). (From ref 9, with permission.)

from cultured endothelial cells in response to exposure to serum from SLE patients correlates with levels of aECA and immune complexes (79). Other causes of pulmonary vascular disease that may lead to pulmonary hypertension in SLE include recurrent thromboembolic disease, in particular in patients with a hypercoagulable state from anti-phospholipid antibodies (such as anticardiolipin antibody present in up to 10 percent of patients with SLE) (80), pulmonary vasculitis, and parenchymal disease (including interstitial lung disease, and the shrinking lung syndrome from myositis of the diaphragm). Combined vasculitis and chronic hypoxia are frequent contributing offenders in these syndromes. In addition, pulmonary venous hypertension can be a consequence of left ventricular dysfunction, myocarditis, or Libman–Sacks endocarditis.

The prevalence of PAH in SLE is unclear but is likely less than in SSc, affecting about 0.5–14 percent of patients with SLE in a large review of the literature encompassing over 100 patients (81). The patients are predominantly female (90 percent), young (average age of 33 at time of diagnosis), and often suffer from Raynaud's phenomenon (underscoring a generalized endothelial dysfunction in these patients with SLE and pulmonary hypertension). The pathological lesions are often indistinguishable from IPAH or SSc-PAH lesions, with intimal hyperplasia, smooth muscle cell hypertrophy, and medial thickening. Survival, which was thought to be quite poor (25–50 percent at 2 years) even compared to SSc-PAH in studies antedating specific pulmonary hypertension treatment, is now estimated at 75 percent (82).

Mixed connective tissue disease

Patients with MCTD have clinical features which overlap between those of SSc, SLE, RA, and polymyositis. The exact prevalence of PAH in MCTD is unknown and has been reported as high as 50 percent (83). PAH in these patients may occasionally respond to immunosuppressive drugs (46).

Rheumatoid arthritis

Both the prevalence and impact of pulmonary hypertension in patients with RA is not well known. PAH is however a rather rare complication of RA.

Primary Sjögren's syndrome

Although primary Sjögren's syndrome (pSS) is a relatively common autoimmune disease with glandular and extraglandular manifestations, it is very rarely complicated by PAH. In a recent review by Launay *et al.* of 28 well-characterized patients with pSS and PAH (84), the mean age at diagnosis of PAH of these almost exclusively female patients (27/28) was 50 years. Patients had severe functional class (FC III and IV) and hemodynamic impairment. Standard therapy (with endothelin receptor antagonists, phosphodiesterase inhibitors or prostanoids) was typically ineffective despite an initial improvement. Some patients were reported to respond to immunosuppressive treatment. However, conclusion regarding treatment is limited by the small size of this case report. Survival rate was low (66 percent at 3 years).

THERAPY FOR PAH RELATED TO CTD

Evidence of chronically impaired endothelial function (85–87), affecting vascular tone and remodeling, has been the basis for current therapy of PAH. Vasodilator therapy using high-dose calcium channel blockers is an effective long-term therapy (88), but only for a minority of patients (less than 7 percent (89) of IPAH patients) who demonstrate acute vasodilation (e.g., to NO or adenosine) during hemodynamic testing, and an even smaller number of patients with PAH related to CTD who typically fail to show a vasodilator response to acute testing (only about 2.6 percent responders in that group in one large study (24)). Therefore, high-dose calcium channel therapy is usually not indicated for patients with PAH associated with CTD such as SSc-PAH although most patients often receive these drugs at low dosage, typically for Raynaud's syndrome.

Anti-inflammatory drugs

As discussed above, it has been increasingly recognized that inflammation may play a significant role in various types of pulmonary hypertension, including IPAH and PAH associated with CTD. Interestingly, some patients with severe PAH associated with some forms of CTD (such as SLE, primary Sjögren's syndrome, and mixed connective tissue diseases) have had dramatic improvement of their pulmonary vascular disease with corticosteroids and/or immunosuppressive therapy (46), emphasizing the relevance of inflammation in these subsets of patients. However, this has not been the case for patients with SSc-PAH whose PAH is usually refractory to immunosuppressive drugs (46).

Prostaglandins

Prostacyclin (epoprostenol) has potent pulmonary vasodilator but also anti-platelet aggregating and antiproliferative properties (90), and has proven effective in improving the exercise capacity, cardiopulmonary hemodynamics, NYHA functional class, symptoms, as well as survival in patients with PAH when given by continuous infusion (91–93). In SSc-PAH, continuous intravenous epoprostenol marginally improves exercise capacity and hemodynamics (94), compared to conventional therapy, and there has been no demonstrable effect on survival.

Treprostinil, an analog of epoprostenol suitable for continuous subcutaneous administration, has been shown to have modest effects on symptoms and hemodynamics in PAH (95). In a small study of 16 patients (among whom six had connective tissue disease related PAH), recently FDA-approved intravenous treprostinil was shown to improve hemodynamics 6MWD, FC, and hemodynamics after 12 weeks of therapy (96). Although the safety profile of this drug is similar to IV epoprostenol, required maintenance doses are usually twice as much as for epoprostenol. However, for patients with SSc-PAH, the lack of requirement of ice packing and less frequent mixing of the drug offer significant advantages.

Several reports of pulmonary edema in SSc-PAH patients treated with prostaglandin derivatives, both in acute and chronic settings, have raised the suspicion of increased prevalence of veno-occlusive disease in these patients (97,98), and concern about usefulness of these drugs for this entity. Nevertheless, intravenous prostaglandin therapy remains an option for patients with SSc-PAH with NYHA class IV. Considering the frequent digital problems and disabilities that these patients often experience, this form of therapy can be quite challenging and may increase the already heavy burden of disease in these patients. In summary, both epoprostenol and treprostinil are FDA approved for PAH, but are cumbersome therapies requiring continuous parenteral administration with the attendant numerous adverse effects (e.g., infection and possibility of pump failure (99)), which make these drugs less than ideal.

Endothelin receptor antagonists

Randomized, placebo-controlled trials of 12–16 weeks duration demonstrated a beneficial effect of bosentan therapy on functional class, 6-minute walk distance, time to clinical worsening and hemodynamics in PAH (100,101). In these studies, roughly one fifth of the population consisted of SSc-PAH patients while a large majority had a diagnosis of IPAH. A subgroup analysis, performed by Rubin et al., reported a non-significant trend towards a positive treatment effect on 6-minute walk distance among the SSc-PAH patients treated with bosentan compared to placebo (101). At most, bosentan therapy prevented deterioration in these patients (as assessed by an increase of 3 m in the 6MWD in the treated group compared to a decrease of 40 m in the placebo group). This less than optimal effect of therapy in patients with SSc-PAH is unclear but may be related to the severity of PAH at time of presentation, as well as other factors such as, hypothetically, more severe RV and pulmonary vascular dysfunction, as compared to patients with other forms of PAH (e.g., IPAH).

In a recent analysis of patients with associated PAH related to connective tissue diseases (e.g., patients with lupus, overlap syndrome, and other rheumatological disorders) included in randomized clinical trials of bosentan, there was a trend toward improvement in 6MWD and improved survival compared to historical cohorts (102). Single-center experience suggests that long-tem outcome of first-line bosentan monotherapy is inferior in SSc-PAH compared to IPAH patients, with no change in functional class and worse survival in the former group (103). Since ET-1 appears to play an important pathogenic role in the development of SSc-PAH, contributing to vascular damage and fibrosis, inhibiting ET-1 remains a rational and viable therapeutic strategy in these patients. In fact, in a small study of 35 patients with SSc (10 of whom had SSc-PAH), bosentan treatment appeared to reduce endothelial cell (as determined by endothelial soluble serum factors such as ICAM-1, VCAM-1, P-selection and PECAM-1) and T cell subset (assessed by expression of lymphocyte function-associated antigen-1, very late antigen-4, and L-selectin on CD3 T cells) activation (104). Aside from improving pulmonary hypertension, ET-1 receptor antagonists (specifically bosentan) cause significant reductions in the occurrence of new digital ulcerations without, however, healing preexisting ulcers (105).

In an effort to target the vasoconstrictive effects of endothelin while preserving its vasodilatory action, selective endothelin-A receptor antagonists have been developed. Sitaxsentan, which is only approved in Europe for treatment of PAH, improved exercise capacity (i.e., change in peak VO_2 at week 12, which was the main end-point of the study) (106). Elevation in liver enzymes was noted in 10 percent of patients at the higher dose tested (300 mg orally once daily). Patients with PAH associated with CTD represented less than quarter of the study group. A *post-hoc* analysis of 42 patients (33 patients who received the drug and nine patients who received placebo) with CTD-PAH demonstrated improved exercise capacity, quality of life and hemodynamics with sitaxsentan although elevated liver enzymes were reported in two patients (107).

It should be noted, however, that sitaxsentan has been withdrawn from the market (2010) because of serious liver toxicity and death. A large placebo-controlled, randomized trial of ambrisentan, the only currently FDA-approved selective endothelin receptor antagonist, improved 6MWD in PAH patients at week 12 of treatment, however, the effect was larger in patients with IPAH compared to patients with CTD-PAH (range of 50–60 m vs. 15–23 m, respectively) (108). Ambrisentan is generally well tolerated although peripheral edema (in up to 20 percent of patients (108)) and congestive heart failure have been reported.

Phosphodiesterase inhibitors

Sildenafil, a phosphodiesterase type V inhibitor that reduces the catabolism of cGMP, thereby enhancing the cellular effects mediated by nitric oxide, has become a widely used and highly efficacious therapy for PAH. A recent clinical trial showed that sildenafil therapy led to an improvement in the 6MWD in patients with IPAH and PAH related to CTD or repaired congenital heart disease (patients were predominantly FC II or III) at all three doses tested (20, 40, and 80 mg, given three times a day) (109). Since there were no significant differences in clinical effects and time to clinical worsening at week 12 between the doses, the FDA recommended a dose of 20 mg three times a day. In a *post-hoc* subgroup analysis of 84 patients with PAH related to CTD (45 percent of whom had SSc-PAH), data from the SUPER study suggest that sildenafil at a dose of 20 mg improved exercise capacity (6MWD), hemodynamic measures and functional class after 12 weeks of therapy (110). However, for reasons that remain unclear (but in part related to the limitations of that study such as *post-hoc* subgroup analysis), there was no effect for the dose of 80 mg three times a day on hemodynamics in this subgroup of patients with CTD-related PAH (110). For this reason and because of the potential of increased side-effects (such as bleeding from arterio-venous malformations) at high doses, a sildenafil dosage of 20 mg three times a day is recommended for SSc-PAH patients (and perhaps patients with PAH associated with other forms of CTD) as standard therapy. Higher doses are occasionally attempted in case of limited response. The impact of long-term sildenafil therapy on survival in these patients remains to be determined. Finally, tadalafil, another phosphodiesterase inhibitor, has now been shown to be effective for PAH although subgroup analysis has not been performed yet and thus its effects on CTD-PAH remain unclear. Tadalafil has the advantage over sildenafil of single daily dosage (111).

Combination therapy

It is now common practice to add drugs when patients fail to improve on monotherapy. Adding inhaled iloprost to patients receiving bosentan has been shown to be beneficial in a small, randomized trial. Combining inhaled iloprost with sildenafil is mechanistically appealing and anecdotally efficacious (112,113) as these drugs target separate, potentially synergistic pathways. Several multicenter trials are now exploring the efficacy of various combinations of two oral drugs or one oral and one inhaled drug. The recently published results of the PACES trial demonstrate that adding sildenafil (at a dose of 80 mg three times a day) to intravenous epoprostenol improves exercise capacity, hemodynamic measurements, time to clinical worsening, and quality of life (114). About 21 percent of these patients had CTD, including 11 percent with SSc-PAH. Although no specific subgroup analysis is provided, improvement was apparently mainly in patients with IPAH. In a smaller one center clinical trial, adding sildenafil to patients with IPAH or scleroderma-related PAH after they failed initial monotherapy with bosentan, demonstrates that combination therapy improved the 6MWD and FC in IPAH patients. The outcome in patients with SSc-PAH was less favorable, although combination therapy may have halted clinical deterioration. In addition, there were more side-effects reported in the SSc-PAH compared to the IPAH patients, including hepatotoxicity that developed after addition of sildenafil to bosentan monotherapy (115).

Anticoagulation

The rationale for the use of anticoagulation in severe PAH is based on pathologic evidence of pulmonary thromboembolic arterial disease and thrombosis *in situ* in patients with IPAH (116), and two clinical studies (a retrospective analysis) (117) and a small, non-randomized prospective study (88) demonstrating a significant beneficial effect of anticoagulation on survival in IPAH. Based essentially on these findings, anticoagulation is routinely recommended in the treatment of IPAH patients. The role of anticoagulation in other forms of PAH, in particular in SSc-PAH or other forms of CTD is much less clear. Theoretically, there is potential for increased bleeding in patients with CTD, particularly with SSc where intestinal telangiectasias may be common. An unpublished review of our experience with anticoagulation in over 100 patients with SSc-PAH suggests that less than 50 percent of these patients remain on long-term anticoagulation therapy. The reason for discontinuing anticoagulation in these patients is often related to occult bleeding in the gastrointestinal tract. In our experience, the source of bleeding is often difficult to diagnose.

Tyrosine kinase inhibitors

The finding that there is pathologically aberrant proliferation of endothelial and smooth muscle cells in PAH, as well as increased expression of secreted growth factors such as VEGF and bFGF, has caused a shift in paradigm in treatment strategies for this disease as some investigators have likened this condition to a neoplastic process reminiscent of advanced solid tumors (118). As a result, antineoplastic drugs have been tested in experimental models (119,120) and some patients (121,122). Two strategies are currently tested for treatment of PAH: disruption of PDGF signaling and disruption of the VEGF signaling pathway. The results of a phase II multicenter trial to evaluate the safety, tolerability, and efficacy of this drug in patients with PAH have recently published and indicate that imatinib is well tolerated in PAH patients. While there was no significant change in 6 minute walk distance (primary end-point) there was a significant decrease in pulmonary vascular resistance and an increase in cardiac output in imatinib-treated patients versus placebo (123). Whether these new antineoplastic drugs with antityrosine kinase activity will have a role in PAH associated with CTD such as SSc-PAH (where there is evidence for both dysregulated proliferation and increased expression of growth factors such as VEGF) remains to be determined.

Lung transplantation

Lung transplantation (LT) is typically offered as a last resort to patients with PAH who fail medical therapy. Although CTD is not an absolute contraindication to lung transplantation, patients with CTD often have associated morbidity and organ dysfunction other than the lung that place them at a specifically high risk for LT. The involvement of the esophagus with severe motility disorder and gastroesophageal reflux in patients with SSc is an example of specific risk that surgeons do not take lightly because of the enhanced postoperative potential of aspiration and damage to the recipient lung. For these reasons, patients with SSc-PAH are often denied the LT option. However, if properly screened and approved for LT, patients with SSc experience similar rates of survival 2 years after the procedure compared with patients who receive LT for pulmonary fibrosis or IPAH (124).

SURVIVAL OF PATIENTS WITH CTD AND PAH

Despite the recent increase in drugs targeting specific pathways in PAH, survival of patients with CTD and PAH remains unacceptably low although there is evidence of mild survival improvement in patients with SSc-PAH (Figure 15.3.3) compared to similar historical controls (75). The reason for a discrepancy in survival between IPAH patients and patients with CTD and PAH, particularly SSc-PAH (Figure 15.3.2), remains poorly understood and may involve more complex disturbances, such as an increased prevalence of pulmonary veno-occlusive lung disease (7) (Figure 15.3.3), or more severe vascular lesions affecting not only proximal and distal pulmonary vessels but also the heart (such as inflammatory myocarditis) in CTD. Thus, a better understanding of the underlying pathophysiology as well as the RV-pulmonary vascular interaction and uncoupling in this disease is needed for better targeted therapy. Whether specific anti-inflammatory agents or drugs targeting tyrosine kinase activity hold any promise of better response is unclear at this time but needs to be explored.

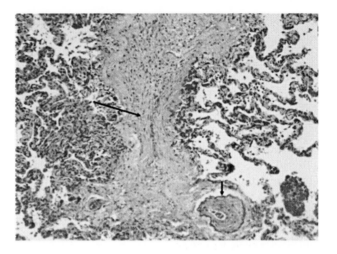

Figure 15.3.3 Evidence of pulmonary veno-occlusive disease in a patient with systemic sclerosis. Histology demonstrates complete occlusion of an interlobular septal vein (arrow) and also partial occlusion of a branch extending into alveolar tissue (short arrow), outlined by Movat staining.

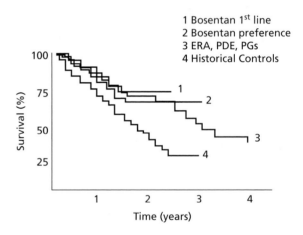

Figure 15.3.4 Survival in SSc-PAH compared to "historical controls." Survival has improved in SSc-PAH patients treated with bosentan (1) as first-line therapy, bosentan preference (2), or various current therapies for PAH (3) including endothelin receptor antagonists (ERA), prostaglandins (PGs) and phosphodiesterase inhibitors (PDE) compared to historical controls (4) treated with conventional therapy +/− PGs. (Adapted from refs 9, 75, and 103.)

CONCLUSION

Pulmonary hypertension is a common complication of CTD, particularly SSc where it has a significantly worse outcome compared to other diseases (such as IPAH) within group 1 of the WHO classification. In addition, modern therapy for PAH appears to be of limited value in SSc-PAH (Figure 15.3.4). Similarly, currently available markers of disease severity or response to therapy in SSc-PAH and other CTD are either limited or lacking. Therefore, there is an urgent need to identify potential genetic causes and novel physiologic, molecular, and imaging biomarkers that will allow a better understanding of the underlying pathogenesis and serve as reliable tools to monitor therapy in this devastating syndrome.

KEY POINTS

- Pulmonary hypertension is a common complication of connective tissue diseases and generally portends a very poor prognosis.
- Prognosis and response to modern therapy for pulmonary hypertension are significantly worse compared to other diseases characterized by pulmonary hypertension.
- There are several clinical markers of pulmonary hypertension in connective tissue diseases which may allow early detection of the disease when followed systematically. Theoretically, early treatment may allow improved survival.
- A search for genetic factors and pathogenic mechanisms involved in connective tissue diseases such as systemic sclerosis is warranted and would allow development of targeted therapy.

REFERENCES

- = Key primary paper
◆ = Major review article

1. D'Alonzo GE, Barst RJ, Ayres SM et al. Survival in patients with primary pulmonary hypertension. Results from a national prospective registry. Ann Intern Med 1991;115(5):343–9.
2. Gaine SP, Rubin LJ. Primary pulmonary hypertension. Lancet 1998;352(9129):719–25.
3. Rich S, Dantzker DR, Ayres SM et al. Primary pulmonary hypertension. A national prospective study. Ann Intern Med 1987;107(2):216–23.
4. Barst RJ, McGoon M, Torbicki A et al. Diagnosis and differential assessment of pulmonary arterial hypertension. J Am Coll Cardiol 2004;43(12 Suppl S):40S–7S.
5. Isern RA, Yaneva M, Weiner E et al. Autoantibodies in patients with primary pulmonary hypertension: association with anti-Ku. Am J Med 1992;93(3):307–12.
6. Humbert M, Monti G, Brenot F et al. Increased interleukin-1 and interleukin-6 serum concentrations in severe primary pulmonary hypertension. Am J Respir Crit Care Med 1995;151(5):1628–31.
7. Do rfmuller P, Humbert M, Perros F et al. Fibrous remodeling of the pulmonary venous system in pulmonary arterial hypertension associated with connective tissue diseases. Hum Pathol 2007;38(6):893–902.
•8. Kawut SM, Taichman DB, Archer-Chicko CL, Palevsky HI, Kimmel SE. Hemodynamics and survival in patients with

pulmonary arterial hypertension related to systemic sclerosis. Chest 2003;123(2):344–50.
•9. Fisher MR, Mathai SC, Champion HC et al. Clinical differences between idiopathic and scleroderma-related pulmonary hypertension. Arthritis Rheum 2006;54(9):3043–50.
◆10. Jimenez SA, Derk CT. Following the molecular pathways toward an understanding of the pathogenesis of systemic sclerosis. Ann Intern Med 2004;140(1):37–50.
11. Tan FK. Systemic sclerosis: the susceptible host (genetics and environment). Rheum Dis Clin North Am 2003;29(2):211–37.
12. LeRoy EC, Black C, Fleischmajer R et al. Scleroderma (systemic sclerosis): classification, subsets and pathogenesis. J Rheumatol 1988;15(2):202–5.
•13. Mayes MD, Lacey JV, Jr., Beebe-Dimmer J et al. Prevalence, incidence, survival, and disease characteristics of systemic sclerosis in a large US population. Arthritis Rheum 2003;48(8):2246–55.
14. Mayes MD. Scleroderma epidemiology. Rheum Dis Clin North Am 2003;29(2):239–54.
15. Silman A, Jannini S, Symmons D, Bacon P. An epidemiological study of scleroderma in the West Midlands. Br J Rheumatol 1988;27(4):286–90.
16. Tamaki T, Mori S, Takehara K. Epidemiological study of patients with systemic sclerosis in Tokyo. Arch Dermatol Res 1991;283(6):366–71.
17. Allcock RJ, Forrest I, Corris PA, Crook PR, Griffiths ID. A study of the prevalence of systemic sclerosis in northeast England. Rheumatology (Oxford) 2004;43(5):596–602.
18. Battle RW, Davitt MA, Cooper SM et al. Prevalence of pulmonary hypertension in limited and diffuse scleroderma. Chest 1996;110(6):1515–9.
19. Stupi AM, Steen VD, Owens GR, Barnes EL, Rodnan GP, Medsger TA, Jr. Pulmonary hypertension in the CREST syndrome variant of systemic sclerosis. Arthritis Rheum 1986;29(4):515–24.
20. Sacks DG, Okano Y, Steen VD, Curtiss E, Shapiro LS, Medsger TA, Jr. Isolated pulmonary hypertension in systemic sclerosis with diffuse cutaneous involvement: association with serum anti-U3RNP antibody. J Rheumatol 1996;23(4):639–42.
21. MacGregor AJ, Canavan R, Knight C et al. Pulmonary hypertension in systemic sclerosis: risk factors for progression and consequences for survival. Rheumatology (Oxford) 2001;40(4):453–9.
•22 Hachulla E, Gressin V, Guillevin L et al. Early detection of pulmonary arterial hypertension in systemic sclerosis: a French nationwide prospective multicenter study. Arthritis Rheum 2005;52(12):3792–800.
•23. Mukerjee D, St George D, Coleiro B et al. Prevalence and outcome in systemic sclerosis associated pulmonary arterial hypertension: application of a registry approach. Ann Rheum Dis 2003;62(11):1088–93.
•24. Humbert M, Sitbon O, Chaouat A et al. Pulmonary arterial hypertension in France: results from a national registry. Am J Respir Crit Care Med 2006;173(9):1023–30.

25. Peacock AJ, Murphy NF, McMurray JJ, Caballero L, Stewart S. An epidemiological study of pulmonary arterial hypertension. Eur Respir J 2007;30(1):104–9.

26. LeRoy EC. Systemic sclerosis. A vascular perspective. Rheum Dis Clin North Am 1996;22(4):675–94.

27. Fleischmajer R, Perlish JS. Capillary alterations in scleroderma. J Am Acad Dermatol 1980;2(2):161–70.

28. Sgonc R, Gruschwitz MS, Boeck G, Sepp N, Gruber J, Wick G. Endothelial cell apoptosis in systemic sclerosis is induced by antibody-dependent cell-mediated cytotoxicity via CD95. Arthritis Rheum 2000;43(11):2550–62.

29. Cerinic MM, Valentini G, Sorano GG et al. Blood coagulation, fibrinolysis, and markers of endothelial dysfunction in systemic sclerosis. Semin Arthritis Rheum 2003;32(5):285–95.

30. Altman RD, Medsger TA, Jr., Bloch DA, Michel BA. Predictors of survival in systemic sclerosis (scleroderma). Arthritis Rheum 1991;34(4):403–13.

31. Denton CP, Bickerstaff MC, Shiwen X et al. Serial circulating adhesion molecule levels reflect disease severity in systemic sclerosis. Br J Rheumatol 1995;34(11):1048–54.

32. Distler O, Del Rosso A, Giacomelli R et al. Angiogenic and angiostatic factors in systemic sclerosis: increased levels of vascular endothelial growth factor are a feature of the earliest disease stages and are associated with the absence of fingertip ulcers. Arthritis Res 2002;4(6):R11.

33. Choi JJ, Min DJ, Cho ML et al. Elevated vascular endothelial growth factor in systemic sclerosis. J Rheumatol 2003;30(7):1529–33.

34. Hebbar M, Peyrat JP, Hornez L, Hatron PY, Hachulla E, Devulder B. Increased concentrations of the circulating angiogenesis inhibitor endostatin in patients with systemic sclerosis. Arthritis Rheum 2000;43(4):889–93.

•35. Okano Y, Steen VD, Medsger TA, Jr. Autoantibody to U3 nucleolar ribonucleoprotein (fibrillarin) in patients with systemic sclerosis. Arthritis Rheum 1992;35(1):95–100.

36. Negi VS, Tripathy NK, Misra R, Nityanand S. Antiendothelial cell antibodies in scleroderma correlate with severe digital ischemia and pulmonary arterial hypertension. J Rheumatol 1998;25(3):462–6.

•37. Tamby MC, Chanseaud Y, Humbert M et al. Anti-endothelial cell antibodies in idiopathic and systemic sclerosis associated pulmonary arterial hypertension. Thorax 2005;60(9):765–72.

38. Fritzler MJ, Hart DA, Wilson D et al. Antibodies to fibrin bound tissue type plasminogen activator in systemic sclerosis. J Rheumatol 1995;22(9):1688–93.

39. Morse JH, Barst RJ, Fotino M et al. Primary pulmonary hypertension, tissue plasminogen activator antibodies, and HLA-DQ7. Am J Respir Crit Care Med 1997;155(1):274–8.

40. Grigolo B, Mazzetti I, Meliconi R et al. Anti-topoisomerase II alpha autoantibodies in systemic sclerosis–association with pulmonary hypertension and HLA-B35. Clin Exp Immunol 2000;121(3):539–43.

41. Nicolls MR, Taraseviciene-Stewart L, Rai PR, Badesch DB, Voelkel NF. Autoimmunity and pulmonary hypertension: a perspective. Eur Respir J 2005;26(6):1110–8.

42. Okawa-Takatsuji M, Aotsuka S, Fujinami M, Uwatoko S, Kinoshita M, Sumiya M. Up-regulation of intercellular adhesion molecule-1 (ICAM-1), endothelial leucocyte adhesion molecule-1 (ELAM-1) and class II MHC molecules on pulmonary artery endothelial cells by antibodies against U1-ribonucleoprotein. Clin Exp Immunol 1999;116(1):174–80.

43. Chizzolini C, Raschi E, Rezzonico R et al. Autoantibodies to fibroblasts induce a proadhesive and proinflammatory fibroblast phenotype in patients with systemic sclerosis. Arthritis Rheum 2002;46(6):1602–13.

44. Tamby MC, Humbert M, Guilpain P et al. Antibodies to fibroblasts in idiopathic and scleroderma-associated pulmonary hypertension. Eur Respir J 2006;28(4):799–807.

45. Terrier B, Tamby MC, Camoin L et al. Identification of target antigens of antifibroblast antibodies in pulmonary arterial hypertension. Am J Respir Crit Care Med 2008;177(10):1128–34.

46. Sanchez O, Sitbon O, Jais X, Simonneau G, Humbert M. Immunosuppressive therapy in connective tissue diseases-associated pulmonary arterial hypertension. Chest 2006;130(1):182–9.

47. Nichols WC, Koller DL, Slovis B et al. Localization of the gene for familial primary pulmonary hypertension to chromosome 2q31–32. Nature Genet 1997;15(3):277–80.

•48 Deng Z, Morse JH, Slager SL et al. Familial primary pulmonary hypertension (gene PPH1) is caused by mutations in the bone morphogenetic protein receptor-II gene. Am J Hum Genet 2000;67(3):737–44.

•49 Lane KB, Machado RD, Pauciulo MW et al. Heterozygous germline mutations in BMPR2, encoding a TGF-beta receptor, cause familial primary pulmonary hypertension. The International PPH Consortium. Nat Genet 2000;26(1):81–4.

50. Newman JH, Trembath RC, Morse JA et al. Genetic basis of pulmonary arterial hypertension: current understanding and future directions. J Am Coll Cardiol 2004;43(12 Suppl S):33S–9S.

51. Koehler R, Grunig E, Pauciulo MW et al. Low frequency of BMPR2 mutations in a German cohort of patients with sporadic idiopathic pulmonary arterial hypertension. J Med Genet 2004;41(12):e127.

52. Morse JH, Deng Z, Knowles JA. Genetic aspects of pulmonary arterial hypertension. Ann Med 2001;33(9):596–603.

53. Trembath RC, Thomson JR, Machado RD et al. Clinical and molecular genetic features of pulmonary hypertension in patients with hereditary hemorrhagic telangiectasia. N Engl J Med 2001;345(5):325–34.

54. Karrer S, Bosserhoff AK, Weiderer P et al. The –2518 promotor polymorphism in the MCP-1 gene is associated with systemic sclerosis. J Invest Dermatol 2005;124(1):92–8.

55. Tsuchiya N, Kuroki K, Fujimoto M et al. Association of a functional CD19 polymorphism with susceptibility to systemic sclerosis. Arthritis Rheum 2004;50(12):4002–7.

56. Tolusso B, Fabris M, Caporali R *et al.* −238 and +489 TNF-alpha along with TNF-RII gene polymorphisms associate with the diffuse phenotype in patients with systemic sclerosis. Immunol Lett 2005;96(1): 103–8.

57. Kawaguchi Y, Tochimoto A, Ichikawa N *et al.* Association of IL1A gene polymorphisms with susceptibility to and severity of systemic sclerosis in the Japanese population. Arthritis Rheum 2003;48(1):186–92.

58. Hutyrova B, Lukac J, Bosak V, Buc M, du Bois R, Petrek M. Interleukin 1alpha single-nucleotide polymorphism associated with systemic sclerosis. J Rheumatol 2004;31(1):81–4.

59. Crilly A, Hamilton J, Clark CJ, Jardine A, Madhok R. Analysis of the 5′ flanking region of the interleukin 10 gene in patients with systemic sclerosis. Rheumatology (Oxford) 2003;42(11):1295–8.

60. Hudson LL, Silver RM, Pandey JP. Ethnic differences in cytotoxic T lymphocyte associated antigen 4 genotype associations with systemic sclerosis. J Rheumatol 2004;31(1):85–7.

61. Zhou X, Tan FK, Wang N *et al.* Genome-wide association study for regions of systemic sclerosis susceptibility in a Choctaw Indian population with high disease prevalence. Arthritis Rheum 2003;48(9):2585–92.

•62 Morse J, Barst R, Horn E, Cuervo N, Deng Z, Knowles J. Pulmonary hypertension in scleroderma spectrum of disease: lack of bone morphogenetic protein receptor 2 mutations. J Rheumatol 2002;29(11):2379–81.

•63 Tew MB, Arnett FC, Reveille JD, Tan FK. Mutations of bone morphogenetic protein receptor type II are not found in patients with pulmonary hypertension and underlying connective tissue diseases. Arthritis Rheum 2002;46(10): 2829–30.

•64 Wipff J, Kahan A, Hachulla E *et al.* Association between an endoglin gene polymorphism and systemic sclerosis-related pulmonary arterial hypertension. Rheumatology (Oxford) 2007;46(4):622–5.

65. Schachna L, Wigley FM, Chang B, White B, Wise RA, Gelber AC. Age and risk of pulmonary arterial hypertension in scleroderma. Chest 2003;124(6):2098–104.

66. Chang B, Schachna L, White B, Wigley FM, Wise RA. Natural history of mild-moderate pulmonary hypertension and the risk factors for severe pulmonary hypertension in scleroderma. J Rheumatol 2006;33(2):269–74.

•67 Steen V, Medsger TA, Jr. Predictors of isolated pulmonary hypertension in patients with systemic sclerosis and limited cutaneous involvement. Arthritis Rheum 2003; 48(2):516–22.

68. Allanore Y, Borderie D, Avouac J *et al.* High N-terminal pro-brain natriuretic peptide levels and low diffusing capacity for carbon monoxide as independent predictors of the occurrence of precapillary pulmonary arterial hypertension in patients with systemic sclerosis. Arthritis Rheum 2008;58(1):284–91.

69. Hsiao SH, Lee CY, Chang SM, Lin SK, Liu CP. Right heart function in scleroderma: insights from myocardial

Doppler tissue imaging. J Am Soc Echocardiogr 2006; 19(5):507–14.

70. Lee CY, Chang SM, Hsiao SH, Tseng JC, Lin SK, Liu CP. Right heart function and scleroderma: insights from tricuspid annular plane systolic excursion. Echocardiography 2007;24(2):118–25.

71. Meune C, Avouac J, Wahbi K *et al.* Cardiac involvement in systemic sclerosis assessed by tissue–Doppler echocardiography during routine care: a controlled study of 100 consecutive patients. Arthritis Rheum 2008;58(6):1803–9.

72. Overbeek MJ, Lankhaar JW, Westerhof N *et al.* Right ventricular contractility in systemic sclerosis-associated and idiopathic pulmonary arterial hypertension. Eur Respir J 2008;31(6):1160–6.

•73 Williams MH, Handler CE, Akram R *et al.* Role of N-terminal brain natriuretic peptide (N-TproBNP) in scleroderma-associated pulmonary arterial hypertension. Eur Heart J 2006;27(12):1485–94.

74. Forfia PR, Mathai SC, Fisher MR *et al.* Hyponatremia predicts right heart failure and poor survival in pulmonary arterial hypertension. Am J Respir Crit Care Med 2008;177(12):1364–9.

•75 Williams MH, Das C, Handler CE *et al.* Systemic sclerosis associated pulmonary hypertension: improved survival in the current era. Heart 2006;92(7):926–32.

76. Koh ET, Lee P, Gladman DD, Abu-Shakra M. Pulmonary hypertension in systemic sclerosis: an analysis of 17 patients. Br J Rheumatol 1996;35(10):989–93.

77. McLaughlin VV, Shillington A, Rich S. Survival in primary pulmonary hypertension: the impact of epoprostenol therapy. Circulation 2002;106(12):1477–82.

◆78 Steen VD, Medsger TA. Changes in causes of death in systemic sclerosis, 1972–2002. Ann Rheum Dis 2007;66(7):940–4.

79. Yoshio T, Masuyama J, Mimori A, Takeda A, Minota S, Kano S. Endothelin-1 release from cultured endothelial cells induced by sera from patients with systemic lupus erythematosus. Ann Rheum Dis 1995;54(5): 361–5.

80. Pope J. An update in pulmonary hypertension in systemic lupus erythematosus – do we need to know about it? Lupus 2008;17(4):274–7.

81. Haas C. Pulmonary hypertension associated with systemic lupus erythematosus. Bull Acad Natl Med 2004; 188(6):985–97; discussion 97.

82. Condliffe R, Kiely DG, Peacock AJ *et al.* Connective tissue disease associated pulmonary arterial hypertension in the modern treatment era. Am J Respir Crit Care Med 2008;179:151–7.

83. Sullivan WD, Hurst DJ, Harmon CE *et al.* A prospective evaluation emphasizing pulmonary involvement in patients with mixed connective tissue disease. Medicine (Baltimore) 1984;63(2):92–107.

◆84 Launay D, Hachulla E, Hatron PY, Jais X, Simonneau G, Humbert M. Pulmonary arterial hypertension: a rare complication of primary Sjogren syndrome: report of

9 new cases and review of the literature. Medicine (Baltimore) 2007;86(5):299–315.

85. Giaid A, Saleh D. Reduced expression of endothelial nitric oxide synthase in the lungs of patients with pulmonary hypertension. N Engl J Med 1995;333(4): 214–21.

86. Tuder RM, Cool CD, Geraci MW et al. Prostacyclin synthase expression is decreased in lungs from patients with severe pulmonary hypertension. Am J Respir Crit Care Med 1999;159(6):1925–32.

87. Giaid A, Yanagisawa M, Langleben D et al. Expression of endothelin-1 in the lungs of patients with pulmonary hypertension. N Engl J Med 1993;328(24):1732–9.

88. Rich S, Kaufmann E, Levy PS. The effect of high doses of calcium-channel blockers on survival in primary pulmonary hypertension. N Engl J Med 1992;327(2): 76–81.

89. Sitbon O, Humbert M, Jais X et al. Long-term response to calcium channel blockers in idiopathic pulmonary arterial hypertension. Circulation 2005;111(23):3105–11.

90. Vane JR, Anggard EE, Botting RM. Regulatory functions of the vascular endothelium. N Engl J Med 1990;323(1): 27–36.

91. Barst RJ, Rubin LJ, Long WA et al. A comparison of continuous intravenous epoprostenol (prostacyclin) with conventional therapy for primary pulmonary hypertension. The Primary Pulmonary Hypertension Study Group. N Engl J Med 1996;334(5):296–302.

92. McLaughlin VV, Genthner DE, Panella MM, Rich S. Reduction in pulmonary vascular resistance with long-term epoprostenol (prostacyclin) therapy in primary pulmonary hypertension. N Engl J Med 1998;338(5):273–7.

93. Rubin LJ, Mendoza J, Hood M et al. Treatment of primary pulmonary hypertension with continuous intravenous prostacyclin (epoprostenol). Results of a randomized trial. Ann Intern Med 1990;112(7):485–91.

•94. Badesch DB, Tapson VF, McGoon MD et al. Continuous intravenous epoprostenol for pulmonary hypertension due to the scleroderma spectrum of disease. A randomized, controlled trial. Ann Intern Med 2000;132(6):425–34.

95. Simonneau G, Barst RJ, Galie N et al. Continuous subcutaneous infusion of treprostinil, a prostacyclin analogue, in patients with pulmonary arterial hypertension: a double-blind, randomized, placebo-controlled trial. Am J Respir Crit Care Med 2002;165(6):800–4.

96. Tapson VF, Gomberg-Maitland M, McLaughlin VV et al. Safety and efficacy of IV treprostinil for pulmonary arterial hypertension: a prospective, multicenter, open-label, 12-week trial. Chest 2006;129(3):683–8.

97. Farber HW, Graven KK, Kokolski G, Korn JH. Pulmonary edema during acute infusion of epoprostenol in a patient with pulmonary hypertension and limited scleroderma. J Rheumatol 1999;26(5):1195–6.

98. Palmer SM, Robinson LJ, Wang A, Gossage JR, Bashore T, Tapson VF. Massive pulmonary edema and death after prostacyclin infusion in a patient with pulmonary veno-occlusive disease. Chest 1998;113(1):237–40.

99. Galie N, Manes A, Branzi A. Emerging medical therapies for pulmonary arterial hypertension. Prog Cardiovasc Dis 2002;45(3):213–24.

100. Channick RN, Simonneau G, Sitbon O et al. Effects of the dual endothelin-receptor antagonist bosentan in patients with pulmonary hypertension: a randomised placebo-controlled study. Lancet 2001;358(9288): 1119–23.

101. Rubin LJ, Badesch DB, Barst RJ et al. Bosentan therapy for pulmonary arterial hypertension. N Engl J Med 2002; 346(12):896–903.

102. Denton CP, Humbert M, Rubin L, Black CM. Bosentan treatment for pulmonary arterial hypertension related to connective tissue disease: a subgroup analysis of the pivotal clinical trials and their open-label extensions. Ann Rheum Dis 2006;65(10):1336–40.

103. Girgis RE, Mathai SC, Krishnan JA, Wigley FM, Hassoun PM. Long-term outcome of bosentan treatment in idiopathic pulmonary arterial hypertension and pulmonary arterial hypertension associated with the scleroderma spectrum of diseases. J Heart Lung Transplant 2005;24(10):1626–31.

104. Iannone F, Riccardi MT, Guiducci S et al. Bosentan regulates the expression of adhesion molecules on circulating T cells and serum soluble adhesion molecules in systemic sclerosis-associated pulmonary arterial hypertension. Ann Rheum Dis 2008;67(8):1121–6.

105. Jain M, Varga J. Bosentan for the treatment of systemic sclerosis-associated pulmonary arterial hypertension, pulmonary fibrosis and digital ulcers. Expert Opin Pharmacother 2006;7(11):1487–501.

106. Barst RJ, Langleben D, Frost A et al. Sitaxsentan therapy for pulmonary arterial hypertension. Am J Respir Crit Care Med 2004;169(4):441–7.

107. Girgis RE, Frost AE, Hill NS et al. Selective endothelin A receptor antagonism with sitaxsentan for pulmonary arterial hypertension associated with connective tissue disease. Ann Rheum Dis 2007;66(11):1467–72.

108. Galie N, Olschewski H, Oudiz RJ et al. Ambrisentan for the treatment of pulmonary arterial hypertension: results of the ambrisentan in pulmonary arterial hypertension, randomized, double-blind, placebo-controlled, multicenter, efficacy (ARIES) study 1 and 2. Circulation 2008;117(23): 3010–9.

109. Galie N, Ghofrani HA, Torbicki A et al. Sildenafil citrate therapy for pulmonary arterial hypertension. N Engl J Med 2005;353(20):2148–57.

110. Badesch DB, Hill NS, Burgess G et al. Sildenafil for pulmonary arterial hypertension associated with connective tissue disease. J Rheumatol 2007;34(12): 2417–22.

111. Galie N, Brundage BH, Ghofrani HA, et al. Tadalafil therapy for pulmonary arterial hypertension. Circulation 2009;119(22):2894–903.

112. McLaughlin VV, Oudiz RJ, Frost A et al. Randomized study of adding inhaled iloprost to existing bosentan in pulmonary arterial hypertension. Am J Respir Crit Care Med 2006;174(11):1257–63.

113. Hoeper MM, Faulenbach C, Golpon H, Winkler J, Welte T, Niedermeyer J. Combination therapy with bosentan and sildenafil in idiopathic pulmonary arterial hypertension. Eur Respir J 2004;24(6):1007–10.

114. Simonneau G, Rubin LJ, Galie N et al. Addition of sildenafil to long-term intravenous epoprostenol therapy in patients with pulmonary arterial hypertension: a randomized trial. Ann Intern Med 2008;149(8):521–30.

115. Mathai SC, Girgis RE, Fisher MR et al. Addition of sildenafil to bosentan monotherapy in pulmonary arterial hypertension. Eur Respir J 2007;29(3):469–75.

116. Pietra GG. Histopathology of primary pulmonary hypertension. Chest 1994;105(2 Suppl):2S–6S.

117. Fuster V, Steele PM, Edwards WD, Gersh BJ, McGoon MD, Frye RL. Primary pulmonary hypertension: natural history and the importance of thrombosis. Circulation 1984;70(4):580–7.

118. Adnot S. Lessons learned from cancer may help in the treatment of pulmonary hypertension. J Clin Invest 2005;115(6):1461–3.

119. Schermuly RT, Dony E, Ghofrani HA et al. Reversal of experimental pulmonary hypertension by PDGF inhibition. J Clin Invest 2005;115(10):2811–21.

120. Moreno-Vinasco L, Gomberg-Maitland M, Maitland ML et al. Genomic assessment of a multikinase inhibitor, sorafenib, in a rodent model of pulmonary hypertension. Physiol Genomics 2008;33(2):278–91.

121. Ghofrani HA, Seeger W, Grimminger F. Imatinib for the treatment of pulmonary arterial hypertension. N Engl J Med 2005;353(13):1412–3.

•122. Patterson KC, Weissmann A, Ahmadi T, Farber HW. Imatinib mesylate in the treatment of refractory idiopathic pulmonary arterial hypertension. Ann Intern Med 2006;145(2):152–3.

123. Ghofrani HA, Morrell NW, Hoeper MM, et al. Imatinib in pulmonary arterial hypertension patients with inadequate response to established therapy. AM J Respir Crit Care Med.

124. Schachna L, Medsger TA, Jr., Dauber JH et al. Lung transplantation in scleroderma compared with idiopathic pulmonary fibrosis and idiopathic pulmonary arterial hypertension. Arthritis Rheum 2006;54(12):3954–61.

Pulmonary hypertension related to appetite suppressants

OLIVIER SITBON, MARC HUMBERT AND GÉRALD SIMONNEAU

INTRODUCTION

The classification of pulmonary hypertension has gone through a series of changes since the first classification was proposed in 1973 at an international conference on pulmonary hypertension endorsed by the World Health Organization (WHO) (1). Twenty-five years later, a new diagnostic classification of pulmonary hypertension was proposed at the 1998 WHO Pulmonary Hypertension Meeting held in Evian, France (2). The "Evian Classification" attempted to create categories of pulmonary hypertension that shared pathological and clinical features as well as similar therapeutic options (2). It reflected advances in the understanding of pulmonary hypertensive diseases, and recognized the similarity between "unexplained" pulmonary hypertension (formerly called "primary" pulmonary hypertension ["PPH"]) and pulmonary arterial hypertension (PAH) associated with several conditions and diseases, such as connective tissue diseases, portal hypertension, congenital left-to-right cardiac shunts, HIV infection, and exposure to toxins and drugs including appetite suppressants. Five years after the Evian conference, a third World Symposium on Pulmonary Arterial Hypertension was held in Venice, Italy. The impact and usefulness of the Evian Classification was reviewed at this conference and modest changes were made (3). During the fourth World Symposium on Pulmonary Hypertension held in 2008 in Dana Point, California, the consensus agreement of experts worldwide was to maintain

the general philosophy and organization of the Evian–Venice classifications (4). Considering the place of anorectic drugs in the diagnostic classification of pulmonary hypertension, no change has been made since the publication of the Evian Classification. Among anorectic drugs, aminorex fumarate and fenfluramine derivatives (Figure 15.4.1) have been reported to be associated with the development of PAH and are considered for many years as definite risk factors for PAH, playing a causal role (Table 15.4.1) (5,6).

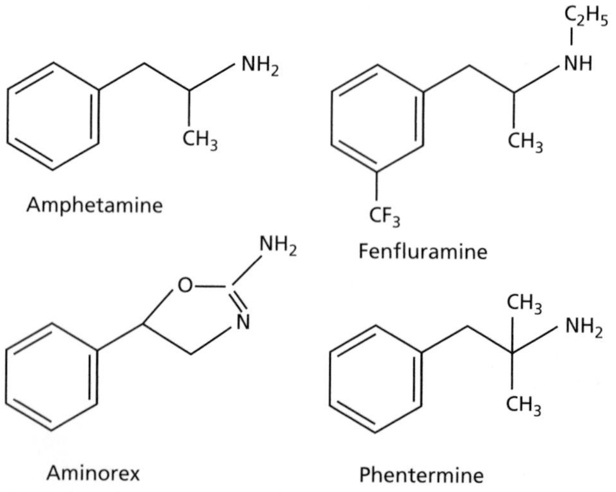

Figure 15.4.1 Chemical structure of amphetamine and other related anorectic drugs (aminorex, fenfluramine, phentermine).

DEFINITION OF A RISK FACTOR FOR PULMONARY ARTERIAL HYPERTENSION

A number of risk factors for the development of PAH have been identified and were included in the Evian, Venice and Dana Point classifications (2–4). A risk factor for PAH is any factor or condition that is suspected to play a causal or facilitating role in the development of the disease (2,5,6). Because risk factors relate to the probability of occurrence of the disease, they must be present prior to the onset of the disease. Risk factors may include drugs, chemical products, diseases or a clinical state (age, gender). When it is not possible to determine whether a factor was present before the onset of pulmonary hypertension, and thus it is unclear whether it played a causal role the term "associated condition" is used (2). Given the fact that the absolute risk is generally low with the known risk factors of PAH, factors of individual susceptibility are likely to play an important role. These elements have been classified according to the strength of the association with pulmonary hypertension and their probable facilitating role (2). "Definite" indicates an association based on several concordant observations, including clear epidemic or large, multicenter epidemiological studies demonstrating an association between the clinical condition or drug and PAH. A "likely" association indicates several concordant observations (including single-center case–control study or multiple case series) that are not attributable to considered biases, or a general consensus among experts. A "possible" association can be suspected,

for example, for drugs with similar mechanisms of action to those in the definite or likely category but which have not been studied yet (association based on case series, registries, or expert opinions). "Unlikely" indicates risk factors that have been proposed but have not been found to have any association from epidemiological studies. The 1998 Evian meeting reviewed this topic and a consensus statement was established (2). This consensus was recently updated in the joint Guidelines of the European Society of Cardiology and European Respiratory Society (5,6). Table 15.4.1 summarizes this consensus.

AMINOREX FUMARATE

The question of a relation between some drug ingestion and pulmonary hypertension was first raised in the late 1960s, when a 20-fold increase of unexplained pulmonary hypertension was reported in Switzerland, Austria, and West Germany (7–9). A dramatic increase in the number of diagnoses of PPH was first noted in a Swiss medical clinic in 1967, which rose from 0.87 percent to 13.5 percent of adults who underwent cardiac catheterization. There were no apparent changes in either size or composition of the population, nor of diagnostic procedures. About half of the patients were more or less overweight, with a female preponderance. Afterwards, 582 cases were identified in a study conducted in Germany, Switzerland, and Austria (8,9). This epidemic just followed the introduction in these countries of the appetite depressant aminorex fumarate (2-amino-5-phenyl-2-oxazoline), and subsided shortly after the drug had been banned from the market (Figure 15.4.2). Approximately only two percent of the population that had

Table 15.4.1 Consensus on drugs and toxins as risk factors for pulmonary arterial hypertension (adapted from refs 5 and 6)

1. **Definite**
   Aminorex
   Fenfluramine
   Dexfenfluramine
   Toxic rapeseed oil
   Benfluorex
2. **Likely**
   Amphetamines
   L-Tryptophan
   Methamphetamines
3. **Possible**
   Cocaine
   Phenylpropanolamine
   St John's wort
   Chemotherapeutic agents
   Selective serotonin reuptake inhibitors
   Pergolide
4. **Unlikely**
   Oral contraceptives
   Estrogen
   Cigarette smoking

See definition of "Definite," "Likely," "Possible" and "Unlikely" risk factors in the text (under "Definition of a risk factor for pulmonary arterial hypertension").

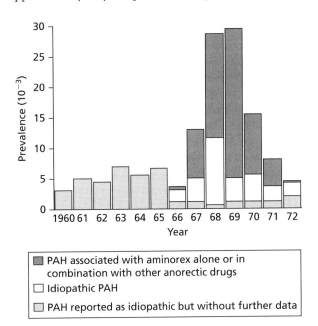

Figure 15.4.2 Prevalence of aminorex-associated pulmonary arterial hypertension in Switzerland, Austria and West Germany. (Adapted from refs 8 and 9.)

taken aminorex developed PAH (7,9,10), but 61 percent of the 582 patients who were identified as new cases of PPH gave a history of aminorex intake, either alone or in combination with other anorectic agents (8,9). In a cohort of 731 patients known to have taken aminorex and who were covered by a single health insurance company, 3 percent developed PPH (11). The number of cases varied geographically, consistent with the marketing, and temporally with the intake of aminorex. The relative risk of developing pulmonary hypertension in aminorex users was estimated to be 52:1 compared with patients without any exposure to the drug (8,9). The clinical manifestations, hemodynamic measures, and pathological changes were reported to be indistinguishable from those of PPH. At that time, controversial conclusions were raised regarding the relationship between the total individual dose and the risk of developing the disease, whereas there was no correlation between the disease severity and the number of tablets each individual patient had taken (8,9). Despite that a dose response effect between aminorex intake and severity of pulmonary hypertension has not been established, and that the evidence has not been substantiated by an animal model, it is widely accepted that the epidemic of pulmonary hypertension was due to aminorex. During follow-up, some authors felt that after discontinuation of the drug, patients with a history of aminorex intake had a better long-term survival than "unexposed" patients with PPH, whereas other authors did not report differences in the survival rates (8,9,11).

Aminorex resembles epinephrine and amphetamine (Figure 15.4.1), and a release of catecholamines from endogenous stores by this drug has been suggested, as well as a mechanism involving lung serotonin release. However, all attempts from experimental work to produce chronic pulmonary hypertension and to demonstrate the effect of the chronic administration of aminorex in any species have failed. This has been explained, first by the low incidence of pulmonary hypertension in test animals as well as in humans, and second by the fact that a prerequisite for the pulmonary circulation to constrict or proliferate when exposed to an offending agent is probably a genetic susceptibility.

FENFLURAMINE DERIVATIVES

Fenfluramine derivatives (DL-fenfluramine and dexfenfluramine) are phenylethylanine derivatives that have been widely prescribed as anorectic drugs since the early 1960s (12).

Many cases of fenfluramine-associated PAH have been reported since 1981 (13–26). For some patients, the condition resolved completely after withdrawal of the drug, although reversibility is debatable (13,14,20). In 1981, Douglas and coworkers published two cases of fenfluramine-associated PAH in women who had taken fenfluramine over 8 months for weight reduction (13). In these patients, symptoms occurred respectively 35 weeks and

18 months after fenfluramine commencement. After drug discontinuation, both symptom and electrocardiographic signs of pulmonary hypertension disappeared within 6 and 3 weeks respectively. In one patient, pulmonary hypertension recurred 6 weeks later after rechallenge with fenfluramine. In 1990, Pouwels reported the case of a 58-year-old woman who developed severe pulmonary hypertension after 11 months of fenfluramine intake; in this patient, symptoms disappeared within 3 weeks after fenfluramine withdrawal and pulmonary artery pressure returned to normal value within 3 months (15).

In 1993, Brenot and coworkers studied a group of 73 PPH patients and found that about 25 percent of them had been exposed to fenfluramine (18). This marked increase followed the large increase in the sales of fenfluramine derivatives in France after the introduction of dexfenfluramine in the market (1985–92). All the 15 patients reported were women who had been exposed to fenfluramine derivatives for at least 3 months with a close temporal relation between fenfluramine derivatives use and development of symptoms related to pulmonary hypertension. Eight patients developed dyspnea approximately 12 months after the beginning of fenfluramine therapy. There were nine current users in whom symptoms suggestive of pulmonary hypertension had appeared or worsened during fenfluramine use, and six previous users whose symptoms developed after fenfluramine discontinuation. The time between onset of symptoms and diagnosis of pulmonary hypertension was about 20 months. The outcome of pulmonary hypertension was not favorable in most of patients, even after drug withdrawal. In fatal cases the lungs showed pulmonary arteriopathy with plexiform lesions (14,16,18).

Finally, the International Primary Pulmonary Hypertension Study (IPPHS) found a clear association between appetite suppressants and pulmonary hypertension, with odds ratio (relative risk estimates) of 6.3 (95 percent CI: 3.0–13.2) (19). Ninety percent of cases for whom a defined product could be traced had used a fenfluramine derivative (19). The risk increased markedly with duration of use (relative risk estimate of 23.1, for more than 3 months, 95 percent CI: 6.9–77.7; Figure 15.4.3) and decreased after cessation of the drug (19). Belgian investigators showed that in the absence of any restriction to the prescription of appetite suppressants more than half of the patients with PPH presented with a history of previous intake of these drugs (23). In this study, patients with previous intake of appetite suppressants appeared to be more severely ill, with a more rapid progression of the disease, and a reduced survival (23). In 1998, our group reported a series of 66 patients with fenfluramine-associated PAH referred between 1986 and 1998 (22). This group of fenfluramine-exposed patients did not differ from a sex-matched idiopathic PAH control group in terms of clinical presentation, severity, hemodynamics at diagnosis and overall survival (22).

In France, the regulations regarding the prescription of appetite suppressants were changed as early as June 1995, leading to a major restriction of their use. In our center, the

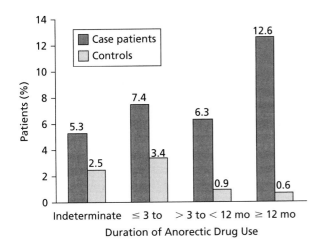

Figure 15.4.3 Duration of exposure to anorectic drugs in patients before the onset of symptoms of pulmonary hypertension. The risk increased markedly with duration of anorectic drug use (relative risk estimate of 23.1, for more than 3 months, 95 percent confidence interval: 6.9–77.7). (Adapted from ref 19.)

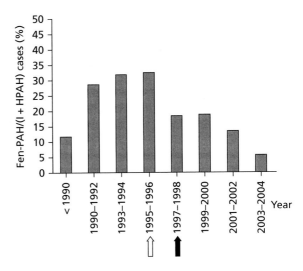

Figure 15.4.4 Percentage of newly-diagnosed fenfluramine-associated pulmonary arterial hypertension (fen-PAH) patients compared with idiopathic and heritable PAH (I + HPAH) patients through time in Paris-Sud 11 University (1986–2004). In France, the regulations regarding the prescription of appetite suppressants were changed as early as June 1995 (white arrow) leading to a major restriction of their use. In September 1997 (black arrow), fenfluramine and dexfenfluramine were recalled from global world market. (Adapted from ref 26.)

annual incidence of fenfluramine-associated PAH increased from 1986 to reach a maximum in 1994. Since the beginning of 1997, the incidence has dropped sharply (Figure 15.4.4) (26). Despite the IPPHS results, dexfenfluramine had been approved for prescription use by the Food and Drug Administration (FDA) for the long-term treatment of obesity. The first cases of fenfluramine- or dexfenfluramine-induced PAH were reported in the United States as early as the beginning of 1997 (20,27–30). Several patients took the off-label combination of fenfluramine and phentermine, commonly called "fen-phen." Fenfluramine and phentermine were approved as individual agents for appetite suppression, with phentermine approved for use in the United States in 1957 and fenfluramine approved in 1973. The total number of prescriptions in the United States exceeded 18 million (31). Following the discovery of valvular heart diseases (31), fenfluramine and dexfenfluramine were removed from the worldwide market in September 1997. After their removal, several North American (Surveillance of North American Pulmonary Hypertension (SNAP) (29) and Surveillance of Pulmonary Hypertension in America (SOPHIA) (32)) and European (26,33) epidemiologic studies showed the association between the use of fenfluramine or dexfenfluramine and PAH and other results consistent with these of IPPHS (19). These provided a better understanding of PAH associated with the use of fenfluramine and dexfenfluramine.

In the French National Registry which included 17 university hospitals, 674 patients with PAH seen between 2002 and 2003 were enrolled. It showed that 9.5 percent of patients had a history of anorexigen exposure mainly with fenfluramine derivatives (77 percent). Two-thirds of them (65 percent) were exposed for more than 6 months. Delay between last appetite suppressant intake and the first symptoms of pulmonary hypertension was more than 2 years

in 76 percent of them, and 44 percent more than 5 years (33). The median duration of fenfluramine exposure was 6 months, with a median of 4.5 years between exposure and onset of symptoms among 109 patients followed up in the French Reference Center Medical for Pulmonary Hypertension (26). The long delay between fenfluramine derivatives exposure and the onset of symptoms highlights the importance of a medical surveillance among patients who have been exposed to fenfluramine derivatives for several years after their discontinuation.

Regarding survival, Rich and coworkers evidenced a poorer survival among patients with fenfluramine-induced PAH compared with patients with idiopathic or familial PAH (median 1.2 vs. 4.1 years) (34). Analyzing a larger sample of patients in our institution, Souza and coworkers did not find a significant difference between patients with fenfluramine-induced PAH compared with patients with idiopathic or familial PAH, with a median survival of 6.4 years (Figure 15.4.5) (26). In both studies, patients were exposed to similar PAH treatment regimen regardless to their exposure status.

The pathogenetic mechanisms of pulmonary hypertension associated to fenfluramine derivatives remain unknown (22). However, it appears that alteration of the serotonin (5-hydroxytryptamine, 5-HT) pathway might be a common denominator (12,35,36). Serotonin is known to be a powerful pulmonary vasoconstrictor and can induce platelet aggregation (36). Moreover, serotonin is also a potent factor stimulating pulmonary smooth muscle proliferation (37). Recent studies support the hypothesis that fenfluramine derivatives may contribute to PAH by

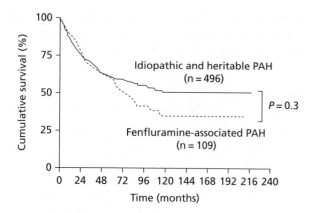

Figure 15.4.5 Survival of patients with fenfluramine-associated pulmonary arterial hypertension (Fen-PAH; n = 109; dashed line) and idiopathic and heritable PAH (I + HPAH; n = 496; solid line). The median survival of the Fen-PAH cohort was 6.4 years. Overall, survival of patients with Fen-PAH did not differ from that of the I + HPAH patients evaluated in the same institution during the same time-frame. (Adapted from ref 26.)

increasing serotonin availability and/or by interacting with serotonin receptors, thus promoting pulmonary vascular smooth muscle proliferation, pulmonary arterial vasoconstriction, and local microthrombosis (36). Under normal conditions, the lung vascular bed is not exposed to excessive serotonin levels, because virtually all blood serotonin is stored in the platelets and free serotonin is rapidly metabolized by the endothelial monoamine oxidase in the liver and the lung endothelium. By interacting with the serotonin transporter, fenfluramine derivatives release serotonin from platelets and inhibit its reuptake into platelet and pulmonary endothelial cells (12). As a consequence blood free serotonin concentration increases with fenfluramine treatment (35). Several evidences indicate that such abnormality in platelet serotonin storage is a trigger factor in the development of PAH in susceptible patients:

1. A decrease in platelet serotonin storage with enhanced blood concentration of free serotonin has been reported in sporadic case of PAH, and in numerous disorders occasionally associated with PAH, including portal hypertension, Raynaud's phenomenon, collagen vascular disease, and platelet storage pool disease (36,38,39).
2. Platelet serotonin storage remains impaired in PAH patients after heart–lung transplantation, whereas it is normal in patients with secondary pulmonary hypertension, indicating that this platelet dysfunction is not secondary to the pulmonary vascular disease (39).
3. The fawn-hooded rat, which has a genetic defect in serotonin platelet storage, develops severe pulmonary hypertension upon exposure to modest hypoxia (36).
4. Fenfluramine in association or not with phentermine has been shown to induce valvular heart disease very similar to that observed after exposure to

serotonin-like drugs such as ergotamine and methysergide, and with increased serotonin levels associated with carcinoid disease (31). Interestingly, one third of these patients with valvular heart disease had coexisting pulmonary hypertension (31). All these observations suggest that fenfluramine may trigger pulmonary hypertension by aggravating or inducing impairment in platelet serotonin storage.

Additional mechanisms seem to be involved in triggering the occurrence of fenfluramine derivatives-associated pulmonary hypertension:

1. Aminorex and fenfluramine derivatives inhibit potassium current flux in rat pulmonary vascular smooth muscle and may therefore stimulate pulmonary vasoconstriction (40). This inhibition is implicated in the pulmonary artery vasoconstriction observed in rat and dog lungs after fenfluramine or serotonin exposure (40,41).
2. Because inhibition of the nitric oxide synthase markedly potentiated the vasoconstrictor effect of fenfluramine in isolated rat lung, it has been speculated that patients who develop pulmonary hypertension while taking an anorectic agent could have a preexisting diminished nitric oxide activity (40). Such a defect has been demonstrated in a small series of patients suffering with severe fenfluramine-associated pulmonary hypertension (42).
3. Lastly, poor metabolizers of fenfluramine derivatives may have a more pronounced exposure to the drug and therefore may be more prone to develop the condition, as recently suggested (43). Fenfluramine and dexfenfluramine are metabolized by cytochrome P450-2D6, an enzyme that shows a marked genetic polymorphism. Lack of the functional enzyme (poor metabolizers), occurs in 8 percent of the general Caucasian population. Higenbottam and colleagues have shown that the frequency of the poor metabolizer genotype of cytochrome P450-2D6 was greater in patients with PAH who had taken fenfluramine or dexfenfluramine (6/26; 23 percent), compared to PPH patients (1/39; 3 percent), pulmonary hypertension associated with other disease (2/26; 8 percent) and healthy control (15/201; 7 percent) (43).

Only a minority of individuals exposed to fenfluramine derivatives will develop pulmonary hypertension, suggesting that this subset of patients could have a genetic susceptibility (19,22). Genetic studies have identified mutations in the bone morphogenetic protein receptor 2 gene (*BMPR2*) – a receptor member of the transforming growth factor-beta (TGF-β) superfamily – in a majority of familial cases of PAH (44). Interestingly, more than 20 percent of patients with idiopathic PAH have mutations in the *BMPR2* gene, emphasizing the relevance of genetic susceptibility for this severe condition (44). Other molecular processes behind the

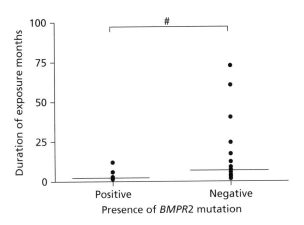

Figure 15.4.6 Comparison of exposure time for fenfluramine derivatives in 40 patients with fenfluramine-related PAH with (n = 9) and without (n = 31) bone morphogenetiprotein receptor type 2 (*BMPR2*) mutation. The duration of exposure to fenfluramine derivatives was significantly shorter in patients with *BMPR2* mutation ($P = 0.007$). (Adapted from ref 26.)

complex vascular changes associated with PAH include vasoconstrictor/vasodilator imbalance, thrombosis, misguided angiogenesis, and inflammation (2,45). In PAH the distinctive vascular changes are found in the precapillary arteries. The same pathology is found in PAH of various origins such as collagen vascular diseases, HIV infection, portal hypertension, congenital systemic to pulmonary shunts, and anorexigen exposure (2). One study sought to determine if patients developing PAH after exposure to appetite suppressants fenfluramine and dexfenfluramine have mutations in the *BMPR2* gene, as reported in heritable PAH (46). *BMPR2* mutations were determined in 33 unrelated patients with idiopathic PAH plus two sisters with heritable PAH, all of whom had taken fenfluramine derivatives, as well as in 130 normal controls. Three new *BMPR2* mutations predicting changes in the primary structure of the *BMPR2* protein were found in three of the 33 unrelated patients (9 percent), and a fourth new mutation was found in the two sisters. No *BMPR2* mutations were identified in the 130 normal controls. This difference in frequency was statistically significant ($P = 0.015$). Moreover, the mutation-positive patients had a somewhat shorter duration of fenfluramine exposure before illness than the mutation-negative patients, a difference that was statistically significant when the two sisters were included in the analysis. *BMPR2* mutations appear to be rare in the general population but may combine with exposure to fenfluramine derivatives to greatly increase the risk of developing severe PAH. The difference in exposure time suggested that these drugs could provide a risk factor for pulmonary hypertension in those patients with mutations even after a short exposure (Figure 15.4.6) (26,46). Nevertheless, most patients had no *BMPR2* mutations suggesting that other genetic or environmental factors could be involved in this condition. The authors further concluded that the onset of disease may require "two events," namely the presence of a heterozygous germline mutation followed

by the use of a fenfluramine derivative. Also, other genes and mechanisms associated with appetite suppressant pulmonary hypertension remain to be characterized.

BENFLUOREX

Benfluorex was approved in Europe as an adjunctive drug for patients with dyslipidemia or diabetes with overweight, and was commonly used in the treatment of metabolic syndrome. This drug, structurally related to amphetamines, was classified by the World Health Organization as an appetite suppressant like fenfluramine and dexfenfluramine, and was sometimes used off-license to help people to lose weight (47). Benfluorex, like fenfluramine and dexfenfluramine, is metabolized into active metabolite norfenfluramine. In France, where benfluorex had been available between 1976 and 2009, Boutet and coworkers reported five cases of severe PAH related to benfluorex consumption (48). All patients were overweight diabetic females, aged from 50 to 57 years, with a body mass index ranging 24.2–49.0 kg m^{-2}. The duration of benfluorex exposure ranged from 3 months to 10 years. Benfluorex was removed from the market in 2003 in Spain and in 2009 in France because cases of valvular heart disease have been observed after its use (49). Therefore, careful assessment of drug exposure in newly diagnosed PAH or valvular heart disease patients is warranted.

AMPHETAMINES

Phentermine has been used as an appetite suppressant since the 1960s. During the aminorex epidemic, a survey found that cases of pulmonary hypertension had used phentermine (50). In the mid-1990s, a large increase in the use of phentermine occurred in the United States due to the popular "phen-fen" combination (28). A few cases of PAH with phentermine use alone have been reported (20,27,30).

Chlorphentermine and phenmetrazine were suggested to contribute to the development of pulmonary hypertension, but no report has been issued in humans since 1972 (51).

In our institution, several patients with an isolated exposure to amphetamine derivatives such as amfepramone and clobenzorex have been clearly identified (52). By contrast with fenfluramine-associated PAH, no close temporal relationship between the onset of amphetamines intake and that of symptoms related to pulmonary hypertension was clearly demonstrated. Furthermore, it is not clear so far whether amphetamines alone can cause the disease (24).

OTHER SEROTONIN REUPTAKE INHIBITORS

The effects of the selective serotonin reuptake inhibitor antidepressant drugs such as fluoxetine on platelets serotonin uptake are very similar to those of fenfluramine (22). However, despite a large worldwide utilization, no case of pulmonary hypertension or valvular heart disease has been yet reported with these drugs. By contrast with fenfluramine derivatives which are serotonin receptors agonists in the brain, these antidepressants do not stimulate serotonin receptors. This suggests that the increase in serotonin availability is not the unique mechanism of fenfluramine-associated pulmonary hypertension, and that fenfluramine derivatives might induce PAH by interacting also with serotonin receptors located in the pulmonary arterial wall (22).

OBESITY

Many detractors of the fact that appetite suppressants could play a role in pulmonary hypertension assumed that obesity by itself was a confounding risk factor for this condition. The IPPHS investigators indeed considered whether the association between the use of appetite suppressants and pulmonary hypertension could be explained by the confounding effect of obesity or that of any hidden factor associated with obesity. However, the odds ratio for anorexic agents was similar whether or not the logistic-regression models were adjusted high body-mass index (19,24,25). The effect of appetite suppressants was the same whether patients had a high body-mass index or not (19,24,25). Neither weight-loss behavior of another type nor the use of thyroid extracts was positively associated with the risk of pulmonary hypertension, as would have been expected if obesity accounted for the odds ratio observed for anorexic agents (19,24,25).

CONCLUSION

The use of fenfluramine derivatives is an established risk factor for PAH. The relative risk is low but does increase markedly in some situations such as long-term use. Therefore, a widespread uncontrolled use of these drugs can lead to an epidemic of PAH. The pathophysiologic link between fenfluramine derivatives intake and the development of PAH remains unclear. However, accumulating evidence suggests a possible role for serotonin. Most patients with fenfluramine-associated PAH had no BMPR2 mutations suggesting that other genetic or environmental factors could be involved in this condition. Unfortunately, the absence of experimental animal models is an important limitation for a better understanding of this condition.

KEY POINTS

- Among anorectic drugs, aminorex fumarate and fenfluramine derivatives are considered as definite risk factors for pulmonary arterial hypertension (PAH), playing a causal role.

- Aminorex was responsible for an epidemic of PAH in the late 1960s.
- Clinical presentation, severity, hemodynamics and overall survival in patients with fenfluramine-associated PAH are very similar to those in patients with idiopathic PAH.
- Reversibility of pulmonary hypertension after appetite-suppressant withdrawal is uncommon.
- The pathogenetic mechanisms of pulmonary hypertension associated to fenfluramine derivatives remain unknown. However, it appears that alteration of the serotonin pathway might be a common denominator. By interacting with the serotonin transporter, fenfluramine derivatives release serotonin from platelets and inhibit its reuptake into platelet and pulmonary endothelial cells.
- Only a minority of individuals exposed to fenfluramine derivatives will develop pulmonary hypertension, suggesting that this subset of patients could have a genetic susceptibility. Bone morphogenetic protein receptor 2 mutations were found in only 9 percent of PAH patients with a history of fenfluramine intake. Nevertheless, most patients had no BMPR2 mutations suggesting that other genetic or environmental factors could be involved in this condition.
- Several cases of amphetamine-associated PAH have been reported. However, it is not clear so far whether amphetamines alone can cause the disease.

REFERENCES

1. Hatano S, Strasser T. Primary Pulmonary Hypertension. Report on a WHO meeting. October 15–17, 1973, Geneva. WHO, 1975.
2. Rich S, ed. Primary Pulmonary Hypertension: Executive Summary from the World Symposium – Primary Pulmonary Hypertension 1998. Available from the World Health Organization via the Internet (http://www.who.int/ncd/cvd/pph.html), 1998.
3. Simonneau G, Galie N, Rubin LJ, Langleben D, Seeger W, Domenighetti G et al. Clinical classification of pulmonary hypertension. J Am Coll Cardiol 2004;43:5S–12S.
4. Simonneau G, Robbins IM, Beghetti M, Channick RN, Delcroix M, Denton CP et al. Updated Clinical Classification of Pulmonary Hypertension. J Am Coll Cardiol 2009;54: S43–54.
5. Galie N, Hoeper MM, Humbert M, Torbicki A, Vachiery JL, Barbera JA et al. Guidelines for the diagnosis and treatment of pulmonary hypertension. The task force for the diagnosis and treatment of pulmonary hypertension of the European Society of Cardiology (ESC) and the European Respiratory Society (ERS), endorsed by the International

Society of Heart and Lung Transplantation (ISHLT). Eur Respir J 2009;34:1219-63.

6. Galie N, Hoeper MM, Humbert M, Torbicki A, Vachiery JL, Barbera JA *et al.* Guidelines for the diagnosis and treatment of pulmonary hypertension: The Task Force for the Diagnosis and Treatment of Pulmonary Hypertension of the European Society of Cardiology (ESC) and the European Respiratory Society (ERS), endorsed by the International Society of Heart and Lung Transplantation (ISHLT). Eur Heart J 2009;30:2493-537.

7. Kay JM, Smith P, Heath D. Aminorex and the pulmonary circulation. Thorax 1971;26:262-70.

8. Gurtner HP. Pulmonary hypertension, plexogenic pulmonary arteriopathy and the appetite depressant drug aminorex: post or propter? Bull Physiopathol Respir (Nancy) 1979;15:897-923.

9. Gurtner HP. Aminorex and pulmonary hypertension. A review. Cor Vasa 1985;27:160-71.

10. Follath F, Burrart F, Schweizer W. Drug-induced pulmonary hypertension? Br Med J 1971;1:265-6.

11. Loogen F, Worth H, Schwan G, Goeckenjan G, Losse B, Horstkotte D. Long-term follow-up of pulmonary hypertension in patients with and without anorectic drug intake. Cor Vasa 1985;27:111-24.

12. McTavish D, Heel RC. Dexfenfluramine. A review of its pharmacological properties and therapeutic potential in obesity. Drugs 1992;43:713-33.

13. Douglas JG, Munro JF, Kitchin AH, Muir AL, Proudfoot AT. Pulmonary hypertension and fenfluramine. Br Med J (Clin Res Ed) 1981;283:881-3.

14. McMurray J, Bloomfield P, Miller HC. Irreversible pulmonary hypertension after treatment with fenfluramine (letter). Br Med J 1986;293:51-2.

15. Pouwels HM, Smeets JL, Cheriex EC, Wouters EF. Pulmonary hypertension and fenfluramine. Eur Respir J 1990;3:606-7.

16. Atanassoff PG, Weiss BM, Schmid ER, Tornic M. Pulmonary hypertension and dexfenfluramine. Lancet 1992;339:436.

17. Roche N, Labrune S, Braun J, Huchon G. Pulmonary hypertension and dexfenfluramine. Lancet 1992;339:436-7.

18. Brenot F, Hervé P, Petitpretz P, Parent F, Duroux P, Simonneau G. Primary pulmonary hypertension and fenfluramine use. Br Heart J 1993;70:537-41.

19. Abenhaim L, Moride Y, Brenot F, Rich S, Benichou J, Kurz X *et al.* Appetite-suppressant drugs and the risk of primary pulmonary hypertension. International Primary Pulmonary Hypertension Study Group. N Engl J Med 1996;335:609-16.

20. Mark EJ, Patalas ED, Chang HT, Evans RJ, Kessler SC. Fatal pulmonary hypertension associated with short-term use of fenfluramine and phentermine. N Engl J Med 1997;337:602-6.

21. Voelkel NF, Clarke WR, Higenbottam T. Obesity, dexfenfluramine, and pulmonary hypertension. A lesson not learned? Am J Respir Crit Care Med 1997;155:786-8.

22. Simonneau G, Fartoukh M, Sitbon O, Humbert M, Jagot JL, Herve P. Primary pulmonary hypertension associated with the use of fenfluramine derivatives. Chest 1998;114:195S-9S.

23. Delcroix M, Kurz X, Walckiers D, Demedts M, Naeije R. High incidence of primary pulmonary hypertension associated with appetite suppressants in Belgium. Eur Respir J 1998;12:271-6.

24. Abenhaim L, Rich S, Benichou J, Bégaud B. Primary pulmonary hypertension and anorectic drugs. N Engl J Med 1999;340:481.

25. Abenhaim L, Humbert M. Pulmonary hypertension related to drugs and toxins. Curr Opin Cardiol 1999;14:437-41.

26. Souza R, Humbert M, Sztrymf B, Jais X, Yaici A, Le Pavec J *et al.* Pulmonary arterial hypertension associated with fenfluramine exposure: report of 109 cases. Eur Respir J 2008;31:343-8.

27. Strother J, Fedullo P, Yi ES, Masliah E. Complex vascular lesions at autopsy in a patient with phentermine-fenfluramine use and rapidly progressing pulmonary hypertension. Arch Pathol Lab Med 1999;123:539-40.

28. Fishman AP. Aminorex to fen/phen: an epidemic foretold. Circulation 1999;99:156-61.

29. Rich S, Rubin L, Walker AM, Schneeweiss S, Abenhaim L. Anorexigens and pulmonary hypertension in the United States: results from the surveillance of North American pulmonary hypertension. Chest 2000;117:870-4.

30. Tomita T, Zhao Q. Autopsy findings of heart and lungs in a patient with primary pulmonary hypertension associated with use of fenfluramine and phentermine. Chest 2002;121:649-52.

31. Connolly HM, Crary JL, McGoon MD, Hensrud DD, Edwards BS, Edwards WD *et al.* Valvular heart disease associated with fenfluramine-phentermine. N Engl J Med 1997;337:581-8.

32. Walker AM, Langleben D, Korelitz JJ, Rich S, Rubin LJ, Strom BL *et al.* Temporal trends and drug exposures in pulmonary hypertension: an American experience. Am Heart J 2006;152:521-6.

33. Humbert M, Sitbon O, Chaouat A, Bertocchi M, Habib G, Gressin V *et al.* Pulmonary arterial hypertension in France: results from a national registry. Am J Respir Crit Care Med 2006;173:1023-30.

34. Rich S, Shillington A, McLaughlin V. Comparison of survival in patients with pulmonary hypertension associated with fenfluramine to patients with primary pulmonary hypertension. Am J Cardiol 2003;92:1366-8.

35. Martin F, Artigas F. Simultaneous effects of P-chloramphetamine, D-fenfluramine, and reserpine on free blood and stored 5-HT in brain and blood. J Neurochem 1992;59:1138-44.

36. Egermayer P, Town GI, Peacock AJ. Role of serotonin in the pathogenesis of acute and chronic pulmonary hypertension. Thorax 1999;54:161-8.

37. Fanburg BL, Lee SL. A new role for an old molecule: serotonin as a mitogen. Am J Physiol 1997;16:795-806.

38. Herve P, Drouet L, Dosquet C, Launay JM, Rain B, Simonneau G *et al.* Primary pulmonary hypertension in a patient with a familial platelet storage pool disease: role of serotonin. Am J Med 1990;89:117-20.

39. Herve P, Launay JM, Scrobohaci ML, Brenot F, Simonneau G, Petitpretz P et al. Increased plasma serotonin in primary pulmonary hypertension. Am J Med 1995;99:249–54.

40. Weir EK, Reeve HL, Huang JM, Michelakis E, Nelson DP, Hampl V et al. Anorexic agents aminorex, fenfluramine, and dexfenfluramine inhibit potassium current in rat pulmonary vascular smooth muscle and cause pulmonary vasoconstriction. Circulation 1996;94:2216–20.

41. Naeije R, Wauthy P, Maggiorini M, Leeman M, Delcroix M. Effects of dexfenfluramine on hypoxic pulmonary vasoconstriction and embolic pulmonary hypertension in dogs. Am J Respir Crit Care Med 1995;151:692–7.

42. Archer SL, Djaballah K, Humbert M, Weir KE, Fartoukh M, Dall'ava-Santucci J et al. Nitric oxide deficiency in fenfluramine- and dexfenfluramine-induced pulmonary hypertension. Am J Respir Crit Care Med 1998;158:1061–7.

43. Higenbottam T, Humbert M, Simonneau G, Machin A, Bidule Z, Truc G et al. Subjects deficient for CYP2D6 expression (poor metabolisers) are over-represented among patients with anorectic associated pulmonary hypertension. Am J Respir Crit Care Med 1999;159:A165.

44. Machado RD, Eickelberg O, Elliott CG, Geraci MW, Hanaoka M, Loyd JE et al. Genetics and genomics of pulmonary arterial hypertension. J Am Coll Cardiol 2009;54:S32–42.

45. Voelkel NF, Tuder RM. Cellular and molecular mechanisms in the pathogenesis of severe pulmonary hypertension. Eur Respir J 1995;8:2129.

46. Humbert M, Deng Z, Simonneau G, Barst RJ, Sitbon O, Wolf M et al. BMPR2 germline mutations in pulmonary hypertension associated with fenfluramine derivatives. Eur Respir J 2002;20:518–23.

47. [No authors listed]. Hidden amphetamines: from smoking cessation to diabetes. Prescrire Int 2004;13:18–20.

48. Boutet K, Frachon I, Jobic Y, Gut-Gobert C, Leroyer C, Carlhant-Kowalski D et al. Fenfluramine-like cardiovascular side-effects of benfluorex. Eur Respir J 2009;33:684–8.

49. Rafel Ribera J, Casanas Munoz R, Anguera Ferrando N, Batalla Sahun N, Castro Cels A, Pujadas Capmany R. [Valvular heart disease associated with benfluorex.] Rev Esp Cardiol 2003;56:215–6.

50. Backman R. Primäre pulmonale hypertonie. In: Steinkopff D, ed. Verhandlungen der deutschen gesellschaft für kreislaufforschungh. Darmstadt: Verlag, 1972:134–41.

51. Fuller RW. Serotonin uptake inhibitors: use in clinical therapy and in laboratory research. Prog Drug Res 1995;45:167–204.

52. Fartoukh M, Sitbon O, Humbert M, Jagot JL, Parent F, Duroux P et al. Primary pulmonary hypertension associated with the use of anorectic drugs. Eur Respir J 1998;12:141s.

Pulmonary hypertension associated with portal hypertension

PHILIPPE HERVÉ, LAURENT SAVALE, ROBERT NAEIJE, GÉRALD SIMONNEAU,
MARC HUMBERT AND OLIVIER SITBON

INTRODUCTION

Liver disease affects the lungs. The most typical pulmonary consequence of liver disease is the "hepatopulmonary syndrome," which is characterized by widespread pulmonary arteriovenous dilatations, *decreased* pulmonary vascular resistance (PVR) and eventual severe hypoxemia caused by a diffusion/perfusion imbalance. However, liver disease is sometimes associated with an *increased* PVR, leading to so-called portopulmonary hypertension (POPAH). The common determinant of both the hepatopulmonary syndrome and POPAH is portal hypertension with portosystemic shunting. Most cases of portal hypertension complicate liver cirrhosis.

In 1951, Mantz and Craig reported on a woman aged 53 years with a history of hematemesis who was admitted for hoarseness and dyspnea, and who died from a refractory right heart failure following an exploratory laparotomy (1). The autopsy disclosed a normal liver, portal thrombosis, extensive portosystemic shunting and right ventricular hypertrophy. Microscopically, there were multiple microthrombi in the small pulmonary arteries, which suggested to the authors that pulmonary hypertension in their patient had been caused by recurrent embolization from the thrombotic portal vein. However, typical aspects of what was at that time called primary pulmonary hypertension, including plexiform lesions, were also found. The notion that portal hypertension could be a predisposing factor to primary pulmonary hypertension was confirmed by Naeye who reported on six cases of "primary pulmonary hypertension" associated with portal hypertension in 1960. The histopathological examination of the lungs of these patients showed a remodeling of the pulmonary arteriolar walls with microthrombi, areas of fibrinoid necrosis and plexiform lesions. The author carefully discussed the possible contributions of high cardiac output and microemboli originating in thrombotic portal veins, and concluded that portal hypertension would be a predisposing factor for primary pulmonary hypertension. From then on, patients with POPAH were included in primary pulmonary hypertension registries (3). Portopulmonary hypertension was placed in the "PAH" category when primary pulmonary hypertension was renamed "PAH" as the WHO-sponsored expert consensus conference held in 1998 in Evian (4), and this was confirmed at the expert consensus conferences of Venice, in 2004, and Dana Point in 2008 (5).

DEFINITION

The diagnosis of POPAH is based on pulmonary hemodynamic criteria obtained via right heart catheterization. Portopulmonary hypertension can be defined as a PAH associated with portal hypertension with or without hepatic disease. Hemodynamic criteria include a mean pulmonary arterial pressure (mPAP) > 25 mmHg at rest, a pulmonary capillary wedge pressure (PCWP) < 15 mmHg, and a PVR > 240 dyne/s cm^{-5} (> 3 Wood units). The criteria applied for the cut-off PVR have been agreed upon by a panel of experts in 2004 (6).

A moderate increase in mPAP (25 to 35 mmHg) is frequent in up to 20 percent of patients with cirrhosis and portal hypertension (7,8). This increase in PAP is mainly passive (with minimum pulmonary vascular remodeling) in relationship with the increases in cardiac output and/or blood volume and is associated with normal or increased PCWP. By contrast, a severe PAH with extensive pulmonary vascular remodeling and elevated PVR is more rarely observed in patients with portal hypertension. This latter condition represents the entity of POPAH and is associated with poor outcome.

EPIDEMIOLOGY

A retrospective study on 17 901 autopsied patients reported a prevalence of PAH of 0.73 percent in patients with portal hypertension or liver cirrhosis, as compared with only 0.13 percent in the general population (9). In the same report, the prevalence of PAH in a clinical series of 2459 patients with biopsy-proved hepatic cirrhosis was 0.61 percent, also significantly higher than in a control population (9). Two prospective hemodynamic studies conducted by Naeije et al. (10) and Hadengue et al. (11) in patients with portal hypertension found a prevalence of 2 percent. More recent studies reported a higher incidence, in the range of 3–5 percent of moderate pulmonary hypertension in patients with severe liver disease (8,12–15). Taken together, these studies suggest an incidence of no more than approximately 2 percent of severe PAH in portal hypertension.

Portopulmonary arterial hypertension is the third form of PAH. Portal hypertension is an associated condition in about 10 percent of the cases of PAH. Among the 674 patients with PAH included in a national French prospective registry (from October 2002 to October 2003), 70 had portal hypertension (10.3 percent). Incidence and prevalence of portal hypertension in these patients with PAH were 14.9 percent and 9.4 percent, respectively (16). POPAH may be more prevalent in developing countries with a high prevalence of hepatosplenic schistosomiasis (17).

ETIOLOGY

In humans and rats with liver cirrhosis, portosystemic shunts and impaired phagocytosis in the liver allow cytokines, circulating bacteria, and bacterial endotoxins from the gastrointestinal tract to enter the pulmonary circulation, where they damage the endothelium and induce extensive recruitment of macrophages to the arterial bed. However POPAH does not develop in cirrhotic animals and affects only a small minority of humans with cirrhosis. On the contrary, PVR is decreased, chiefly as a result of pulmonary

vasodilation mediated mainly by nitric oxide (NO) (6,18). In liver cirrhosis, the pulmonary arteries are continuously exposed to mediators of inflammation but are usually protected against pulmonary hypertension. Cirrhosis has been shown to improve monocrotaline-induced pulmonary hypertension in rats (19). Therefore, it has been suspected that some particular gene expression would be associated with predominantly pro-remodeling effects of systemic inflammatory changes and increased vascular wall shear stress in portal hypertension. The genetic counterpart of this particular susceptibility to PAH in some patients with portal hypertension has not been yet identified.

Mutations in *BMPR-2* and *ALK-1*, genes that encode members of the transforming growth factor-beta (TGF-β) receptor superfamily, reported in familial and idiopathic PAH have not been found in patients with POPAH (6). Compared with controls, patients with idiopathic PAH more frequently carry the LL variant of serotonin transporter. This was not found in POPAH (20). A recent study has reported 29 single nucleotide polymorphisms in 15 candidate genes associated with the risk of POPAH, including genes coding for estrogen receptor 1, aromatase, phosphodiesterase-5, angiopoietin-1, and calcium binding protein A4. The clinical relevance of these genetic variations in estrogen signaling and cell growth regulators is unclear (21).

It has been hypothesized that the pulmonary vascular bed needs something to control angiogenesis, which exits the liver via the hepatic veins. Patients with congenital heart disease develop diffuse pulmonary arteriovenous malformations after anastomosis of the superior vena cava to the right pulmonary artery (22). No such abnormalities have been reported after total cavopulmonary anastomosis, which directs the entire systemic venous return including hepatic venous blood to the pulmonary arterial bed. Moreover, redirection of hepatic venous flow to the pulmonary bed either by surgical inclusion of hepatic vein (23) or by heart transplantation can reverse these vascular abnormalities (24). These findings suggest that the absence of a hepatic agent in the pulmonary vasculature by virtue of either poor hepatic synthetic function or decreased hepatic venous blood flow result in exaggerated angiogenesis. This factor could be the angiogenesis inhibitor endostatin because the liver is the major source of collagen XVIII, the precursor of the endostatin (25).

CLINICAL PRESENTATION

We recently reported the largest population of patients with POPAH (26). The study included 154 patients. Our patients with POPAH were older than those previously reported (7) in relation with a higher prevalence of alcoholic cirrhosis. However, when compared with the sex ratio in the cirrhotic population without PAH, the proportion of female patients was relatively higher in POPAH. This female predominance is also found in other types of PAH, underlying the potential role of a hormonal influence in the pathogenesis of PAH. In this study the etiology of cirrhosis was mainly alcohol consumption and hepatitis virus infection, and the severity of the cirrhosis showed a Child–Pugh class A predominance. Another recent multicenter case–control study identified two risk factors for the development of POPAH: female sex and autoimmune hepatitis (27). Interestingly, hepatitis C infection was associated with a decreased risk. These results may suggest that autoimmunity could contribute to the pathogenesis of PAH in the setting of portal hypertension, as has been demonstrated in idiopathic PAH.

A non-hepatic cause of portal hypertension was present in 11 percent of our patients, including three Budd–Chiari syndromes. This is consistent with other series and case-reports (1,2,7) indicating that portal hypertension rather than liver disease is the key factor for the development of POPAH. The severity of liver failure as estimated by the Child–Pugh score, was not correlated with PVR in our experience as well as in the study by Hadengue et al. (11). In most series, the diagnosis of portal hypertension antedated that of POPAH in the majority of the patients.

In the study of Hadengue et al. (11), 60 percent of patients with POPAH were asymptomatic, and PVR values were lower in asymptomatic patients. In our series, NYHA grades of dyspnea were lower in the patients with portal hypertension than in those with idiopathic PAH. There were no significant differences in the frequency of chest pain, syncope, or hemoptysis.

Mean PAP was lower for patients with POPAH than with idiopathic PAH (55 ± 11 vs. 63 ± 12 mmHg, respectively, $P = 0.02$), whereas cardiac index and mixed venous oxygen saturation were higher (2.9 ± 0.7 vs. 2.2 ± 0.6 L/min/m^2, and 66 ± 10 vs. 58 ± 8 percent, $P = 0.0004$), yielding lower calculated total PVR values (30 ± 9 vs. 21 ± 7 mmHg/L/min/m^2). The other hemodynamic values were similar in the two groups. These findings are comparable to those previously reported. An increased lung NO production may explain these differences. Indeed, exhaled NO concentrations are increased in POPAH and decreased in idiopathic PAH, compared to normal individuals (Le Pavec, personal communication).

Only one of our POPAH patients had a positive response to acute vasodilator testing. This low percentage of responders (0.6 percent) vs. about 10 percent in idiopathic PAH could be related to persistent lung NO overproduction in POPAH.

Patients with POPH are generally believed to have substantially shorter survival rate than idiopathic PAH patients (7). By contrast, actuarial survival rates in our series at 1, 3, and 5 years were 88, 75, and 68 percent, respectively. Similar findings were reported in a recent study (13). Only the absence of cirrhosis, Child–Pugh scores B and C, and cardiac index were identified as independent prognostic factors (Figure 15.5.1). In our study, half of deaths were attributed to PAH and half to liver disease. This indicates that not only the hemodynamic profile but also the severity

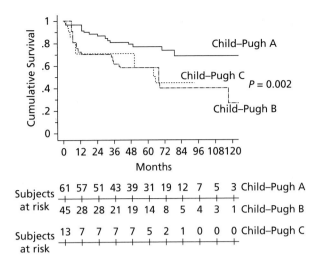

Subjects at risk	61	57	51	43	39	31	19	12	7	5	3	Child–Pugh A
	45	28	28	21	19	14	8	5	4	3	1	Child–Pugh B
Subjects at risk	13	7	7	7	7	5	2	1	0	0	0	Child–Pugh C

Figure 15.5.1 Survival in patients with portopulmonary hypertension according to the Child–Pugh score in patients with cirrhosis. Survival rates at 1, 3, and 5 years were 97, 79, and 71 percent, respectively, in patients with a Child–Pugh score A; 76, 59, and 55 percent in patients with a Child–Pugh score B; and 73, 73, and 58 percent in patients with a Child–Pugh score C ($P = 0.02$, log-rank test).

of the liver disease are the major independent prognostic factors in this population.

The diagnosis of POPAH based on clinical presentation is challenging because many symptoms are common to advanced liver disease and severe pulmonary hypertension. Moreover, many POPAH patients are asymptomatic at the time of diagnosis. Two-dimensional and Doppler echocardiography should be routinely performed as primary screening procedure especially in patients undergoing a preoperative liver transplant evaluation. When suspected of POPAH, these patients should undergo right heart catheterization.

MANAGEMENT

At the present time, there are no randomized, controlled clinical studies or guidelines on the use of vasodilator therapies in POPAH. Thus, treatment of POPAH has been empirical. The usual approach in treating POPAH has been to initiate therapy when the patient is both symptomatic and has an elevated mPAP (> 35 mmHg) as well as an increased PVR.

Anticoagulation is not recommended in the POPAH patients with high risk of bleeding from the gastrointestinal tract. Contrary to occasional recommendations (28), β-blockers, which are used to decrease portal pressure and lower the risk of bleeding from esophageal varices, are contraindicated as well. Provencher et al. reported a marked improvement in pulmonary hemodynamics and exercise capacity after withdrawal of β-blocker therapies in

POPAH patients (29). This is explained by the deleterious negative inotropic and chronotropic effects exerted by β-blockers on the overloaded right ventricle, limiting cardiac output responses to peripheral oxygen demand.

Calcium channel blockers are contraindicated in POPH, because they may further increase the hepatic venous pressure gradient and the risk of bleeding from esophageal varices.

Although randomized controlled trials have not been performed, case series have shown substantial improvement of exercise capacity with compassionate use of intravenous epoprostenol in NYHA class III or IV POPAH patients (30,31). A possible complication of this treatment may be the development of splenomegaly with aggravated thrombocytopenia and leukopenia (32). Other uncontrolled studies have shown improvement in exercise capacity and functional state with inhaled iloprost (33), the endothelin receptor antagonist bosentan (33,34) and the phosphodiesterase-5 inhibitor sildenafil (35). Because of a concern of possible hepatic toxicity, the administration of endothelin receptor antagonists to POPAH is limited to those with associated to Child A cirrhosis or extrahepatic portal hypertension (36). Although evidence-based guidelines are lacking, based on the successful experiences with other PAH categories, treatment of POPAH patients with parenteral prostanoids, endothelin receptor antagonists and phosphodiesterase-5 inhibitors, or a combination of these agents, appears reasonable.

Liver transplantation is associated with a slow improvement of the hepatopulmonary syndrome, but has not been convincingly reported to reverse POPAH (26). On the other hand, both pulmonary vascular complications of portal hypertension increase the mortality of the procedure (6,37,38). The mortality of liver transplantation has been shown to increase in proportion to mPAP, reaching 100 percent for a mPAP > 50 mmHg, 50 percent for a mPAP between 35 and 50 mmHg and a PVR > 250 dyne/s cm^{-5}, and down to 0 percent for a mPAP < 35 mmHg (37). Pretreatment of POPAH with endothelin receptor antagonists, phosphodiesterase-5 inhibitors or prostacyclins may improve the prognosis of liver transplantation in POPAH patients, but controlled evidence of this is still lacking. In patients with refractory POPAH, combined liver and (heart–) lung transplantation remains the only therapeutic option (39).

HEPATOPULMONARY SYNDROME AND POPAH

Hypoxemia is not a feature of POPAH (40,41). However, some POPAH patients become hypoxemic because of shunting through a patent foramen ovale (42). On the other hand, POPAH may complicate a pre-existing hepatopulmonary syndrome. In these patients, there has been report of improved arterial oxygenation and decreased dyspnea symptomatology (43–45).

KEY POINTS

- Pulmonary artery pressure is often increased in patients with advanced liver cirrhosis as a consequence of a high cardiac output.
- The diagnosis of portopulmonary arterial hypertension (POPAH) requires a right heart catheterization.
- POPAH is defined by a mean pulmonary artery pressure higher than 25 mmHg and a pulmonary vascular resistance higher than 250 dyn/s cm^{-5} in a patient with portal hypertension and no causal cardiac or pulmonary disease and no pulmonary embolism.
- POPAH occurs in approximately 2 percent of patients with advanced liver disease.
- The histopathology of POPAH is indistinguishable from that of PAH, and medical treatment options are similar.
- The prognosis of POPAH is affected by the severity of liver disease.
- POPAH has not convincingly been shown to regress after liver transplantation.
- POPAH increases the mortality of liver transplantation in proportion to increased pulmonary artery pressure.
- Treating POPAH with prostacyclins, endothelin receptor antagonists or phosphodiesterase-5 inhibitors may improve the outcome of liver transplantation.
- However, there have been no randomized controlled trials of these medical treatments on POPAH.

REFERENCES

● = Key primary paper

1. Mantz FA, Craig E. Portal axis thrombosis with spontaneous porto-caval shunt and resultant cor pulmonale. Arch Pathol 1951;52:91–97.
2. Naeije RL. Primary pulmonary hypertension with coexisting portal hypertension. a retrospective study of six cases. Circulation 1960;22:376–84.
3. Rich S, Dantzker DR, Ayres SM, Bergofsky EH et al. Primary pulmonary hypertension: a national prospective study. Ann Intern Med 1987;107:216–23.
4. Fishman AP. Clinical classification of pulmonary hypertension. Clin Chest Med 2001;22;385–91.
●5. Simonneau G, Robbins IM, Beghetti M et al. Updated classification of pulmonary hypertension. J Am Coll Cardiol 2009;54(1 Suppl):S43–54.
●6. Rodriguez-Roisin R, Rodríguez-Roisin R, Krowka MJ, Hervé P, Fallon MB. ERS Task Force Pulmonary-Hepatic Vascular

Disorders (PHD) Scientific Committee. Pulmonary vascular hepatic disorders. Eur Respir J 2004;24:861–80.

•7. Mandell SM, Groves BM. Pulmonary hypertension in liver disease. Clin Chest Med 1996;17:17–33.

8. Krowka, MJ. Hepatopulmonary syndrome and portopulmonary hypertension: distinctions and dilemmas. Hepatology 1997;25:1282–4.

9. McDonnell PJ, Toye PA, Hutchins GM. Primary PH and cirrhosis: are they related? Am Rev Respir Dis 1983;127:437–41.

10. Naeije R, Melot C, Hallemans R, Mols P, Lejeune P. Pulmonary hemodynamics in liver cirrhosis. Semin Respir Med 1985;7:164–70.

11. Hadengue A, Benhayoun MK, Lebrec D, Benhamou JP. Pulmonary hypertension complicating portal hypertension: prevalence and relation to splanchnic hemodynamics. Gastoenterology 1991;100:520–28.

12. Tamara P, Garcia-Valdecasas JC, Beltran J et al. Moderate primary pulmonary hypertension in patients undergoing liver transplantation. Anaesth Analg 1996;83:675–80.

13. Yang YY, Lin HC, Hou MC, Lee FY, Chang FY, Lee SD. Portopulmonary hypertension: distinctive hemodynamic and clinical manifestations. J Gastroenterol 2001;36:181–6.

14. Toregrossa M, Genesca J, Gonzalez A, Evangelista A, Mora A, Margarit C, Esteban R, Guardia J. Role of Doppler echocardiography in the assessment of portopulmonary hypertension liver transplantation candidates. Transplantation 2001;71:572–4.

15. Taura P, Garcia-Valdecasas JC, Beltran J et al. Moderate primary pulmonary hypertension in patients undergoing liver transplantation. Anesth Analg 1996;83:675–80.

16. Humbert M, Sitbon O, Chaouat A et al. Pulmonary arterial hypertension in France: results from a national registry. Am J Respir Crit Care Med 2006;173:1023–30.

17. Lapa M, Dias B, Jardim C et al. Cardiopulmonary manifestations of hepatosplenic schistosomiasis. Circulation 2009;119:1518–23.

18. Nunes H, Lebrec D, Mazmanian M et al. Role of nitric oxide in HPS in cirrhotic rats. Am J Respir Crit Care Med 2001;164:879–85.

19. Le Pavec J, Perros F, Eddahibi S et al. Cirrhosis ameliorates monocrotaline-induced pulmonary hypertension in rats. Eur Respir J 2009; 34:731–9.

20. Roberts KE, Fallon MB, Krowka MJ et al. Serotonin transporter polymorphisms in patients with portopulmonary hypertension Chest 2009;135:1470–5.

21. Roberts KE, Fallon MB, Krowka MJ et al. Genetic risk factors for portopulmonary hypertension in patients with advanced liver disease. Am J Respir Crit Care Med 2009; 179:835–42.

22. Srivastava D, Preminger T, Lock JE, Mandell V, Keane JF, Mayer JE, Kozakewich H, Spevak PJ. Hepatic venous blood and the development of pulmonary arteriovenous malformations in congenital heart disease. Circulation 1995;92:1217–22.

23. Shah MJ, Rychick J, Fogel MA, Murphy JD, Jacobs ML. Pulmonary arteriovenous malformations after superior cavopulmonary connection: resolution after inclusion of hepatic veins in the pulmonary circulation. Ann Thorac Surg 1997;63:960–3.

24. Graham K, Sonheimer H, Schaffer M. Resolution of cavopulmonary shunt-associated pulmonary arteriovenous malformation after heart transplantation. J Heart Transpl 1997;16:1271–4.

25. Clement B, Musso O, Lietard J, Theret N. Homeostatic control of angiogenesis: a newly identified function of the liver? Hepatology 1999;29:621–3.

•26. Le Pavec J, Souza R, Herve P et al. Portopulmonary hypertension: survival and prognostic factors. Am J Respir Crit Care Med 2008;178:637–43.

27. Kawut SM, Krowka MJ, Trotter F et al. Pulmonary Vascular Complications of Liver Disease Study Group. Clinical risk factors for portopulmonary hypertension. Hepatology 2008;48:196–203.

28. Budhiraja R, Hassoun P. Portopulmonary hypertension: a tale of two circulations. Chest 2003;123:562–76.

•29. Provencher S, Herve P, Jais X, Lebrec D, Humbert M, Simonneau G, Sitbon O. Deleterious effects of beta-blockers on exercise capacity and hemodynamics in patients with portopulmonary hypertension. Gastroenterology 2006;130:120–6.

30. Krowka MJ, Frantz RP, McGoon MD, Severson C, Plevak DJ, Wiesner RH. Improvement in pulmonary hemodynamics during intravenous epoprostenol (prostacyclin): a study of 15 patients with moderate to severe portopulmonary hypertension. Hepatology 1999;30:641–8.

31. Kuo PC, Johnson LB, Plotkin JS, Howell CD, Bartlett ST, Rubin LJ. Continuous intravenous infusion of epoprostenol for the treatment of portopulmonary hypertension. Transplantation 1997;63:604–6.

32. Findlay JY, Plevak DJ, Krowka MJ, Sack EM, Porayko MK. Progressive splenomegaly after epoprostenol therapy in portopulmonary hypertension. Liver Transpl Surg 1999;5:362–5.

33. Hoeper MM, Seyfarth HJ, Hoeffken G et al. Experience with inhaled iloprost and bosentan in portopulmonary hypertension. Eur Respir J 2007;30:1096–102.

34. Hoeper MM, Halank M, Marx C, Hoeffken G, Seyfarth HJ, Schauer J, Niedermeyer J, Winkler J. Bosentan therapy for portopulmonary hypertension. Eur Respir J 2005;25:502–8.

35. Reichenberger F, Voswinckel R, Steveling E et al. Sildenafil treatment for portopulmonary hypertension. Eur Respir J 2006;28:563–7.

36. Hoeper MM, Galie N, Simonneau G, Rubin LJ. New treatments for pulmonary arterial hypertension. Am J Respir Crit Care Med 2002;165:1209–16.

•37. Krowka MJ, Plevak DJ, Findlay JY, Rosen CB, Wiesner RH, Krom RA. Pulmonary hemodynamics and perioperative cardiopulmonary-related mortality in patients with portopulmonary hypertension undergoing liver transplantation. Liver Transpl 2000;6:443–50.

38. Starkel P, Vera A, Gunson B, Mutimer D. Outcome of liver transplantation for patients with pulmonary hypertension. Liver Transpl 2002;8:382–8.

39. Pirenne J, Verleden G, Nevens F *et al*. Combined liver and heart–lung transplantation in liver transplant candidates with refractory portoPH. Transplantation 2002;73:140–2.

40. Vachiery F, Moreau R, Hadengue A, Gadano A, Soupison T, Valla D, Lebrec D. Hypoxemia in patients with cirrhosis: relationship with liver failure and hemodynamic alterations. J Hepatol 1997;492–5.

41. Swanson KL, Krowka MJ. Arterial oxygenation associated with portopulmonary hypertension. Chest 2002;121:1869–75.

42. Raffy O, Sleiman C, Vachiery F *et al*. Refractory hypoxemia during liver cirrhosis: hepatopulmonary syndrome or primary pulmonary hypertension. Am J Respir Crit Care Med 1996;153:1169–71.

43. Mal H, Burgiere O, Durand F, Fartoukh M, Cohen-Solal A, Fournier M. Pulmonary hypertension following hepatopulmonary syndrome in a patient with cirrhosis. J Hepatol 1999;31:360–4.

44. Kaspar MD, Ramsay MA, Shuey CB Jr, Levy MF, Klintmalm GG. Severe pulmonary hypertension and amelioration of hepatopulmonary syndrome after liver transplantation. Liver Transpl Surg 1998;4:177–9.

45. Jones FD, Kuo PC, Johnson LB, Njoku MJ, Dixon-Ferguson MK, Plotkin JS. The coexistence of portopulmonary hypertension and hepatopulmonary syndrome. Anesthesiology 1999;90:626–9.

Pulmonary arterial hypertension associated with HIV infection

RUDOLF SPEICH

INTRODUCTION

Human immunodeficiency virus (HIV) infection is associated with numerous infectious and non-infectious complications. During the first years of the epidemic non-infectious conditions remained mostly undetected because they were overshadowed by HIV-related opportunistic infections and malignancies. With the advent of highly active antiretroviral therapy (HAART) and the increased survival time of HIV-infected patients, non-infectious complications such as cardiovascular diseases including dilated cardiomyopathy, pericardial effusion, bacterial or non-bacterial thrombotic endocarditis and accelerated atherosclerosis have emerged.

In 1987, pulmonary hypertension was reported for the first time in a 40-year-old homosexual white man with AIDS and membranoproliferative glomerulonephritis by Kim and Factor (1). Autopsy of the lungs revealed plexiform lesions. An immune-mediated pathogenesis was suggested, but in contrast to the findings of the glomerular immunohistochemistry, no IgG deposits were found in the pulmonary vessels. One year later, Goldsmith *et al.* described "primary" pulmonary hypertension in five HIV-infected hemophiliacs and suggested a possible pathogenic role of treatment with low-purity factor VIII (2).

Subsequently, two groups reported six cases each with pulmonary hypertension clinically and pathologically resembling idiopathic pulmonary hypertension (IPAH) out of a cohort of 1200 HIV-infected patients, thus both estimating a cumulative incidence of 0.5 percent (3,4). In consideration of the annual incidence of IPAH of 1 to 2 per million in the general population these findings strongly suggested an association between HIV infection and pulmonary arterial hypertension (PAH). Further case series (5,6), an analytic review of 131 cases (7), and the occurrence of the disorder in patients without other possible confounding factors such as portal hypertension or use of intravenous drugs, or amphetamine prompted the WHO conference in Evian to conclude that HIV infection is a definite risk factor for the development of pulmonary arterial hypertension (HIV-PAH).

DEFINITIONS AND INVESTIGATIONS

Although many of the early cases were diagnosed solely by echocardiography, by now right heart catheterization has become the standard diagnostic tool. As in other conditions, PAH is defined by a mean pulmonary artery pressure (mPAP) $>25\,$mmHg at rest and a pulmonary capillary wedge pressure or left ventricular end diastolic pressure $\leq 15\,$mmHg (8).

Invasive hemodynamic assessment is especially important in order to exclude other known causes for pulmonary hypertension including congenital or left-sided valvular heart disease, and HIV-associated myocardial disease. Lung function testing and computed tomography are essential to exclude HIV-associated emphysema, idiopathic interstitial pneumonitis, pulmonary veno-occlusive disease, and other pulmonary complications. A lung perfusion scan should be performed, since these patients may also have an increased risk of venous thromboembolism (9), possibly due to the increased incidence of antiphospholipid antibodies and decreased levels of protein S and C (10). Whether acute vasodilator testing should be performed in HIV-PAH is a matter of debate, since according to the French expert center, none of the patients was a responder to acute nitric oxide testing (11). Liver function tests, viral hepatitis serology and abdominal ultrasound should be performed, if liver cirrhosis is suspected.

The diagnosis HIV infection is based on standard serological testing. For classification, the 1993 Revised Centers for Disease Control and Prevention (CDC) Classification System for HIV-Infection is still widely used (12).

EPIDEMIOLOGY

The National French Registry has shown that HIV-PAH accounted for 6.2 percent of all patients with PAH (13). The risk for the development of PAH is clearly increased in HIV-infected subjects. A large case–control study involving 3349 HIV-infected patients over a period of 5.5 years demonstrated a cumulative incidence of PAH of 0.57 percent, resulting in an annual incidence of about 0.1 percent (5). Compared with the annual incidence of IPAH in the general population of 1 to 2 per million, HIV infection carries a relative risk for PAH of 500 to 1000.

The prevalence of HIV-PAH of around 0.5 percent now has been confirmed by multiple studies. A recent large French series analyzing 7648 HIV-infected patients reported a percentage of 0.46 percent (14) comparable to the Swiss experience (15).

Based on data from the Swiss HIV cohort (Figure 15.6.1), the annual incidence of HIV-PAH showed a median value of 0.1 percent (range 0.04 percent to 0.21 percent) until about 2001. Subsequently, there was a significant trend towards a lower incidence of HIV-PAH ($P < 0.001$). The reason for the declining incidence of HIV-PAH is not clear. Although the occurrence of the disease is independent of the CD4 cell count (see below), quite unexpectedly, patients diagnosed during recent years had significantly lower levels of CD4 cells (15). Thus, other factors than the advent of HAART must be responsible for the decreased incidence of HIV-PAH.

CLINICAL PRESENTATION

The clinical presentation of the HIV-PAH patients from the French cohort (11,43) is shown in Table 15.6.1. In contrast to IPAH, there is a slight male preponderance, probably reflecting the sex distribution of the HIV population. Overall, the most frequent mode of HIV infection in

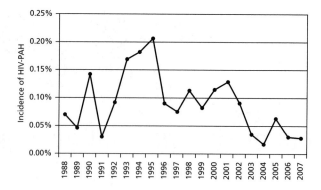

Figure 15.6.1 Yearly incidence of new PAH diagnoses as percentage of the total number of Swiss HIV Cohort Study participants with a follow-up visit during that year. Number of patients was 1433 in 1988, increasing to 7037 in 2007. The total prevalence was 0.47%. Since 2001 there was a significantly decreasing incidence by about 13% per year (Poisson regression: incidence rate ratio 0.87 (95% CI 0.80–0.94; $P < 0.001$). Courtesy of the Swiss HIV Cohort Study (Opravil M and Ledergerber B).

Table 15.6.1 Clinical characteristics of patients with HIV-PAH

Age (years)	40 (34)
Males (%)	63
Mode of HIV infection (%)	
Intravenous drug use	32 (59)
Heterosexual contact	34 (11)
Man having sex with men	27 (17)
Others	7
Duration of HIV infection (years)	6
Time interval from onset of symptoms to diagnosis of PAH (mo)	9
CD4 cell counts, /μL	437 (269)
CD4 cell counts < 200/μL, %	20 (52)
CDC stage C/symptomatic AIDS (%)	(37)
Undetectable viral load (%)	51
Receiving HAART at time of diagnosis of HIV-PAH (%)	83 (48)
Mean pulmonary artery pressure (mmHg)	49
Cardiac Index (L/min^{-1} m^{-2})	2.9
Pulmonary vascular resistance, dyn/sec cm^{-5}	749
Mixed venous saturation (%)	60
Acute responder to inhaled nitric oxide (%)	0

Data compiled from the French cohort (11,43). Values are given from their 59 HIV-PAH patients treated with first-line bosentan between 2002 and 2007 (11). If different, the data of their initial report of 82 cases admitted between 1986 and 2000 are indicated in brackets (11,43).

HIV-PAH patients is intravenous drug use (6,7,11,16). An epidemiological survey from France revealed that this transmission mode was significantly higher compared to the general HIV population (51 percent vs. 22 percent,

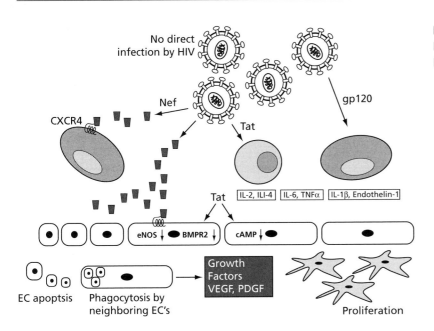

Figure 15.6.2 Suggested pathogenesis of HIV-PAH (see text). EC, endothelial cells; Lyc, lymphocytes; MΦ, macrophages.

$P < 0.001$) (14). While heterosexual and homosexual contacts seem to become an increasingly important HIV risk factor, infection through blood products and congenital transmission is exceedingly rare.

Symptoms and signs of HIV-PAH are comparable to those of the other forms of PAH. Progressive shortness of breath is the presenting symptom in more than 90 percent of the patients. Less common symptoms are peripheral edema or syncope in about 30 percent, non-productive cough, chest pain or Raynaud phenomenon in about 15 percent (7,16). The interval between onset of symptoms and diagnosis is only 10 to 14 months in the HIV-PAH group (6,11) compared to 30 months in sporadic IPAH (6). This might be due to a higher awareness with respect to HIV-PAH and/or a more aggressive course of the disease in HIV-infected patients.

The findings on physical examination were described only sporadically in the case reports (7,16). Electrocardiogram and chest radiograph findings were reported in about half of the patients, and both demonstrated the typical features of pulmonary hypertension in only 25 to 70 percent.

The duration of HIV infection before diagnosis is usually several years. However, there are cases in which PAH was the first indicator of HIV infection. It is important to note that patients in all stages of HIV infection can be affected by PAH. Less than one-third have CD4 cell counts below $200/\mu L$, and a quarter even had values greater than $500/\mu L$ (7,16). Nowadays, most of the patients are on treatment with HAART at the time PAH is diagnosed, and half of them have an undetectable viral load (11).

ETIOLOGY

HIV-PAH is characterized clinically and pathologically by the features of IPAH. Histopathologic findings were available from 43 literature cases. Of these, 36 patients (83 percent) demonstrated plexiform lesions (7). In addition, there are three literature reports of pulmonary veno-occlusive disease in HIV-infected patients (7).

In almost half of the cases described in the literature (7,14), HIV infection was the sole potential risk factor for PAH. Hence, it was hypothesized that infection by HIV could play a direct role in the pathogenesis of HIV-PAH. However, the virus itself could never be detected in the affected pulmonary vessels (17,18). In this context it has to be emphasized that neither does human herpesvirus-8 play a role in the pathogenesis of IPAH or HIV-PAH (19).

The absence of HIV in the vascular lesions suggests that the mechanisms underlying HIV-PAH may be due to indirect actions of HIV proteins and/or the associated immune dysregulation present in patients with HIV infection (Figure 15.6.2). In fact, Marecki *et al.* could show that in macaques infected by the simian immunodeficiency virus (SIV), complex plexiform-like lesions could be found exclusively in the animals infected by a chimeric viral construct containing the HIV *nef* gene in an SIV backbone (20). *Nef* enters macrophages and lymphocytes via the chemokine receptor CXCR4 very early during HIV infection. From there it is released and taken up into endothelial cells by the same receptor. The impact of endothelial *Nef* may be twofold. First, the HIV *Nef* protein induces disruption and apoptosis in endothelial cell layers, and the engulfment of these cells by surrounding endothelial cells may lead to an apoptosis-resistant population with increased secretion of cytokines and growth factors such as vascular endothelial growth factor and platelet-derived growth factor (PDGF) (20). It is well known that the expression of the latter is significantly increased in perivascular cells of patients with HIV-PAH (17). PDGF has the ability to induce the proliferation and migration of smooth muscle cells and fibroblasts, and it has been proposed to be a key mediator of fibroproliferation in PAH. Second, *Nef* is known as an important regulator of intracellular trafficking (21) and thus, for instance, might decrease transmembrane BMPR2 or cause trapping of eNOS in the Golgi complexes. This could also be the reason for the impressive tubuloreticular structures found in very early studies of HIV-PAH (18).

The essential and potential activator of HIV transcription, Tat, has been demonstrated to reduce BMPR2 promoter activity in a dose-dependent manner by up to 80 percent, resulting in a decreased activation of SMAD1, -5 and -6 (22). In addition, Tat upregulates TNF-α, IL-2, IL-4 and IL-6 (23). The importance of the latter in the pathogenesis of PAH has been underscored by Humbert et al., who found significantly increased IL-6 levels in IPAH patients compared to COPD and normal controls (24). Tat itself can function like an exogenous cytokine by the activation of endothelial cells and selectively upregulating E-selectin expression and enhances the secretion of IL-6 (25). Other effects of Tat are the reduction of cyclic AMP in rat microglia cultures (26) and the growth of abnormally large pleomorphic endothelial cells resembling Kaposi's sarcoma (27).

Another important HIV protein involved in the pathogenesis of HIV-PAH is the HIV-1 gp120 protein. It has been shown to cause apoptosis of human lung endothelial cells (28). In addition, the same authors found a dose-dependent up to 10-fold increase in endothelin-1 (ET-1) secretion by these cells. Gp120 can also stimulate ET-1 secretion by macrophages (29). Other groups have shown that HIV-1 gp120 induces the proliferation of vascular smooth muscle cells (30) and has the intrinsic capacity to stimulate monokine secretion including TNF-α, IL-1 β, and IL-6 (31); its importance in the pathogenesis has been shown previously by others (24).

Further evidence for a pathogenic role of endogenous vasoactive substances stems from a study which showed a marked reduction in the expression of prostacyclin synthase in two patients with HIV-PAH, comparable to the findings in IPAH (32).

Concomitant conditions present in the HIV population have to be considered as risk factors for the development of HIV-PAH. Even though intravenous drug use is significantly more frequent HIV-PAH (51 percent vs. 22 percent; $P < 0.001$) (14), according to the second WHO conference only the use of amphetamines is a very likely risk factor for PAH (33). In contrast, cocaine is regarded merely as a possible risk factor by these experts. The occurrence of pulmonary hypertension in HIV negative cocaine users is very rare. There are only nine cases reported in the literature. In all of them the hemodynamic changes were mild (34) and transient (35). Injection of small particles containing talc may cause granulomas within small pulmonary arteries and lead to increased pulmonary vascular resistance, as evidenced in autopsy studies (36). However, several studies conducted in the pre-AIDS era have clearly demonstrated that ordinary heroin does not contain enough crystalline debris to induce pulmonary angiothrombosis (37). This observation was also confirmed by autoptic studies on intravenous drug users (38). Moreover, histological specimens

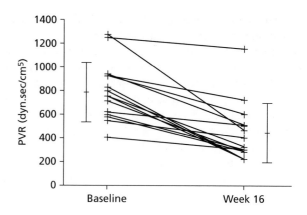

Figure 15.6.3 Individual change in pulmonary vascular resistance (PVR) from baseline to Week 16 of treatment with bosentan (n = 15). The mean value decreased from 781 + 250 dyn/sec cm^{-5} at baseline to 442 + 246 at Week 16 ($P < 0.001$). Reproduced from Sitbon et al. (47) with permission of the American Thoracic Society.

from patients with HIV-PAH showed only occasional birefringent talc particles that were usually located adjacent to and not within the plexiform lesions (Figure 15.6.3). In addition, their amount was incongruous with the severity of the vascular changes (39).

Liver cirrhosis was present in at least 11 of the literature cases of HIV-PAH. Since there is a very likely association between PAH and portal hypertension secondary to liver cirrhosis with a reported co-incidence of up to 2 percent (40), liver disease might have contributed at least in part to the development of PAH in some patients. However, no such case has been reported in literature so far.

MANAGEMENT

There are no guidelines for the treatment of HIV-PAH. In analogy to IPAH, oral anticoagulation is usually recommended in compliant patients without contraindications. The response to calcium antagonists in HIV-PAH is even poorer than in IPAH. None of the 41 cases in the National French Registry was an acute vasodilator responder (13). Serious adverse events including a case of cardiogenic shock have been reported (41).

Previous small series suggested that continuous intravenous epoprostenol might have a beneficial effect in HIV-PAH (42,43). Nunes et al. found an improved 3-year survival of 59 percent compared with 17 percent in historical cases on conventional therapy (43). However, the need of a permanent central venous access was hampered by the associated potential for infectious complications, particularly in these immunocompromised patients (43). Only single case reports have described the efficacy of sildenafil in patients with HIV-PAH (44,45). However, serious drug interactions with protease inhibitors may limit the use of sildenafil in these patients (46).

Fortunately, the management of HIV-PAH has been revolutionized during the past few years. After an initial study from the Swiss cohort suggested a benefit for patients receiving zidovudine (5), the subsequent retrospective analysis revealed a significant benefit for patients treated with HAART (15). Whereas untreated patients and those receiving only nucleoside reverse transcriptase inhibitors had a median survival of 1.5 and 1.7 years, respectively, only three of the 19 patients (16 percent) treated with HAART died after a mean follow-up of 3.4 years. Hence, it can be concluded that modern HAART is the mainstay treatment of HIV-PAH.

An open "proof of concept" 4-month study (BREATHE-4) involving 16 patients with severe HIV-PAH (mPAP 52 mmHg) demonstrated that bosentan increased the 6-minute walking distance by 91 meters, and in all but one stable patient also improved their NYHA/WHO functional class (47). Also most parameters of quality of life measured by the EQ-5D and the SF-36 improved significantly. Particularly impressive was the reduction of the PVR by –43 percent from 781 to 442 dyn/sec cm^{-5} (Figure 15.6.3).

Recently, the results of an open long-term observational study in 59 HIV-PAH patients receiving first-line bosentan monotherapy have been published (11). After 4 months the improvement was comparable to that in the BREATHE-4 study. After a mean follow-up time of 28 months, only five of 44 patients needed a combination therapy. In the 38 patients treated for more than 1 year, the 6-minute walking distance improved from 357 to 449 meters and the PVR decreased from 769 to 444 dyn/sec cm^{-5}. Notably, 10 patients had normalized their hemodynamics and improved to NYHA/WHO functional class I. Their baseline characteristics were comparable to those of the whole cohort. In four patients bosentan could be withdrawn without any adverse sequelae. In three of them bosentan had to be stopped because of elevated liver enzymes. However, as shown in a recent large-scale post-marketing surveillance (48), the frequency of liver enzyme elevations was no higher in HIV-PAH than in patients with PAH due to other aetiologies. In addition, in both trials bosentan had no influence on the control of HIV infection.

Hence, it can be concluded that the actual management of HIV-PAH consists of suppression of the HIV viral load by effective HAART and specific therapy of HIV-PAH by bosentan.

PROGNOSIS

During earlier years, HIV-PAH contributed significantly to mortality of HIV-infected patients. A case–control study comparing 19 cases of HIV-PAH with a well-matched HIV-infected group of patients without HIV-PAH demonstrated a median survival of 1.3 years in the HIV-PAH cases versus 2.6 years in the control subjects (5).

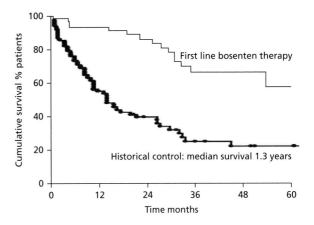

Figure 15.6.4   Kaplan–Meier estimates of survival in 59 patients with HIV-PAH treated with first-line bosenta (11) compared with historical control patients compiled from untreated historical controls (5,7,15,43). Reproduced and adapted from Degano *et al.* (11) with permission of the European Respiratory Society.

Fortunately, these dismal figures are outdated by now. The long-term study of Degano *et al.* demonstrated survival rates of 93, 86, and 66 percent at 1, 2, and 3 years, respectively (Figure 15.6.4) (11). So far, no consistent predictive factor for survival could be identified. Whereas in the earlier cohorts about half of the patients died because of right heart failure (5), in the bosentan long-term experience this was the case in only 7 percent (11).

KEY POINTS

- PAH is definitely associated with HIV infection with an annual incidence of about 0.1 percent and a prevalence around 0.5 percent.
- Hence, the relative risk of PAH in HIV-infected subjects is 500 to 1000 compared with the general population.
- The clinical and pathological presentation of HIV-PAH is comparable to IPAH.
- HIV-PAH occurs at any HIV stage independently of the CD4 cell count.
- While there are many new clinical and experimental data, the pathogenesis of HIV-PAH still remains unknown.
- The current optimal management strategy consists of effective HAART and treatment of HIV-PAH with the endothelin receptor antagonist bosentan.
- Although HIV-PAH initially had a worse prognosis than IPAH, with modern therapy its survival data approach that of IPAH patients.
- Screening with echocardiography of all HIV-infected subjects with unexplained shortness of breath or syncope is mandatory.

REFERENCES

• = Key primary paper

•1. Kim KK, Factor SM. Membranoproliferative glomerulonephritis and plexogenic pulmonary arteriopathy in a homosexual man with acquired immunodeficiency syndrome. Hum Pathol 1987;18:1293–6.

•2. Goldsmith GH, Jr., Baily RG, Brettler DB, Davidson WR, Jr., Ballard JO, Driscol TE et al. Primary pulmonary hypertension in patients with classic hemophilia. Ann Intern Med 1988;108:797–9.

•3. Himelman RB, Dohrmann M, Goodman P, Schiller NB, Starksen NF, Warnock M et al. Severe pulmonary hypertension and cor pulmonale in the acquired immunodeficiency syndrome. Am J Cardiol 1989;64: 1396–9.

•4. Speich R, Jenni R, Opravil M, Pfab M, Russi EW. Primary pulmonary hypertension in HIV infection. Chest 1991;100:1268–71.

•5. Opravil M, Pechere M, Speich R, Joller-Jemelka HI, Jenni R, Russi EW et al. HIV-associated primary pulmonary hypertension. A case control study. Swiss HIV Cohort Study. Am J Respir Crit Care Med 1997;155:990–5.

•6. Petitpretz P, Brenot F, Azarian R, Parent F, Rain B, Herve P et al. Pulmonary hypertension in patients with human immunodeficiency virus infection. Comparison with primary pulmonary hypertension. Circulation 1994; 89:2722–7.

•7. Mehta NJ, Khan IA, Mehta RN, Sepkowitz DA. HIV-related pulmonary hypertension: analytic review of 131 cases. Chest 2000;118:1133–41.

8. Barst RJ, McGoon M, Torbicki A, Sitbon O, Krowka MJ, Olschewski H et al. Diagnosis and differential assessment of pulmonary arterial hypertension. J Am Coll Cardiol 2004;43:40S–47S.

9. Maliakkal R, Friedman SA, Sridhar S. Progressive pulmonary thromboembolism in association with HIV disease. NY State J Med 1992;92:403–4.

10. Shen YM, Frenkel EP. Thrombosis and a hypercoagulable state in HIV-infected patients. Clin Appl Thromb Hemost 2004;10:277–80.

11. Degano B, Yaici A, Le Pavec J, Savale L, Jais X, Camara B et al. Long-term effects of bosentan in patients with HIV-associated pulmonary arterial hypertension. Eur Respir J 2009;33:92–8.

12. Centers for Disease Control and Prevention. 1993 revised classification system for HIV infection and expanded surveillance case definition for AIDS among adolescents and adults. MMWR 1992;41:1–17.

•13. Humbert M, Sitbon O, Chaouat A, Bertocchi M, Habib G, Gressin V et al. Pulmonary arterial hypertension in France: results from a national registry. Am J Respir Crit Care Med 2006;173:1023–30.

•14. Sitbon O, Lascoux-Combe C, Delfraissy JF, Yeni PG, Raffi F, De Zuttere D et al. Prevalence of HIV-related pulmonary arterial hypertension in the current antiretroviral therapy era. Am J Respir Crit Care Med 2008;177:108–13.

15. Zuber JP, Calmy A, Evison JM, Hasse B, Schiffer V, Wagels T et al. Pulmonary arterial hypertension related to HIV infection: improved hemodynamics and survival associated with antiretroviral therapy. Clin Infect Dis 2004;38:1178–85.

16. Krings P, Konorza T, Neumann T, Erbel T, on behalf of the Competence Network of Heart Failure. Pulmonary arterial hypertension related to HIV infection: a systematic review of the literature comprising 192 cases. Curr Med Res Opin 2007;23:S63–9.

•17. Humbert M, Monti G, Fartoukh M, Magnan A, Brenot F, Rain B et al. Platelet-derived growth factor expression in primary pulmonary hypertension: comparison of HIV seropositive and HIV seronegative patients. Eur Respir J 1998;11:554–9.

18. Mette SA, Palevsky HI, Pietra GG, Williams TM, Bruder E, Prestipino AJ et al. Primary pulmonary hypertension in association with human immunodeficiency virus infection. A possible viral etiology for some forms of hypertensive pulmonary arteriopathy. Am Rev Respir Dis 1992;145: 1196–200.

19. Montani D, Marcelin AG, Sitbon O, Calvez V, Simonneau G, Humbert M. Human herpes virus 8 in HIV and non-HIV infected patients with pulmonary arterial hypertension in France. Aids 2005;19:1239–40.

•20. Marecki JC, Cool CD, Parr JE, Beckey VE, Luciw PA, Tarantal AF et al. HIV-1 Nef is associated with complex pulmonary vascular lesions in SHIV-nef-infected macaques. Am J Respir Crit Care Med 2006;174:437–45.

21. Sehgal PB, Mukhopadhyay S. Dysfunctional intracellular trafficking in the pathobiology of pulmonary arterial hypertension. Am J Respir Cell Mol Biol 2007;37: 31–7.

22. Caldwell RL, Gadipatti R, Lane KB, Shepherd VL. HIV-1 TAT represses transcription of the bone morphogenic protein receptor-2 in U937 monocytic cells. J Leukoc Biol 2006; 79:192–201.

23. Sharma V, Knobloch TJ, Benjamin D. Differential expression of cytokine genes in HIV-1 tat transfected T and B cell lines. Biochem Biophys Res Commun 1995;208:704–13.

24. Humbert M, Monti G, Brenot F, Sitbon O, Portier A, Grangeot-Keros L et al. Increased interleukin-1 and interleukin-6 serum concentrations in severe primary pulmonary hypertension. Am J Respir Crit Care Med 1995;151:1628–31.

25. Hofman FM, Wright AD, Dohadwala MM, Wong-Staal F, Walker SM. Exogenous tat protein activates human endothelial cells. Blood 1993;82:2774–80.

26. Patrizio M, Colucci M, Levi G. Human immunodeficiency virus type 1 Tat protein decreases cyclic AMP synthesis in rat microglia cultures. J Neurochem 2001;77:399–407.

27. Vogel J, Hinrichs SH, Reynolds RK, Luciw PA, Jay G, Overland ES et al. The HIV tat gene induces dermal lesions resembling Kaposi's sarcoma in transgenic mice. Nature 1988;335:606–11.

28. Kanmogne GD, Primeaux C, Grammas P. Induction of apoptosis and endothelin-1 secretion in primary human lung endothelial cells by HIV-1 gp120 proteins. Biochem Biophys Res Commun 2005;333:1107–15.

29. Ehrenreich H, Rieckmann P, Sinowatz F, Weih KA, Arthur LO, Goebel FD et al. Potent stimulation of monocytic endothelin-1 production by HIV-1 glycoprotein 120. J Immunol 1993;150:4601–9.

30. Kim J, Ruff M, Karwatowska-Prokopczuk E, Hunt L, Ji H, Pert CB et al. HIV envelope protein gp120 induces neuropeptide Y receptor-mediated proliferation of vascular smooth muscle cells: relevance to AIDS cardiovascular pathogenesis. Regul Pept 1998;75–76:201–5.

31. Ameglio F, Capobianchi MR, Castilletti C, Cordiali Fei P, Fais S, Trento E et al. Recombinant gp120 induces IL-10 in resting peripheral blood mononuclear cells; correlation with the induction of other cytokines. Clin Exp Immunol 1994;95:455–8.

32. Tuder RM, Cool CD, Geraci MW, Wang J, Abman SH, Wright L et al. Prostacyclin synthase expression is decreased in lungs from patients with severe pulmonary hypertension. Am J Respir Crit Care Med 1999;159:1925–32.

33. Simonneau G, Galie N, Rubin LJ, Langleben D, Seeger W, Domenighetti G et al. Clinical classification of pulmonary hypertension. J Am Coll Cardiol 2004;43:5S–12S.

34. Yakel DL, Jr., Eisenberg MJ. Pulmonary artery hypertension in chronic intravenous cocaine users. Am Heart J 1995;130:398–9.

35. Collazos J, Martinez E, Fernandez A, Mayo J. Acute, reversible pulmonary hypertension associated with cocaine use. Respir Med 1996;90:171–4.

36. Kringsholm B, Christoffersen P. Lung and heart pathology in fatal drug addiction: a consecutive autopsy study. Forensic Sci Int 1987;34:39–51.

37. Overland ES, Nolan AJ, Hopewell PC. Alteration of pulmonary function in intravenous drug abusers. Prevalence, severity, and characterization of gas exchange abnormalities. Am J Med 1980;68:231–7.

38. Tomashefski JE, Hirsch CS. The pulmonary vascular lesions of intravenous drug abuse. Hum Pathol 1980;11:133–45.

39. Polos PG, Wolfe D, Harley RA, Strange C, Sahn SA. Pulmonary hypertension and human immunodeficiency virus infection. Two reports and a review of the literature. Chest 1992;101:474–8.

40. Hadengue A, Benhayoun MK, Lebrec D, Benhamou JP. Pulmonary hypertension complicating portal hypertension: prevalence and relation to splanchnic hemodynamics. Gastroenterology 1991;100:520–8.

41. Louis M, Thorens JB, Chevrolet JC. Calcium-channel blockers testing for primary pulmonary hypertension associated with HIV infection (abstract). Am Rev Respir Dis 1993;147:A536.

42 Aguilar RV, Farber HW. Epoprostenol (prostacyclin) therapy in HIV-associated pulmonary hypertension. Am J Respir Crit Care Med 2000;162:1846–50.

•43. Nunes H, Humbert M, Sitbon O, Morse JH, Deng Z, Knowles JA et al. Prognostic factors for survival in human immunodeficiency virus-associated pulmonary arterial hypertension. Am J Respir Crit Care Med 2003;167:1433–9.

44. Schumacher YO, Zdebik A, Huonker M, Kreisel W. Sildenafil in HIV-related pulmonary hypertension. Aids 2001;15:1747–8.

45. Alp S, Schlottmann R, Bauer TT, Schmidt WE, Bastian A. Long-time survival with HIV-related pulmonary arterial hypertension: a case report. Aids 2003;17:1714–5.

46. Highleyman L. Protease inhibitors and sildenafil (Viagra) should not be combined. Beta 1999;12:3.

•47. Sitbon O, Gressin V, Speich R, Macdonald PS, Opravil M, Cooper DA et al. Bosentan for the treatment of human immunodeficiency virus-associated pulmonary arterial hypertension. Am J Respir Crit Care Med 2004;170:1212–7.

48. Humbert M, Segal ES, Kiely DG, Carlsen J, Schwierin B, Hoeper MM. Results of European post-marketing surveillance of bosentan in pulmonary hypertension. Eur Respir J 2007;30:338–44.

Pulmonary hypertension associated with congenital systemic-to-pulmonary shunts

MAURICE BEGHETTI

INTRODUCTION

Congenital heart defects (CHD) are among the most common major malformations at birth with an incidence of approximately 8 per 1000 live births. These defects are characterized by a heterogeneous group of abnormal communications and connections between the cardiac chambers and vessels with different hemodynamic consequences and hence, varying need for follow-up and intervention(s). The most common forms are congenital systemic-to-pulmonary shunts (i.e., ventricular septal defects, atrial septal defects, atrioventricular septal defects or patent ductus arteriosus) that account for almost 60 percent of the malformations.

Pulmonary hypertension remains a major complicating factor of many types of congenital heart disease characterized by a systemic-to-pulmonary shunt either by causing increased morbidity and mortality during or immediately after surgical repair, or even preventing complete repair for those with advanced pulmonary vascular disease (PVD) (1).

When uncorrected, left-to-right shunting can lead to pulmonary vascular injury due to elevated pulmonary blood flow and shear stress (2). Vascular remodeling ensues, leading to increased pulmonary vascular resistance (PVR) and PVD: 15 percent of the CHD population is thought to develop PVD (3). These include those patients whose PVR may exceed systemic vascular resistance resulting in

reversed shunting (Eisenmenger's syndrome (ES)), with consequent chronic hypoxemia (4). For the patients with the most advanced form (ES), considered inoperable, histological lesions are very similar to idiopathic pulmonary arterial hypertension (PAH). One may argue that we do not know whether these are exactly similar, as a progression of the lesions is described only with a left-to-right shunt. Based on this assumption new targeted therapies have emerged as a potential treatment for ES. However, cardiac surgery (closure of the systemic-to-pulmonary shunt) performed at an early age is the treatment of choice for PAH associated with CHD (PAH-CHD) but the timing of surgery is crucial (5). Early intervention and protection of the pulmonary circulation is therefore a major determinant of prognosis for patients with PAH-CHD and screening of patients with CHD and systemic-to-pulmonary shunts for the presence of pulmonary vascular disease is essential.

DEFINITION

According to the currently accepted definition, PAH is characterized by a mean pulmonary arterial pressure (PAP) $>25\,mmHg$ at rest with a left atrial pressure $<15\,mmHg$ and a PVR >3 Wood units (6). However, in the setting of congenital heart disease, it is of utmost importance to

---

> **BOX 15.7.1: Simplified Therapeutic Approach of Systemic-to-pulmonary Shunts Based on Pulmonary Vascular Resistance**
>
> - Left to right shunt with high pulmonary blood flow and low pulmonary vascular resistance
>   - Therapy: surgical repair
> - Bidirectional shunt with normal or slightly increase pulmonary blood flow and moderate increase in pulmonary vascular resistance (considered inoperable)
>   - Therapy: conventional treatment or trial of targeted therapies (experimental)
> - Eisenmenger's syndrome: Right to left shunt with decreased pulmonary blood flow and high pulmonary vascular resistance
>   - Therapy: conventional treatment and trial of targeted therapies

appraise the hemodynamic cause of the increase in pulmonary arterial pressure. In CHD with left-to-right shunt, the increase in mean pulmonary arterial pressure may be due to an increase in pulmonary blood flow and/or an increase in PVR. PVR cannot be directly measured and is defined as the ratio of the mean fall of pressure across the pulmonary vascular bed divided by the pulmonary blood flow. PVR is thus derived from the formula PA-LA/Q, where PA is the mean pulmonary arterial pressure, LA is the left atrial pressure, and Q the pulmonary blood flow. From this formula, it appears clear that an increase in PAP may either be due to an increase in pulmonary blood flow (i.e., a left-to-right shunt), an increase in PVR or an increase in pulmonary venous pressure. It is consequently understandable that an accurate etiological diagnosis must be done before embarking on treatment, as patients with increased pulmonary blood flow and low PVR benefit from corrective surgery (closure of the shunt). In the opposite, namely those with decreased pulmonary blood flow, increased PVR and right-to-left shunt (Eisenmenger's syndrome), patients show generally advanced pulmonary vascular lesions and are denied corrective surgery as the risk of death is extremely high. For patients with moderate increase in PVR and who are considered inoperable (based on clinical and/or hemodynamic criteria) the role of targeted therapies has to be defined (Box 15.7.1). It should be noted that there are still no definite criteria to decide on operability.

EPIDEMIOLOGY AND CLASSIFICATION

A wide range of CHD can lead to PAH, but the most important group is left-to-right shunt lesions. This group includes many different defects that have different evolutions and this is of importance. One major difference is between pre- and post-tricuspid shunts, the latter developing PVD more rapidly.

Advances in pediatric cardiology and surgery have increased the number of CHD patients surviving into adulthood, and helped to prevent the onset of ES in many patients in the western world, resulting in a reduction of approximately 50 percent in prevalence over the past 50 years (7). However, there are still a growing number of patients presenting with malformations characterized by a so-called single ventricle physiology requiring a particular surgical approach (partial or total cavopulmonary anastomosis). Although they do not present pulmonary hypertension as per the classical definition, these patients may have pulmonary vascular lesions that either preclude surgery or carry a high level of morbidity.

Structural changes in the pulmonary vasculature in all forms of PAH, including ES, are qualitatively similar, although there is some variation in the distribution and prevalence of pathological changes within different underlying etiologies. According to the Venice classification, pulmonary hypertension resulting from CHD is grouped with IPAH, drug-related PAH, PAH associated with connective tissue diseases and HIV-related PAH (8). However, CHD is, as mentioned above, a complex group of pathologies that may differ from other forms of PAH with regards to cardiac anatomy, hemodynamic and natural history. This is one of the reasons why subclassifications have been developed to better define PAH-CHD patients. Subclassifications have been suggested by Galie (9) and Berger (10), both of them taking into account several factors important for describing the lesions, but also factors important in the development of PVD such as type and size of defects, hemodynamics, presence of extracardiac anomalies and repair status (unrepaired, palliated or repaired). Based on these suggestions and further understanding of the disease, several modifications have been introduced in the updated clinical classification of pulmonary hypertension (Dana Point, 2008) (11). These modifications include a specific subclassification for PAH-CHD allowing for a clinical classification of congenital systemic-to-pulmonary shunt, including ES; pre-Eisenmenger's considered inoperable; PAH with small defects that are not considered the cause of PAH; and PAH after successful corrective surgery (Box 15.7.2). An updated pathologic and physiopathologic classification has also been compiled that should satisfy both the CHD expert and non-expert (Box 15.7.3). The latter allows definition of all characteristics of the systemic-to-pulmonary shunt.

PATHOBIOLOGY AND PATHOPHYSIOLOGY

Intense research activity has led to a better understanding of the pathophysiology of the development of pulmonary vascular disease in congenital cardiac shunt.

In congenital heart disease with significantly increased pulmonary blood flow, progressive anatomic and functional abnormalities of the pulmonary vascular bed occur. This state is characterized by progressive smooth muscle hypertrophy and hyperplasia, intimal proliferation and pulmonary

BOX 15.7.2: Clinical Classification of Congenital Systemic-to-pulmonary Shunts Associated with PAH. (With permission of the Journal of American College of Cardiology, ref 11 and 39.)

- Eisenmenger's syndrome
  - Includes all systemic-to-pulmonary shunts due to large defects, leading to a severe increase of PVR and resulting in a reversed (pulmonary-to-systemic) or bidirectional shunt. Cyanosis, erythrocytosis and multiple organs involvement are present.
- Pulmonary arterial hypertension associated with systemic-to-pulmonary shunts
  - In these patients with moderate to large septal defects the increase of PVR is mild to moderate, systemic-to-pulmonary shunt is still largely prevalent and no cyanosis is present at rest.
- Pulmonary arterial hypertension with small septal defects
  - In these cases with small defects (usually ventricular septal defects < 1 cm and atrial septal defect < 2 cm of effective diameter assessed by echo) the clinical picture is very similar to idiopathic PAH.
- Pulmonary arterial hypertension after corrective cardiac surgery
  - In these cases congenital heart disease has been corrected but PAH either is still present immediately after surgery or has recurred several months or years after surgery in the absence of significant immediate postoperative residual lesions.

BOX 15.7.3: Pathological–pathophysiological Classification of Congenital Systemic-to-pulmonary Shunts Associated with PAH (Modified from Venice 2003; with Permission of the Journal of American College of Cardiology, ref 11 and 39.)

1. Type
   1.1 Simple Pre-tricuspid Shunts
      1.1.1 Atrial septal defect (ASD)
         1.1.1.1 Ostium stecundum
         1.1.1.2 Sinus venosus
      1.1.2 Total or partial unobstructed anomalous pulmonary venous return
   1.2 Simple Post-tricuspid Shunts
      1.2.1 Ventricular septal defect (VSD)
      1.2.2 Patent ductus arteriosus
   1.3 Combined Shunts
      Describe combination and define predominant defect
   1.4 Complex CHD
      1.4.1 Atrioventricular septal defects
         1.4.1.1 Partial (Ostium primum ASD)
         1.4.1.2 Complete
      1.4.2 Truncus arteriosus
      1.4.3 Single ventricle physiology with unobstructed pulmonary blood flow
      1.4.4 Transposition of the great arteries with VSD (without pulmonary stenosis) and/or patent ductus arteriosus
      1.4.5 Other

2. Dimension **(specify for each defect if more than one congenital heart defect)**
   2.1 Hemodynamic
      2.1.1 Restrictive (pressure gradient across the defect)
      2.1.2 Non-restrictive
   2.2 Anatomic
      2.2.1 Small to moderate (ASD $\leq$ 2.0 cm and VSD $\leq$ 1.0 cm)
      2.2.2 Large (ASD $>$ 2.0 cm and VSD $>$ 1.0 cm)

3. Direction of shunt
   3.1 Predominantly systemic-to-pulmonary
   3.2 Predominantly pulmonary-to-systemic
   3.3 Bidirectional

4. Associated extracardiac abnormalities

5. Repair status
   5.1 **Unoperated**
   5.2 **Palliated (specify type of operation/s, age at surgery)**
   5.3 **Repaired (specify type of operation/s, age at surgery)**

vasoconstriction. In addition, there are changes in extracellular matrix and adventitia with synthesis and deposition of collagen and elastin. The role of hemodynamics in the development of pulmonary vascular disease has been clearly demonstrated. Endothelial dysfunction occurs before the onset of pulmonary hypertension or histological evidence of smooth muscle dysfunction (12).

Complex interactions between vasoactive substances produced by the vascular endothelium may explain in part the changes in pulmonary vascular tone (13). Shear stress has been shown to alter the production of vasoactive substances. Endothelial shear stress is directly proportional to blood flow velocity and is inversely proportional to the radius of the vessel. A high blood flow rate alters the mean shear stress and may directly damage the endothelial cell; this in turn may impair the balance of vasoconstrictor/vasodilator, as well as promitotic and antimitotic functions, and lead to smooth muscle cell hypertrophy and proliferation (14).

The pulmonary vascular remodeling process is reversible in the early stages of the disease but may progress, with continuous stress, to smooth muscle cell proliferation in small arteries. It provokes changes in the extracellular

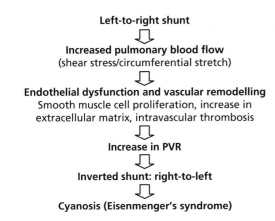

Left-to-right shunt

⇩

Increased pulmonary blood flow
(shear stress/circumferential stretch)

⇩

Endothelial dysfunction and vascular remodelling
Smooth muscle cell proliferation, increase in
extracellular matrix, intravascular thrombosis

⇩

Increase in PVR

⇩

Inverted shunt: right-to-left

⇩

Cyanosis (Eisenmenger's syndrome)

Figure 15.7.1 Natural history of congenital systemic-to-pulmonary shunts.

matrix and adventitia with synthesis and deposition of collagen and elastin; this progression renders the vessels relatively unresponsive to vasodilators and may preclude corrective surgery (Figure 15.7.1). The age at which congenital heart lesions cause inoperable pulmonary vascular disease varies. The consequences of increased pulmonary blood flow are more severe in the immature than mature animal. Endothelial cell morphology is modified as early as 2 months after birth in children with increased pulmonary blood flow. The development of irreversible lesions is also associated with the type of heart defect, and it seems that a combination of high pressure and high flow causes more rapid and more severe remodeling (5). Thus, surgical correction should be performed early in life in children with massive increase in pulmonary blood flow; before 2 years of age for ventricular septal defects (15) and even earlier (< 6 months) for atrioventricular septal defects, transposition of the great arteries with ventricular septal defect (16) or truncus arteriosus.

CLINICAL PRESENTATION

Young patients with systemic-to-pulmonary shunt present first, for the vast majority, with signs of congestive heart failure secondary to volume overload of the pulmonary vasculature and left side heart cavities. This is associated with feeding difficulties, tachypnea and/or dyspnea, recurrent chest infections and failure to thrive. As pulmonary vascular lesions progress and PVR increases, systemic-to-pulmonary shunt decrease and signs of congestive cardiac failure disappear. This is misleading as the patient seems indeed to improve, but this is related to the development of pulmonary vascular disease that will lead to inoperability and what was called fixed pulmonary vascular lesions. The natural history as shown in Figure 15.7.1 is a progressive increase in PVR until it reaches systemic vascular resistance (SVR); the shunt inverts and becomes right-to-left; and the patient develops central cyanosis. This is the classical definition of ES.

Physical findings of patients with ES show some similarities, but also some differences with other forms of PAH. The most striking difference is central cyanosis secondary to the right-to-left shunt. This cyanosis is responsible for numerous clinical findings or problems presented by ES patients. Clubbing, secondary erythrocytosis and hemoptysis are particular to these patients. Exercise intolerance is particularly severe as demonstrated by Diller *et al.* (7). Cerebrovascular incidents, thrombocytopenia, renal dysfunction, glomerular abnormalities, hyperuricemia, cholelithiasis and cholecystitis are potential clinical problems. Finally, if signs of cardiac failure reappear, they underscore advanced disease and high risk of mortality. Cardiac examination may show a right ventricular impulse, an accentuated second heart sound (pulmonary), and eventually a pulmonary and/or tricuspid regurgitant murmur.

INVESTIGATIONS

Chest x–ray

In operable patients, the chest radiograph shows cardiomegaly and increased pulmonary vascular markings characteristic of increased pulmonary blood flow, thus underscoring the low PVR. In the opposite in ES, there is a hyper-translucent periphery due to a decrease in pulmonary vascular markings as well as a dilatation of hilar and proximal vessels.

Electrocardiogram

In a simple lesion such as a ventricular septal defect, it may be easy to detect increased PVR as there will be clear signs of right ventricular hypertrophy. However, electrocardiogram features are more related to the underlying cardiac anatomy, and it is thus difficult to draw rules because of the complexity of some malformations, but there is usually hypertrophy of the subpulmonary ventricle.

Echocardiography

Echocardiography is essential in congenital cardiology, particularly in pediatric cardiology. Cardiac anatomy can almost always be clearly defined in experienced hands. Measurements of right and left atria and ventricles can be assessed as well as systolic and diastolic function. However, this should be assessed in relation to the cardiac malformation. Doppler interrogation of all valves or shunts can be performed and pulmonary arterial pressures measured using the Bernoulli equation, either for the systolic pulmonary arterial pressure with the Doppler interrogating the peak velocity of a tricuspid regurge or the velocity of blood flow at the level of the shunt, or the mean and diastolic pulmonary arterial pressure using the pulmonary valve regurgitation velocity.

Cardiac catheterization

For many years, cardiac catheterization was the most important investigation for cardiac malformations both for anatomical and hemodynamic assessment, but with the improvement in non-invasive methods such as echocardiography and magnetic resonance imaging, its role for defining anatomy has dramatically decreased. It still remains the gold standard for hemodynamics and particularly for PVR calculations, even if some inaccuracies in measurement of flow and resistance are difficult to avoid (17). A conventional study should assess the direction of the shunt, its magnitude (the ratio of pulmonary blood flow over systemic blood flow also called Qp/Qs) and the systemic and pulmonary vascular resistance. When the PVR is increased over the limit accepted for considering a low-risk surgical correction (there is indeed no accepted consensus limit but over 6 Wood units) a careful assessment of pulmonary vascular reactivity should be performed to evaluate the lowest PVR and pulmonary arterial pressure achieved during the test. It is used as a guide to decide for surgical repair. If PVR < 6 Wood units or the ratio of PVR over SVR < 0.3 the patient is still considered operable. This is based on the previous description of the histological lesion in congenital systemic-to-pulmonary shunt. A positive vasodilatory test indicates predominant vasoconstriction (medial hypertrophy and increased muscularization) that may regress after corrective surgery and closure of the shunt. Failure to induce a decrease in PVR indicates advanced lesions that will not regress after surgery and which carry a very high risk of immediate or short-term postoperative mortality. The test can be performed with the same drugs as the those used for other forms of PAH (6), but a preference is given to inhaled nitric oxide because of its selectivity for the pulmonary vascular bed, particularly when a shunt is present.

It is essential to remember that patients with intracardiac and extracardiac shunt represent a challenge when pulmonary and systemic blood flows need to be measured. The use of simple techniques such as thermodilution are not accurate and the Fick formula should be used. For this purpose it is suggested that measured instead of assumed oxygen consumption should be used (17,18). Several pressure and oxygen saturations have to be measured in all cavities and vessels. If the patient requires a vasodilatory testing, this should be performed in similar conditions to allow for comparisons. As conditions should be exactly similar pre and during testing, all confounding factors should be avoided. These factors are numerous: changes in sedation, pH, oxygenation, sampling errors, failure to account for dissolved oxygen if required, are only a few examples. This is the reason why this testing is difficult, long and requires experienced centers in which to be performed.

Should the patient present with PAH after correction of a systemic-to-pulmonary shunt, vasodilatory testing can be performed similarly to idiopathic PAH.

Magnetic resonance imaging

Magnetic resonance imaging is increasingly used in CHD. It allows a very accurate anatomic diagnosis even in complex malformations. Magnetic resonance imaging allows us to measure ventricular dimension and function. It can also detect the presence of intravascular thrombi. Several groups are currently studying the possibility of assessing hemodynamics in patients with CHD-PAH or idiopathic PAH using velocity encoding imaging and other methods (19,20). Even if it is not possible in current clinical practice, these studies are promising and it may be possible in the near future to perform a complete hemodynamic assessment non-invasively with this technique.

Open lung biopsy

Open lung biopsy is only seldom used nowadays. It was indeed a common practice to assess pulmonary vascular lesions in the 1980s. Assessment of pulmonary vascular lesions was based on the classification proposed by Heath and Edwards (21). This classification describes the patterns of microscopic lesions of the lung vessels. It includes six grades where grades I and II are considered reversible, and thus the patient operable, whereas grades IV to VI are considered irreversible. Grade III may or may not be reversible, and as for catheterization, this remains a grey area for potential operability. However, the lack of homogeneity of the lesions through the lung is a problem and progressively operability has been assessed through dynamic assessment as described before. Haworth and Reid (22) as well as Rabinovitch et al. (23) have tried to better the approach with improved descriptions, but currently very few centers base their decisions on lung biopsies.

With better understanding of the lung lesions, biopsies may gain favor again. Recently, Levy et al. described correlations between lung biopsy and circulating factors that may identify patients who are still operable (24).

Exercise capacity

Exercise capacity, particularly the 6-minute walk distance, has become of major interest in patients with PAH, as it has been the primary endpoint of numerous studies for this disease. It may be of interest in patients with ES; it has been reported that in these patients exercise capacity is particularly poor (25). The assessment of exercise capacity in patients with severe cyanosis and longstanding disease may also be biased by deconditioning and this should be taken into account in these patients.

Biological markers

Biological markers are of interest in this population as they are in the other forms of PAH. They are probably not of interest for diagnosis except for some circulating factors (endothelial progenitor cells) that may be related to endo-thelial function, but this requires further study. Their interest is more for follow-up. Clearly BNP and Nt-proBNP need studies to assess their role in the follow-up of these patients, particularly for the therapeutic approach and maybe for transplant listing.

TREATMENT

As already mentioned, when possible closure of the shunt either by surgery or interventional catheterization is cura-tive for congenital systemic-to-pulmonary shunts. Even if clear-cut numbers cannot be given to define operability, PVR > 10 Wood units or a PVR/SVR ratio > 0.7 are a con-traindication for closure. Conversely, a PVR < 3 Wood units and a ratio of < 0.3 is a clear indication for surgery. The problem arises in between these values and each center has its own limits. A consensus is difficult as there is still a need for better understanding of the operability contraindica-tions. However, it is of major importance to define the limit adequately, as patients who had surgery and presented with recurrent or persistent PAH showed a dismal prognosis as demonstrated by the report of Haworth *et al.* (26).

ACUTE POSTOPERATIVE PULMONARY HYPERTENSION

Even though this chapter is dedicated to chronic PAH in the setting of a congenital systemic-to-pulmonary shunt, it is important to discuss briefly the acute pulmonary hyper-tension presented by some patients immediately after adequate surgical repair.

In the immediate postoperative period of shunt cor-rection, the child is vulnerable to a sudden or sustained increase in PVR. Following surgery, pulmonary vascular reactivity is heightened and vasospastic stimuli may result in sudden increases in pulmonary arterial pressure and resistance resulting in acute right heart failure, tricuspid regurgitation, systemic hypotension, myocardial ischemia and increased airway resistance. These episodes, called pul-monary hypertensive crises, may be lethal events. Further-more, mildly stimulating events precipitate similar crises, and the crises tend to last longer and cluster (27,28).

Clearly, the pathophysiology of such events is complex and incompletely understood by the analysis or measure-ment of a single vasoactive mediator. Postoperative pulmo-nary hypertension represents a complex interplay between the preoperative condition of the patient (importantly age at repair, type of lesion and presence of a syndrome) and the inevitable disruption in the endocrine and vasoactive peptide (endothelin-1, nitric oxide and prostacyclin) milieu that results from surgery. Important contributors of enhanced vasoconstriction are cardiopulmonary bypass, hypothermia and circulatory arrest. Residual cardiac lesions and the sequelae of the stress response, hypoxia, metabolic and respiratory acidosis may all contribute additional

imbalances favoring pulmonary vasoconstriction. Cur-rently, endothelial cell dysfunction, presenting preoperatively and exacerbated by preoperative influences is considered a unifying hypothesis (29–31). However, improvements in surgical and perioperative technique and perhaps most importantly the trend towards performing surgical repair early, have resulted in a marked decrease in the incidence of symptomatic postoperative pulmonary hypertension in countries with privileged referral patterns. The incidence of postoperative pulmonary hypertensive events decreased from 31 percent in the 1980–84 era to 6.8 percent before the routine use of inhaled nitric oxide (32). Series reflective of contemporary practice suggest that pulmonary hyper-tension complicates 2.0 percent of patients undergoing congenital heart surgery with crises occurring in 0.75 per-cent (33). However, the mortality in those suffering a crisis remains high at 20 percent and pulmonary vascular disease is identified as a major contributor to hospital length of stay and need for prolonged mechanical ventilation (34,35).

EISENMENGER'S SYNDROME

As already mentioned, the most advanced form of PAH-CHD in the presence of a systemic-to-pulmonary shunt is ES. PAH associated with high pulmonary blood flow and low PVR is cured in the vast majority with surgical correc-tion and is not discussed further. Patients who present with persistent or recurrent PAH after surgical correction are indeed treated as idiopathic PAH, the hemodynamic pat-tern being similar. Borderline patients considered inoper-able due to moderate increase in PVR but not real ES will be discussed below.

In 1897, Viktor Eisenmenger described a patient who had suffered cyanosis and dyspnea since infancy and who subsequently died of massive hemoptysis at 32 years of age. Postmortem examination revealed a large ventricular septal defect and severe pulmonary vascular disease (36). Almost 60 years later, Paul Wood coined the term ES to describe pulmonary hypertension with reversed (pulmonary-to-systemic) shunt due to a range of cardiac defects including atrial septal defects, ventricular septal defects, patent duc-tus arteriosus, or aortopulmonary window (37).

ES represents the most advanced form of pulmonary arterial hypertension (PAH) associated with congenital heart disease (CHD). The signs and symptoms of ES usually result from low blood oxygen saturation and include cya-nosis, dyspnea, fatigue, dizziness, syncope, and arrhythmia. Symptoms may not arise until childhood or early adult-hood. In general, patients with ES have reduced life expect-ancy, although many survive into their third to fifth decade, with some even surviving into their seventh decade with appropriate management (38). Of all patients with CHD, those with ES are the most severely compromised in terms of exercise intolerance (25). Exercise intolerance in these patients has been identified as a predictor of hospitali-zation or death, independent of age, gender, World Health

Organization (WHO) functional class or underlying cardiac defect (25). Anecdotal evidence suggests that patients with ES adapt their lifestyle around their exercise capabilities, and that they tend to under-report their limitations. Despite this, ES clearly and severely affects a patient's exercise capacity and so decreases their quality of life.

Until recently, management options have been limited to palliative and supportive treatment alone for those patients who present with established disease. Increased understanding of the pathophysiology of ES and the success of disease-specific therapy in the treatment of other forms of PAH offers new hope for patients with ES (39).

Eisenmenger's syndrome compared with other forms of PAH

The structural changes in the pulmonary vasculature seen in all forms of PAH, including ES, are qualitatively similar, although there is some variation in the distribution and prevalence of pathological changes with different underlying etiologies (40). According to the Venice classification system, pulmonary hypertension resulting from CHD is grouped in the PAH category which also includes IPAH, drug-related PAH, PAH associated with connective tissue disease and HIV-related PAH. These forms of PAH are considered to have similar morphological findings, and to share similar responsiveness to treatment with continuous infusion of eproprostenol (41).

Although ES and IPAH share similar morphological findings, notable clinical differences do exist between these etiologies. In addition to morbidities typically seen in patients with IPAH such as dyspnea, cyanosis, fatigue and dizziness, patients with ES also suffer from a range of atypical problems including hemoptysis, cerebrovascular incidents, brain abscesses, secondary erythrocytosis and coagulation abnormalities, as well as sudden death, cardiac arrhythmia, and other problems associated with insufficient tissue oxygenation (38,42). Although both IPAH and ES are associated with reduced life expectancy, adults with ES have a more favorable hemodynamic profile and prognosis than adults with IPAH (43). Patients with ES have increased survival compared to patients with IPAH, with a reported 3-year survival rate of 77 percent compared with 35 percent for untreated IPAH.

It is thought that improved survival in patients with ES compared with patients with IPAH results from initial preservation of right ventricular function (44). In addition, some of the excess pressure in the right ventricle is relieved by the shunt to the left ventricle which develops in ES, although this is at the expense of hypoxia and cyanosis. Consequently, patients with ES have a better life expectancy than IPAH patients because of delayed appearance of heart failure.

Management options for patients with ES have been limited and the condition has generally been considered to be less amenable to therapy than IPAH. It has been long thought that, because of prolonged life expectancy, the best approach was primum non nocere! Despite the above described differences, the major similarities in vascular pathology between ES and IPAH imply that similar mechanisms and mediators may be active in both. For example, as discussed earlier, vasoactive factors have been recognized to be implicated as a key pathogenic mediator in IPAH and PAH associated with connective tissue disease and ES (45). Recent successes with new therapies targeted against the pathways implicated in the development of IPAH therefore offer potential benefits for patients with ES.

Treatment of Eisenmenger's syndrome

Advances in surgical technique for repair of cardiac defects mean that the development of ES can be prevented in most pediatric patients. However, when patients present with established disease, treatment has generally been limited to symptomatic management or heart–lung transplantation in a small, selected subgroup of patients.

CONVENTIONAL THERAPY

A summary of background therapy is given in Box 15.7.4. Treatment options for patients with ES were historically limited to palliative measures and heart–lung transplantation. Treatment most commonly involved the use of digitalis, diuretics, antiarrhythmics, and/or anticoagulants. However, none of these classes of drugs significantly modifies survival or significantly affects the risk of deterioration in ES (38). Digoxin has been used in palliative therapy for right heart failure in ES, although available evidence supporting its use for this indication is particularly weak. Digoxin may still be useful in patients with arrhythmias.

The use of anticoagulants in patients with ES is controversial, as ES patients have a high incidence of pulmonary artery thrombosis and stroke but of hemoptysis and hemorrhage also (46). One recent study estimated the prevalence of pulmonary artery thrombosis in ES to be 20 percent, the risk correlating with increasing age, biventricular dysfunction, dilatation of the pulmonary arteries, and concomitantly

---

BOX 15.7.4: Conventional Approach for Eisenmenger's Syndrome

PRIMUM NON NOCERE
- Regular follow-up in experienced centers
- Patient education
- Keep the physiological balance
- Prevent complications
- Endocarditis prophylaxis
- Avoid unnecessary non-cardiac surgery or if mandatory perform it in expert center with trained anesthetist and cardiac staff
- Contraception and avoid pregnancy
- Avoid strenuous but allow mild to moderate exercise
- Maintain fluid balance, avoid dehydration
- Annual immunization (influenza, pneumococcus)
- Oxygen: tailored approach
- Anticoagulation: tailored approach

decreased pulmonary flow velocity (47). Although evidence suggests a benefit of such treatment in patients with IPAH, no data exist in ES, and the associated hemorrhagic risks of treatment in these patients may outweigh potential benefits. No general recommendations for the use of anti-coagulants in patients with ES can therefore be given and patients should be assessed individually, with decisions guided by history and potential risk of bleeding.

The efficacy of calcium channel blockers in patients with ES is neither proven nor generally recommended, as their use can result in an acute decrease in systemic arterial pressure and increased right-to-left shunting, which may lead to syncope and sudden death (42).

Long-term oxygen therapy at home for a minimum of 12–15 hours per day may improve symptoms, but has not been shown to modify survival (7,46). As with anticoagulant use, each patient should be evaluated individually for oxygen therapy.

Patient education, behavioral modifications and awareness of potential medical risk factors are all important aspects of management. Patients with ES are at particular risk during cardiac and non-cardiac surgery and anesthesia, and as a result of dehydration, chest infections, high altitude and intravenous lines. It is also recommended to avoid strenuous exercise and not to participate in competitive sports (7) but regular activity is probably beneficial.

Pregnancy carries a high risk for both the mother and fetus and should therefore be discouraged (7).

Surgery, preferably heart–lung transplantation (HLT) or lung transplantation with heart surgery in very specific cases, is an option only for a small, selected subgroup of patients, and is severely limited by the availability of donor organs. Overall, transplantation in patients with ES is associated with high perioperative mortality (48). However, studies suggest that short- and long-term survival rates following HLT are similar to those reported in non-ES recipients, although the postoperative course tends to be more complicated in patients with ES (49). The prolonged estimated survival of patients with ES in comparison to idiopathic PAH, however, makes it very difficult to address if and when ES patients should be listed for transplant surgery. Studies to identify and define risk factors in this population are therefore required.

Given the paucity of suitable donor organs, the small number of suitable recipients and the poor prognosis following HLT, any treatment to delay the need for HLT in ES patients would be very welcome. One recent retrospective analysis suggests that ES patients who received novel, advanced therapies including prostacyclin analogs and endothelin receptor antagonists may benefit from significantly longer mean times to death or active listing for transplantation, by comparison with non-treated patients (50).

TARGETED THERAPY

Three major pathways (endothelin, nitric oxide and prostacyclin) are thought to be involved in the abnormal cellular proliferation and contraction seen in the pulmonary arteries of patients with PAH (45). All etiologies of PAH,

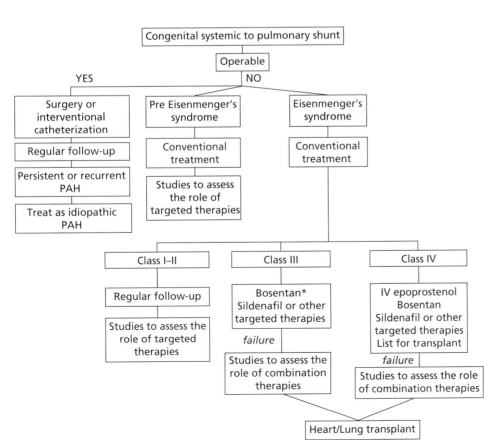

Figure 15.7.2 Suggested therapeutic approach of congenital systemic-to-pulmonary shunts. *Bosentan is the only approved targeted therapy in Eisenmenger's syndrome NHYA class III.

including PAH-CHD, share this similar pathology (9). These three pathophysiological pathways represent important signaling cascades in PAH, with current emerging therapies interacting with specific targets within these pathways. In view of the marked similarities between the pulmonary vascular changes observed in ES and other forms of PAH, disease-targeting therapies that have proved successful in IPAH have recently been investigated for the management of patients with ES.

Endothelin receptor antagonists (ERAs)

The endothelin-1 system plays a role in the structural and functional abnormalities in the pulmonary vasculature and the progression of PAH in all forms of the condition, including PAH-CHD (51,52). Given that treatment with ERAs has been successful in treating patients with other forms of PAH, they would be expected to have similar beneficial effects in patients with PAH-CHD. The first randomized, double-blind, placebo-controlled study in patients with ES was BREATHE-5 (Bosentan Randomized Trial of Endothelin Antagonist-5) which investigated the efficacy of the dual ERA, bosentan, in 54 adult patients with ES. During this 16-week study, bosentan significantly reduced PVR and mean PAP and improved exercise capacity compared with the placebo group, without adversely affecting systemic arterial oxygen saturation (53). This safety finding is of particular importance in patients with ES given the potential for aggravation of the overall shunt due to the possibility of a fall in systemic resistance in response to vasodilatory therapies. Longer follow-up data from the open-label follow-up study of patients enrolled in the original 16-week double-blind trial showed that improvements in exercise capacity continued over a further 24 weeks of treatment (54). Functional class also improved over this period, and treatment was well tolerated.

These findings are supported by a number of small-scale, open-label studies, which also demonstrate improvements in functional class, oxygen saturation, clinical status and pulmonary hemodynamics in pediatric and adult patients with ES (55–59). Long-term data suggest that improvements are maintained for as long as two years of treatment, without safety or tolerability issues (56,60,61). Others have controversial data showing return to baseline status (62,63). The findings from these studies challenge the dogma that pulmonary vascular disease in patients with ES is not amenable to treatment. On the other hand, ES is not a stable disease as it has been assumed, but progressive deterioration occurs, as demonstrated by the increase in PVR seen in patients from the placebo arm of the BREATHE-5 study (53).

Published data with sitaxentan* and ambrisentan are so far not available, but congress reports suggest beneficial effect in small uncontrolled data.

*Sitaxsentan was withdrawn in December 2010.

Prostacyclin and prostacyclin analogs

Overall, there are few data and no large trials concerning the use of prostanoids in ES. Long-term intravenous prostacyclin improved hemodynamics and functional class in 20 patients with PAH associated with a range of CHD, although none of the patients had an acute hemodynamic response (41). Continuous intravenous epoprostenol significantly improved functional class, arterial saturation and 6-minute walk distance, and decreased PVR in eight patients with ES after three months therapy (64). Two single case studies suggested that continuous prostacyclin therapy may improve hemodynamics sufficiently to enable ES patients with ASD to undergo surgical repair of the cardiac lesion (65,66). Clearly the potential benefits and risks of potent preoperative vasodilator therapy in what would be deemed "inoperable cases" merits further investigation. In addition, a number of adverse events have been recorded, including cerebrovascular accidents which probably resulted from the use of a central venous catheter in the presence of a right-to-left shunt. Given the relatively longer median survival in patients with ES compared to those with IPAH, the potential risks of long-term catheter use is especially important when analyzing the risk-to-benefit ratio of treatment. Data on other forms of prostanoid therapy in ES, including inhaled and intravenous iloprost, oral beraprost or subcutaneous treprostinil are limited to case reports and small studies (67–70). Inhaled and oral prostanoids offer obvious advantages over epoprostenol in terms of safety of long-term administration, but their efficacy and safety has not yet been fully studied in ES.

Phosphodiesterase type 5 inhibitors

There are no randomized controlled data regarding the use of the phosphodiesterase type 5 (PDE-5) inhibitors in patients with ES. After six months of treatment, WHO functional class, oxygen saturation, mean and systolic PAP and PVR were significantly improved in seven patients with ES who participated in a prospective, open-label trial of sildenafil, but although there was a trend towards improvement, changes in 6-minute walk distance (6MWD) did not reach significance (71). There were few significant side effects, and, although there was a theoretical possibility of reduced pulmonary blood flow due to reduced systemic resistance, cyanosis actually improved in these patients. Functional class, exercise capacity and pulmonary hemodynamics also improved without significant side effects in 21 patients with ES treated with sildenafil in a prospective, non-randomized, uncontrolled study (72).

Other small studies of PDE-5 inhibitors, alone and in combination with prostanoids, also showed improvements in exercise capacity, functional class and some hemodynamic parameters without safety issues (70,73,74). One study has been performed with tadalafil with similar results (73). In one study which was presented as an abstract at the last

European Society of Cardiology meeting, Palazzini and colleagues evaluated sildenafil in 24 patients with PAH-CHD. In this cohort, significant improvements were observed in both 6MWD and cardiopulmonary hemodynamics, with no important side effects. Taken together, these data increase confidence in the safety of PDE-5 inhibitors in ES. Results with regard to efficacy, although encouraging, need validation in large randomized, placebo-controlled trials. Such a trial – to investigate the effects of sildenafil on exercise capacity and cardiopulmonary hemodynamics in patients with ES – is currently recruiting participants in Germany.

INOPERABLE PATIENTS/PRE-EISENMENGER'S

Since the introduction of new targeted therapies for ES, major interest has focused on the potential of treating borderline patients in order to de-remodel the pulmonary vascular bed and enable successful corrective surgery. So far only a few case reports have been published on this subject and no definite proof of this potential has been recorded (65,66). One must remember that no cure has been offered with the current therapies in other forms of PAH, particularly idiopathic PAH that would support the role of regression of the lesions. However this needs to be trialed in this group of patients with careful assessment of long-term follow-up. The prolonged survival seen in ES compared to the dismal prognosis reported in patients with sustained or recurrent PAH after closure of the shunt must be kept in mind when this approach is evoked.

FUTURE ASPECTS

Although abnormalities in vasoconstriction may be clinically relevant in some patients, for those with more advanced vascular pathology changes in vessel structure, arterial narrowing and loss of the pulmonary microcirculation are likely to limit its contribution. Therapeutic approaches aimed at reversing vascular structural changes and regenerating pulmonary microvasculature may be of benefit in improving hemodynamics in such patients. There are currently no data as to whether targeted therapies result in significant improvement in the pathologic changes in the pulmonary arterial bed seen in ES along with other forms of PAH.

Concomitantly to clinical research and evaluation of new therapies, focus should remain on better understanding of the cause of pulmonary vascular remodeling in the setting of congenital systemic-to-pulmonary shunt.

Systemic endothelial dysfunction has been demonstrated in patients with cyanotic CHD, including ES, which is characterized by a markedly reduced vasodilatory response (75). A number of factors may be associated with this dysfunction, including the effects of prolonged hypoxia, cyanosis, and secondary erythrocytosis The clinical relevance of this systemic endothelial dysfunction in PAH-CHD – and therefore in ES – is unclear, although potentially this may

contribute to cardiovascular and cerebrovascular events seen in adults with these conditions (75). Whether current PAH therapies may also have a positive effect on the systemic circulation, and hence on other complications in ES, remains to be elucidated.

The potential use of regimens comprising combinations of targeted oral therapies is becoming increasingly common for treatment of PAH, and may offer an alternative treatment strategy for patients with ES. One group reported that a combination of bosentan with sildenafil was an efficacious treatment strategy in a small cohort of patients with IPAH or PAH-CHD (76). Clearly, these early data will need to be investigated in the context of randomized, controlled trials in larger PAH-CHD populations.

In addition, it is becoming increasingly apparent that the early diagnosis and treatment of PAH may underlie its optimal management. The key question facing physicians treating patients with ES is at which stage of disease should treatment start? A slow but clinically apparent progression of ES has been observed in the placebo-treated group of World Health Organization functional class III patients in the BREATHE-5 trial. Results from the randomized, double-blind, placebo-controlled EARLY trial, which enrolled PAH patients in World Health Organization functional class II exclusively, including those with PAH-CHD, indicate that early treatment with bosentan delays disease progression (77).

Finally, the role of new therapies currently studied in other forms of PAH such as guanylate cyclase stimulators, PDGF inhibitors, vasoactive intestinal peptide and statins, need to be specifically tested in the PAH-CHD populations.

CONCLUSIONS

ES is a severe and devastating condition which is associated with considerable morbidity, especially with regards to exercise capacity, and increased mortality. Patients with ES require meticulous management – preferably in a dedicated established CHD center connected with a pulmonary hypertension center – to enable the multisystemic nature of their disease to be addressed by a multidisciplinary approach. Research into the underlying pathophysiology of PAH has identified, and continues to identify, a number of important pathways and mechanisms which are involved in the vascular changes characteristic of the disease, and has led to the development of successful, targeted therapies. Results from clinical trials of these therapies in patients with ES are challenging the notion that ES is a stable disease, not amenable to treatment. To date, a number of targeted therapies including endothelin receptor antagonists, phosphodiesterase type 5 inhibitors, prostacyclin and prostacyclin analogs have shown to be effective in ES patients, offering improvements in exercise capacity, functional class and hemodynamics without compromising oxygen saturation. Future studies may seek to evaluate combined regimens of targeted therapies, or investigate if the pulmonary vascular remodeling in PAH-CHD can be specifically targeted and reversed.

KEY POINTS

- In the presence of congenital systemic-to-pulmonary shunt there is a progressive increase of pulmonary vascular lesions leading to advanced pulmonary vascular disease that finally precludes corrective surgery.
- The role of endothelial dysfunction in PAH associated with congenital systemic-to-pulmonary shunt has been clearly demonstrated.
- Early surgical repair avoids the progression of the lesions and is curative for the vast majority of patients.
- Even in the presence of adequate surgical repair, patients may present with acute pulmonary hypertensive crisis in the immediate postoperative setting and require aggressive therapy.
- Persistent or recurrent pulmonary arterial hypertension after surgical repair carries a dismal prognosis.
- Guidelines as well as new tools to define operability are required.
- For the most advanced form, Eisenmenger's syndrome, the new targeted treatments offer a potential new therapeutic approach, but long-term follow-up is required to understand the definite role of these drugs.
- For borderline patients, considered inoperable, the role of new targeted therapies needs to be assessed.
- New therapies should aim at de-remodeling the pulmonary vascular bed to potentially allow for surgical repair.

REFERENCES

- • = Key primary paper
- ◆ = Major review article
- ∗ = Management guideline

◆1. Beghetti M. Congenital heart disease and pulmonary hypertension. Rev Port Cardiol 2004;23(2):273–81.

◆2. Granton JT, Rabinovitch M. Pulmonary arterial hypertension in congenital heart disease. Cardiol Clin 2002;20(3): 441–57, vii.

•3. Kidd L, Driscoll DJ, Gersony WM et al. Second natural history study of congenital heart defects. Results of treatment of patients with ventricular septal defects. Circulation 1993;87(2 Suppl):I38–51.

•4. Diller GP, Dimopoulos K, Broberg CS et al. Presentation, survival prospects, and predictors of death in Eisenmenger

syndrome: a combined retrospective and case–control study. Eur Heart J 2006;27(14):1737–42.

5. Haworth SG. Pulmonary vascular disease in different types of congenital heart disease. Br Heart J 1984;52: 557–71.

∗6. Galie N, Torbicki A, Barst R et al. Guidelines on diagnosis and treatment of pulmonary arterial hypertension. The Task Force on Diagnosis and Treatment of Pulmonary Arterial Hypertension of the European Society of Cardiology. Eur Heart J 2004;25(24):2243–78.

◆7. Diller GP, Gatzoulis MA. Pulmonary vascular disease in adults with congenital heart disease. Circulation 2007;115(8):1039–50.

∗8. Simonneau G, Galie N, Rubin LJ et al. Clinical classification of pulmonary hypertension. J Am Coll Cardiol 2004; 43(12 Suppl S):5S–12S.

◆9. Galie N, Manes A, Palazzini M et al. Management of pulmonary arterial hypertension associated with congenital systemic-to-pulmonary shunts and Eisenmenger's syndrome. Drugs 2008;68(8):1049–66.

10. van Albada ME, Berger RM. Pulmonary arterial hypertension in congenital cardiac disease – the need for refinement of the Evian–Venice classification. Cardiol Young 2008;18(1):10–7.

∗11. Simonneau G, Robbin IM, Beghetti M et al. Updated clinical classification of pulmonary hypertension. J Am Coll Cardiol 2009 (in press).

12. Celermajer DS, Cullen S, Deanfield JE. Impairment of endothelium-dependent pulmonary artery relaxation in children with congenital heart disease and abnormal pulmonary hemodynamics. Circulation 1993;87(2): 440–6.

13. Rabinovitch M, Bothwell T, Hayakawa B et al. Pulmonary artery endothelial abnormalities in patients with congenital heart defects and pulmonary hypertension. Lab Inv 1986;55(6):632–53.

14. Rabinovitch M. Pulmonary hypertension: pathophysiology as a basis for clinical decision making. J Heart Lung Transplant 1999;18(11):1041–53.

•15. Haworth SG. Pulmonary vascular disease in ventricular septal defect: structural and functional correlations in lung biopsies from 85 patients, with outcome of intracardiac repair. J Pathol 1987;152(3):157–68.

16. Newfeld EA, Paul MM, Muster AJ, Idriss FS. Pulmonary vascular disease in complete transposition of the great arteries: a study of 200 patients. Am J Cardiol 1974;34(1):75–82.

17. Berger RM. Possibilities and impossibilities in the evaluation of pulmonary vascular disease in congenital heart defects. Eur Heart J 2000;21(1):17–27.

18. Fakler U, Pauli C, Hennig M, Sebening W, Hess J. Assumed oxygen consumption frequently results in large errors in the determination of cardiac output. J Thorac Cardiovasc Surg 2005;130(2):272–6.

19. Kuehne T, Yilmaz S, Schulze-Neick I et al. Magnetic resonance imaging guided catheterisation for assessment of pulmonary vascular resistance: in vivo validation and

clinical application in patients with pulmonary hypertension. Heart 2005;91(8):1064–9.

•20. Muthurangu V, Taylor A, Andriantsimiavona R *et al.* Novel method of quantifying pulmonary vascular resistance by use of simultaneous invasive pressure monitoring and phase-contrast magnetic resonance flow. Circulation 2004;110(7):826–34.

•21. Heath D, Edwards JE. The pathology of hypertensive pulmonary vascular disease; a description of six grades of structural changes in the pulmonary arteries with special reference to congenital cardiac septal defects. Circulation 1958;18(4 Part 1):533–47.

22. Haworth SG, Reid L. A morphometric study of regional variation in lung structure in infants with pulmonary hypertension and congenital cardiac defect. A justification of lung biopsy. Br Heart J 1978;40(8):825–31.

23. Rabinovitch M, Haworth S, Castaneda A, Nadas A, Reid L. Lung biopsy in congenital heart disease: a morphometric approach to pulmonary vascular disease. Circulation 1978;58:1107–22.

•24. Smadja DM, P. G, Mauge L *et al.* Circulating endothelial cells: a new candidate biomarker of irreversible pulmonary hypertension secondary to congenital heart disease. Circulation 2009;119:374–81.

•25. Diller GP, Dimopoulos K, Okonko D *et al.* Exercise intolerance in adult congenital heart disease: comparative severity, correlates, and prognostic implication. Circulation 2005;112(6):828–35.

•26. Haworth SG, Hislop AA. Treatment and survival in children with pulmonary arterial hypertension: the UK Pulmonary Hypertension Service for Children 2001–2006. Heart 2009;95(4):312–7.

27. Wheller J, George BL, Mulder DG, Jamarkani JM. Diagnosis and management of postoperative pulmonary hypertensive crisis. Circulation 1979;60(7):1640–4.

28. Hopkins RA, Bull C, Haworth SG, de Leval MR, Stark J. Pulmonary hypertensive crises following surgery for congenital heart defects in young children. Eur J Cardiothorac Surg 1991;5(12):628–34.

29. Adatia I, Barrow S, Stratton P, Ritter J, Haworth S. Effect of intracardiac repair on biosynthesis of thromboxane A2 and prostacyclin in children with a left-to-right shunt. Br Heart J 1994;72:452–6.

30. Komai H, Adatia I, Elliott MJ, Leval MRD, Haworth SG. Increased plasma levels of endothelin-1 after cardiopulmonary bypass in patients with pulmonary hypertension and congenital heart disease. J Thorac Cardiovasc Surg 1993;106:473–8.

•31. Wessel DL, Adatia I, Giglia TM, Thompson JE, Kulik TJ. Use of inhaled nitric oxide and acetylcholine in the evaluation of pulmonary hypertension and endothelial function after cardiopulmonary bypass. Circulation 1993;88(5 Pt 1): 2128–38.

32. Bando K, Turrentine MW, Sharp TG *et al.* Pulmonary hypertension after operations for congenital heart disease: analysis of risk factors and management. J Thorac Cardiovasc Surg 1996;112(6):1600–7; discussion 7–9.

33. Lindberg L, Olsson AK, Jogi P, Jonmarker C. How common is severe pulmonary hypertension after pediatric cardiac surgery? J Thorac Cardiovasc Surg 2002;123(6):1155–63.

34. Schulze-Neick I, Li J, Penny DJ, Redington AN. Pulmonary vascular resistance after cardiopulmonary bypass in infants: effect on postoperative recovery. J Thorac Cardiovasc Surg 2001;121(6):1033–9.

35. Brown KL, Ridout DA, Goldman AP, Hoskote A, Penny DJ. Risk factors for long intensive care unit stay after cardiopulmonary bypass in children. Crit Care Med 2003;31(1):28–33.

•36. Eisenmenger V. Die Angeborenen Defects des Kammerscheidewand des Herzen. Z Klin Med 1897; 32(1–28).

•37. Wood P. The Eisenmenger syndrome or pulmonary hypertension with reversed central shunt. I. Br Med J 1958;46(5098):701–9.

38. Daliento L, Somerville J, Presbitero P *et al.* Eisenmenger syndrome. Factors relating to deterioration and death. Eur Heart J 1998;19(12):1845–55.

◆39. Beghetti M, Galiè N. Eisenmenger syndrome. A clinical perspective in a new therapeutic era of pulmonary arterial hypertension. J Am Coll Cardiol 2009;53:733–40.

40. Pietra GG. The pathology of pulmonary hypertension. In: Primary Pulmonary Hypertension. Rubin LJ, Rich S, eds. New York: Marcel Dekker, 1997, Chapter 2, pp. 19–61.

•41. Rosenzweig EB, Kerstein D, Barst RJ. Long-term prostacyclin for pulmonary hypertension with associated congenital heart defects. Circulation 1999;99(14):1858–65.

42. Vongpatanasin W, Brickner ME, Hillis LD, Lange RA. The Eisenmenger syndrome in adults. Ann Intern Med 1998;128(9):745–55.

43. Hopkins WE, Ochoa LL, Richardson GW, Trulock EP. Comparison of the hemodynamics and survival of adults with severe primary pulmonary hypertension or Eisenmenger syndrome. J Heart Lung Transplant 1996; 15(1 Pt 1):100–5.

◆44. Hopkins WE. The remarkable right ventricle of patients with Eisenmenger syndrome. Coron Artery Dis 2005;16(1):19–25.

◆45. Humbert M, Morrell NW, Archer SL *et al.* Cellular and molecular pathobiology of pulmonary arterial hypertension. J Am Coll Cardiol 2004;43(12 Suppl S):13S–24S.

46. Deanfield J, Thaulow E, Warnes C *et al.* Management of grown up congenital heart disease. Eur Heart J 2003;24(11):1035–84.

47. Broberg CS, Ujita M, Prasad S *et al.* Pulmonary arterial thrombosis in Eisenmenger syndrome is associated with biventricular dysfunction and decreased pulmonary flow velocity. J Am Coll Cardiol 2007;50(7):634–42.

48. Berman EB, Barst RJ. Eisenmenger's syndrome: current management. Prog Cardiovasc Dis 2002;45(2):129–38.

49. Stoica SC, McNeil KD, Perreas K *et al.* Heart–lung transplantation for Eisenmenger syndrome: early and long-term results. Ann Thorac Surg 2001;72(6):1887–91.

50. Adriaenssens T, Delcroix M, Van Deyk K, Budts W. Advanced therapy may delay the need for transplantation in patients

with the Eisenmenger syndrome. Eur Heart J 2006;27(12): 1472–7.

◆51. Beghetti M, Black SM, Fineman JR. Endothelin-1 in congenital heart disease. Pediatr Res 2005;57(5 Pt 2): 16R–20R.

52. Galie N, Manes A, Branzi A. The endothelin system in pulmonary arterial hypertension. Cardiovasc Res 2004;61(2):227–37.

●53. Galie N, Beghetti M, Gatzoulis MA et al. Bosentan therapy in patients with Eisenmenger syndrome: a multicenter, double-blind, randomized, placebo-controlled study. Circulation 2006;114(1):48–54.

54. Gatzoulis MA, Beghetti M, Galie N et al. Longer-term bosentan therapy improves functional capacity in Eisenmenger syndrome: results of the BREATHE-5 open-label extension study. Int J Cardiol 2008;127(1):27–32.

55. Brun H, Thaulow E, Fredriksen PM, Holmstrom H. Treatment of patients with Eisenmenger's syndrome with Bosentan. Cardiol Young 2007;17(3):288–94.

56. Benza RL, Rayburn BK, Tallaj JA et al. Efficacy of bosentan in a small cohort of adult patients with pulmonary arterial hypertension related to congenital heart disease. Chest 2006;129(4):1009–15.

57. Schulze-Neick I, Gilbert N, Ewert R et al. Adult patients with congenital heart disease and pulmonary arterial hypertension: first open prospective multicenter study of bosentan therapy. Am Heart J 2005;150(4):716.

58. Gatzoulis MA, Rogers P, Li W et al. Safety and tolerability of bosentan in adults with Eisenmenger physiology. Int J Cardiol 2005;98(1):147–51.

59. Christensen DD, McConnell ME, Book WM, Mahle WT. Initial experience with bosentan therapy in patients with the Eisenmenger syndrome. Am J Cardiol 2004;94(2):261–3.

60. Diller GP, Dimopoulos K, Kaya MG et al. Long-term safety, tolerability and efficacy of bosentan in adults with pulmonary arterial hypertension associated with congenital heart disease. Heart 2007;93(8):974–6.

61. D'Alto M, Vizza CD, Romeo E et al. Long term effects of bosentan treatment in adult patients with pulmonary arterial hypertension related to congenital heart disease (Eisenmenger physiology): safety, tolerability, clinical, and haemodynamic effect. Heart 2007;93(5):621–5.

62. van Loon RL, Hoendermis ES, Duffels MG et al. Long-term effect of bosentan in adults versus children with pulmonary arterial hypertension associated with systemic-to-pulmonary shunt: does the beneficial effect persist? Am Heart J 2007;154(4):776–82.

63. Apostolopoulou SC, Manginas A, Cokkinos DV, Rammos S. Long-term oral bosentan treatment in patients with pulmonary arterial hypertension related to congenital heart disease: a 2-year study. Heart 2007;93(3):350–4.

64. Fernandes SM, Newburger JW, Lang P et al. Usefulness of epoprostenol therapy in the severely ill adolescent/adult

with Eisenmenger physiology. Am J Cardiol 2003;91(5): 632–5.

65. Frost AE, Quinones MA, Zoghbi WA, Noon GP. Reversal of pulmonary hypertension and subsequent repair of atrial septal defect after treatment with continuous intravenous epoprostenol. J Heart Lung Transplant 2005;24(4):501–3.

66. Schwerzmann M, Zafar M, McLaughlin PR, Chamberlain DW, Webb G, Granton J. Atrial septal defect closure in a patient with "irreversible" pulmonary hypertensive arteriopathy. Int J Cardiol 2006;110(1):104–7.

67. Limsuwan A, Pienvichit P, Khowsathit P. Beraprost therapy in children with pulmonary hypertension secondary to congenital heart disease. Pediatr Cardiol 2005;26(6):787–91.

●68. Ivy DD, Doran AK, Smith KJ et al. Short- and long-term effects of inhaled iloprost therapy in children with pulmonary arterial hypertension. J Am Coll Cardiol 2008;51(2):161–9.

69. Agapito AF, Sousa L, Oliveira JA, Feliciano J, Cacela D, Quininha J. Eisenmenger syndrome in the adult – experience with new drugs for the treatment of pulmonary hypertension. Rev Port Cardiol 2005;24(3):421–31.

70. Okyay K, Cemri M, Boyac B, Yalcn R, Cengel A. Use of long-term combined therapy with inhaled iloprost and oral sildenafil in an adult patient with Eisenmenger syndrome. Cardiol Rev 2005;13(6):312–4.

71. Chau EM, Fan KY, Chow WH. Effects of chronic sildenafil in patients with Eisenmenger syndrome versus idiopathic pulmonary arterial hypertension. Int J Cardiol 2007; 120(3):301–5.

72. Garg N, Sharma MK, Sinha N. Role of oral sildenafil in severe pulmonary arterial hypertension: clinical efficacy and dose response relationship. Int J Cardiol 2007;120(3):306–13.

●73. Mukhopadhyay S, Sharma M, Ramakrishnan S et al. Phosphodiesterase-5 inhibitor in Eisenmenger syndrome: a preliminary observational study. Circulation 2006; 114(17):1807–10.

74. Lim ZS, Salmon AP, Vettukattil JJ, Veldtman GR. Sildenafil therapy for pulmonary arterial hypertension associated with atrial septal defects. Int J Cardiol 2007;118(2): 178–82.

●75. Oechslin E, Kiowski W, Schindler R, Bernheim A, Julius B, Brunner-La Rocca HP. Systemic endothelial dysfunction in adults with cyanotic congenital heart disease. Circulation 2005;112(8):1106–12.

76. Lunze K, Gilbert N, Mebus S et al. First experience with an oral combination therapy using bosentan and sildenafil for pulmonary arterial hypertension. Eur J Clin Invest 2006;36 Suppl 3:32–8.

●77. Galie N, Rubin L, Hoeper M et al. Treatment of patients with mildly symptomatic pulmonary arterial hypertension with bosentan (EARLY study): a double-blind, randomised controlled trial. Lancet 2008;371(9630):2093–100.

Hemolysis-associated pulmonary hypertension in sickle cell disease and thalassemia

CLAUDIA R MORRIS AND MARK T GLADWIN

INTRODUCTION

The hemoglobinopathies are among the most common genetic disorders in the world. An estimated 5 percent of the global population are carriers of variants in either α or β globin genes resulting in two major red blood cell disorders, the thalassemia syndromes and sickle cell disease (SCD). These are autosomal recessive conditions that affect over 30 million people worldwide (1–5).

SCD occurs in individuals of African, Caribbean, Mediterranean, Arab and other Middle Eastern descent, and affects nearly 100,000 people in the US. Although an accurate account of the global burden of SCD is unknown, recent newborn screening analysis for hemoglobinopathies in the state of California revealed an incidence of 1/393 African-American infants born with SCD over an 8.5-year time period (6) whereas in sub-Saharan Africa, it is estimated that 1–4 percent of the population is born with this disease (4). Of interest, 12.5 percent of sickle-beta thalassemia infants born in California were of Hispanic origin (6).

Genetically, SCD is caused by an amino acid substitution of valine for glutamic acid in the sixth position of the β subunits of hemoglobin. This structural change results in intracellular polymerization of the deoxygenated hemoglobin molecules under hypoxic conditions. Intracellular polymer increases erythrocyte rigidity and ultimately damages and distorts the erythrocyte membrane. This produces a rigid "sickled" red cell with altered rheological and adhesive properties that becomes entrapped in the microcirculation and gives rise to the vaso-occlusive events characteristic of the disease (7).

Cycles of ischemia and reperfusion produce inflammation associated with increased expression of adhesion molecules on erythrocytes and endothelial cells. Adhesive interactions between erythrocytes, leukocytes, and endothelium, increased levels of circulating inflammatory cytokines, reduced blood flow from increased viscosity and vasoconstriction, hemostatic activation, and endothelial damage are all thought to contribute to obstruction of the microvasculature by sickled erythrocytes (8,9). Ultimately these red cell changes initiate a cascade of events that results in episodic vaso-occlusion and subsequent ischemia-reperfusion injury, leading to clinical sequelae (10).

The clinical phenotype of SCD varies widely, and is characterized by anemia, severe pain, and potentially life-threatening complications such as bacterial sepsis, splenic sequestration, acute chest syndrome (pneumonia), stroke and chronic organ damage. These and other manifestations result from chronic hemolysis and intermittent episodes of vascular occlusion that cause tissue injury and organ dysfunction (7,11,12).

The thalassemia syndromes are a heterogeneous group of inherited hemoglobin disorders resulting from unbalanced production of the alpha and beta globin subunits of the hemoglobin tetramer (13). Over 125 different genetic lesions can cause β-thalassemia, which is characterized by decreased (β^+-thalassemia) or absent (B0-thalassemia) synthesis of the β-globin chain (14). Thalassemia is most common in individuals whose ancestors originated from the Mediterranean region, Africa, southern China, Southeast Asia, and India (1). An estimated 900,000 births with clinically significant thalassemia disorders are expected in the next 20 years (15). The clinical spectrum is a consequence of imbalanced globin chain accumulation, resulting in impaired erythropoiesis and hemolytic anemia (16). The two clinically significant phenotypes of β-thalassemia have been designated thalassemia major and thalassemia intermedia. Thalassemia major is characterized by severe anemia starting during the first year of life, requiring life-long transfusion therapy for survival, while thalassemia intermedia has a later clinical onset with a milder anemia, does not typically require chronic transfusions, and offers a longer life expectancy (16). Heart failure is the most common cause of death in both forms of the disease (17–19). Thalassemia heart disease involves mainly left ventricular dysfunction caused by transfusion-induced iron overload. However, recent studies suggest that both thalassemia major and intermedia patients have a unique hemodynamic pattern consistent with right ventricular cardiomyopathy and pulmonary hypertension (PH), in addition to the left ventricular abnormalities (20). PH in β-thalassemia represents a common (21–26), yet less well explored complication in the cardiopulmonary spectrum of the disease.

Intravascular or intramedullary hemolysis, chronic anemia, oxidative stress, and a high frequency of PH are common features of both SCD and thalassemia (26–29). Secondary PH is emerging as one of the leading causes of mortality and morbidity in patients with hemolytic anemias (3,12,29–32); the consequence of complex and multifactorial mechanisms that will be addressed in this chapter. Current recommendations for the management of this newly appreciated category of PH will also be summarized.

HEMOLYSIS–ASSOCIATED PULMONARY HYPERTENSION: PREVALENCE AND EPIDEMIOLOGY

PH is an increasingly recognized complication of chronic hemolytic anemia, including the SCD and thalassemia syndromes (Box 15.8.1). Autopsy studies in both SCD and thalassemia reveal plexiform and concentric medial hyperplastic pulmonary vascular lesions, and in situ pulmonary artery thrombosis (33–37), which are common to all forms of PH. However, PH in patients with hemolytic disease exhibits unique features compared with other forms of PH, despite overlapping appearances. Patients with idiopathic pulmonary arterial hypertension (PAH) for example, tend to be young, lack comorbid organ dysfunction, and do not have critical anemia (38). In SCD, the presence of chronic anemia requires a high resting cardiac output (typically around 10 L/min) to compensate for a decrease

---

BOX 15.8.1: Hemolytic Disorders Associated with Pulmonary Hypertension

Sickle cell disease
Thalassemia intermedia and major
Paroxysmal nocturnal hemoglobinuria
Malaria
Glucose-6-phosphate dehydrogenase deficiency
Hereditary spherocytosis and stomatocytosis (and other red cell membrane disorders)
Hb-Mainz hemolytic anemia (and other unstable hemoglobin variants)
Alloimmune hemolytic anemia
Pyruvate kinase deficiency
Microangiopathic hemolytic anemia (hemolytic uremic syndrome, thrombotic thrombocytopenic purpura)
Hemolysis from mechanical heart valves
Left ventricular assist devices and cardio-pulmonary bypass procedures

---

in blood oxygen carrying capacity. Even mild elevations of pulmonary artery pressures in SCD appear to be poorly tolerated and are associated with significant morbidity and mortality (32).

Sickle cell disease

Much of what is known about the epidemiology of PH in SCD has emerged over the past decade as a consequence of several relatively large screening studies (4,5,32,39,40). Echocardiography has been successfully used to screen sickle cell populations for PH and to exclude underlying cardiac disease (12,32,41–44). Pulmonary pressures can be estimated by Doppler-echocardiographic assessment of the tricuspid regurgitant jet velocity (TRV). Using the Bernoulli equation, the TRV can allow one to calculate the right ventricular and pulmonary artery systolic pressures (PASP $\approx$ 4*TRV2) after adding an estimate of the central venous pressure. In SCD patients, this echocardiographic estimate correlates well with measured PASP by right heart catheterization (32). Using a definition of PH of a TRV $\geq$ 2.5 m/sec identifies approximately 30 percent of adult patients at risk for pulmonary artery systolic hypertension (PASP $\geq$ 35 mmHg); using a definition of PH of a TRV $\geq$ 3.0 m/sec identifies approximately 9 percent of adult patients at risk for pulmonary artery systolic hypertension (32).

While controversy surrounds the inclusion of a mildly elevated TRV between 2.5–2.9 m/sec in this definition (45,46), this value is approximately 2 standard deviations greater than normal. In SCD patients, the mortality risk associated with high TRV rises linearly and even values between 2.5–2.9 m/sec are associated with a high risk of death with an odds ratio for death of 4.4 (95 percent CI, 1.6–12.2; $P < 0.001$); a TRV $\geq$ 3 m/sec is associated with an odds ratio for death of 10.6 (95 percent CI, 3.3–33.6; $P < 0.001$) (Figure 15.8.1) (32). This association between increased TRV and mortality is significant, and has been confirmed in multiple studies (42,43,47–50). A TRV ≥ 2.5 m/sec carries a 40 percent mortality risk within 40 months of diagnosis in SCD (32) and is also associated with high risk of death in other conditions, such as congestive heart failure (51–53). While the presence of an elevated TRV is an independent risk factor for mortality (32,42,43, 48,49), it remains to be determined if this measurement reflects true PH per se, or a biomarker of disease severity and systemic vasculopathy in SCD.

It is increasingly clear that pulmonary pressures rise acutely during vaso-occlusive crisis (54) and even more so during the acute chest syndrome (55). A recent study examined 84 consecutive hospitalized patients with the acute chest syndrome and found that 13 percent had clinical manifestations of right heart failure placing them at the highest risk for mechanical ventilation and death (55). These data suggest that acute PH and right heart dysfunction represent major co-morbidities during the acute chest syndrome.

Although not as well characterized as the homozygous sickle cell population (HbSS), studies of SCD patients with a milder hemoglobin genotype (HbSC) demonstrate a high TRV in approximately 10–15 percent. Of interest, the mortality risk associated with an elevated TRV is similar, and possibly worse than observed with the HbSS population (56,57).

Early retrospective reports on the prevalence of Doppler-defined PH in children with SCD were similar to adults (49,58–61), however the consequences of PH in younger patients remain to be determined and are the topic of active research. The Pulmonary Hypertension and the Hypoxic Response in Sickle Cell Disease (PUSH) study is currently being conducted to evaluate this population prospectively; interim analysis of the first 399 SCD patients between the ages of 3 and 20 enrolled suggests a slightly lower prevalence of TRV elevation above 2.5 m/sec of 22 percent (62–64). However, based on the mean TRV + 2 SD in age- and gender-matched control children, the PUSH study has defined an elevated TRV in children as ≥ 2.6 m/sec. Using this definition, the prevalence of an elevated TRV is actually 11 percent in the PUSH study (62). More recently, a study focused on younger primarily African children (mean age 6.2 years) found a 21.6 percent prevalence of a TRV ≥ 2.5 m/sec which was associated with a history of acute chest syndrome. Children as young as 3 years old were found to have a TRV ≥ 2.5 m/sec. Longitudinal follow-up of eight patients within this cohort revealed persistent and often increasing elevations in TRV suggesting that, even in early childhood, an abnormal echocardiogram can be a useful study to screen for a higher risk population (65). Correlating right heart catheterization data, the gold standard diagnostic test for PH, are lacking in children, aside from case reports (66). However, the PUSH studies demonstrates that an elevated TRV in children is associated with increased hemolytic rate, oxygen desaturation during 6-minute walk test (62), and with decline in exercise capacity over 2 years (67). Although a different clinical phenotype has been described in children with Doppler-defined PH compared to adults (49), it appears that an elevated TRV may identify children at risk for cardiopulmonary dysfunction. Preliminary studies suggest that short-term mortality risk in SCD may not be as great in children with an elevated TRV compared to adults (49,68), however these children may still be at greater risk for complications in young adulthood and warrant close observation.

With the mortality risk in adults similar to that of other forms of PH despite the apparently mild elevation of pulmonary artery pressures, universal annual Doppler echocardiography screening of adults with SCD is recommended in order to identify a high-risk group that may be responsive to intervention (32). Routine screening of children should be strongly considered, particularly those with evidence of a high hemolytic rate. Annual screening is also warranted for the thalassemia syndromes.

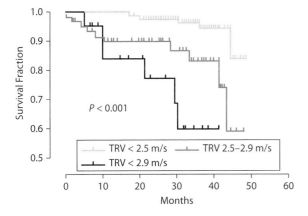

Figure 15.8.1 Survival of patients with SCD according to tricuspid regurgitant jet velocity (TRV). Survival of 247 patients in the NIH SCD cohort is shown from time of screening echocardiogram. Median follow-up is 30 months, results significant by logrank test for trend. Significantly greater survival is demonstrated in patients with normal pulmonary artery pressures (indicated by a TRV < 2.5 m/sec). A TRV between 2.5–2.9 m/sec is associated with an odds ratio for death of 4.4 (95 percent CI, 1.6–12.2; $P < 0.001$); a TRV ≥ 3 m/sec is associated with an odds ratio for death of 10.6 (95 percent CI, 3.3–33.6; $P < 0.001$).

DIASTOLIC DYSFUNCTION

The presence of left-sided heart disease detected either by echocardiogram or by right heart catheterization in up to 40 percent of these patients suggests an overlap, in some, of PAH and pulmonary venous hypertension (32,38,56). Left-sided heart disease in SCD is primarily due to diastolic dysfunction (present in approximately 13 percent of patients), although cases of systolic dysfunction and mitral or aortic valvular disease can occur as well (present in approximately 2 percent of patients) (48). The presence of diastolic dysfunction alone in SCD patients is an independent risk factor for mortality (48). Importantly, patients with both pulmonary vascular disease and echocardiographic evidence of diastolic dysfunction are at a particularly high risk of death (odds ratio for death of 12.0; 95 percent CI, 3.8 to 38.1; $P < 0.001$) (48).

FINDINGS ON RIGHT HEART CATHETERIZATION

Right heart catheterization studies of patients with SCD and PH reveal a hyperdynamic state similar to the hemodynamic profile of porto-pulmonary hypertension (12,38,50). The mean pulmonary artery pressure in patients with SCD and PH catheterized at the NIH is approximately 40 mmHg with a pulmonary vascular resistance (PVR) > 200 dynes/sec cm^{-5} (Table 15.8.1). The relatively low pulmonary vascular resistance observed in these patients is reflective of the high cardiac output of anemia. As hemoglobin level decreases, cardiac output increases, filling pressures tend to decrease and systemic and pulmonary vascular resistances decrease. In the above referenced NIH cohort of SCD patients undergoing right heart catheterization, the mean cardiac output and pulmonary vascular resistance for patients without PH were 10.9 L/min and 68 dynes/sec/cm^{-5}, respectively (38). It is within the context of these data that one must consider the impact of PH in chronically anemic patients with hemolytic disorders. Therefore, it is appropriate to consider a lower upper limit of "normal" pulmonary vascular resistance (such as < 160 dynes/sec/cm^{-5}) in these patients. Note that because PVR decreases as cardiac output rises, for an SCD patient with a "normal" cardiac output of 10 L/min

and a mean pulmonary artery pressure of 35 mmHg, the cardiac output would have to drop by more than 50 percent to increase the PVR above 3 Woods units.

In contrast to patients with traditional forms of pulmonary arterial hypertension (e.g. idiopathic, scleroderma-associated), who are symptomatic with mean pulmonary arterial pressures in the range of 50–60 mmHg, in patients with hemolytic disorders the degree of elevation in mean pulmonary pressures is mild to moderate, in the range of 30–40 mmHg, with mild elevations in pulmonary vascular resistance. Of catheterized SCD patients in the NIH cohort, approximately 60 percent with a TRV ≥ 3.0 m/sec meet the definition of PAH, indicating that the vasculopathy primarily involves the pulmonary arterial system. In the remaining 40 percent, the left ventricular end diastolic pressures are greater than 15 mmHg, indicating a component of left ventricular diastolic dysfunction. Figure 15.8.2 highlights a flow diagram for prevalence estimates of pulmonary systolic hypertension and pulmonary arterial and venous hypertension diagnosed by cardiac catheterization (12). A recently presented study of a French cohort of patients with SCD revealed slightly different results but confirmed the multifactorial etiology of elevated pulmonary artery pressures in this population (69). They reported that 6 percent of their screened cohort had a mean PAP of greater than or equal to 25 mmHg on right heart catheterization, even after excluding patients with chronic renal insufficiency, low total lung capacity, and evidence of liver dysfunction, which are all common complication of SCD (a likely explanation for their lower prevalence compared to the NIH cohort). Of the patients with MPAP greater than or equal to 25 mmHg, 55 percent of patients had pulmonary venous hypertension,

Table 15.8.1 Echocardiographic and hemodynamic measurements in patients with sickle cell disease

	Without PH	With PH	P value
Number of patients	17	26	
Age	41 ± 2	43 ± 2	NS
Gender (M/F)	8/9	11/15	
Hb (g/dL)	8.1 ± 0.3	8.3 ± 0.2	NS
TRV (m/sec)	2.4 ± 0.1	3.4 ± 0.1	< 0.001
6MWT	435 ± 31	320 ± 20	0.002
PAP mean (mmHg)	21.1 ± 0.4	36.6 ± 1.5	< 0.001
RAP (mmHg)	6.2 ± 0.5	10.7 ± 1.1	0.020
PCWP (mmHg)	12.1 ± 0.6	16.6 ± 1	0.009
CO (L/min)	10.9 ± 0.6	8.6 ± 0.5	0.017
Ejection fraction	65 ± 2	61 ± 2	NS
PVR (dynes/sec/cm^{-5})	68.3 ± 6	206.1 ± 29	< 0.001
TPR (dynes/sec/cm^{-5})	157 ± 10	370 ± 26	< 0.001
Pulmonary capacitance (mL/mmHg)	8.5 ± 0.8	4.3 ± 1.3	< 0.001
SVo$_2$	73 ± 1.5	66 ± 1.3	0.010

M/F, male/female; Hb, hemoglobin; TRV, tricuspid regurgitant jet velocity; 6MWT, 6-minute walk test; PA, pulmonary artery pressure; RAP, right atrial pressure; PCWP, pulmonary capillary wedge pressure; CO, cardiac output; PVR, Pulmonary vascular resistance; TPR, total pulmonary resistance; SVo$_2$, mixed venous oxygen saturation. Data are presented as mean ± SD; modified with permission (38).

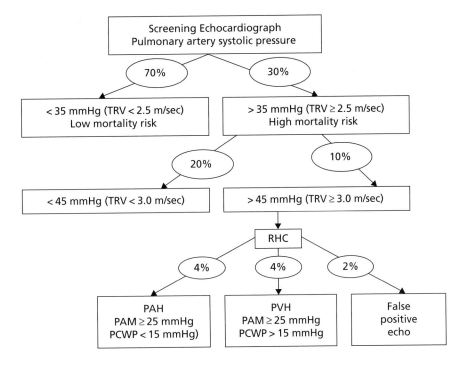

Figure 15.8.2 Overview of the epidemiology of pulmonary hypertension in the Hemoglobin SS adult population. These data are derived from the NIH population. Approximately 30 percent of HbSS adults will have a TRV of ≥ 2.5 m/sec (PASP ≥ 35 mmHg). Of those subjects, two thirds (20 percent of the total number of patients) will have PASP between 35 and 45 mmHg (TRV between 2.5 and 2.9 m/sec). The remaining 10 percent will have an estimated PASP of ≥ 45 mmHg (TRV ≥ 3.0 m/sec) and should proceed to right heart catheterization. At right heart catheterization (RHC), 4 percent of the original population will have pulmonary arterial hypertension, while 4 percent will have pulmonary venous hypertension. The remaining 2 percent will have normal right heart catheterizations, reflective of a false-positive echocardiogram.

22.5 percent had pulmonary arterial hypertension and 22.5 percent had PH secondary to a hyperdynamic state (69).

Thalassemia

Asymptomatic PH is a leading factor in heart failure and death in thalassemia (13–17,26). Studies in both thalassemia intermedia and major demonstrate that adults frequently have undetected PH, with a prevalence of 15–75 percent reported (18–22,25,70,71). In a study of thalassemia major, pulmonary systolic pressure above 30 mmHg was found in all patients over 22 years (21). A more recent study that included asymptomatic adults and children with thalassemia major over 10 years of age identified Doppler-defined PH in 20 percent of patients screened, 14 percent of adults, and 25 percent of children (71). Although the high prevalence of PH in non-transfused thalassemia intermediate patients has now been well documented (70,72,73), mild to moderate PH was diagnosed in over 50 percent of patients with β-thalassemia despite transfusion (21,24,73). Recent PH studies in more uniformly treated thalassemia patients have shown a lower frequency of increased pulmonary pressure in chronically transfused patients (19,22,74). A study of 202 thalassemia major patients concluded that strict compliance with chronic transfusion and chelation therapy to prevent iron overload reduces the occurrence of heart failure, and prevents PH (74). Although more aggressive transfusion programs may provide greater protection from the development of PH, the occurrence of intramedullary hemolysis, thrombocytosis, iron deposits and a resultant vasculopathy may still be able to induce PH which likely progresses slower. Nevertheless, these findings highlight the beneficial effect of regular transfusion in either prevention or slowing down the progression of PH in thalassemia (75).

RISK FACTORS

Sickle cell disease

Clinical risk factors for PH in adults include SS genotype, advancing age, a high hemolytic rate (elevated LDH, low hemoglobin, high bilirubin and reticulocyte counts), relative systemic hypertension, iron overload and priapism in men (5,32,44,49,59,76–78). Gender, fetal hemoglobin level, white-cell count, platelet count and the use of hydroxyurea therapy were unrelated to PH (32). Please see refs 79–91 for further details.

Thalassemia

Advancing age and a history of splenectomy are risk factors for PH in patients with thalassemia (26,70,73,92,93). In one study, the degree of anemia, number of transfusions and serum ferritin levels did not appear to correlate with risk (24). However, since strict compliance with chronic transfusion and chelation therapy to prevent iron overload reduces the occurrence of heart failure, and prevents PH (19,22,70,74), insufficiently transfused thalassemia patients may be at greater risk for the development of PH.

ETIOLOGY

A variety of abnormalities common to both SCD and thalassemia contribute to elevations in PASP and involve a complex interaction of platelets, the coagulation system, erythrocytes and endothelial cells along with inflammatory and vascular mediators. Although overlap in mechanisms contributing to vasculopathy occur in both hemoglobinopathies, the pathophysiology of PH is fundamentally different in patients with thalassemia intermedia compared to thalassemia major. Hemolysis is likely a driving force towards PH in non-transfused thalassemia intermedia patients, while the consequences of iron overload, splenectomy, and oxidative stress play a more significant role in thalassemia major patients on transfusion therapy. However, the biologic consequences of chronic hypoxia, long-term sequelae of splenectomy (93,94), red cell membrane pathology (95), coagulation abnormalities (96–99), low nitric oxide (NO) bioavailability (100), excess arginase activity (77,101,102), platelet activation (73,103,104), oxidative stress (78,105), iron overload (20–22,72,106–108), and chronic hemolysis (31,100) will simultaneously contribute in various degrees to PH in both SCD and the thalassemia syndromes. Ultimately the etiology of PH in these hemoglobinopathies is complex and multifactorial (Figure 15.8.3). Since the majority of these mechanisms are covered in other chapters, we will focus on the evolving appreciation of the role of hemolysis, and its contribution to vasculopathy and the pathophysiology of PH in SCD and thalassemia.

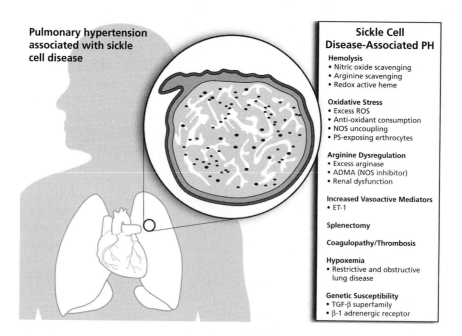

Figure 15.8.3 Mechanisms of vasculopathy and pulmonary hypertension in sickle cell disease. Hemolysis, arginine dysregulation, splenectomy, coagulopathy, oxidative stress, hypoxemia and genetic susceptibility are key mechanisms that contribute to the complex vascular pathophysiology of sickle cell disease (SCD). These events limit nitric oxide (NO) bioavailability through several paths that ultimately provoke increased consumption and decreased production of the potent vasodilator, NO. Although often discussed independently, there is significant overlap closely linking these pathways of endothelial dysfunction that prohibit determining cause and effect. The contribution of inflammation coupled with antioxidant depletion, ischemia-reperfusion injury, and acute as well as chronic end organ damage obscure mechanistic boundaries further. The end result is vascular smooth muscle proliferation, chronic pulmonary vasoconstriction, elevated pulmonary vascular resistance and an increase in pulmonary artery pressures. Overabundant thrombin generation and altered red cell membrane lipid biology contributes to a chronic hypercoagulable state. As this becomes more long-standing, vascular smooth muscle hyperplasia begins to create a relatively fixed lesion, compounded in later stages by irregular, activated endothelium with expression of adhesion molecules. In situ thrombosis further occludes the vessel lumen, and results in plexogenic changes, further accelerating the progression of the pulmonary artery hypertension.

Disruption of the arginine–nitric oxide pathway by intravascular hemolysis: A novel paradigm

A new paradigm of hemolysis-associated endothelial dysfunction has been hypothesized to contribute to the development of PH in the hemoglobinopathies (3,12,31,32,76,100–102,109–111). Rapid consumption and decreased production of NO is a fundamental aspect of this model.

According to this hypothesis, hemoglobin is decompartmentalized from the erythrocyte during the process of hemolysis and released into plasma where it rapidly reacts with and destroys NO (112). This results in abnormally high NO consumption, the formation of reactive oxygen species, and a state of NO resistance (31,113). The simultaneous release of erythrocyte arginase, an enzyme that metabolizes arginine, the obligate substrate for NO production during hemolysis (77) further diminished NO bioavailability (Figure 15.8.4). Formation of superoxide from

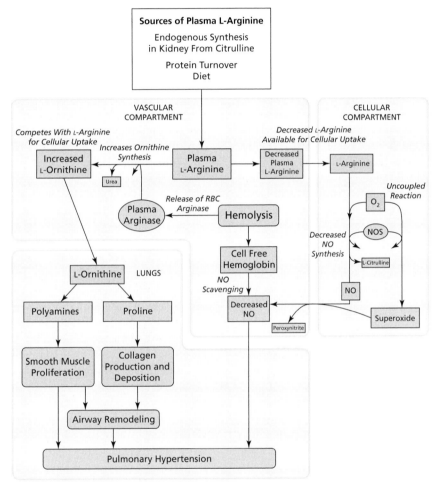

© American Medical Association. JAMA 2005;294:81–90.

Figure 15.8.4 Disruption of the arginine-nitric oxide pathway in hemolytic disorders. Arginine is synthesized endogenously from citrulline primarily via the intestinal-renal axis. Arginase and nitric oxide synthase (NOS) compete for arginine, their common substrate. In sickle cell disease (SCD), bioavailability of arginine and nitric oxide (NO) are decreased by several mechanisms linked to hemolysis, and similar mechanisms are postulated for thalassemia and other hemolytic disorders. The release of erythrocyte arginase during hemolysis increases plasma arginase levels and shifts arginine metabolism towards ornithine production, decreasing the amount available for NO production. The bioavailability of arginine is further decreased by increased ornithine levels because ornithine and arginine compete for the same transporter system for cellular uptake. Endogenous synthesis of arginine from citrulline may be compromised by renal dysfunction, commonly associated with SCD. Despite an increase in NOS in SCD, NO bioavailability is low due to low substrate availability, NO scavenging by cell-free hemoglobin released during hemolysis, and through reactions with free radicals such as superoxide. Superoxide is elevated in SCD due to low superoxide dismutase activity, high xanthine oxidase activity and potentially as a result of uncoupled NOS in an environment of low arginine and/or tetrahydrobiopterin concentration. Endothelial dysfunction resulting from NO depletion and increased levels of the downstream products of ornithine metabolism (polyamines and proline) likely contribute to the pathogenesis of lung injury, fibrosis and pulmonary hypertension. This new disease paradigm has implications for all hemolytic processes. Reproduced with permission from the American Medical Association (77).

enzymatic oxidases such as NADPH oxidase (114), xanthine oxidase (115,116) and uncoupled endothelial NO synthase (110,113) will also react with and scavenge NO, contributing to a state of NO resistance. Consequently, smooth muscle guanylyl cyclase is not activated and vasodilation is inhibited. NO destruction by hemoglobin can also cause further impairment in vascular endothelial function via transcriptional activation of adhesion molecules, and potent vasoconstrictors such as endothelin-1 (31). Intravascular hemolysis also has the potential to drive a pro-coagulant state, as NO has properties that inhibits platelet activation, tissue factor expression and thrombin generation (31).

PH has been definitively linked to hemolytic rate and low NO bioavailability in both human (3,31,32,76,111) and sickle cell transgenic mouse studies (110,117). Endothelial dysfunction is also a result of an impaired arginine-NO pathway, oxidative stress and tissue damage, which enhances hypercoagulability and *in situ* thrombus formation within the pulmonary artery walls, contributing to functional and structural alterations of pulmonary vessels (118). Oxidative stress is exacerbated by hemolysis (78,104), the presence of iron overload (105) and through cycles of ischemia and reperfusion. Iron overload, present in transfused thalassemia and SCD patients, also affects PH by other mechanisms. It induces interstitial pulmonary fibrosis (107) as well as left and right cardiac hemosiderosis which subsequently results in cardiac dysfunction and affects pulmonary vascular resistance (107). Chronic anemia and hypoxemia lead to further vasoconstriction and increase of pulmonary vascular resistance. Hypoxia is also shown to alter the von Willebrand factor (vWF) released by endothelial cells in secondary PH, affecting platelet activation and consumption (119).

Alterations in the arginine metabolome and elevated arginase activity have been implicated in the pathogenesis of PH in both hemolytic (27,77,120,121,89,101,102,121, 122) and non-hemolytic disorders (123,124). Once released into circulation, arginase will convert arginine to ornithine, which in turn is the precursor to proline, an amino acid involved in collagen formation, lung fibrosis, airway remodeling, asthma and vascular smooth muscle proliferation (77). These are common features of pulmonary dysfunction in both SCD (38,49,91,125,126) and thalassemia (127). By creating a shift towards ornithine metabolism, arginase triggers a process that contributes to a proliferative vasculopathy regardless of the initiating trigger (27,28,77).

CLINICAL PRESENTATION

Early stages of PH in chronic hemolytic disorders may be asymptomatic or associated with mild symptoms. Classic symptoms of PH like exertional dypsnea overlap with those of chronic anemia, often delaying clinical suspicion until late in the course of disease. In addition, the multi-organ complications of hemolytic anemias may limit exercise tolerance independent of elevations in pulmonary vascular resistance (30). Asthma may also be a co-founding complication with overlapping symptoms that requires screening (49,128). Hypoxemia, which could also be the result of restrictive lung disease, may be an early sign of PH. Although cardiac function is frequently compromised due to iron overload, chronic anemia and hypoxemia, liver disease and a hypercoagulable state, more specific symptoms of PH such as angina, syncope and lower extremity edema are uncommon and are associated with severe and advanced PH. Physical findings suggestive of right ventricular dysfunction, including jugular venous distention, right ventricular S3 gallop, an accentuated pulmonary component of S2, oxygen desaturation, ascites, peripheral edema should raise suspicion, and a high prevalence of clubbing in sickle cell and thalassemia patients with PH has been observed. Other conditions commonly found in these patients, such as left ventricular systolic or diastolic function, pulmonary fibrosis, and cirrhosis of the liver also contribute to the pathogenesis of PH (30).

Adults with SCD and PH tend to be older, have higher systolic arterial blood pressure, lower hemoglobin levels, higher indices of hemolytic rate, lower oxygen saturations, a greater degree of renal and liver dysfunction, and higher number of lifetime red blood cell transfusions, (5,32,44, 49,59,76,77) suggesting a greater burden of disease and a generalized vasculopathy associated with intravascular hemolysis (12,28,32,129). A high TRV in children is also associated with an increased hemolytic rate (58,61,62,130,131) with a normal TRV. Young patients have few clinical symptoms of PH and less end-organ damage than their adult counterpart, but a history of acute chest syndrome (49,65), asthma and/or sepsis is more common than children (49).

Intravascular hemolysis is associated with a growing list of clinical complications of SCD, including multi-organ failure (132), priapism (76,133), leg ulcers (76,133,134) and stroke (135) in addition to PH and mortality and constitute what is now considered the hemolytic subphenotypes of SCD (111). These patients as a group, often have less frequent vaso-occlusive pain events and a hyperhemolysis phenotype (136) coupled with elevated lactate dehydrogenase (LDH) levels (76). Serum LDH is released from the erythrocyte along with free hemoglobin and arginase. As such, LDH represents a convenient biomarker of intravascular hemolysis and NO bioavailability associated with mortality in SCD (76) that Kato and colleagues found helpful in identifying the clinical subphenotypes of hemolysis-associated vasculopathy (Figure 15.8.5) (111). Following steady-state LDH levels may be a convenient means to monitor these patients and intensify therapy when chronic hyper-hemolysis is identified (76,111,136,137). Priapism and cutaneous leg ulcers have also been reported in patients with thalassemia intermedia and other hemolytic anemias in addition to SCD (111). Similar to SCD, PH is often diagnosed at late stages in the thalassemia syndromes. Therefore, clinical suspicion should be high in all hemolytic disorders.

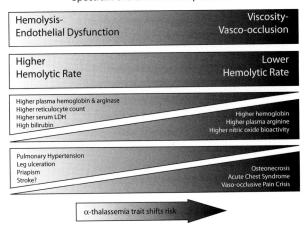

Spectrum of Sickle Cell Complications

Figure 15.8.5 Spectrum of sickle cell subphenotypes affected by hemolytic rate. The viscosity-vaso-occlusion subphenotype is associated with a lower hemolytic rate, marked by a higher hemoglobin level, and low plasma hemoglobin, lactate dehydrogenase (LDH), bilirubin and arginase levels. Patients with these features have a higher incidence of vaso-occlusive pain crisis, acute chest syndrome, and osteonecrosis. In contrast, patients with the hemolysis-endothelial dysfunction subphenotype exhibit markers of high hemolytic rate, including low hemoglobin level, high plasma hemoglobin, LDH, bilirubin, and arginase, culminating in low nitric oxide bioavailability and high prevalence of pulmonary hypertension, leg ulceration, priapism, and stroke. Co-inheritance of α–thalassemia trait with sickle cell disease reduces the hemolytic rate, minimizes the risk of hemolysis-associated complications and increases the risk of viscosity-related complications. Adapted with permission (111).

INVESTIGATIONS

Echocardiography can identify patients at high risk of PH in patients with a detectable TRV, however the gold standard for diagnosis of PH is right-sided cardiac catheterization with measure of the pulmonary artery pressure. Diagnostic evaluations for PH in patients with hemolytic disorders should follow the same guidelines established for other causes of PAH. Symptoms evaluation should include the World Health Organization classification and a Borg Dypsnea Score. Vital signs should include monitoring of systolic and diastolic blood pressure as well as oxygen saturation by pulse-oximetry. History and laboratory assessment should be performed to exclude other conditions associated with PH, including collagen vascular disorders, HIV, viral hepatitis, particularly hepatitis C, pregnancy and stimulant use. Liver and renal function tests, biomarkers of hemolytic rate (LDH, reticulocyte count, hemoglobin/hematocrit, bilirubin) (62), NT-proBNP levels (80), and severity of iron-overload should also monitored. An electrocardiogram should be performed given association with prolonged QTc that has been identified in patients with

SCD and PH (138). Since abnormal pulmonary function is common in both SCD and thalassemia (38,49,91,125–127,139–145), a comprehensive pulmonary evaluation should also incorporate annual pulmonary function testing to include spirometry, lung volumes and diffusion capacity (DL_{CO}) corrected for hemoglobin. In SCD, an association of TRV with lung fibrosis (146) and restrictive (125) as well as obstructive lung disease (60) has been described. Measurements of reversible airway reactivity should also be performed given increased risk of mortality in patients with SCD and asthma (141), and can be determined by clinical history alone (95) and through bronchodilator responsiveness or metacholine challenge (142,143).

Six-minute walk test (6MWT)

The 6MWT, the most commonly used exercise test in patients with PH, was recently validated in adults with SCD as an index of PH and cardiopulmonary function. 6MWT correlates directly with peak oxygen consumption and TRV by Doppler echocardiography, and inversely with pulmonary vascular resistance and mean pulmonary artery pressure on cardiac catheterization (38). A high degree of oxygen desaturation during the 6MWT in children with SCD might serve as an early biomarker for PH and is associated with blood biomarkers of hemolysis (62).

Doppler echocardiography

The use of echocardiography to estimate PASP (32) has been validated in patients with SCD, and correlates well with the measurement of pulmonary arterial pressures by right heart catheterization (38,48) and exercise capacity (38). To avoid the more subjective estimation of central venous pressures, PH can be defined by a specific TRV value ≥ 2.5 m/sec and moderate-to-severe PH defined by a TRV ≥ 3.0 m/sec (32). More severe disease is also suggested by evidence of right ventricular failure, such as paradoxical septal motion, a flattened interventricular septum, a dilated right ventricle and atrium, and a pericardial effusion. Exercise echocardiograms will identify patients with significant exertional dyspnea despite a normal resting TRV (54). Screening for PH in SCD should be performed at baseline and in the absence of disease exacerbation, because pulmonary pressures increase transiently during acute chest syndrome (55), pain episodes and with exercise (54).

It is important to evaluate for indications of left ventricular systolic and diastolic dysfunction (48), either of which may be found alone or in combination with PH (38,56). The presence of diastolic dysfunction can be assessed by tissue Doppler or conventional assessment of the E/A ratio.

Atrial ejection fraction in thalassemia major patients may serve as a valuable marker of pre-clinical cardiac dysfunction, as depressed values occur in patients with heavy cardiac iron burden (147).

Right heart catheterization

The most reliable diagnostic procedure for PH is right-sided cardiac catheterization, which can confirm the diagnosis and assess severity while excluding other contributors such as left heart disease. Experts in the field recommend that hemoglobinopathy patients with a TRV ≥ 3.0 m/sec measured by Doppler echocardiography undergo cardiac catheterization (12).

Cardiac magnetic resonance imaging (MRI)

Heart failure due to iron overload remains a chief cause of death in β-thalassemia major and other transfusion-dependent anemias (19), and contributes to the high frequency of PH in these disorders (22,101,107,148). MRI is effective in detecting iron in the heart and liver. It is routinely used in chronically transfused thalassemia patients to screen for iron cardiotoxicity, and experience in SCD is accumulating (149–152). Cardiac MRI is a noninvasive tool that also reliably determines other hemodynamic indices in addition to iron burden, such as right and left ventricular volume and ejection fraction, left ventricular mass, and cardiac output. Cardiac MRI can accurately qualify left ventricular function (independent of septal geometry) and measure cardiac output. Combined with a peripheral blood pressure measurement, total vascular resistance (mean blood pressure/cardiac output) can be determined. Cardiac MRI may be a helpful assessment tool in the management of PH in hemolytic anemias.

TREATMENT/MANAGEMENT

Guidelines for the assessment and management of hemolysis-associated PH are currently being established through the American Thoracic Society. Much of what is being done clinically with PH in patients with hemoglobinopathies is based upon the PAH literature, case reports (153,154) and small open-label studies (82,155,156). General recommendations include intensification of thalassemia and sickle cell-directed therapies, treatment of causal factors or associated diseases, general supportive measures, and use of PH-specific pharmacologic agents (12).

Insufficient data are available for recommendations regarding treatment specifically targeting pulmonary arterial hypertension and the choice of agents is largely empirical. For further details, see refs 157–164.

In the absence of clinical guidelines and paucity of placebo-controlled therapeutic trials for the evaluation and treatment of PH in the sickle cell population, a diagnostic and therapeutic approach based on accumulating clinical experience is summarized below.

Patients with mild PH (TRV 2.5–2.9 m/sec)

- Hydroxyurea treatment at the maximum tolerated dose as defined by the Multicenter Study of Hydroxyurea,

with erythropoietin therapy considered if reticulocytopenia limits hydroxyurea therapy. Erythropoietin is often needed in combination with hydroxyurea because many of the adult patients presenting with PH have coexistent renal insufficiency that limits hydroxyurea dose escalation (165).
- Monthly transfusion therapy may be considered for patients with poor responses to hydroxyurea, accompanied by chelation therapy, if indicated. Anecdotally, the TRV has declined in some patients with institution of these treatment measures (161), especially in children and young adults, although this has not been studied to date.
- Consultation with a pulmonologist or cardiologist experienced in PH is recommended, the latter especially if the echocardiogram shows evidence of left or right ventricular dysfunction.
- Identify and treat risk factors associated with PH such as rest, exercise and nocturnal hypoxemia, sleep apnea, pulmonary thromboembolic disease, restrictive lung disease/fibrosis, left ventricular systolic and diastolic dysfunction, severe anemia and iron overload.

Patients with TRV ≥ 3 m/sec

- All recommendations for TRV 2.5–2.9 m/sec.
- Right heart catheterization to assess left ventricular diastolic and systolic function.
- A CT-pulmonary angiogram, V/Q scan, and or pulmonary angiogram to exclude chronic thromboembolic PH.
- Consider systemic anticoagulation (improves outcomes in patients with primary PH and in-situ thrombosis but no data available in patients with SCD).

Consider specific therapy with selective pulmonary vasodilator and remodeling drugs, particularly if the patient has symptomatic dyspnea on exertion which has progressed in recent months or years. Drugs which are FDA-approved for primary PH include the endothelin receptor antagonists (bosentan and ambrisentan), various forms of prostaglandin therapy (epoprostenol, treprostinol and iloprost), and the phosphodiesterase-5 inhibitors (sildenafil, tadalafil and vardenafil). Few published randomized studies in the SCD population exist for any of these agents. Although the Walk-PHaSST trial was stopped early due to increased hospitalization for pain in the treatment group, no final conclusions can be made from these data regarding contraindications. Treatment should be individually tailored by a cardiopulmonary expert with PH experience. Appropriate consultation and right heart catheterization is recommended at baseline and repeated annually for patients on such therapy.

Many of these recommendations can be applied to the treatment of PH in thalassemia. Since strict compliance with chronic transfusion and chelation therapy was found to prevent PH (19,22,74) early transfusion to keep the hemoglobin > 10 g/dL and iron chelation should be offered to all thalassemia patients with PH, even those with thalassemia intermedia. Given the contributory role of thromboembolism and a hypercoagulable state to PH in the thalassemia syndromes (28,73,98,99,101,102,152,166), long-term anticoagulation and/or antiplatelet therapy, although controversial, should be considered. The potential benefits of such therapies in SCD must be weighed against the risk of hemorrhagic stroke, however it can be argued that the relatively low risk of hemorrhagic stroke (167) compared with the high risk of death in patients with moderate to severe PH (32,42,43,48–50,79) supports use of anticoagulation in patients demonstrating evidence of thromboemolism (97) unless other contraindications are present.

FUTURE DIRECTIONS

Therapy

Randomized trials evaluating the effects of specific therapy for hemolysis-associated PH are clearly indicated (168,169). Combination therapies targeting multiple mechanisms including hemolysis and oxidative stress may surpass benefits of any single strategy (28,78,169,170).

Children with hemoglobinopathies who have an HLA-compatible sibling can be cured by allogeneic bone marrow transplantation before they have a chance to develop chronic organ damage and PH (152,171–175). Alternative sources of donor hematopoietic cells that include HLA-matched unrelated donor and umbilical cord blood are being pursued for hemoglobinopathies, with promising initial results (175), while promising advances in gene replacement therapy (176,177) bringing hope for the elusive cure to these devastating disorders.

KEY POINTS

- Approximately 30 per cent of adults with sickle cell disease (SCD), and > 30 per cent of patients with a thalassemia syndrome have an elevated tricuspid regurgitant jet velocity of 2.5 m/sec or higher, which is 2-SD above the mean. These patients are at high risk of death. 9 per cent of the SCD adult population has a TRV greater than or equal to 3 m/sec, which is 3-SD above the mean. Right heart catheterization studies suggest that 6–11 per cent of adults with SCD have pulmonary hypertension (PH) defined by a mean pulmonary artery pressure greater than or equal to 25 mmHg (3-SD above the mean). Approximately half of these cases are pulmonary artery hypertension, and half are pulmonary venous hypertension. Pediatric studies using Doppler-echocardiography suggest PH is mild with only 11 percent having TRV > 2.5 m/sec (PUSH study in steady state) (62) and few have TRV > 3 m/sec. Whether these children are at risk of developing PH as they age is

an area of active investigation. Studies in children with thalassemia and PH are needed.
- Etiology of PH in SCD and thalassemia is complex and multifactorial, including hemolysis and its effect on the arginine-NO pathway, oxidative stress, splenic dysfunction/asplenia, thrombosis, hypoxia, chronic lung disease, and iron overload.
- Early clinical manifestations of PH are mild and difficult to recognize in hemolytic disorders as they overlap with signs and symptoms of chronic anemia.
- PH in hemolytic disease is a different disorder than other forms of PH, with lower pulmonary pressures, and higher cardiac output from anemia.
- Doppler echocardiography reliably identifies SCD patients at high risk for early death, and those at higher risk for PH, however a right heart cardiac catheterization is required for a PH diagnosis; a TRV ≥ 2.5 m/sec is the strongest predictor of early mortality in SCD, with a risk ratio > 10. Mild elevations in pulmonary pressures are poorly tolerated in this patient population.
- Annual to semi-annual routine screening for PH by Doppler echocardiogram is recommended in adults and children with hemolytic disorders.
- Diastolic dysfunction is present in 18 percent of SCD patients, is a co-morbid finding in 11 percent of PH patients, and is an independent risk factor of mortality.
- An intensive transfusion program and adequate iron chelation is protective against the development of PH in thalassemia patients.
- Guidelines for the management of hemolysis-associated PH are currently being established through the American Thoracic Society. Recommendations include intensification of thalassemia and sickle cell-directed therapies, treatment of causal factors or associated diseases, general supportive measures, and use of PH-specific pharmacologic agents.

REFERENCES

• = Key primary paper
♦ = Major review article

1. Loukopolous D, Kollia P. Worldwide distribution of beta-thalassemia. In: Steinberg MH, Forget BG, Higgs DR et al., eds. Disorders of Hemoglobin Genetics, Pathophysiology, and Clinical Management. Cambridge: Cambridge University Press, 2001:861–984.
♦2. Steinberg MH. Sickle cell anemia, the first molecular disease: overview of molecular etiology, pathophysiology, and therapeutic approaches. Sci World J 2008;8:1295–324.

•3. Barnett CF, Hsue PY, Machado RF. Pulmonary hypertension: an increasingly recognized complication of hereditary hemolytic anemias and HIV infection. JAMA 2008;299: 324–31.

◆4. Aliyu ZY, Kato GJ, Taylor JT, Babadoko A *et al.* Sickle cell disease and pulmonary hypertension in Africa: a global perspective and review of epidemiology, pathophysiology, and management. Am J Hematol 2008;83:63–70.

•5. Aliyu ZY, Gordeuk V, Sachdev V, Babadoko A *et al.* Prevalence and risk factors for pulmonary artery systolic hypertension among sickle cell disease patients in Nigeria. Am J Hematol 2008;83:485–90.

6. Michlitsch J, Aximi M, Hoppe C, Walters MC *et al.* Newborn screening for hemoglobinopathies in California. Pediatr Blood Cancer 2009;52:486–90.

◆7. Bunn HF. Pathogenesis and treatment of sickle cell disease. N Engl J Med 1997;337:762–9.

8. Frenette PS. Sickle cell vaso-occlusion: multistep and multicellular paradigm. Curr Opin Hematol 2002;9:101–6.

9. Parise LV, Telen MJ. Erythrocyte adhesion in sickle cell disease. Curr Hematol Rep 2003;2:102–8.

10. Hagar W, Vichinsky E. Advances in clinical research in sickle cell disease. Br J Haematol 2008;141:346–56.

◆11. Stuart MJ, Nagel RL. Sickle-cell disease. Lancet 2004;364:1343–60.

◆12. Gladwin MT, Vichinsky E. Pulmonary complications of sickle cell disease. N Engl J Med 2008;359:2254–65.

13. Cohen AR, Galanello R, Pennell DJ, Cunningham MJ *et al.* Thalassemia. Hematology (Am Soc Hematol Educ Program) 2004;14–34.

14. Forgot BG. Molecular mechanisms of beta-thalassemia. In: Steinberg MH, Forgot BG, Higgs DR *et al.*, eds. Disorders of hemoglobin genetics, pathophysiology and clinical management. Cambridge: Cambridge University Press, 2001:252–76.

15. Vichinsky EP. Changing patterns of thalassemia worldwide. Ann NY Acad Sci 2005;1054:18–24.

◆16. Olivieri NF. The beta-thalassemias. N Engl J Med 1999;341:99–109.

17. Borgna-Pignatti C, Rugolotto S, De Stefano P, Piga A *et al.* Survival and disease complications in thalassemia major. Ann NY Acad Sci 1998;850:227–31.

18. Aessopos A, Stamatelow G, Skoumas V, Vassilopoulos G *et al.* Pulmonary hypertension and right heart failure in patients with B-thalassemia intermedia. Chest 1995;107:50–3.

•19. Aessopos A, Farmakis D, Deftereos S, Tsironi M *et al.* Thalassemia heart disease: a comparative evaluation of thalassemia major and thalassemia intermedia. Chest 2005;127:1523–30.

20. Hahalis G, Alexopoulos D, Kremastinos DT, Zoumbos NC. Heart failure in beta-thalassemia syndromes: a decade of progress. Am J Med 2005;118:957–67.

21. Du ZD, Roguin N, Milgram E, Saab K *et al.* Pulmonary hypertension in patients with thalassemia major. Am Heart J 1997;134:532–7.

22. Aessopos A, Farmakis D. Pulmonary hypertension in beta-thalassemia. Ann NY Acad Sci 2005;1054:342–9.

23. Tam DH, Farber HW. Pulmonary hypertension and beta-thalassemia major: report of a case, its treatment, and a review of the literature. Am J Hematol 2006;81:443–7.

24. Hagar RW, Morris CR, Vichinsky EP. Pulmonary hypertension in thalassaemia major patients with normal left ventricular systolic function. Br J Haematol 2006;133:433–5.

25. Grisaru D, Rachmilewitz EA, Mosseri M, Gotsman M *et al.* Cardiopulmonary assessment in beta-thalassemia major. Chest 1990;5:1138–42.

◆26. Morris CR, Vichinsky EP. Pulmonary hypertension in thalassemia. Ann NY Acad Sci 2010;1202:205–13.

◆27. Morris CR, Gladwin MT, Kato G. Nitric oxide and arginine dysregulation: a novel pathway to pulmonary hypertension in hemolytic disorders. Curr Mol Med 2008;8:81–90.

◆28. Morris CR. Mechanisms of vasculopathy in sickle cell disease and thalassemia. Hematology Am Soc Hematol Educ Program 2008;2008:177–85.

◆29. Machado RF, Gladwin MT. Pulmonary hypertension in hemolytic disorders: pulmonary vascular disease: the global perspective. Chest 2010;137:30S–8S.

30. Machado RF, Gladwin MT. Hemolytic anemia association pulmonary hypertension. In: Mandel J, Taichman D, eds. Pulmonary Vascular Disease. Philadelphia, PA: Saunders Elsevier, 2006:170–87.

◆31. Rother RP, Bell L, Hillmen P, Gladwin MT. The clinical sequelae of intravascular hemolysis and extracellular plasma hemoglobin: A novel mechanism of human disease. JAMA 2005;293:1653–62.

•32. Gladwin M, Sachdev V, Jison M, Shizukuda Y *et al.* Pulmonary hypertension as a risk factor for death in patients with sickle cell disease. N Engl J Med 2004;350:22–31.

33. Haque AK, Grinberg AR, Lencioni M, Molina MM *et al.* Pulmonary hypertension in sickle cell hemoglobinopathy: A clinicopathologic study of 20 cases. Hum Pathol 2002;33:1037–43.

34. Manci EA, Culberson DE, Yang YM, Gardner TM *et al.* Causes of death in sickle cell disease: an autopsy study. Br J Haematol 2003;123:359–65.

35. Sonakul D, Fucharoen S. Pulmonary thromboembolism in thalassemic patients. Southeast Asian J Trop Med Public Health 1992;23 Suppl 2:25–8.

36. Sonakul D, Pacharee P, Thakerngpol K. Pathologic findings in 76 autopsy cases of thalassemia. Birth Defects Orig Artic Ser 1988;23:157–76.

37. Sonakul D, Suwanagool P, Sirivaidyapong P, Fucharoen S. Distribution of pulmonary thromboembolic lesions in thalassemic patients. Birth Defects Orig Artic Ser 1987;23:375–84.

•38. Anthi A, Machado RF, Jison ML, Taveira-Dasilva AM *et al.* Hemodynamic and functional assessment of patients with sickle cell disease and pulmonary hypertension. Am J Respir Crit Care Med 2007;175:1272–9.

39. Aessopos A, Farmakis D, Trompoukis C, Tsironi M *et al.* Cardiac involvement in sickle beta-thalassemia. Ann Hematol 2009;88:557–64.

40. Voskaridou E, Tsetsos G, Tsoutsias A, Spyropoulou E *et al.* Pulmonary hypertension in patients with sickle cell/beta thalassemia: incidence and correlation with serum N-terminal pro-brain natriuretic peptide concentrations. Haematologica 2007;92:738–43.

41. Lindsay J Jr, Meshel JC, Patterson RH. The cardiovascular manifestations of sickle cell disease. Arch Intern Med 1974;133:643–51.

•42. Ataga KI, Moore CG, Jones S, Olajide O *et al.* Pulmonary hypertension in patients with sickle cell disease: a longitudinal study. Br J Haematol 2006;134:109–15.

•43. De Castro LM, Jonassaint JC, Graham FL, Ashley-Koch A *et al.* Pulmonary hypertension associated with sickle cell disease: clinical and laboratory endpoints and disease outcomes. Am J Hematol 2008;83:19–25.

44. Gordeuk VR, Sachdev V, Taylor JG, Gladwin MT *et al.* Relative systemic hypertension in patients with sickle cell disease is associated with risk of pulmonary hypertension and renal insufficiency. Am J Hematol 2008;83:15–8.

45. Gladwin MT, Barst RJ, Castro OL, Gordeuk VR *et al.* Pulmonary hypertension and NO in sickle cell. Blood 2010;116:852–4.

46. Bunn HF, Nathan DG, Dover GJ, Hebbel RP *et al.* Pulmonary hypertension and nitric oxide depletion in sickle cell disease. Blood 2010;116:687–92.

47. Darbari DS, Kple-Faget P, Kwagyan J, Rana S *et al.* Circumstances of death in adult sickle cell disease patients. Am J Hematol 2006;81:858–63.

•48. Sachdev V, Machado RF, Shizukuda Y, Rao YN *et al.* Diastolic dysfunction is an independent risk factor for death in patients with sickle cell disease. J Am Coll Cardiol 2007;49:472–9.

49. Hagar RW, Michlitsch JG, Gardner J, Vichinsky EP *et al.* Clinical differences between children and adults with pulmonary hypertension and sickle cell disease. Br J Haematol 2008;140:104–12.

•50. Castro O, Hoque M, Brown M. Pulmonary hypertension in sickle cell disease: cardiac catheterization results and survival. Blood 2003;101:1257–61.

51. Farzaneh-Far R, Na B, Whooley MA, Schiller NB. Usefulness of noninvasive estimate of pulmonary vascular resistance to predict mortality, heart failure, and adverse cardiovascular events in patients with stable coronary artery disease (from the Heart and Soul Study). Am J Cardiol 2008;101:762–6.

52. Tedrow UB, Kramer DB, Stevenson LW, Stevenson WG *et al.* Relation of right ventricular peak systolic pressure to major adverse events in patients undergoing cardiac resynchronization therapy. Am J Cardiol 2006;97:1737–40.

53. Thohan V. Prognostic implications of echocardiography in advanced heart failure. Curr Opin Cardiol 2004;19:238–49.

•54. Machado RF, Kyle Mack A, Martyr S, Barnett C *et al.* Severity of pulmonary hypertension during vaso-occlusive pain crisis and exercise in patients with sickle cell disease. Br J Haematol 2007;136:319–25.

•55. Mekontso Dessap A, Leon R, Habibi A, Nzouakou R *et al.* Pulmonary hypertension and cor pulmonale during severe acute chest syndrome in sickle cell disease. Am J Respir Crit Care Med 2008;177:646–53.

56. Klings ES, Anton Bland D, Rosenman D, Princeton S *et al.* Pulmonary arterial hypertension and left-sided heart disease in sickle cell disease: clinical characteristics and association with soluble adhesion molecule expression. Am J Hematol 2008;83:547–53.

•57. Taylor JGt, Ackah D, Cobb C, Orr N *et al.* Mutations and polymorphisms in hemoglobin genes and the risk of pulmonary hypertension and death in sickle cell disease. Am J Hematol 2008;83:6–14.

◆58. Kato GJ, Onyekwere OC, Gladwin MT. Pulmonary hypertension in sickle cell disease: relevance to children. Pediatr Hematol Oncol 2007;24:159–70.

59. Pashankar FD, Carbonella J, Bazzy-Asaad A, Friedman A. Prevalence and risk factors of elevated pulmonary artery pressures in children with sickle cell disease. Pediatrics 2008;121:777–82.

60. Onyekwere OC, Campbell A, Teshome M, Onyeagoro S *et al.* Pulmonary hypertension in children and adolescents with sickle cell disease. Pediatr Cardiol 2008;29:309–12.

61. Ambrusko SJ, Gunawardena S, Sakara A, Windsor B *et al.* Elevation of tricuspid regurgitant jet velocity, a marker for pulmonary hypertension in children with sickle cell disease. Pediatr Blood Cancer 2006;47:907–13.

•62. Minniti CP, Sable C, Campbell A, Rana S *et al.* Elevated tricuspid regurgitant jet velocity in children and adolescents with sickle cell disease: association with hemolysis and hemoglobin oxygen desaturation. Haematologica 2009;94:340–7.

•63. Dham N, Ensing G, Minniti C, Campbell A *et al.* Prospective echocardiography assessment of pulmonary hypertension and its potential etiologies in children with sickle cell disease. Am J Cardiol 2009;104:713–20.

64. Gordeuk VR, Campbell A, Rana S, Nouraie M *et al.* Relationship of erythropoietin, fetal hemoglobin, and hydroxyurea treatment to tricuspid regurgitation velocity in children with sickle cell disease. Blood 2009;114:4639–44.

•65. Colombatti R, Maschietto N, Varotto E, Grison A *et al.* Pulmonary hypertension in sickle cell disease children under 10 years of age. Br J Haematol 150:601–9.

66. Villavicencio K, Ivy D, Cole L, Nuss R. Symptomatic pulmonary hypertension in a child with sickle cell disease. J Pediatr 2008;152:879–81.

•67. Gordeuk VR, Minniti C, Nouraie M, Campbell A *et al.* Elevated tricuspid regurgitation velocity and decline in exercise capacity over 22 months of follow-up in children and adolescents with sickle cell anemia. Haematologica (in press).

•68. Lee MT, Small T, Khan MA, Rosenzweig EB *et al.* Doppler-defined pulmonary hypertension and the risk of death in children with sickle cell disease followed for a mean of three years. Br J Haematol 2009;146:437–41.

69. Bachir D, Parent F, Hajji L, Inamo J *et al.* Prospective multicentric survey on pulmonary hypertension (PH) in adults with sickle cell disease. Blood 2009;114:Abstract 572.

●70. Taher AT, Musallam KM, Karimi M, El-Beshlawy A et al. Overview on practices in thalassemia intermedia management aiming for lowering complication rates across a region of endemicity: the OPTIMAL CARE study. Blood 2010;115:1886–92.

71. Kiter G, Balci YI, Ates A, Hacioglu S et al. Frequency of pulmonary hypertension in asymptomatic beta-thalassemia major patients and the role of physiological parameters in evaluation. Pediatr Hematol Oncol 2010;27:597–607.

72. Aessopos A, Farmakis D, Karagiorga M, Voskaridou E et al. Cardiac involvement in thalassemia intermedia: a multicenter study. Blood 2001;97:3411–6.

73. Singer ST, Kuypers FA, Styles L, Vichinsky EP et al. Pulmonary hypertension in thalassemia: association with platelet activation and hypercoagulable state. Am J Hematol 2006;81:670–5.

●74. Aessopos A, Farmakis D, Hatziliami A, Fragodimitri C et al. Cardiac status in well-treated patients with thalassemia major. Eur J Haematol 2004;73:359–66.

75. Atichartakarn V, Chuncharunee S, Chandanamattha P, Likittanasombat K et al. Correction of hypercoagulability and amelioration of pulmonary arterial hypertension by chronic blood transfusion in an asplenic hemoglobin E/beta-thalassemia patient. Blood 2004;103:2844–6.

●76. Kato GJ, McGowan V, Machado RF, Little JA et al. Lactate dehydrogenase as a biomarker of hemolysis-associated nitric oxide resistance, priapism, leg ulceration, pulmonary hypertension, and death in patients with sickle cell disease. Blood 2006;107:2279–85.

●77. Morris CR, Kato GJ, Poljakovic M, Wang X et al. Dysregulated arginine metabolism, hemolysis-associated pulmonary hypertension and mortality in sickle cell disease. JAMA 2005;294:81–90.

●78. Morris CR, Suh JH, Hagar W, Larkin S et al. Erythrocyte glutamine depletion, altered redox environment, and pulmonary hypertension in sickle cell disease. Blood 2008;140:104–12.

79. Sebastiani P, Nolan VG, Baldwin CT, Abad-Grau MM et al. A network model to predict the risk of death in sickle cell disease. Blood 2007;110:2727–35.

●80. Machado RF, Anthi A, Steinberg MH, Bonds D et al. N-terminal pro-brain natriuretic peptide levels and risk of death in sickle cell disease. JAMA 2006;296:310–8.

81. Isma'eel H, Chafic AH, Rassi FE, Inati A et al. Relation between iron-overload indices, cardiac echo-Doppler, and biochemical markers in thalassemia intermedia. Am J Cardiol 2008;102:363–7.

●82. Morris CR, Morris SM, Jr., Hagar W, van Warmerdam J et al. Arginine Therapy: A new treatment for pulmonary hypertension in sickle cell disease? Am J Respir Crit Care Med 2003;168:63–9.

83. Tang WH, Wang Z, Cho L, Brennan DM et al. Diminished global arginine bioavailability and increased arginine catabolism as metabolic profile of increased cardiovascular risk. J Am Coll Cardiol 2009;53:2061–7.

84. Vallance P. The asymmetrical dimethylarginine/dimethylarginine dimethylaminohydrolase pathway in the regulation of nitric oxide generation. Clin Sci 2001;100:159–60.

●85. Schnog JB, Teerlink T, van der Dijs FP, Duits AJ et al. Plasma levels of asymmetric dimethylarginine (ADMA), an endogenous nitric oxide synthase inhibitor, are elevated in sickle cell disease. Ann Hematol 2005;84:282–6.

86. Kielstein JT, Bode-Boger SM, Hesse G, Martens-Lobenhoffer J et al. Asymmetrical dimethylarginine in idiopathic pulmonary arterial hypertension. Arterioscler Thromb Vasc Biol 2005;25:1414–8.

87. Pullamsetti S, Kiss L, Ghofrani HA, Voswinckel R et al. Increased levels and reduced catabolism of asymmetric and symmetric dimethylarginines in pulmonary hypertension. Faseb J 2005;19:1175–7.

88. Cooke JP. ADMA: its role in vascular disease. Vasc Med 2005;10 Suppl 1:S11–7.

●89. Landburg PP, Teerlink T, van Beers EJ, Muskiet FA et al. Association of asymmetric dimethylarginine with sickle cell disease-related pulmonary hypertension. Haematologica 2008;93:1410–2.

●90. Ashley-Koch AE, Elliott L, Kail ME, De Castro LM et al. Identification of genetic polymorphisms associated with risk for pulmonary hypertension in sickle cell disease. Blood 2008;111:5721–6.

◆91. Morris CR. Asthma management: reinventing the wheel in sickle cell disease. Am J Hematol 2009;84:234–41.

92. Wu KH, Chang JS, Su BH, Peng CT. Tricuspid regurgitation in patients with beta-thalassemia major. Ann Hematol 2004;83:779–83.

93. Phrommintikul A, Sukonthasarn A, Kanjanavanit R, Nawarawong W. Splenectomy: a strong risk factor for pulmonary hypertension in patients with thalassaemia. Heart 2006;92:1467–72.

94. Atichartakarn V, Likittanasombat K, Chuncharunee S, Chandanamattha P et al. Pulmonary arterial hypertension in previously splenectomized patients with beta-thalassemic disorders. Int J Hematol 2003;78:139–45.

95. Kuypers FA. Membrane lipid alterations in hemoglobinopathies. Hematology Am Soc Hematol Educ Program 2007;2007:68–73.

96. Borgna Pignatti C, Carnelli V, Caruso V, Dore F et al. Thromboembolic events in beta thalassemia major: an Italian multicenter study. Acta Haematol 1998;99:76–9.

◆97. Singer ST, Ataga KI. Hypercoagulability in sickle cell disease and beta-thalassemia. Curr Mol Med 2008;8:639–45.

98. Eldor A, Rachmilewitz EA. The hypercoagulable state in thalassemia. Blood 2002;99:36–43.

◆99. Ataga KI, Cappellini MD, Rachmilewitz EA. Beta-thalassaemia and sickle cell anaemia as paradigms of hypercoagulability. Br J Haematol 2007;139:3–13.

100. Gladwin MT, Kato GJ. Cardiopulmonary complications of sickle cell disease: role of nitric oxide and hemolytic anemia. Hematology (Am Soc Hematol Educ Program) 2005:51–7.

◆101. Morris CR, Vichinsky E, Singer ST. Pulmonary hypertension in thalassemia: Association with hemolysis, arginine metabolism dysregulation and a hypercoaguable state. Adv Pulm Hypertens 2007;5:31–8.

●102. Morris C, Kuypers F, Kato G, Lavrisha L et al. Hemolysis-associated pulmonary hypertension in thalassemia. An NY Acad Sci 2005;1054:481–5.

●103. Villagra J, Shiva S, Hunter LA, Machado RF et al. Platelet activation in patients with sickle disease, hemolysis-associated pulmonary hypertension and nitric oxide scavenging by cell-free hemoglobin. Blood 2007;110:2166–72.

●104. Ataga KI, Moore CG, Hillery CA, Jones S et al. Coagulation activation and inflammation in sickle cell disease-associated pulmonary hypertension. Haematologica 2008;93:20–6.

●105. Walter PB, Fung EB, Killilea DW, Jiang Q et al. Oxidative stress and inflammation in iron-overloaded patients with beta-thalassaemia or sickle cell disease. Br J Haematol 2006;135:254–63.

106. Fung EB, Harmatz PR, Lee PD, Milet M et al. Increased prevalence of iron-overload associated endocrinopathy in thalassaemia versus sickle-cell disease. Br J Haematol 2006;135:574–82.

107. Zakynthinos E, Vassilakopoulos T, Kaltsas P, Malagari E et al. Pulmonary hypertension, interstitial lung fibrosis, and lung iron deposition in thalassaemia major. Thorax 2001;56:737–9.

●108. Fung EB, Harmatz P, Milet M, Ballas SK et al. Morbidity and mortality in chronically transfused subjects with thalassemia and sickle cell disease: A report from the multi-center study of iron overload. Am J Hematol 2007;82:255–65.

109. Kato GJ, Hsieh M, Machado R, Taylor JT et al. Cerebrovascular disease associated with sickle cell pulmonary hypertension. Am J Hematol 2006;81:503–10.

●110. Hsu LL, Champion HC, Campbell-Lee SA, Bivalacqua TJ et al. Hemolysis in sickle cell mice causes pulmonary hypertension due to global impairment in nitric oxide bioavailability. Blood 2007;109:3088–98.

◆111. Kato GJ, Gladwin MT, Steinberg MH. Deconstructing sickle cell disease: Reappraisal of the role of hemolysis in the development of clinical subphenotypes. Blood Rev 2007; 21:37–47.

●112. Reiter C, Wang X, Tanus-Santos J, Hogg N et al. Cell-free hemoglobin limits nitric oxide bioavailability in sickle cell disease. Nat Med 2002;8:1383–9.

◆113. Wood KC, Hsu LL, Gladwin MT. Sickle cell disease vasculopathy: a state of nitric oxide resistance. Free Radic Biol Med 2008;44:1506–28.

114. Wood KC, Hebbel RP, Granger DN. Endothelial cell NADPH oxidase mediates the cerebral microvascular dysfunction in sickle cell transgenic mice. Faseb J 2005;19:989–91.

●115. Aslan M, Ryan TM, Adler B, Townes TM et al. Oxygen radical inhibition of nitric oxide-dependent vascular function in sickle cell disease. Proc Natl Acad Sci USA 2001;98:15215–20.

116. Aslan M, Freeman BA. Oxidant-mediated impairment of nitric oxide signaling in sickle cell disease – mechanisms

and consequences. Cell Mol Biol (Noisy-le-Grand) 2004;50:95–105.

●117. Kaul DK, Zhang X, Dasgupta T, Fabry ME. Arginine therapy of transgenic-knockout sickle mice improves microvascular function by reducing non-nitric oxide vasodilators, hemolysis, and oxidative stress. Am J Physiol Heart Circ Physiol 2008;295:H39–47.

118. Lopes AA, Caramuru LH, Maeda NY. Endothelial dysfunction associated with chronic intravascular coagulation in secondary pulmonary hypertension. Clin Appl Thromb Hemost 2002;8:353–8.

119. Caramuru LH, Soares R de P, Maeda NY, Lopes AA. Hypoxia and altered platelet behavior influence von Willebrand factor multimeric composition in secondary pulmonary hypertension. Clin Appl Thromb Hemost 2003;9:251–8.

120. Schnog JB, Jager EH, van der Dijs FP, Duits AJ et al. Evidence for a metabolic shift of arginine metabolism in sickle cell disease. Ann Hematol 2004;83:371–5.

121. Janka JJ, Koita OA, Traore B, Traore JM et al. Increased pulmonary pressures and myocardial wall stress in children with severe malaria. J Infect Dis 2010;202:791–800.

122. Omodeo-Sale F, Cortelezzi L, Vommaro Z, Scaccabarozzi D et al. Dysregulation of L-arginine metabolism and bioavailability associated to free plasma heme. Am J Physiol Cell Physiol 2010;299:C148–54.

123. Xu W, Kaneko TF, Zheng S, Comhair SA et al. Increased arginase II and decreased NO synthesis in endothelial cells of patients with pulmonary arterial hypertension. FASEB 2004;18:1746–8.

124. Morris CR, Teehankee C, Kato G, Gardner J et al. Decreased arginine bioavailability contributes to the pathogenesis of pulmonary artery hypertension. American College of Cardiology Annual Meeting, Orlando, Florida, 2005.

●125. Klings ES, Wyszynski DF, Nolan VG, Steinberg MH. Abnormal pulmonary function in adults with sickle cell anemia. Am J Respir Crit Care Med 2006;173:1264–9.

126. Field JJ, Glassberg J, Gilmore A, Howard J et al. Longitudinal analysis of pulmonary function in adults with sickle cell disease. Am J Hematol 2008;83:574–6.

127. Piatti G, Allegra L, Fasano V, Gambardella C et al. Lung function in beta-thalassemia patients: a longitudinal study. Acta Haematol 2006;116:25–9.

128. Morris CR. Asthma Management: Re-inventing the wheel in sickle cell disease. Am J Hematol 2009;84:234–41.

129. Klings ES. Pulmonary hypertension of sickle cell disease: more than just another lung disease. Am J Hematol 2008;83:4–5.

130. Onyekwere OC, Campbell A, Teshome M, Onyeagoro S et al. Pulmonary hypertension in children and adolescents with sickle cell disease. Pediatr Cardiol 2008;29:309–12.

●131. Liem RI, Young LT, Thompson AA. Tricuspid regurgitant jet velocity is associated with hemolysis in children and young adults with sickle cell disease evaluated for pulmonary hypertension. Haematologica 2007;92:1549–52.

●132. Kato GJ, Martyr S, Blackwelder WC, Nichols JS et al. Levels of soluble endothelium-derived adhesion molecules in patients with sickle cell disease are associated with pulmonary hypertension, organ dysfunction, and mortality. Br J Haematol 2005;130:943–53.

133. Nolan VG, Wyszynski DF, Farrer LA, Steinberg MH. Hemolysis-associated priapism in sickle cell disease. Blood 2005;106:3264–7.

134. Nolan VG, Adewoye A, Baldwin C, Wang L et al. Sickle cell leg ulcers: associations with haemolysis and SNPs in Klotho, TEK and genes of the TGF-beta/BMP pathway. Br J Haematol 2006;133:570–8.

•135. Lezcano NE, Odo N, Kutlar A, Brambilla D et al. Regular transfusion lowers plasma free hemoglobin in children with sickle-cell disease at risk for stroke. Stroke 2006; 37:1424–6.

•136. Taylor JG, Nolan VG, Mendelsohn L, Kato GJ et al. Chronic hyper-hemolysis in sickle cell anemia: association of vascular complications and mortality with less frequent vasoocclusive pain. PLoS ONE 2008;3:e2095.

137. O'Driscoll S, Height SE, Dick MC, Rees DC. Serum lactate dehydrogenase activity as a biomarker in children with sickle cell disease. Br J Haematol 2008;140:206–9.

138. Akgul F, Seyfeli E, Melek I, Duman T et al. Increased QT dispersion in sickle cell disease: effect of pulmonary hypertension. Acta Haematol 2007;118:1–6.

139. Field JJ, Stocks J, Kirkham FJ, Rosen CL et al. Airway hyper-responsiveness in children with sickle cell anemia. Chest 2010 [epub ahead of print].

140. Tai DY, Wang YT, Lou J, Wang WY et al. Lungs in thalassaemia major patients receiving regular transfusion. Eur Respir J 1996;9:1389–94.

•141. Boyd JH, Macklin EA, Strunk RC, Debaun MR. Asthma is associated with increased mortality in patients with sickle cell anemia. Haematologica 2007;92:1115–8.

142. Ozbek OY, Malbora B, Sen N, Yazici AC et al. Airway hyperreactivity detected by methacholine challenge in children with sickle cell disease. Pediatr Pulmonol 2007;42:1187–92.

143. Strunk RC, Brown MS, Boyd JH, Bates P et al. Methacholine challenge in children with sickle cell disease: a case series. Pediatr Pulmonol 2008;43:924–9.

144. Caboot JB, Allen JL. Pulmonary complications of sickle cell disease in children. Curr Opin Pediatr 2008;20:279–87.

145. Carnelli V, D'Angelo E, Pecchiari M, Ligorio M. Pulmonary dysfunction in transfusion-dependent patients with thalassemia major. Am J Respir Crit Care Med 2003;168:180–4.

146. Nielson VG, Tan S, Weinbroum A, McCammon AT et al. Lung injury after hepatoenteric ischemia-reperfusion: role of xanthine oxidase. Am J Respir Crit Care Med 1996;154:1364–9.

147. Li W, Coates T, Wood JC. Atrial dysfunction as a marker of iron cardiotoxicity in thalassemia major. Haematologica 2008;93:311–2.

148. Koren A, Garty I, Antonelli D, Katzuni E. Right ventricular cardiac dysfunction in beta-thalassemia major. Am J Dis Child 1987;141:93–6.

149. Wood JC, Ghugre N. Magnetic resonance imaging assessment of excess iron in thalassemia, sickle cell disease and other iron overload diseases. Hemoglobin 2008;32:85–96.

150. Westwood MA, Shah F, Anderson LJ, Strange JW et al. Myocardial tissue characterization and the role of chronic anemia in sickle cell cardiomyopathy. J Magn Reson Imaging 2007;26:564–8.

151. Wood JC. Cardiac iron across different transfusion-dependent diseases. Blood Rev 2008;22 Suppl 2:S14–21.

152. Morris CR, Singer ST, Walters MC. Clinical hemoglobinopathies: iron, lungs and new blood. Curr Opin Hematol 2006;13:407–18.

•153. Derchi G, Forni GL, Formisano F, Cappellini MD et al. Efficacy and safety of sildenafil in the treatment of severe pulmonary hypertension in patients with hemoglobinopathies. Haematologica 2005;90:452–8.

154. Littera R, La Nasa G, Derchi G, Cappellini MD et al. Long-term treatment with sildenafil in a thalassemic patient with pulmonary hypertension. Blood 2002;100:1516–7.

•155. Machado RF, Martyr S, Kato GJ, Barst RJ et al. Sildenafil therapy in patients with sickle cell disease and pulmonary hypertension. Br J Haematol 2005;130:445–53.

156. Little JA, Hauser KP, Martyr SE, Harris A et al. Hematologic, biochemical, and cardiopulmonary effects of L-arginine supplementation or phosphodiesterase 5 inhibition in patients with sickle cell disease who are on hydroxyurea therapy. Eur J Haematol 2009;82:315–21.

157. Barst RJ, Langleben D, Frost A, Horn EM et al. Sitaxsentan therapy for pulmonary arterial hypertension. Am J Respir Crit Care Med 2004;169:441–7.

158. Akoglu S, Kaya H, Seyfeli E, Babayigit C et al. The effectiveness of long-term inhaled iloprost in addition to oral sildenafil treatment in severe pulmonary hypertension associated with sickle cell disease. Turkish Respir J 2007;8:23–6.

•159. Karimi M, Borzouee M, Mehrabani A, Cohan N. Echocardiographic finding in beta-thalassemia intermedia and major: absence of pulmonary hypertension following hydroxyurea treatment in beta-thalassemia intermedia. Eur J Haematol 2009;82:213–8.

•160. El-Beshlawy A, Youssry I, El-Saidi S, El Accaoui R et al. Pulmonary hypertension in beta-thalassemia major and the role of L-carnitine therapy. Pediatr Hematol Oncol 2008;25:734–43.

161. Claster S, Hammer M, Hagar W, Ataga K et al. Treatment of pulmonary hypertension in sickle cell disease with transfusion. In: Ohene-Frempong K, ed. 24th Annual Meeting of the National Sickle Cell Disease Program, Philadelphia, Pennsylvania, 2000:46a.

•162. Minniti CP, Machado RF, Coles WA, Sachdev V et al. Endothelin receptor antagonists for pulmonary hypertension in adult patients with sickle cell disease. Br J Haematol 2009;147:737–43.

•163. Barst RJ, Mubarak KK, Machado RF, Ataga KI et al. Exercise capacity and haemodynamics in patients with sickle cell disease with pulmonary hypertension treated with bosentan: results of the ASSET studies. Br J Haematol 2010;149:426–35.

164. Machado R, Barst RJ, Yovetich N, Hassell K et al. Safety and efficacy of sildenafil therapy for Doppler-defined pulmonary hypertension in patients

with sickle cell disease: preliminary results of the Walk-PHaSST clinical trial. Blood 2009;114:Abstract 571.

165. Little JA, McGowan VR, Kato GJ, Partovi KS *et al.* Combination erythropoietin-hydroxyurea therapy in sickle cell disease: experience from the National Institutes of Health and a literature review. Haematologica 2006;91:1076–83.

166. Cappellini MD, Robbiolo L, Bottasso BM, Coppola R *et al.* Venous thromboembolism and hypercoagulability in splenectomized patients with thalassaemia intermedia. Br J Haematol 2000;111:467–73.

167. Ohene-Frempong K, Weiner SJ, Sleeper LA, Miller ST *et al.* Cerebrovascular accidents in sickle cell disease: rates and risk factors. Blood 1998;91:288–94.

◆168. Kato GJ, Gladwin MT. Evolution of novel small-molecule therapeutics targeting sickle cell vasculopathy. JAMA 2008;300:2638–46.

169. Kato GJ. Novel small molecule therapeutics for sickle cell disease: nitric oxide, carbon monoxide, nitrite, and apolipoprotein a-I. Hematology Am Soc Hematol Educ Program 2008;2008:186–92.

◆170. Steinberg MH. Clinical trials in sickle cell disease: adopting the combination chemotherapy paradigm. Am J Hematol 2008;83:1–3.

171. Giardini C, Lucarelli G. Bone marrow transplantation for beta-thalassemia. Hematol Oncol Clin North Am 1999;13:1059–64, viii.

172. Fixler J, Vichinsky E, Walters MC. Stem cell transplantation for sickle cell disease: can we reduce the toxicity? Pediatr Pathol Mol Med 2001;20:73–86.

173. Walters MC, Patience M, Leisenring W, Rogers ZR *et al.* Collaborative multicenter investigation of marrow transplantation for sickle cell disease: current results and future directions. Biol Blood Marrow Transplant 1997;3:310–5.

174. Hoppe CC, Walters MC. Bone marrow transplantation in sickle cell anemia. Curr Opin Oncol 2001;13:85–90.

◆175. Michlitsch JG, Walters MC. Recent advances in bone marrow transplantation in hemoglobinopathies. Curr Mol Med 2008;8:675–89.

●176. Hanna J, Wernig M, Markoulaki S, Sun CW *et al.* Treatment of sickle cell anemia mouse model with iPS cells generated from autologous skin. Science 2007;318:1920–3.

◆177. Townes TM. Gene replacement therapy for sickle cell disease and other blood disorders. Hematology Am Soc Hematol Educ Program 2008;2008:193–6.

15.9

Pulmonary hypertension in pregnancy

LAURA PRICE, XAVIER JAÏS AND MARC HUMBERT

INTRODUCTION

Pulmonary arterial hypertension (PAH) is defined as a mean pulmonary artery pressure (mPAP) greater than 25 mmHg in the setting of normal or reduced cardiac output and normal pulmonary capillary wedge pressure (≤ 15 mmHg) (1). PAH is a disease of the small pulmonary arteries characterized by vascular proliferation and remodeling (2). It results in a progressive increase in pulmonary vascular resistance, right ventricular failure and ultimately death. PAH can be characterized as idiopathic (IPAH), heritable, or may be associated with other conditions including collagen vascular disease, congenital heart disease, portal hypertension, HIV infection, and the use of certain drugs (3). PAH most commonly presents in women of childbearing age, and is more common in women overall (4,5). Specific advanced therapies have been developed for PAH during the last decade, which have improved quality of life and outcome for patients with PAH, however there remains no cure for this devastating condition (6). We are limited to the discussion of PAH and non-operable chronic thromboembolic pulmonary hypertension (CTEPH) as there are no pregnancy data on patients with non-PAH PH, for example in patients secondary to chronic respiratory disease. It may be hypothesized that some of the principles may be extrapolated, but it is important to note that there are no outcome data in this non-PAH subgroup.

Pregnancy in women with PAH including IPAH or PAH associated with congenital heart disease or other conditions is reported to be associated with a high maternal mortality, historically between 30 and 56 percent (7). The major hemodynamic changes that occur during pregnancy and especially during labor and birth are poorly tolerated by these patients. This is reflected in the timing of clinical deterioration and the increased mortality in the late stages of pregnancy when the maximum increase in blood volume and cardiac output occurs, and also during delivery and in the puerperium (8). Patients may present with previously undiagnosed, subclinical PAH that is unmasked by pregnancy. Current clinical recommendations are therefore that all pregnancies should be strongly discouraged, with effective contraceptive methods recommended in women of childbearing age (9). If this fails, early pregnancy termination is advised, although this procedure is not without risk. There are increasing advanced PAH therapies that have improved outcomes in patients with PAH, with more women of childbearing age considering pregnancy (6). The care of the pregnant woman with PAH requires a highly planned, multidisciplinary approach, involving obstetricians, pulmonary hypertension specialists, anesthetists and intensivists, preferably in a dedicated PH referral center. This allows formulation of an agreed and documented management strategy for delivery. This chapter will focus on the management of PAH during pregnancy, delivery considerations and the resulting impact on pregnancy outcomes.

EPIDEMIOLOGY: PROGNOSIS AND PREGNANCY OUTCOMES

Maternal outcomes

PAH pregnancies are rare. A 2002–2004 US-wide analysis reported 182 patients with IPAH out of 11.2 million deliveries (10) and an ongoing UK prospective study has reported 16 cases in 1.37 million maternities (11). Currently, the available outcome data are retrospective in nature, derived from case reports and case series (7,8,12,13). The first of two major series (7) reviewed 125 reported pregnancies between 1978 and 1996 in mothers with CHD-PAH, IPAH, and what was at that time termed "secondary PH" (anorexigen-induced PAH, connective tissue disease PAH, sickle cell disease PAH, portopulmonary hypertension and CTEPH). Maternal mortality was found to be 36 percent in CHD-PAH, 30 percent in IPAH and was 56 percent in secondary PH. Except for three prepartum deaths due to Eisenmenger's syndrome, all fatalities occurred within 35 days after delivery. Late diagnosis of PAH and timing of hospital admission (risk increasing by 9 percent with each week of pregnancy) were independent risk factors of maternal mortality. Moreover, operative delivery, severity of pulmonary hypertension and number of previous pregnancies and deliveries were contributing factors. A comparative study of parturients has been recently repeated since the era of new advanced therapies with cases from 1997 to 2007 (13). In this series, overall mortality has fallen from 38 percent to 25 percent ($P = 0.047$) compared to the previous decade, with a substantial although nonsignificant reduction in the subgroups: IPAH mortality had reduced from 30 percent to 17 percent, CHD-PAH from 36 percent to 28 percent, and secondary PH 56 percent to 33 percent. Most deaths again occurred due to right ventricular failure within the first month following delivery, and other reported maternal complications included thromboembolism, peripartum bleeding or a fall in hemoglobin requiring transfusion (13).

Studies have suggested that CHD-PAH patients have worse outcomes when compared to those with IPAH (7,13). Previous reviews of Eisenmenger's pregnancies both from the late 1940s to 1978 (14) and more recently (12,13,15,16) report maternal mortality rates of 30–40 percent, although these appear to be lower in single-center studies (17). The two major comparative case series report higher death rates in CHD-PAH compared to IPAH, at 36 percent in the 1978 to 1996 era, and 28 percent in the more recent era. Suggested causes for the increased mortality include increased bleeding and thrombotic tendencies, arrhythmias and multisystem involvement (18).

Fetal outcomes

Fetal mortality in IPAH mothers has been reported as 10 percent in the most recent retrospective case series (13) and is strongly influenced by maternal outcome, with 4–9 percent perinatal deaths in maternal survivors overall, compared with 25 percent in mothers who died (7). In the ongoing prospective UK series, there have been no perinatal deaths thus far in 15 maternal survivors (11). Elective delivery prior to term (< 37 weeks) is frequently described, in 85–100 percent reported pregnancies (12,13), which is likely to be at least in part because of the anticipated increase in maternal complications, pregnancies are usually not allowed to proceed to full term. The incidence of intrauterine growth retardation (IUGR) may be up to 33 percent (13), especially in patients with antiphospholipid antibodies and lupus-associated PAH (19,20). In mothers with Eisenmenger's syndrome (12,14), poor fetal outcomes are thought to be related to the level of maternal hypoxemia (21), with the likelihood of a live birth being much reduced if the resting arterial saturation is less than 85 percent (21).

ETIOLOGY

Hemodynamic changes in normal pregnancy

Important changes occur as early as 5–8 weeks in pregnancy, and gradually return to normal 2–12 weeks postpartum 22, and are summarized in Table 15.9.1. These changes follow the estrogen- and prostaglandin-induced relaxation of vascular smooth muscle, leading to an increase in venous capacitance and reduced systemic vascular resistance (SVR).

Total blood volume rises above pre-pregnant level by 10 percent, 30 percent, and 45 percent over the first, second, and third trimesters, respectively (23). This increases end diastolic volume and heart rate (by 10–20 beats/minute) while cardiac output (CO) increases by 50 percent by the second trimester during a normal pregnancy (24) mostly due to an increase in stroke volume (22,25). In contrast, there is no change in central venous pressure (CVP) or pulmonary capillary wedge pressure (PCWP) as both SVR and pulmonary vascular resistance (PVR) are reduced (25). The 20–30 percent fall in SVR is a fundamental physiological change in pregnancy and is a consequence of systemic vasodilatation and the development of the low resistance utero-placental circulation. Pulmonary pressures remain normal due to a similar decrease in PVR to accommodate the increased cardiac output (26). The CO usually exceeds the non-pregnant level by 50 percent at weeks 20–24

Table 15.9.1 Hemodynamic changes in normal pregnancy

Parameter	Effect of normal pregnancy
Heart rate (32 weeks)	Increased 10–20 beats/min
SVR	Decreased by 20%
PVR	Decreased by 20–30%
Cardiac output (25 weeks)	Increased by 30–50%
Blood volume	Increased by 40%
Plasma volume	Increased by 45–50%
Red cell mass	Increased by 20–30%
PCWP	No change
CVP	No change

SVR, systemic vascular resistance; PVR, pulmonary vascular resistance; PCWP, pulmonary capillary wedge pressure; CVP, central venous pressure.

(22,25,27). Mild myocardial hypertrophy and remodeling are characteristic in the late stages of pregnancy (28).

The most significant cardiovascular challenges occur at the time of labor, delivery and in the post-partum period. Cardiac output increases further during labor, up to 15 percent in the first stage and by 50 percent in the second stage, especially during contractions, when oxygen consumption is greatly increased (29) but also between contractions. The sympathetic response to pain and anxiety further elevate heart rate and blood pressure. Uterine contractions lead to an autotransfusion of a total of 300–500 mL, and following delivery of the baby, up to 1 L of placental blood may be returned to the circulation following aortocaval decompression and further contraction of the uterus. Intra-thoracic blood volume rises, and cardiac output increases by up to 80 percent of pre-term values (30). Women with PAH are therefore most at risk during the second stage of labor and the immediate postpartum period. Postpartum, most of these changes revert quite rapidly during the first week, with rapid reduction in heart rate and CO within hours of delivery then slower normalization over the following six weeks (28,31).

Physiological consequences of gestational hemodynamic changes

The increased blood volume and CO throughout pregnancy, and especially the fluid shifts following delivery, present an extreme maternal challenge in PAH patients, with their high and fixed resistance to pulmonary vascular flow (32). This is reflected in the high maternal mortality in the later stages of pregnancy, at the time of delivery and during the puerperium (7,8,30). In normal subjects, the low-resistance pulmonary vascular bed copes with the large increases in blood flow in pregnancy (such as occurs during exercise) through vasodilatation and recruitment of pulmonary capillaries. This allows the capacity for large changes in pulmonary blood flow with little change in pulmonary artery pressure. In PAH, obliteration of pulmonary vessels reduces the total area of the pulmonary vascular bed, and remodeled pulmonary vessels have reduced ability to vasodilate, hence the capacity for pulmonary vascular recruitment is diminished. The resulting excessive afterload on the right ventricle (RV) will be poorly tolerated, and with increasing right ventricular pressure overload, a downwards spiral of RV failure will follow (33).

Additionally, in mothers with Eisenmenger's syndrome, the pregnancy-induced fall in systemic vascular resistance (SVR) can increase the right-to-left shunt, reduce pulmonary blood flow and worsen hypoxemia, which may also precipitate cardiovascular collapse (34).

CLINICAL PRESENTATION

Patients with PAH typically deteriorate at 20–24 weeks of pregnancy (8) with increasing symptoms of exercise intolerance, chest pain, syncope and fatigue and with signs of RV dysfunction (35). Patients are likely to be admitted antenatally due to clinical deterioration (10). Hemoptysis and syncope may be pre-morbid events. The examination findings of normal pregnancy should be remembered (Table 15.9.2). Patients with ES have more marked cyanosis and polycythemia, and are at increased risk of paradoxical emboli and strokes. Patients with CHD-PAH are more likely to have a pre-existing PAH diagnosis prior to pregnancy, compared to those with IPAH (7,13). In the most recent case series, 55 percent of patients with IPAH were *de novo* presentations during pregnancy (13). In this setting, dyspnea, excessive peripheral edema and weight gain, for example, may be difficult to distinguish from that of normal pregnancy, and diagnosis can easily be delayed.

Investigations

BASIC CLINICAL INVESTIGATIONS

Plasma expansion in pregnancy leads to a normocytic anemia, urea and creatinine are lowered and there is usually a mild leukocytosis. Levels of BNP rise throughout normal pregnancy (25 ± 2 in the first trimester compared to 49 ± 9 pg/mL at term, $P < 0.01$) (36). When interpreting arterial blood gases, it should be remembered that the progesterone-driven increase in minute ventilation may lead to a respiratory alkalosis with mild hypocapnia, and higher PaO_2 in early pregnancy (37,38). Oxygen saturations are unchanged (39), although the risk of hypoxemia is much greater, especially in later pregnancy as the increased oxygen demand by the fetoplacental unit may exceed oxygen stores due to the reduction in functional residual capacity. The electrocardiographic axis is shifted upwards in late pregnancy as the heart lies in a more horizontal position. Atrial and ventricular ectopic beats, small Q-waves and T-wave inversion in the right precordial leads are often seen.

RADIOLOGY

Ventilation perfusion (VQ) scanning delivers a higher fetal radiation dose than CT pulmonary angiography (CTPA),

Table 15.9.2 Cardiovascular examination in normal pregnancy

Cardiovascular signs in normal pregnancy
Loud S1
Exaggerated splitting S2
Physiological S3 at apex
Systolic ejection murmur LSE (common, may extend all over precordium)
Venous hums
Bounding pulse
Ectopic beats common

S1, First heart sound; LSE left sternal edge.

although CTPA delivers a higher maternal dose than to the fetus. This is especially a consideration to the maternal breast in late pregnancy: CTPA increases the lifetime breast cancer risk by 13 percent above the risk from VQ scanning (40). Furthermore, suboptimal CTPA images are more likely during pregnancy (41). For suspected pulmonary embolism, limited perfusion scans only are therefore performed in some centers as the first line test (42). Magnetic resonance imaging is considered safe in pregnancy.

ECHOCARDIOGRAPHY AND RIGHT–HEART CATHETERIZATION

As in the non-pregnancy setting, echocardiography is a very useful screening technique to detect patients with suspected pulmonary hypertension (PH). During pregnancy, however, it may be more difficult to view the inferior vena cava because of the effects of gravid uterus, and right atrial pressure (RAP) may therefore be overestimated (43). A study of 11 critically ill obstetric patients using simultaneous echo and right heart catheterization (RHC) showed good correlation between the two techniques in the estimation of cardiac index, intracardiac pressures and pulmonary artery systolic pressures (44). A more recent study evaluating the correlation of estimated pulmonary artery pressures (PAP) by echocardiography with RHC measurements in pregnant women (43) again showed a good correlation between right ventricular systolic pressure (estimated by echocardiography) and PAP measured by RHC, however, in 30 percent of cases, RHC eliminated the diagnosis of PH when echocardiography suspected the presence of PH. In a further study comparing the accuracy of echocardiography versus RHC in pregnant women with suspected PH, echocardiography similarly overestimated RVSP in 30 percent of cases compared to RHC (59.6 vs. 54.8 mmHg; $P < 0.004$). In addition, 32 percent of the patients had PH when estimated by echocardiography, but had normal PAP on subsequent catheterization (45). Therefore, RHC remains the gold standard to confirm the presence of PAH, to assess the severity of the disease and to guide treatment decisions such as pregnancy interruption or preterm delivery.

Roberts et al. have been able to provide some prognostic data on pregnant patients with PAH, using RHC values demonstrating an improvement in survival, with a cardiac index of > 4 L/min, right atrial pressure < 10 mmHg, and PVR < 1000 dyne/s cm^{-5} (32). There are no formal studies suggesting improved survival in pregnant women who are positive vasoresponders, although several case reports have described successful outcomes in these patients (46–49).

MANAGEMENT

General measures

Despite the observed reduction in mortality in the last decade, the maternal risk remains significant (13). Most

PH specialists therefore strongly discourage pregnancy, giving specific contraceptive advice to women of child-bearing age and advising termination in existing pregnancies when indicated, preferably before 22 weeks gestation. Women continuing with pregnancy should be assessed monthly, ideally in a PAH referral center, and, in addition to full clinical evaluation, should undergo echocardiography (50). Monitoring of fetal growth is recommended to assess for IUGR.

General measures include limitation of physical activity to minimize additional cardiac demands. Periods of bed rest are therefore thought to be advisable to avoid additional strain. At gestations beyond 24 weeks, mothers should be nursed in a lateral position to avoid supine hypertension, whereby compression of their vena cava by the gravid uterus can impede venous return, leading to potentially significant symptoms including syncope.

Conventional medical therapy

OXYGEN THERAPY

Moderate hypoxemia is common in PAH in the non-pregnant setting where the low CO results in a low mixed venous oxygen saturation (SvO_2), or by right-to-left shunting whereby a patent foramen ovale or other small septal defect acts as a "pressure relief valve." More severe alveolar hypoxia induces hypoxic pulmonary vasoconstriction at a partial pressure of oxygen (pO_2) below 60 mmHg in normoxic subjects (51), and this may increase PVR. Beneficial pulmonary vasodilating effects result from oxygen therapy in hypoxic (52) and non-hypoxic patients with PAH, so avoiding further increases in pulmonary vascular resistance. The effects of maternal hypoxia on fetal well-being are well described, with higher rates of IUGR and prematurity (21), although oxygen therapy during labor to non-hypoxic otherwise healthy mothers is not recommended (53). Current recommendations are therefore that oxygen therapy is administered to these patients when hypoxic during pregnancy, with suggested recommendations to maintain pO_2 above 70 mmHg (50).

DIURETICS

Diuretics may be useful during pregnancy to relieve the increased intravascular volume and also to reduce hepatic congestion resulting from RV failure. Furosemide is safe in pregnancy, and the dose may be escalated as required. Spironolactone should be avoided because of its fetal anti-androgenic effects.

ANTICOAGULATION

Lifelong anticoagulation is recommended in patients with IPAH to reduce the risk of in-situ thrombosis and thromboembolism (54,55), with improved survival seen in those treated with anticoagulants (56,57). Because of similar microthrombotic lesions in other types of PAH (58,59), these patients are also anticoagulated. Pregnancy itself induces a hypercoagulable state, and the risk of thromboembolism is increased, especially during the first postpartum week and also following operative deliveries. Pulmonary embolism (PE) is the leading direct cause of maternal mortality in the developed world (60,61). The occurrence of ongoing pulmonary vascular thrombosis or a new onset pulmonary thromboembolism may worsen RV function during pregnancy, and contribute to the increased maternal mortality (13,62). In several series of maternal PAH deaths (7,63,64), no post mortem evidence of a new pulmonary thromboembolic event was evident, perhaps suggesting that at least these mothers died primarily of pre-existing PAH rather than a new thrombotic event.

Warfarin is contraindicated during the first trimester as it may lead to fetal craniofacial malformations. Heparins are safe throughout pregnancy, although there are no current guidelines in terms of heparin dosage (thromboprophylaxis versus treatment dose) or management around the time of delivery. In mothers receiving prostacyclins, the additional short-lived antiplatelet effect should be considered (65) at the time of delivery, although these agents should not be stopped. One study has shown that prophylactic anticoagulation did not improve pregnancy survival in patients with Eisenmenger's syndrome, where it in fact increased postoperative PPH (63), although this was inconsistent with other studies. In the most recent series, peripartum bleeding was present in half of the CHD-PAH deaths, although pulmonary embolism was the cause of death in some of these patients (13).

Current recommendations are to anticoagulate patients with PAH throughout pregnancy, usually with low molecular weight (LMW) heparin. It should be remembered that because of increased renal excretion, the half-life of LMW heparins falls in pregnancy, and appropriate dose increases should be made (66,67). The current recommendation for mothers with Eisenmenger's syndrome is to use a prophylactic rather than treatment dose regime, given the concurrent risk of increased bleeding (64). In any case, planned elective delivery would allow for prior temporary cessation of anticoagulation. The peripartum management should be considered individually, and the risks and benefits considered. All teams should be made aware of the anticoagulation plan and the potential risks of PPH. When stable, LMW heparins can usually be restarted 12 hours after delivery, in the absence of persistent bleeding (68), and warfarin restarted when the risk of PPH abated (50,69).

PAH-specific therapy

Several case reports have described the successful use of pulmonary antiproliferative and vasodilator therapy in this patient population in pregnancy (8,19,69–83). Increased mortality has been associated with both severe PH and late diagnosis (7), therefore early treatment with PAH therapies is indicated. In the most recent large series, where 60 percent of patients were in NYHA III-IV during pregnancy, 72 percent of IPAH patients and 52 percent of those with CHD-PAH received specific PAH therapy during pregnancy (13).

CALCIUM CHANNEL BLOCKERS

In those patients who are positive vasoresponders to inhaled nitric oxide (iNO), high-dose calcium channel blockers (CCB) are indicated (84), and both nifedipine and diltiazem are safe to use during pregnancy (85,86). Sometimes, in those "responders" to iNO, high-dose CCB may produce near-normalization of pulmonary arterial pressure and right ventricular function after long-term use (84). This patient group may be the only subgroup of PAH patients in whom pregnancy can be allowed to progress to term (8,86).

PROSTANOIDS

Epoprostenol

Prostanoids are potent pulmonary vasodilators and inhibitors of platelet aggregation. Intravenous epoprostenol (prostaglandin I2, prostacyclin) was first used to treat PAH in the 1980s, and remains the first-line therapy for the most severe patients with PAH (6). Reproductive studies in rats and rabbits have shown no impaired fertility or fetal harm at 2.5–4.8 times the recommended human dose (87). There have been several cases reports documenting its successful use in pregnancy with no reported adverse fetal outcomes when used during the first (19,71,80,86) or the second trimester (72,75,76,81). It has also been used to manage acute perioperative PH crises without adverse fetal outcomes (8,20,72,77,82). There remain, however, reported maternal deaths despite treatment with epoprostenol (20,82) which may reflect delayed recognition and treatment when PAH presents in late pregnancy (70,86), as well as the real risk of late maternal death despite maximal treatment.

Iloprost

Iloprost is a stable analogue of prostacyclin that is an effective pulmonary vasodilator when given by intermittent inhalation. There are conflicting reports of congenital anomalies following iloprost use in animal studies. There have, however, been several successful pregnancies using inhaled iloprost in early pregnancy (69,74,88), with at least five reported cases in NYHA II-III patients, with no congenital abnormalities reported.

PHOSPHODIESTERASE TYPE 5 INHIBITORS

Sildenafil, a phosphodiesterase type 5 inhibitor, is effective in several types of PH (89) through a reduction in cyclic GMP breakdown, increasing the sensitivity of pulmonary vascular smooth muscle to nitric oxide (90). There have been at least three reports of its use in early pregnancy (72,78,79) with no reported adverse fetal outcomes.

ENDOTHELIN RECEPTOR ANTAGONISTS

Bosentan, sitaxsentan* and ambrisentan are endothelin receptor antagonists (ERAs), used extensively in PAH treatment. Endothelin-1 (ET-1) plays an important role in fetal development (91), and bosentan is a potent teratogen in animal studies. Pregnancy must always therefore be excluded prior to starting treatment with ERAs, and pregnant women stable on these agents should be switched to alternative agents. Despite the risk, there have been two reported pregnancies in women who were stable on bosentan and sildenafil combination therapy, without congenital abnormalities (72,79).

NITRIC OXIDE

Inhaled nitric oxide is mostly used diagnostically to assess pulmonary vasoreactivity (6). It has been used as treatment during pregnancy (83) but is more often used as an acute pulmonary vasodilator in the peripartum setting (73,92).

Current treatment recommendations

Establishment on prostanoid therapy is indicated as early as possible in patients that progress with pregnancy (8,69,71,80). Intravenous epoprostenol should be the recommended treatment for patients in NYHA functional class III or IV (8,19,87). Nebulized iloprost (69,74) or oral sildenafil (78,79) may be suitable treatment options for patients in NYHA functional class II with more stable PAH. A proposed treatment algorithm is shown in Figure 15.9.1.

Peripartum management

Multidisciplinary care and good planning is central to the overall care of these patients, and ideally their peripartum management should be managed in a center with suitable facilities and expertise (93,94).

METHOD OF DELIVERY

The timing and optimum mode of delivery (vaginal versus cesarean section (CS)) remains debated (7,8,13,50,95–97). Successful CS (8,47,70,74,80,98–100) and vaginal deliveries (8) have both been reported. In the USA 2002–2004 report, 57.9 percent of IPAH cases were delivered under CS compared to 31.1 percent in controls ($P < 0.05$) (10). There has also been a temporal increase in CS in mothers with IPAH (44 to 70 percent) when compared to the previous series of cases reported prior to 1996 (13). Vaginal delivery is associated with fewer infections, reduced blood loss and thromboembolic risk (101), although the latter is reduced with thromboprophylaxis. There are also less abrupt hemodynamic changes during vaginal delivery, particularly when assisted by effective analgesia and a short second stage of labor. However, prolonged, difficult and painful labors can exacerbate pre-existing tachycardia, tachypnea, with detrimental pulmonary vascular effects (102). The lack of predictable delivery time where the team can be fully prepared makes a case for the planned induction of labor. Full anticoagulation, if used, also needs to be withheld prior to delivery, and this requires a degree of planning ahead. There also needs to be a carefully considered strategy regarding the perioperative management of intravenous heparin and prostacyclin, especially if regional anesthesia is planned. Elective CS has the advantage of taking place during the day and avoiding the risk of an urgent CS out of hours. The timing is usually 32–34 weeks for planned deliveries to allow sufficient fetal maturity while avoiding maternal physiological deterioration and unplanned emergency deliveries.

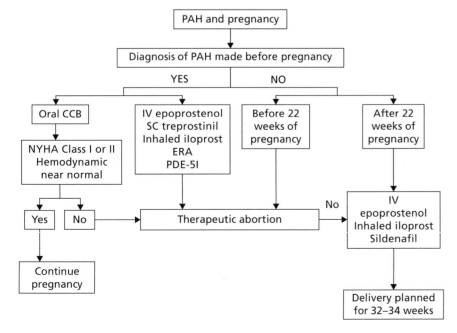

Figure 15.9.1 Algorithm for the management of pregnant women with PAH. CCB, calcium channel blocker; ERA, endothelin receptor antagonist; PDE-5I, phosphodiesterase type 5 inhibitors.

*Sitaxsentan was withdrawn in December 2010.

PERIPARTUM MONITORING

Intraoperative monitoring at delivery is always advocated with ECG, pulse oximetry and invasive arterial blood pressure monitoring (47,70,86,99,100,103). Central venous pressure (CVP) (17) and a form of cardiac output (CO) monitoring are advisable to detect the onset of low CO and rising CVP, characteristic of RV failure. Forms of CO monitoring include echocardiography, lithium dilution techniques (LIDCO) and the pulmonary arterial catheter (PAC), which also gives detailed information regarding right-sided cardiac pressures. Use of a PAC is however debated because of the increased risk of pulmonary artery thrombosis, rupture or perforation (104) and also of both atrial and ventricular arrhythmias in PAH (105,106). There is also no current evidence that PAC use improves outcomes in parturients with PAH (7,8). Atrial arrhythmias occur in 43–87 percent of patients with PH following PAC insertion (107) and can lead to rapid decompensation in these patients (108). In a 2005 single-center series, standard access in all cases included arterial line monitoring, a CVP line, and a large-bore venous catheter, and in only three of the 15 cases was a PAC used (8).

ANESTHETIC TECHNIQUE

The presence of pulmonary hypertension increases the risk of death in patients undergoing both cardiac and noncardiac surgery (109–112). Decompensation is thought to occur following minor stimulation leading to tachycardia or increased pulmonary vascular resistance (PVR) with resulting RV failure and ultimately cardiovascular collapse (98). The risk of these events is increased further by the hemodynamic challenges during late pregnancy and the puerperium (28). Rises in PVR may occur due to hypoxemia, hypercapnia, acidosis (113), pulmonary emboli and also due to elevated catecholamine levels during painful labor (102). The hemodynamic principles of anesthetic management include the maintenance of oxygenation, normovolemia, normotension, minimizing catecholamine surges with adequate analgesia and reducing ventricular preload in the immediate postpartum period, and may be difficult to achieve in these patients. Deliveries by CS may be performed under general anesthesia (GA) (8,17,70,98), even utilizing extracorporeal membrane oxygenation in some cases (114,115), although there is an increasing body of evidence suggesting that CS under incremental regional anesthesia (RA) in these patients is preferable (8,112). A systematic review of all PAH pregnancies published between 1997 and 2007 found that parturient women who received GA for CS were at higher risk of death (13). Contributing factors that may exacerbate RV dysfunction during general anesthesia may include the adverse pulmonary vascular effects of laryngeal stimulation, increased airway plateau pressure during positive pressure ventilation (103) and potentially negative RV effects of volatile anesthetic agents (116,117). In patients where incremental RA

techniques are used, however, the hemodynamic challenges appear to be reduced (8,47,118–121). These techniques describe the use of gradual doses of epidural anesthesia, with or without a small single spinal dose. Historically, larger "single-shot" spinal doses were used more frequently, risking more marked sympathetic blockade and systemic hypotension following the reduction in RV preload, and are now effectively contraindicated in these patients (103,122). Hypotension following sympathetic blockade may also worsen shunt and increase hypoxemia in Eisenmenger's patients (123). Vasopressors are often used for this spinal hypotension, and norepinephrine is preferable to phenylephrine in these patients (124).

RA is contraindicated in the presence of significant coagulopathy because of the risk of epidural hematomas, and also in the presence of severe hemodynamic instability or local sepsis. The use of neuraxial blockade therefore requires cessation of anticoagulation with LMW heparin. The potential additional bleeding risk due to the antiplatelet effects of intravenous prostacyclin should be considered, although as far as we are aware, there have as yet been no reported cases of this potential complication when heparinization is temporarily discontinued in the peripartum period (8,19).

UTEROTONICS

Some of the agents used to reduce the risk of PPH may themselves have adverse cardiac effects, and methods to improve surgical hemostasis, such as the B-Lynch suture, may be considered in women at high risk. Prostaglandin F2alpha causes pulmonary vasoconstriction (125,126) and should be avoided. Syntocinon, the synthetic analogue of oxytocin, is an important part of obstetric management used both as infusions to induce labor, and also as a bolus dose usually followed by an infusion to contract the uterus following delivery and reduce the risk of PPH. It however, has untoward dose-related hemodynamic effects including systemic vasodilatation with reflex tachycardia (127) that is usually compensated for by an increase in CO in healthy women, and it may increase PVR (128). The use of bolus doses has been associated with hemodynamic instability in patients with PAH (82,98,129), although, as suggested in the non-PAH setting, this may be reduced with lower doses. If required at all, the omission of a bolus altogether and use of a low-dose syntocinon infusion may be the most hemodynamically stable compromise (120), remembering that large volumes of infused fluid following delivery may be poorly tolerated.

Postpartum management

Most maternal deaths occur in the 2nd to 30th day following delivery (7), mostly due to intractable RV failure and also PPH. Contributing factors to RV failure include placental autotransfusion volume-loading a failing RV, excessive PVR due to any cause leading to PH crises, adverse hemodynamic effects of oxytocin and new thromboembolic events (72,98,130). The increased risk should be anticipated by the multidisciplinary team and ideally a management plan preconceived. Current recommendations are to continue close maternal monitoring for 72 hours postpartum, ideally in an intensive care unit (8,33,98,101).

MANAGEMENT OF RV FAILURE IN PREGNANCY

The principles of management of RV failure always include minimization of RV afterload, maintenance of appropriate RV preload with sufficient SVR for adequate coronary perfusion, and "off-loading" of the RV, as appropriate (131). In the setting of a PH crisis, with equalization of systemic and pulmonary vascular pressures, the minimization of RV afterload with maximal pulmonary vasodilator therapy is absolutely crucial. Therapies for postpartum PH crises have included iNO (8,70), intravenous epoprostenol (8,19,71) and inhaled iloprost (8,72). Systemic vasopressors and inotropes may also be needed, with dobutamine (72) being a good choice of inotrope as it increases contractility but not PVR:SVR ratio (132,133), and norepinephrine a commonly used vasopressor. Other suitable inotropes include milrinone and levosimendan although their use has not been described in pregnancy. In the setting of an intractable PH crisis, there may be a role for low-dose vasopressin, which may have a relatively selective vasopressor activity more specific to the systemic rather than pulmonary circulation (124,134–136).

Birth control

PREGNANCY TERMINATION

Therapeutic abortion should be offered, particularly when early deterioration occurs (137). The earlier the procedure can be performed, the lower the theoretical maternal risk. Maternal counseling should always be offered (95,138). In one series of patients with ES, fifteen pregnancies were surgically terminated in patients between 6–20 weeks without complications (64). From other studies, perioperative mortality rates up to 4–6 percent are reported in women undergoing interruption of pregnancy and/or laparoscopic, open or transvaginal sterilization (139). Late surgical termination is certainly associated with increased hemodynamic challenge and risk (115). Non-surgical methods for late termination such as the anti-progestogen RU486 may be an alternative, although this has not been described in this patient population.

CONTRACEPTION

Effective contraception is clearly very important in this patient group, however it may be particularly challenging because of drug interactions. Furthermore, estrogen-containing agents are contraindicated because of the increased risk of venous and arterial thromboses, and fluid retention, precluding use of the combined oral contraceptive pill (COCP) (64). Intra-uterine devices are also contraindicated in patients with PAH because the vagal simulation that often follows cervical manipulation (in 5 percent of cases) is thought to induce too great a hemodynamic disturbance. Therefore the realistic available choices in these patients lie between sterilization and progesterone-only hormonal contraceptives.

Progestogen-only contraception is thought not to increase the risk of venous or arterial thrombosis (140,141), except perhaps in polycythemic patients with ES (142), so are safer than estrogens in this patient group. Progestogens do, however, interact with warfarin, and increased INR monitoring is needed. Cerazette (desgestrel 75 μg) is a new formulation of progestogen-only pill (POP) that has a similar efficacy to COCPs and has a similar 12-hour window if missed (95). The p450 enzyme-inducing effect of bosentan reduces the efficacy of POPs, however, and higher doses are needed. The 12-weekly injectable progesterone implant, Depot-Provera, is not affected by bosentan and may be useful, although the deep intramuscular injections may lead to hematomas in those on warfarin.

For emergency contraception, the commonly used agent, levonorgestrel, contains no estrogens, and is therefore safe in patients with PAH. It is administered as a single dose, and when used within 72 hours of exposure has a 1 percent failure rate, although side effects including nausea are common. Patients on bosentan will need to increase the dose by 50–100 percent.

STERILIZATION

Sterilization can be performed at the time of CS, avoiding the risk of a separate procedure, however the failure rate is reportedly higher in this setting (143). In ES, in expert hands, nine tubal ligations were performed using either RA or GA with or without CVP monitoring without adverse complications (94). The role of awake hysteroscopic sterilization is not currently clear (144), but is an appealing alternative and would avoid the risks of general anesthesia and laparoscopy in these patients.

INFERTILITY

Further to the risks of pregnancy itself, the risks precipitated by general anesthesia required for egg retrieval for in-vitro fertilization (IVF) in these patients are high. Furthermore, hormonal therapies are likely to have detrimental side effects (64,142).

KEY POINTS

- Despite the recent advances in the management of pregnant women with PAH, maternal mortality remains high, and pregnancy should continue to be strongly discouraged.

- Pregnant patients should be informed of the very high maternal risk, and early termination, when it is possible, should be discussed.
- Those patients who choose to continue pregnancy should be treated early with targeted PAH therapies including IV epoprostenol and/or sildenafil.
- The management of the pregnant woman with PAH can be challenging and is ideally undertaken at PAH referral centers with an experienced multidisciplinary team. This allows formulation of an agreed and documented management strategy for planned delivery and postpartum monitoring.

ACKNOWLEDGMENTS

The authors would like to thank Professor Frédéric Mercier (Antoine Béclère Hospital, Clamart, France) and Dr Paul Forrest (Royal Prince Alfred Hospital, Sydney, Australia) for their helpful comments.

REFERENCES

1. Barst RJ, McGoon M, Torbicki A, Sitbon O, Krowka MJ, Olschewski H et al. Diagnosis and differential assessment of pulmonary arterial hypertension. J Am Coll Cardiol 2004;43(12 Suppl S):40S–47S.
2. Rubin LJ. Primary pulmonary hypertension. N Engl J Med 1997;336(2):111–7.
3. Simonneau G, Galie N, Rubin LJ, Langleben D, Seeger W, Domenighetti G et al. Clinical classification of pulmonary hypertension. J Am Coll Cardiol 2004;43(12 Suppl S):5S–12S.
4. Humbert M, Sitbon O, Chaouat A, Bertocchi M, Habib G, Gressin V et al. Pulmonary arterial hypertension in France: results from a national registry. Am J Respir Crit Care Med 2006;173(9):1023–30.
5. D'Alonzo GE, Barst RJ, Ayres SM, Bergofsky EH, Brundage BH, Detre KM et al. Survival in patients with primary pulmonary hypertension. Results from a national prospective registry. Ann Intern Med 1991;115(5):343–9.
6. Humbert M, Sitbon O, Simonneau G. Treatment of pulmonary arterial hypertension. N Engl J Med 2004;351(14):1425–36.
7. Weiss BM, Zemp L, Seifert B, Hess OM. Outcome of pulmonary vascular disease in pregnancy: a systematic overview from 1978 through 1996. J Am Coll Cardiol 1998;31(7):1650–7.
8. Bonnin M, Mercier FJ, Sitbon O, Roger-Christoph S, Jais X, Humbert M et al. Severe pulmonary hypertension during pregnancy: mode of delivery and anesthetic management of 15 consecutive cases. Anesthesiology 2005;102(6):1133–7; discussion 5A–6A.
9. Badesch DB, Abman SH, Ahearn GS, Barst RJ, McCrory DC, Simonneau G et al. Medical therapy for pulmonary arterial hypertension: ACCP evidence-based clinical practice guidelines. Chest 2004;126(1 Suppl):35S–62S.
10. Chakravarty EF, Khanna D, Chung L. Pregnancy outcomes in systemic sclerosis, primary pulmonary hypertension, and sickle cell disease. Obstet Gynecol 2008;111(4):927–34.
11. Knight M KJ, Sprak P, Brocklehurst. UK Obstetric Surveillance System (UKOSS) Annual Report 2008. National Perinatal Epidemiology Unit, Oxford, 2008.
12. Yentis SM, Steer PJ, Plaat F. Eisenmenger's syndrome in pregnancy: maternal and fetal mortality in the 1990s. Br J Obstet Gynaecol 1998;105(8):921–2.
13. Bedard E, Dimopoulos K, Gatzoulis MA. Has there been any progress made on pregnancy outcomes among women with pulmonary arterial hypertension? Eur Heart J 2009;30(3):256–65.
14. Gleicher N, Midwall J, Hochberger D, Jaffin H. Eisenmenger's syndrome and pregnancy. Obstet Gynecol Surv 1979;34(10):721–41.
15. Pitkin RM, Perloff JK, Koos BJ, Beall MH. Pregnancy and congenital heart disease. Ann Intern Med 1990;112(6):445–54.
16. Achouh L, Montani D, Garcia G, Jais X, Hamid AM, Mercier O et al. Pulmonary arterial hypertension masquerading as severe refractory asthma. Eur Respir J 2008;32(2):513–6.
17. Smedstad KG, Cramb R, Morison DH. Pulmonary hypertension and pregnancy: a series of eight cases. Can J Anaesth 1994;41(6):502–12.
18. Diller GP, Gatzoulis MA. Pulmonary vascular disease in adults with congenital heart disease. Circulation 2007;115(8):1039–50.
19. Bendayan D, Hod M, Oron G, Sagie A, Eidelman L, Shitrit D et al. Pregnancy outcome in patients with pulmonary arterial hypertension receiving prostacyclin therapy. Obstet Gynecol 2005;106(5 Pt 2):1206–10.
20. McMillan E, Martin WL, Waugh J, Rushton I, Lewis M, Clutton-Brock T et al. Management of pregnancy in women with pulmonary hypertension secondary to SLE and antiphospholipid syndrome. Lupus 2002;11(6):392–8.
21. Presbitero P, Somerville J, Stone S, Aruta E, Spiegelhalter D, Rabajoli F. Pregnancy in cyanotic congenital heart disease. Outcome of mother and fetus. Circulation 1994;89(6):2673–6.
22. Capeless EL, Clapp JF. Cardiovascular changes in early phase of pregnancy. Am J Obstet Gynecol 1989;161(6 Pt 1):1449–53.
23. Ueland K. Maternal cardiovascular dynamics. VII. Intrapartum blood volume changes. Am J Obstet Gynecol 1976;126(6):671–7.
24. Thornburg KL, Jacobson SL, Giraud GD, Morton MJ. Hemodynamic changes in pregnancy. Semin Perinatol 2000;24(1):11–4.
25. Robson SC, Boys RJ, Hunter S, Dunlop W. Maternal hemodynamics after normal delivery and delivery complicated by postpartum hemorrhage. Obstet Gynecol 1989;74(2):234–9.
26. Ueland K. Pregnancy and cardiovascular disease. Med Clin North Am 1977;61(1):17–41.

27. van Oppen AC, Stigter RH, Bruinse HW. Cardiac output in normal pregnancy: a critical review. Obstet Gynecol 1996;87(2):310–8.

28. Clapp JF, 3rd, Capeless E. Cardiovascular function before, during, and after the first and subsequent pregnancies. Am J Cardiol 1997;80(11):1469–73.

29. Robson SC, Dunlop W, Boys RJ, Hunter S. Cardiac output during labor. Br Med J (Clin Res Ed) 1987; 295(6607):1169–72.

30. McCaffrey RM, Dunn LJ. Primary pulmonary hypertension in pregnancy. Obstet Gynecol Surv 1964;19:567–91.

31. Duvekot JJ, Peeters LL. Maternal cardiovascular hemodynamic adaptation to pregnancy. Obstet Gynecol Surv 1994;49(12 Suppl):S1–14.

32. Roberts NV, Keast PJ. Pulmonary hypertension and pregnancy – a lethal combination. Anaesth Intensive Care 1990;18(3):366–74.

33. Budev MM, Arroliga AC, Emery S. Exacerbation of underlying pulmonary disease in pregnancy. Crit Care Med 2005;33(10 Suppl):S313–8.

34. Midwall J, Jaffin H, Herman MV, Kupersmith J. Shunt flow and pulmonary hemodynamics during labor and delivery in the Eisenmenger syndrome. Am J Cardiol 1978;42(2): 299–303.

35. Sugishita Y, Ito I, Kubo T. Pregnancy in cardiac patients: possible influence of volume overload by pregnancy on pulmonary circulation. Jpn Circ J 1986;50(4):376–83.

36. Yoshimura T, Yoshimura M, Yasue H, Ito M, Okamura H, Mukoyama M et al. Plasma concentration of atrial natriuretic peptide and brain natriuretic peptide during normal human pregnancy and the postpartum period. J Endocrinol 1994;140(3):393–7.

37. Templeton A, Kelman GR. Maternal blood-gases, PAO$_2$–PaO$_2$), physiological shunt and VD/VT in normal pregnancy. Br J Anaesth 1976;48(10):1001–4.

38. Campbell LA, Klocke RA. Implications for the pregnant patient. Am J Respir Crit Care Med 2001;163(5):1051–4.

39. Van Hook JW, Harvey CJ, Anderson GD. Effect of pregnancy on maternal oxygen saturation values: use of reflectance pulse oximetry during pregnancy. South Med J 1996; 89(12):1188–92.

40. RCOG. Royal College Obstetricians and Gynecologists: Thromboembolic Disease in Pregnancy and the Puerperium: Acute Management. Green Top Guideline no. 28, 2007.

41. JM UK-I, Freeman SJ, Boylan T, Cheow HK. Quality of CT pulmonary angiography for suspected pulmonary embolus in pregnancy. Eur Radiol 2008;18(12):2709–15.

42. Scarsbrook AF, Bradley KM, Gleeson FV. Perfusion scintigraphy: diagnostic utility in pregnant women with suspected pulmonary embolic disease. Eur Radiol 2007;17(10):2554–60.

43. Wylie BJ, Epps KC, Gaddipati S, Waksmonski CA. Correlation of transthoracic echocardiography and right heart catheterization in pregnancy. J Perinat Med 2007;35(6):497–502.

44. Belfort MA, Rokey R, Saade GR, Moise KJ, Jr. Rapid echocardiographic assessment of left and right heart hemodynamics in critically ill obstetric patients. Am J Obstet Gynecol 1994;171(4):884–92.

45. Penning S, Robinson KD, Major CA, Garite TJ. A comparison of echocardiography and pulmonary artery catheterization for evaluation of pulmonary artery pressures in pregnant patients with suspected pulmonary hypertension. Am J Obstet Gynecol 2001;184(7):1568–70.

46. Breen TW, Janzen JA. Pulmonary hypertension and cardiomyopathy: anaesthetic management for caesarean section. Can J Anaesth 1991;38(7):895–9.

47. Weiss BM, Maggiorini M, Jenni R, Lauper U, Popov V, Bombeli T et al. Pregnant patient with primary pulmonary hypertension: inhaled pulmonary vasodilators and epidural anesthesia for cesarean delivery. Anesthesiology 2000;92(4):1191–4.

48. Slomka F, Salmeron S, Zetlaoui P, Cohen H, Simonneau G, Samii K. Primary pulmonary hypertension and pregnancy: anesthetic management for delivery. Anesthesiology 1988;69(6):959–61.

49. Decoene C, Bourzoufi K, Moreau D, Narducci F, Crepin F, Krivosic-Horber R. Use of inhaled nitric oxide for emergency Cesarean section in a woman with unexpected primary pulmonary hypertension. Can J Anaesth 2001;48(6):584–7.

50. Madden BP. Pulmonary hypertension and pregnancy. Int J Obstet Anesth 2009;18(2):156–64.

51. Melot C, Naeije R, Hallemans R, Lejeune P, Mols P. Hypoxic pulmonary vasoconstriction and pulmonary gas exchange in normal man. Respir Physiol 1987;68(1):11–27.

52. Morgan JM, Griffiths M, du Bois RM, Evans TW. Hypoxic pulmonary vasoconstriction in systemic sclerosis and primary pulmonary hypertension. Chest 1991;99(3):551–6.

53. O'Driscoll BR, Howard LS, Davison AG. BTS guideline for emergency oxygen use in adult patients. Thorax 2008;63 Suppl 6:vi1–68.

54. Palevsky HI, Schloo BL, Pietra GG, Weber KT, Janicki JS, Rubin E et al. Primary pulmonary hypertension. Vascular structure, morphometry, and responsiveness to vasodilator agents. Circulation 1989;80(5):1207–21.

55. Bjornsson J, Edwards WD. Primary pulmonary hypertension: a histopathologic study of 80 cases. Mayo Clin Proc 1985;60(1):16–25.

56. Fuster V, Steele PM, Edwards WD, Gersh BJ, McGoon MD, Frye RL. Primary pulmonary hypertension: natural history and the importance of thrombosis. Circulation 1984;70(4):580–7.

57. Rich S, Dantzker DR, Ayres SM, Bergofsky EH, Brundage BH, Detre KM et al. Primary pulmonary hypertension. A national prospective study. Ann Intern Med 1987;107(2):216–23.

58. Naeye RL. Pulmonary vascular lesions in systemic scleroderma. Dis Chest 1963;44:374–9.

59. Sato T, Matsubara O, Tanaka Y, Kasuga T. Association of Sjogren's syndrome with pulmonary hypertension: report of two cases and review of the literature. Hum Pathol 1993;24(2):199–205.

60. Marik PE, Plante LA. Venous thromboembolic disease and pregnancy. N Engl J Med 2008;359(19):2025–33.

61. Lewis G. The Confidential Enquiry into Maternal and Child Health (CEMACH). Saving Mothers' Lives: Reviewing maternal deaths to make motherhood safer, 2003–5. The Seventh Report of the Confidential Enquiries into Maternal Deaths in the United Kingdom. London, CEMACH, 2007.

62. Tsou E, Waldhorn RE, Kerwin DM, Katz S, Patterson JA. Pulmonary venoocclusive disease in pregnancy. Obstet Gynecol 1984;64(2):281–4.

63. Pitts JA, Crosby WM, Basta LL. Eisenmenger's syndrome in pregnancy: does heparin prophylaxis improve the maternal mortality rate? Am Heart J 1977;93(3):321–6.

64. Daliento L, Somerville J, Presbitero P, Menti L, Brach-Prever S, Rizzoli G et al. Eisenmenger syndrome. Factors relating to deterioration and death. Eur Heart J 1998;19(12):1845–55.

65. Beghetti M, Reber G, de MP, Vadas L, Chiappe A, Spahr-Schopfer I et al. Aerosolized iloprost induces a mild but sustained inhibition of platelet aggregation. Eur Respir J 2002;19(3):518–24.

66. Casele HL, Laifer SA, Woelkers DA, Venkataramanan R. Changes in the pharmacokinetics of the low-molecular-weight heparin enoxaparin sodium during pregnancy. Am J Obstet Gynecol 1999;181(5 Pt 1):1113–7.

67. Sephton V, Farquharson RG, Topping J, Quenby SM, Cowan C, Back DJ et al. A longitudinal study of maternal dose response to low molecular weight heparin in pregnancy. Obstet Gynecol 2003;101(6):1307–11.

68. Duhl AJ, Paidas MJ, Ural SH, Branch W, Casele H, Cox-Gill J et al. Antithrombotic therapy and pregnancy: consensus report and recommendations for prevention and treatment of venous thromboembolism and adverse pregnancy outcomes. Am J Obstet Gynecol 2007;197(5):457 e1–21.

69. Elliot CA, Stewart P, Webster VJ, Mills GH, Hutchinson SP, Howarth ES et al. The use of iloprost in early pregnancy in patients with pulmonary arterial hypertension. Eur Respir J 2005;26(1):168–73.

70. Monnery L, Nanson J, Charlton G. Primary pulmonary hypertension in pregnancy; a role for novel vasodilators. Br J Anaesth 2001;87(2):295–8.

71. Stewart R, Tuazon D, Olson G, Duarte AG. Pregnancy and primary pulmonary hypertension: successful outcome with epoprostenol therapy. Chest 2001;119(3):973–5.

72. Price LC, Forrest P, Sodhi V, Adamson DL, Nelson-Piercy C, Lucey M et al. Use of vasopressin after Caesarean section in idiopathic pulmonary arterial hypertension. Br J Anaesth 2007;99(4):552–5.

73. Lam GK, Stafford RE, Thorp J, Moise KJ, Jr., Cairns BA. Inhaled nitric oxide for primary pulmonary hypertension in pregnancy. Obstet Gynecol 2001;98(5 Pt 2):895–8.

74. Wong PS, Constantinides S, Kanellopoulos V, Kennedy CR, Watson D, Shiu MF. Primary pulmonary hypertension in pregnancy. J R Soc Med 2001;94(10):523–5.

75. Avdalovic M, Sandrock C, Hoso A, Allen R, Albertson TE. Epoprostenol in pregnant patients with secondary pulmonary hypertension: two case reports and a review of the literature. Treat Respir Med 2004;3(1):29–34.

76. Bildirici I, Shumway JB. Intravenous and inhaled epoprostenol for primary pulmonary hypertension during pregnancy and delivery. Obstet Gynecol 2004;103(5 Pt 2):1102–5.

77. Geohas C, McLaughlin VV. Successful management of pregnancy in a patient with Eisenmenger syndrome with epoprostenol. Chest 2003;124(3):1170–3.

78. Lacassie HJ, Germain AM, Valdes G, Fernandez MS, Allamand F, Lopez H. Management of Eisenmenger syndrome in pregnancy with sildenafil and L-arginine. Obstet Gynecol 2004;103(5 Pt 2):1118–20.

79. Molelekwa V, Akhter P, McKenna P, Bowen M, Walsh K. Eisenmenger's syndrome in a 27 week pregnancy – management with bosentan and sildenafil. Ir Med J 2005;98(3):87–8.

80. Badalian SS, Silverman RK, Aubry RH, Longo J. Twin pregnancy in a woman on long-term epoprostenol therapy for primary pulmonary hypertension. A case report. J Reprod Med 2000;45(2):149–52.

81. Mojoli F, Zanierato M, Campana C, Braschi A. Inhaled nitric oxide test in a pregnant patient with severe pulmonary hypertension. Anaesthesia 2006;61(9):912.

82. Takeuchi T, Nishii O, Okamura T, Yaginuma T. Primary pulmonary hypertension in pregnancy. Int J Gynaecol Obstet 1988;26(1):145–50.

83. Robinson JN, Banerjee R, Landzberg MJ, Thiet MP. Inhaled nitric oxide therapy in pregnancy complicated by pulmonary hypertension. Am J Obstet Gynecol 1999;180(4):1045–6.

84. Sitbon O, Humbert M, Jais X, Ioos V, Hamid AM, Provencher S et al. Long-term response to calcium channel blockers in idiopathic pulmonary arterial hypertension. Circulation 2005;111(23):3105–11.

85. Chamaidi A, Gatzoulis MA. Heart disease and pregnancy. Hellenic J Cardiol 2006;47(5):275–91.

86. Easterling TR, Ralph DD, Schmucker BC. Pulmonary hypertension in pregnancy: treatment with pulmonary vasodilators. Obstet Gynecol 1999;93(4):494–8.

87. Huang S, DeSantis ER. Treatment of pulmonary arterial hypertension in pregnancy. Am J Health Syst Pharm 2007;64(18):1922–6.

88. Cotrim C, Simoes O, Loureiro MJ, Cordeiro P, Miranda R, Silva C et al. Acute resynchronization with inhaled iloprost in a pregnant woman with idiopathic pulmonary artery hypertension. Rev Port Cardiol 2006;25(5):529–33.

89. Galie N, Ghofrani HA, Torbicki A, Barst RJ, Rubin LJ, Badesch D et al. Sildenafil citrate therapy for pulmonary arterial hypertension. N Engl J Med 2005;353(20):2148–57.

90. Zhao L, Mason NA, Morrell NW, Kojonazarov B, Sadykov A, Maripov A et al. Sildenafil inhibits hypoxia-induced pulmonary hypertension. Circulation 2001;104(4):424–8.

91. Coceani F, Kelsey L. Endothelin-1 release from lamb ductus arteriosus: relevance to postnatal closure of the vessel. Can J Physiol Pharmacol 1991;69(2):218–21.

92. Goodwin TM, Gherman RB, Hameed A, Elkayam U. Favorable response of Eisenmenger syndrome to inhaled nitric oxide during pregnancy. Am J Obstet Gynecol 1999;180(1 Pt 1):64–7.

93. Landzberg MJ, Murphy DJ, Jr., Davidson WR, Jr., Jarcho JA, Krumholz HM, Mayer JE, Jr. et al. Task force 4: organization

of delivery systems for adults with congenital heart disease. J Am Coll Cardiol 2001;37(5):1187–93.

94. Ammash NM, Connolly HM, Abel MD, Warnes CA. Noncardiac surgery in Eisenmenger syndrome. J Am Coll Cardiol 1999;33(1):222–7.

95. Thorne S, Nelson-Piercy C, MacGregor A, Gibbs S, Crowhurst J, Panay N et al. Pregnancy and contraception in heart disease and pulmonary arterial hypertension. J Fam Plann Reprod Health Care 2006;32(2):75–81.

96. Siu SC, Sermer M, Colman JM, Alvarez AN, Mercier LA, Morton BC et al. Prospective multicenter study of pregnancy outcomes in women with heart disease. Circulation 2001;104(5):515–21.

97. Song YB, Park SW, Kim JH, Shin DH, Cho SW, Choi JO et al. Outcomes of pregnancy in women with congenital heart disease: a single center experience in Korea. J Korean Med Sci 2008;23(5):808–13.

98. O'Hare R, McLoughlin C, Milligan K, McNamee D, Sidhu H. Anaesthesia for caesarean section in the presence of severe primary pulmonary hypertension. Br J Anaesth 1998;81(5):790–2.

99. Olofsson C, Bremme K, Forssell G, Ohqvist G. Cesarean section under epidural ropivacaine 0.75 percent in a parturient with severe pulmonary hypertension. Acta Anaesthesiol Scand 2001;45(2):258–60.

100. Ghai B, Mohan V, Khetarpal M, Malhotra N. Epidural anesthesia for cesarean section in a patient with Eisenmenger's syndrome. Int J Obstet Anesth 2002;11(1):44–7.

101. Uebing A, Steer PJ, Yentis SM, Gatzoulis MA. Pregnancy and congenital heart disease. BMJ 2006;332:401–6.

102. Power KJ, Avery AF. Extradural analgesia in the intrapartum management of a patient with pulmonary hypertension. Br J Anaesth 1989;63(1):116–20.

103. Blaise G, Langleben D, Hubert B. Pulmonary arterial hypertension: pathophysiology and anesthetic approach. Anesthesiology 2003;99(6):1415–32.

104. Barash PG, Nardi D, Hammond G, Walker-Smith G, Capuano D, Laks H et al. Catheter-induced pulmonary artery perforation. Mechanisms, management, and modifications. J Thorac Cardiovasc Surg 1981;82(1):5–12.

105. George RB, Olufolabi AJ, Muir HA. Critical arrhythmia associated with pulmonary artery catheterization in a parturient with severe pulmonary hypertension. Can J Anaesth 2007;54(6):486–7.

106. Chou WR, Kuo PH, Shih JC, Yang PC. A 31-year-old pregnant woman with progressive exertional dyspnea and differential cyanosis. Chest 2004;126(2):638–41.

107. Ermakov S, Hoyt JW. Pulmonary artery catheterization. Crit Care Clin 1992;8(4):773–806.

108. Tongers J, Schwerdtfeger B, Klein G, Kempf T, Schaefer A, Knapp JM et al. Incidence and clinical relevance of supraventricular tachyarrhythmias in pulmonary hypertension. Am Heart J 2007;153(1):127–32.

109. Ramakrishna G, Sprung J, Ravi BS, Chandrasekaran K, McGoon MD. Impact of pulmonary hypertension on the outcomes of noncardiac surgery: predictors of perioperative morbidity and mortality. J Am Coll Cardiol 2005;45(10):1691–9.

110. Reich DL, Bodian CA, Krol M, Kuroda M, Osinski T, Thys DM. Intraoperative hemodynamic predictors of mortality, stroke, and myocardial infarction after coronary artery bypass surgery. Anesth Analg 1999;89(4):814–22.

111. Reich DL, Wood RK, Jr., Emre S, Bodian CA, Hossain S, Krol M et al. Association of intraoperative hypotension and pulmonary hypertension with adverse outcomes after orthotopic liver transplantation. J Cardiothorac Vasc Anesth 2003;17(6):699–702.

112. Martin JT, Tautz TJ, Antognini JF. Safety of regional anesthesia in Eisenmenger's syndrome. Reg Anesth Pain Med 2002;27(5):509–13.

113. Richter JA, Barankay A. Pulmonary hypertension and right ventricular dysfunction after operations for congenital heart disease. Acta Anaesthesiol Scand Suppl 1997;111:31–3.

114. Sugioka J, Nakajima T, Ohsumi H, Kuro M, Sasako Y. [Anesthetic management using percutaneous cardiopulmonary support for cesarean section in a patient with severe pulmonary hypertension]. Masui 1995;44(4):574–8.

115. Satoh H, Masuda Y, Izuta S, Yaku H, Obara H. Pregnant patient with primary pulmonary hypertension: general anesthesia and extracorporeal membrane oxygenation support for termination of pregnancy. Anesthesiology 2002;97(6):1638–40.

116. Ewalenko P, Brimioulle S, Delcroix M, Lejeune P, Naeije R. Comparison of the effects of isoflurane with those of propofol on pulmonary vascular impedance in experimental embolic pulmonary hypertension. Br J Anaesth 1997;79(5):625–30.

117. Ciofolo MJ, Reiz S. Circulatory effects of volatile anesthetic agents. Minerva Anestesiol 1999;65(5):232–8.

118. Spinnato JA, Kraynack BJ, Cooper MW. Eisenmenger's syndrome in pregnancy: epidural anesthesia for elective cesarean section. N Engl J Med 1981;304(20):1215–7.

119. Rosenberg B, Simon K, Peretz BA, Roguin N, Birkhahn HJ. [Eisenmenger's syndrome in pregnancy. Controlled segmental epidural block for cesarean section]. Reg Anaesth 1984;7(4):131–3.

120. Cole PJ, Cross MH, Dresner M. Incremental spinal anaesthesia for elective Caesarean section in a patient with Eisenmenger's syndrome. Br J Anaesth 2001;86(5):723–6.

121. Tibaldi G, Marchi L, Huscher M, Forlini G. [Anesthesia for cesarean section in a pregnant woman with Eisenmenger's syndrome. Description of a clinical case]. Minerva Ginecol 1988;40(2):145–6.

122. Weeks SK, Smith JB. Obstetric anaesthesia in patients with primary pulmonary hypertension. Can J Anaesth 1991;38(7):814–6.

123. Foster JM, Jones RM. The anaesthetic management of the Eisenmenger syndrome. Ann R Coll Surg Engl 1984;66(5):353–5.

124. Price LC, Brett SJ, Howard LS. The use of vasopressors in pulmonary hypertension on the intensive care unit. Br J Hosp Med (Lond) 2007;68(5):280.

125. Secher NJ, Thayssen P, Arnsbo P, Olsen J. Effect of prostaglandin E2 and F2alpha on the systemic and

pulmonary circulation in pregnant anesthetized women. Acta Obstet Gynecol Scand 1982;61(3):213–8.

126. Lange AP, Westergaard JG, Secher NJ, Pedersen GT. Labor induction with prostaglandins. Acta Obstet Gynecol Scand Suppl 1983;113:177–85.

127. Secher NJ, Arnsbo P, Wallin L. Haemodynamic effects of oxytocin (syntocinon) and methyl ergometrine (methergin) on the systemic and pulmonary circulations of pregnant anaesthetized women. Acta Obstet Gynecol Scand 1978;57(2):97–103.

128. Roberts NV, Keast PJ, Brodeky V, Oates A, Ritchie BC. The effects of oxytocin on the pulmonary and systemic circulation in pregnant ewes. Anaesth Intensive Care 1992;20(2):199–202.

129. Duggan AB, Katz SG. Combined spinal and epidural anaesthesia for caesarean section in a parturient with severe primary pulmonary hypertension. Anaesth Intensive Care 2003;31(5):565–9.

130. Lust KM, Boots RJ, Dooris M, Wilson J. Management of labor in Eisenmenger syndrome with inhaled nitric oxide. Am J Obstet Gynecol 1999;181(2):419–23.

131. Mebazaa A, Karpati P, Renaud E, Algotsson L. Acute right ventricular failure – from pathophysiology to new treatments. Intensive Care Med 2004;30(2):185–96.

132. Kerbaul F, Rondelet B, Motte S, Fesler P, Hubloue I, Ewalenko P et al. Effects of norepinephrine and dobutamine on pressure load-induced right ventricular failure. Crit Care Med 2004;32(4):1035–40.

133. Pagnamenta A, Fesler P, Vandinivit A, Brimioulle S, Naeije R. Pulmonary vascular effects of dobutamine in experimental pulmonary hypertension. Crit Care Med 2003;31(4):1140–6.

134. Smith AM, Elliot CM, Kiely DG, Channer KS. The role of vasopressin in cardiorespiratory arrest and pulmonary hypertension. QJM 2006;99(3):127–33.

135. Evora PR, Pearson PJ, Schaff HV. Arginine vasopressin induces endothelium-dependent vasodilatation of the pulmonary artery. V1-receptor-mediated production of nitric oxide. Chest 1993;103(4):1241–5.

136. Forrest P. Anaesthesia and right ventricular failure. Anaesth Intensive Care 2009;37(3):370–85.

137. Sanchez O, Marie E, Lerolle U, Wermert D, Israel-Biet D, Meyer G. [Pulmonary arterial hypertension in women]. Rev Mal Respir 2008;25(4):451–60.

138. Stout K. Pregnancy in women with congenital heart disease: the importance of evaluation and counselling. Heart 2005;91(6):713–4.

139. Weiss BM, Hess OM. Pulmonary vascular disease and pregnancy: current controversies, management strategies, and perspectives. Eur Heart J 2000;21(2):104–15.

140. Vasilakis C, Jick H, del Mar Melero-Montes M. Risk of idiopathic venous thromboembolism in users of progestagens alone. Lancet 1999;354(9190):1610–1.

141. Heinemann LA, Assmann A, DoMinh T, Garbe E. Oral progestogen-only contraceptives and cardiovascular risk: results from the Transnational Study on Oral Contraceptives and the Health of Young Women. Eur J Contracept Reprod Health Care 1999;4(2):67–73.

142. Somerville J. The Denolin Lecture: The woman with congenital heart disease. Eur Heart J 1998;19(12):1766–75.

143. RCOG. Royal College Obstetricians and Gynecologists: Male and Female Sterilization, Green Top Guideline No 4, RCOG Press, 2003.

144. Kerin JF, Cooper JM, Price T, Herendael BJ, Cayuela-Font E, Cher D et al. Hysteroscopic sterilization using a micro-insert device: results of a multicenter Phase II study. Hum Reprod 2003;18(6):1223–30.

PART 5

DRUG AND NON DRUG TREATMENT OF PULMONARY HYPERTENSION

Conventional medical therapies: General measures, supportive treatments and calcium channel blockers

NAZZARENO GALIÈ, ALESSANDRA MANES, MASSIMILIANO PALAZZINI AND ENRI LECI

INTRODUCTION

The suggested initial approach after the diagnosis of pulmonary arterial hypertension (PAH) is the adoption of the general measures, the initiation of the supportive therapy and referral to an expert center for the vasoreactivity testing.

General measures are recommendations on general activities of daily living, including physical activity, birth control and pregnancy, travel, psychosocial support, infection prevention and elective surgery.

Supportive therapies include oral anticoagulants, diuretics, oxygen, digoxin and other inotropic drugs. These treatments are recommended even if no formal randomized controlled trials (RCTs) have been performed in PAH. Supportive therapies are largely used in PAH patients as demonstrated by the baseline treatment of PAH patients included in the RCTs, testing the efficacy of modern targeted treatments (1). Even if the results of the trials with new compounds have substantially changed the current algorithms of treatment of PAH, the role of supportive treatments has not yet been challenged. In fact, it can be argued that the efficacy of the new compounds has been demonstrated when added "on top of" supportive treatments (including oral anticoagulants and diuretics) and no information is available if the investigational treatments were used alone.

Calcium channel blockers agents (CCBs) are included in this chapter because they represent the first class of drugs developed for the treatment of a minority of patients with PAH, namely, those responders to the acute vasoreactivity test. In these cases, the clear favorable response of the long-term treatment with high doses of CCBs has discouraged the performance of RCTs for ethical reasons.

GENERAL MEASURES

Patients with PAH require sensible advice about general activities of daily living and need to adapt to the uncertainty associated with a serious chronic life-threatening disease. The diagnosis usually confers a degree of social isolation (2). Encouraging patients and their family members to join patient support groups can have positive effects on coping, confidence and outlook.

Physical activity and supervised rehabilitation

Patients should be encouraged to be active within symptom limits. Mild breathlessness is acceptable, but patients should avoid exertion that leads to severe breathlessness, exertional dizziness or chest pain. Patients should therefore avoid excessive physical activity that leads to distressing symptoms, but when physically deconditioned may undertake supervised exercise rehabilitation.

One recent study has demonstrated an improvement in exercise capacity in patients with PAH who took part in a training program (3). More data are required to fully understand the clinical impact of supervised rehabilitation programs on the outcome of PAH patients.

There is growing evidence supporting loss of peripheral muscle mass in patients with advanced PAH, and this may be corrected by a defined rehabilitation program.

RECOMMENDATIONS

- Excessive physical activity that leads to distressing symptoms is not recommended in patients with PAH.
- Physically deconditioned PAH patients should be considered for supervised exercise rehabilitation.

Pregnancy, birth control and postmenopausal hormonal therapy

There is consistency from the WHO, existing guidelines and the Expert Consensus Document of the ESC (4) that pregnancy is associated with a 30–50 percent mortality in patients with PAH (5) and as a consequence PAH is a contraindication to pregnancy. There is less consensus relating to the most appropriate methods of birth control. Barrier contraceptive methods are safe for the patient, but with an unpredictable effect. Progesterone-only preparations such as medroxyprogesterone acetate and etonogestrel are effective approaches to contraception and avoid potential issues of estrogens as were included in the old generation mini-pill (6). It should be remembered that the endothelin receptor antagonist (ERA) bosentan may reduce the efficacy of oral contraceptive agents. The Mirena coil is also effective, but rarely leads to a vasovagal reaction when inserted, which may be poorly tolerated in severe PAH (6). A combination of two methods may also be utilized. The patient who becomes pregnant should be informed of the high risk of pregnancy and termination of pregnancy discussed. Those patients who choose to continue pregnancy should be treated with disease targeted therapies, planned elective delivery and effective close collaboration between obstetricians and the PAH team (7,8).

It is not clear if the use of hormonal therapy in postmenopausal women with PAH is advisable or not. It may be considered in cases of intolerable menopausal symptoms in conjunction with oral anticoagulation.

RECOMMENDATIONS

- It is recommended that patients with PAH should avoid pregnancy.
- Hormonal therapy in postmenopausal women with PAH may be considered in cases of intolerable menopausal symptoms in conjunction with oral anticoagulation.

Travel/altitude

Air travel is considered to be of potential harm for patients with underlying pulmonary hypertension because of the generalized pulmonary vasoconstriction at O_2 concentration < 21 percent in the breathing air (9). It is conceivable that the potential dangerous effect is directly proportional to the length of the flight.

There are no studies using flight simulation to determine the need for supplemental O_2 during prolonged flights in patients with PAH. The known physiological effects of hypoxia suggest that in flight O_2 administration should be considered for patients in WHO-FC III and IV and those with arterial blood O_2 pressure consistently less than 8 kPa (60 mmHg). A flow rate of 2 liters per minute will raise inspired O_2 pressure to values seen at sea level. Similarly, such patients should avoid going to altitudes above 1500 to 2000 meters without supplemental O_2. Patients should be advised to travel with written information about their PAH and be advised how to contact local PH clinics in close proximity to where they are traveling.

Prolonged air travel is considered a risk factor for deep venous thrombosis and acute pulmonary embolism (10) mainly caused by immobilization and local venous flow deficiency. In PAH patients who are not treated with oral anticoagulants and have potential risk factors such as WHO FC III and IV or obesity, preventive measures (low-molecular-weight heparin, leg exercises) on long-haul flights over 5000 km may be considered.

RECOMMENDATIONS

- In flight O_2 administration should be considered for PAH patients in WHO-FC III and IV and those with arterial blood O_2 pressure consistently less than 8 kPa (60 mmHg).
- In PAH patients who are not treated with oral anticoagulants and have potential risk factors such as WHO FC III and IV or obesity, preventive measures (low-molecular-weight heparin, leg exercises) on long-haul flights may be considered.

Psychosocial support

Many PAH patients develop anxiety and depression leading to impairment in quality of life. Timely referral to a psychiatrist or psychologist should be made when appropriate. Information on the severity of the disease is available from many non-professional sources and an important role of the PAH multidisciplinary team is to support patients with accurate and up-to-date information. Patient support groups may also play an important role in this area and patients should be advised to join such groups.

RECOMMENDATION

- Psycho-social support should be considered in patients with PAH.

Infection prevention

Patients with PAH are susceptible to developing pneumonia, which is the cause of death in 7 percent of cases (11).

Whilst there are no controlled trials, it is recommended to vaccinate against influenza and pneumococcal pneumonia.

RECOMMENDATIONS

- Immunization of PAH patients against influenza and pneumococcal infection is recommended.

Elective surgery

Elective surgery is expected to have an increased risk in patients with PAH. It is not clear as to which form of anesthesia is preferable, but epidural is probably better tolerated than general anesthesia. Patients usually maintained on oral therapy may require temporary conversion to i.v. or nebulized treatment until they are able to both swallow and absorb drugs taken orally. Oral anticoagulant treatment, if performed, should be withdrawn for the shortest possible time and deep venous thrombosis prophylaxis should be systematically adopted.

RECOMMENDATIONS

- Epidural anesthesia instead of general anesthesia should be utilized, if possible for elective surgery.

Hemoglobin levels

PAH patients are highly sensitive to reduction of hemoglobin levels. Any kind of anemia, even milder degrees, should be corrected. On the other hand, patients with long-standing hypoxemia like those with right-to-left shunts tend to develop erythrocytosis with elevated levels of hematocrit. In these circumstances, venesections are indicated only if hematocrit is above 65 percent and hyperviscosity symptoms are present (12).

RECOMMENDATIONS

- Anemia of any degree should be avoided in patients with PAH.

Concomitant medications

Currently three classes of drugs are approved in PAH (endothelin-receptor antagonists, phosphodiesterase type-5 inhibitors and prostanoid) and care is needed to avoid drug–drug interactions between them and with any other drug which may be utilized (13). Although non-steroid anti-inflammatory drugs did not seem to be associated with PAH in a case-control study (14), their use may further reduce glomerular filtration rate in patients with low cardiac output and pre-renal azotemia. Anorexigens that have been linked to the development of PAH are no longer available on the market in most countries. The effects of the new generation serotonin-related compounds (e.g.

antidepressants) are unknown, but no clear relationships with PAH have yet been demonstrated. The efficacy of current treatments for chronic "biventricular" heart failure like ace-inhibitors and beta-blockers has not been tested in patients with PAH. In addition, the use of these compounds may favor hypotension and progression of right heart failure in PAH patients due to vasodilatation and negative inotropic effects.

SUPPORTIVE THERAPY

Oral anticoagulants

There is a high prevalence of vascular thrombotic lesions at post mortem in patients with idiopathic PAH (IPAH) (15,16). Abnormalities in coagulation and fibrinolytic pathways have also been reported (17–19). It is not clear if the presence of microthrombotic lesions in the small pulmonary arteries (20,21) of PAH patients represents the consequence of or the cause of PAH, but in any case the thrombotic changes likely contribute to the progression of the disease. Mural thrombi have been shown in central elastic pulmonary arteries of patients with IPAH (16) and Eisenmenger's syndrome patients (12,22) as a consequence of several factors including prothrombotic abnormalities, vessel dilatation, atherosclerotic intimal lesions and low cardiac output. It is possible that the peripheral embolization from proximal thrombi may favor the progression of the obstructive changes in smaller vessels.

All the above factors together with the nonspecific increased risk for venous thromboembolism, including heart failure and immobility, may represent the rationale for oral anticoagulation in PAH.

Evidence in favor of oral anticoagulation is confined to patients with IPAH, heritable PAH and PAH due to anorexigens; it is generally retrospective and based on single-center experience (15,23,24).

The survival of PAH patients treated with oral anticoagulant treatment on the basis of clinical judgment, was improved as compared to a concurrent (not randomized) population that was not treated. Three-year survival improved from 21 percent to 49 percent in the series reported by Fuster et al. (15) and from 31 percent to 47 percent in the series of Rich et al. (23). Interestingly, in this second report the survival improvement was observed either in the presence or in the absence of a concomitant treatment with calcium channel antagonists. The design of these studies was not randomized and one can argue that the lower survival of the control groups could be related to comorbidities that prevented the use of anticoagulation in the untreated patients. In addition, only IPAH and anorexigen-related PAH patients were included in the above studies. Nevertheless, the uniformity of the results and the rationale discussed before have convinced the experts to recommend oral anticoagulant treatment in PAH patients in the absence of bleeding risk factors. In recent clinical trials, oral anticoagulant treatment was present at inclusion in a fraction of patients ranging from 50 percent to 80 percent (25).

The potential benefits of oral anticoagulation should be weighed against the risks in patients with other forms of PAH, especially when there is an increased risk of bleeding such as PAH associated with Eisenmenger's syndrome and hemoptysis, with connective tissue diseases and gastrointestinal tract abnormalities (predisposing to bleeding), with portal hypertension (severe esophageal varices, coagulation abnormalities, low platelet count) and with HIV infection (low platelet count poor compliance). Generally, patients with PAH receiving therapy with long-term i.v. prostaglandins are anticoagulated in the absence of contraindications due in part to the additional risk of catheter-associated thrombosis. Also patients with PAH and supraventricular arrhythmias should be anticoagulated. Further research into the role of oral anticoagulation and PAH is encouraged.

Doses of oral anticoagulants are adjusted according to the levels of international normalized ratio (INR) and the therapeutic range varies in different cardiovascular conditions (26). Increased risk for thrombosis is present if the INR consistently falls below 2, while there is no detectable increase of risk for bleeding as long as the INR remains below 3.

Advice regarding the target INR in patients with IPAH varies from 1.5 to 2.5 in most centers of North America to 2.0 to 3.0 in European centers. The aim is to maintain the traditional INR therapeutic range of 2 to 3 in the absence of any bleeding risk factors. A lower level of anticoagulation (INR of 1.5 to 2.5) may be adopted in cases of bleeding predisposition and clear indications for oral anticoagulation (such as heart failure, presence of central venous catheters, supraventricular arrhythmias and local pulmonary artery thrombosis).

RECOMMENDATIONS

- Oral anticoagulant treatment should be considered in patients with IPAH, familial PAH and PAH associated with anorexigen use.
- Oral anticoagulant treatment may be considered in associated PAH forms.
- In patients with Eisenmenger's syndrome, in the absence of significant hemoptysis, oral anticoagulant treatment should be considered in cases with PA thrombosis or signs of heart failure.
- In patients with PAH associated with connective tissue diseases, oral anticoagulation should be considered on an individual basis.
- Anticoagulation is not recommended in patients with PAH associated with portal hypertension or HIV infection and increased risk of bleeding.

Diuretics

Decompensated right heart failure leads to fluid retention, raised central venous pressure, hepatic congestion, peripheral edema and ascites (in advanced cases) (27). Increased intra- and extravascular volumes can markedly impair symptoms and exercise capacity. In WHO functional class III and IV patients hepatic congestion and, occasionally, ascites may reduce diaphragmatic respiratory dynamics compromising lung volumes.

Although there are no RCTs of diuretics in PAH, clinical experience shows clear symptomatic benefit in fluid overloaded patients treated with this therapy. In the recent clinical trials of new treatments about 50 percent to 70 percent of patients were treated with diuretics.

The choice and dose of diuretic therapy may be left to the PAH physician. The appropriate diuretic dose is strictly individual and theoretically should be the lowest dose that is able to maintain an optimal fluid balance and minimize symptoms of congestion. The reasons for variation in diuretic requirement include varying salt and water intake, neuro-hormonal profile, right ventricular performance and different bioavailability of the drugs (27,28). Proper fluid balance can be facilitated by a controlled salt and water intake. Intravenous administration of diuretics is temporary preferred in cases of important fluid retention to overcome the reduced oral bioavailability. Loop diuretics are generally used and furosemide oral doses may vary from 20–25 mg/day up to 500 mg/day. Loop diuretics with better bioavailability may present some advantages (28). The addition of aldosterone antagonists should also be considered. The combination of loop diuretics with thiazides may be temporarily used in selected cases with refractory edema for the synergistic effects of the two compounds. In fact, the mid- to long-term combination of these two classes of diuretics increases the incidence of severe electrolyte disturbances.

It is important to monitor renal function and blood biochemistry in patients to avoid hypokalemia and hyponatremia and the effects of decreased intravascular volume leading to pre-renal failure.

RECOMMENDATIONS

- Diuretic treatment is indicated in PAH patients with signs of RV failure and fluid retention.
- The appropriate diuretic dose is strictly individual and theoretically should be the lowest dose that is able to maintain an optimal fluid balance and minimize symptoms of congestion.

Oxygen

The oxygen content of arterial blood and oxygen delivery to tissues are generally not reduced unless the PaO_2 falls < 60 mmHg (29). Most patients with lung diseases are hypoxemic because of altered ventilation-perfusion matching (30). In contrast, most patients with PAH (except those with associated congenital heart disease) present with only mild degrees of arterial hypoxemia at rest. The pathophysiologic mechanisms in this case include a low mixed venous oxygen saturation caused by low cardiac output and only minimally altered ventilation-perfusion matching. In some patients with hypoxemia a patent foramen ovale can be found. In patients with PAH associated with congenital cardiac defects, hypoxemia is related to right-to-left shunting. Shunt-induced hypoxemia is refractory to increased inspired oxygen.

Oxygen therapy improves quality of life and decreases mortality in patients with pulmonary hypertension related to chronic respiratory insufficiency (31,32) and it is currently indicated in patients with chronic lung disease and arterial oxygen pressure repeatedly measured below 55 to 60 mmHg, or in patients with sleep-associated or exercised-induced hypoxemia (33). No consistent data are currently available on the effect of long-term oxygen treatment in patients with PAH. Although O_2 administration has been demonstrated to reduce the pulmonary vascular resistance in patients with PAH (34) there are no randomized data to suggest that long-term O_2 therapy is beneficial. Most patients with PAH except those with congenital heart diseases and pulmonary-to-systemic shunts have minor degrees of arterial hypoxemia at rest unless they have a patent foramen ovale. There are data showing that nocturnal O_2 therapy does not modify the natural history of advanced Eisenmenger's syndrome (35). Guidance may be based on evidence in patients with COPD; when arterial blood O_2 pressure is consistently less than 8 kPa (60 mmHg) patients are advised to take O_2 to achieve an arterial blood O_2 pressure of over 8 kPa (36). Ambulatory O_2 may be considered in patients when there is evidence of symptomatic benefit and correctable desaturation on exercise.

Experts suggest that the same strategy may also be performed in patients with PAH. Patients who have severe right heart failure and resting hypoxemia caused by low cardiac output and low mixed venous oxygen saturation may benefit from continuous oxygen therapy. The symptomatic improvement related to the use of portable oxygen equipment should be confirmed in the clinical practice by objective assessment of functional capacity. In fact, psychological dependency and mobility limitations related to these devices may overcome the benefits of supplemental oxygen.

There is little rationale to treat patients with hypoxemia predominantly due to right-to-left shunt through a patent foramen ovale, atrial or ventricular septal defects or patent ductus arteriosus with long-term oxygen therapy. In these cases a consistent increase of oxygen saturation and symptomatic improvement on oxygen therapy should be demonstrated.

RECOMMENDATIONS

- Continuous long-term O_2 therapy is indicated in PAH patients when arterial blood O_2 pressure is consistently less than 8 kPa (60 mmHg).
- In patients with Eisenmenger's syndrome use of supplemental O_2 therapy should be considered in cases in which it produces a consistent increase in arterial oxygen saturation and reduces symptoms.

Inotropic drugs

In patients with PAH, the consequent increase in pulmonary vascular resistance leads to right ventricular overload, hypertrophy and dilatation and eventually to right failure and premature death. The importance of the progression of right heart failure on the outcome of idiopathic PAH patients is testified by the prognostic impact of right atrial pressure, cardiac index and pulmonary artery pressure (37), three main parameters of right ventricular pump function. Since the depression of myocardial contractility seems to be one of the primary events in the progression of heart failure, the drugs that increase the force of contraction of myocytes, defined as inotropic agents, have been considered as a logical approach to the treatment of this condition. However, in patients with precapillary pulmonary hypertension excessive afterload seems to be the leading determinant of heart failure. In fact, its removal, for instance after successful pulmonary thromboendoarterectomy or lung transplantation (38), leads almost invariably to a sustained recovery of right ventricular function. On the other hand, changes in the adrenergic pathways of right ventricular myocytes leading to reduced contractility have been shown in idiopathic PAH patients (39). In addition, the response of the overloaded right ventricle, may also be influenced by genetic determinants (40).

ADRENERGIC INOTROPIC DRUGS

The effects of adrenergic inotropic drugs on the failing right ventricle have received little attention by the investigators. From a theoretical point of view and from some experimental studies (41) it emerges that the inotropic stimulation of these compounds is similar on the right and left ventricular myocardium. Data on humans are available mostly for the prevalent beta 2-adrenergic receptor agonist isoproterenol (42) that was administered to IPAH patients for its supposed effects of vasodilatation on the pulmonary circulation (43,44). Isoproterenol induced increase of cardiac output and heart rate and in some cases reduction of blood pressure.

Dobutamine (42) is a prevalent beta 1-adrenergic receptor agonist that exerts inotropic and vasodilator effects comparable to isoproterenol, but it has a less pronounced chronotropic activity. Dobutamine is widely used in the acute deterioration of patients with chronic biventricular failure. No data are available on the acute and long-term administration of dobutamine in PAH patients, but it is likely that its effects are comparable to those of isoproterenol.

Dopamine (42) is a beta-, alpha- and dopaminergic-receptor agonist and its profile of action may present some advantages over the prevalent beta-receptor agonists. In fact, the alpha-adrenergic activity allows us to preserve the blood pressure levels and even to increase them. The stimulation of beta 1-adrenergic receptors induces a consistent increase of cardiac output while the dopaminergic stimulation increases the renal blood flow facilitating diuresis. The dopaminergic effect is present at low doses (2 μg/kg/min) while the stimulation of beta 1-adrenergic receptors increases progressively up to 10–15 μg/kg/min and a consistent alpha-adrenergic effect is detectable at high doses (10–20 μg/kg/min). A possible effect of pulmonary vasoconstriction seems not to be present at doses < 20 μg/kg/min.

In severe, decompensated right heart failure the use of intravenous adrenergic support may help the recovery of blood pressure and renal function. The absence of systemic hypotensive effects together with the renal blood flow increase suggest the use of dopamine alone or in combination with dobutamine as the inotropic strategy of choice in PAH patients. In critical cases dopamine can be used together with intravenous prostanoids for its synergistic activity on cardiac output and its antagonistic effect on blood pressure decrease.

DIGOXIN

Even if digoxin increases indices of right ventricular contractility (45) its clinical impact in PAH patients is still unknown. The effects of digoxin have been analyzed in patients with cor pulmonale secondary to chronic airflow obstruction (46–48) and in this setting no consistent results have been obtained. In fact, some investigators claimed a reduction in right sided filling pressures and an increase of cardiac output after the administration of digitalis (33,34) while others did not confirm these findings (48). Moreover, the acute administration of digoxin may induce pulmonary vasoconstriction (49) and the presence of hypoxia and electrolyte imbalance could increase the incidence of digitalis toxicity. On the other hand, short-term intravenous administration of digoxin in IPAH patients induces a modest increase of cardiac output and a significant reduction in circulating norepinephrine (50). In chronic "biventricular" heart failure patients, digoxin treatment has no influence on mortality, but it reduces the rate of hospitalization for acute decompensation. For all these reasons, the use of digitalis in PAH patients is based mostly on the personal experience and "feelings" of the expert rather than on clear scientific evidence of efficacy.

Although digoxin has been shown to improve cardiac output acutely in IPAH, its efficacy is unknown when administered chronically (50). It may be given to slow ventricular rate in patients with PAH who develop atrial tachyarrhythmias.

In PAH clinical trials digoxin was administered at entry to a percentage of patients variable from 15 percent to 50 percent.

RECOMMENDATIONS

- Inotropic adrenergic support may be considered in patients with severe decompensated right heart failure.
- Digoxin may be considered in patients with PAH who develop atrial tachyarrhythmias to slow ventricular rate.

CALCIUM CHANNEL BLOCKERS

The evidence for medial hypertrophy in the small pulmonary arteries together with the reduction of pulmonary vascular resistance obtained by vasodilator drugs led Paul Wood many years ago (51) to elaborate the "vasoconstrictive" hypothesis as the basis for understanding the pathogenesis and the pathophysiology of primary pulmonary hypertension. He suggested that the active vasoconstriction of small muscular pulmonary arteries and arterioles was the main determinant of the hemodynamics and subsequent evolution of primary pulmonary hypertension. Since then, many attempts to reduce pulmonary vascular resistance and improve symptoms have been performed in a small series of PAH patients in both acute and long-term studies. A variety of vasodilators have been used including tolazoline, acetylcholine, diazoxide, hydralazine, phentolamine, isoproterenol, nitrates, verapamil, nifedipine and diltiazem (23,43,51,52,53–55,56). It soon became clear that a meaningful reduction of pulmonary artery pressure associated with a reduction of pulmonary vascular resistance could only be obtained in a minority of patients with primary pulmonary hypertension on acute vasoreactivity tests. In addition, favorable results of long-term treatments were confirmed in larger scale trials only with CCBs, in particular with nifedipine and diltiazem (23,56).

Acute vasoreactivity tests

In PAH, vasoreactivity testing should be performed at the time of diagnostic right heart catheterization to identify patients who may benefit from long-term therapy with CCBs (23,57). Acute vasodilator challenge should only be performed with short-acting, safe and easy to administer drugs with no or limited systemic effects. Currently the agent most used in acute testing is nitric oxide (Table 16.1.1) (57). Based on previous experience (23,58,59) intravenous (i.v.) epoprostenol or i.v. adenosine may also be used as an alternative (but risk of systemic vasodilator effects) (Table 16.1.1).

Inhaled iloprost and oral sildenafil may be associated with significant vasodilator effects. Their role in the prediction of the response to CCB therapy has not yet been demonstrated. Due to the risk of potentially life-threatening complications, the use of CCB given orally or i.v. as an acute test is discouraged. A positive acute response (positive acute responders) is defined as a reduction of mean PAP ≥ 10 mmHg to reach an absolute value of mean PAP ≤ 40 mmHg with an increased or unchanged CO (57). Only about 10 percent of patients with IPAH will meet these criteria. Positive acute responders are most likely to show a sustained response to long-term treatment with high doses of CCB and they are the only patients that can safely be treated with this type of therapy. About half of IPAH positive acute responders are also positive long-term responders to CCBs (57) and only in these cases is the continuation of

Table 16.1.1 Route of administration, half-life, dose ranges, increments and duration of administration of the most commonly used agents for pulmonary vasoreactivity tests

Drug	Route	Half–life	Dose range*	Increments[†]	Duration[‡]
Nitric oxide	Inhaled	15–30 sec	10–20 ppm	–	5 min[§]
Epoprostenol	Intravenous	3 min	2–12 ng/kg/min	2 ng/kg/min	10 min
Adenosine	Intravenous	5–10 sec	50–350 µg/kg/min	50 µg/kg/min	2 min

*Initial dose and maximal dose suggested.
[†]Increments of dose by each step; [‡]duration of administration on each step.
[§]For NO a single step within the dose range is suggested.

CCB as a single treatment warranted. The usefulness of acute vasoreactivity tests and long-term treatment with CCBs in patients with other PAH types, such as heritable PAH, connective tissues diseases, and HIV infection patients is less clear than IPAH. Nevertheless, experts recommend performing acute vasoreactivity studies in these patients and to look for a long-term response to CCB in those in which the test is positive. No data are available on the usefulness of long-term CCB therapy in patients with PH associated with congenital heart diseases and therefore the value of performing a vasoreactivity test in this setting is controversial. Acute vasoreactivity studies to identify patients with a long-term favorable response to CCB is not recommended in pulmonary hypertension associated with left heart disease, lung diseases, chronic thromboembolic pulmonary hypertension and pulmonary hypertension due to multiple mechanisms.

Long-term treatment with calcium–channel blockers

Smooth muscle cell hypertrophy, hyperplasia and vasoconstriction have long been known to contribute to the pathogenesis of IPAH and this has led to the use of CCBs. It has been recognized that only a small number of patients with IPAH who demonstrate a favorable response to acute vasodilator testing at the time of RHC do well with CCB (23,57).

The CCBs that have been predominantly used in reported studies are nifedipine, diltiazem and amlodipine with particular emphasis on the first two (23,57). The choice of CCB is based upon the patient's heart rate at baseline with a relative bradycardia favoring nifedipine and amlodipine and a relative tachycardia favoring diltiazem. The daily doses of these drugs that have shown efficacy in IPAH are relatively high, 120–240 mg for nifedipine, 240–720 mg for diltiazem and up to 20 mg for amlodipine. It is advisable to start with a low dose, e.g. 30 mg of slow release nifedipine twice a day, or 60 mg of diltiazem three times a day, or 2.5 mg of amlodipine once a day and increase cautiously and progressively to the maximum tolerated dose. Limiting factors for dose increase are usually systemic hypotension and lower limb peripheral edema. Patients with IPAH who meet the criteria for a positive vasodilator response and are

treated with CCB should be followed closely for both safety and efficacy with an initial reassessment after 3–4 months of therapy including RHC.

If the patient does not show an adequate response defined as being in WHO-FC I or II and with a marked hemodynamic improvement, additional PAH therapy should be instituted. Patients who have not undergone a vasoreactivity study or those with a negative study should not be started on CCB because of potential severe side-effects (e.g. hypotension, syncope and RV failure).

Vasodilator responsiveness does not appear to predict a favorable long-term response to CCB therapy in patients with PAH in the setting of connective tissue diseases, and high doses of CCB are often not well tolerated in such patients (60).

No clear data support the use of CCB in patients with Eisenmenger's syndrome and the empirical use of CCB is dangerous and should be avoided.

RECOMMENDATIONS

- Vasoreactivity testing is indicated in patients with IPAH, heritable PAH and PAH associated with anorexigen used to detect patients who can be treated with high doses of CCB.
- A positive response to vasoreactivity testing is defined as a reduction of mean pulmonary arterial pressure ≥ 10 mmHg to reach an absolute value of mean PAP ≤ 40 mmHg with an increased or unchanged cardiac output.
- Vasoreactivity testing should be performed only in referral centers.
- Vasoreactivity testing should be performed using nitric oxide as vasodilator.
- Vasoreactivity testing may be performed in other types of PAH.
- Vasoreactivity testing may be performed using i.v. epoprostenol or i.v. adenosine.
- The use of oral or i.v. CCB in acute vasoreactivity testing is not recommended.
- Vasoreactivity testing to detect patients who can be safely treated with high doses of CCB is not recommended in patients with pulmonary hypertension associated with left heart disease, lung diseases, chronic

thromboembolic pulmonary hypertension and pulmonary hypertension due to multiple mechanisms.

- CCBs treatment is not recommended in patients with Eisenmenger's syndrome patients.

KEY POINTS

- Excessive physical activity that leads to distressing symptoms is not recommended in patients with PAH.
- It is recommended that patients with PAH should avoid pregnancy.
- Epidural anesthesia instead of general anesthesia should be utilized, if possible for elective surgery.
- Oral anticoagulant treatment should be considered in patients with IPAH, familial PAH and PAH associated with anorexigen use.
- Diuretic treatment is indicated in PAH patients with signs of RV failure and fluid retention.
- Continuous long-term O_2 therapy is indicated in PAH patients when arterial blood O_2 pressure is consistently less than 8 kPa (60 mmHg).
- Digoxin may be considered in patients with PAH who develop atrial tachyarrhythmias to slow ventricular rate.
- Vasoreactivity testing with NO performed in referral centers is indicated in patients with IPAH, heritable PAH, and PAH associated with anorexigen use to detect patients who can be treated with high doses of CCB.
- A positive response to vasoreactivity testing is defined as a reduction of mean pulmonary arterial pressure $\geqslant 10$ mmHg to reach an absolute value of mean PAP $\leqslant 40$ mmHg with an increased or unchanged cardiac output.
- CCBs teratment is not recommended in patients with Elsenmenger's syndrome.

REFERENCES

1. Galie N, Manes A, Negro L, Palazzini M, Bacchi Reggiani ML, Branzi A. A meta-analysis of randomized controlled trials in pulmonary arterial hypertension. Eur Heart J 2009;30(4):394–403.
2. Loewe B, Graefe K, Ufer C et al. Anxiety and depression in patients with pulmonary hypertension. Psychosom Med 2004;66:831–6.
3. Mereles D, Ehlken N, Kreuscher S et al. Exercise and respiratory training improve exercise capacity and quality of life in patients with severe chronic pulmonary hypertension. Circulation 2006;114(14):1482–9.
4. Expert consensus document on management of cardiovascular diseases during pregnancy: The Task Force on the Management of Cardiovascular Diseases During Pregnancy of the European Society of Cardiology. Eur Heart J 2003;24(8):761–81.
5. Bedard E, Dimopoulos K, Gatzoulis MA. Has there been any progress made on pregnancy outcomes among women with pulmonary arterial hypertension? Eur Heart J 2009;30(3):256–65.
6. Thorne S, Nelson-Piercy C, MacGregor AJ et al. Pregnancy and contraception in heart disease and pulmonary arterial hypertension. J Fam Plann Reprod Health Care 2006;32:75–81.
7. Bendayan D, Hod M, Oron G et al. Pregnancy outcome in patients with pulmonary arterial hypertension receiving prostacyclin therapy. Obstet Gynecol 2005;106:1206–10.
8. Bonnin M, Mercier FJ, Sitbon O et al. Severe pulmonary hypertension during pregnancy: mode of delivery and anesthetic management of 15 consecutive cases. Anesthesiology 2005;102:1133–7.
9. Mohr LCM. Hypoxia During Air Travel in Adults With Pulmonary Disease. [Article]. Am J Med Sci 2008;335(1):71–9.
10. Lehmann R, Suess C, Leus M, Luxembourg B, Miesbach W, Lindhoff-Last E, Zeiher AM, Spyridopoulos I. Incidence, clinical characteristics, and long-term prognosis of travel-associated pulmonary embolism. Eur Heart J 2009;30(2):233–41.
11. Rich S, Dantzker DR, Ayres SM et al. Primary pulmonary hypertension. A national prospective study. Ann Intern Med 1987;107(2):216–23.
12. Galiè N, Manes A, Palazzini M et al. Management of pulmonary arterial hypertension associated with congenital systemic-to-pulmonary shunts and Eisenmenger's syndrome. Drugs 2008;68:1049–66.
13. Galiè N, Hoeper M, Humbert M et al. Guidelines on diagnosis and treatment of pulmonary hypertension: The Task Force on Diagnosis and Treatment of Pulmonary Hypertension of the European Society of Cardiology and of the European Respiratory Society. Eur Heart J 2009;30:2493–537.
14. Abenhaim L, Moride Y, Brenot F et al. Appetite-suppressant drugs and the risk of primary pulmonary hypertension. International Primary Pulmonary Hypertension Study Group [see comments]. N Engl J Med 1996;335(9):609–16.
15. Fuster V, Steele PM, Edwards WD, Gersh BJ, McGoon MD, Frye RL. Primary pulmonary hypertension: natural history and the importance of thrombosis. Circulation 1984;70(4):580–7.
16. Moser KM, Fedullo PF, Finkbeiner WE, Golden J. Do patients with primary pulmonary hypertension develop extensive central thrombi? Circulation 1995;91(3):741–5.
17. Herve P, Humbert M, Sitbon O et al. Pathobiology of pulmonary hypertension: the role of platelets and thrombosis. Clin Chest Med 2001;22:451–8.
18. Hoeper MM, Sosada M, Fabel H. Plasma coagulation profiles in patients with severe primary pulmonary hypertension. Eur Respir J 1998;12(6):1446–9.
19. Huber K, Beckmann R, Frank H et al. Fibrinogen, t-PA, and PAI-1 plasma levels in patients with pulmonary hypertension. Am J Respir Crit Care Med 1994;150(4):929–33.

20. Pietra GG, Edwards WD, Kay JM *et al*. Histopathology of primary pulmonary hypertension. A qualitative and quantitative study of pulmonary blood vessels from 58 patients in the National Heart, Lung, and Blood Institute, Primary Pulmonary Hypertension Registry [see comments]. Circulation 1989;80(5):1198–206.

21. Wagenvoort CA, Mulder PG. Thrombotic lesions in primary plexogenic arteriopathy. Similar pathogenesis or complication? [see comments]. Chest 1993;103(3):844–9.

22. Beghetti M, Galiè N. Eisenmenger syndrome: a clinical perspective in a new therapeutic era of pulmonary arterial hypertension. J Am Coll Cardiol 2009;53(9):733–40.

23. Rich S, Kaufmann E, Levy PS. The effect of high doses of calcium-channel blockers on survival in primary pulmonary hypertension [see comments]. N Engl J Med 1992;327(2):76–81.

24. Frank H, Mlczoch J, Huber K, Schuster E, Gurtner HP, Kneussl M. The effect of anticoagulant therapy in primary and anorectic drug-induced pulmonary hypertension. Chest 1997;112(3):714–21.

25. Nomenclature Committee. Nomenclature and Classification of Pulmonary Hypertension. Primary Pulmonary Hypertension: Executive Summary from the World Symposium-Primary Pulmonary Hypertension 1998.

26. Ansell J, Hirsh J, Dalen J, Bussey H, Anderson D, Poller L, Jacobson A, Deykin D, Matchar D. Managing oral anticoagulant therapy. Chest 2001;119(1 Suppl):22S–38S.

27. Cohn JN. Optimal diuretic therapy for heart failure. Am J Med 2001;111(7):577.

28. Murray MD, Deer MM, Ferguson JA *et al*. Open-label randomized trial of torsemide compared with furosemide therapy for patients with heart failure. Am J Med 2001;111(7):513–20.

29. Hales CA. The site and mechanisms of oxygen sensing for the pulmonary vessels. Circulation 1985;88:235s–240s.

30. West JB. Ventilation/perfusion relationships. Am Rev Respir Dis 1977;116:919–43.

31. Continuous or nocturnal oxygen therapy in hypoxemic chronic obstructive lung disease: a clinical trial. Nocturnal Oxygen Therapy Trial Group. Ann Intern Med 1980;93(3):391–8.

32. Long term domiciliary oxygen therapy in chronic hypoxic cor pulmonale complicating chronic bronchitis and emphysema. Report of the Medical Research Council Working Party. Lancet 1981;1(8222):681–6.

33. Tarpy SP, Celli BR. Long-term oxygen therapy. N Engl J Med 1995;333(11):710–4.

34. Roberts DH, Lepore JJ, Maroo A, Semigran MJ, Ginns LC. Oxygen therapy improves cardiac index and pulmonary vascular resistance in patients with pulmonary hypertension. Chest 2001;120(5):1547–55.

35. Sandoval J, Aguirre JS, Pulido T, Martinez-Guerra ML, Santos E, Alvarado P, Rosas M, Bautista E. Nocturnal oxygen therapy in patients with the Eisenmenger syndrome. Am J Respir Crit Care Med 2001;164(9):1682–7.

36. Weitzenblum E, Sautegeau A, Ehrhart M, Mammosser M, Pelletier A. Long-term oxygen therapy can reverse the progression of pulmonary hypertension in patients with chronic obstructive pulmonary disease. Am Rev Respir Dis 1985;131(4):493–8.

37. D'Alonzo GE, Barst RJ, Ayres SM *et al*. Survival in patients with primary pulmonary hypertension. Results from a national prospective registry. Ann Intern Med 1991;115(5):343–9.

38. Ritchie M, Waggoner AD, Dávila RV, Barzilai B, Trulock EP, Eisenberg PR. Echocardiographic characterization of the improvement in right ventricular function in patients with severe pulmonary hypertension after single-lung transplantation. J Am Coll Cardiol 1993;22(4):1170–4.

39. Bristow MR, Minobe W, Rasmussen R *et al*. Beta-adrenergic neuroeffector abnormalities in the failing human heart are produced by local rather than systemic mechanisms. J Clin Invest 1992;89(3):803–15.

40. Abraham WT, Raynolds MV, Gottschall B *et al*. Importance of angiotensin-converting enzyme in pulmonary hypertension. Cardiology 1995;10 (Suppl1):9–15.

41. Schmidt HD, Hoppe H, Hedenreich L. Direct effects of dopamine, orciprenaline and norepinephrine on the right and left ventricle of isolated canine hearts. Cardiology 1979;64:133–48.

42. Leier CV. Acute inotropic support. In: Leier CV, ed. Cardiotonic Drugs. New York: Marcel Dekker, 1986:49–84.

43. Shettigar UR, Hultgren HN, Specter M, Martin R, Davies DH. Primary pulmonary hypertension: favorable effect of isoproterenol. N Engl J Med 1976;295(25):1414–5.

44. Pietro DA, LaBresh KA, Shulman RM, Folland ED, Parisi AF, Sasahara AA. Sustained improvement in primary pulmonary hypertension during six years of treatment with sublingual isoproterenol. N Engl J Med 1984;19;310(16):1032–4.

45. Green L, Smith T. The use of digitalis in patients with pulmonary disease. Ann Intern Med 1977;87:459–65.

46. Gray FD, Williams MH, Gray FG. The circulatory and ventilatory changes in chronic pulmonary disease as affected by lanatoside C. Am Heart J 1952;44:517–30.

47. Ferrer MI, Harvey RM, Cathcart RT, Webster CA, Richards DW, Cournand A. Some effects of digoxin in chronic cor pulmonale. Circulation 1950;1:161–86.

48. Berglund E, Widminsky J, Malmberg R. Lack of effect of digitalis in patients with pulmonary disease with and without heart failure. Am J Cardiol 1963;11:447.

49. Kim YS, Aviado DM. Digitalis and the pulmonary circulation. Am Heart J 1961;62:680–6.

50. Rich S, Seidlitz M, Dodin E, Osimani D, Judd D, Genthner D, McLaughlin V, Francis G. The short-term effects of digoxin in patients with right ventricular dysfunction from pulmonary hypertension. Chest 1998;114(3):787–92.

51. Wood P. Primary pulmonary hypertension, with special reference to the vasoconstrictive factor. Br Heart J 1958; 20(4):557–65.

52. Dresdale DT, Schultz M, Michtom RJ. Primary Pulmonary Hypertension. I. Clinical and Hemodynamic Study. Am J Med 1951;11:686–705.

53. Rubin LJ, Peter RH. Oral hydralazine therapy for primary pulmonary hypertension. N Engl J Med 1980;302(2):69–73.

54. Reeves JT, Groves BM, Turkevich D. The case for treatment of selected patients with primary pulmonary hypertension. Am Rev Respir Dis 1986;134(2):342–6.

55. Weir EK, Rubin LJ, Ayres SM *et al*. The acute administration of vasodilators in primary pulmonary hypertension. Experience from the National Institutes of Health Registry on Primary Pulmonary Hypertension. Am Rev Respir Dis 1989;140(6):1623–30.

56. Barst RJ, Maislin G, Fishman AP. Vasodilator therapy for primary pulmonary hypertension in children. Circulation 1999;99(9):1197–208.

57. Sitbon O, Humbert M, Jais X *et al*. Long-term response to calcium channel blockers in idiopathic pulmonary arterial hypertension. Circulation 2005;111(23):3105–11.

58. Galie N, Ussia G, Passarelli P, Parlangeli R, Branzi A, Magnani B. Role of pharmacologic tests in the treatment of primary pulmonary hypertension. Am J Cardiol 1995;75(3):55A–62A.

59. McLaughlin VV, Genthner DE, Panella MM, Rich S. Reduction in pulmonary vascular resistance with long-term epoprostenol (prostacyclin) therapy in primary pulmonary hypertension [see comments]. N Engl J Med 1998;338(5):273–7.

60. Mukerjee D, St George D, Coleiro B, Knight C, Denton CP, Davar J, Black CM, Coghlan JG. Prevalence and outcome in systemic sclerosis associated pulmonary arterial hypertension: application of a registry approach. Ann Rheum Dis 2003;62(11):1088–93.

Prostacyclins: Intravenous, subcutaneous, inhaled and oral

VALLERIE MCLAUGHLIN AND MELVYN RUBENFIRE

INTRODUCTION

Prostacyclin therapy has transformed the care of patients with pulmonary arterial hypertension (PAH), an orphan disease for which there was no effective treatment option for the great majority of patients until 15 years ago (1). Over 25 years ago epoprostenol (PGI_2), a stable freeze-dried preparation of prostacyclin, was shown to reduce symptoms and improve hemodynamics in a woman with severe primary pulmonary hypertension (PPH) awaiting lung transplant (2). Following relatively small clinical trials and a pivotal trial that established the safety and efficacy in a uniformly fatal disease, intravenous epoprostenol (Flolan®) was approved for clinical use in PAH by the US Food and Drug Administration (FDA) in 1995 (3–7). The effectiveness of prostacyclin, a vasodilator and inhibitor of platelet aggregation, reflects the mechanisms believed to contribute substantially to the development of PAH. The evolution of prostanoid therapies with FDA approval has been rapid and now includes intravenous epoprostenol (Flolan® and generic), intravenous and subcutaneous treprostinil (Remodulin®), and inhaled iloprost (Ventavis®), and inhaled treprostinil (Tyvaso®).

PATHOPHYSIOLOGICAL BASIS FOR PROSTACYCLIN USE

The complex pathobiology of PAH is thought to begin with endothelial dysfunction that results in chronically impaired production of vasodilators including nitric oxide (NO) and prostacyclin (PGI_2), and overexpression of the endogenous vasoconstrictor endothelin (ET)-1 and the prothrombotic thromboxane A_2 (8,9). Prostacyclin synthase expression is decreased in lungs from patients with severe PAH (10), and smooth muscle proliferation and medial hypertrophy is associated with a decrease in smooth muscle cell PGI_2 receptor activity (11). Each of the pathways involved in the pathogenesis of PAH are potential pharmacological targets (12).

Initially described in 1976 by Moncada and Vane, prostacyclin (epoprosentol, PGI_2, PGX) is a member of the prostaglandin family produced by vascular endothelial cells (13,14). They described a substance isolated from arterial tissue with potent antiplatelet and vasodilating effects that was distinct from the known arachidonic acid metabolites at that time. The authors prophetically stated that "a deficiency of PGX could, therefore underlie some forms of hypertension." Shortly thereafter, PGX was reported to be prostacyclin, or PGI_2, and unlike most prostaglandins which are rapidly inactivated by the pulmonary circulation, PGI_2 was generated by the lungs and released into the systemic circulation as a circulating hormone.

PGI_2 is a potent direct vasodilator of both the pulmonary and systemic vascular beds, as well as an inhibitor of platelet aggregation. There is also evidence that it has antiproliferative effects. Prostacylin analogs have been shown *in vitro* to inhibit smooth muscle cell growth (15). The mechanism by which prostacyclins mediate vasodilation is via ligand binding to a G-protein-coupled receptor with subsequent signal transduction inducing relaxation of vascular smooth muscle. Signal transduction via adenylate cyclase increases intracellular cyclic adenosine monophosphate (cAMP).

Why are the prostanoids so effective in PAH?

The benefit of PGI_2 in PAH was initially assumed to be related to the vasodilating effect produced by activating membrane-bound adenylate cyclase to increase cyclic adenosine monophosphate (AMP) which results in smooth muscle cell relaxation (16). Considering there is no relationship between the acute vasodilating response to epoprostenol and long-term benefit, vasodilatation is not the sole or even predominant benefit. Other putative benefits of prostacyclin each targeting factors involved in the pathogenesis of PAH that could improve symptoms and survival by reducing rate of progression and possibly regression include: (i) reduction in rate of remodeling by antiproliferative and anti-secretive effects on smooth muscle cells (15,17,18); (ii) reduced endothelial cell dysfunction (19); (iii) reduced platelet aggregation (19); (iv) anti-thrombotic effects (20); (v) decrease in extracellular matrix secretion by endothelial and SMC (21); (vi) reverse remodeling with reduction in smooth muscle mass (11); and (vii) increase in right heart inotropy (22,23).

INTRAVENOUS EPOPROSTENOL

Epoprostenol sodium (Flolan®, GlaxoSmithKline, Research Triangle Park, North Carolina Veletri®, Actelion Pharmaceuticals. South San Francisco, California, and generic epoprostenol sodium, Teva Pharmaceuticals, North Wales, Pennsylvania) is the intravenous formulation of PGI2. Intravenous (IV) epoprostenol was FDA approved in 1995 for IPAH (then referred to as primary pulmonary hypertension) and subsequently the indication was expanded to include PAH related to the scleroderma spectrum of diseases. IV epoprostenol is commonly used for many forms of WHO Group I PAH. IV epoprostenol is the PAH therapy for which the longest term and most robust data exists, and is considered the gold standard in patients with more advanced (functional class III and IV) disease. While originally thought to be simply a bridge to heart-lung or lung transplantation, long-term outcomes with IV epoprostenol have established it as a chronic therapy.

Pharmacokinetics

Epoprostenol is rapidly degraded in blood at a neutral pH into two primary metabolites (6-keto-$PGF_{1\alpha}$ and 6,15-diketo-13,14-dihydro-$PGF_{1\alpha}$), both of which are relatively biologically inactive and excreted in the urine. The half-life of epoprostenol in humans is approximately 6 minutes.

The two major pharmacologic actions of epoprostenol are inhibition of platelet aggregation and potent vasodilation of systemic and pulmonary vascular beds, both of which are mediated via stimulation of adenylate cyclase and increased production of cyclic adenosine monophosphate (cAMP).

Drug delivery

Epoprostenol sodium for injection is supplied as a sterile freeze-dried powder in glass vials, available in 0.5 mg (500 000 ng) and 1.5 mg (1 500 000 ng), which must be stored at 59–77 degrees Farenheit. Epoprostenol sodium must be diluted with sterile diluent for Flolan. Because of the need to maintain an uninterrupted infusion, and because of the high pH (10.2–10.8) after reconstitution, long-term infusion is maintained via a tunneled, cuffed central venous catheter, although it may be given via a peripheral line temporarily (e.g. in emergency situations). IV epoprostenol is administered continuously via an ambulatory portable, battery-operated infusion pump, most commonly the CADD-Legacy pump (Simms-Deltec). The pump has low-battery, end of infusion, and occlusion alarms, and is positive-pressure driven with intervals between pulses not exceeding 3 minutes to deliver the prescribed medication rate.

In most instances, insurance approval is obtained prior to the commencement of therapy. Most centers hospitalize patients for initiation of IV epoprostenol for monitoring as well as extensive teaching regarding sterile preparation of the medication, operation of the ambulatory infusion pump, and care of the central venous catheter.

Clinical trial data – randomized and observational

In 1982, Rubin et al. investigated the hemodynamic effects of escalating doses of intravenous epoprostenol (2–12 ng/kg/min) in seven patients with idiopathic pulmonary arterial hypertension (IPAH) and severe hemodynamic compromise (24). At a mean dose of 5.7 ng/kg/min, epoprostenol reduced total pulmonary resistance by approximately 43 percent while cardiac output increased by 56 percent. Longer term infusions (1–25 months) led to hemodynamic improvement, clinical stabilization, and improved exercise capacity in patients with severe IPAH who were refractory to oral vasodilators, digoxin, and diuretic therapy (2). These early observational studies led to the first randomized trail with epoprostenol in 1990 (25). Patients with IPAH ($n = 23$) were randomized to epoprostenol (mean dose 7.1 ng/kg/min) or conventional therapy, and functional classification, six-minute walk distance (6MWD), and cardiopulmonary hemodynamics were compared at baseline and two months after therapy. All 10 patients treated with epoprostenol improved by at least one functional class, and on average increased their 6MWD from 246 to 378 meters. Total pulmonary resistance fell from 21.6 to 13.9 mmHg/L/min and cardiac output rose from 3.3 to 3.9 L/min. In contrast, the majority of placebo-treated patients did not symptomatically improve, had a lesser increase in walk distance, with no significant changes in hemdoynamics. Of note, three patients in the placebo arm died over the 8-week study period vs. one subject treated with epoprostenol. These findings also provided the impetus for the first prospective multicenter open label trial, which randomized 81 IPAH patients, functional class III or IV, to epoprostenol plus conventional therapy vs. conventional therapy alone (4). At 12 weeks, the epoprostenol-treated group (mean dose 9.2 ng/kg/min) had improved quality of life scores, improved functional class, and increased their median 6MWD (+31 meters vs. −29 meters in conventional therapy group) vs. conventional therapy alone. Pulmonary vascular resistance fell by approximately 25 percent (placebo increased 9 percent) and cardiac index rose by 15 percent while mean systemic arterial pressure fell by only 5 percent. Patients with the greatest hemodynamic improvements over the study period tended to have the largest improvements in 6MWD. Eight patients died during the 12-week study period, all of whom had been randomized to the conventional therapy group. Importantly, the hemodynamic and clinical improvements seen in the epoprostenol treated patient were not predicted by short-term hemodynamic responsiveness to epoprostenol prior to randomization, confirming previous observations that the longer term effects of epoprostenol are not well predicted by short-term acute vasodilator responsiveness. The results of this study led to FDA approval of epoprostenol in 1995 for patients with IPAH.

Epoprostenol has also been studied specifically in a population with PAH related to the scleroderma spectrum of diseases. Badesch et al. studied epoprostenol in 111 such patients in a randomized, open-label trial conducted over a 12-week period (7). The patients in the epoprostenol treatment group were quite ill at baseline, with a mean 6MWD of only 272 meters, right atrial pressure of 13 mmHg and cardiac index of 1.9 L/min^{-1} m^{-2}. In response to epoprostenol (mean dose 11.2 ng/kg^{-1} min^{-1}), PVR declined by 32 percent and cardiac index increased 0.5 L/min^{-1} m^{-2}, while 6MWD increased (270 to 316 meters). In patients treated with conventional therapy the 6MWD declined (240 to 192 meters), for an impressive placebo-corrected 6MWD difference of +108 meters. Unlike the in IPAH, there were no survival differences detected (four deaths in epoprostenol group, five deaths in conventional treatment group) over this relatively short follow-up period, although neither study was powered to detect a survival benefit.

Longer term observational studies have demonstrated improved outcomes in IPAH patients treated with epoprostenol. Long-term survival on epoprostenol was assessed in a prospective cohort of 69 IPAH patients with functional class III and IV patients who were followed 330–770 days (5). Survival at 1, 2, and 3 years was 80 percent, 76 percent, and 49 percent, respectively. In a smaller, observational study of patients treated with IV epoprostenol for over a year, 26 of 27 patients had an improvement in functional

class (6). Improvements in exercise duration (142 percent), mean PAP (decreased by 22 percent) and cardiac output (increased by 67 percent) were noted. Interestingly, significant improvements in hemodynamics occurred in most patients despite the absence of an acute response to IV adenosine during acute vasodilator testing. In 2002, McLaughlin et al. reported on the long-term clinical outcomes of 162 patients with IPAH treated with epoprostenol (median follow-up 36 months) (26). The observed survival at 1, 2, 3, and 5 years was 88 percent, 76 percent, 63 percent, and 47 percent and was significantly greater than the expected survival 1, 2, and 3-year survivals of 59 percent, 46 percent, and 35 percent as predicted by the NIH survival. Baseline predictors of survival included exercise capacity, right atrial pressure and vasodilator responsiveness in response to adenosine. On follow-up, subjects who remained functional class I–II fared far better (3, 5-year survival 89 percent, 73 percent) than those who were class III (62 percent, 35 percent); patients who remained class IV did especially poorly (survival 42 percent at 2 years, 0 percent at 3 years). A total of 70 episodes of sepsis were reported, four of which were fatal; one patient died due to interruption of epoprostenol therapy. Similarly, Sitbon et al. reported an overall survival rate at 1, 2, 3, and 5 years of 85 percent, 70 percent, 63 percent, and 55 percent, respectively in 178 patients with IPAH treated with continuous intravenous epoprostenol (27). After three months on therapy, a history of right heart failure, persistence of class III or IV functional status and a < 30 percent fall in total pulmonary resistance were associated with poor survival. These findings provide the basis for the recommendation for referral for lung transplantation in PAH patients who remain class III or IV despite prostacyclin therapy. Observational series have also demonstrated beneficial effects of epoprostenol in associated forms of PAH including congenital heart disease, HIV, and portopulmonary hypertension, in addition to sarcoid related and chronic thromboembolic pulmonary hypertension (28–33).

Dosing/dose titration

The optimal long-term dosing protocol for epoprostenol had not been established by randomized controlled trials. At the end of the 12-week randomized trials, patients were being treated with 9–11 ng/kg/min. In the Sitbon series, mean dose at 12 weeks was 14 ng/kg/min, and at 1 year was 21 ng/kg/min. In the McLaughlin series, the dose was 34.5 and 51.7 ng/kg/min at 17 and 30 months, respectively, although in patients who began treatment after 1998 these values were 21.9 and 27.2 ng/kg/min. Epoprostenol overdose can occur, typically manifesting clinically with stereotypical, but excessive prostanoid side effects (diarrhea, flushing) and a high cardiac output state by right heart catheterization (34).

In general, IV epoprostenol is initiated in a monitored at 2 ng/kg/min. In a stable patient who is starting therapy

Table 16.2.1 Hospital initiation and titration of IV epoprostenol

Initiate at 2 ng/kg/min.	Clinical nurse specialist calls weekly for first several months post-discharge.	Dose at 1 year generally 20–40 ng/km/min.
Titrate up by 2 ng/kg/min daily as tolerated.	IV epoprostenol increased by 2 ng/kg/min once or twice weekly as tolerated.	Functional class and 6MW with each clinic visit.
First visit at 6–8 weeks; if patient lives far away, first visit at 3 months.	First return visit 4–12-weeks, depending on clinical status of the patient, subsequently approximately every 3 months.	Right heart catheterization at 1 year.
Hospital stay generally 3–5 days, depending on patient ability to mix the epoprostenol and operate the pump.	Dose increases continue based on symptoms of PAH and side effects of IV epoprostenol.	

The actual dose varies depending on concentration and delivery rate options based upon pump characteristics.

electively, we typically titrate up by 2 ng/kg/min on a daily basis until side effects become intolerable or interfere with teaching sessions. The majority of our patients are discharged on 4–8 ng/kg/min. If the patient is critically ill, dosing uptitration is more aggressive. See Table 16.2.1.

Dosing is highly individualized and needs to be assessed for each patient based on their symptoms of pulmonary hypertension and side effects of IV epoprostenol. The nurse clinician plays a pivotal role in chronic outpatient management.

Adverse effects

The most common acute adverse effects noted during the clinical trials include flushing, headache, nausea/vomiting, and systemic hypotension. Jaw pain, often described as occurring with the first bite or two of food, is nearly universal and diarrhea is common also. These side effects associated with acute dosing can be present intermittently and tend to become less intense with the duration of therapy. Other side effects that may occur with longer term therapy include leg and foot pain, thrombocytopenia, weight loss, and rarely, ascites.

Serious complications related to the delivery system include local catheter infections, blood stream infections, catheter-related thrombosis, and paradoxical embolism. Symptoms of severe pulmonary hypertension may recur after abrupt discontinuation of the infusion, and this can be fatal.

SUBCUTANEOUS TREPROSTINIL

Treprostinil sodium (Remodulin®, United Therapeutics Corporation, Research Triangle Park, North Carolina) is a chemically stable, tricyclic benzindene analog of prostacyclin (21). Subcutaneous (SC) treprostinil received a provisional FDA approval in 2002 for PAH in WHO class II–IV and full approval in 2006 after demonstration of short-term equivalency to IV epoprostenol (35). The potential advantages of SC treprostinil compared to intravenous prostanoids include: no need for central venous access; small cassette pump; no risk of catheter occlusion and less risk of

catheter fracture; no risk of bacteremia or endocarditis; and no risk of catheter or venous thrombosis or thromboembolism; and compared to IV epoprostenol, because of the relatively long half-life there is minimal risk for sudden clinical deterioration from transient loss of access.

Pharmacokinetics

SC treprostinil is rapidly and completely absorbed with complete bioavailability (36). A dose of 10–15 ng/kg/min results in rapid rise in plasma concentration and reaches maximum plasma concentration (C_{max}) within 2 to 3 hours of onset of infusion, and elimination half-life in healthy volunteers is 2.9 to 4.6 hours (37). SC treprostinil steady-state pharmacokinetics studies in PAH patients demonstrates dose linearity within a range from 10 to 125 ng/kg/min (38). In very early studies designed to test the relative hemodynamic effects of prostanoids in patients with PPH, McLaughlin et al. found that at short-term maximal tolerated doses, intravenous epoprostenol and intravenous treprostinil resulted in a similar reduction in pulmonary vascular resistance acutely (22 percent and 20 percent, respectively). Intravenous treprostinil and subcutaneous treprostinil also demonstrated comparable short-term decrease in pulmonary vascular resistance (23 percent and 28 percent, respectively) (39).

Drug delivery

Treprostinil sodium is a sterile sodium salt with the same formulation for subcutaneous and intravenous administration, and is stable at room temperature with neutral pH. It is supplied in 20 mL multi-use vials in four strengths: 1 mg/mL, 2.5 mg/mL, 5 mg/mL or 10 mg/mL of treprostinil. During use, a single reservoir (syringe) of undiluted treprostinil can be administered up to 72 hours at 37°C.

SC treprostinil is administered by continuous infusion via a self-inserted subcutaneous catheter using an infusion pump designed for subcutaneous drug delivery (e.g. MiniMed, Sylmar, CA). The ambulatory infusion pump should be: (i) small and lightweight; (ii) adjustable to approximately 0.002 mL/h; (iii) have occlusion/no delivery, low battery, programming error and motor malfunction alarms; (iv) have delivery accuracy of ±6 percent or better; and (v) be positive pressure driven. The reservoir should be made of polyvinyl chloride, polypropylene or glass.

As with other prostacyclins, once insurance approved has been secured, extensive patient education is provided. In contrast to intravenous prostanoids, SC treprostinil can be started at home, although some patients are hospitalized for 2 or 3 days.

Clinical trial data – randomized and observational

The efficacy and safety of SC treprostinil was established in a pivotal 12-week double-blind, placebo-controlled study, conducted in 24 PH centers throughout the US, Europe, and Australia (40). A total of 470 patients with PAH were randomized to receive SC treprostinil or placebo in addition to standard care. The primary efficacy endpoint of change in 6MWD was modestly greater with treprostinil than with placebo (between-group difference in median 6MWD, 16 m, $P = 0.006$). Compared to placebo, SC treprostinil treatment also improved the Borg dyspnea index score ($P < 0.0001$). The improvement in 6MWD was highly correlated with dose (36 m when dose at 12 weeks was > 13.8 ng/kg/min).

The largest open-label, observational study of SC treprostinil was reported by Barst et al. in 2006. The observational study was conducted in 860 patients with PAH who had participated in one of three placebo-controlled trials of SC treprostinil or were de novo patients with standard criteria for treprostinil. Patients continued in the study until one of the following: (i) death; (ii) transplantation; (iii) initiation of IV, inhaled or oral prostaglandins or their analogs; or (iv) an intolerable adverse event (AE). In the 860 patients who received SC treprostinil for up to 4.5 years, Kaplan–Meier estimates for survival at 1, 2, 3, and 4 years were 87 percent, 78 percent, 71 percent, and 68 percent, respectively. The treatment was discontinued in 23 percent of patients because of adverse events, and 11 percent were switched to another prostanoid. A second PAH-specific treatment was added in 130 patients.

A subset of 90 of 470 patients (majority WHO FC III) participating in two placebo-controlled 12-week trials of SC treprostinil had PAH associated with a connective tissue disease (SLE, scleroderma, or MCTD/overlap). Treatment was associated with improved exercise capacity, reduced symptoms, and improved hemodynamics including a decrease in PVR and increase in CI (41). Two open-labeled studies support a role for SC treprostinil in inoperable CTEPH (42,43).

A multicenter withdrawal study was designed to assess the efficacy of SC treprostinil compared to IV epoprostenol. Patients with stable PAH receiving IV epoprostenol were hospitalized for 2 weeks to provide a safe environment for transition to SC treprostinil or placebo. Twenty-two patients were randomized in a 2 to 1 ratio (SC treprostinil and SC placebo). Patients were assessed on a daily basis regarding effort tolerance and examined by an experienced nurse and physician unaware of the treatment (35). The mean epoprostenol dose at baseline was 22.3 ± 3.3 ng/kg/min in the treprostinil treatment group, and the mean maximum treprostinil dose over the 8-week study was 32.2 ± 4.9 ng/kg/min. Safety and tolerability results for patients transitioning to SC treprostinil were consistent with findings in de novo patients. The results of this trial led to the US Food and Drug Administration amendment of this agent to include patients transitioning from epoprostenol treatment to treprostinil therapy. Vachiery et al. demonstrated that successful transitions can be done over short periods of time in the hospital setting. Transitions between prostacyclins should only be considered by physicians with extensive experience with both agents (44).

Dosing/dose titration

Optimization of SC treprostinil dosing regimens has not been subjected to clinical trials. The FDA-approved package insert recommends the rate be initiated at 1.25 ng/kg/min, which if necessary is reduced to 0.625 ng/kg/min. Infusion rate is increased in increments of 1.25 ng/kg/min per week for the first four weeks and then 2.5 ng/kg/min per week depending on clinical response. The goal of gradual chronic dosage adjustments is to establish a dose at which PAH symptoms are improved (optimally to WHO FC I–II), while minimizing excessive side effects (headache, nausea, emesis, restlessness, anxiety and infusion site pain or reaction). These recommendations are based on the pivotal trial in which SC treprostinil was initiated at 1.25 ng/kg/min and up-titrated slowly to a maximum dose of 22.5 ng/kg/min (40).

The safety and efficacy of rate of titration was recently described in a randomized prospective study comparing a slow versus a rapid dose-escalation protocol in 23 patients with PAH (45). The SC treprostinil slow-escalation group was initiated at 2 ng/kg/min, and increased weekly if tolerated by 1.25–2.0 ng/kg/min. The rapid-escalation group was initiated at 2.5 ng/kg/min, and increased by 2.5 ng/kg/min twice in the first week, and an additional increase of 2.5 ng/kg/min every 1 or 2 weeks. At week 12, the mean dose had reached 12.9 ± 2.7 ng/kg/min in the slow-escalation group (similar to the pivotal trial) and 20.3 ± 5.8 ng/kg/min in the rapid-escalation group. Improvements in exercise capacity at week 12 were significantly greater in the rapid-escalation group compared with the slow-escalation group ($P = 0.03$), and contrary to initial thought, infusion site pain was more common in the slow-escalation group (81.8 percent) compared with the rapid-escalation group (58.3 percent; $P = 0.04$).

Our protocol at the University of Michigan includes a rapid home or hospital titration and relatively rapid subsequent titration (see Table 16.2.2). Rapid titration facilitates the evaluation of clinical response to SC treprostinil within several months whether as monotherapy or as 2nd or 3rd agent combination therapy.

Table 16.2.2 Home or hospital initiation and titration of SC treprostinil

Initiate at 1.5 ng/kg/min.	After first visit, increase dose 2.5 ng/kg/min every 1–2 weeks as tolerated by side effects with target improvement to WHO FC I–II.	Clinic visits every 3 months.
Increase by 2.5 ng/kg/min twice weekly until first visit, provided patient tolerates dosage.	Average dose after 6 months is about 60 ng/kg/min.	BNP and 6MWD at each visit.
First visit at 6–8 weeks; if patient lives far away, first visit at 3 months.	Range 15–125 ng/kg/min.	Repeat right heart catheterization at 1 year.
Hospital initiates 2.5 ng/kg/min day 1 and considers increase by 2.5 ng/kg/min prior to discharge.		Consider further dose titration depending on hemodynamic response.

The actual dose varies depending on concentration and delivery rate options based upon pump characteristics.

Table 16.2.3 Best subcutaneous treprostinil infusion sites depend on SC fat

Preferred	Sites to avoid
Abdomen (first site)	Stretch marks and scar tissue
Upper lateral buttocks	Edematous areas (pannus) and areas with erythema or induration
Lower flanks	Underneath waistbands or beltlines
Thigh and underside of upper arm if adequate fat	Sites with nodular or rubbery texture or previous abscess
	Boney prominences

While the half-life is about 4 hours, patients and caregivers are told that abrupt cessation of SC treprostinil infusion should be avoided. Restarting the SC infusion within a few hours after an interruption can be done using the same dose rate. Interruptions for longer periods may require the dose to be re-titrated.

The absorption of drug does not appear dependent on site or site duration. The standard recommendation is site change every 3 days. However, experienced patients will use sites for up to 30 days without difficulty. The latter are considered "good sites" and may be reused months later. Sites in which pain is intense within the first day and there is no relief by day 3 are considered "bad sites." Optimal sites vary between individuals. It is best to rotate to a distant site until site pain and inflammation is resolved. Examples of typical effective and ineffective sites are provided in Table 16.2.3.

Adverse effects

The most common adverse events reported for treprostinil and placebo in the 12-week study were infusion site pain (85 percent), infusion site reaction (83 percent), and infusion site bleeding/bruising (34 percent) (40). Other common adverse events were consistent with prostacyclin therapy and included diarrhea, jaw pain, flushing, and lower-limb edema. Safety and tolerability during long-term treatment were comparable with observations during the placebo-controlled studies.

Table 16.2.4 Local, topical, and systemic options to manage infusion site pain

Local/topical	Systemic
Ice	Ibuprofen
Warm bath with Epsom salt	Gabapentin
PLO gel compounds* (current or old sites)	Pregabalin
Lidocaine 5% patches (current or old sites)	Loratadine
Diphenhydramine HCl, topical	Hydroxyzine pamoate (for severe itching)
Hemorrhoid ointment	Amitriptyline HCl and other antidepressants
Aloe vera gel	Tramadol HCl
Triamcinolone acetonide	Fexofenadine HCl
Fluticasone propionate nasal spray	Cetirizine HCl
Lidocaine/prilocaine cream	Ranitidine HCl
Hydrocortisone cream	Famotidine
Pimecrolimus cream 1%	If fentanyl or other narcotics are required more than occasionally, consider IV treprostinil, epoprostenol, or aerosolized iloprost
Clobetasol propionate cream	

*Contain ketoprofen, lidocaine, and gabapentin and may also contain ketamine, amitriptyline, and clonidine.
PLO gel = pluronic lecithin organogel.
Courtesy of United Therapeutics.

The most common cause of treatment failure is intolerable site pain, which can be minimized if the patients are properly prepared by their health care providers. Table 16.2.4 describes the methods of reducing pain and increasing site duration.

INTRAVENOUS TREPROSTINIL

Given the limitation of site pain/reaction from subcutaneous infusion, and that SC and IV treprostinil have virtually the same bioavailability and hemodynamic effects, long-term IV treprostinil has also been studied in PAH (38). The pharmacology of intravenous treprostinil is identical to that described above for subcutaneous treprostinil. The continuous intravenous infusion is similar to that described above for IV epoprostenol. Based on bioequivalence data, IV treprostinil is indicated in PAH for those unable to tolerate subcutaneous infusion, although it is used as the initial parenteral prostacyclin in some patients due to the convenience of the longer half-life and its stability at room temperature, obviating the need for ice packs.

Clinical trial data – randomized and observational

An investigator-initiated, open-label, uncontrolled trial with IV treprosinil in PAH patients has led to important observations in both naïve and IV epoprostenol transition patients. Tapson *et al.* reported on 16 patients with PAH treated with IV treprostinil as their initial therapy in an open-label, uncontrolled series (46). Over 12 weeks, the primary endpoint, 6MWD, improved from 319 to 400 meters. There were also significant improvements in secondary endpoints including Naughton–Balke protocol treadmill time, Borg-dyspnea score, and hemodynamics. In an open-label uncontrolled trial, Gomberg-Maitland transitioned 31 patients with PAH on intravenous epoprostenol to intravenous treprostinil (47). Four patients were transitioned back to eproprostenol over the 12-week study. Among those 27 who remained on intravenous treprostinil, the 6MWD was unchanged, although the mean PAP was slightly higher, and the cardiac output was slightly lower than baseline. At week 12, the mean dose of treprostinil was more than twice the dose of epoprostenol.

A placebo-controlled trial of intravenous treprostinil (2:1 randomization) was conducted in 44 patients with PAH at 14 sites in India (48). Treprostinil increased the 6MWD by a placebo-corrected median of 83 meters ($P = 0.008$; mean increase 93 ± 42 meters). Notably, this study was terminated early after the independent Rescue Therapy and Safety Committee reviewed all catheter-related complications, deaths, and other serious adverse events and recommended suspension of the trial pending implementation of a series of recommendations to increase patient safety.

Intravenous treprostinil may also be administered via "low-flow" pumps at rates as low as 0/1 mL/h. In a 12-week study pump complications occurred in 5 of 12 patients receiving such therapy, although no catheter occlusions occurred (49). Notably, patients were anticoagulated to an INR of at least 2.0 throughout that study.

Dosing/dose titration

Like IV epoprostenol, IV treprostinil is initiated in a monitored setting in the hospital. Like IV epoprostenol, it is generally started at a dose of 2 ng/kg/min and in the stable patient, titrated up at a dose of 2 ng/kg/min on a daily basis. Chronic outpatient care is similar to that described for epoprostenol, although generally doses are about twice as high as those for IV epoprostenol.

Adverse effects

With the exception of the local site reactions, the adverse effects for IV treprostinil include those listed above for subcutaneous treprostinil. In addition, the adverse effects of the continuous intravenous delivery system described above for IV epoprostenol may occur with IV treprostinil. While blood stream infection is a concern with intravenous agents, a concern for an increased risk of Gram-negative infections has been raised with intravenous treprostinil (50).

ILOPROST

Iloprost (Ventavis®, Berlimed, Madrid, Spain), the first inhaled or aerosolized therapy for PAH, was approved by the FDA in December 2004 for PAH WHO FCC III–IV, and is approved for chronic thromboembolic pulmonary hypertension (CTEPH) in other countries. Iloprost is a stable synthetic analog of prostacyclin (PGI_2) with a longer half-life of 20 to 30 min. The inhaled formulation was developed as an alternative to epoprostenol with the promise of greater pulmonary vascular selectivity and less systemic vasodilator effect, no indwelling intravenous infusion catheter requirement, no risk of sudden rebound from catheter dislodgement or occlusion, and marked decrease in risk of hypoxemia from increasing perfusion through poorly ventilated lung tissue.

Pharmacokinetics

Iloprost is delivered by specifically designed nebulizers that aerosolize the drug to particles of about 3 μm in diameter, which diffuse from the terminal airways – alveoli to adjacent intra-acinar pulmonary arterioles. Following a 5 μg dose of iloprost via inhalation, the peak serum level is 150 pg/mL and not detectable in the plasma 30 minutes to 1 hour after inhalation. The drug is completely metabolized (cytochrome P450 plays only a minor role) and excretion of metabolites is primarily via the kidneys; the elimination half-life of iloprost is 20 to 30 minutes. The blood level is not influenced by hepatic function or renal function. Clinical studies suggest a 1:5 dose equivalency with prostacyclin (e.g. 10 μg/mL blood level of iloprost is ~50 μg/mL of prostacyclin) (51).

Drug delivery

Ventavis® (iloprost) inhalation solution is a clear, colorless, sterile solution containing 10 μg/mL iloprost in 1 mL or

2 mL single use glass ampules formulated for inhalation via either of two pulmonary drug delivery devices: the I-neb™ AAD® (Adaptive Aerosol Delivery) System or the Prodose® AAD® System. Each mL of the aqueous solution contains 0.01 mg iloprost, 0.81 mg ethanol, 0.121 mg tromethamine, 9.0 mg sodium chloride, and approximately 0.51 mg hydrochloric acid (for pH adjustment to 8.1) in water for injection. Ventavis® should not come in contact with skin or eyes.

Clinical trial data – randomized and observational

The major pivotal trial demonstrating the clinical efficacy of inhaled iloprost in PH is the AIR study (The Aerosolized Iloprost Randomized Study), a 12-week placebo-controlled study which was reported by Olschewski et al. in 2002 (52). A total of 203 patients WHO FC III–IV with PAH or CTEPH (about one-third) were randomized to either 2.5 μg or 5 μg of iloprost or placebo dosed six to nine times daily. The primary end point was an improvement by at least one functional class and a 10 percent or greater increase in the 6MWD without clinical deterioration or death. The combined clinical end point was met by 16.8 percent of the patients receiving iloprost and 4.9 percent on placebo ($P = 0.007$). The iloprost group had an average of 36.4 m placebo corrected increase in 6 MWD ($P = 0.004$). In an open-labeled 2-year continuation of inhaled iloprost in 63 participants in the AIR study, iloprost increased 1-year survival in IPAH compared to historical controls (53).

An open-label observational trial suggested beneficial effects of aerosolized iloprost on exercise capacity and hemodynamic variables over a 1-year period in 24 patients with IPAH (54). Contrary to this, another group observed an event-free survival at 12 months of only 53 percent, at 2 years 29 percent, and at 5 years 13 percent and concluded that inhaled iloprost has only limited role as a first-line monotherapy (55). The safety of inhaled iloprost in addition to bosentan has been demonstrated in a randomized controlled trial (56).

Dosing/dose titration

Treatments are given 6–9 times per day to obtain optimal benefits, but experience is that the majority of patients average 5–6 treatments. The initial dose of aerosolized iloprost is 2.5 μg every 2–3 hours during waking hours. If the low dose is tolerated, the dose is increased to 5 μg per treatment. There is no need for treatment at night. Taking a treatment prior to strenuous activity improves performance. Care should be taken in patients with low blood pressure and not initiated if the systolic pressure is < 85 mmHg.

Adverse effects

In the clinical trials, placebo subtracted side effects with > 5 percent incidence were as follows: flushing 18 percent; cough 13 percent; headache 10 percent, jaw claudication or trismus 9 percent, insonia 6 percent. An increase in breathlessness associated with iloprost should be evaluated with consideration for bronchitis/pneumonia or interstitial lung disease in PAH associated with scleroderma.

INHALED TREPROSTINIL

Treprostinil, discussed above given intravenously and subcutaneously, has more recently been studied as an inhaled therapy. In 2009 inhaled treprostinil (Tyvaso®) received FDA approval for the treatment of PAH patients with functional class III symptoms.

Pharmacokinetics

In a study of 12 patients with PAH, maximum plasma concentration and half-life of inhaled treprostinil demonstrated that, when inhaled, treprostinil reached the systemic circulation in a dose-dependent fashion. The maximum concentration of the 30 μg and 45 μg groups was 0.33 ng/mL and 0.96 ng/mL, respectively. Similarly, the time until maximum concentration for the 30 μg and 45 μg groups was 15 and 45 minutes, respectively, with a half-life of 44–52 minutes (57).

Drug delivery

Inhaled treprostinil is delivered via a hand-held ultrasonic, single-breath nebulizer OPTINEB™ device (Nebu-Tec; Elsenfeld, Germany). Sterile solution for oral inhalation is provided in 2.9 mL ampules containing 1.74 mg of treprostinil (0.6 mg per mL). Patients are taught how to prepare and operate the nebulizer device. Treatments are given four times daily, with each treatment lasting approximately 3 minutes.

Clinical trial data – randomized and observational

In an open-label, observational trial of 12 PAH patients treated with inhaled treprostinil, 6-minute walk distance improved from 339 ± 86 meters at baseline to 406 ± 121 meters at 12-weeks, measured 1 hour post-inhalation (57).

In a placebo-controlled trial of 235 patients with PAH on oral monotherapy with either bosentan or sildenafil, treatment with inhaled treprostinil resulted in an improvement in 6MWD. The placebo-corrected median change from baseline in peak 6MWD was 19 meters at Week 6 ($P = 0.0001$) and 20 meters at Week 12 ($P = 0.0004$). Placebo-corrected trough 6MWD at Week 12 improved by 14 meters ($P = 0.0066$). QOL measures and NT pro-BNP improved on active therapy. There were no improvements in other secondary end points including time to clinical worsening, Borg Dyspnea Score, NYHA functional class, and PAH signs and symptoms (58).

Adverse effects

The most common adverse effects noted with inhaled treprostinil during the clinical trials included cough, headache, throat irritation, nausea, flushing, and syncope.

Dosing/dose titration

During the clinical trials, inhaled treprostinil was initiated at three breaths (18 µg) four times daily. Doses were increased by three breaths every one to two weeks to a maximum dose of nine breaths (54 µg) four times daily.

ORAL PROSTACYCLINS

The success of prostacylin therapy coupled with the complex delivery systems of the intravenous and subcutaneous routes of delivery have served as the impetus to develop less invasive means of administering prostacyclins. The oral prostacyclin analog, beraprost, is available in Japan and parts of Europe for the treatment of PAH.

Pharmacokinetics and drug delivery

Beraprost is an orally active prostacyclin analog with a stable structure due to its cyclopentabenzofuranyl skeleton (59). Beraprost is rapidly absorbed in the fasting condition with peak plasma concentrations reached after 30 minutes and elimination half-life of 35–40 minutes after a single oral administration (60). When administered with a meal, peak concentration is lower and the half-life is prolonged to approximately 3–3.5 hours.

Clinical trial data – randomized and observational

Observational series have suggested improved hemodynamics, functional class, and 6MWD with beraprost (61–64). However, two randomized, placebo-controlled trials have reported conflicting results. In a European trial of 130 PAH patients randomized to beraprost or placebo for 12 weeks, a 25.1-meter ($P = 0.036$) improvement in 6 MWD was observed in the patients randomized to active therapy (65). However, in a double-blind randomized, placebo-controlled study in the US, there were improvements in 6MWD at 3 and 6 months which were not sustained at 9 and 12 months (66).

Adverse effects

The most common adverse effects of beraprost reported in the above cited studies include headache, flushing, jaw pain, diarrhea, leg pain and nausea. Side effects can be minimized when the drug is taken with a meal.

Dosing/dose titration

Beraprost is generally commenced at a dose of 20 µg four times daily and increased by 20 µg each week based on side effects. The maximum dose in the above cited clinical trials ranged from 120–200 µg four times daily.

THE CLINICAL PERSPECTIVE

Using the prostanoids in PAH requires a thorough understanding of the diagnosis and natural history of the disease, the pharmacology, experience in monitoring response, and other treatment options including transplant. Despite the advances in oral and parenteral treatment options for PAH, the 5-year mortality remains high, and the majority of participants in placebo-controlled trials of oral PAH-specific therapies were WHO FC II and III.

Treatment options for PAH have been formulated into guidelines by consensus of US and European expert panels (67–70). There is general agreement within the cardiology, pulmonology, and rheumatology communities that prior to treatment decisions, the diagnosis and prognosis needs to be assessed and/or confirmed by physicians experienced in PH. PH centers have multidisciplinary groups of physicians and unique support by nurses in both the outpatient and inpatient settings.

Patients who have advanced symptoms (WHO FC IV), who fail an oral PAH-specific drug after a 3-month trial and remain WHO FC III, or those who progress on oral therapy should be referred to an experienced center for consideration of prostanoid therapy. Other poor prognostic indicators, including high right atrial pressure, low cardiac index, and low 6MWD influence the decision to proceed to parenteral prostacyclin therapy (12,67). Much of the clinical trial results and metrics for risk stratification in PAH are based upon IPAH and scleroderma, but apply to other associated diseases with the exception of congenital heart disease that generally has a better prognosis. Monitoring of the response to a given strategy and decision for advancing therapies requires a considerable amount of clinical experience and ability to interpret testing including the 6-minute hall walk, echo-Doppler, chest computed tomography, pulmonary function tests, cardiopulmonary exercise testing, biomarkers (BNP, NT-BNP), renal and hepatic function, and baseline and on-treatment hemodynamic indices.

Criteria for initiating the prostanoids

Prior to considering prostanoids the patient and family members and participating physician(s) need to consider the patient's physical and emotional status, support system, and provider issues, which are listed in Table 16.2.5.

The most essential are an understanding of prognosis, treatment options, and availability of insurance. It is essential that patients and family members understand there is no cure for PAH, and not be given undue expectations.

Table 16.2.5 Considerations prior to choosing prostanoid

Patient related
- Understanding prognosis
- Understanding treatment options and expectations
- Understanding complexity and potential complications of treatment
- Adequate physical ability (e.g. scleroderma)
- Emotional stability
- Bleeding risk
- End of life decisions
- Insurance coverage

Support system
- Significant other or available close friend
- Proximity to a local hospital and physician
- Experienced home health care agency
- Local PH support group

Treating physician
- Experience in prostanoid therapy
- Experienced nursing team
- Reliable testing facilities

Table 16.2.6 Educational requirement for patient and significant other prior to discharge

Response to emergencies
- Catheter dislodgement or pump alarm
- Worsening of symptoms
- Use of local hospital and emergency services
- Home health care agency
- 24/7 contact and access with PH office staff

Use of the pump
- Rate adjustments
- Requirement for dry ice
- Need for back-up pump

Central access site
- Sterile techniques
- Signs of infections
- Securing sutures

Prostacyclin
- Reconstitution of epoprostenol
- Handling of vials with treprostinil
- Handling tubing/connect/disconnect
- Site care for sub-Q treprostinil
- Plans for dose titration

Expected side effects
- Minor
- Major

They are told that prostacyclin therapy may improve symptoms within days to months, and if so, will likely prolong life expectancy. In those without a lung transplant option (e.g. age and associated diseases), the patient and family member need to have an understanding that end of life decisions in PAH are complex and the hospice option may not be possible on parenteral prostacyclins. Despite those messages, it is the rare patient who is unwilling to accept a treatment trial, and experience is that they are grateful having been made totally aware.

The choice between parenteral prostanoids depends on patient preference, physician experience, and hemodynamic instability. Because of the short half-life (4 to 6 min) and experience with rapid dose titration in critically ill patients, IV epoprostenol is preferred over IV treprostinil in hemodynamically unstable patients, and those rapidly deteriorating to WHO class IV requiring emergent hospitalization. The need for ice packs and short half-life of epoprostenol are reasons patients and physicians may prefer IV treprostinil. There are less clinical trial data and a slightly higher rate of catheter infection with treprostinil than epoprostenol, a risk that needs to be balanced with the potential advantages (50). The alternative of subcutaneous treprostinil may have advantages in WHO class III patients who may want to avoid the central venous catheter.

The education requirements for patients and family members are summarized in Table 16.2.6.

IV prostacyclin can be initiated via a mid-line or peripherally inserted central catheter (PICC), but long-term treatment requires a central catheter. The infusion catheter should be single lumen, tunneled, and placed no farther than the superior vena cava under fluoroscopic guidance. The exit site should be in the subclavicular–pectoral region on the non-dominant side to allow for patient use of the dominant arm/hand. When patients are not certain about

BOX 16.2.1: Complications of Indwelling Infusion Catheter

- Air embolism
- Bleeding
- Brachial plexus injury
- Pneumothorax
- Cardiac arrhythmia
- Catheter erosion
- Catheter fractures between clavicle and first rib
- Catheter thrombosis
- Catheter kinking
- Catheter dislodgement and extravasation
- Catheter infection/bacteremia
- Exit site infection or necrosis
- Endocarditis
- Subclavian or internal jugular thrombosis
- Superior vena cava syndrome
- Pulmonary embolism
- Paradoxical embolism via PFO or ASD

long-term use or a trial is necessary to determine safety, a PICC line is preferable and can be used for up to a few months. The complications of the indwelling catheter are listed in Box 16.2.1.

Titration of prostacyclins is often begun in the hospital as discussed above. Prior to discharge the other adjunctive treatment should be considered including salt restricted diet, diuretics, oxygen requirement, and warfarin anticoagulation. Because of increased bleeding risk, if anticoagulation is used the target INR should be reduced to 1.5 to 2.5, and there is no need for transition with heparin or low molecular weight heparin, the exception being in the setting of CTEPH or anti-phospholipid antibody syndrome.

Long-term management of patients on parenteral prostacyclin

This includes a 4- to 6-week post-initiation visit to assess clinical response, infusion catheter exit site or subcutaneous site, emotional and educational needs, and dose adjustment of ancillary therapies. Subsequent visits at 3- to 6-month intervals depend on travel distance, local physician support and clinical status. In addition to the clinical assessment there is evidence and clinical experience that progress is best monitored with 6MW and BNP or NT-BNP at each visit (71,72).

Prostacyclin, the pump, and catheter are generally well tolerated. The monitoring team must have a high index of suspicion for catheter-associated bacteremia, the only sign of which can be loss of energy and mild increase in dyspnea. Practice guidelines for prevention of catheter-related infection associated with the prostanoids have been developed (73).

KEY POINTS

- Prostacyclin synthase is deficient in PAH patients.
- Prostacyclin is a potent vasodilator, inhibitor of platelet aggregation, and has antiproliferative effects.
- Intravenous epoprostenol improves exercise tolerance, hemodynamics, and survival in IPAH.
- Treprostinil is a prostacyclin analogue which can be administered via continuous subcutaneous or intravenous infusion, or intermittent inhalation available for the treatment of PAH.
- Iloprost is a prostacyclin analogue administered by intermittent inhalation available for the treatment of PAH.
- Beraprost is an oral prostacyclin analogue available in some countries, although the clinical trial data are mixed with respect to efficacy.
- Common prostacyclin side effects include flushing, headache, diarrhea, and jaw pain.
- Side effects related to the delivery system may include bloodstream infections, infusion site pain and erythema and cough.
- Whilst very effective, the delivery of prostacyclin therapy is complex and is best managed by experienced clinicians.

REFERENCES

1. D'Alonzo GE et al. Survival in patients with primary pulmonary hypertension. Results from a national prospective registry. Ann Intern Med 1991;115(5):343-9.
2. Higenbottam T et al. Long-term treatment of primary pulmonary hypertension with continuous intravenous epoprostenol (prostacyclin). Lancet 1984;1(8385): 1046-7.
3. Barst RJ et al. Survival in primary pulmonary hypertension with long-term continuous intravenous prostacyclin. Ann Intern Med 1994;121:409-15.
4. Barst RJ et al. A comparison of continuous intravenous epoprostenol (prostacyclin) with conventional therapy for primary pulmonary hypertension. N Engl J Med 1996;334:296-301.
5. Shapiro SM et al. Primary pulmonary hypertension: improved long-term effects and survival with continuous intravenous epoprostenol infusion. J Am Coll Cardiol 1997;30:343-9.
6. McLaughlin VV et al. Reduction in pulmonary vascular resistance with long-term epoprostenol (prostacyclin) therapy in primary pulmonary hypertension. N Engl J Med 1998;338:273-7.
7. Badesch DB et al. Continuous intravenous epoprostenol for pulmonary hypertension due to the scleroderma spectrum of disease. Ann Intern Med 2000;132:425-34.
8. Christman BW et al. An imbalance between the excretion of thromboxane and prostacyclin metabolites in pulmonary hypertension. N Engl J Med 1992;327:70-5.
9. Humbert M et al. Cellular and molecular pathobiology of pulmonary arterial hypertension. J Am Coll Cardiol 2004;43(12 Suppl S):13S-24S.
10. Tuder RM et al. Prostacyclin synthase expression is decreased in lungs from patients with severe pulmonary hypertension. AJRCCM 1999;159(6):1925-32.
11. Hoshikawa Y et al. Prostacyclin receptor-dependent modulation of pulmonary vascular remodeling. Am J Respir Crit Care Med 2001;164(2):314-8.
12. McLaughlin VV, McGoon MD. Pulmonary arterial hypertension. Circulation 2006;114(13):1417-31.
13. Moncada S et al. An enzyme isolated from arteries transforms prostaglandin endoperoxides to an unstable substance that inhibits platelet aggregation. Nature 1976;263(5579):663-5.
14. Moncada S, Vane JR. Arachidonic acid metabolites and the interactions between platelets and blood-vessel walls. N Engl J Med 1979;300(20):1142-7.
15. Clapp LH et al. Differential effects of stable prostacyclin analogs on smooth muscle proliferation and cyclic AMP generation in human pulmonary artery. Am J Respir Cell Mol Biol 2002;26(2):194-201.
16. Best LC et al. Prostacyclin increases cyclic AMP levels and adenylate cyclase activity in platelets. Nature 1977;267(5614):850-2.
17. Jeffery TK, Morrell N. Molecular and cellular basis of pulmonary vascular remodeling in pulmonary hypertension. Progr Cardiovasc Dis 2002;45(3):173-202.

18. Fetalvero KM, Martin KA, Hwa J. Cardioprotective prostacyclin signaling in vascular smooth muscle. Prostaglandins Other Lipid Mediat 2007;82(1–4):109–18.

19. Friedman R, Mears JG, Barst RJ. Continuous infusion of prostacyclin normalizes plasma markers of endothelial cell injury and platelet aggregation in primary pulmonary hypertension. Circulation 1997;96:2782–4.

20. Boyer-Neumann C et al. Continuous infusion of prostacyclin decreases plasma levels of t-PA and PAI-1 in primary pulmonary hypertension. Thromb Haemost 1995;73(4):735–6.

21. Olschewski H et al. Prostacyclin and its analogs in the treatment of pulmonary hypertension. Pharmacol Ther 2004;102(2):139–53.

22. Fassina G, Tessari F, Dorigo P. Positive inotropic effect of a stable analog of PGI2 and of PGI2 on isolated guinea pig atria. Mechanism of action. Pharmacol Res Commun 1983;15(8):735–49.

23. Fontana M et al. Treprostinil potentiates the positive inotropic effect of catecholamines in adult rat ventricular cardiomyocytes. Br J Pharmacol 2007;151(6):779–86.

24. Rubin LJ et al. Prostacyclin-induced acute pulmonary vasodilation in primary pulmonary hypertension. Circulation 1982;66(2):334–8.

25. Rubin LJ et al. Treatment of primary pulmonary hypertension with continuous intravenous prostacyclin (epoprostenol). Results of a randomized trial. Ann Intern Med 1990;112(7):485–91.

26. McLaughlin VV, Shillington A, Rich S. Survival in primary pulmonary hypertension: the impact of epoprostenol therapy. Circulation 2002;106:1477–82.

27. Sitbon O et al. Long-term intravenous epoprostenol infusion in primary pulmonary hypertension: prognostic factors and survival. J Am Coll Cardiol 2002;40:780–8.

28. Robbins IM et al. Epoprostenol for treatment of pulmonary hypertension in patients with systemic lupus erythematosus. Chest 2000;117:14–8.

29. McLaughlin VV et al. Compassionate use of continuous prostacyclin in the management of secondary pulmonary hypertension: a case series. Ann Intern Med 1999;130:740–3.

30. Petitpretz P et al. Pulmonary hypertension in patients with human immunodeficiency virus infection: comparison with primary pulmonary hypertension. Circulation 1994;89:2722–7.

31. Aguilar RV, Farber HW. Epoprostenol (prostacyclin) therapy in HIV-associated pulmonary hypertension. Am J Respir Crit Care Med 2000;162(5):1846–50.

32. Rosenzweig EB, Kerstein D, Barst RJ. Long-term prostacyclin for pulmonary hypertension with associated congenital heart defects. Circulation 1999;99:1858–65.

33. Kuo PC et al. Continuous intravenous infusion of epoprostenol for the treatment of portopulmonary hypertension. Transplantation 1997;63:604–16.

34. Rich S, McLaughlin VV. The effects of chronic prostacyclin therapy on cardiac output and symptoms in primary pulmonary hypertension. J Am Coll Cardiol 1999;34:1184–7.

35. Rubenfire M et al. Transition from IV epoprostenol to subcutaneous treprostinil in pulmonary arterial hypertension: a controlled trial. Chest 2007;132(3):757–63.

36. Wade M et al. Absolute bioavailability and pharmacokinetics of treprostinil sodium administered by acute subcutaneous infusion. J Clin Pharmacol 2004;44(1):83–8.

37. Wade M et al. Pharmacokinetics of treprostinil sodium administered by 28-day chronic continuous subcutaneous infusion. J Clin Pharmacol 2004;44(5):503–9.

38. McSwain CS et al. Dose proportionality of treprostinil sodium administered by continuous subcutaneous and intravenous infusion. J Clin Pharmacol 2008;48(1): 19–25.

39. McLaughlin VV et al. Efficacy and safety of treprostinil: an epoprostenol analog for primary pulmonary hypertension. J Cardiovasc Pharmacol 2003;41(2):293–9.

40. Simonneau G et al. Continuous subcutaneous infusion of treprostinil, a prostacyclin analog, in patients with pulmonary arterial hypertension. Am J Respir Crit Care Med 2002;165:800–4.

41. Oudiz R et al. Treprostinil, a prostacyclin analog, in pulmonary arterial hypertension associated with connective tissue disease. Chest 2004;126:420–7.

42. Skoro-Sajer N et al. Treprostinil for severe inoperable chronic thromboembolic pulmonary hypertension. J Thromb Haemost 2007;5(3):483–9.

43. Lang I et al. Efficacy of long-term subcutaneous treprostinil sodium therapy in pulmonary hypertension. Chest 2006;129(6):1636–43.

44. Vachiery JL et al. Transitioning from IV epoprostenol to subcutaneous treprostinil in pulmonary arterial hypertension. Chest 2002;121:1561–5.

45. Skoro-Sajer N et al. A clinical comparison of slow- and rapid-escalation treprostinil dosing regimens in patients with pulmonary hypertension. Clin Pharmacokinet 2008;47(9):611–8.

46. Tapson VF et al. Safety and efficacy of IV treprostinil for pulmonary arterial hypertension: a prospective, multicenter, open-label, 12-week trial. Chest 2006;129(3):683–8.

47. Gomberg-Maitland M et al. Transition from intravenous epoprostenol to intravenous treprostinil in pulmonary hypertension. Am J Respir Crit Care Med 2005;172(12):1586–9.

48. Hiremath J et al. Exercise improvement and plasma biomarker changes with intravenous treprostinil therapy for pulmonary arterial hypertension: a placebo-controlled trial. J Heart Lung Transplant 2010;29:137–49.

49. Tapson VF et al. Delivery of intravenous treprostinil at low infusion rates using a miniaturized infusion pump in patients with pulmonary arterial hypertension. J Vasc Access 2006;7(3):112–7.

50. Kallen AJ et al. Bloodstream infections in patients given treatment with intravenous prostanoids. Infect Control Hosp Epidemiol 2008;29(4):342–9.

51. Olschewski H. *et al.* Aerosolized prostacyclin and iloprost in severe pulmonary hypertension. Ann Int Med 1996; 124:820–4.

52. Olschewski H *et al.* Inhaled iloprost for severe pulmonary hypertension. N Engl J Med 2002;347:322–9.

53. Badesch DB *et al.* Prostanoid therapy for pulmonary arterial hypertension. J Am Coll Cardiol 2004;43(12 Suppl S): 56S–61S.

54. Hoeper MM *et al.* Long-term treatment of primary pulmonary hypertension with aerosolized iloprost, a prostacyclin analog. N Engl J Med 2000;342:1866–70.

55. Opitz CF *et al.* Clinical efficacy and survival with first-line inhaled iloprost therapy in patients with idiopathic pulmonary arterial hypertension. Eur Heart J 2005; 26(18):1895–902.

56. McLaughlin VV *et al.* Randomized study of adding inhaled iloprost to existing bosentan in pulmonary arterial hypertension. Am J Respir Crit Care Med 2006;174(11): 1257–63.

57. Channick RN *et al.* Safety and efficacy of inhaled treprostinil as add-on therapy to bosentan in pulmonary arterial hypertension. J Am Coll Cardiol 2006;48(7):1433–7.

58. McLaughlin V *et al.* Triumph I: efficacy and safety of inhaled treprostinil sodium in patients with pulmonary arterial hypertension (PAH). (abstr). Am J Respir Crit Care Med 2008;117:A965.

59. Sim AK *et al.* Effect of a stable prostacyclin analog on platelet function and experimentally-induced thrombosis in the microcirculation. Arzneimittelforschung 1985;35(12):1816–8.

60. Yuge T *et al.* Pharmacokinetics and biotransformation of beraprost sodium 2: absorption, distribution and excretion after single administration of beraprost sodium in rat. Xenobio Metabol Dispos 1989;4:101–16.

61. Saji T *et al.* Short-term hemodynamic effect of a new oral PGI2 analog, beraprost, in primary and secondary pulmonary hypertension. Am J Cardiol 1996;78(2):244–7.

62. Okano Y *et al.* Orally active prostacyclin analog in primary pulmonary hypertension. Lancet 1997;349:1365.

63. Nagaya N *et al.* Effect of orally active prostacyclin analog on survival of outpatients with primary pulmonary hypertension. J Am Coll Cardiol 1999;34:1188–92.

64. Vizza CD *et al.* Long-term treatment of pulmonary arterial hypertension with beraprost, an oral prostacyclin analog. Heart 2001;86:661–5.

65. Galie N *et al.* Effects of beraprost sodium, an oral prostacyclin analog, in patients with pulmonary arterial hypertension: a randomized, double-blind, placebo-controlled trial. J Am Coll Cardiol 2002;39:1496–502.

66. Barst RJ *et al.* Beraprost therapy for pulmonary arterial hypertension. J Am Coll Cardiol 2003;41(12):2119–25.

67. McLaughlin VV *et al.* ACCF/AHA 2009 expert consensus document on pulmonary hypertension a report of the American College of Cardiology Foundation Task Force on Expert Consensus Documents and the American Heart Association developed in collaboration with the American College of Chest Physicians; American Thoracic Society, Inc.; and the Pulmonary Hypertension Association. J Am Coll Cardiol 2009;53(17):1573–619.

68. Badesch DB *et al.* Medical therapy for pulmonary arterial hypertension: updated ACCP evidence-based clinical practice guidelines. Chest 2007;131(6): 1917–28.

69. Galie N *et al.* Guidelines for the diagnosis and treatment of pulmonary hypertension: The Task Force for the Diagnosis and Treatment of Pulmonary Hypertension of the European Society of Cardiology (ESC) and the European Respiratory Society (ERS), endorsed by the International Society of Heart and Lung Transplantation (ISHLT). Eur Heart J 2009;30:2493-537.

70. Barst RJ *et al.* Updated evidence-based treatment algorithm in pulmonary arterial hypertension. J Am Coll Cardiol 2009;54(1 Suppl):S78-84.

71. Gilbert C *et al.* Estimating a minimally important difference in pulmonary arterial hypertension following treatment with sildenafil. Chest 2009;135(1):137–42.

72. Fijalkowska A *et al.* Serum N-terminal brain natriuretic peptide as a prognostic parameter in patients with pulmonary hypertension. Chest 2006;129(5): 1313–21.

73. Doran AK *et al.* Guidelines for the prevention of central venous catheter-related blood stream infections with prostanoid therapy for pulmonary arterial hypertension. Int J Clin Pract Suppl 2008;(160):5–9.

Inhaled nitric oxide and nitric oxide donors

ROBERTO F MACHADO

INTRODUCTION

Ever since endothelium-derived relaxing factor was pharmacologically defined as identical to nitric oxide (NO) activity, NO has been proposed as the major physiologic regulator of blood vessel tone. Specifically, NO plays a central role in vascular homeostasis by maintaining basal and stimulated vasomotor tone, limiting platelet aggregation and ischemia–reperfusion/radical oxygen species injury, and modulating endothelial proliferation. Several experimental models also report antibacterial and anti-inflammatory effects of NO.

Inhaled NO has been shown to selectively dilate the pulmonary circulation and improve oxygenation by redistributing pulmonary blood flow to well-ventilated lung units in several pathologic states. As such, these physiologic effects have led to the use of NO-based therapies in several clinical settings. Despite such potential beneficial effects, the role of inhaled NO in adults is not well established. In this chapter we will discuss the role of this gaseous molecule in the physiology and pathology of the pulmonary circulation.

CHEMICAL BIOLOGY OF NITRIC OXIDE

NO is a colorless gas at room temperature and pressure. Like oxygen it is somewhat lipophilic and possesses 6–8-fold higher solubility in nonpolar solvents and lipid membranes than water (1). NO has one unpaired electron and therefore is a free radical species that can react with other free radicals such as oxygen, superoxide, amino acids and transition metal ions (2). In fact the *in vivo* properties of NO are determined by its chemistry and the multiple reactions it can undergo either directly with its biological targets or indirectly by its interactions with other radical species (3).

NO is subject to rapid inactivation reactions with hemoglobin that greatly limit its lifetime in blood. The affinity of NO for oxyhemoglobin (HbO_2) is at least 1000 times greater than that of oxygen (4,5). NO is oxidized to the inert metabolite nitrate by its reaction with oxyhemoglobin, while reaction of NO with deoxyhemoglobin results in the formation of iron-nitrosyl hemoglobin (6). NO can also react with thiol groups in proteins such as hemoglobin or albumin to form S-nitrosothiols, which may have vasoactive properties or serve to store NO bioactivity (7). Finally, NO can be oxidized in blood to nitrite and several studies suggest that hemoglobin possesses an allosterically regulated nitrite reductase activity that reduces nitrite to NO along the physiological oxygen gradient, potentially contributing to hypoxic vasodilation (recently reviewed by Gladwin *et al.* (8).

PHYSIOLOGY AND MECHANISM OF ACTION OF INHALED NITRIC OXIDE

Nitric oxide synthases (NOS) are enzymes responsible for synthesis of endogenous NO. These enzymes convert L-arginine to NO and L-citrulline in a reaction that requires oxygen and NADPH. These enzymes can be divided into two groups: constitutive and inducible isoforms. The endothelial (NOS1) and neuronal (NOS3) constitutively

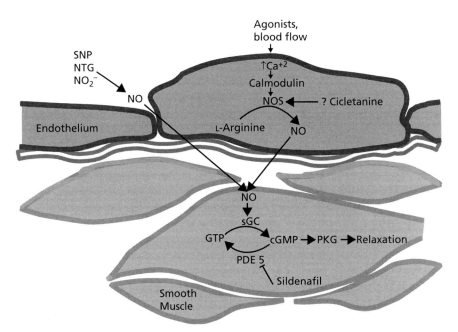

Figure 16.3.1 The nitric oxide (NO) axis and NO-based therapeutic targets. NO produced by endothelial nitric oxide synthase (NOS) with arginine as a substrate diffuses into smooth muscle to activate soluble guanylyl cyclase (sGC) to form cyclic guanosine monophosphate and maintain basal vascular tone. These effects can be harnessed therapeutically by direct administration of inhaled NO or by compounds that can release NO to tissues or enhance the effects of NO by increasing its enzymatic production or by inhibiting its metabolism. SNP: sodium nitroprusside, NTG: nitroglycerin, PDE-5: phosphodiesterase type 5.

expressed NOS depend on increases in calcium to bind calmodulin, leading to enzyme activation and picomolar levels of NO production (9). The inducible isoform (NOS2) is induced in diverse cell types by cytokines and contains calmodulin as a subunit, allowing the production of nanomolar levels of NO at resting levels of intracellular calcium (9). All isoforms are present in the lung (10,11). Endothelial NOS-derived NO production is stimulated by several chemical and physical stimuli including neurohormonal mediators such as acetylcholine, ADP and bradykinin or the shear stress induced in the vessel wall by blood flow.

NO stimulates soluble guanylate cyclase (sGC) to synthesize cyclic guanosine monophosphate (cGMP), which activates cGMP-dependent protein kinase G (PKG), which, in turn, promotes vascular smooth muscle relaxation. The action of cGMP is limited by its hydrolysis by phosphodiesterases. As previously stated, NO can interact with other heme containing-molecules, protein containing thiol groups and other radical species to exert effects that are cGMP independent. Further, in addition to its effects on vascular tone NO can limit platelet aggregation and ischemia-reperfusion/radical oxygen species injury, modulate endothelial proliferation and exert antibacterial and anti-inflammatory effects (recently reviewed in refs 12 and 13).

Endothelial NOS-derived NO appears to play an important role in maintaining a low pulmonary vascular tone under normoxic conditions (14). As such, infusion of the NOS inhibitor L-LMMA in the pulmonary circulation of healthy humans results in an increase in pulmonary vascular resistance and decreased pulmonary blood flow velocity. (15,16). In contrast, NO inhalation has minimal effects on pulmonary blood flow in healthy individuals suggesting that a healthy pulmonary circulation is typically fully dilated (17). In this context, abnormalities in vasodilator substances such as NO have been proposed as important in

the development of pulmonary arterial hypertension (PAH). Although there is controversy as to whether the expression of endothelial NOS in the pulmonary circulation of patients with PAH is decreased (18) or normal when compared to controls (19,20) several lines of evidence suggest that a state of decreased NO bioavailability occurs in the pathologic state of pulmonary hypertension. NO and NO biochemical reaction products are lower in the lungs and the exhaled breath of individuals with PAH (21,22) than healthy controls and these levels increase with therapy (23,24). Further, increased NO consumption due to oxidant stress (21) or decreased production due to increased arginase activity (20) (which depletes L-arginine, the substrate for NO synthesis) have also been demonstrated in patients with PAH.

When given by inhalation NO appears to selectively dilate the pulmonary vasculature, as upon reaching the systemic circulation it would be scavenged by hemoglobin. In an experimental study of thromboxane or hypoxia-induced pulmonary hypertension, Frostel *et al.* demonstrated that inhalation of NO decreased pulmonary arterial pressure (PAP) and pulmonary vascular resistance (PVR) in a dose-dependent matter (25). A similar effect was first reported in 1991 in patients with pulmonary hypertension (26). These effects of inhaled NO can also maximize V/Q matching and consequently improve gas exchange by eliciting vasodilation in well-ventilated lung units. However, this positive effect depends on the extent to which pulmonary vasoconstriction and V/Q mismatching are contributing to impaired oxygenation (27). By causing increased pulmonary arterial flow, inhaled NO can increase left ventricular end diastolic pressure and consequently precipitate pulmonary edema in patients with left ventricular dysfunction (28,29). Finally, the rapid withdrawal of inhaled NO can induce rebound pulmonary hypertension and hypoxemia (30,31).

Most studies suggest a lack of systemic effects of NO inhalation, but recent data have challenged this contention.

In experimental models inhaled NO has been shown to decrease systemic vascular resistance (32,33), improve mesenteric perfusion after NOS inhibition (34) and to decrease systemic vascular resistance in a model of hemolysis associated endothelial dysfunction (35). Further, in a study of healthy volunteers Cannon et al. (36) have shown that inhaled NO can increase forearm blood flow during blockade of regional NO synthesis, suggesting that NO can be transported in the systemic circulation to modulate blood flow peripherally.

DELIVERY OF INHALED NITRIC OXIDE

NO readily reacts with oxygen to form nitrogen dioxide (NO_2), which is a pulmonary irritant. Therefore, NO must be stored and administered with an inert gas such as nitrogen to minimize its reaction with oxygen, and delivery systems continuously monitor NO_2 concentrations. Because of its short half-life NO has to be administered continuously via a tight fitting face mask in spontaneously breathing patients or through the ventilator circuit in patients undergoing mechanical ventilation. Pulse delivery systems (which deliver a higher concentration bolus of NO with inspiration via nasal cannula) have been developed and are in use in studies evaluating the role of chronic ambulatory inhaled NO therapy in pulmonary vascular diseases.

Given the nature of its physiologic effects most of the potential clinical applications of inhaled NO are related to pulmonary vascular disorders and/or diseases that are characterized by abnormalities in gas exchange. Inhaled NO has emerged as a potential therapy for a variety of disorders such as neonatal pulmonary disorders, acute respiratory distress syndrome (ARDS) and pulmonary hypertension (Table 16.3.1). However, despite a large amount of clinical studies, the therapeutic role of inhaled NO is relatively uncertain and only well established in neonatal disorders such as persistent pulmonary hypertension of the newborn (PPHN).

NO may have the following applications:

- Pulmonary arterial hypertension (37–45).
- Pulmonary hypertension associated with lung diseases (46–51).
- Acute lung injury in adults (52–64).
- Acute right ventricular dysfunction (65–76).
- Lung transplantation (77–83).
- High altitude pulmonary edema (84–86).
- Sickle cell disease (13,87,89).

Neonatal and pediatric use of inhaled nitric oxide

Infants who fail to achieve the normal decrement in PVR at birth develop severe respiratory distress and hypoxemia

Table 16.3.1 Clinical use of inhaled nitric oxide

Indication	Effects	Supporting evidence
Acute vasoreactivity testing in patients with PAH	Acute vasoreactivity during RHC associated with responsiveness to chronic calcium channel blocker therapy and a favorable prognosis	Uncontrolled case series
Chronic treatment of PAH	Inhaled NO well tolerated	Uncontrolled case series
Chronic treatment of PH related to lung disease	No adverse effect on oxygenation when used in combination with oxygen Improvement in PAP, PVR and CO	Uncontrolled case series One RCT
Acute lung injury/ARDS	Improvement in systemic oxygenation No improvement in morbidity or mortality	Multiple RCTs
Acute pulmonary hypertension and right ventricular dysfunction	Improvement in hemodynamic parameters/right ventricular function	Uncontrolled case series
Lung transplantation	Improvement in systemic oxygenation No effect of prophylactic use on the incidence of acute graft dysfunction	Uncontrolled case series Two RCTs
High altitude pulmonary edema	Improvement in systemic oxygenation and hemodynamic parameters	Uncontrolled case series
Sickle cell disease	Improvement in systemic oxygenation Improved severity of vaso-occlusive pain crisis	Uncontrolled case series One RCT
Neonatal respiratory failure	Improvement in systemic oxygenation and decreased need for ECMO in PPHN Decrease in the incidence of BPD in premature infants weighing > 1000 g	Multiple RCTs

(characterized by right to left extrapulmonary shunting), a syndrome referred to as persistent pulmonary hypertension of the newborn (PPHN) that is a major cause of morbidity and mortality in neonates (90). It is well established that inhaled NO (typical doses 5–20 ppm) improves oxygenation in neonates with PPHN (91–94). Although randomized trials have not shown a beneficial effect of this therapy on mortality, the use of inhaled NO decreases the need for ECMO in near-term newborns (>34 weeks) whereas the effect in pre-term newborns (<34 weeks) is less established.

Bronchopulmonary dysplasia (BPD) is a chronic lung disease that most commonly affects premature infants who have received mechanical ventilation and oxygen therapy for acute respiratory distress (95). There are emerging data suggesting that inhaled NO may have a role in the prevention of BPD. Recent large randomized trials suggest that in premature infants weighing $>1000\,g$ the use in inhaled NO improves systemic oxygenation and reduces the incidence of BPD or the combined end point of death/BPD (96–99). Although the results of these trials are encouraging these effects were not demonstrated in infants with birth weight $\leqslant 1000\,g$.

TOXICITY OF INHALED NITRIC OXIDE

At high inspired levels NO is toxic to tissues and an acute inhaled overdose (500–1000 ppm) can lead to NO_2 formation, methemoglobinemia, pulmonary edema, alveolar hemorrhage and death (100,101). NO inhalation leads to the formation of methemoglobin and methemoglobin levels should be monitored in patients undergoing NO therapy. However, clinically used doses, typically up to 80 ppm, are generally not associated with clinically significant methemoglobinemia, which when it occurs is readily responsive to dose reduction. Methemoglobinemia appears to be more common in neonates and in individuals with methemoglobin reductase deficiency (102). Overall, there have been no reports of sequelae of methemoglobinemia in published clinical studies.

NO inhibits platelet aggregation thus suggesting that inhaled NO therapy could be associated with an increased risk of bleeding. This potential risk has not been demonstrated in the majority of randomized studies of adults and pediatric patients. However, in one study of inhaled NO therapy in neonates with respiratory failure, a higher risk of intracerebral hemorrhage was seen in infants weighing $\leqslant 1000\,g$ (99). These findings have not been reproduced in other similar studies and their significance is uncertain. A recent meta-analysis of the use of inhaled NO in patients with ALI/ARDS suggests that patients receiving NO have an increased risk of developing renal dysfunction (64).

Finally, it is important to point out that most of the data related to the toxicities of inhaled NO are derived form relatively short-term studies. In the few case series reporting longer exposure times no significant adverse effects have been reported.

NITRIC OXIDE DONORS AND THERAPIES THAT ENHANCE THE EFFECTS OF NITRIC OXIDE

The use of inhaled NO is expensive, requires continuous inhalation and relatively complicated delivery systems. Therefore the development of alternative agents that can deliver or enhance the effects of NO in more practical ways is highly desirable. NO donors are pharmacologically active compounds that can release NO to tissues. Other agents can enhance the effects of NO by increasing its enzymatic production or by inhibiting its metabolism. Several agents have been evaluated in experimental studies of pulmonary hypertension but data on their clinical use are very limited.

Nitric oxide donors

Sodium nitroprusside and nitroglycerin exert their vasodilatory effects by enzymatic release of NO and when given by inhalation can cause selective pulmonary vasodilation. In animal models of pulmonary hypertension, sodium nitroprusside produces dose-dependent selective pulmonary vasodilation comparable to the effect of inhaled NO, with loss of selectivity and decreased systemic arterial pressures being observed at higher doses (103,104). There is one report of the clinical use of inhaled sodium nitroprusside (105). Ten cyanotic newborns were treated with aerosolized sodium nitroprusside, at a concentration of $0.25\,mg/mL$ in distilled water. Nine of the newborns responded with a significant increase in their ratio of PaO_2 to fraction of inspired oxygen fraction after 1 hour of therapy (mean increase from 32 to 94 mmHg). Inhaled nitroglycerin produced selective pulmonary vasodilation in animal models of pulmonary hypertension (106), in children with congenital heart disease and pulmonary hypertension (107,108) and in patients with pulmonary hypertension undergoing mitral valve surgery (109).

Recent studies have demonstrated that the nitrite anion acts as a vasodilator by generating NO in tissues with lower oxygen tension and pH (8). In a sheep model of PPHN, inhaled nitrite was converted to NO gas in the lung and selectively vasodilated in the pulmonary circulation (110). If these data are confirmed in clinical studies of diseases such as PAH which are characterized by regional hypoxia and vasoconstriction, nitrite may provide an ideal stable therapeutic NO donor.

Details of the following therapies may be found in the references quoted:

- Phosphodiesterase inhibitors and soluble guanylate cyclase agonists (112–117).
- Arginine (118–120).
- Cicletanine (121–126).

KEY POINTS

- NO plays a central role in vascular homeostasis by maintaining basal and stimulated vasomotor tone, limiting platelet aggregation and ischemia-reperfusion/radical oxygen species injury, and modulating endothelial proliferation.

- Several lines of evidence suggest that a state of decreased NO bioavailability occurs in the pathologic state of pulmonary hypertension.

- When given by inhalation NO selectively dilates the pulmonary vasculature with decreases in pulmonary arterial pressure and pulmonary vascular resistance in a dose-dependent matter. These effects of inhaled NO can also maximize V/Q matching and consequently improve gas exchange by eliciting vasodilation in well-ventilated lung units.

- Most studies suggest a lack of systemic effects of NO inhalation, but emerging data suggest that NO can be transported in the systemic circulation to modulate blood flow peripherally.

- Inhaled NO has been used as a potential therapy for a variety of cardiopulmonary disorders. However, despite a large amount of clinical studies, the therapeutic role of inhaled NO is relatively uncertain and only well established in neonatal disorders such as persistent pulmonary hypertension of the newborn.

- Given the complexities associated with the delivery of inhaled NO, the development of alternative agents that can deliver or enhance the effects of NO in more practical ways such as NO donors, or agents that can enhance the effects of NO is highly desirable. Several agents have been evaluated in experimental studies of pulmonary hypertension but with the exception of phosphodiesterase-5 inhibitors, data on their clinical use are very limited.

REFERENCES

● = Key primary paper
◆ = Major review article

1. Shaw AW, Vosper AJ. Solubility of nitric oxide in aqueous and non aqueous solvents. J Chem Soc, Faraday Trans 1 1977;73:1239–44.
2. McCleverty JA. Chemistry of nitric oxide relevant to biology. Chem Rev 2004;104:403–18.
3. Espey MG, Miranda KM, Feelisch M et al. Mechanisms of cell death governed by the balance between nitrosative and oxidative stress. Ann NY Acad Sci 2000;899:209–21.
4. Carlsen E, Comroe JH, Jr. The rate of uptake of carbon monoxide and of nitric oxide by normal human erythrocytes and experimentally produced spherocytes. J Gen Physiol 1958;42:83–107.
5. Huang KT, Han TH, Hyduke DR et al. Modulation of nitric oxide bioavailability by erythrocytes. Proc Natl Acad Sci USA 2001;98:11771–6.
6. Liu X, Miller MJ, Joshi MS, Sadowska-Krowicka H, Clark DA, Lancaster JR, Jr. Diffusion-limited reaction of free nitric oxide with erythrocytes. J Biol Chem 1998;273:18709–13.
◆7. Gladwin MT, Crawford JH, Patel RP. The biochemistry of nitric oxide, nitrite, and hemoglobin: role in blood flow regulation. Free Radic Biol Med 2004;36:707–17.
◆8. Gladwin MT, Raat NJ, Shiva S et al. Nitrite as a vascular endocrine nitric oxide reservoir that contributes to hypoxic signaling, cytoprotection, and vasodilation. Am J Physiol Heart Circ Physiol 2006;291:H2026–35.
9. Stuehr DJ. Mammalian nitric oxide synthases. Biochim Biophys Acta 1999;1411:217–30.
10. Kobzik L, Bredt DS, Lowenstein CJ et al. Nitric oxide synthase in human and rat lung: immunocytochemical and histochemical localization. Am J Respir Cell Mol Biol 1993;9:371–7.
11. Sanders SP. Nitric oxide in asthma. Pathogenic, therapeutic, or diagnostic? Am J Respir Cell Mol Biol 1999;21:147–9.
12. Bogdan C. Nitric oxide and the immune response. Nat Immunol 2001;2:907–16.
◆13. Reiter CD, Gladwin MT. An emerging role for nitric oxide in sickle cell disease vascular homeostasis and therapy. Curr Opin Hematol 2003;10:99–107.
●14. Fagan KA, Tyler RC, Sato K et al. Relative contributions of endothelial, inducible, and neuronal NOS to tone in the murine pulmonary circulation. Am J Physiol 1999;277:L472–8.
●15. Celermajer DS, Dollery C, Burch M, Deanfield JE. Role of endothelium in the maintenance of low pulmonary vascular tone in normal children. Circulation 1994;89:2041–4.
●16. Stamler JS, Loh E, Roddy MA, Currie KE, Creager MA. Nitric oxide regulates basal systemic and pulmonary vascular resistance in healthy humans. Circulation 1994;89:2035–40.
●17. Brett SJ, Chambers J, Bush A, Rosenthal M, Evans TW. Pulmonary response of normal human subjects to inhaled vasodilator substances. Clin Sci (Lond) 1998;95:621–7.
●18. Giaid A, Saleh D. Reduced expression of endothelial nitric oxide synthase in the lungs of patients with pulmonary hypertension. N Engl J Med 1995;333:214–21.
●19. Xue C, Johns RA. Endothelial nitric oxide synthase in the lungs of patients with pulmonary hypertension. N Engl J Med 1995;333:1642–4.
●20. Xu W, Kaneko FT, Zheng S et al. Increased arginase II and decreased NO synthesis in endothelial cells of patients with pulmonary arterial hypertension. FASEB J 2004;18:1746–8.
●21. Kaneko FT, Arroliga AC, Dweik RA et al. Biochemical reaction products of nitric oxide as quantitative markers of primary pulmonary hypertension. Am J Respir Crit Care Med 1998;158:917–23.

• 22. Machado RF, Londhe Nerkar MV, Dweik RA et al. Nitric oxide and pulmonary arterial pressures in pulmonary hypertension. Free Radic Biol Med 2004;37:1010-7.

• 23. Girgis RE, Champion HC, Diette GB, Johns RA, Permutt S, Sylvester JT. Decreased exhaled nitric oxide in pulmonary arterial hypertension: response to bosentan therapy. Am J Respir Crit Care Med 2005;172:352-7.

• 24. Ozkan M, Dweik RA, Laskowski D, Arroliga AC, Erzurum SC. High levels of nitric oxide in individuals with pulmonary hypertension receiving epoprostenol therapy. Lung 2001;179:233-43.

• 25. Frostell C, Fratacci MD, Wain JC, Jones R, Zapol WM. Inhaled nitric oxide. A selective pulmonary vasodilator reversing hypoxic pulmonary vasoconstriction. Circulation 1991;83:2038-47.

• 26. Pepke-Zaba J, Higenbottam TW, Dinh-Xuan AT, Stone D, Wallwork J. Inhaled nitric oxide as a cause of selective pulmonary vasodilatation in pulmonary hypertension. Lancet 1991;338:1173-4.

• 27. Scherrer U, Vollenweider L, Delabays A et al. Inhaled nitric oxide for high-altitude pulmonary edema. N Engl J Med 1996;334:624-9.

• 28. Loh E, Stamler JS, Hare JM, Loscalzo J, Colucci WS. Cardiovascular effects of inhaled nitric oxide in patients with left ventricular dysfunction. Circulation 1994;90: 2780-5.

• 29. Bocchi EA, Bacal F, Auler Junior JO, Carmone MJ, Bellotti G, Pileggi F. Inhaled nitric oxide leading to pulmonary edema in stable severe heart failure. Am J Cardiol 1994;74:70-2.

• 30. Lavoie A, Hall JB, Olson DM, Wylam ME. Life-threatening effects of discontinuing inhaled nitric oxide in severe respiratory failure. Am J Respir Crit Care Med 1996;153: 1985-7.

◆ 31. Rossaint R, Falke KJ, Lopez F, Slama K, Pison U, Zapol WM. Inhaled nitric oxide for the adult respiratory distress syndrome. N Engl J Med 1993;328:399-405.

32. Kubes P, Payne D, Grisham MB, Jourd-Heuil D, Fox-Robichaud A. Inhaled NO impacts vascular but not extravascular compartments in postischemic peripheral organs. Am J Physiol 1999;277:H676-82.

33. Takahashi Y, Kobayashi H, Tanaka N, Sato T, Takizawa N, Tomita T. Nitrosyl hemoglobin in blood of normoxic and hypoxic sheep during nitric oxide inhalation. Am J Physiol 1998;274:H349-57.

34. Fox-Robichaud A, Payne D, Hasan SU et al. Inhaled NO as a viable antiadhesive therapy for ischemia/reperfusion injury of distal microvascular beds. J Clin Invest 1998; 101:2497-505.

• 35. Minneci PC, Deans KJ, Zhi H et al. Hemolysis-associated endothelial dysfunction mediated by accelerated NO inactivation by decompartmentalized oxyhemoglobin. J Clin Invest 2005;115:3409-17.

• 36. Cannon RO, 3rd, Schechter AN, Panza JA et al. Effects of inhaled nitric oxide on regional blood flow are consistent with intravascular nitric oxide delivery. J Clin Invest 2001;108:279-87.

• 37. Hoeper MM, Olschewski H, Ghofrani HA et al. A comparison of the acute hemodynamic effects of inhaled nitric oxide and aerosolized iloprost in primary pulmonary hypertension. German PPH study group. J Am Coll Cardiol 2000;35: 176-82.

• 38. Jolliet P, Bulpa P, Thorens JB, Ritz M, Chevrolet JC. Nitric oxide and prostacyclin as test agents of vasoreactivity in severe precapillary pulmonary hypertension: predictive ability and consequences on haemodynamics and gas exchange. Thorax 1997;52:369-72.

• 39. Ricciardi MJ, Knight BP, Martinez FJ, Rubenfire M. Inhaled nitric oxide in primary pulmonary hypertension: a safe and effective agent for predicting response to nifedipine. J Am Coll Cardiol 1998;32:1068-73.

• 40. Sitbon O, Brenot F, Denjean A et al. Inhaled nitric oxide as a screening vasodilator agent in primary pulmonary hypertension. A dose-response study and comparison with prostacyclin. Am J Respir Crit Care Med 1995;151:384-9.

• 41. Sitbon O, Humbert M, Jagot JL et al. Inhaled nitric oxide as a screening agent for safely identifying responders to oral calcium-channel blockers in primary pulmonary hypertension. Eur Respir J 1998;12:265-70.

• 42. Channick RN, Newhart JW, Johnson FW et al. Pulsed delivery of inhaled nitric oxide to patients with primary pulmonary hypertension: an ambulatory delivery system and initial clinical tests. Chest 1996;109:1545-9.

43. Channick RN, Yung GL. Long-term use of inhaled nitric oxide for pulmonary hypertension. Respiratory Care 1999;44:212-9.

44. Snell GI, Salamonsen RF, Bergin P, Esmore DS, Khan S, Williams TJ. Inhaled nitric oxide used as a bridge to heart-lung transplantation in a patient with end-stage pulmonary hypertension. Am J Respir Crit Care Med 1995;151:1263-6.

45. Koh E, Niimura J, Nakamura T, Yamakage H, Takahashi H. Long-term inhalation of nitric oxide for a patient with primary pulmonary hypertension. Jpn Circ J 1998;62: 940-2.

◆ 46. Behr J, Ryu JH. Pulmonary hypertension in interstitial lung disease. Eur Respir J 2008;31:1357-67.

◆ 47. Chaouat A, Naeije R, Weitzenblum E. Pulmonary hypertension in COPD. Eur Respir J 2008;32:1371-85.

• 48. Barbera JA, Roger N, Roca J, Rovira I, Higenbottam TW, Rodriguez-Roisin R. Worsening of pulmonary gas exchange with nitric oxide inhalation in chronic obstructive pulmonary disease. Lancet 1996;347:436-40.

49. Channick RN, Hoch RC, Newhart JW, Johnson FW, Smith CM. Improvement in pulmonary hypertension and hypoxemia during nitric oxide inhalation in a patient with end-stage pulmonary fibrosis. Am J Respir Crit Care Med 1994;149:811-4.

• 50. Ghofrani HA, Wiedemann R, Rose F et al. Sildenafil for treatment of lung fibrosis and pulmonary hypertension: a randomised controlled trial. Lancet 2002;360:895-900.

• 51. Vonbank K, Ziesche R, Higenbottam TW et al. Controlled prospective randomised trial on the effects on pulmonary haemodynamics of the ambulatory long term use of nitric oxide and oxygen in patients with severe COPD. Thorax 2003;58:289–93.

●52. Day RW, Allen EM, Witte MK. A randomized, controlled study of the 1-hour and 24-hour effects of inhaled nitric oxide therapy in children with acute hypoxemic respiratory failure. Chest 1997;112:1324–31.

●53. Dellinger RP, Zimmerman JL, Taylor RW *et al*. Effects of inhaled nitric oxide in patients with acute respiratory distress syndrome: results of a randomized phase II trial. Inhaled Nitric Oxide in ARDS Study Group. Crit Care Med 1998;26:15–23.

●54. Dobyns EL, Cornfield DN, Anas NG *et al*. Multicenter randomized controlled trial of the effects of inhaled nitric oxide therapy on gas exchange in children with acute hypoxemic respiratory failure. J Pediatr 1999;134:406–12.

●55. Gerlach H, Keh D, Semmerow A *et al*. Dose–response characteristics during long-term inhalation of nitric oxide in patients with severe acute respiratory distress syndrome: a prospective, randomized, controlled study. Am J Respir Crit Care Med 2003;167:1008–15.

●56. Lundin S, Mang H, Smithies M, Stenqvist O, Frostell C. Inhalation of nitric oxide in acute lung injury: results of a European multicentre study. The European Study Group of Inhaled Nitric Oxide. Intensive Care Med 1999;25:911–9.

●57. Mehta S, Simms HH, Levy MM, Hill NS, Schwartz W, Nelson D. Inhaled nitric oxide improves oxygenation acutely but not chronically in acute respirator distress syndrome. J Appl Res 2001;1:73–84.

●58. Michael JR, Barton RG, Saffle JR *et al*. Inhaled nitric oxide versus conventional therapy: effect on oxygenation in ARDS. Am J Respir Crit Care Med 1998;157:1372–80.

●59. Park KJ, Lee YJ, Oh YJ, Lee KS, Sheen SS, Hwang SC. Combined effects of inhaled nitric oxide and a recruitment maneuver in patients with acute respiratory distress syndrome. Yonsei Med J 2003;44:219–26.

60. Payen D, Vallet B, l'ARDS GdedNd. Results of the French prospective multicentric randomized double-blind– placebo-controlled trial of inhlade nitric oxide (NO) in ARDS. Intensive Care Med 1999;25:S166.

61. Schwebel C, Beuret P, Pedrix JP, Jospe R, Dueperret S, Fogliani J. Early inhaled nitric oxide inhalation in acute lung injury: results of a double-blind randomized study. Intensive Care Med 1997;23:S2.

●62. Taylor RW, Zimmerman JL, Dellinger RP *et al*. Low-dose inhaled nitric oxide in patients with acute lung injury: a randomized controlled trial. JAMA 2004;291:1603–9.

●63. Troncy E, Collet JP, Shapiro S *et al*. Inhaled nitric oxide in acute respiratory distress syndrome: a pilot randomized controlled study. Am J Respir Crit Care Med 1998;157: 1483–8.

◆64. Adhikari NK, Burns KE, Friedrich JO, Granton JT, Cook DJ, Meade MO. Effect of nitric oxide on oxygenation and mortality in acute lung injury: systematic review and meta–analysis. BMJ 2007;334:779.

65. Fullerton DA, McIntyre RC, Jr. Inhaled nitric oxide: therapeutic applications in cardiothoracic surgery. Ann Thorac Surg 1996;61:1856–64.

66. Journois D, Pouard P, Mauriat P, Malhere T, Vouhe P, Safran D. Inhaled nitric oxide as a therapy for pulmonary hypertension after operations for congenital heart defects. J Thorac Cardiovasc Surg 1994;107:1129–35.

67. Sharma R, Raizada N, Choudhary SK *et al*. Does inhaled nitric oxide improve survival in operated congenital disease with severe pulmonary hypertension? Indian Heart J 2001;53:48–55.

68. Ardehali A, Hughes K, Sadeghi A *et al*. Inhaled nitric oxide for pulmonary hypertension after heart transplantation. Transplantation 2001;72:638–41.

69. Auler Junior JO, Carmona MJ, Bocchi EA *et al*. Low doses of inhaled nitric oxide in heart transplant recipients. J Heart Lung Transplant 1996;15:443–50.

70. Gardeback M, Larsen FF, Radegran K. Nitric oxide improves hypoxaemia following reperfusion oedema after pulmonary thromboendarterectomy. Br J Anaesth 1995;75:798–800.

71. Imanaka H, Miyano H, Takeuchi M, Kumon K, Ando M. Effects of nitric oxide inhalation after pulmonary thromboendarterectomy for chronic pulmonary thromboembolism. Chest 2000;118:39–46.

72. Pinelli G, Mertes PM, Carteaux JP *et al*. Inhaled nitric oxide as an adjunct to pulmonary thromboendarterectomy. Ann Thorac Surg 1996;61:227–9.

73. Dang NC, Topkara VK, Mercando M *et al*. Right heart failure after left ventricular assist device implantation in patients with chronic congestive heart failure. J Heart Lung Transplant 2006;25:1–6.

●74. Argenziano M, Choudhri AF, Moazami N *et al*. Randomized, double-blind trial of inhaled nitric oxide in LVAD recipients with pulmonary hypertension. Ann Thorac Surg 1998;65: 340–5.

75. Inglessis I, Shin JT, Lepore JJ *et al*. Hemodynamic effects of inhaled nitric oxide in right ventricular myocardial infarction and cardiogenic shock. J Am Coll Cardiol 2004;44:793–8.

76. Szold O, Khoury W, Biderman P, Klausner JM, Halpern P, Weinbroum AA. Inhaled nitric oxide improves pulmonary functions following massive pulmonary embolism: a report of four patients and review of the literature. Lung 2006;184:1–5.

●77. Guidot DM, Hybertson BM, Kitlowski RP, Repine JE. Inhaled NO prevents IL-1-induced neutrophil accumulation and associated acute edema in isolated rat lungs. Am J Physiol 1996;271:L225–9.

●78. Guidot DM, Repine MJ, Hybertson BM, Repine JE. Inhaled nitric oxide prevents neutrophil-mediated, oxygen radical- dependent leak in isolated rat lungs. Am J Physiol 1995; 269:L2–5.

79. Struber M, Harringer W, Ernst M *et al*. Inhaled nitric oxide as a prophylactic treatment against reperfusion injury of the lung. Thorac Cardiovasc Surg 1999;47:179–82.

80. Ardehali A, Laks H, Levine M *et al*. A prospective trial of inhaled nitric oxide in clinical lung transplantation. Transplantation 2001;72:112–5.

81. Date H, Triantafillou AN, Trulock EP, Pohl MS, Cooper JD, Patterson GA. Inhaled nitric oxide reduces human lung

allograft dysfunction. J Thorac Cardiovasc Surg 1996;111:913–9.

•82. Meade MO, Granton JT, Matte-Martyn A *et al.* A randomized trial of inhaled nitric oxide to prevent ischemia-reperfusion injury after lung transplantation. Am J Respir Crit Care Med 2003;167:1483–9.

•83. Botha P, Jeyakanthan M, Rao JN *et al.* Inhaled nitric oxide for modulation of ischemia–reperfusion injury in lung transplantation. J Heart Lung Transplant 2007;26: 1199–205.

•84. Hyers TM, Scoggin CH, Will DH, Grover RF, Reeves JT. Accentuated hypoxemia at high altitude in subjects susceptible to high-altitude pulmonary edema. J Appl Physiol 1979;46:41–6.

•85. Maggiorini M, Melot C, Pierre S *et al.* High-altitude pulmonary edema is initially caused by an increase in capillary pressure. Circulation 2001;103:2078–83.

•86. Anand IS, Prasad BA, Chugh SS *et al.* Effects of inhaled nitric oxide and oxygen in high-altitude pulmonary edema. Circulation 1998;98:2441–5.

◆87. Machado RF, Gladwin MT. Chronic sickle cell lung disease: new insights into the diagnosis, pathogenesis and treatment of pulmonary hypertension. Br J Haematol 2005;129:449–64.

88. Sullivan KJ, Goodwin SR, Evangelist J, Moore RD, Mehta P. Nitric oxide successfully used to treat acute chest syndrome of sickle cell disease in a young adolescent. Crit Care Med 1999;27:2563–8.

•89. Weiner DL, Hibberd PL, Betit P, Cooper AB, Botelho CA, Brugnara C. Preliminary assessment of inhaled nitric oxide for acute vaso-occlusive crisis in pediatric patients with sickle cell disease. JAMA 2003;289:1136–42.

◆90. Abman SH. Recent advances in the pathogenesis and treatment of persistent pulmonary hypertension of the newborn. Neonatology 2007;91:283–90.

•91. Inhaled nitric oxide in full-term and nearly full-term infants with hypoxic respiratory failure. The Neonatal Inhaled Nitric Oxide Study Group. N Engl J Med 1997;336:597–604.

•92. Clark RH, Kueser TJ, Walker MW *et al.* Low-dose nitric oxide therapy for persistent pulmonary hypertension of the newborn. Clinical Inhaled Nitric Oxide Research Group. N Engl J Med 2000;342:469–74.

•93. Davidson D, Barefield ES, Kattwinkel J *et al.* Inhaled nitric oxide for the early treatment of persistent pulmonary hypertension of the term newborn: a randomized, double-masked, placebo-controlled, dose–response, multicenter study. The I-NO/PPHN Study Group. Pediatrics 1998; 101:325–34.

•94. Roberts JD, Jr., Fineman JR, Morin FC, 3rd *et al.* Inhaled nitric oxide and persistent pulmonary hypertension of the newborn. The Inhaled Nitric Oxide Study Group. N Engl J Med 1997;336:605–10.

◆95. Kinsella JP, Greenough A, Abman SH. Bronchopulmonary dysplasia. Lancet 2006;367:1421–31.

•96. Ballard RA, Truog WE, Cnaan A *et al.* Inhaled nitric oxide in preterm infants undergoing mechanical ventilation. N Engl J Med 2006;355:343–53.

•97. Kinsella JP, Cutter GR, Walsh WF *et al.* Early inhaled nitric oxide therapy in premature newborns with respiratory failure. N Engl J Med 2006;355:354–64.

•98. Schreiber MD, Gin-Mestan K, Marks JD, Huo D, Lee G, Srisuparp P. Inhaled nitric oxide in premature infants with the respiratory distress syndrome. N Engl J Med 2003; 349:2099–107.

•99. Van Meurs KP, Wright LL, Ehrenkranz RA *et al.* Inhaled nitric oxide for premature infants with severe respiratory failure. N Engl J Med 2005;353:13–22.

100. Clutton-Brock J. Two cases of poisoning by contamination of nitrous oxide with higher oxides of nitrogen during anaesthesia. Br J Anaesth 1967;39:388–92.

101. Greenbaum R, Bay J, Hargreaves MD *et al.* Effects of higher oxides of nitrogen on the anaesthetized dog. Br J Anaesth 1967;39:393–404.

102. Young JD, Dyar O, Xiong L, Howell S. Methaemoglobin production in normal adults inhaling low concentrations of nitric oxide. Intensive Care Med 1994;20:581–4.

•103. Adrie C, Ichinose F, Holzmann A, Keefer L, Hurford WE, Zapol WM. Pulmonary vasodilation by nitric oxide gas and prodrug aerosols in acute pulmonary hypertension. J Appl Physiol 1998;84:435–41.

•104. Schreiber MD, Dixit R, Rudinsky B *et al.* Direct comparison of the effects of nebulized nitroprusside versus inhaled nitric oxide on pulmonary and systemic hemodynamics during hypoxia-induced pulmonary hypertension in piglets. Crit Care Med 2002;30:2560–5.

105. Palhares DB, Figueiredo CS, Moura AJ. Endotracheal inhalatory sodium nitroprusside in severely hypoxic newborns. J Perinat Med 1998;26:219–24.

106. Bando M, Ishii Y, Kitamura S, Ohno S. Effects of inhalation of nitroglycerin on hypoxic pulmonary vasoconstriction. Respiration 1998;65:63–70.

107. Goyal P, Kiran U, Chauhan S, Juneja R, Choudhary M. Efficacy of nitroglycerin inhalation in reducing pulmonary arterial hypertension in children with congenital heart disease. Br J Anaesth 2006;97:208–14.

108. Omar HA, Gong F, Sun MY, Einzig S. Nebulized nitroglycerin in children with pulmonary hypertension secondary to congenital heart disease. W V Med J 1999;95:74–5.

109. Yurtseven N, Karaca P, Uysal G *et al.* A comparison of the acute hemodynamic effects of inhaled nitroglycerin and iloprost in patients with pulmonary hypertension undergoing mitral valve surgery. Ann Thorac Cardiovasc Surg 2006;12:319–23.

•110. Hunter CJ, Dejam A, Blood AB *et al.* Inhaled nebulized nitrite is a hypoxia-sensitive NO-dependent selective pulmonary vasodilator. Nat Med 2004;10:1122–7.

•111. Galie N, Ghofrani HA, Torbicki A *et al.* Sildenafil citrate therapy for pulmonary arterial hypertension. N Engl J Med 2005;353:2148–57.

•112. Ghofrani HA, Wiedemann R, Rose F *et al.* Combination therapy with oral sildenafil and inhaled iloprost for severe pulmonary hypertension. Ann Intern Med 2002;136:515–22.

•113. Lepore JJ, Maroo A, Bigatello LM *et al.* Hemodynamic effects of sildenafil in patients with congestive heart failure and pulmonary hypertension: combined administration with inhaled nitric oxide. Chest 2005;127:1647–53.

•114. Lepore JJ, Maroo A, Pereira NL *et al.* Effect of sildenafil on the acute pulmonary vasodilator response to inhaled nitric oxide in adults with primary pulmonary hypertension. Am J Cardiol 2002;90:677–80.

•115. Namachivayam P, Theilen U, Butt WW, Cooper SM, Penny DJ, Shekerdemian LS. Sildenafil prevents rebound pulmonary hypertension after withdrawal of nitric oxide in children. Am J Respir Crit Care Med 2006;174:1042–7.

•116. Evgenov OV, Ichinose F, Evgenov NV *et al.* Soluble guanylate cyclase activator reverses acute pulmonary hypertension and augments the pulmonary vasodilator response to inhaled nitric oxide in awake lambs. Circulation 2004;110:2253–9.

•117. Evgenov OV, Kohane DS, Bloch KD *et al.* Inhaled agonists of soluble guanylate cyclase induce selective pulmonary vasodilation. Am J Respir Crit Care Med 2007;176:1138–45.

•118. Mehta S, Stewart DJ, Langleben D, Levy RD. Short-term pulmonary vasodilation with L-arginine in pulmonary hypertension. Circulation 1995;92:1539–45.

•119. Nagaya N, Uematsu M, Oya H *et al.* Short-term oral administration of L-arginine improves hemodynamics and exercise capacity in patients with precapillary pulmonary hypertension. Am J Respir Crit Care Med 2001;163:887–91.

•120. Morris CR, Morris SM, Jr., Hagar W *et al.* Arginine therapy: a new treatment for pulmonary hypertension in sickle cell disease? Am J Respir Crit Care Med 2003;168:63–9.

121. Akamatsu N, Sawada S, Komatsu S *et al.* Effect of cicletanine on the nitric oxide pathway in human umbilical vein endothelial cells. J Cardiovasc Pharmacol 2001;38:174–82.

122. Chamiot-Clerc P, Choukri N, Legrand M, Droy-Lefaix MT, Safar ME, Renaud JF. Relaxation of vascular smooth muscle by cicletanine in aged wistar aorta under stress conditions: importance of nitric oxide. Am J Hypertens 2000;13:208–13.

123. Kalinowski L, Dobrucki IT, Malinski T. Cicletanine stimulates nitric oxide release and scavenges superoxide in endothelial cells. J Cardiovasc Pharmacol 2001;37:713–24.

124. Szilvassy Z, Csont T, Pali T, Droy-Lefaix MT, Ferdinandy P. Nitric oxide, peroxynitrite and cGMP in atherosclerosis-induced hypertension in rabbits: beneficial effects of cicletanine. J Vasc Res 2001;38:39–46.

•125. Saadjian A, Philip-Joet F, Paganelli F, Arnaud A, Levy S. Long-term effects of cicletanine on secondary pulmonary hypertension. J Cardiovasc Pharmacol 1998;31:364–71.

126. Waxman AB, Lawler L, Cornett G. Cicletanine for the treatment of pulmonary arterial hypertension. Arch Intern Med 2008;168:2164–6.

Endothelin receptor antagonists

RICHARD N CHANNICK*

INTRODUCTION

The endothelins are a family of 21-amino acid peptides that play a key role in the regulation of vascular tone. The first member of this family identified was endothelin-1 (ET-1), a 2492 dalton peptide with potent vasoconstrictor properties, isolated by Yanagisawa and colleagues in 1988 (1). Two additional endothelin isopeptides: endothelin-2 (ET-2) and endothelin-3 (ET-3), were subsequently discovered (2). All three of these proteins share a high degree of amino acid homology. They also bear structural similarity to a family of peptides labeled sarafotoxins which are isolated from the venom of the snake *Atractaspis engaddensis*, suggesting a possible shared evolutionary origin (3).

Vascular endothelial cells are the major source of endothelins in humans. However, genes encoding the endothelin peptides are also found in a wide range of additional cell types including bronchial epithelium, macrophages, cardiac myocytes, glomerular mesangium, and glial cells to name a few (4–7).

The years following the discovery of endothelins have seen an explosion of basic research into these compounds (8). This has led clinicians to postulate numerous potential applications to the manipulation of the endothelin system: including the treatment of renal diseases, systemic hypertension and cerebral vasospasm (8,9).

It is in the therapy of pulmonary vascular disease, however, that endothelin biology has, thus far, shown its greatest penetration into the clinical arena. This chapter will review the current understanding of the role of endothelins in the physiology and pathophysiology of the pulmonary circulation, as well as the clinical experiences gained from the use of endothelin receptor antagonists in the treatment of pulmonary arterial hypertension.

PHYSIOLOGY

Although marked structural similarity amongst the endothelins results in significant areas of overlapping biologic function, these compounds are not as similar as they first may appear. The human genes for ET-1, ET-2 and ET-3 are each located on different chromosomes (8). Furthermore, the distribution of the three endothelin proteins throughout different tissues appears to be quite heterogeneous. Endothelial cells, including those of the pulmonary circulation, predominantly generate ET-1. Kidney cells appear to express higher levels of ET-2 (10). ET-3 has been found in high concentrations in the intestine and brain (11,12). Each of these three compounds seems to have a distinct physiologic role that guides their site(s) of expression. Our understanding of these unique yet overlapping roles remains incomplete.

*Abbreviations: ET-1, Endothelin-1; ET-2, Endothelin-2; ET-3, Endothelin-3; ECE-1, Endothelin-1 converting enzyme; ET_A receptor, Endothelin receptor A; ET_B receptor, Endothelin receptor B; G protein, Guanine-nucleotide-binding protein; IP_3, 1,4,5-inositol triphosphate; mRNA, messenger ribonucleic acid; Ca^{2+}, ionized calcium; IPAH, primary pulmonary hypertension; PAH, pulmonary arterial hypertension; NYHA, New York Heart Association; CTEPH, chronic thromboembolic pulmonary hypertension; IPAHN, persistent pulmonary hypertension of the newborn; 6MWT, 6-minute walk test; mmHg, millimeters of mercury; ALT, alanine aminotransferase; AST, aspartate aminotransferase.

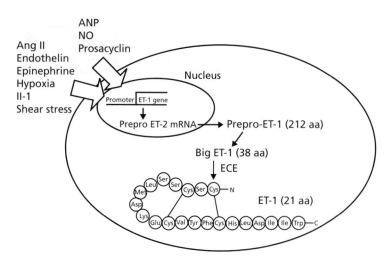

Figure 16.4.1 Schematic illustration of production of ET-1 by pulmonary artery endothelial cells. PPET-1, preproendothelin-1; MRNA, messenger ribonucleic acid; Big ET-1, big endothelin-1; ECE-1, endothelin-1 converting enzyme; ET-1, endothelin-1; *rate limiting step.

Investigators have focused in particular on the physiology of ET-1, due to its prominent role in vascular control. The molecular mechanisms of ET-1 activity merit review (even in a clinical text) not only because of their emerging clinical relevance but also because they represent novel pathways in the regulation of the pulmonary circulation.

Endothelin-1 production

The human ET-1 gene is located on the telomeric region of chromosome 6p (8). The ET-1 gene includes five exons that encode mRNA for a large precursor protein: preproendothelin-1 (PPET-1). The intermediate steps between transcription of PPET-1 and release of ET-1 from the endothelial cell are summarized in Figure 16.4.1.

Unlike some other proteins, ET-1 is not kept in secretory granules (13) within cells. The rate-limiting step in the biosynthesis of ET-1 occurs at the level of transcription (1). Many stimuli that regulate ET-1 production have evolved through direct action upon transcription factors (Table 16.4.1). It appears that vascular endothelial cells are able to rapidly increase or inhibit ET-1 production to regulate vascular tone (14).

The majority of ET-1 secreted from cultured endothelial cells occurs from the abluminal side of the cells towards the adjacent vascular smooth muscle cells, which contain specific endothelin receptors (15). Thus, it is important to note that although circulating ET-1 can be detected in the plasma, and may have important clinical correlations with pulmonary vascular disease, these plasma levels may not necessarily reflect the paracrine action of ET-1 on adjacent smooth muscle cells.

Endothelin receptors

There are two distinct receptors for the endothelin family of peptides, endothelin receptor A (ET_A) and endothelin receptor B (ET_B). The endothelin receptors belong to the

Table 16.4.1   Transcriptional regulation of ET-1 production

Upregulating factors
- Angiotensin II (65)
- Norepinephrine (12)
- Vasopressin (65)
- TGF β (66)
- TNF α (67)
- Thrombin (68)
- Interleukin-1 (69)
- Bradykinin (70)
- Low shear stress (71)
- Oxidated LDL (72)
- Hypoxia (12)

Inhibiting factors
- Nitric oxide (12)
- Atrial natriuretic peptide (73)
- Brain natriuretic peptide (73)
- Prostacyclin (12)
- Prostaglandin E2 (12)
- Endothelin-3 (12)

family of receptors connected to guanine nucleotide-binding (G) proteins (16). The two receptors have unique locations (17) and binding affinities (10) for the endothelin peptides. ET_A receptors are expressed on pulmonary vascular smooth muscle cells, and have high affinity for ET-1 and ET-2, with less affinity for ET-3. ET_B receptors are located on both pulmonary vascular endothelial cells and smooth muscle cells. ET_B receptors bind all three endothelin isoforms with nearly equal affinity.

When activated, the ET_A receptor located in pulmonary vascular smooth muscle cells mediates vasoconstriction. The mechanism is thought to occur via G protein-induced phospholipase C activation; 1,4,5-inositol triphosphate (IP_3) formation; and the consequent release of Ca^{2+} from intracellular stores (16). There is some evidence that ET_A

receptor may also increase intracellular calcium by activating non-selective calcium channels on the surface of the smooth muscle cell (18). The vasoconstriction induced by ET_A has been shown to persist even after ET-1 is removed from the receptor, likely due to persistently elevated concentrations of intracellular Ca^{2+} (19).

In addition to its powerful vasoconstricting effects, ET-1 is known to be a potent mitogen, with the ability to induce cell proliferation in a number of cell types, including vascular smooth muscle cells (20). It has been shown that the mitogenic actions of ET-1 are mediated by both the ET_A (21) and ET_B (22) receptors.

In the pulmonary vasculature, ET_B receptors are predominantly expressed on endothelial cells (23,24). ET_B receptors on endothelial cells mediate vasodilation via increased production of nitric oxide and prostacyclin (24–26). Nitric oxide and prostacyclin also negatively feedback on ET-1 activity by inhibition of PPET-1 transcription (see Figure 16.4.1).

ET_B receptors contribute to the clearance of circulating ET-1, likely due to internalization of the ET-1/ET_B receptor complex into the cell after binding (27).

It has been observed that the normal human lung removes roughly 50 percent of circulating ET-1, and that it releases a similar quantity, resulting in the lack of an arterial-to-venous ET-1 gradient across the pulmonary vasculature in the normal state (28).

There are data suggesting that the ET_B receptor does not exclusively mediate pulmonary vasodilation. Under some circumstances it may actually contribute to pulmonary vasoconstriction, through a population of ET_B receptors located on vascular smooth muscle cells (29). The vasoconstrictive actions of ET_B receptors may become more pronounced in the pathologic setting of pulmonary hypertension (30) than in the normal pulmonary vasculature. It has been postulated that this action may result from downregulation of ET_A receptors in states of pulmonary hypertension, possibly as an adaptive response to high levels of circulating ET-1 (31).

The vasoconstrictive actions of the ET_B receptor may confer a therapeutic advantage to the strategy of dual ET_A/ET_B receptor blockade over selective ET_A receptor blockade in the treatment of pulmonary arterial hypertension.

PATHOPHYSIOLOGY

The endothelins are thought to participate in the pathophysiology of a spectrum of pulmonary vascular diseases. The extent to which the endothelin system is involved in each disease affecting the pulmonary circulation is not completely understood, however similarities in the pathogenesis of this family of disorders suggest that endothelin biology has broad applicability. The evidence for the role of the endothelin system in the pathophysiology of several individual pulmonary vascular diseases will be subsequently reviewed.

Idiopathic pulmonary arterial hypertension

Patients with idiopathic pulmonary arterial hypertension (IPAH) demonstrate higher serum levels of ET-1 and higher arterial-to-venous ratios of ET-1 than healthy controls (32). This phenomenon may represent increased production of ET-1 by the lung, reduced clearance by the lung, or a combination of these processes. Lung specimens from patients with IPAH, when compared to those from patients without pulmonary hypertension, exhibit increased ET-1 staining of the muscular pulmonary arteries and increased expression of PPET-1 in the endothelial cells of the same vessels (33). There is furthermore a correlation between the intensity of staining for ET-1 and the patients' hemodynamic measurements of pulmonary vascular resistance. Recent studies have shown increased ECE-1 in the pulmonary vascular endothelial cells of IPAH patients (34), and increased net pulmonary clearance of ET-1 in patients with IPAH treated with continuous intravenous epoprostenol (35).

Other pulmonary vascular diseases

PULMONARY HYPERTENSION FROM CHRONIC HYPOXIA

Pulmonary hypertension from chronic hypoxia has been shown in animal models to be associated with increased ET-1 and ET_A expression (36,37). In these models, it is also notable that dual ET_A/ET_B receptor blockade resulted in amelioration of pulmonary hypertensive changes (38). Interestingly, rat models have also demonstrated regional differences in endothelin expression throughout the lung, leading some authors to suggest that heterogeneity of the endothelin system may help to regulate local responses to hypoxia in the pulmonary circulation (39,40). Detailed human investigations into the role of the endothelin system in chronic hypoxemia have not been reported to date.

PULMONARY HYPERTENSION FROM CONGENITAL CARDIAC DISEASE

Pulmonary hypertension from congenital cardiac disease has been shown in human investigations to correlate with high levels of ET_A receptor density and circulating ET-1, which in some instances decreased following surgical correction of the cardiac lesions (41–43). The development of hypoxemia in patients with congenital shunts may be an additional factor which magnifies the detrimental effects of ET-1 (44).

CHRONIC THROMBOEMBOLIC PULMONARY HYPERTENSION

Chronic thromboembolic pulmonary hypertension (CTEPH) has been associated with increased activity of the ET-1 system in both animal (45,46) and human (47) pathologic studies. Pulmonary hypertensive changes were attenuated in the presence of dual ET_A/ET_B receptor blockade in a canine model of CTEPH (45). It is known that many patients with CTEPH have a concomitant small vessel vasculopathy which can limit the hemodynamic improvement following pulmonary thromboendarterectomy. These data suggest that endothelin may play a role in this process.

PERSISTENT PULMONARY HYPERTENSION OF THE NEWBORN

Persistent pulmonary hypertension of the newborn (IPAHN) has been associated with increased ET-1 expression and ETA receptor activity in a number of animal studies, involving several different models of IPAHN (48–51). Clinical studies of human babies with IPAHN (52–55) have also revealed elevated levels of circulating ET-1, which appear to correlate with other markers of disease severity.

CLINICAL USE OF ENDOTHELIN RECEPTOR ANTAGONISTS

There are currently three endothelin receptor antagonists commercially available for the treatment of PAH, ambrisentan, sitaxsentan* (not approved in the USA), and bosentan. These agents were all approved based on results of 12–16-week randomized, placebo-controlled trials demonstrating their efficacy in improving exercise capacity, as measured by the 6-minute walk test. Long-term, open-label studies have confirmed the benefits of this class of medication.

Ambrisentan

Ambrisentan is a specific ET-A receptor antagonist approved for PAH, functional classes II and III at doses of 5 mg or 10 mg once daily. Following a Phase 2 dosing study showing favorable pulmonary hemodynamic effects (56), two RCTs (ARIES 1 and ARIES 2) of ambrisentan (ARIES 1: 5 mg, 10 mg, placebo; ARIES 2: 2.5 mg, 5 mg, placebo) were performed, enrolling a total of 394 patients (57). Both trials achieved the primary endpoint of placebo-corrected improvement in 6-minute walk distance. In ARIES-2, there was a significant improvement in time to clinical worsening in the treatment group as compared with placebo. There was a trend towards improvement in time to clinical worsening in the ARIES-1 study, but it was not statistically significant ($P = 0.307$). WHO functional class improvement was significant in ARIES-1 and there was a trend towards improvement in ARIES-2 but did not reach statistical significance ($P = 0.117$). A total of 298 patients were enrolled and followed in the long-term extension study over 48 weeks. Eighteen patients required additional therapies (prostanoids or PD-5 inhibitors). Of the 280 patients continued on ambrisentan monotherapy, the improvement in 6MWT at 12 weeks was 40 meters and maintained at 39 meters. Although there were no patients with elevations in serum aminotransferases > 3 times upper limit of

*Sitaxsentan was withdrawn in December 2010.

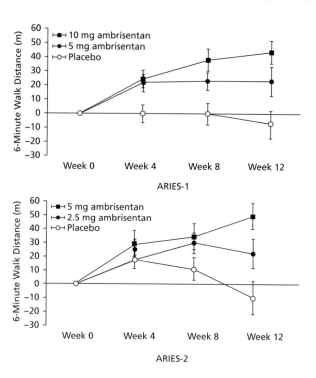

Figure 16.4.2 Effects of ambrisentan vs. placebo on 6-minute walk distance, from the two pivotal trials. (From ref 57.)

normal while on ambrisentan, in the trials, long-term follow-up has revealed cases of transaminase elevations which resolve upon discontinuation of ambrisentan.

Sitaxsentan

Sitaxsentan, a selective ETA receptor antagonist was studied in two pivotal randomized, controlled studies (58,59). The first trial, STRIDE 1, failed to demonstrate a benefit of this agent on the primary endpoint of improvement in maximal oxygen consumption (58). The STRIDE 2 study, which used 6-minute walk distance as the primary endpoint, was significant, with a placebo-corrected improvement of 31 meters (59). Subgroup analysis has shown a benefit of sitaxsentan in patients with PAH associated with connective tissue diseases (60). Sitaxsentan was not approved by the Food and Drug Administration (FDA), but did receive approval in other countries, including Canada and the European Union.

Bosentan

Bosentan is a potent, non-peptide, oral endothelin A and B receptor antagonist, with higher affinity for the ET_A subtype receptor. Bosentan received FDA approval in November 2001 for patients with WHO functional class III or IV PAH. The first double-blind, placebo-controlled trial randomized 32 patients with IPAH (84 percent) or PH associated with scleroderma with NYHA class III to bosentan or placebo for 12 weeks (61). The primary endpoint was the

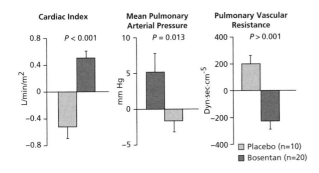

Figure 16.4.3 Hemodynamic effects of bosentan vs. placebo from study 351. (From ref 61.)

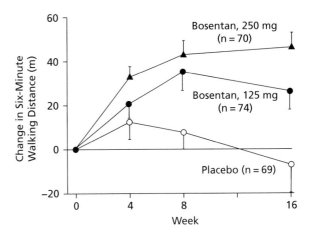

Figure 16.4.4 Change in 6-minute walk distance in patients treated with bosentan 125 mg bid compared to placebo. (From ref 62.)

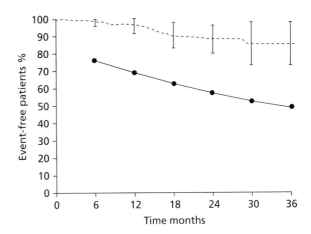

Figure 16.4.5 Survival in patients treated with first-line bosentan in two pivotal trials, compared to predicted survival. (From ref 65.)

placebo-corrected change in 6MWT, with secondary endpoints including change in pulmonary hemodynamics, WHO functional class, Borg dyspnea index and clinical worsening. The placebo-corrected improvement in 6MWT was 76 meters in favor of the bosentan group. In addition, pulmonary hemodynamics, especially cardiac index and pulmonary vascular resistance were favorably affected by bosentan (Figure 16.4.3). There were asymptomatic increases in liver aminotransferases in two patients on bosentan, but these returned to baseline without discontinuing or changing the dose.

The larger BREATHE-1 (bosentan randomized trial of endothelin antagonist therapy) trial, which randomized 213 patients with IPAH (70 percent) and pulmonary hypertension associated with connective tissue disease with WHO functional class III and IV to placebo or bosentan at 125 mg or 250 mg twice daily, confirmed the efficacy and safety of bosentan over 16 weeks (62). At 16 weeks, a placebo-corrected 6MWD improvement of 44 meters was noted ($P < 0.001$). There were also improvements in the Borg dyspnea score and time to clinical worsening in both bosentan groups. Increases in liver aminotransferases greater than eight times upper limit of normal was again noted in the bosentan group and was dose-dependent with two patients in the 125 mg group and five patients in the 250 mg group.

In addition to the above "pivotal" trials of bosentan, a recently published RCT of bosentan in PAH patients less functional impaired (WHO Class II), the EARLY trial demonstrated a benefit in reducing pulmonary vascular resistance and preventing clinical worsening at 6 months. No statistically significant effect on 6-minute walk distance was seen, although baseline walk distance was greater than 400 meters, confirming that this cohort had better baseline exercise capacity (63).

Bosentan has also been studied in a controlled fashion in patients with congenital heart disease (64). The BREATHE 5 study demonstrated that, compared to placebo, bosentan improved 6-minute walk distance without worsening hypoxemia.

Long-term survival data in patients on bosentan, although uncontrolled, have been published. Of the 169 IPAH patients enrolled in the two pivotal trials of bosentan, estimated survival at 1 and 2 years was 96 percent and 89 percent, respectively, as compared to the predicted survival of 69 percent and 57 percent (65) (based on a validated NIH equation calculating predicted survival from baseline hemodynamics). It should be acknowledged that there are no prospective controlled survival data with the newer agents, given obvious ethical concerns about such trials in the era of existing therapy.

FUTURE DIRECTIONS

The next steps in the research of endothelin receptor antagonists for the therapy of PAH appear to have great promise. Questions which remain to be answered include the role of endothelin receptor antagonists in: (a) long-term efficacy on morbidity and mortality of ERAs in combination with other agents; (b) upfront combination therapies, for example with epoprostenol or sildenafil; and (c) expanded disease indications, such as CTEPH or fibrotic lung disease.

The ease of oral administration and relatively well-tolerated side effect profile of endothelin receptor antagonists will likely allow them to provide continued advances in the therapy of a range of diseases of the pulmonary circulation.

KEY POINTS

- Endothelin receptor antagonists (ETRA) were the first orally available therapies for PAH and remain the mainstay of treatment.
- ETRA may be selective for A or B endothelin receptors or non-selective. At present there is no clear advantage for selectivity.
- All ETRA carry the risk of liver failure and patients must therefore have monthly liver function tests. Sitaxsentan has now been withdrawn because of unacceptable liver toxicity.

REFERENCES

1. Yanagisawa M *et al*. A novel potent vasoconstrictor peptide produced by vascular endothelial cells. Nature 1988;332: 411–5.
2. Inoue A *et al*. The human endothelin family: three structurally and pharmacologically distinct isopeptides predicted by three separate genes. Proceedings of the Natl Acad Sci USA 1989;86:2863–7.
3. Takasaki C *et al*. Sarafotoxins S6: several isotoxins from Atractaspis engaddensis (burrowing asp) venom that affect the heart. Toxicon 1988;26(6):543–8.
4. Mattoli S *et al*. Specific binding of endothelin on human bronchial smooth muscle cells in culture and secretion of endothelin-like material from bronchial epithelial cells. Am J Respir Cell Mol Biol 1990;3:145–51.
5. Yu J, Davenport A. Secretion of endothelin-1 and endothelin-3 by human cultured vascular smooth muscle cells. Br J Pharmacol 1995;114:551–7.
6. Ehrenreich H *et al*. Endothelins, peptides with potent vasoactive properties, are produced by human macrophages. J Exp Med 1990;172:1741–8.
7. Miyauchi T, Masaki T. Pathophysiology of endothelin in the cardiovascular system. Ann Rev Physiol 1999;61:391–415.
8. Michael J, Markewitz B. Endothelins and the lung. Am J Respir Crit Care Med 1996;154:555–81.
9. Benigni A, Remuzzi G. Endothelin antagonists. Lancet 1999;353:133–8.
10. Masaki T. The discovery of endothelins. Cardiovasc Res 1998;39:530–3.
11. Shinmi O *et al*. Endothelin-3 is a novel neuropeptide: isolation and sequence determination of endothelin-1 and endothelin-3 in porcine brain. Biochem Biophys Res Commun 1989;164(1):587–93.
12. Levin E. Endothelins. N Engl J Med 1995;333(6):356–63.
13. Nakamura S *et al*. Immunocytochemical localization of endothelin in cultured bovine endothelial cells. Histochemistry 1990;94:475–7.
14. Inoue A *et al*. The human preproendothelin-1 gene. J Biol Chem 1989;264(25):14954–9.
15. Yoshimoto S *et al*. Effect of carbon dioxide and oxygen on endothelin production by cultured porcine cerebral endothelial cells. Stroke 1991;22:378–83.
16. Takuwa Y *et al*. Endothelin receptor is coupled to phospholipase C via pertussis toxin insensitive guanine nucleotide binding regulatory protein in vascular smooth muscle cells. J Clin Invest 1990;85:653–8.
17. Benigni A. Defining the role of endothelins in renal pathophysiology on the basis of selective and unselective endothelin receptor antagonist studies. Curr Opin Nephrol Hypertens 1995;4:349–53.
18. Iwamuro Y *et al*. Activation of three types of voltage-independent Ca^{2+} channel in A7r5 cells by endothelin-1 as revealed by a novel Ca^{2+} channel blocker LOE 908. Br J Pharmacol 1999;126:1107–14.
19. Clarke J *et al*. Endothelin is a potent long-lasting vasoconstrictor in men. Am J Physiol 1989;257:H2033–5.
20. Chua B *et al*. Endothelin stimulates protein synthesis in smooth muscle cells. Am J Physiol 1992;262:E412–6.
21. Davie N *et al*. ETA and ETB receptors modulate the proliferation of human pulmonary artery smooth muscle cells. Am J Respir Crit Care Med 2002;165:398–405.
22. Sugawara F *et al*. Endothelin-1-induced mitogenic responses of Chinese hamster ovary cells expressing human endothelin A: the role of a wortmannin-sensitive signalling pathway. Mol Pharmacol 1996;49(3):447–57.
23. Sakurai T *et al*. Cloning of a cDNA encoding a non-isopeptide-selective subtype of the endothelin receptor. Nature 1990;348:732–5.
24. Hirata Y, Emori T, Eguchi S. Endothelin receptor subtype B mediates synthesis of nitric oxide by cultured bovine endothelial cells. J Clin Invest 1993;91:1367–3.
25. De Nucci G *et al*. Pressor effects of circulating endothelin are limited by its removal in the pulmonary circulation and by the release of prostacyclin and endothelium-derived relaxing factor. Proc Natl Acad Science USA 1988;85: 9797–800.
26. Filep J *et al*. Antiaggregatory and hypotensive effects of endothelin-1 in beagle dogs: role for prostacyclin. J Cardiovasc Pharmacol 1991;17(Suppl 7):S216–8.
27. Dupuis J, Goresky C, Fournier A. Pulmonary clearance of circulating endothelin-1 in dogs in vivo: exclusive role of ETB receptors. J Appl Physiol 1996;81(4):1510–5.
28. Dupuis J *et al*. Human pulmonary circulation is an important site for both clearance and production of endothelin-1. Circulation 1996;94:1578–84.
29. Masaki T. Possible role of endothelin in endothelial regulation of vascular tone. Ann Rev Pharmacol Toxicol 1995;35:235–55.
30. Dupuis J *et al*. Importance of local production of endothelin-1 and of the ETB receptor in the regulation of pulmonary vascular tone. Pulm Pharmacol Therapeut 2000;13:135–40.

31. Kuc R, Davenport A. Endothelin-A-receptors in human aorta and pulmonary arteries are downregulated in patients with cardiovascular disease: an adaptive response to increased levels of endothelin-1? J Cardiovasc Pharmacol 2000;36(Suppl 1):S377–9.

32. Stewart D et al. Increased plasma endothelin-1 in pulmonary hypertension: marker or mediator of disease? Ann Intern Med 1991;114:464–9.

33. Giaid A et al. Expression of endothelin-1 in the lungs of patients with pulmonary hypertension. N Engl J Med 1993;328:1732–9.

34. Giaid A. Nitric oxide and endothelin-1 in pulmonary hypertension. Chest 1998;114(3):S208–12.

35. Langleben D et al. Continuous infusion of epoprostenol improves the net balance between pulmonary endothelin-1 clearance and release in primary pulmonary hypertension. Circulation 1999;99:3266–71.

36. Chen Y, Oparil S. Endothelin and pulmonary hypertension. J Cardiovasc Pharmacol 2000;35(Suppl 2):S49–53.

37. Chen S et al. The orally active nonpeptide endothelin A-receptor antagonist A-127722 prevents and reverses hypoxia-induced pulmonary hypertension and pulmonary vascular remodelling in Sprague–Dawley rats. J Cardiovasc Pharmacol 1997;29:713–25.

38. Eddahibi S et al. Protection from pulmonary hypertension with an orally active endothelin receptor antagonist in hypoxic rats. Am J Physiol 1995;268:H828–35.

39. Takahashi H et al. Upregulation of ET-1 and its receptors and remodelling in small pulmonary veins under hypoxic conditions. Am J Physiol 2001;280:L1104–14.

40. Takahashi H et al. Discrepant distribution of big endothelin (ET)-1 and ET receptors in the pulmonary artery. Eur Respir J 2001;18:5–14.

41. Bando K et al. Dynamic changes of endothelin-1, nitric oxide, and cyclic GMP in patients with congenital heart disease. Circulation 1997;96(9 Suppl): II 346–51.

42. Ishikawa S et al. Elevated levels of plasma endothelin-1 in young patients with pulmonary hypertension caused by congenital heart disease are decreased after successful surgical repair. J Thorac Cardiovasc Surg 1995;110:271–3.

43. Lutz J et al. Endothelin-1 and endothelin receptors in lung biopsies of patients with pulmonary hypertension due to congenital heart disease. Clin Chem Lab Med 1999;37(4):423–8.

44. Allen S et al. Circulating immunoreactive endothelin-1 in children with pulmonary hypertension. Association with acute hypoxic pulmonary vasoreactivity. Am Rev Respir Dis 1993;148:519–22.

45. Kim H et al. Endothelin mediates pulmonary vascular remodelling in a canine model of chronic embolic pulmonary hypertension. Eur Respir J 2000;15:640–8.

46. Kim H et al. Pulmonary vascular remodeling distal to pulmonary artery ligation is accompanied by upregulation of endothelin receptors and nitric oxide synthase. Exp Lung Res 2000;26(4):287–301.

47. Bauer M et al. Selective upregulation of endothelin B receptor gene expression in severe pulmonary hypertension. Circulation 2002;105:1034–6.

48. Ivy D et al. Increased lung preproET-1 and decreased ETB receptor gene expression in fetal pulmonary hypertension. Am J Physiol 1998;274:L535–41.

49. Ivy D, Kinsella J, Abman S. Physiologic characterization of endothelin A and B receptor activity in the ovine fetal pulmonary circulation. J Clin Invest 1994;93:2141–8.

50. Okazaki T et al. Pulmonary vascular balance in congenital diaphragmatic hernia: enhanced endothelin-1 gene expression as a possible cause of pulmonary vasoconstriction. J Pediatr Surg 1998;33(1):81–4.

51. Shima H et al. Antenatal dexamethasone enhances endothelin receptor B expression in hypoplastic lung in nitrofen-induced diaphragmatic hernia in rats. J Pediatr Surg 2000;35(2):203–7.

52. Christou H. et al. Effect of inhaled nitric oxide on endothelin-1 and cyclic guanosine 5′-monophosphate plasma concentrations in newborn infants with persistent pulmonary hypertension. J Pediatr 1997;130:603–11.

53. Kumar P, Kazzi N, Shankaran S. Plasma immunoreactive endothelin-1 concentrations in infants with persistent pulmonary hypertension of the newborn. Am J Perinatol 1996;13(6):335–41.

54. MacDonald P et al. Endothelin-1 levels in infants with pulmonary hypertension receiving extracorporeal membrane oxygenation. J Perinat Med 1999;27:216–20.

55. Rosenberg A et al. Elevated immunoreactive endothelin-1 levels in newborn infants with persistent pulmonary hypertension. J Pediatr 1993;123:109–14.

56. Galie N, Badesch D, Oudiz R et al. Ambrisentan therapy for pulmonary arterial hypertension. J Am Coll Cardiol 2005;46:529–35.

57. Galie N, Olschewki H, Oudiz RJ et al. Ambrisentan in Pulmonary Arterial Hypertension, Randomized, Double-Blind, Placebo-Controlled, Multicenter, Efficacy Studies (ARIES) Group. Circulation 2008;117(23):3010–9.

58. Barst RJ, Langleben D, Frost A et al.; STRIDE-1 Study Group. Sitaxsentan therapy for pulmonary arterial hypertension. Am J Respir Crit Care Med 2004;169(4):441–7.

59. Barst RJ, Langleben D, Badesch D, Frost A, Lawrence EC, Shapiro S, Naeije R, Galie N; STRIDE-2 Study Group Treatment of pulmonary arterial hypertension with the selective endothelin-A receptor antagonist sitaxsentan. J Am Coll Cardiol 2006;47(10):2049–56.

60. Girgis RE, Frost AE, Hill NS et al. Selective endothelin A receptor antagonism with sitaxsentan for pulmonary arterial hypertension associated with connective tissue disease. Ann Rheum Dis 2007;66(11):1467–72.

61. Channick R et al. Effects of the dual endothelin-receptor antagonist bosentan in patients with pulmonary hypertension: a randomized placebo controlled study. Lancet 2001;358:1119–23.

62. Rubin L et al. Bosentan therapy for pulmonary arterial hypertension. N Engl J Med 2002;346(12):896–903.

63. Galiè N, Rubin LJ, Hoeper M *et al.* Treatment of patients with mildly symptomatic pulmonary arterial hypertension with bosentan (EARLY study): A double-blind, randomized controlled trial. Lancet 2008;37:2093–100.

64. Galiè N, Beghetti M, Gatzoulis MA, Granton J, Berger RM, Lauer A, Chiossi E, Landzberg M; Bosentan Randomized Trial of Endothelin Antagonist Therapy-5 (BREATHE-5) Investigators. Bosentan therapy in patients with Eisenmenger syndrome: a multicenter, double-blind, randomized, placebo-controlled study. Circulation 2006;114(1):48–54.

65. McLaughlin VV, Sitbon O, Badesch DB *et al.* Survival with first-line bosentan in patients with primary pulmonary hypertension. Eur Respir J 2005;25:244–9.

The nitric oxide and cyclic guanosine monophosphate pathway

COLIN CHURCH AND ANDREW PEACOCK

Nitric oxide (NO) is an important signaling molecule which underlies many key biological processes. In recent years its importance in the regulation of cardiovascular hemostasis has become clear and a great deal more about the molecular signaling pathways which are involved has become elucidated.

NITRIC OXIDE SYNTHASES

NO is synthesized from an amino acid L-arginine which is oxidized by one of three isoforms of nitric oxide synthase which differ in their tissue distribution pattern. Endothelial NOS (eNOS or NOS_3) is expressed in the endothelial cells and is the main source of NO in the pulmonary circulation, although under conditions of stress such as inflammatory cytokines, inducible NOS (iNOS or NOS_2) is also upregulated in the pulmonary vasculature [1,2]. The relative contributions have been elegantly demonstrated by knockout mice [3]. The final isoenzyme is neuronal NOS or NOS_1 which is most abundantly found, as its name would suggest, in neurons particularly Purkinje cells in the brain.

NOS are active as homodimers and each subunit has a reductase domain and an oxygenase domain. The production of NO requires a heme moiety binding to the oxygenase domain and there is transfer of molecular oxygen to the L-arginine to produce NO and L-citrulline [2]. Important co-factors in this process include zinc and tetrahydrobiopterin (BH4), the latter of which has a role in the stabilization and prevention of uncoupling of the NOS enzyme which if not prevented can lead to the development of reactive oxygen species [4].

THE CLASSICAL NO PATHWAY

The main target for diffusible NO is the soluble guanylate cyclase (sGC) and can be activated by nanomolar concentrations of NO. These are widely expressed enzymes which when activated convert GTP into the second messenger cyclic GMP (cGMP). These are heterodimers with two subunits – α and β, of which the $\alpha_1\beta_2$ and $\alpha_2\beta_1$ are most well characterized [5]. The smaller β subunit contains an evolutionary conserved amino-terminal heme binding domain which is critical for the sensing of NO [6,7]. However, the $\alpha1$ subunit has been shown to be of particular importance in limiting the degree of pulmonary vascular remodeling seen in mice which are deficient in this subunit [8].

Of further importance to the functioning of the enzyme is that the heme moiety requires a reduced ferrous Fe^{2+} state in order to sense and bind the NO; indeed removal of the ferrous state removes the ability of NO to activate the enzyme [9]. Currently it is felt that the ferrous iron interacts with the four nitrogens of the heme group and a histidine residue on the β-subunit. The binding of NO forms a hexacoordinated unstable complex which leads to cleavage of the heme–histidine bond and this acts as a key molecular switch with conformational change which activates the enzyme (10). Thus the redox state of the cell is an important predictor of the action of NO on the sGC. If there is oxidative stress in the cell with production of free radicals (O_2^- or peroxynitrite) then this can lead to an NO-insensitive sGC and interruption of the normal NO cellular effects such as vasorelaxation (11). As a direct consequence of this agents which increase NO levels will still not be able to stimulate the sGC. The pharmacological importance of this will be explained later with the development of two new classes of agents which can activate sGC independently of NO (so-called sGC activators) or enhance the enzymes sensitivity to low levels of NO (so-called sGC stimulators).

The downstream effects of cGMP are mediated by three biological mechanisms: cGMP-dependent protein kinase (protein kinase G; PKG); cGMP-gated ion channels; and cGMP-regulated phosphodiesterases. There is evidence that depending on the cell type the cGMP leads to vasorelaxation, inhibition of platelet aggregation, antiremodeling (12), promotion of apoptosis, and an anti-inflammatory effect. Particularly in the smooth muscle cell cGMP acts to hyperpolarize the cell membrane and prevent further calcium influx to the cell. It also leads to activation of myosin light chain phosphatase which reduces the sensitivity of the myofilaments to calcium thereby inhibiting contraction. Furthermore PKG inactivates RhoA and the Rho-kinase mediated inhibition of myosin light chain phosphatize (13).

ALTERNATIVE NO PATHWAY

There is increasing evidence that NO can also signal through conversion by oxidation to nitrite or reaction with protein thiol groups to produce so called S-nitrosothiols (SNO). These compounds can act as vasodilators or lead to protein posttranslational modifications and alter cellular function (14,15). New studies have also suggested that these compounds may pay a role in homeostatic control of the peripheral circulation. Perhaps the main scavenger for NO in the pulmonary circulation is hemoglobin and binding of NO to the iron in the heme group leads to its inactivation. SNOs can bind to hemoglobin through a conserved cysteine residue on the β-subunit (reviewed in ref 16). This is favored in the oxygenated state of Hb and once the oxygen is released by the Hb molecule the SNO is also released to other thiol groups. The hypothesis is that the circulating Hb releases the oxygen to hypoxic peripheral tissues and the SNO act as a vasodilatory agent to further increase the delivery of oxygen to those tissues.

In addition nitrite when injected into the peripheral circulation can lead to vasodilation (17). The main source of nitrite may be dietary and the nitrite accumulates in the red blood cell cytoplasm. This then becomes reduced to NO in the periphery and released on the local vasculature resulting in their dilatation. In terms of the pulmonary circulation the red blood cells would be expected to have a vasodilatory effect from release of the nitrite or SNOs (reviewed in ref 2).

Indeed it has been shown that increasing the SNO-Hb content of red blood cells led to a reduction in the pulmonary vascular resistance. The role of this in terms of the balance between hypoxic vasoconstriction and vasodilation in the pulmonary vascular bed is as yet unclear (18).

PHOSPHODIESTERASE BIOLOGY IN PULMONARY VASCULATURE

The control of cGMP signaling is by the action of cGMP-dependent phosphodiesterases (PDE) which act to hydrolyse the second messengers. There are 11 PDE families which have been identified currently and they differ in terms of tissue distribution, the messengers which control them and their resultant actions. PDE1, PDE5 and PDE3/4 seem to be particularly involved in the pulmonary circulation. In particular PDE5 inhibitors sildenafil and tadalafil have made substantial improvements in the treatment of patients with PAH.

PDE1

There are three different isoforms of this calcium/calmodulin responsive enzyme (PDE1A-C) and they can hydrolyse both cGMP and cAMP but with different efficacy. There are further splice variants of these individual isoforms. Studies have shown that in humans with PAH and animal models of PAH and individual pulmonary artery smooth muscle cells there are upregulated levels of PDE1A and PDE1C (19). In proliferating pulmonary artery smooth muscle cells there are elevated levels of PDE1C and inhibition can reduce DNA synthesis and proliferation in these cells (19,20). In addition inhibition of PDE1 using 8-methoxymethyl-isobutyl-1-methylxanthine(8MM-IBMX) has been shown in vivo to improve hemodynamics, right ventricular hypertrophy and pulmonary vascular remodeling in both monocrotaline and chronic hypoxic animal models of PAH (19).

An interesting point to notice is that although sildenafil, the main phosphodiesterase inhibitor in clinical practice, is said to be specific for PDE5 isoenzyme it actually also acts on PDE1 at the therapeutic doses used (21). Thus blockade of PDE1 may become an important concurrent pathway to block in PAH.

PDE3/4

These two isoenzymes are predominantly cAMP selective, although they can act on cGMP. PDE3 has been shown to be present and indeed upregulated in pulmonary vessels in the MCT rat model and PDE3 and 4 have been shown to exist in the cytoplasm of pulmonary artery smooth muscle cells (22). Moreover, experiments using two separate mixed selective PDE3/4 blockers have shown improvement in hemodynamics and pulmonary vascular remodeling in

Color Plates

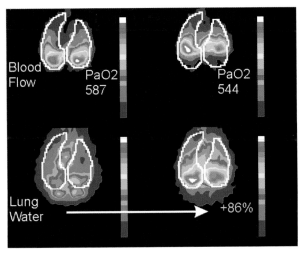

Figure 1.7a

Figure 1.7b

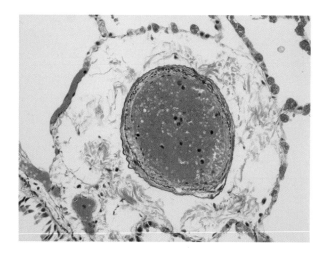

Figure 3.1a

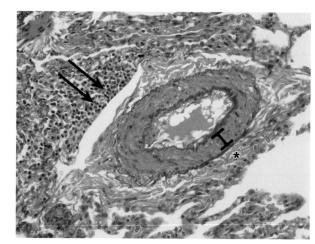

Figure 3.1b

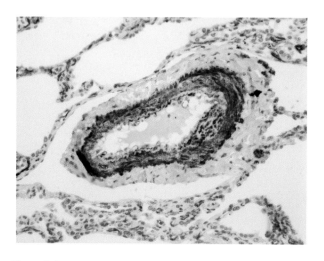

Figure 3.1c

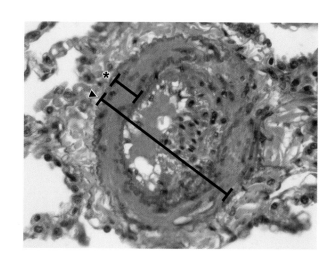

Figure 3.1d

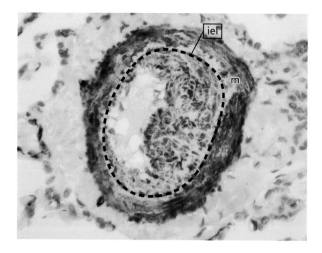

Figure 3.1e

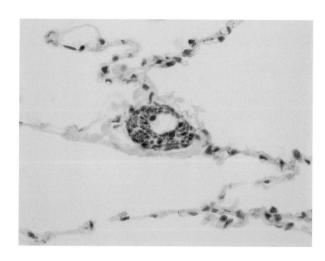

Figure 3.1f

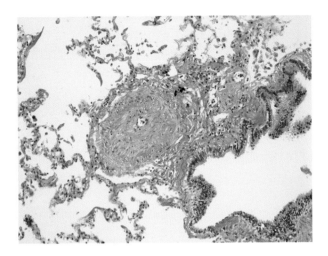

Figure 3.2a

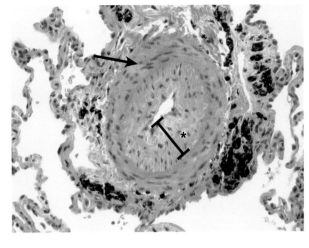

Figure 3.2b

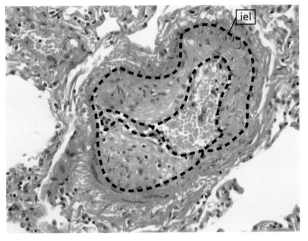

Figure 3.2c

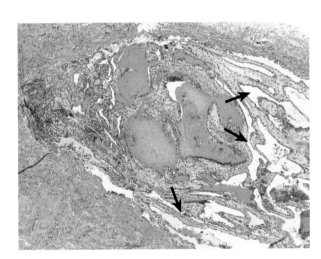

Figure 3.2d

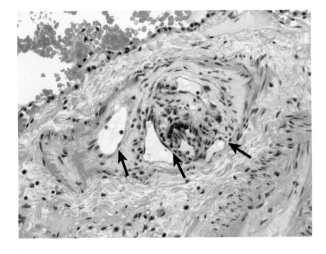

Figure 3.2e

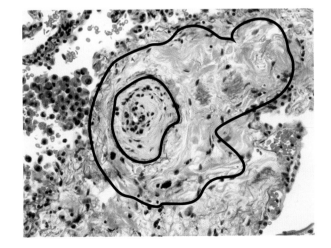

Figure 3.2f

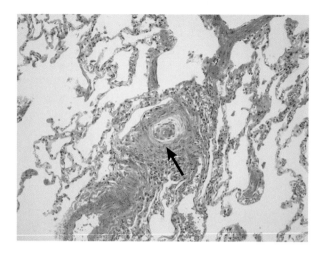

Figure 3.3a

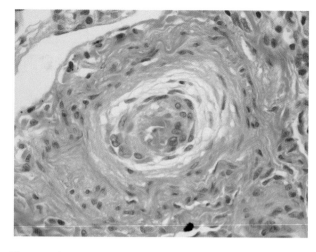

Figure 3.3b

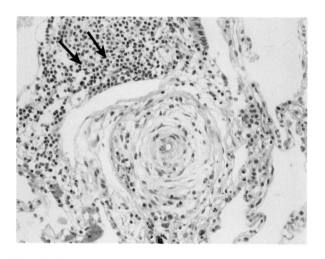

Figure 3.3c

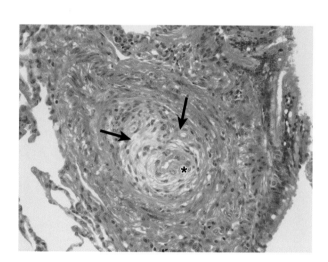

Figure 3.3d

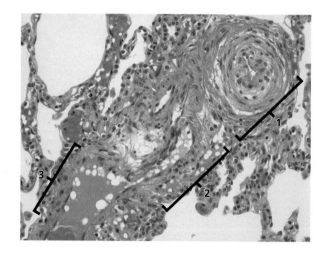

Figure 3.3e

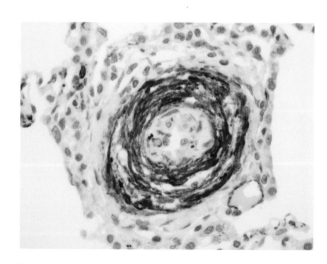

Figure 3.3f

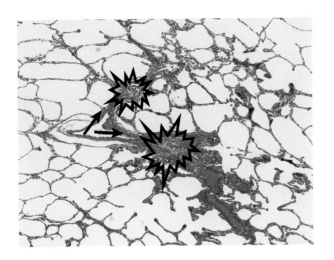

Figure 3.4a

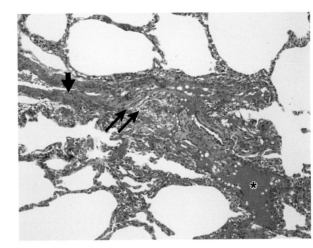

Figure 3.4b

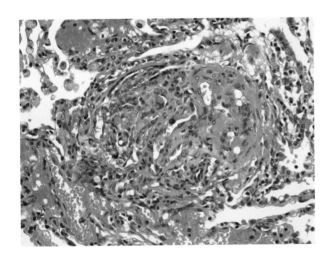

Figure 3.4c

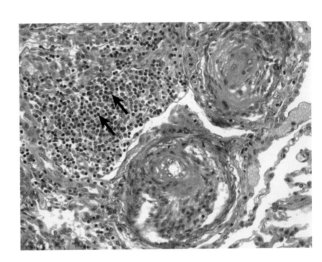

Figure 3.4d

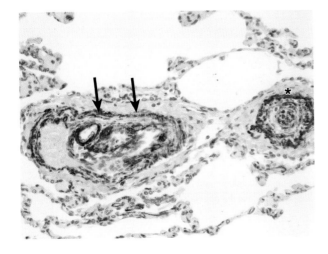

Figure 3.4e

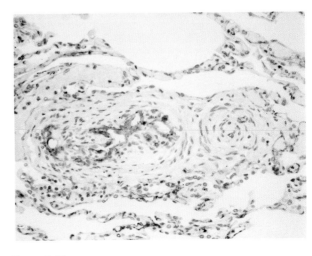

Figure 3.4f

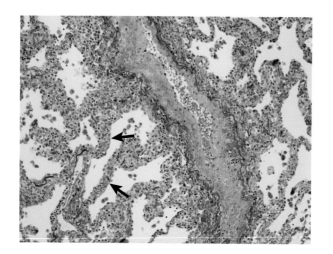

Figure 3.5a

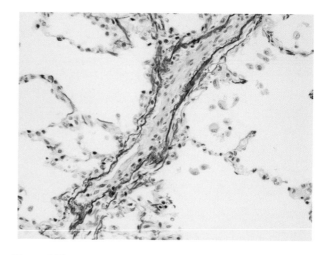

Figure 3.5b

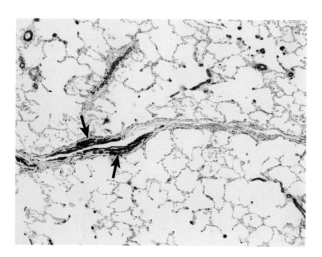

Figure 3.5c

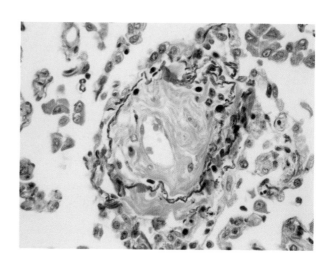

Figure 3.5d

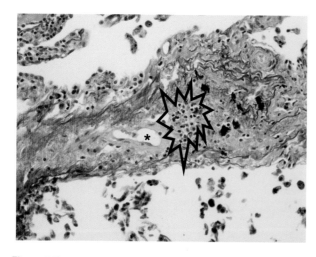

Figure 3.5e

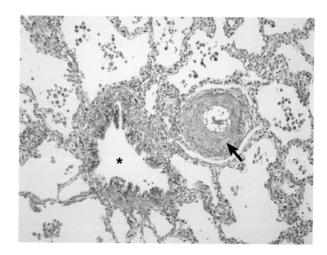

Figure 3.5f

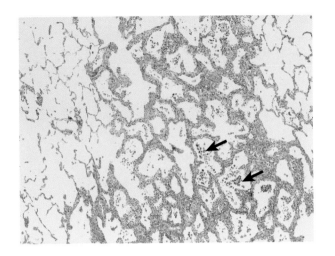

Figure 3.6a

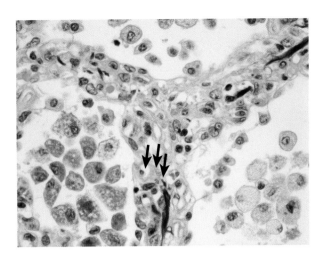

Figure 3.6b

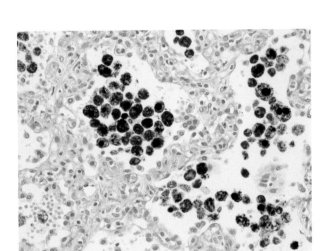

Figure 3.6c

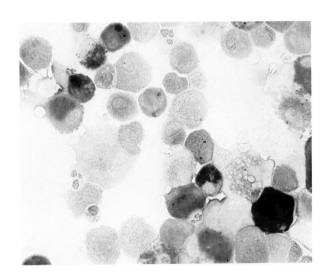

Figure 3.6d

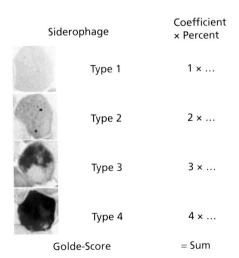

Siderophage	Coefficient × Percent
Type 1	1 × …
Type 2	2 × …
Type 3	3 × …
Type 4	4 × …
Golde-Score	= Sum

Figure 3.6e

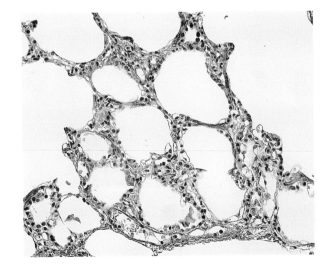

Figure 3.6f

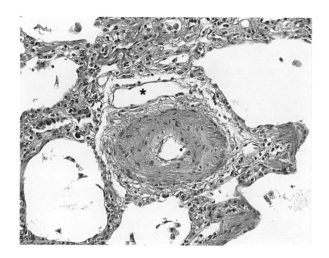

Figure 3.7a

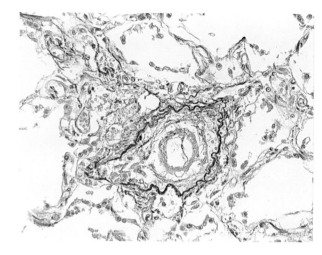

Figure 3.7b

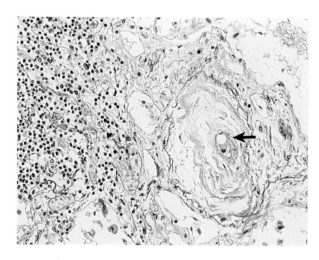

Figure 3.7c

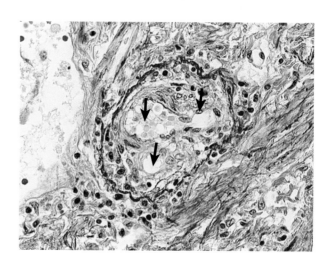

Figure 3.7d

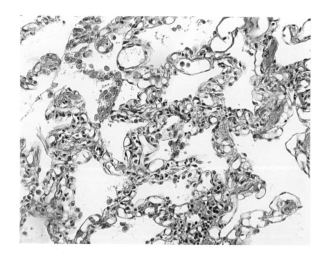

Figure 3.7e

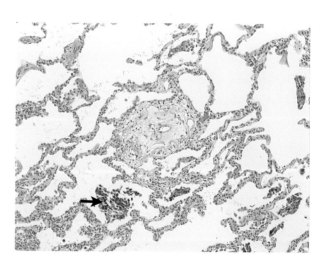

Figure 3.7f

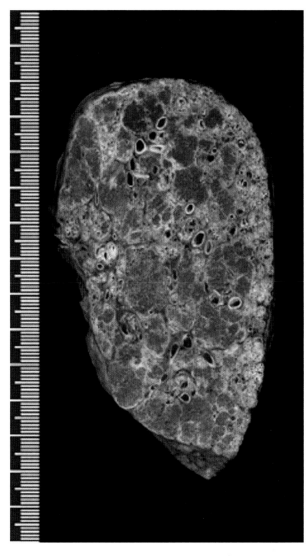

Figure 3.8a

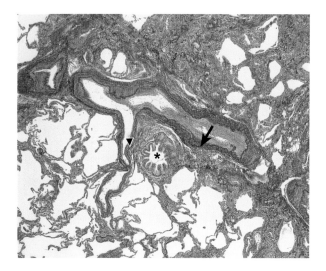

Figure 3.8a2

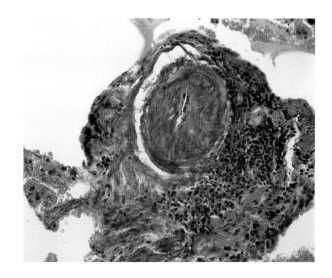

Figure 3.8b

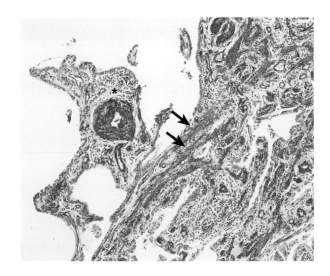

Figure 3.8c

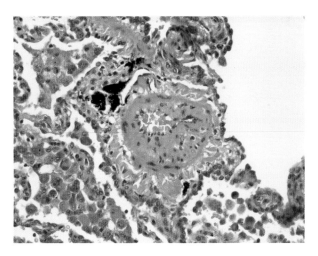

Figure 3.8d

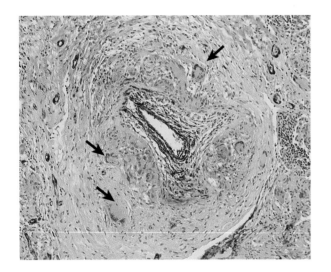

Figure 3.8e

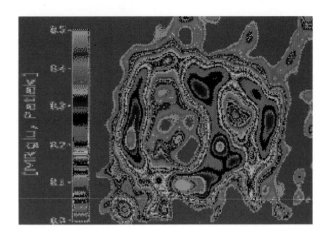

Figure 9.6a

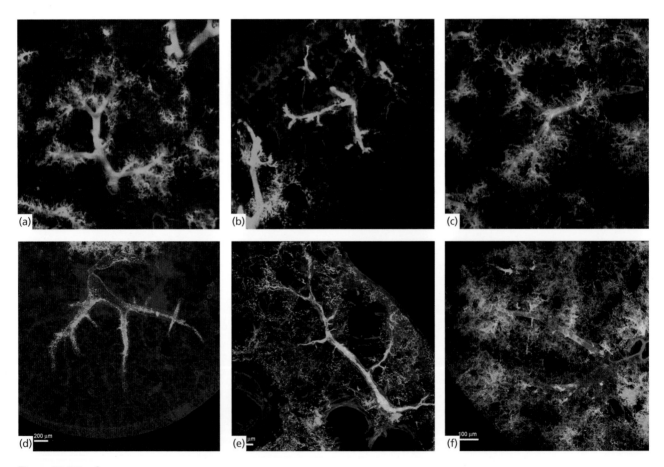

Figure 16.7.2a–f

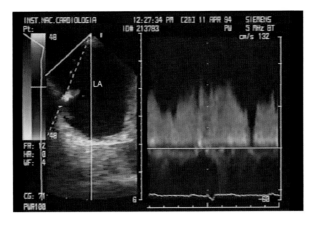

Figure 17.2.5

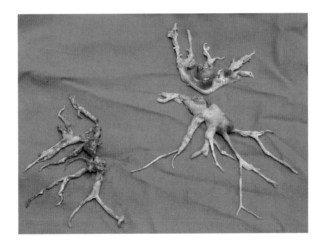

Figure 17.3.4

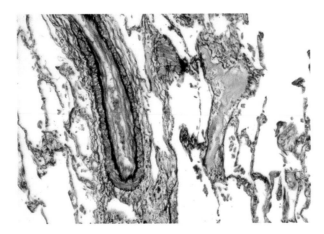

Figure 19.2.3

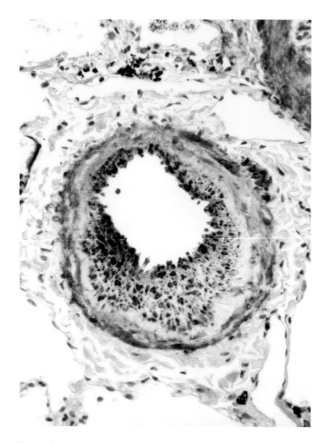

Figure 20.1.3a

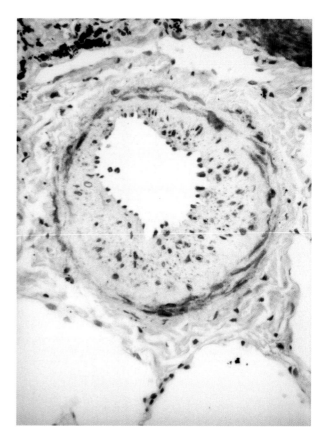

Figure 20.1.3b

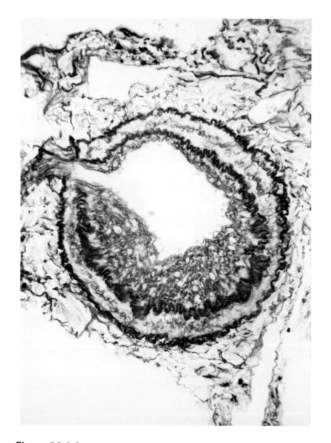

Figure 20.1.3c

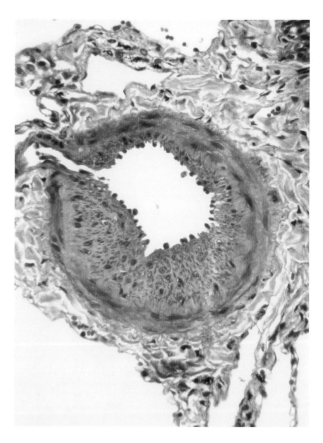

Figure 20.1.3d

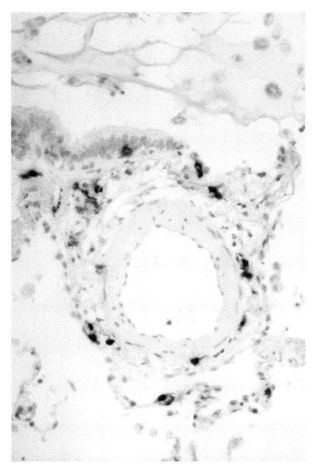

Figure 20.1.3e

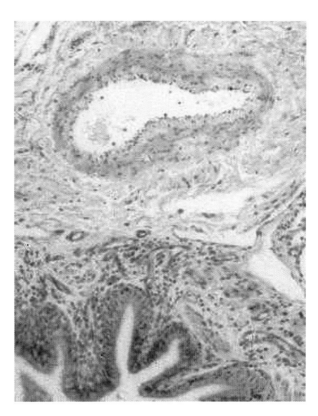

Figure 20.1.3f

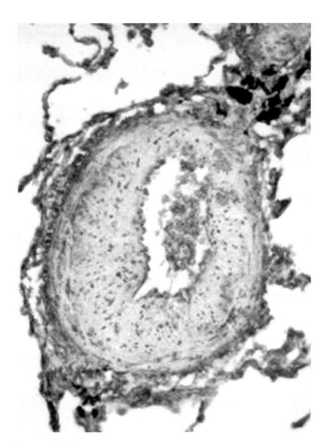

Figure 20.1.3g

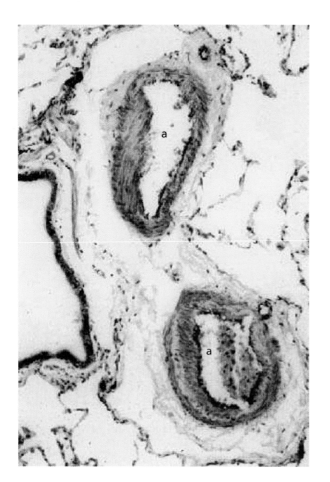

Figure 20.1.3h

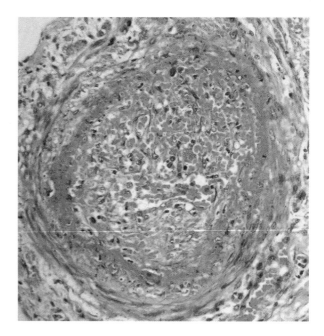

Figure 21.2

the MCT rat (22). However, a recent study has raised concerns that PDE3 inhibitors in chronic usage may increase mortality (23).

PDE5

This enzyme has been the main focus of research and manipulation in terms of the NO pathway in PAH. Similar to other PDE, the enzyme has a conserved catalytic domain at the C-terminus which acts to bind and hydrolyse cGMP. The regulatory domains are found at the N-terminus and contain so-called GAF domains which bind cGMP and result in a 10-fold increase in activation of the enzyme (24). This is an example of positive feedback where the actual substrate of the enzyme can actually activate it. Furthermore the downstream signaling effector of cGMP, PKG, can also phosphorylate a serine residue on the GAF domain and lead to activation of the enzymatic activity.

The gene for PDE5 allows the generation of three splice variants called PDE5A1–3. PDE5 is expressed in most tissues although large levels are identified in vascular smooth muscle and the lung; however there are differences with the splice variants with the PDE5A3 expression being limited to smooth muscle (25). Importantly the level of PDE5 was found to be greater in lung homogenates and laser microdissected pulmonary vessels in patients with PAH (12,19,26). The promoter region of the PDE5 gene also contains cyclic nucleotide responsive binding sites which can allow upregulation of the transcription of the enzyme (27).

The rationale for using PDE5 inhibitors has been established in animal models of PAH, namely the monocrotaline and chronic hypoxic rat model. In isolated rat lungs they inhibit the vasoconstriction induced by hypoxia and thromboxane antagonism (28,30). In both animal models, chronic sildenafil administration has both attenuated the development of pulmonary hypertension and also been used to partially reverse the pathology when used as a treatment strategy (31,32). Furthermore, *in vitro* studies have shown that the cGMP pathway can inhibit cellular proliferation in distal pulmonary artery smooth muscle cells and this can be effected by use of PDE5 blockers such as sildenafil. Evidence of beneficial effects of combination therapy of the PDE5 inhibitors with either prostanoids or endothelin receptor antagonists have also shown been demonstrated (33,34).

PHOSPHODIESTERASE BIOLOGY IN RIGHT VENTRICLE

Initial work on the cardiomyocyte showed that there was very little PDE5 expressed under normal basal conditions and enzyme activity is low (35). Indeed some evidence suggests repression of PDE5 expression during embryonic development (36). However, more recent studies have suggested that this might not be the case and that PDE5 may actually have a physiological role to play (37,38). Indeed PDE5 inhibition can lead to blunting of acute beta-adrenergic stimulation of the heart (39,40). Excitingly, a recent report found that in patients with pulmonary hypertension and right ventricular hypertrophy PDE5 was expressed in higher levels compared to normal hearts in humans and rats (41). Furthermore the inhibition of PDE5 led to elevated cGMP levels and cAMP levels which resulted in a net effect of improving right ventricular function, suggesting a direct effect on the ventricle and therefore a therapeutic role in patients with RV dysfunction (41). It has also been demonstrated that sildenafil can increase the cardiac output compared to inhaled NO, suggesting a direct effect on the RV contractility with sildenafil (42).

In the myocardium there is also believed to be an interaction with the PDE3 enzyme which acts to preferentially reduce levels of cAMP. The increased levels of cGMP generated by the inhibition of PDE5 can lead to inhibition of PDE3 which in turn results in increased cAMP levels and protein kinase A activation. The result is increased ventricular contraction (41).

The investigation of the role of PDE in cardiac function is at an early stage, yet the initial findings are encouraging in that PDE inhibition may help RV function. (For extended review of PDE in cardiovascular function see ref 24.)

NATRIURETIC-MEDIATED cGMP PRODUCTION

The natriuretic peptides ANP, BNP and CNP can also produce cGMP through receptor or particulate-mediated guanylate cyclase. These are transmembrane receptors which have an extracellular domain which binds the NO and an intracellular domain which acts to hydrolyse GTP to cGMP (43,44). Mice lacking one of the natriuretic receptors NPR-A have been shown to demonstrate an extreme response when exposed to a hypoxic environment (45).

RELEVANCE OF NO TO PULMONARY VASCULAR CONTROL AND PULMONARY HYPERTENSION

Various genetic and pharmacological interventions have demonstrated the importance of the NO system in the maintenance and control of the pulmonary vasculature. Genetic knockouts of mice (for example eNOS and GTP-cyclohydrase-1, a key enzyme in BH4 synthesis; refs 46,47) have been implicated in the development of elevated pulmonary pressures. In addition knockout of one allele of DDAH1 (dimethylarginine dimethylaminohydrolase) which is an enzyme involved in the degradation of an endogenous NOS inhibitor called ADMA, has demonstrated an increase in the right ventricular systolic pressure and thickened walls of pulmonary arterioles in mice exposed to hypoxia (48). In normal humans the use of specific NOS antagonists has demonstrated an increase in resting pulmonary vascular resistance (49). Thus it seems clear that NO plays a pivotal role in the homeostasis of pulmonary vascular tone.

Evidence also exists of the importance of lack of NO in the pulmonary system as playing an etiological role in pulmonary hypertension. In animal models there is documented reduction in cGMP activity in the pulmonary vasculature and increasing NO levels in animals can also ameliorate the rise in pulmonary artery pressure (50–52). In humans, studies have shown a lower level of NO in patients with pulmonary hypertension. Patients with idiopathic pulmonary hypertension have lower exhaled breath levels of NO and decreased levels of eNOS have been seen in pulmonary vessels from explanted lungs in IPAH patients, although plexiform lesions do seem to have higher expressed levels (53,54). At altitude the degree in which dwellers are able to maintain or increase their NO levels has been shown to be important in the development of pulmonary hypertension (55). In addition levels of ADMA are higher in patients with IPAH and these are potent NOS inhibitors and may play a role in the elevated pressures (56).

Evidence has also shown that in the disease state homeostatic mechanisms attempt to utilize the NO pathway in order to normalize the pulmonary pressures. For example in patients with IPAH there are higher levels of the natriuretic peptides such as BNP and ANP which are released from the stressed right ventricle and can activate the sGC pathway as described above (57).

These findings described above have provided the rationale for utilizing the NO pathway in pulmonary hypertension.

PHOSPHODIESTERASE INHIBITORS

There are currently three PDE5 inhibitors which have been used to treat pulmonary arterial hypertension: sildenafil, tadalafil and vardenafil (58). Currently the most commonly prescribed is sildenafil. The drugs differ in chemical structure, but also in terms of pharmacokinetics. They all inhibit PDE5 in the nanomolar range.

Sildenafil

PHARMACOKINETICS

Sildenafil is rapidly absorbed orally, although it is subject to first pass metabolism, and has peak effects at 2 hours. It has a plasma half-life of 4 hours and is principally cleared by hepatic metabolism. The cytochrome CYP3A4 is mainly involved in this and interactions with other drugs which inhibit or induce CYP3A4 are seen. Of particular clinical importance are erythromycin, ketoconazole and saquinavir which act to inhibit CYP3A4 while bosentan induces this enzyme and can lead to up to 50 percent reduction in

plasma levels of sildenafil when co-administered (59). Moreover, sildenafil itself is an inhibitor of the CYP3A4 system and as a result in its own right can inhibit bosentan metabolism and increase plasma levels of bosentan. However, it is as yet unclear as to whether these interactions have any clinical relevance. Sildenafil is lipophilic and the bioavailability can be reduced if taken with a high fat meal.

Because of effects of vasodilation in the systemic circulation certain agents should not be co-administered with sildenafil. These principally include nitrates used in management of ischemic heart disease as the combined vasodilatory effect can be significant and lead to syncope.

PHARMACODYNAMICS

Acute effects in PAH

When administered as a single dose sildenafil has been shown to reduce the pulmonary vascular resistance, and the magnitude is dose-dependent (60). It is also relatively selective for the pulmonary circulation with effects similar to inhaled NO although drops in the systemic blood pressure have been seen with high oral doses of sildenafil. Indeed intravenous infusion of up to 40 mg of sildenafil at rest or following maximal exercise can lead to net reduction in systolic systemic pressure by 6 percent (60).

Acute effects on the pulmonary circulation of the three PDE5 agents currently used have been studied. Hemodynamics and oxygenation were measured over 120 minutes following the administration to patients with PAH of varying doses of either sildenafil (50 mg), vardenafil (10 or 20 mg) and tadalafil (20, 40 or 60 mg) (61). It was clear that although all the agents inhibit the same enzyme and caused pulmonary vasodilatation, the effects in terms of clinical response vary amongst them. Vardenafil had the most rapid onset of action, while sildenafil and tadalafil had the most selectivity for the pulmonary circulation.

In combination with inhaled NO, sildenafil augments the pulmonary vasodilatory action of NO showing a greater reduction in the pulmonary vascular resistance than using either agent individually. Furthermore sildenafil prevented the acute hypoxic vasoconstriction which can be seen when inhaled nitric oxide is withdrawn.

Chronic effects in PAH

Sildenafil is a specific PDE5 inhibitor which was originally licensed for erectile dysfunction. However, uncontrolled case reports suggested that patients with PAH benefited from sildenafil.

The initial study to look at the use of sildenafil in PAH came when 22 patients were treated in a prospective randomized double-blind crossover trial. In this trial the exercise capacity as measured by time on the treadmill and hemodynamics as assessed by echocardiography showed a statistically significant improvement (62).

These findings were confirmed in the pivotal sildenafil use in the Pulmonary Arterial Hypertension (SUPER) trial which demonstrated improvement in exercise, functional class and reduction in the mean pulmonary artery pressure (63). A total of 278 patients with either idiopathic, connective tissue disease-related or surgically corrected congenital heart disease-related PAH were randomized to placebo or sildenafil in varying doses (20, 40 or 80 mg three times daily) and followed up for 12 weeks. The primary endpoint in this study was the change in 6-minute walk distance at the end of 12 weeks and all doses of sildenafil showed a statistically significant increase in this parameter ranging from +45–50 m over placebo. In addition all doses improved the hemodynamics including cardiac index and the functional class. However, there was no statistically significant change in terms of incidence of clinical worsening when compared to placebo. Sildenafil in the dosage of 20 mg three times a day was subsequently approved for the treatment of PAH.

However, higher doses were not approved for clinical use. Yet importantly in an open-label study in which 222 patients participated and were all uptitrated to 80 mg three times daily, the benefit in 6-minute walk was maintained to at least 12 months. The long-term outcome in patients on 20 mg is not clear. Furthermore the hemodynamic improvements seen in the SUPER-1 study were dose-dependent with the greatest fall in pulmonary vascular resistance being in the 80 mg group. Thus some physicians continue to increase the sildenafil dosage up to 80 mg three times daily in their patients when they become less well, although this remains an "off-label" use (64).

In a direct head-to-head comparison trial of sildenafil versus bosentan there were found to be no significant differences between the treatment groups in terms of 6-minute walk distance, echocardiography and plasma BNP (65). However, patients in the sildenafil group had a reduction in the mass of the right ventricle as compared to the bosentan group when assessed by cardiac MRI. The clinical relevance is unclear, but as described above there is increasing evidence that PDE5 may play an important role in cardiac function.

Along with the PAH conditions included in the above trials, sildenafil has been investigated in portopulmonary hypertension. In agreement with some case reports, a retrospective study has shown that patients on sildenafil improved their 6-minute walk distance at 3 and 12 months (66). This was accompanied with a fall in the level in NT-proBNP. Interestingly the PDE5 inhibitors may also have a direct effect on the portal hypertension, with vardenafil and tadalafil having been shown to reduce the hepatovenous pressure gradient (67,68).

Sildenafil is very well tolerated with 86 percent completing the 1-year open-label study. Side effects include flushing, epistaxis, heartburn and headache. There is a potential interaction with bosentan in the route of metabolism (see above) and the drug exacerbates hypotension caused by nitrates so should be avoided in patients receiving nitrates. There is a risk of visual problems such as blurred vision, altered color perception, developing which is reflected by the action of sildenafil on PDE type 6 which is predominantly expressed in retinal tissue. This is reported in 7 percent of patients who were taking the higher dose of 80 mg (69).

SILDENAFIL IN CHRONIC THROMBOEMBOLIC PULMONARY HYPERTENSION

There have been a few studies which have suggested that sildenafil can improve symptoms and hemodynamics in patients who have inoperable chronic thromboembolic pulmonary hypertension (CTEPH). Pathological analysis of patients with inoperable CTEPH have shown similar changes to those patients with IPAH, thus giving a rationale for using disease-targeted therapy. In a pilot randomized double-blind placebo-controlled study in 19 patients at 12 months there were improvements seen in terms of pulmonary vascular resistance, cardiac index, and 6-minute walk test in those treated with sildenafil (70).

Similarly, an open-label study of sildenafil 50 mg three times a day showed an improvement in 6-minute walk distance at 3 and 12 months of treatment in 104 patients (71). In addition, pulmonary vascular resistance was found to be lower at 3 months.

Taken together, these studies have shown that sildenafil can be an appropriate treatment for patients with chronic thromboembolic disease.

Tadalafil and PAH

Tadalafil is a selective PDE5 inhibitor and has a longer half-life of 17.5 hours compared to sildenafil. As such it has a once-daily pharmacokinetic profile which is more likely to be favored by patients. Initial case reports suggested efficacy in the treatment of PAH (72).

The PHIRST trial was a double-blind placebo-controlled multicenter trial which tested the effect of four different dosage schemes (2.5, 10, 20, 40 mg) of tadalafil on patients with IPAH or connective tissue disease-related PAH and used change in 6-minute walk as a primary endpoint (73). A total of 405 patients were followed up for 16 weeks. Tadalafil increased the 6-minute walk distance when compared to placebo by 33 m overall, but this only reached the predetermined level of statistical significance in the 40 mg dose. Treatment-naive patients improved by 44 m, while those patients who were already on bosentan increased their distance by 23 m.

Statistically significant improvements were also seen in quality of life scores and importantly in the time to clinical worsening, which is being proposed as a primary endpoint for future PAH clinical trials. However, no effect was seen on functional class. In terms of hemodynamics mean pulmonary artery pressure, pulmonary vascular resistance and cardiac index all improved and the drug was well tolerated with only headaches, flushing and myalgia being reported as significant adverse effects. As many as 83 percent of patients who had been enrolled were followed up to 10 months on treatment and showed that the 6-minute walk distance improvement was maintained. The improvement in quality of life parameters has been shown in other analyses (74).

This trial is interesting for a number of reasons. It again confirms the efficacy of PDE5 inhibitors in treatment of pulmonary hypertension. It probably also represents the last placebo-controlled trial which will be conducted in PAH as ethically this is now unacceptable. In addition the trial included a large cohort (53 percent) of patients who were already established on an endothelin receptor antagonist and with the addition of tadalafil received sequential combination therapy. These patients further improved their 6-minute walk distance despite being on disease-targeted therapy, suggesting perhaps further rationale to the use of combination therapy in PAH.

Vardenafil and PAH

Vardenafil is a more potent inhibitor of PDE5, but has only recently become a focus of attention in PAH (61). It has also been shown to produce vasorelaxation of isolated vascular rings through an inhibitory effect on calcium channels in vascular smooth muscle separate from the PDE5 inhibition (75). This effect has not been seen in sildenafil or tadalafil.

Initial clinical studies with vardenafil in five patients with pulmonary arterial hypertension suggested that hemodynamics may be improved over 3 months of treatment (76). As mentioned previously, Ghofrani had showed that in the acute administration of vardenafil there did not seem to be any pulmonary selectivity (61). This new study showed that at 3 months in these patients there was a fall in the pulmonary vascular resistance/systemic vascular resistance ratio by 20 percent suggesting with time the effect may become more pulmonary selective (76).

An open-label uncontrolled study of 45 patients with PAH was conducted and has confirmed that at 12 months the pulmonary selectivity remains (77). Furthermore, exercise tolerance measured by 6-minute walk improved by a mean of 70 m at 3 months and this was maintained at 14 months, although this was not corrected by a placebo group. Functional class and hemodynamics also improved.

A further interesting report is that vardenafil acts to increase the number of circulating endothelial progenitor cells in patients with PAH (78). These cells are currently felt to be important in repairing damaged endothelium although recent reports have raised doubts on this and may actually suggest that they could play a role in the disease pathogenesis (79).

SOLUBLE GUANYLATE CYCLASE STIMULATORS/ACTIVATORS

As explained above, the functioning of the soluble guanylate cyclase enzyme in response to NO is dependent on the presence of a reduced ferrous moiety on the heme group in the enzyme. Thus in conditions in which oxidative stress exists such as pulmonary hypertension, the heme group can be oxidized and become unresponsive to NO. Novel dugs have been developed and are now entering clinical trial phase which can stimulate the sGC independent of NO. There are two defined groups – the heme-dependent sGC stimulators which require the heme moiety to be in a reduced state and the heme-independent sGC activators which can still activate the enzyme independent of the redox state of the enzyme.

Heme-dependent sGC stimulators

These agents, of which there are now a number, act by stimulating the sGC in its reduced heme state and also have potent synergistic effects in the presence of NO. They can be viewed as NO sensitizers in that the sGC produces a greater cGMP response for any given concentration of NO when in the presence of the sGC stimulator. The initial drug developed was called YC-1 and now derivatives from this agent (BAY41-2272) and from newer unrelated structural molecules (A-350619) are available (80,81). The exact mechanism of activation by these drugs is unclear, but suggestions include the binding to the catalytic domain of sGC resulting in a conformational change which leads to activation. BAY41-2272 is more potent than YC-181. Infusion of BAY41-2272 into sheep model of persistent pulmonary hypertension of the newborn showed a reduction in the mean pulmonary artery pressure and pulmonary vascular resistance, a finding which was further confirmed in sheep that had been treated with a thromboxane analogue to replicate acute pulmonary hypertension (82,83). Interestingly at higher doses there was systemic vasodilation and increased cardiac output in this model which was abolished by the administration of L-NAME, a NOS inhibitor (83). However, the pulmonary vasodilation effects remained. This suggests that the pulmonary effect of BAY41-2272 may be actually independent of NO, but the systemic effects require endogenous NO. These agents have also shown prolongation of the pulmonary vasodilatory effect of NO. However, this drug did not lead to a fall in the right atrial pressure, a feature which would be attractive in patients with right heat dysfunction (84). As a result, a derivative which did was developed and this is now called Riociguat (BAY63-2521).

These agents have also been tested in animal models of PAH and have shown that the right ventricular systolic pressure and the vascular remodeling can be reduced (84–86). Furthermore, *in vitro* testing has shown that they also have anti-proliferative effects on vascular smooth muscle and reduce the secretion of matrix metalloproteinases (87). This may add an anti-mitogenic and anti-matrix remodeling dimension to these agents. Work is ongoing in this area.

A recent study using larger than clinically relevant doses has demonstrated an inhibitory effect on PDE5 which tantalizingly may suggest a further mechanism by which these agents increase the cGMP levels (88). However, it is unlikely that this will translate into a clinically relevant action.

CLINICAL APPLICATIONS OF SGC STIMULATORS

Riociguat (BAY 63-2521) is a derivative of the drug BAY 41-2272. It has been shown to be efficacious in reducing pulmonary hemodynamics and improved cardiac index in 19 patients with moderate to severe PAH and was well tolerated (89). It also had a more prolonged effect on pulmonary hemodynamics than inhaled NO. These clinical findings have led to the setting up of two clinical trials which are currently recruiting. The CHEST trial (NCT00855465) is a phase III, double-blind, placebo-controlled trial to assess the efficacy and safety in patients with chronic thromboembolic pulmonary hypertension, while PATENT (NCT00810693) will assess these variables in patients with pulmonary arterial hypertension.

Heme-independent sGC activators

These compounds have been found to activate sGC when it has the heme group in its oxidized and therefore NO unresponsive state (83,90). The most potent currently is BAY58-2667 which actually preferentially binds to oxidized sGC with the mechanistic argument that the drug actually replaces the heme moiety and binds directly to the catalytic subunit and activates it. This has been supported by some recent experiments (90). Moreover, the dissociation of the heme group from sGC leads to the degradation of the enzyme and so the binding of these sGC activators helps to stabilize the enzyme.

Furthermore, as seen in the sGC stimulators, these agents can reverse pulmonary vascular remodeling and reduce pulmonary hemodynamics in animal models of PAH. Although NO is not required for the direct activation of the sGC by these drugs it seems endogenous NO is still needed in some role to allow reversal of the PAH animal models. This has been demonstrated by the loss of effects on reversing the pulmonary vascular remodeling when these agents were administered to NOS_3 knockout mice (85).

Importantly it has been shown that these novel agents act on nitrate tolerant vessels. Isolated vessels with time become tolerant to the effects on NO as a result of reduction of NO-responsive nonoxidized sGC11. However, this is the redox state that these agents act on, and so as the sensitivity to NO decreases, the efficacy of the sGC activators increases.

CLINICAL APPLICATIONS OF SGC ACTIVATORS

BAY 28-2667 has been named Cinaciguat, and has been shown to be well tolerated in healthy volunteers with a reduction in the pre and afterload in the cardiovascular system (91). In addition a recently published study has shown favorable effects in patients with pulmonary venous hypertension with a fall in the pulmonary vascular resistance and mean pulmonary artery pressure and increase in cardiac output (92).

KEY POINTS

- The manipulation of the nitric oxide pathway in the treatment of pulmonary hypertension is well established.
- Blockade of phosphodiesterases in the pulmonary vasculature leads to vasorelaxation and may be anti-proliferative.
- Sildenafil has become a recognized first-line therapy for many PAH conditions, although newer PDE5 inhibitors are also now available and in some respects have shown some benefit over sildenafil.
- Novel agents such as the soluble guanylate cyclase activators and stimulators have renewed the interest in the biology of this enzyme and are currently undergoing clinical trials. Time will tell whether these agents will fulfil the promise they have shown in animal models.

REFERENCES

- • = Key primary paper
- ◆ = Major review article

1. Shaul PW, North AJ, Brannon TS et al. Prolonged in vivo hypoxia enhances nitric oxide synthase type I and type III gene expression in adult rat lung. Am J Respir Cell Mol Biol 1995;13(2):167–74.

◆2. Coggins MP, Bloch KD. Nitric oxide in the pulmonary vasculature. Arterioscler Thromb Vasc Biol 2007;27(9): 1877–85.

•3. Fagan KA, Tyler RC, Sato K et al. Relative contributions of endothelial, inducible, and neuronal NOS to tone in the murine pulmonary circulation. Am J Physiol 1999; 277(3 Pt 1):L472–8.

4. Venema RC, Ju H, Zou R, Ryan JW, Venema VJ. Subunit interactions of endothelial nitric-oxide synthase. Comparisons to the neuronal and inducible nitric-oxide synthase isoforms. J Biol Chem 1997;272(2):1276–82.

5. Zabel U, Weeger M, La M, Schmidt HH. Human soluble guanylate cyclase: functional expression and revised isoenzyme family. Biochem J 1998;335(Pt 1):51–7.

•6. Pellicena P, Karow DS, Boon EM, Marletta MA, Kuriyan J. Crystal structure of an oxygen-binding heme domain related to soluble guanylate cyclases. Proc Natl Acad Sci USA 2004;101(35):12854–9.

7. Iyer LM, Anantharaman V, Aravind L. Ancient conserved domains shared by animal soluble guanylyl cyclases and bacterial signaling proteins. BMC Genom 2003;4(1):5.

•8. Vermeersch P, Buys E, Pokreisz P et al. Soluble guanylate cyclase-alpha1 deficiency selectively inhibits the pulmonary vasodilator response to nitric oxide and increases the pulmonary vascular remodeling response to chronic hypoxia. Circulation 2007;116(8):936–43.

9. Ignarro LJ, Adams JB, Horwitz PM, Wood KS. Activation of soluble guanylate cyclase by NO-hemoproteins involves NO-heme exchange. Comparison of heme-containing and heme-deficient enzyme forms. J Biol Chem 1986;261(11): 4997–5002.

10. Ignarro LJ, Wood KS, Wolin MS. Activation of purified soluble guanylate cyclase by protoporphyrin IX. Proc Natl Acad Sci USA 1982;79(9):2870–3.

•11. Stasch JP, Schmidt PM, Nedvetsky PI et al. Targeting the heme-oxidized nitric oxide receptor for selective vasodilatation of diseased blood vessels. J Clin Invest 2006;116(9):2552–61.

12. Wharton J, Strange JW, Moller GM et al. Antiproliferative effects of phosphodiesterase type 5 inhibition in human pulmonary artery cells. Am J Respir Crit Care Med 2005;172(1):105–13.

13. Sauzeau V, Le Jeune H, Cario-Toumaniantz C et al. Cyclic GMP-dependent protein kinase signaling pathway inhibits RhoA-induced Ca^{2+} sensitization of contraction in vascular smooth muscle. J Biol Chem 2000;275(28): 21722–9.

14. Kim-Shapiro DB, Schechter AN, Gladwin MT. Unraveling the reactions of nitric oxide, nitrite, and hemoglobin in physiology and therapeutics. Arterioscl Thromb Vasc Biol 2006;26(4):697–705.

15. Hess DT, Matsumoto A, Kim SO, Marshall HE, Stamler JS. Protein S-nitrosylation: purview and parameters. Nat Rev Mol Cell Biol 2005;6(2):150–66.

16. Gaston B, Singel D, Doctor A, Stamler JS. S-nitrosothiol signaling in respiratory biology. Am J Respir Crit Care Med 2006;173(11):1186–93.

•17. Cosby K, Partovi KS, Crawford JH et al. Nitrite reduction to nitric oxide by deoxyhemoglobin vasodilates the human circulation. Nature Med 2003;9(12):1498–505.

18. McMahon TJ, Ahearn GS, Moya MP et al. A nitric oxide processing defect of red blood cells created by hypoxia: deficiency of S-nitrosohemoglobin in pulmonary hypertension. Proc Natl Acad Sci USA 2005;102(41):14801–6.

19. Schermuly RT, Pullamsetti SS, Kwapiszewska G et al. Phosphodiesterase 1 upregulation in pulmonary arterial hypertension: target for reverse-remodeling therapy. Circulation 2007;115(17):2331–9.

20. Rybalkin SD, Rybalkina I, Beavo JA, Bornfeldt KE. Cyclic nucleotide phosphodiesterase 1C promotes human arterial smooth muscle cell proliferation. Circulation Res 2002;90(2):151–7.

◆21. Wilkins MR, Wharton J, Grimminger F, Ghofrani HA. Phosphodiesterase inhibitors for the treatment of pulmonary hypertension. Eur Respir J 2008;32(1):198–209.

22. Dony E, Lai YJ, Dumitrascu R et al. Partial reversal of experimental pulmonary hypertension by phosphodiesterase-3/4 inhibition. Eur Respir J 2008;31(3):599–610.

23. Amsallem E, Kasparian C, Haddour G, Boissel JP, Nony P. Phosphodiesterase III inhibitors for heart failure. Cochrane database of systematic reviews (Online) 2005(1):CD002230.

◆24. Kass DA, Champion HC, Beavo JA. Phosphodiesterase type 5: expanding roles in cardiovascular regulation. Circulation Res 2007;101(11):1084–95.

25. Lin CS, Chow S, Lau A, Tu R, Lue TF. Human PDE5A gene encodes three PDE5 isoforms from two alternate promoters. Internatl J Impotence Res 2002;14(1): 15–24.

26. Corbin JD, Beasley A, Blount MA, Francis SH. High lung PDE5: a strong basis for treating pulmonary hypertension with PDE5 inhibitors. Biochem Biophys Res Commun 2005;334(3):930–8.

27. Lin CS, Chow S, Lau A, Tu R, Lue TF. Identification and regulation of human PDE5A gene promoter. Biochem Biophys Res Commun 2001;280(3):684–92.

•28. Cohen AH, Hanson K, Morris K et al. Inhibition of cyclic 3'-5'-guanosine monophosphate-specific phosphodiesterase selectively vasodilates the pulmonary circulation in chronically hypoxic rats. J Clin Invest 1996;97(1):172–9.

•29. Zhao L, Mason NA, Morrell NW et al. Sildenafil inhibits hypoxia-induced pulmonary hypertension. Circulation 2001;104(4):424–8.

30. Braner DA, Fineman JR, Chang R, Soifer SJ. M&B 22948, a cGMP phosphodiesterase inhibitor, is a pulmonary vasodilator in lambs. Am J Physiol 1993;264(1 Pt 2): H252–8.

31. Schermuly RT, Kreisselmeier KP, Ghofrani HA et al. Chronic sildenafil treatment inhibits monocrotaline-induced pulmonary hypertension in rats. Am J Respir Crit Care Med 2004;169(1):39–45.

32. Sebkhi A, Strange JW, Phillips SC, Wharton J, Wilkins MR. Phosphodiesterase type 5 as a target for the treatment of hypoxia-induced pulmonary hypertension. Circulation 2003;107(25):3230–5.

33. Itoh T, Nagaya N, Fujii T et al. A combination of oral sildenafil and beraprost ameliorates pulmonary hypertension in rats. Am J Respir Crit Care Med 2004;169(1):34–8.

34. Clozel M, Hess P, Rey M, Iglarz M, Binkert C, Qiu C. Bosentan, sildenafil, and their combination in the monocrotaline model of pulmonary hypertension in rats. Exp Biol Med 2006;231(6):967–73.

35. Corbin J, Rannels S, Neal D et al. Sildenafil citrate does not affect cardiac contractility in human or dog heart. Curr Med Res Opin 2003;19(8):747–52.

36. Sanchez LS, de la Monte SM, Filippov G, Jones RC, Zapol WM, Bloch KD. Cyclic-GMP-binding, cyclic-GMP-specific phosphodiesterase (PDE5) gene expression is regulated during rat pulmonary development. Pediatr Res 1998;43(2):163–8.

•37. Das A, Xi L, Kukreja RC. Phosphodiesterase-5 inhibitor sildenafil preconditions adult cardiac myocytes against necrosis and apoptosis. Essential role of nitric oxide signaling. J Biol Chem 2005;280(13):12944–55.

38. Chen Y, Traverse JH, Hou M, Li Y, Du R, Bache RJ. Effect of PDE5 inhibition on coronary hemodynamics in pacing-induced heart failure. Am J Physiol Heart Circ Physiol 2003;284(5):H1513–20.

39. Takimoto E, Champion HC, Belardi D et al. cGMP catabolism by phosphodiesterase 5A regulates cardiac adrenergic stimulation by NOS3-dependent mechanism. Circulation Res 2005;96(1):100–9.

40. Senzaki H, Smith CJ, Juang GJ et al. Cardiac phosphodiesterase 5 (cGMP-specific) modulates beta-adrenergic signaling in vivo and is down-regulated in heart failure. Faseb J 2001;15(10):1718–26.

•41. Nagendran J, Archer SL, Soliman D et al. Phosphodiesterase type 5 is highly expressed in the hypertrophied human right ventricle, and acute inhibition of phosphodiesterase type 5 improves contractility. Circulation 2007;116(3): 238–48.

42. Tedford RJ, Hemnes AR, Russell SD et al. PDE5A inhibitor treatment of persistent pulmonary hypertension after mechanical circulatory support. Circ Heart Fail 2008;1(4):213–9.

43. Richards AM. Natriuretic peptides: update on peptide release, bioactivity, and clinical use. Hypertension 2007;50(1):25–30.

44. Piggott LA, Hassell KA, Berkova Z, Morris AP, Silberbach M, Rich TC. Natriuretic peptides and nitric oxide stimulate cGMP synthesis in different cellular compartments. J Gen Physiol 2006;128(1):3–14.

45. Zhao L, Mason NA, Strange JW, Walker H, Wilkins MR. Beneficial effects of phosphodiesterase 5 inhibition in pulmonary hypertension are influenced by natriuretic peptide activity. Circulation 2003;107(2):234–7.

46. Steudel W, Ichinose F, Huang PL et al. Pulmonary vasoconstriction and hypertension in mice with targeted disruption of the endothelial nitric oxide synthase (NOS$_3$) gene. Circulation Res 1997;81(1):34–41.

47. Khoo JP, Zhao L, Alp NJ et al. Pivotal role for endothelial tetrahydrobiopterin in pulmonary hypertension. Circulation 2005;111(16):2126–33.

48. Leiper J, Nandi M, Torondel B et al. Disruption of methylarginine metabolism impairs vascular homeostasis. Nature Med 2007;13(2):198–203.

•49. Stamler JS, Loh E, Roddy MA, Currie KE, Creager MA. Nitric oxide regulates basal systemic and pulmonary vascular resistance in healthy humans. Circulation 1994;89(5):2035–40.

50. Champion HC, Bivalacqua TJ, Greenberg SS, Giles TD, Hyman AL, Kadowitz PJ. Adenoviral gene transfer of endothelial nitric-oxide synthase (eNOS) partially restores normal pulmonary arterial pressure in eNOS-deficient mice. Proc Natl Acad Sci USA 2002;99(20):13248–53.

51. Steudel W, Scherrer-Crosbie M, Bloch KD et al. Sustained pulmonary hypertension and right ventricular hypertrophy after chronic hypoxia in mice with congenital deficiency of nitric oxide synthase 3. J Clin Invest 1998;101(11):2468–77.

52. Fagan KA, Fouty BW, Tyler RC et al. The pulmonary circulation of homozygous or heterozygous eNOS-null mice is hyperresponsive to mild hypoxia. J Clin Invest 1999; 103(2):291–9.

53. Girgis RE, Champion HC, Diette GB, Johns RA, Permutt S, Sylvester JT. Decreased exhaled nitric oxide in pulmonary arterial hypertension: response to bosentan therapy. Am J Respir Crit Care Med 2005;172(3):352–7.

54. Mason NA, Springall DR, Burke M et al. High expression of endothelial nitric oxide synthase in plexiform lesions of pulmonary hypertension. J Pathol 1998;185(3):313–8.

55. Beall CM, Laskowski D, Strohl KP et al. Pulmonary nitric oxide in mountain dwellers. Nature 2001;414(6862):411–2.

56. Pullamsetti S, Kiss L, Ghofrani HA et al. Increased levels and reduced catabolism of asymmetric and symmetric dimethylarginines in pulmonary hypertension. Faseb J 2005;19(9):1175–7.

57. Leuchte HH, Holzapfel M, Baumgartner RA et al. Clinical significance of brain natriuretic peptide in primary pulmonary hypertension. J Am Coll Cardiol 2004;43(5): 764–70.

◆58. Archer SL, Michelakis ED. Phosphodiesterase type 5 inhibitors for pulmonary arterial hypertension. N Engl J Med 2009;361(19):1864–71.

59. Paul GA, Gibbs JS, Boobis AR, Abbas A, Wilkins MR. Bosentan decreases the plasma concentration of sildenafil when coprescribed in pulmonary hypertension. Br J Clin Pharmacol 2005;60(1):107–12.

60. Jackson G, Benjamin N, Jackson N, Allen MJ. Effects of sildenafil citrate on human hemodynamics. Am J Cardiol 1999;83(5A):13C–20C.

61. Ghofrani HA, Voswinckel R, Reichenberger F et al. Differences in hemodynamic and oxygenation responses to three different phosphodiesterase-5 inhibitors in patients with pulmonary arterial hypertension: a randomized prospective study. J Am Coll Cardiol 2004;44(7):1488–96.

62. Sastry BK, Narasimhan C, Reddy NK, Raju BS. Clinical efficacy of sildenafil in primary pulmonary hypertension: a randomized, placebo-controlled, double-blind, crossover study. J Am Coll Cardiol 2004;43(7):1149–53.

•63. Galie N, Ghofrani HA, Torbicki A et al. Sildenafil citrate therapy for pulmonary arterial hypertension. N Engl J Med 2005;353(20):2148–57.

64. Hoeper MM, Welte T. Sildenafil citrate therapy for pulmonary arterial hypertension. N Engl J Med 2006;354(10):1091–3; author reply, p. 3.

65. Wilkins MR, Paul GA, Strange JW et al. Sildenafil versus Endothelin Receptor Antagonist for Pulmonary Hypertension (SERAPH) study. Am J Respir Crit Care Med 2005;171(11):1292–7.

66. Reichenberger F, Voswinckel R, Steveling E et al. Sildenafil treatment for portopulmonary hypertension. Eur Respir J 2006;28(3):563–7.

67. Deibert P, Schumacher YO, Ruecker G et al. Effect of vardenafil, an inhibitor of phosphodiesterase-5, on portal

haemodynamics in normal and cirrhotic liver – results of a pilot study. Aliment Pharmacol Therapeut 2006;23(1):121–8.

68. Deibert P, Bremer H, Roessle M, Kurz-Schmieg AK, Kreisel W. PDE-5 inhibitors lower portal and pulmonary pressure in portopulmonary hypertension. Eur Respir J 2007;29(1): 220–1.

69. Agency EM. Revatio: product information. http://wwwemeaeuropaeu 2009.

70. Suntharalingam J, Treacy CM, Doughty NJ et al. Long-term use of sildenafil in inoperable chronic thromboembolic pulmonary hypertension. Chest 2008;134(2):229–36.

•71. Reichenberger F, Voswinckel R, Enke B et al. Long-term treatment with sildenafil in chronic thromboembolic pulmonary hypertension. Eur Respir J 2007;30(5):922–7.

72. de Carvalho AC, Hovnanian AL, Fernandes CJ, Lapa M, Jardim C, Souza R. Tadalafil as treatment for idiopathic pulmonary arterial hypertension. Arq Brasil Cardiol 2006;87(5):e195–7.

•73. Galie N, Brundage BH, Ghofrani HA et al. Tadalafil therapy for pulmonary arterial hypertension. Circulation 2009; 119(22):2894–903.

74. Pepke-Zaba J, Beardsworth A, Chan M, Angalakuditi M. Tadalafil therapy and health-related quality of life in pulmonary arterial hypertension. Curr Med Res Opin 2009;25(10):2479–85.

75. Toque HA, Teixeira CE, Priviero FB, Morganti RP, Antunes E, De Nucci G. Vardenafil, but not sildenafil or tadalafil, has calcium-channel blocking activity in rabbit isolated pulmonary artery and human washed platelets. Br J Pharmacol 2008;154(4):787–96.

76. Aizawa K, Hanaoka T, Kasai H et al. Long-term vardenafil therapy improves hemodynamics in patients with pulmonary hypertension. Hypertens Res 2006;29(2):123–8.

77. Jing ZC, Jiang X, Wu BX et al. Vardenafil treatment for patients with pulmonary arterial hypertension: a multicenter, open-label study. Heart (Br Cardiac Soc) 2009;95(18):1531–6.

78. Foresta C, Lana A, Cabrelle A et al. PDE-5 inhibitor, Vardenafil, increases circulating progenitor cells in humans. Internatl J Impotence Res 2005;17(4):377–80.

79. Toshner M, Voswinckel R, Southwood M et al. Evidence of dysfunction of endothelial progenitors in pulmonary arterial hypertension. Am J Respir Crit Care Med 2009;180(8):780–7.

80. Ko FN, Wu CC, Kuo SC, Lee FY, Teng CM. YC-1, a novel activator of platelet guanylate cyclase. Blood 1994;84(12): 4226–33.

81. Stasch JP, Becker EM, Alonso-Alija C et al. NO-independent regulatory site on soluble guanylate cyclase. Nature 2001; 410(6825):212–5.

82. Deruelle P, Grover TR, Abman SH. Pulmonary vascular effects of nitric oxide-cGMP augmentation in a model of chronic pulmonary hypertension in fetal and neonatal sheep. Am J Physiol 2005;289(5):L798–806.

83. Evgenov OV, Ichinose F, Evgenov NV et al. Soluble guanylate cyclase activator reverses acute pulmonary hypertension and augments the pulmonary vasodilator response to inhaled nitric oxide in awake lambs. Circulation 2004;110(15):2253–9.

84. Boerrigter G, Costello-Boerrigter LC, Cataliotti A et al. Cardiorenal and humoral properties of a novel direct soluble guanylate cyclase stimulator BAY 41-2272 in experimental congestive heart failure. Circulation 2003;107(5):686–9.

•85. Dumitrascu R, Weissmann N, Ghofrani HA et al. Activation of soluble guanylate cyclase reverses experimental pulmonary hypertension and vascular remodeling. Circulation 2006;113(2):286–95.

86. Deruelle P, Balasubramaniam V, Kunig AM, Seedorf GJ, Markham NE, Abman SH. BAY 41-2272, a direct activator of soluble guanylate cyclase, reduces right ventricular hypertrophy and prevents pulmonary vascular remodeling during chronic hypoxia in neonatal rats. Biol Neonate 2006;90(2):135–44.

87. Tulis DA. Novel therapies for cyclic GMP control of vascular smooth muscle growth. Am J Therapeut 2008; 15(6):551–64.

88. Mullershausen F, Russwurm M, Friebe A, Koesling D. Inhibition of phosphodiesterase type 5 by the activator of nitric oxide-sensitive guanylyl cyclase BAY 41-2272. Circulation 2004;109(14):1711–3.

•89. Grimminger F, Weimann G, Frey R et al. First acute haemodynamic study of soluble guanylate cyclase stimulator riociguat in pulmonary hypertension. Eur Respir J 2009; 33(4):785–92.

90. Stasch JP, Schmidt P, Alonso-Alija C et al. NO- and haem-independent activation of soluble guanylyl cyclase: molecular basis and cardiovascular implications of a new pharmacological principle. Br J Pharmacol 2002;136(5): 773–83.

91. Frey R, Muck W, Unger S, Artmeier-Brandt U, Weimann G, Wensing G. Pharmacokinetics, pharmacodynamics, tolerability, and safety of the soluble guanylate cyclase activator cinaciguat (BAY 58-2667) in healthy male volunteers. J Clin Pharmacol 2008;48(12):1400–10.

92. Lapp H, Mitrovic V, Franz N et al. Cinaciguat (BAY 58-2667) improves cardiopulmonary hemodynamics in patients with acute decompensated heart failure. Circulation 2009;119(21):2781–8.

Combination therapy for pulmonary arterial hypertension

STEVEN M KAWUT AND HAROLD I PALEVSKY

INTRODUCTION

The combination of multiple therapies is basic to the treatment of complex chronic diseases. Modern clinical approaches to asthma, coronary artery disease, congestive heart failure (CHF), and cancer are predicated on using multiple drugs with different mechanisms of action (sometimes sequentially and sometimes together "up front"). Considering the multitude of disease pathways which contribute to these conditions, it makes sense that while monotherapy may impact on one pathophysiologic process (and subsequent morbidity or mortality), targeting one or several pathways with multiple therapies might lead to greater benefit (1,2).

For many years, intravenous epoprostenol was the only available effective therapy for PAH, limiting the controversy around combination therapy. However, the recent proliferation of oral and inhaled drugs shown to be useful as single agents in short-term randomized clinical trials (RCTs) has made the possibility of combination therapy in PAH a reality. Clinical effects could be additive or synergistic if drug classes were combined. Other potential benefits of combination therapy include the ability to limit doses of individual drugs (and possibly side-effects). The use of multiple chemotherapies below toxicity-limiting dosages in oncologic disease is an example of this approach.

Combination therapy is not without risk however, as "The better is the enemy of the good" (3). Multiple medications increase the complexity of both the management of the patient and the patient's self-care. Combination therapies may heighten the risk of side effects and toxicity; a more complicated medical regimen makes it more difficult to identify the culprit if there are overlapping side-effect profiles. Multiple drug regimens may of course increase health care expenditures.

The most important current problem with combination therapy is its unconstrained widespread use without a sufficient evidence base, therefore engendering possible risks without clear clinical benefit to patients. Of course, the drawbacks of combination therapy (side-effects, complexity, and cost) would be more than justifiable given a clearly documented impact on a surrogate or intermediate end point or mortality in double-blind, placebo-controlled RCTs. Such data are just being gathered for different combinations and different approaches, which are imperative to support an evidence-based approach.

COMBINATION THERAPY STRATEGIES

There are several distinct approaches to combination therapy. Initial or "up-front" combination therapy entails starting multiple drugs simultaneously in the treatment-naive patient on the premise that multiple drugs will improve clinical response, prevent failure of monotherapy, result in less side-effects, or ultimately save money. The "add-on" approach entails sequential addition of therapeutic agents with maintenance of others, triggered by any of several indicators. Failure of a single drug (in terms of progressive symptoms or worsening exercise function or hemodynamics) might warrant additional therapy.

Some have touted "suboptimal response" as another indication. While some response targets may be obvious (e.g., no improvement in a dangerously low cardiac index with severe symptoms), others are less so. Epidemiologic studies have demonstrated strong associations between functional class, 6-minute walk distance (6MWD), and plasma brain natriuretic peptide (BNP) concentration and long-term outcome in PAH (4–6). Less consistent have been associations between oxygen consumption at peak exercise and survival (7–9). It has been tempting to interpret these epidemiologic risk factors as therapeutic "goals" to be pursued with sequential addition of medications, in the hopes of achieving better long-term outcomes (10). Of course, making the leap from epidemiologic studies to "goal-directed" treatment strategies assumes that (i) multiple medications can help achieve these targets and (ii) achieving these targets will translate into improved long-term outcome. Neither assumption has thus far been proven in PAH (11).

The track record of plasma BNP-guided therapy in CHF testifies to the problem with making such assumptions. Despite more than 2500 papers published in English on BNP in CHF (12), with many showing strong and consistent associations between higher plasma BNP level and worse outcomes, recent RCTs of the use of BNP-guided medical therapy (including combination therapy) in CHF showed mixed results, including no significant impact on all-cause hospitalization or mortality (13,14). The unclear role of BNP-guided treatment in CHF should serve as a caveat against adopting goal-directed combination therapy in PAH before RCTs demonstrate the safety and efficacy of this approach.

COMBINATION THERAPY PARADIGM AND STUDY DESIGN

Endothelin-1 levels, nitric oxide signaling, and endogenous prostacyclin production are abnormal in PAH and regulatory board-approved therapies for PAH target these pathways, as discussed in detail in other chapters. RCTs of the combination of pathway-specific therapies face a few specific issues in terms of design and interpretation of results.

Placebo-controlled RCTs of up-front or add-on combination therapy conducted with all subjects receiving some background effective PAH treatment avoid the controversy of the ethics and safety of allowing PAH patients to go untreated in a placebo-controlled RCT, since all patients will receive at least one standard therapy (15). This feature allows for RCTs of sufficient duration (6–12 months) to show convincing effects on exercise performance, functional status, and clinically important outcomes. Unfortunately, most completed, active, and planned studies of combination therapy have been ≤ 4 months in duration, greatly limiting the potential insights into the efficacy of long-term combination therapy. The enrolment of subjects into such trials of limited research value may challenge the ethical stance of these studies (15).

The other important issue faced by all RCTs in PAH is the use of surrogate, intermediate, and definitive clinical end points (11,16,17). Virtually all RCTs in PAH have been predicated on showing differences in 6MWD over the short term (3–4 months), viewed by regulatory boards as an intermediate end point (i.e., the difference in changes in 6MWD over time implies a clinical benefit for patients). Most monotherapy studies of untreated PAH patients have demonstrated differences around 30–40 m.

Up-front combination therapy RCTs compare two active drugs to one (two-arm) (or the other [three-arm]), likely producing a smaller incremental benefit compared to studies of one drug versus placebo. Add-on therapy in an already-treated PAH population (with lower mean pulmonary artery pressure (mPAP) and pulmonary vascular resistance (PVR) and higher cardiac index) will also likely result in a smaller incremental benefit. Rather than a "ceiling effect" specific to PAH, such studies of patients with less severe physiologic derangements (as in treated disease) often show changes of a lesser magnitude, as in the case of treated patients with diabetes mellitus, systemic hypertension, or CHF who enter a clinical trial of a new drug.

Unfortunately, the minimally important difference in an intermediate end point (18) or the increment in change of a surrogate end point which reliably predicts a change in long-term outcome in a combination therapy trial are undefined. A smaller treatment effect is expected, so that even a 10–20 m difference between changes in 6MWD may have significant implications regarding long-term outcome in a combination therapy trial, whereas such a difference may not in a monotherapy trial. Studies of the validity and minimally important differences of surrogate and intermediate end points are therefore necessary for combination therapy studies in PAH.

ENDOTHELIN RECEPTOR ANTAGONISTS (ERAs) AND PROSTACYCLIN ANALOGS

Bosentan and epoprostenol

There is one published double-blind, placebo-controlled RCT of the initiation of intravenous epoprostenol with or without oral bosentan (Bosentan Randomized Trial of Endothelin Antagonist Therapy for PAH [BREATH-2]) (19). Patients with PAH that was idiopathic or associated with connective tissue disease in New York Heart Association (NYHA) functional class III–IV were randomized to bosentan 62.5 mg po bid or placebo in a 2:1 ratio two days after initiation of intravenous epoprostenol.

Bosentan was uptitrated to 125 mg po bid after four weeks. The primary end point of this study was the change in total pulmonary resistance (TPR) after 16 weeks of study treatment, powered to detect a mean difference of 28 percent between study groups.

The median reduction in the TPR was 39.6 percent in the active treatment group and 14.3 percent in the placebo group ($P = 0.08$). There were no other significant differences between changes in other hemodynamic parameters, including PVR. The median changes in 6MWD in bosentan and placebo groups were similar, but these analyses were limited by missing data. Interestingly, epoprostenol side-effects were reported less frequently in patients receiving bosentan than in those receiving placebo. Three patients died during the trial (or soon after withdrawal), all in the combined therapy group. In summary, this trial does not support the routine addition of bosentan at epoprostenol initiation; the imbalance in deaths in the trial raises some concern regarding safety as well.

Bosentan and iloprost

Two RCTs of the addition of inhaled iloprost to background treatment with oral bosentan have been published. The Combination Therapy of Bosentan and Aerosolized Iloprost in IPAH (COMBI) trial was an open-label, randomized, non-placebo-controlled multicenter trial performed in Germany (NCT00120380) (20). Idiopathic PAH patients in NYHA functional class III were eligible if they had received bosentan for >3 months with a 6MWD between 150–425 m and were deemed clinically stable. The primary end point was the difference in change in 6MWD between the two groups after 12 weeks. Bosentan was administered at 125 mg bid and inhaled iloprost was administered six times daily at 5 µg per inhalation. Thirty-six patients in each group were required to detect a mean difference of 45 m between the changes of 6MWD in the two groups. The trial was stopped for futility after a planned interim analysis with 19 patients in the iloprost group and 21 in the control group. The median change in 6MWD in the control group was $+5$ m whereas the median change in the iloprost group was $+25$ m ($P = 0.65$). There were no differences in secondary end points and minimal side-effects associated with the study treatment.

The Safety and Pilot Efficacy Trial in Combination with Bosentan for Evaluation of PAH (STEP) trial also studied the addition of inhaled iloprost to patients receiving oral bosentan 125 mg twice daily (NCT00086463) (21). Patients had PAH which was idiopathic or associated with connective tissue disease, repaired congenital left to right cardiac shunts, HIV infection, or anorexigen use. They were between 10–80 years of age, had symptoms despite bosentan therapy for ≥ 4 months (mean: 18 months), and had 6MWD between 100–425 m, resting mPAP >25 mmHg, PVR ≥ 240 dyne/sec cm^{-5}, and pulmonary capillary wedge pressure <15 mmHg. Eligible patients were randomized in

a double-blind fashion to iloprost 5 µg or placebo six to nine times daily while awake. Randomization was blocked and stratified by diagnosis with 32 iloprost and 33 placebo patients in the final analysis. Formal power calculations were not performed.

The post-dose mean changes in 6MWD over 12 weeks for iloprost and placebo were not significantly different ($+30$ m and $+4$ m, respectively; Figure 16.6.1) ($P = 0.051$). Neither were there significant differences in the pre-dose 6MWD ($+29$ m and $+11$ m, respectively, $P = 0.14$). On the other hand, significantly more patients in the iloprost group (34 percent) improved one NYHA functional class from baseline compared to the placebo group (6 percent) ($P = 0.002$). Time to clinical worsening (PAH-related death, hospitalization or discontinuation, initiation of new PAH therapy, lung transplantation or atrial septostomy) was significantly longer in the iloprost group compared to the placebo group (Figure 16.6.2) ($P = 0.02$). No patients in the iloprost group had a clinical deterioration by 12 weeks compared to 15 percent of the placebo group. There were

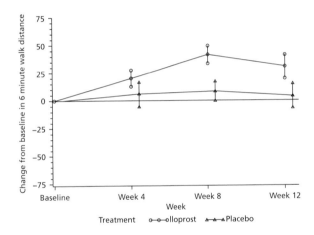

Figure 16.6.1 Mean ($\pm$ standard error) change in post-inhalation 6MWD from baseline to Week 12 in the placebo and iloprost groups. $P = 0.051$ at Week 12.

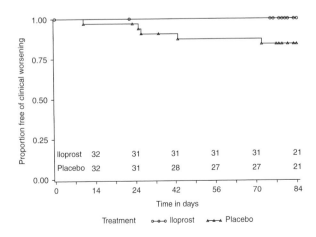

Figure 16.6.2 Time to clinical worsening for the iloprost group and the placebo group. $P = 0.02$ by log rank test.

four hospitalizations and one addition of PAH therapy in the placebo group. While decreases in mPAP and PVR post-dose were significantly greater in the iloprost group compared to the placebo group, there were no differences in the changes in pre-dose hemodynamics at Week 12. Side-effects typical for prostacyclin analogs (headache, jaw pain, and flushing) as well as cough and chest pain were more common with active drug compared to placebo.

In summary, there is one study which supports the use of inhaled iloprost in patients receiving bosentan with a positive effect on functional class, post-inhalation hemodynamics, and time to clinical end points. The role of upfront combined treatment of bosentan and inhaled iloprost has not been studied.

ERAs and treprostinil

The 16-Week, International, Multicenter, Double-Blind, Randomized, Placebo-Controlled Comparison of the Efficacy and Safety of Oral Treprostinil in Combination with an ERA and/or a PDE5 Inhibitor in Subjects with PAH (FREEDOM-C) has been presented without peer-review (NCT00325442) (22). This study enrolled 354 patients (of whom 350 received study drug) who were at least 12 years of age with PAH that was idiopathic, familial, or associated with anorexigen use, connective tissue disease, or congenital systemic to pulmonary cardiac shunts. Patients receiving either an ERA or PDE5 inhibitor for at least three months with a stable dose for 30 days who had a 6MWD between 140–450 m were included. Patients were randomized 1:1 to oral treprostinil (started at 1 mg twice daily with up-titration every five days for four weeks to the maximally tolerated dose) or placebo. The primary end point for this study was the median difference in the change in 6MWD at 16 weeks after randomization adjusted for baseline 6MWD and background treatment. The study was planned with 90 percent power to detect a treatment effect of 35 m.

The median change in 6MWD in the treprostinil group was $+14.5$ m and in the placebo group was $+4.8$ m, with a median treatment effect of treprostinil of $+11$ m at 16 weeks ($P = 0.072$). Patients receiving ERAs only showed a treatment effect of $+8$ m and those receiving ERAs and PDE5 inhibitors showed a treatment effect of $+11$ m, neither of which were statistically significant. There was no difference in the time to clinical events (defined as death, lung transplantation, atrial septostomy, or clinical deterioration) between the groups ($P = 0.46$) or in WHO functional class ($P = 0.94$). Headache, nausea, vomiting, flushing, jaw pain, and extremity pain were more frequent in the active drug group compared to placebo.

The Double-Blind Placebo-Controlled Clinical Investigation Into the Efficacy and Tolerability of Inhaled Treprostinil Sodium in Patients With Severe PAH (TRIUMPH 1) study compared the efficacy of inhaled treprostinil to placebo in addition to background treatment

with oral bosentan or sildenafil (NCT00147199) (23). This study enrolled 235 patients who were 18–75 years of age with PAH that was idiopathic, familial, or associated with anorexigen use, connective tissue disease, or HIV infection. Patients receiving either bosentan or sildenafil for at least three months who had a 6MWD between 200–450 m were included. Patients were randomized 1:1 to four inhalations of active drug or placebo daily over 12 weeks. The primary end point for this study was the median difference in the change in post-dose 6MWD at 12 weeks after randomization adjusted for baseline 6MWD and disease etiology.

The median difference between inhaled treprostinil and placebo groups in post-dose change in 6MWD was $+20$ m at 12 weeks ($P < 0.0005$). The median pre-dose difference was $+14$ m ($P < 0.007$). Patients receiving background therapy with bosentan showed a treatment effect of $+25$ m ($P < 0.0002$) (n = 165) (results for subjects receiving background therapy with sildenafil are discussed below). There was no difference in the time to clinical events between the groups. Cough, headache, flushing, and throat irritation were more frequent in the active drug group compared to the placebo group.

In summary, trials of the addition of treprostinil to oral bosentan treatment have been completed, but only preliminary data are available. The addition of oral treprostinil did not have a significant impact on change in 6MWD and was possibly difficult to tolerate. On the other hand, inhaled treprostinil had a greater impact on 6MWD which was statistically significant, but had no effect on time to clinical events.

ERAs and PDE5 inhibitors

The ability to combine two approved oral therapies acting on different components of the mechanistic pathway of PAH offers considerable appeal. The drawbacks to this approach include potential metabolic interactions between such drugs. Sildenafil inhibits CYP3A4 leading to increased plasma concentrations of bosentan, theroretically leading to a potential increase in toxicity (specifically liver). Tadalafil does not affect bosentan metabolism (24). Alternatively, bosentan induces CYP3A4, potentially reducing sildenafil and other PDE5 inhibitor plasma levels (24,25). These interactions have been evaluated in short-term studies with unclear implications for long-term therapy.

Bosentan and tadalafil

A double-blind, placebo-controlled RCT of tadalafil (Tadalafil in the Treatment of Pulmonary Arterial Hypertension [PHIRST-1]) included a subset of patients already treated with bosentan (NCT00125918) (26). The study included PAH patients (idiopathic, familial, or related to anorexigen use, connective tissue disease, HIV infection, or congenital systemic-to-pulmonary cardiac shunts) at least 12 years of age. Patients who were untreated or who had been using oral bosentan 125 mg twice daily for at least 12 weeks at the time of screening were randomized to one of four doses of tadalafil or placebo. A total of 405 patients were randomized of whom 216 were using bosentan at enrolment. The primary end point was the difference in change in 6MWD from baseline to Week 16. Randomization was stratified by 6MWD, type of PAH, and bosentan use.

The placebo-corrected mean differences in 6MWD at Week 16 are shown in Figure 16.6.3 stratified by the use of bosentan at screening. Tadalafil resulted in statistically and clinically significant placebo-corrected mean differences in 6MWD in patients who were not receiving bosentan (+32 m and +44 m for the tadalafil 20 mg and 40 mg doses, respectively). On the other hand, while there was a monotonic relationship between increasing tadalafil dose and the placebo-corrected differences in 6MWD, these differences were not statistically significant and were overall of a smaller magnitude (but not statistically significantly so) (+23 m for the tadalafil 20 mg and 40 mg doses) in patients who were treated with bosentan. The effect of tadalafil on the time to clinical worsening in the subgroup of patients receiving bosentan therapy was not presented.

Bosentan and sildenafil

There are several RCTs of the combination of bosentan and sildenafil which are ongoing. One is a double-blind, placebo-controlled RCT of sildenafil 20 mg tid in patients receiving bosentan (Assess the Efficacy and Safety of Sildenafil when Added to Bosentan in the Treatment of PAH) (NCT00323297). The other (Effects of the Combination of Bosentan and Sildenafil Versus Sildenafil Monotherapy on Pulmonary Arterial Hypertension (PAH) (COMPASS-2)) will enrol patients receiving sildenafil 20 mg TID for at least 12 weeks and randomize them to bosentan 125 mg bid or placebo in a double-blind fashion (NCT00303459). One randomized, placebo-controlled double-blind cross-over study of the addition of sildenafil to baseline bosentan therapy has been completed in patients with Eisenmenger's syndrome but results have not been published (NCT00303004).

Other ERAs and PDE5 inhibitors

The Randomized, Multicenter Study of Ambrisentan and Sildenafil Combination Therapy in Subjects with PAH Who Have Demonstrated a Suboptimal Response to Sildenafil (ATHENA) is randomizing individuals with a "suboptimal" response to sildenafil (defined as NYHA functional class III, mPAP > 25 mmHg, and PVR > 400 dyne/sec cm^{-5}) to ambrisentan or placebo (NCT00617305). The primary end point of this study is the change in PVR from baseline to 24 weeks. Another study (Sitaxsentan Efficacy and Safety Trial With a Randomized Prospective Assessment of Adding Sildenafil [SR-PAAS]) is examining the addition of sildenafil to sitaxsentan* (NCT00795639).

In summary, the available data are insufficient to support an incremental benefit of the combination of ERAs and PDE5 inhibitors, however there are several ongoing trials which are specifically designed and powered to address this issue.

PDE5 INHIBITORS AND PROSTACYCLIN ANALOGS

Sildenafil and epoprostenol

The Pulmonary Arterial Hypertension Combination Study of Epoprostenol and Sildenafil (PACES) Study enrolled 267 patients who were at least 16 years of age with PAH that was idiopathic, familial, or associated with anorexigen use, connective tissue disease, or congenital systemic to pulmonary cardiac shunts (NCT00159861) (27). Patients receiving intravenous epoprostenol for more than three months (and without a dose change within four weeks) and not receiving ERAs who had a 6MWD between 100 and 450 m were eligible. Randomization was 1:1 stratified by baseline 6MWD and idiopathic PAH vs. other form of PAH. Sildenafil was started at 20 mg three times daily for four weeks, then uptitrated to 40 mg three times daily for four weeks, before receiving 80 mg three times daily for the remainder of the 16- week trial. The primary end point for this study was the difference in the change in 6MWD over 16 weeks after randomization.

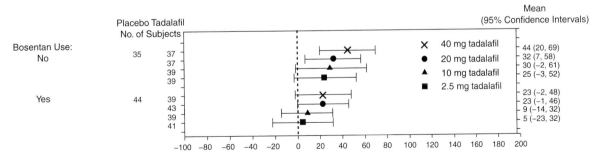

Figure 16.6.3 Placebo-corrected effect of tadalafil treatment on the 6MWD from baseline to Week 16. The treatment effects, with 95% CIs, are presented for each tadalafil dose.

*Sitaxsentan was withdrawn in December 2010.

The adjusted difference in 6MWD for the sildenafil group was 29.8 m and for the placebo group was 1.0 m, giving an adjusted treatment effect of +28.8 m (Figure 16.6.4) ($P < 0.001$). There were also statistically significant differences in the changes in mean right atrial pressure, mPAP, PVR, and cardiac output favoring the use of sildenafil. The group assigned to sildenafil showed a significant increase in the time to clinical events (defined as death, lung transplantation, hospitalization due to PAH, change in epoprostenol dose due to clinical deterioration, or initiation of bosentan therapy) compared to the group assigned to placebo (Figure 16.6.5) ($P = 0.002$). Seven (5.3 percent) of the subjects in the placebo group died compared to none in the sildenafil group. Sildenafil also improved health-related quality of life measured by the Short Form-36. Headache was more common with the sildenafil group, but otherwise adverse events were similar between the two groups.

These results appear generalizable to the relatively small subset of PAH patients worldwide receiving intravenous epoprostenol (28). Change in epoprostenol dose was the most common event defining "clinical worsening" in the placebo group, however the clinical significance of a change in epoprostenol dosing after relative stability is not well established. With these *caveats*, this trial is the first RCT of combination therapy which has shown significant

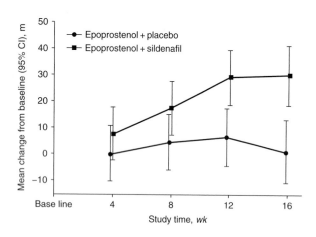

Figure 16.6.4   Change from baseline in 6MWD, by treatment group (model-adjusted estimates).

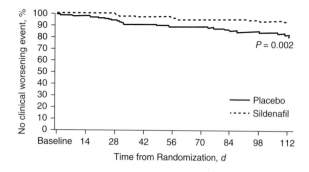

Figure 16.6.5   Kaplan–Meier plot of time to clinical worsening.

effects on both the 6MWD as well as time to prespecified clinical worsening end points.

Sildenafil and iloprost

The Ventavis Inhalation with Sildenafil to Improve and Optimize Pulmonary Arterial Hypertension (VISION) trial assessed the impact of inhaled iloprost in idiopathic and familial PAH patients receiving a stable dose of sildenafil (NCT00302211). This study was terminated in 2008 due to slow enrolment, and results have not yet been released.

Sildenafil and treprostinil

The TRIUMPH-1 and FREEDOM-C studies included subjects receiving sildenafil who were randomized to oral and inhaled treprostinil, respectively (discussed in detail above). TRIUMPH-1 and FREEDOM-C showed median differences in the change in 6MWD conferred by treprostinil with sildenafil background therapy of +17 m and +9 m, respectively, neither of which was statistically significant (22,23).

In summary, the use of sildenafil in patients currently being treated with intravenous epoprostenol results in benefit in terms of 6MWD and time to clinical worsening over 16 weeks. The currently available data do not support the use of oral treprostinil in addition to sildenafil, whereas the addition of inhaled treprostinil to either bosentan or sildenafil may be effective.

NOVEL AGENTS

Investigators are planning a double-blind, placebo-controlled RCT of imatinib, a tyrosine kinase inhibitor, for patients with severe PAH (PVR > 1000 dyne/sec cm^{-5}) despite treatment with two or more PAH therapies (Imatinib in Pulmonary Arterial Hypertension, a Randomized, Efficacy Study (IMPRES)-NCT00902174). The primary end point of this trial is the difference in the change in 6MWD between the groups at six months. Two Phase II double-blind, placebo-controlled RCTs of simvastatin on background therapy are ongoing. One is randomizing patients with idiopathic or connective tissue disease-associated PAH who are receiving sildenafil or bosentan to simvastatin 40 mg daily or placebo with the primary end point of change in right ventricular mass measured by cardiac magnetic resonance imaging at six months (Simvastatin as a Treatment for Pulmonary Hypertension- NCT00180713). A Clinical Trial of Aspirin and Simvastatin in PAH (ASA-STAT) is a placebo-controlled 2×2 factorial trial of simvastatin and aspirin conducted on background PAH therapy with the primary end point of 6MWD at six months (NCT00384865).

GUIDELINES

In 2004, a European Society of Cardiology Task Force gave combination therapy for PAH its lowest class recommendation based on the lowest level of evidence, although this predated most of the data discussed in this chapter (29). A British Thoracic Society/British Rheumatology Society consensus statement recommended that individuals with idiopathic PAH, familial PAH, or anorexigen-associated PAH who demonstrate an inadequate response to monotherapy (such as WHO functional class IV symptoms, progression of breathlessness, 6MWD < 380 m, refractory heart failure, or syncope) should be considered for combination therapy. The criteria for combination therapy in connective tissue disease-associated PAH included WHO functional class III or IV, progression of breathlessness, 6MWD not improved, refractory heart failure, or syncope on monotherapy. This guideline emphasized the importance of using a goal-oriented strategy but also recommended that combination therapy should first and foremost be used in the setting of a clinical trial. In the absence of an ongoing clinical trial, there was considered to be sufficient evidence to proceed with combination therapy with careful monitoring of the response to treatment.

The updated American College of Chest Physicians guidelines included combination therapy for PAH as a therapeutic option given no improvement or deterioration for patients in functional class III–IV receiving monotherapy but also recommended enrolment in RCTs (30). The American College of Cardiology and American Heart Association consensus document recommended considering combination therapy after reassessing the PAH patient started on monotherapy and provided general guidelines for what constituted an adequate response (31). The Proceedings from the Fourth World Symposium on Pulmonary Hypertension recommended that combination therapy should be considered for patients who fail to show improvement or who deteriorate with monotherapy, but considered the available combinations to be investigational (32).

CONCLUSIONS

The use of combination therapy in PAH follows a paradigm well established in other chronic medical conditions. However, the recent availability of multiple therapies for PAH has greatly outpaced the RCTs necessary to understand their use in this rare disease. Current data support the addition of inhaled iloprost to PAH patients treated with bosentan with persistent hemodynamic abnormalities and symptoms and the use of sildenafil in patients receiving intravenous epoprostenol. RCTs are currently underway to provide answers regarding the safety and efficacy of the many other possible drug combinations now available to clinicians and patients with PAH.

KEY POINTS

- Combination therapy is a standard approach in a variety of chronic medical conditions.
- Several studies are ongoing or planned to assess the use of currently approved PAH therapies in a variety of combinations.
- Studies of combination therapy in PAH are limited by short duration and lack of an accepted minimally important difference and validated surrogate end points.
- Data support the use of inhaled iloprost in addition to background bosentan therapy to prolong time to clinical worsening. Similarly, the use of sildenafil in patients who are on a stable dose of intravenous epoprostenol improves exercise tolerance, hemodynamics, and time to clinical worsening.

REFERENCES

• = Key primary paper

•1. O'Callaghan DS, Gaine SP. Combination therapy and new types of agents for pulmonary arterial hypertension. Clin Chest Med 2007;28:169–85, ix.
2. Benza RL, Park MH, Keogh A, Girgis RE. Management of pulmonary arterial hypertension with a focus on combination therapies. J Heart Lung Transplant 2007;26:437–6.
3. Voltaire. La Bégueule, 1772.
4. Sitbon O, Humbert M, Nunes H, Parent F, Garcia G, Herve P, Rainisio M, Simonneau G. Long-term intravenous epoprostenol infusion in primary pulmonary hypertension: prognostic factors and survival. J Am Coll Cardiol 2002;40:780–8.
5. McLaughlin VV, Shillington A, Rich S. Survival in primary pulmonary hypertension: the impact of epoprostenol therapy. Circulation 2002;106:1477–82.
6. Nagaya N, Nishikimi T, Uematsu M et al. Plasma brain natriuretic peptide as a prognostic indicator in patients with primary pulmonary hypertension. Circulation 2000;102:865–70.
7. Opitz CF, Wensel R, Winkler J et al. Clinical efficacy and survival with first-line inhaled iloprost therapy in patients with idiopathic pulmonary arterial hypertension. Eur Heart J 2005;26:1895–902.
8. Wensel R, Opitz CF, Anker SD et al. Assessment of survival in patients with primary pulmonary hypertension: importance of cardiopulmonary exercise testing. Circulation 2002;106:319–24.
9. Kawut SM, Horn EM, Berekashvili KK et al. New predictors of outcome in idiopathic pulmonary arterial hypertension. Am J Cardiol 2005;95:199–203.

10. Hoeper MM, Markevych I, Spiekerkoetter E, Welte T, Niedermeyer J. Goal-oriented treatment and combination therapy for pulmonary arterial hypertension. Eur Respir J 2005;26:858–63.

11. Ventetuolo CE, Benza RL, Peacock AJ, Zamanian RT, Badesch DB, Kawut SM. Surrogate and combined end points in pulmonary arterial hypertension. Proc Am Thorac Soc 2008;5:617–22.

12. Pubmed. http://www.ncbi.nlm.nih.gov/pubmed/. Accessed June 15, 2009.

13. Jourdain P, Jondeau G, Funck F et al. Plasma brain natriuretic peptide-guided therapy to improve outcome in heart failure: the STARS-BNP Multicenter Study. J Am Coll Cardiol 2007;49:1733–9.

14. Pfisterer M, Buser P, Rickli H et al. BNP-guided vs. symptom-guided heart failure therapy: the Trial of Intensified vs Standard Medical Therapy in Elderly Patients With Congestive Heart Failure (TIME-CHF) randomized trial. JAMA 2009;301:383–92.

15. Halpern SD, Doyle R, Kawut SM. The ethics of randomized clinical trials in pulmonary arterial hypertension. Proc Am Thorac Soc 2008;5:631–5.

16. Snow JL, Kawut SM. Surrogate end points in pulmonary arterial hypertension: assessing the response to therapy. Clin Chest Med 2007;28:75–89, viii.

17. Hoeper MM, Oudiz RJ, Peacock A et al. End points and clinical trial designs in pulmonary arterial hypertension: clinical and regulatory perspectives. J Am Coll Cardiol 2004;43:48S–55S.

18. Gilbert C, Brown MC, Cappelleri JC, Carlsson M, McKenna SP. Estimating a minimally important difference in pulmonary arterial hypertension following treatment with sildenafil. Chest 2009;135:137–42.

19. Humbert M, Barst RJ, Robbins IM et al. Combination of bosentan with epoprostenol in pulmonary arterial hypertension: BREATHE-2. Eur Respir J 2004;24:353–9.

20. Hoeper MM, Leuchte H, Halank M et al. Combining inhaled iloprost with bosentan in patients with idiopathic pulmonary arterial hypertension. Eur Respir J 2006;28:691–4.

21. McLaughlin VV, Oudiz RJ, Frost A et al. Randomized study of adding inhaled iloprost to existing bosentan in pulmonary arterial hypertension. Am J Respir Crit Care Med 2006;174:1257–63.

22. Tapson VF, Torres F, Kermeen F, Keogh A, Allen RP. Results of the FREEDOMC Study: A pivotal study of oral treprostinil used adjunctively with an ERA and/or PDE5-inhibitor for the treatment of PAH. Paper presented at the International Conference of the American Thoracic Society, 2009, San Diego.

23. McLaughlin VV, Rubin LJ, Benza RL et al. TRIUMPH I: Efficacy and safety of inhaled treprostinil Sodium in patients with pulmonary arterial hypertension. Paper presented at the International Conference of the American Thoracic Society, 2008, Toronto.

24. http://dailymed.nlm.nih.gov/dailymed/drugInfo.cfm?id=9812. Accessed June 25, 2009.

25. Paul GA, Gibbs JS, Boobis AR, Abbas A, Wilkins MR. Bosentan decreases the plasma concentration of sildenafil when coprescribed in pulmonary hypertension. Br J Clin Pharmacol 2005;60:107–12.

26. Galie N, Brundage BH, Ghofrani HA et al. Tadalafil therapy for pulmonary arterial hypertension. Circulation 2009;119:2894–903.

27. Simonneau G, Rubin LJ, Galie N et al. Addition of sildenafil to long-term intravenous epoprostenol therapy in patients with pulmonary arterial hypertension: a randomized trial. Ann Intern Med 2008;149:521–30.

28. Taichman DB. Therapy for pulmonary arterial hypertension: the more, the merrier? Ann Intern Med 2008;149:583–5.

29. Galie N, Torbicki A, Barst R et al. Guidelines on diagnosis and treatment of pulmonary arterial hypertension. The Task Force on Diagnosis and Treatment of Pulmonary Arterial Hypertension of the European Society of Cardiology. Eur Heart J 2004;25:2243–78.

30. Badesch DB, Abman SH, Simonneau G, Rubin LJ, McLaughlin VV. Medical therapy for pulmonary arterial hypertension: updated ACCP evidence-based clinical practice guidelines. Chest 2007;131:1917–28.

31. McLaughlin VV, Archer SL, Badesch DB et al. ACCF/AHA 2009 expert consensus document on pulmonary hypertension: a report of the American College of Cardiology Foundation Task Force on Expert Consensus Documents and the American Heart Association: developed in collaboration with the American College of Chest Physicians, American Thoracic Society, Inc., and the Pulmonary Hypertension Association. Circulation 2009;119:2250–94.

32. Barst R, Gibbs S, Ghofrani HA et al. Updated evidence-based treatment algorithm in pulmonary arterial hypertension. J Am Coll Cardiol 2009;54:S78–84.

Stem cell therapy

MARK L ORMISTON, DAVID W COURTMAN AND DUNCAN J STEWART

INTRODUCTION

As described in the preceding chapters, the introduction of new vasodilatory therapies for the treatment of pulmonary arterial hypertension (PAH) over the last decade has had a significant impact on the clinical management of this disease and the quality of life of those suffering from its devastating effects. However, while prostanoids, endothelin receptor antagonists and phosphodiesterase inhibitors have all been shown to improve the functional status and, to a lesser extent, the hemodynamic parameters of patients with PAH (1), the capacity of these vasodilatory therapies to significantly extend survival remains uncertain. A recent meta-analysis, reviewing 16 randomized controlled trials of the three classes of vasodilatory therapies, demonstrated that currently approved treatments, when analyzed together, do not provide a significant survival benefit when compared to controls (2). Of the trials cited in this meta-analysis, only the 1996 epoprostenol trial provided long-term (9 month) follow-up and demonstrated a reduced mortality in the treatment group (3).

The lack of a more profound survival benefit with current therapies has been attributed to the fact that, while excessive vasoconstriction may be a contributing factor to the progression of PAH, vasodilatory agents do little to address the occlusive vascular remodeling and microvascular loss that are now recognized as the major driving forces behind elevated pulmonary vascular resistance (PVR). Accordingly, the focus of the scientific community has shifted over the last decade towards the investigation of therapeutic strategies that target and reverse pathological vascular remodeling (4). One of the strategies currently being investigated is the use of cell-based therapy as a means of regenerating a functional pulmonary microvasculature. While established PAH is characterized by the development of occlusive vascular lesions, associated with the excessive proliferation of both endothelial cells (ECs) (5,6) and smooth muscle cells (SMCs) (7), there are several lines of evidence supporting a role for EC apoptosis in the initiation of PAH (8). It has been proposed that recurring periods of endothelial injury and apoptosis, particularly at the level of the precapillary arterioles, may lead to the initial loss of microvessels and, over time, the generation of occlusive vascular lesions through the preferential selection of apoptosis resistant, hyperproliferative ECs (6,9).

Early work investigating cell-based therapies for PAH aimed to address this endothelial loss through cell-based gene therapy, and the use of somatic cells (smooth muscle cells or fibroblasts) as vectors for the delivery of endothelial survival factors, including vascular endothelial growth factor (VEGF), angiopoeitin-1 or endothelial nitric oxide synthase (eNOS) (10–12). In these studies, experimental pulmonary hypertension (PH), induced in the rat model by the injection of the plant alkaloid monocrotaline (MCT), was either inhibited or reversed by delivery of genetically altered somatic cells into the pulmonary circulation. More recently, several groups have moved towards the investigation of autologous stem or progenitor cell populations, such as endothelial progenitor cells (EPCs) (13) or mesenchymal stem cells (MSCs) (14), which have been reported to possess an innate capacity to regenerate or repair damaged endothelium (15,16). A summary of

Table 16.7.1   Summary of reports investigating stem cell therapy for PAH

Cell type	Source	Model	Result	Reference
EPCs	Human, umbilical cord blood	MCT rat, prevention	Improved PVR, pulmonary arterial muscularization and survival. Transfection with adrenomedullin-enhanced protection	(44)
	Autologous dog blood	Dehydro-MCT dog	Improved mean PAP, cardiac output and PVR	(45)
	Syngeneic rat bone marrow	MCT rat, prevention and reversal	Near complete prevention of elevated RVSP and RV hypertrophy and halted progression of established disease eNOS transfection allowed for reversal of established disease	(13)
	Human peripheral blood	Human IPAH	Improved 6-min walk, mean PAP, cardiac output and PVR	(32, 33)
MSCs	Syngeneic rat bone marrow	MCT rat, prevention	Improved RVSP and RV hypertrophy eNOS transfection-enhanced protection and survival	(14)

reports investigating the application of stem cell therapy for the treatment of PAH is shown in Table 16.7.1.

ENDOTHELIAL PROGENITOR CELLS

Until recently, the conventional belief in vascular biology was that the *de novo* generation of blood vessels from mesodermal angioblasts was limited to the period of embryo development (17). Following birth, angiogenesis, or the sprouting of new capillaries from the ECs of pre-existing vessels, was believed to govern vascular regeneration (18). However, this belief was challenged as early as 1963, when a report by Stump and colleagues proposed that ECs lining dacron vascular grafts were derived from circulating blood cells, and not from the pre-existing endothelium (19). Over three decades later, the concept of postnatal vasculogenesis was reaffirmed by Shi and colleagues (20), who used a canine bone marrow transplant model to demonstrate that the endothelial cells lining dacron grafts were indeed bone marrow-derived. In the years since this report, several groups have used bone marrow transplant models (21–23), or the study of peripheral blood cultures from sex-mismatched bone marrow transplant recipients (24), to demonstrate the capacity of bone marrow-derived, circulating cells to contribute to vascular regeneration by homing to areas of vascular injury and differentiating into mature endothelium.

Confirmation of the existence of bone marrow-derived endothelial progenitors in the circulation also led numerous groups to isolate putative EPCs for use in applications of therapeutic revascularization. The first isolation and characterization of EPCs from peripheral blood is credited to Asahara and colleagues (25), who in 1997 demonstrated that endothelial-like cells could be derived in culture from a CD34+-enriched fraction of peripheral

blood mononuclear cells (PBMNCs). After 7 days, cultures of CD34-enriched PBMNCs gave rise to spindle-shaped cells that possessed several characteristics of endothelial cells, including expression of the endothelial surface markers, VEGF receptor II (VEGFR2), CD31 and Tie-2, as well as eNOS expression, uptake of acetylated low-density lipoprotein (acLDL), binding of Ulex (UEA-1) lectin and the ability to form tube-like structures *in vitro*. Subsequent *in vivo* studies also confirmed the capacity of these endothelial-like cells to incorporate into areas of vascular regeneration.

This initial characterization resulted in a definition for EPCs as circulating, bone marrow-derived cells, positive for the markers CD34 and VEGFR2. A later report identified CD133 (or prominin), which is expressed on a subset of CD34+ cells, as an additional marker of circulating EPCs (26). While the enumeration of EPCs in the circulation using some or all of these surface markers has been employed as a prognostic indicator in a range of cardiovascular diseases, including coronary artery disease (27), diabetic vasculopathy (28) and PAH (29), these CD34+/CD133+/VEGFR2+ cells exist at extremely low levels in the circulation, and, as such, are of limited value for most applications of autologous cell therapy. Instead, the majority of studies investigating the regenerative capacity of EPCs in models of vascular injury have made use of "*ex vivo* expanded" EPCs, generated through the application of specific EPC culture techniques applied to PBMNCs or bone marrow isolates, which are not enriched for CD34+ cells (13,15). These cultures yield a large of number cells that, after 7 days in culture, possess many of the endothelial-like characteristics of the CD34+ EPCs described originally by Asahara.

Ex vivo expanded EPCs have been shown to induce enhanced vascular regeneration when transplanted into several models of cardiovascular injury, including acute myocardial infarction (30), hind-limb ischemia (15) and MCT-induced PH (13). Success in animal models also led to the initiation of a number of clinical trials, some of which have shown modest yet significant benefits for BM-derived cells or peripheral blood-derived EPCs in cases of acute myocardial infarction (31) and PAH (32,33). Despite these successes, uncertainty remains regarding the mechanism(s) by which the beneficial effects of EPC therapy are achieved. The suggestion from the earliest studies investigating EPC-based therapy was that *ex vivo* expanded EPCs, like their circulating counterparts, act by homing to areas of vascular injury, where they differentiate into mature endothelium and initiate the formation of new capillaries. However, subsequent reports failed to support this hypothesis, demonstrating instead that transplanted, bone marrow-derived cells, including EPCs, can enhance vascular regeneration by mechanisms that do not require long-term cell retention (34).

It has been proposed that *ex vivo* expanded EPCs induce therapeutic revascularization through the release of paracrine factors, and the induction of a localized angiogenic response (35–37). This concept is supported by a number of studies demonstrating the similarity of *ex vivo* expanded EPCs to monocytes and macrophages, which have a well-documented capacity to stimulate vessel growth through the release of angiogenic factors (38). Unlike Asahara's original classification of EPCs from CD34+ PBMNCs (25), EPCs derived from cultures of total PBMNCs initially express CD34 only at very low levels (39), and are positive for the monocytic and panleukocyte markers, CD14 and CD45 (35,40). A review by Schatteman also highlighted the fact that many of the surface markers, such as CD31, VEGFR2, VE-cadherin and Tie-2, and functional characteristics, including lectin binding and acLDL uptake, used to identify culture-derived cells as "endothelial-like" are not exclusive to ECs, and are shared by circulating cells, including monocytes and monocyte-derived macrophages (34). Additional studies have demonstrated that peripheral blood-derived, CD14+ monocytes can give rise to cells in culture that display the phenotypic characteristics of endothelial cells, but retain the expression of monocytic antigens (41–43), leading some to question whether the cells generated from *ex vivo* EPC cultures are truly endothelial-like, or simply a subset of hematopoietic cells which express a number of characteristics usually attributed to ECs.

EPCs IN EXPERIMENTAL PULMONARY HYPERTENSION

Regardless of the uncertainty surrounding their characterization and mode of action, the capacity of exogenously generated EPCs to regenerate injured or dysfunctional vessels has made them an attractive possibility for the treatment of PAH, which is marked by extensive microvascular loss and endothelial dysfunction. The first reported investigation of EPCs for the treatment of PAH is attributed to Nagaya and colleagues, who tested the therapeutic capacity of human, umbilical cord blood-derived EPCs in an athymic nude rat model of MCT-induced PH (44). In this study, EPCs were shown to incorporate into the vascular walls of MCT-treated rats, but demonstrated only a modest capacity to prevent the onset of MCT-induced PH, as evidenced by a 16 percent reduction in pulmonary vascular resistance versus sham treated controls. Despite this limited benefit, EPC therapy significantly decreased pulmonary arterial muscularization and enhanced survival in MCT-challenged rats. This therapeutic effect was enhanced following transfection of the EPCs with a plasmid encoding the vasodilatory peptide, adrenomedullin.

The results of this initial investigation were supported by a later study reporting the capacity of autologous, blood-derived EPCs to prevent dehydromonocrotaline-induced PH in a dog model (45). While these first studies demonstrated some promise for EPCs in the treatment of PAH, they were limited to the prevention of PH in experimental models, and thus did not test the ability of these cells to reverse established disease. Since PAH patients generally do not present until late in the course of disease progression, long after the development of advanced symptoms and severe abnormalities in vascular structure and function (46), the reversal of established disease represents a more clinically relevant target than disease prevention. A later work by the Stewart group addressed this concern by testing the capacity of syngeneic, bone marrow-derived EPCs to both prevent and reverse established PH in the MCT-induced rat model (13). This work demonstrated that syngeneic EPCs integrate into the vessel walls of distal precapillary arterioles and provide near complete prevention of MCT-induced increases in right ventricular systolic pressure (RVSP) and right ventricular hypertrophy when delivered 3 days after the initiation of disease. When delivered 21 days post-MCT, after the development of established PH and the associated vascular remodeling, EPCs were shown to halt disease progression, but were unable to reverse the established disease (see Figure 16.7.1). However, transfection of EPCs with a plasmid encoding the gene for eNOS significantly enhanced their therapeutic efficacy, allowing for the reversal of established PH by 35 days post-MCT.

In addition to the assessment of RVSP and right ventricular hypertrophy, this work made use of a 3-dimensional fluorescence microangiography technique to image the distal pulmonary microvasculature. This technique involves the perfusion of the pulmonary vasculature with low-melting point agarose loaded with fluorescent microspheres (0.2 μm). Following perfusion, thick sections (100 to 200 μm) of rat lung tissue were imaged using confocal microscopy to generate a 3-dimensional reconstruction of the pulmonary microvasculature. As seen in Figure 16.7.2, this technique allowed for the visualization of extensive microvascular pruning in MCT-challenged rats and the capacity of EPCs to prevent this microvascular remodeling when delivered at 3 days post-MCT. For the reversal model, MCT-challenged rats given eNOS transfected EPCs at 21 days demonstrated near normal microvascular circulation at 35 days post-MCT, providing further evidence to suggest that these cells function by stimulating microvascular regeneration.

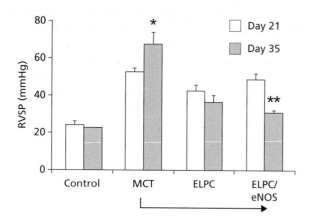

Figure 16.7.1 In a reversal model of MCT-induced PH, RVSP was measured at 21 days after MCT and again 14 days after cell therapy or control saline injections (day 35) in the same animals. In MCT-saline-injected rats, a significant elevation of RVSP was observed between days 21 and 35 post-MCT. Treatment on day 21 with endothelial-like progenitor cells (ELPCs) halted disease progression, and eNOS transduced ELPC treatment resulted in reversal of PAH with significantly lower RVSP values at day 35. (Reproduced with permission from ref 13.)

MESENCHYMAL STEM CELLS FOR PAH

In addition to EPCs, mesenchymal stem cells (MSCs) have also been investigated for their efficacy in the treatment of experimental PAH. MSCs, sometimes referred to as multipotent mesenchymal stromal cells, are bone marrow-derived, non-hematopoietic, pluripotent cells, characterized by their adherence to tissue culture polystyrene and their capacity to differentiate into at least three mesenchymal lineages: osteoblasts, chondroblasts and adipocytes (47). In addition to these basic characterization criteria, MSCs are also defined by the expression of certain surface markers, including CD105, CD73 and CD90, and the lack of typical hematopoietic markers, such as CD14, CD34 and CD45 (47). Beyond the capacity to differentiate into the mesenchymal cell types listed above, work by Jiang and colleagues demonstrated that multipotent MSCs can also differentiate into endothelial cells both *in vitro* and *in vivo* (48), suggesting the possibility that these cells, like EPCs, could be used to regenerate the pulmonary microvasculature in the treatment of PAH.

The application of MSCs to the treatment of PAH is limited to a single study investigating their capacity to

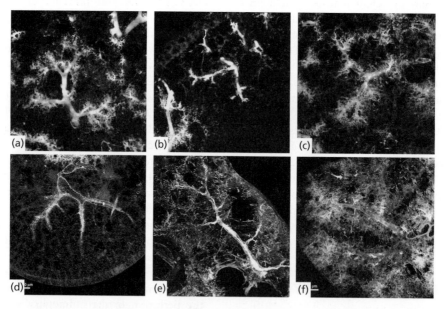

Figure 16.7.2 Representative confocal projection images of lung sections perfused with fluorescent microspheres (green) suspended in agarose and immunostained for smooth muscle α-actin (red). Normal filling of the microvasculature was observed in control rats (a), whereas rats treated with MCT showed a marked loss of microvascular perfusion and widespread precapillary occlusion 21 (b) and 35 (d) days after MCT injection. In the prevention model, animals receiving EPCs displayed improved microvascular perfusion and preserved continuity of the distal vasculature (c). In the reversal model, eNOS-transduced EPCs dramatically improved the appearance of the pulmonary microvasculature (f), whereas progenitor cells alone resulted in more modest increases in perfusion and little noticeable reduction in arteriolar muscularization (e, scale bar = 100 μm). (Reproduced with permission from ref 13.)

prevent MCT-induced PH in the rat model (14). In this study, syngeneic MSCs were shown to prevent the onset of MCT-induced PH, as demonstrated by reduced elevation of RVSP and diminished RV hypertrophy. In agreement with previously discussed reports for EPCs transfected to overexpress eNOS or adrenomedullin, transfection of MSCs with eNOS enhanced the therapeutic benefit of MSCs. Furthermore, eNOS-transfected MSCs, but not MSCs alone, extended the survival of MCT-challenged rats when compared to vehicle-treated controls.

While this study did not elaborate on the mechanism by which MSCs were achieving these therapeutic effects, and did not investigate the long-term retention of transplanted MSCs within the lung, the suggestion from the authors was that the transplanted cells held the potential to differentiate into endothelial cells *in vivo* and regenerate the pulmonary vasculature. A later study by Yue and colleagues supported this claim by demonstrating the capacity of transplanted MSCs to incorporate into an injured vascular wall and take on an endothelial phenotype in a rat model of vein grafting (16). However, other studies have suggested that MSCs could be acting through alternate mechanisms. Patel and colleagues demonstrated that MSC-conditioned media could reverse hypoxic pulmonary vasoconstriction, suggesting that MSCs regulate vascular tone through the production of secreted factors (49). MSCs have also been shown to possess a potent capacity to reduce the inflammatory response to injury (50), which has been at least partially credited with their efficacy in other models of lung disease, such as LPS-induced acute lung injury (51). Considering the well-established link between PAH and immune dysfunction, including the prominence of chronic inflammation in both clinical cases of PAH and the MCT model (52), the capacity of MSCs to modulate the inflammatory response may be critical to their mode of therapeutic action.

CLINICAL APPLICATIONS OF CELL THERAPY

The favorable results from animal studies suggested that the clinical application of blood or bone marrow-derived progenitor cells, with or without transfection with a therapeutic transgene, may provide a viable strategy for halting or reversing the progression of PAH. Recently, two randomized controlled trials explored the therapeutic capacity of EPCs in PAH patients. In the first published report by Wang and colleagues (32), the intravenous administration of autologous, peripheral blood-derived EPCs resulted in a significantly greater increase in 6-minute walk distance at 12 weeks after injection (from 263 ± 42 m to 312 ± 44 m) in PAH patients receiving cells versus those treated with conventional therapy (from 264 ± 42 m to 270 ± 44 m), with a mean difference between the two groups of 42.5 m ($P < 0.001$). In this study, patients receiving cell therapy also demonstrated a significant improvement in mean pulmonary arterial pressure, PVR and cardiac output versus control patients. However, it should be noted that, in this non-blinded trial, it is not possible to exclude placebo effects or other sources of bias that could have contributed to these rather modest benefits.

The favorable results from this first study were followed up by a second, open-label study by the same group, exploring the safety and efficacy of autologous EPC transplantation in children with idiopathic PAH (33). In this study, EPCs derived from PBMNC cultures were once again delivered systemically by intravenous injection. As with the first study, patients given cell therapy demonstrated significant improvements in 6-minute walk distance, mean PAP, PVR, cardiac output and NYHA functional class. While both trials demonstrated a beneficial effect for EPC therapy in the treatment of PAH, this benefit was achieved following only a single dose of a relatively small number of cells ($1.1 \pm 0.6 \times 10^7$ cells for adults (32) and $0.6 \pm 0.33 \times 10^7$ cells for children (33)). The optimization of EPC therapy in future studies may require an increased number of cells or a dosing regime that allows for multiple injections. Moreover, the previously described work in the MCT rat model also demonstrated that the therapeutic capacity of EPCs could be enhanced following genetic manipulation to induce eNOS overexpression (13). In accordance with these results, the Stewart group has initiated the early phase, dose-ranging Pulmonary Hypertension Assessment of Cell Therapy (PHACeT) trial, investigating the treatment of PAH patients using autologous, peripheral blood-derived EPCs, transfected to overexpress eNOS. This study is the world's first clinical trial combining both gene and cell therapy for the treatment of cardiovascular disease.

FUTURE DIRECTIONS

While the initial reports investigating the use of stem cell therapies for the treatment of PAH have shown great promise, the field remains in its infancy. Translation of this therapeutic strategy into viable clinical treatments will depend upon the completion of a series of studies defining the appropriate cell phenotype, dose, and delivery mechanism. Advancement is also limited by a lack of knowledge surrounding the mode of action by which the therapeutic cells induce tissue regeneration. It has been suggested that both MSCs and EPCs act by differentiating into endothelial cells and regenerating the damaged pulmonary microvasculature. However, the current body of preclinical studies have not generated sufficient evidence to support this claim. As stem cell therapies for PAH progress from preclinical studies to small-scale clinical trials, the future success of this novel treatment platform will depend on an improved characterization of the therapeutic cell types, a greater understanding of how these cells induce regenerative vascular remodeling and what cellular attributes can be enhanced to positively influence their therapeutic efficacy.

KEY POINTS

- Stem cell-based therapies for PAH are being investigated with the goal of reversing pathological vascular remodeling and stimulating microvascular regeneration.
- Both EPCs and MSCs have been shown to produce endothelial-like cells in culture, suggesting a capacity to enact vascular regeneration *in vivo*.
- Both EPCs and MSCs have been shown to provide a therapeutic benefit in experimental models of PAH, which can be enhanced following transfection with eNOS or adrenomedullin.
- Initial clinical trials have demonstrated a modest yet significant benefit for EPCs in the treatment of IPAH patients.
- Uncertainty remains regarding both the characterization of these cell types as stem cells and their mode of action in the treatment of PAH.

REFERENCES

• = Key primary paper

1. Chin KM, Rubin LJ. Pulmonary arterial hypertension. J Am Coll Cardiol 2008;51(16):1527–38.
2. Macchia A, Marchioli R, Marfisi R, Scarano M, Levantesi G, Tavazzi L et al. A meta-analysis of trials of pulmonary hypertension: a clinical condition looking for drugs and research methodology. Am Heart J 2007;153(6):1037–47.
3. Barst RJ, Rubin LJ, Long WA, McGoon MD, Rich S, Badesch DB et al. A comparison of continuous intravenous epoprostenol (prostacyclin) with conventional therapy for primary pulmonary hypertension. The Primary Pulmonary Hypertension Study Group. N Engl J Med 1996;334(5): 296–302.
4. Rubin LJ. Therapy of pulmonary hypertension: the evolution from vasodilators to antiproliferative agents. Am J Respir Crit Care Med 2002;166(10):1308–9.
5. Tuder RM, Groves B, Badesch DB, Voelkel NF. Exuberant endothelial cell growth and elements of inflammation are present in plexiform lesions of pulmonary hypertension. Am J Pathol 1994;144(2):275–85.
6. Masri FA, Xu W, Comhair SA, Asosingh K, Koo M, Vasanji A et al. Hyperproliferative apoptosis-resistant endothelial cells in idiopathic pulmonary arterial hypertension. Am J Physiol Lung Cell Mol Physiol 2007;293(3):L548–54.
7. Jones PL, Cowan KN, Rabinovitch M. Tenascin-C, proliferation and subendothelial fibronectin in progressive pulmonary vascular disease. Am J Pathol 1997;150(4):1349–60.
8. Voelkel NF, Cool C. Pathology of pulmonary hypertension. Cardiol Clin 2004;22(3):343–51.
9. Lee SD, Shroyer KR, Markham NE, Cool CD, Voelkel NF, Tuder RM. Monoclonal endothelial cell proliferation is present in primary but not secondary pulmonary hypertension. J Clin Invest 1998;101(5):927–34.
10. Campbell AI, Zhao Y, Sandhu R, Stewart DJ. Cell-based gene transfer of vascular endothelial growth factor attenuates monocrotaline-induced pulmonary hypertension. Circulation 2001;104(18):2242–8.
11. Zhao YD, Campbell AI, Robb M, Ng D, Stewart DJ. Protective role of angiopoietin-1 in experimental pulmonary hypertension. Circ Res 2003;92(9):984–91.
12. Zhao YD, Courtman DW, Ng DS, Robb MJ, Deng YP, Trogadis J et al. Microvascular regeneration in established pulmonary hypertension by angiogenic gene transfer. Am J Respir Cell Mol Biol 2006;35(2):182–9.
•13. Zhao YD, Courtman DW, Deng Y, Kugathasan L, Zhang Q, Stewart DJ. Rescue of monocrotaline-induced pulmonary arterial hypertension using bone marrow-derived endothelial-like progenitor cells: efficacy of combined cell and eNOS gene therapy in established disease. Circ Res 2005;96(4):442–50.
14. Kanki-Horimoto S, Horimoto H, Mieno S, Kishida K, Watanabe F, Furuya E et al. Implantation of mesenchymal stem cells overexpressing endothelial nitric oxide synthase improves right ventricular impairments caused by pulmonary hypertension. Circulation 2006;114(1 Suppl):I181–5.
15. Kalka C, Masuda H, Takahashi T, Kalka-Moll WM, Silver M, Kearney M et al. Transplantation of ex vivo expanded endothelial progenitor cells for therapeutic neovascularization. Proc Natl Acad Sci USA 2000; 97(7):3422–7.
16. Yue WM, Liu W, Bi YW, He XP, Sun WY, Pang XY et al. Mesenchymal stem cells differentiate into an endothelial phenotype, reduce neointimal formation, and enhance endothelial function in a rat vein grafting model. Stem Cells Dev 2008;17(4):785–93.
17. Flamme I, Frolich T, Risau W. Molecular mechanisms of vasculogenesis and embryonic angiogenesis. J Cell Physiol 1997;173(2):206–10.
18. Yancopoulos GD, Klagsbrun M, Folkman J. Vasculogenesis, angiogenesis, and growth factors: ephrins enter the fray at the border. Cell 1998;93(5):661–4.
19. Stump MM, Jordan GL Jr., Debakey ME, Halpert B. Endothelium grown from circulating blood on isolated intravascular Dacron hub. Am J Pathol 1963;43:361–7.
20. Shi Q, Rafii S, Wu MH, Wijelath ES, Yu C, Ishida A et al. Evidence for circulating bone marrow-derived endothelial cells. Blood 1998;92(2):362–7.
•21. Asahara T, Takahashi T, Masuda H, Kalka C, Chen D, Iwaguro H et al. VEGF contributes to postnatal neovascularization by mobilizing bone marrow-derived endothelial progenitor cells. Embo J 1999;18(14):3964–72.
22. Takahashi T, Kalka C, Masuda H, Chen D, Silver M, Kearney M et al. Ischemia- and cytokine-induced mobilization of bone marrow-derived endothelial progenitor cells for neovascularization. Nat Med 1999;5(4):434–8.
23. Spring H, Schuler T, Arnold B, Hammerling GJ, Ganss R. Chemokines direct endothelial progenitors into tumor neovessels. Proc Natl Acad Sci USA 2005;102(50):18111–6.

24. Lin Y, Weisdorf DJ, Solovey A, Hebbel RP. Origins of circulating endothelial cells and endothelial outgrowth from blood. J Clin Invest 2000;105(1):71–7.

25. Asahara T, Murohara T, Sullivan A, Silver M, van der Zee R, Li T et al. Isolation of putative progenitor endothelial cells for angiogenesis. Science 1997;275(5302):964–7.

26. Gehling UM, Ergun S, Schumacher U, Wagener C, Pantel K, Otte M et al. In vitro differentiation of endothelial cells from AC133-positive progenitor cells. Blood 2000;95(10):3106–12.

27. Vasa M, Fichtlscherer S, Aicher A, Adler K, Urbich C, Martin H et al. Number and migratory activity of circulating endothelial progenitor cells inversely correlate with risk factors for coronary artery disease. Circ Res 2001;89(1):E1–7.

28. Fadini GP, Sartore S, Albiero M, Baesso I, Murphy E, Menegolo M et al. Number and function of endothelial progenitor cells as a marker of severity for diabetic vasculopathy. Arterioscler Thromb Vasc Biol 2006;26(9):2140–6.

29. Diller GP, van Eijl S, Okonko DO, Howard LS, Ali O, Thum T et al. Circulating endothelial progenitor cells in patients with Eisenmenger syndrome and idiopathic pulmonary arterial hypertension. Circulation 2008;117(23):3020–30.

30. Kawamoto A, Gwon HC, Iwaguro H, Yamaguchi JI, Uchida S, Masuda H et al. Therapeutic potential of ex vivo expanded endothelial progenitor cells for myocardial ischemia. Circulation 2001;103(5):634–7.

31. Schachinger V, Assmus B, Britten MB, Honold J, Lehmann R, Teupe C et al. Transplantation of progenitor cells and regeneration enhancement in acute myocardial infarction: final one-year results of the TOPCARE-AMI Trial. J Am Coll Cardiol 2004;44(8):1690–9.

32. Wang XX, Zhang FR, Shang YP, Zhu JH, Xie XD, Tao QM et al. Transplantation of autologous endothelial progenitor cells may be beneficial in patients with idiopathic pulmonary arterial hypertension: a pilot randomized controlled trial. J Am Coll Cardiol 2007;49(14):1566–71.

33. Zhu JH, Wang XX, Zhang FR, Shang YP, Tao QM, Zhu JH et al. Safety and efficacy of autologous endothelial progenitor cells transplantation in children with idiopathic pulmonary arterial hypertension: Open-label pilot study. Pediatr Transplant 2008;12(6):650–5.

◆34. Schatteman GC, Dunnwald M, Jiao C. Biology of bone marrow-derived endothelial cell precursors. Am J Physiol Heart Circ Physiol 2007;292(1):H1–18.

35. Hur J, Yoon CH, Kim HS, Choi JH, Kang HJ, Hwang KK et al. Characterization of two types of endothelial progenitor cells and their different contributions to neovasculogenesis. Arterioscler Thromb Vasc Biol 2004;24(2):288–93.

36. Gnecchi M, He H, Liang OD, Melo LG, Morello F, Mu H et al. Paracrine action accounts for marked protection of ischemic heart by Akt-modified mesenchymal stem cells. Nat Med 2005;11(4):367–8.

37. Cho HJ, Lee N, Lee JY, Choi YJ, Ii M, Wecker A et al. Role of host tissues for sustained humoral effects after endothelial progenitor cell transplantation into the ischemic heart. J Exp Med 2007;204(13):3257–69.

38. Dirkx AE, Oude Egbrink MG, Wagstaff J, Griffioen AW. Monocyte/macrophage infiltration in tumors: modulators of angiogenesis. J Leukoc Biol 2006;80(6):1183–96.

39. Romagnani P, Annunziato F, Liotta F, Lazzeri E, Mazzinghi B, Frosali F et al. CD14+ CD34 low cells with stem cell phenotypic and functional features are the major source of circulating endothelial progenitors. Circ Res 2005;97(4): 314–22.

40. Gulati R, Jevremovic D, Peterson TE, Chatterjee S, Shah V, Vile RG et al. Diverse origin and function of cells with endothelial phenotype obtained from adult human blood. Circ Res 2003;93(11):1023–5.

41. Fernandez Pujol B, Lucibello FC, Gehling UM, Lindemann K, Weidner N, Zuzarte ML et al. Endothelial-like cells derived from human CD14 positive monocytes. Differentiation 2000;65(5):287–300.

42. Harraz M, Jiao C, Hanlon HD, Hartley RS, Schatteman GC. CD34-blood-derived human endothelial cell progenitors. Stem Cells 2001;19(4):304–12.

43. Schmeisser A, Garlichs CD, Zhang H, Eskafi S, Graffy C, Ludwig J et al. Monocytes coexpress endothelial and macrophagocytic lineage markers and form cord-like structures in Matrigel under angiogenic conditions. Cardiovasc Res 2001;49(3):671–80.

●44. Nagaya N, Kangawa K, Kanda M, Uematsu M, Horio T, Fukuyama N et al. Hybrid cell-gene therapy for pulmonary hypertension based on phagocytosing action of endothelial progenitor cells. Circulation 2003;108(7):889–95.

45. Takahashi M, Nakamura T, Toba T, Kajiwara N, Kato H, Shimizu Y. Transplantation of endothelial progenitor cells into the lung to alleviate pulmonary hypertension in dogs. Tissue Eng 2004;10(5–6):771–9.

46. Humbert M, Sitbon O, Chaouat A, Bertocchi M, Habib G, Gressin V et al. Pulmonary arterial hypertension in France: results from a national registry. Am J Respir Crit Care Med 2006;173(9):1023–30.

47. Pittenger MF, Mackay AM, Beck SC, Jaiswal RK, Douglas R, Mosca JD et al. Multilineage potential of adult human mesenchymal stem cells. Science 1999;284(5411):143–7.

48. Jiang Y, Jahagirdar BN, Reinhardt RL, Schwartz RE, Keene CD, Ortiz-Gonzalez XR et al. Pluripotency of mesenchymal stem cells derived from adult marrow. Nature 2002; 418(6893):41–9.

49. Patel KM, Crisostomo P, Lahm T, Markel T, Herring C, Wang M et al. Mesenchymal stem cells attenuate hypoxic pulmonary vasoconstriction by a paracrine mechanism. J Surg Res 2007;143(2):281–5.

50. Jones BJ, McTaggart SJ. Immunosuppression by mesenchymal stromal cells: from culture to clinic. Exp Hematol 2008;36(6):733–41.

51. Mei SH, McCarter SD, Deng Y, Parker CH, Liles WC, Stewart DJ. Prevention of LPS-induced acute lung injury in mice by mesenchymal stem cells overexpressing angiopoietin 1. PLOS Med 2007;4(9):e269.

52. Dorfmuller P, Perros F, Balabanian K, Humbert M. Inflammation in pulmonary arterial hypertension. Eur Respir J 2003;22(2):358–63.

Novel anti-proliferative strategies

SONI SAVAI PULLAMSETTI, FRIEDRICH GRIMMINGER AND RALPH THEO SCHERMULY

INTRODUCTION

Overview of pulmonary hypertension

Pulmonary hypertension (PH) is a progressive disease with a poor prognosis that results in right heart dysfunction and right heart failure (1). Characterized by increased pulmonary vascular resistance (PVR), PH includes a heterogeneous group of clinical entities that have been subcategorized into five categories based on association with other diseases according to the currently accepted PH classification (2). Among these, class 1 represents the so-called pulmonary arterial hypertension (PAH), which includes a mixture of diseases that have several pathophysiological, histological as well as prognostic features in common. Idiopathic PAH (IPAH), formerly known as primary PH (PPH), familial PAH in which loss-of-function mutations in the TGF-β/BMP superfamily have been identified as one underlying mechanism, PH associated with other diseases such as connective tissue diseases (e.g. systemic sclerosis), porto pulmonary hypertension and PH related to HIV infection, drugs and toxins. Class 2 encompasses patients with PH due to left heart diseases and represents the large group of pulmonary venous hypertension. Class 3, also a very large group, includes all forms of PH associated with alveolar hypoxia and/or disorders of the respiratory system. All (thrombo)embolic diseases leading to PH are summarized in class 4. Class 5 comprises a group of diseases directly affecting pulmonary vessels, which are rare in the western world, but may be of prominent importance in many underdeveloped countries (e.g. *Schistosomiasis* infection) (3).

It is estimated that, taken together, all variants of PH affect up to 100 million people worldwide.

Pathophysiology of PH

The pathogenesis of PH is a complicated, multifactorial process. Increased pulmonary arterial pressure (PAP) in PH patients may result from a combination of pulmonary vasoconstriction, in ward vascular wall remodeling and *in situ* thrombosis, leading to increased vascular stiffness as well as narrowing of the vascular lumen (4). However, what triggers PH has not been identified yet, but the initial insult either by chronic hypoxia, inflammation, viral infection, mechanical stretch, shear stress, and/or unknown factors occurring in the setting of a genetic predisposition is considered to activate or dysfunction the endothelium resulting in altered production of endothelial mediators has been increasingly implicated in PH (5–7). Since most of these mediators affect the growth of smooth muscle cells (SMC), an alteration in their production may facilitate the development of pulmonary vascular remodeling characteristic of PH.

Of those local mediators, nitric oxide, prostacyclin, thromboxane, serotonin and endothelin-1 are among the best studied and most commonly implicated in the pathogenesis of PAH (8). As a result, three of the currently approved therapeutic modalities for the treatment of PAH, such as prostacyclins, phosphodiesterase inhibitors, and endothelin receptor antagonists emerged in part from restoring the balance between these mediators (9–11). With current therapies progression of disease is slowed, but not halted. Lung transplantation remains the only treatment option for patients with progressive PH.

PULMONARY VASCULAR REMODELING

Pulmonary vascular remodeling is a hallmark of severe, advanced PH, presenting histologically as neointimal proliferation, intimal fibrosis, medial and adventitial hyperplasia and hypertrophy (8,12). Intimal changes include endothelial injury, endothelial cell proliferation, invasion of the intima by (myo)-fibroblast-like cells, enhanced matrix deposition with intimal fibrosis and – in some cases – obstruction of the vascular lumen by unique plexiform lesions (13). Pulmonary arterial smooth muscle cell (PASMC) proliferation is a prominent feature in virtually all PH entities, causing medial hypertrophy of the intra-acinar muscular resistance vessels, muscularization of the normally non-muscular precapillary arterioles and an increase in connective tissue deposition in the medial layer. In several forms of PH, these structural abnormalities are accompanied by marked hypertrophy of the adventitia, with (myo)-fibroblast proliferation/invasion and enhanced matrix deposition representing the predominant finding (8,14,15). Overall, these structural changes suggest a switch from "quiescent" towards proliferative, "apoptosis resistant" cellular phenotypes. In addition to the local expansion of the pre-existent "physiological" cell types, there is remarkable appearance of myofibroblasts, which may originate from (de)differentiated SMC/fibroblasts, local or recruited circulating progenitor cells, or endothelial- or epithelial-mesenchymal transition (15,16). In addition, the lung vascular remodeling process in PH may be preceded and/or accompanied by features of chronic inflammatory events, including enhanced adhesion and invasion of different leukocyte forms observed in some types of PH such as infection-linked (e.g. human immunodeficiency virus) or autoimmune-linked (e.g. systemic lupus erythematosus) variants of PH. In addition, various progenitor cell types may be recruited to the sites of lung vascular remodeling, both "fueling" the proliferative change and thereby contributing to disease etiology (e.g. circulating fibrocytes and mesenchymal progenitor cells) (17), or exerting an "antiproliferative" function and therefore offering for therapeutic intervention (e.g. endothelial progenitor cells) (18).

Of note, vascular remodeling is a response of blood vessels to both physiological and pathological stimuli (19). Vascular remodeling can be a physiological response, reversible, likely adaptive in nature and occurs to strengthen the vascular wall to alterations in hemodynamic environment (flow and pressure). On the other hand, it can be maladaptive and can compromise organ function, contributing to the fatal course of severe PH (20,21). The maladaptive response results in an inappropriate increased pulmonary vascular resistance and consequently, sustained PH. Severe PH increases right ventricular afterload and eventually leads to the clinical syndrome of right heart failure with systemic congestion and inability to adapt right ventricular output to peripheral demand (22,23). Hence, increased awareness of cellular and molecular mechanisms driving vascular remodeling may provide new therapeutic insights for the future.

CELLULAR AND MOLECULAR MECHANISMS OF PROLIFERATION IN PULMONARY VASCULAR REMODELING

As it has been mentioned before, pulmonary vascular remodeling is a complex process involving cell proliferation (hyperplasia, an increase in cell number associated with DNA synthesis), hypertrophy (an increase in cell size without change in DNA content), cell migration, phenotypic switching, or apoptosis, as well as production, degradation, and realignment of the extracellular matrix (24).

Because most vascular cells in the adult pulmonary circulation are in a quiescent state and have low baseline levels of proliferation, the development of vascular remodeling requires cells arrested in G0 or G1 to enter the cell cycle (25). As depicted in Figure 16.8.1, progression through the cell cycle requires the coordinated interaction of cyclin-dependent kinases (CDKs) that form holoenzymes with their regulatory subunits, the cyclins. Cyclin-CDK complexes activate transcription factors (p53, E2F, GAX, GATA-6 etc.) important in cell cycle progression (26). Furthermore, cell cycle progression is regulated by cyclin-dependent kinase inhibitors (CKIs) such as INK and Cip/Kip, which bind to CDKs and prevent their activation (27).

In response to mitogenic signals, cyclin D/CDK4/6/Cip/Kip complexes assemble, sequestering Cip/Kip proteins from cyclin E-CDK2. Cyclin D- and E-dependent kinases phosphorylate the retinoblastoma protein (Rb), resulting in release of E2F, which is necessary for transcription of genes required for S-phase progression, including cyclin E, cyclin A and CDK1. Importantly, CKI such as p27Kip1, belonging to the family of Cip/Kip has been shown to be an important regulator of PASMC proliferation in vitro (28–30) and to limit vascular remodeling in vivo in the experimental models of PH.

The list of factors known to trigger or influence PASMC proliferation has been extensively studied over the past 20 years, and includes growth factors, cytokines, chemokines, hypoxia and reactive oxygen species (ROS) and others (31–34). Additional growth effects mediated by changes in cell matrix are delineated (35). The temporal and spatial coordination of these events are shown to modulate the environment in which other growth factors initiate cell cycle events. However, the cellular source of these factors that stimulate PASMC is not clear, as vascular wall injury can induce humoral, autocrine and paracrine growth factors from endothelial cells, adventitial fibroblasts, and invasive cells such as monocytes and lymphocytes (36,37). Furthermore, cyclic stretch and laminar shear stress might be present after vessel injury, resulting in increased FGF-2

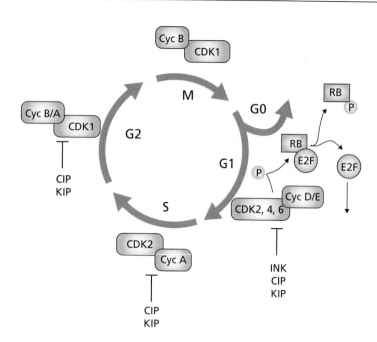

Figure 16.8.1 Schematic representation of cell cycle. Progression through mitotic cycle involves the successive formation, activation and subsequent inactivation of cyclin-dependent protein kinases (CDK). The kinases bind sequentially to a series of cyclins (Cyc), which are responsible for differential activation of the kinase during the cell cycle. The G1 to S phase transition is thought to be controlled by CDKs containing D- and E-type cyclins (Cyc D/E) that phosphorylate the retinoblastoma (RB) protein, releasing E2F transcription factors. E2F is involved in the transcription of genes needed for the G1 to S transition such as Cyc E, Cyc A etc. CKI (p27kip1, p21kip1, p57kip1) and INK bind to and inhibit the activation of cyclin-CDK complexes.

promoter activity, and intracellular and extracellular FGF-2 protein levels and results in PASMC proliferation (38). These factors stimulate several signaling cascades such as the Ras/MAPK and PI3K/Akt pathways that regulate cell proliferation. Signaling cascades mediated by individual factors are described in Figure 16.8.2.

Since the net balance between proliferation and apoptosis determines the extent of SMC growth, apoptosis of vascular smooth muscle cells (SMCs) also plays a prominent role in pulmonary vascular remodeling (19,25,39). For instance, compared with PASMCs from normal subjects and patients with SPH, PASMCs from PPH patients exhibited a significant resistance to apoptotic inducers such as BMP2 and BMP7 (40), suggesting that increased PASMC proliferation and decreased PASMC apoptosis can concurrently mediate thickening of the pulmonary vasculature, which subsequently reduces the inner-lumen diameter of pulmonary arteries, thus increasing pulmonary vascular resistance (PVR).

In recent years, PASMC dedifferentiation and phenotype change is thought to be an important aspect of vascular wall remodeling during PH (41,42). Differentiated PASMCs have a spindle shape, low proliferation rate and physiological contractile functions; dedifferentiated PASMCs exhibit a phenotypic change characterized by loss of contractility and abnormal proliferation, migration, and matrix secretion. Recently, BMP signaling is shown to modulate PASMC phenotype via cross-talk with the RhoA/myocardin-related transcription factor (MRTF) pathway, and may contribute to the development of the pathological characteristics observed in patients with PAH and other obliterative vascular diseases (43). However, more studies are necessary to define the role of vascular SMC phenotypic and functional heterogeneity in both normal homeostatic functions as well as in pathophysiologic responses to injury.

ANTI-PROLIFERATION AS A THERAPEUTIC APPROACH FOR PATIENTS WITH PH

The list of factors known to trigger or influence vascular growth has lengthened extensively over the past 20 years, ranging from growth factors to cytokines, chemokines, hypoxia, reactive oxygen species and others. Growth factors are proteins that bind to receptors on cell membranes and elicit biological responses leading to cell proliferation and differentiation. Four major signaling pathways were characterized in PASMC proliferation as shown in Figure 16.8.2, involving the receptor tyrosine kinase signaling, the small G-protein coupled receptors, receptor serine/threonine kinase signaling and cytokine receptor signaling (44–46). Tyrosine phosphorylation is considered one of the most important characteristic features of several growth factors.

Growth factor/growth factor receptors

TYROSINE KINASE RECEPTORS

Receptor tyrosine kinases (RTKs) are a subclass of cell-surface growth-factor receptors with an intrinsic, ligand-controlled tyrosine-kinase activity (47). Receptor tyrosine kinases have an extracellular ligand-binding domain, a transmembrane domain, and an intracellular catalytic domain. When a ligand (mostly a growth factor) binds to its receptor, it induces both receptor dimerization and an increase in the activity of the kinase (48,49). The intracellular region of the activated receptor then becomes extensively autophosphorylated and these phosphorylated tyrosines form specific docking sites for intracellular molecules that contain Src homology 2 (SH2)- and phosphotyrosine-binding (PTB) domain-containing proteins. Molecules recruited via these binding motifs are either enzymes that are tyrosine

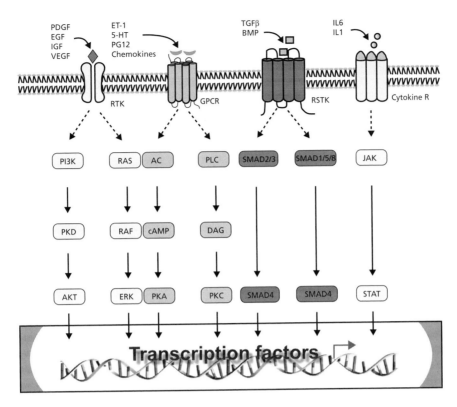

Figure 16.8.2 Major signaling pathways regulating PASMC proliferation. Four major signaling pathways were characterized, involving receptor tyrosine kinase (RTK) signaling, G-protein coupled receptors (GPCR), receptor serine/threonine kinase (RSTK) signaling and cytokine receptor (cytokine R) signaling. In general ligand binding (PDGF, EGF, IGF, VEGF, ET-1, 5-HT, PGI2, chemokines, TGFβ, BMP, IL1, IL6) activates the receptors and initiates multiple intracellular cascades, substrates and finally transcription factors that leads to changes in gene expression. The biochemistry of intracellular signaling has been very widely studied. The diagram summarizes the key reactions. PDGF: platelet derived growth factor; EGF: epidermal growth factor; VEGF: vascular endothelial growth factor; FGF: fibroblast growth factor; ET-1: endothelin-1; 5-HT: 5-hydroxytryptamine; PGI2: prostacyclin; TGF-β: transforming growth factor-β; BMP: bone morphogenic protein; IL6: interleukin 6; IL1: interleukin 1; PI3K: phosphatidylinositol kinase; PDK: phosphoinositide-dependent protein kinase; AKT: oncogenic kinase initially isolated from a transforming mouse retrovirus; Ras: oncogene first isolated in rat sarcomas; Raf: oncogenic kinase initially isolated from a transforming mouse virus; ERK: extracellular-regulated kinase; AC: adenylyl cyclase; cAMP: cyclicAMP; PKA: protein kinase A; PLC: phospholipase C; DAG: diacylglycerol; PKC: protein kinase C; SMAD: mothers against drosophila protein homolog; JAK: janus kinase; STAT: signal transducer and activator of transcription.

phosphorylated and activated, such as Src and phospholipase Cγ, or adaptor molecules (Shc, Grb2, or Cbl) that link RTK activation to downstream signaling pathways (50). These proteins then recruit additional effector molecules containing SH2, SH3, PTB, and Pleckstrin-homology domains to the activated receptor, which results in the assembly of signaling complexes at the membrane and the activation of intracellular downstream signaling cascades. The most important downstream signaling cascades activated by RTKs include the Ras-extracellular regulated kinase (ERK)-mitogen activated (MAP) kinase pathway, the phosphoinositide 3-kinase (PI 3-kinase)-Akt, and the JAK/STAT pathway. Ultimately, the complex signaling network triggered by RTKs leads either to activation or repression of various subsets of genes and thus defines and regulates intercellular communication controlling cell growth, proliferation, differentiation, survival, and metabolism. Conversely, RTK activity in resting and normal cells is tightly controlled. Concomitant with the initiation of signal transduction, activated receptors are either internalized

rapidly by the endocytic pathway or ubiquitinated by a proteasome-dependent pathway leading to attenuation of the signal-transduction cascades (49).

Based on their extracellular structural characteristics and ligand-binding properties, RTKs can be classified into approximately 20 families (51). Some examples of receptors are listed here: family I, EGF receptor and its homologs with two cysteine-rich domains; family III, PDGF receptors with five immunoglobulin-like domains; family IV, FGF receptors with three immunoglobulin-like domains; family V, VEGF receptors with seven immunoglobulin domains; family VI, the HGF receptor and its homologs that have a heterodimeric structure; family XIV, the Ret receptor with a cadherin repeat and a cysteine-rich region.

Recently, several growth factors and RTKs have been implicated in the abnormal proliferation and migration of pulmonary vascular cells, including platelet-derived growth factor (PDGF), basic fibroblast growth factor (b-FGF), epidermal growth factor (EGF), and vascular endothelial growth factor (VEGF), suggesting that the PH shares features of cancer, and anti-neoplastic drugs can potentially control vascular remodeling in PH.

The following receptors in this subclass may affect the development and progression of PH:

- PDGF receptors (52–60).
- VEGF receptors (61–68).
- EGF receptors (69–76).

SERINE/THREONINE KINASE RECEPTORS

TGF–β/BMP receptors

The TGF-β superfamily comprises a multitude of pleiotropic and pluripotent growth factors, including the TGF-β ligands themselves, bone morphogenetic proteins (BMPs), growth and differentiation factors (GDFs), activins and nodal. Signaling begins with the binding of a TGF beta superfamily ligand to a TGF beta type II receptor. The type II receptor is a serine/threonine receptor kinase, which catalyses the phosphorylation of the type I receptor. The type I receptor then phosphorylates receptor-regulated SMADs (R-SMADs) which can now bind the coSMAD SMAD4. R-SMAD/coSMAD complexes accumulate in the nucleus where they act as transcription factors and participate in the regulation of target gene expression (77,78). Genetic studies of FPAH patients revealed a germline mutation in one copy of BMPR2, loss-of-function mutations of TGF-β receptor I, Alk1, and a markedly reduced expression of BMPR2 in the pulmonary vasculature of patients with mutations in the BMPR2 gene (79–81). BMPR2 expression and the main downstream signaling pathway i.e., phosphorylation of SMAD1/5 was also significantly reduced in the pulmonary vasculature of patients with IPAH and experimental models of PAH in whom no mutation in the BMPR2 gene was identified, suggesting a critical role of BMP signaling to the pathogenesis of PAH (82). In further studies, the PASMC from patients with IPAH or FPAH showed resistance to the anti-proliferative effects of BMP and TGF-β (83) and transgenic overexpression of a dominant-negative kinase domain mutant BMPR-II in SMCs cause increased pulmonary vascular remodeling and PH (84).

On the other hand, there is an evidence of increased expression of TGF-β isoforms, TGF-β and BMP receptors, and enhanced TGF-β-dependent signaling in both familial PAH and IPAH lungs. These findings suggest that PH might develop due to unbalanced TGF-β signaling in pulmonary vascular cells. In support of this concept, inhibition of TGF-β signaling with SD-208 significantly attenuated the development of the PH and reduced pulmonary vascular remodeling (85).

G-PROTEIN COUPLED RECEPTORS

Work on G-protein coupled receptors includes:

- ET receptors (86–93).
- PGI$_2$ receptors (94–97).
- Chemokine receptors (33,98–101).

SECRETED FACTORS COUPLED TO OTHER RECEPTORS

IL receptors

Elevated serum IL-1β and IL-6 concentrations have been reported in patients with most forms of human PAH, suggesting a role for inflammation in development of PAH (102). Indeed, previous studies suggest that IL-6 stimulates vessel-wall remodeling mediated either by direct stimulation of vascular SMC migration or by indirect effects on PASMC proliferation (103).

Extracellular matrix regulation of growth factors

MATRIX METALLOPROTEASES (MMP)

The MMPs are a family of matrix-degrading enzymes that have been implicated in two important processes in vessel wall repair: cellular migration (104), and regulating extracellular matrix composition and content (105). Based on their substrate specificity, MMPs were subdivided into four groups, interstitial collagenases, type IV collagenases, stromelysins and membrane type-MMPs. Besides catabolism of the ECM, MMPs release growth factors from ECM-bound stores thereby promoting vascular remodeling. For example, it has been shown that during the development and progression of PAH, members of the matrix metalloprotease (MMP) family are activated in concert with the pro-proliferative ECM glycoprotein tenascin-C (TN-C) within the SMC medial layer of hypertensive pulmonary arteries (106,107). In fact, direct inhibition of MMPs, including gelatinolytic activity attributable to MMP-2, or of serine elastases, leads to reduced TN-C, reduced PASMC proliferation, induction of PASMC apoptosis, loss of ECM, and regression of pulmonary arterial hypertension (108).

Intracellular signaling molecules

RAF

The Raf is a serine threonine kinase family consisting of three isoforms, Raf-1 (C-Raf), A-Raf, and B-Raf. Each isoform has three conserved regions in common: CR1, CR2, and CR3 that includes several regulatory phosphorylation sites. Importantly, Raf isoforms vary in their cell-specific expression, potency of kinase activity, and show both overlapping and unique regulatory functions (109). The activation of Raf is a complex multistep process that begins with the recruitment of inactive Raf (complexed with 14-3-3 and heat shock proteins) from the cytosol to the plasma membrane by activated Ras. The effector domain of Ras, binds to Raf at the Ras-binding domain and cysteine rich domains of the CR1 region (110). Once recruited to the cell membrane, Raf must then undergo several further modifications before being rendered active. After activation, Raf kinase then phosphorylates and activates MEK1 and MEK2, which then phosphorylates and activates ERK1 and ERK2. The activated ERK1 and ERK2 translocates to the nucleus where they induce phosphorylation of both cytoplasmic (p90RSK: ribosomal 6 kinase) and nuclear targets (C-FOS, CMYC, Elk-1, Ets, Sp1, and HIF-1) leading to cell cycle checkpoints, aberrant growth, dedifferentiation, and cell survival (111).

Screening for Raf-MEK-ERK signaling cascade in experimental models of PH suggested increased levels of p-ERK and p-MEK1/2 in both hypoxia and hypoxia/SU-5416-exposed rats compared with normoxia, with no changes in the total amount of MAPK components (112). Similarly, increased phosphorylation of Raf-1 and ERK1/2 in the lungs as well as in the right ventricle was observed in MCT induced PH rats. In both studies, administration of a Raf kinase inhibitor, sorafenib (tosylate salt of BAY 43-9006; Nexavar) prevented hemodynamic changes and demonstrated dramatic attenuation of PH-associated vascular remodeling. In addition, sorafenib exerted direct myocardial antihypertrophic effects, which appear to be mediated via inhibition of the Raf kinase pathway (113). Although, initially developed as an inhibitor of Raf-1, sorafenib also showed very potent inhibitory activity for other protein kinases *in vitro* and *in vivo*, in particular, for the proangiogenic

RTKs such as VEGFR-2, VEGFR-3, PDGFR-β, Flt-3, c-Kit and FGFR-1 (114).

PDE

Phosphodiesterases (PDEs) are enzymes that hydrolyse the secondary messengers, cAMP and/or cGMP. They encompass eleven distinct families and play an important role in the regulation of vascular tone and vascular remodeling (115). In structurally remodeled pulmonary arteries and isolated PASMCs from patients with PAH and in animal models of PAH, the expression and activities of PDE1, PDE3 and PDE5 are increased compared to healthy controls (116,117). Furthermore, a selective PDE5 inhibitor and PDE1 inhibitor dose dependently inhibited the DNA synthesis of human PASMCs (117,118). Similarly, treatment with PDE1 inhibitor in hypoxic mice and MCT injected rats with fully established PH reversed the pulmonary artery pressure elevation, structural remodeling of the lung vasculature and right heart hypertrophy (117).

Transcription factors

NFAT

NFAT is a family of transcription factors activated by calcineurin and comprised of four well-characterized members, NFATc1 (NFAT2/c), NFATc2 (NFAT1/p), NFATc3

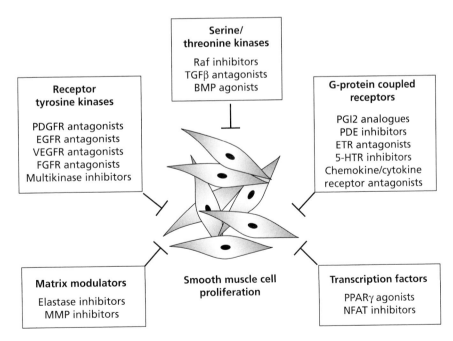

Figure 16.8.3 Therapies targeting the pro-proliferative component in PH. Analogues, agonists, antagonists or inhibitors of several key players involved in anti-proliferative actions against pulmonary arterial smooth muscle cell proliferation is depicted here. PDGFR: platelet derived growth factor receptor; EGFR: epidermal growth factor receptor; VEGFR: vascular endothelial growth factor receptor; FGFR: fibroblast growth factor receptor; Raf: oncogenic kinase initially isolated from a transforming mouse virus; TGF-β: transforming growth factor-β; BMP: bone morphogenic protein; PGI2: prostacyclin; ETR: endothelin receptor; 5-HT: 5-hydroxytryptamine; 5-HTR: 5-hydroxytryptamine receptor; PPARγ: peroxisome proliferator-activated receptor gamma; NFAT: Nuclear factor of activated T-cells.

(NFAT4/x), and NFATc4 (NFAT3) (119). Although first identified in activated T cells, NFAT has since been shown to play a role in non-immune cells, including vascular smooth muscle and myocardial cells (120). Most interestingly, NFAT activation and NFAT nuclear accumulation, as well as increased levels of NFAT-regulated cytokines, were found in both human and experimental models of PAH. Indeed, pharmacological inhibition of calcineurin activation of NFAT by cyclosporine or genetic ablation of NFATc3 prevents chronic hypoxia-induced arterial wall thickness and right ventricular hypertrophy (121). In another study, Michelakis and colleagues also found that inhibition of NFAT by VIVIT peptide (which blocks the docking of calcineurin on NFAT) or cyclosporine decreased proliferation and increased apoptosis *in vitro* and *in vivo*; cyclosporine decreased established rat MCT induced PAH (122).

PPARγ

Peroxisome proliferator-activated receptor gamma (PPARγ) is a member of the nuclear hormone receptor superfamily, which regulates transcription of target genes in a ligand-dependent manner. Ligands for PPARγ have been shown to attenuate proliferation of vascular smooth muscle cells, and to induce apoptosis in several cell lines *in vitro* (123,124). PPARγ ligands reduce MCT-induced PH and pulmonary vascular wall thickening in rats. Inhibition of MCT-induced cell proliferation and induction of apoptosis in the pulmonary arterial walls may account for this effect (125).

CONCLUSION

In summary, the current therapeutic approach (prostacyclin analogs, endothelin receptor antagonists and phosphodiesterase type 5 inhibitors) for the treatment of PH mainly provides symptomatic relief, as well as improvement of prognosis. However, they do not appear to reverse or modify the disease. The successful outcome of anti-proliferative approaches described in Figure 16.8.3, signifies a paradigm shift in PH therapy from a vasodilatory to anti-proliferative and pro-apoptotic therapies. Apart from few hurdles such as diversity of targets involved in pulmonary vascular remodeling, complex interplay of signal transduction pathways and challenges in designing effective treatment regimens, anti-proliferative strategies provide a new hope for the treatment of severe PH.

KEY POINTS

- Pulmonary hypertension (PH) is a progressive disease with a poor prognosis that results in right heart dysfunction and right heart failure. It is estimated that, taken together, all variants of PH affect up to 100 million people worldwide. With current therapies progression of disease is slowed, but not halted.
- The pathogenesis of PH is a complicated, multifactorial process. Increased pulmonary arterial pressure in PH patients results from pulmonary vascular remodeling, a hallmark of severe, advanced PH, presenting histologically as neointimal proliferation, intimal fibrosis, medial and adventitial hyperplasia and hypertrophy.
- Pulmonary arterial smooth muscle cell (PASMC) proliferation is a prominent feature in virtually all PH entities, causing medial hypertrophy of the intra-acinar muscular resistance vessels, muscularization of the normally non-muscular precapillary arterioles and an increase in connective tissue deposition in the medial layer.
- The list of factors known to trigger or influence vascular growth has lengthened extensively over the past 20 years, ranging from growth factors to cytokines, chemokines, hypoxia, reactive oxygen species, extracellular matrix and others.
- Major families of growth factor receptors are the tyrosine kinases (PDGF, EGF, VEGF, FGF), serine/threonine kinases (TGFβ, BMP), the small G-protein-associated receptors (ET-1, PGI2, chemokines), intracellular signaling molecules (Raf, PDE) and transcription factors (PPARγ, NFAT) have been implicated in the abnormal proliferation of PASMCs, suggesting that the PH shares features of cancer, and anti-neoplastic drugs can potentially control vascular remodeling in PH.
- Indeed, preclinical evaluation of drug candidates that target the above signaling has reversed established experimental PH, signifying a paradigm shift in PH therapy from a vasodilatory to antiproliferative therapies.

REFERENCES

1. Rubin LJ. Pulmonary arterial hypertension. Proc Am Thorac Soc 2006;3:111–5.
2. Simonneau G, Galie N, Rubin LJ *et al*. Clinical classification of pulmonary hypertension. J Am Coll Cardiol 2004;43: 5S–12S.
3. Butrous G, Ghofrani HA, Grimminger F. Pulmonary vascular disease in the developing world. Circulation 2008;118: 1758–66.
4. Barst RJ, McGoon M, Torbicki A *et al*. Diagnosis and differential assessment of pulmonary arterial hypertension. J Am Coll Cardiol 2004;43:40S–7S.
5. Budhiraja R, Tuder RM, Hassoun PM. Endothelial dysfunction in pulmonary hypertension. Circulation 2004;109:159–65.

6. Lopes AA, Maeda NY, Goncalves RC, Bydlowski SP. Endothelial cell dysfunction correlates differentially with survival in primary and secondary pulmonary hypertension. Am Heart J 2000;139:618–23.

7. Tuder RM, Cool CD, Yeager M et al. The pathobiology of pulmonary hypertension. Endothelium. Clin Chest Med 2001;22:405–18.

8. Humbert M, Morrell NW, Archer SL et al. Cellular and molecular pathobiology of pulmonary arterial hypertension. J Am Coll Cardiol 2004;43:13S–24S.

9. Barst RJ, Rubin LJ, Long WA et al. A comparison of continuous intravenous epoprostenol (prostacyclin) with conventional therapy for primary pulmonary hypertension. The Primary Pulmonary Hypertension Study Group. N Engl J Med 1996;334:296–302.

10. Galie N, Ghofrani HA, Torbicki A et al. Sildenafil citrate therapy for pulmonary arterial hypertension. N Engl J Med 2005;353:2148–57.

11. Rubin LJ, Badesch DB, Barst RJ et al. Bosentan therapy for pulmonary arterial hypertension. N Engl J Med 2002; 346:896–903.

12. Pietra GG, Capron F, Stewart S et al. Pathologic assessment of vasculopathies in pulmonary hypertension. J Am Coll Cardiol 2004;43:25S–32S.

13. Rabinovitch M. Pathobiology of pulmonary hypertension. Annu Rev Pathol 2007;2:369–99.

14. Rabinovitch M. Molecular pathogenesis of pulmonary arterial hypertension. J Clin Invest 2008;118:2372–9.

15. Stenmark KR, Fagan KA, Frid MG. Hypoxia-induced pulmonary vascular remodeling: cellular and molecular mechanisms. Circ Res 2006;99:675–91.

16. Arciniegas E, Frid MG, Douglas IS, Stenmark KR. Perspectives on endothelial-to-mesenchymal transition: potential contribution to vascular remodeling in chronic pulmonary hypertension. Am J Physiol Lung Cell Mol Physiol 2007;293:L1–8.

17. Frid MG, Brunetti JA, Burke DL et al. Hypoxia-induced pulmonary vascular remodeling requires recruitment of circulating mesenchymal precursors of a monocyte/macrophage lineage. Am J Pathol 2006;168:659–69.

18. Zhao YD, Courtman DW, Deng Y et al. Rescue of monocrotaline-induced pulmonary arterial hypertension using bone marrow-derived endothelial-like progenitor cells: efficacy of combined cell and eNOS gene therapy in established disease. Circ Res 2005;96: 442–50.

19. Gibbons GH, Dzau VJ. The emerging concept of vascular remodeling. N Engl J Med 1994;330:1431–8.

20. Mulvany MJ. Small artery remodeling and significance in the development of hypertension. News Physiol Sci 2002;17:105–9.

21. Rizzoni D, Porteri E, Boari GE et al. Prognostic significance of small-artery structure in hypertension. Circulation 2003;108:2230–5.

22. Naeije R. Pulmonary hypertension and right heart failure in chronic obstructive pulmonary disease. Proc Am Thorac Soc 2005;2:20–2.

23. Pries AR, Secomb TW, Gaehtgens P. Structural autoregulation of terminal vascular beds: vascular adaptation and development of hypertension. Hypertension 1999;33:153–61.

24. Mandegar M, Fung YC, Huang W et al. Cellular and molecular mechanisms of pulmonary vascular remodeling: role in the development of pulmonary hypertension. Microvasc Res 2004;68:75–103.

25. Voelkel NF, Tuder RM. Cellular and molecular biology of vascular smooth muscle cells in pulmonary hypertension. Pulm Pharmacol Ther 1997;10:231–41.

26. Sherr CJ, Roberts JM. Inhibitors of mammalian G1 cyclin-dependent kinases. Genes Dev 1995;9:1149–63.

27. Sherr CJ, Roberts JM. CDK inhibitors: positive and negative regulators of G1-phase progression. Genes Dev 1999;13:1501–12.

28. Fouty BW, Grimison B, Fagan KA et al. p27(Kip1) is important in modulating pulmonary artery smooth muscle cell proliferation. Am J Respir Cell Mol Biol 2001;25:652–8.

29. Tanner FC, Boehm M, Akyurek LM et al. Differential effects of the cyclin-dependent kinase inhibitors p27(Kip1), p21(Cip1), and p16(Ink4) on vascular smooth muscle cell proliferation. Circulation 2000;101:2022–5.

30. Tanner FC, Yang ZY, Duckers E et al. Expression of cyclin-dependent kinase inhibitors in vascular disease. Circ Res 1998;82:396–403.

31. Dempsey EC, Frid MG, Aldashev AA et al. Heterogeneity in the proliferative response of bovine pulmonary artery smooth muscle cells to mitogens and hypoxia: importance of protein kinase C. Can J Physiol Pharmacol 1997;75:936–44.

32. Pak O, Aldashev A, Welsh D, Peacock A. The effects of hypoxia on the cells of the pulmonary vasculature. Eur Respir J 2007;30:364–72.

33. Schober A, Zernecke A. Chemokines in vascular remodeling. Thromb Haemost 2007;97:730–7.

34. Wedgwood S, Black SM. Role of reactive oxygen species in vascular remodeling associated with pulmonary hypertension. Antioxid Redox Signal 2003;5:759–69.

35. Rabinovitch M. Elastase and cell matrix interactions in the pathobiology of vascular disease. Acta Paediatr Jpn 1995;37:657–66.

36. Jeffery TK, Morrell NW. Molecular and cellular basis of pulmonary vascular remodeling in pulmonary hypertension. Prog Cardiovasc Dis 2002;45:173–202.

37. Stenmark KR, Orton EC, Reeves JT et al. Vascular remodeling in neonatal pulmonary hypertension. Role of the smooth muscle cell. Chest 1988;93:127S–33S.

38. Wedgwood S, Devol JM, Grobe A et al. Fibroblast growth factor-2 expression is altered in lambs with increased pulmonary blood flow and pulmonary hypertension. Pediatr Res 2007;61:32–6.

39. Stenmark KR, Mecham RP. Cellular and molecular mechanisms of pulmonary vascular remodeling. Annu Rev Physiol 1997;59:89–144.

40. Zhang S, Fantozzi I, Tigno DD et al. Bone morphogenetic proteins induce apoptosis in human pulmonary vascular

smooth muscle cells. Am J Physiol Lung Cell Mol Physiol 2003;285:L740–54.

41. Mitani Y, Ueda M, Komatsu R *et al*. Vascular smooth muscle cell phenotypes in primary pulmonary hypertension. Eur Respir J 2001;17:316–20.

42. Stenmark KR, Frid MG. Smooth muscle cell heterogeneity: role of specific smooth muscle cell subpopulations in pulmonary vascular disease. Chest 1998;114:82S–90S.

43. Lagna G, Ku MM, Nguyen PH *et al*. Control of phenotypic plasticity of smooth muscle cells by bone morphogenetic protein signaling through the myocardin-related transcription factors. J Biol Chem 2007;282:37244–55.

44. Khan TA, Bianchi C, Ruel M *et al*. Mitogen-activated protein kinase pathways and cardiac surgery. J Thorac Cardiovasc Surg 2004;127:806–11.

45. Luttrell DK, Luttrell LM. Signaling in time and space: G protein-coupled receptors and mitogen-activated protein kinases. Assay Drug Dev Technol 2003;1:327–38.

46. Muto A, Fitzgerald TN, Pimiento JM *et al*. Smooth muscle cell signal transduction: implications of vascular biology for vascular surgeons. J Vasc Surg 2007;(45 Suppl A):A15–24.

47. Yarden Y, Ullrich A. Growth factor receptor tyrosine kinases. Annu Rev Biochem 1988;57:443–78.

48. Heldin CH. Dimerization of cell surface receptors in signal transduction. Cell 1995;80:213–23.

49. Ullrich A, Schlessinger J. Signal transduction by receptors with tyrosine kinase activity. Cell 1990;61:203–12.

50. Pawson T. Protein modules and signalling networks. Nature 1995;373:573–80.

51. Robinson DR, Wu YM, Lin SF. The protein tyrosine kinase family of the human genome. Oncogene 2000;19:5548–57.

52. Humbert M, Monti G, Fartoukh M *et al*. Platelet-derived growth factor expression in primary pulmonary hypertension: comparison of HIV seropositive and HIV seronegative patients. Eur Respir J 1998;11:554–9.

53. Perros F, Montani D, Dorfmuller P *et al*. Platelet-derived growth factor expression and function in idiopathic pulmonary arterial hypertension. Am J Respir Crit Care Med 2008;178:81–8.

54. Schermuly RT, Dony E, Ghofrani HA *et al*. Reversal of experimental pulmonary hypertension by PDGF inhibition. J Clin Invest 2005;115:2811–21.

55. Balasubramaniam V, Le Cras TD, Ivy DD *et al*. Role of platelet-derived growth factor in vascular remodeling during pulmonary hypertension in the ovine fetus. Am J Physiol Lung Cell Mol Physiol 2003;284:L826–33.

56. Katayose D, Ohe M, Yamauchi K *et al*. Increased expression of PDGF A- and B-chain genes in rat lungs with hypoxic pulmonary hypertension. Am J Physiol 1993;264:L100–6.

57. Capdeville R, Buchdunger E, Zimmermann J, Matter A. Glivec (STI571, imatinib), a rationally developed, targeted anticancer drug. Nat Rev Drug Discov 2002;1:493–502.

58. Ghofrani HA, Seeger W, Grimminger F. Imatinib for the treatment of pulmonary arterial hypertension. N Engl J Med 2005;353:1412–3.

59. Patterson KC, Weissmann A, Ahmadi T, Farber HW. Imatinib mesylate in the treatment of refractory idiopathic pulmonary arterial hypertension. Ann Intern Med 2006;145:152–3.

60. Souza R, Sitbon O, Parent F *et al*. Long term imatinib treatment in pulmonary arterial hypertension. Thorax 2006;61:736.

61. Voelkel NF, Vandivier RW, Tuder RM. Vascular endothelial growth factor in the lung. Am J Physiol Lung Cell Mol Physiol 2006;290:L209–21.

62. Ferrara N, Gerber HP, LeCouter J. The biology of VEGF and its receptors. Nat Med 2003;9:669–76.

63. Geiger R, Berger RM, Hess J *et al*. Enhanced expression of vascular endothelial growth factor in pulmonary plexogenic arteriopathy due to congenital heart disease. J Pathol 2000;191:202–7.

64. Partovian C, Adnot S, Raffestin B *et al*. Adenovirus-mediated lung vascular endothelial growth factor overexpression protects against hypoxic pulmonary hypertension in rats. Am J Respir Cell Mol Biol 2000;23:762–71.

65. Grover TR, Parker TA, Markham NE, Abman SH. rhVEGF treatment preserves pulmonary vascular reactivity and structure in an experimental model of pulmonary hypertension in fetal sheep. Am J Physiol Lung Cell Mol Physiol 2005;289:L315–21.

66. Campbell AI, Zhao Y, Sandhu R, Stewart DJ. Cell-based gene transfer of vascular endothelial growth factor attenuates monocrotaline-induced pulmonary hypertension. Circulation 2001;104:2242–8.

67. Le Cras TD, Markham NE, Tuder RM *et al*. Treatment of newborn rats with a VEGF receptor inhibitor causes pulmonary hypertension and abnormal lung structure. Am J Physiol Lung Cell Mol Physiol 2002;283:L555–62.

68. Taraseviciene-Stewart L, Kasahara Y, Alger L *et al*. Inhibition of the VEGF receptor 2 combined with chronic hypoxia causes cell death-dependent pulmonary endothelial cell proliferation and severe pulmonary hypertension. FASEB J 2001;15:427–38.

69. Singh AB, Harris RC. Autocrine, paracrine and juxtacrine signaling by EGFR ligands. Cell Signal 2005;17:1183–93.

70. Jones PL, Crack J, Rabinovitch M. Regulation of tenascin-C, a vascular smooth muscle cell survival factor that interacts with the alpha v beta 3 integrin to promote epidermal growth factor receptor phosphorylation and growth. J Cell Biol 1997;139:279–93.

71. Le Cras TD, Hardie WD, Fagan K *et al*. Disrupted pulmonary vascular development and pulmonary hypertension in transgenic mice overexpressing transforming growth factor-alpha. Am J Physiol Lung Cell Mol Physiol 2003;285:L1046–54.

72. Merklinger SL, Jones PL, Martinez EC, Rabinovitch M. Epidermal growth factor receptor blockade mediates smooth muscle cell apoptosis and improves survival in rats with pulmonary hypertension. Circulation 2005; 112:423–31.

73. Eswarakumar VP, Lax I, Schlessinger J. Cellular signaling by fibroblast growth factor receptors. Cytokine Growth Factor Rev 2005;16:139–49.

74. Li P, Oparil S, Sun JZ et al. Fibroblast growth factor mediates hypoxia-induced endothelin – a receptor expression in lung artery smooth muscle cells. J Appl Physiol 2003;95:643–51; discussion 863.

75. Quinn TP, Schlueter M, Soifer SJ, Gutierrez JA. Cyclic mechanical stretch induces VEGF and FGF-2 expression in pulmonary vascular smooth muscle cells. Am J Physiol Lung Cell Mol Physiol 2002;282:L897–903.

76. Izikki M, Guignabert C, Fadel E et al. Endothelial-derived FGF2 contributes to the progression of pulmonary hypertension in humans and rodents. J Clin Invest 2009;119:512–23.

77. Attisano L, Wrana JL. Signal transduction by the TGF-beta superfamily. Science 2002;296:1646–7.

78. Kawabata M, Imamura T, Miyazono K. Signal transduction by bone morphogenetic proteins. Cytokine Growth Factor Rev 1998;9:49–61.

79. Atkinson C, Stewart S, Upton PD et al. Primary pulmonary hypertension is associated with reduced pulmonary vascular expression of type II bone morphogenetic protein receptor. Circulation 2002;105:1672–8.

80. Harrison RE, Flanagan JA, Sankelo M et al. Molecular and functional analysis identifies ALK-1 as the predominant cause of pulmonary hypertension related to hereditary haemorrhagic telangiectasia. J Med Genet 2003;40:865–71.

81. Lane KB, Machado RD, Pauciulo MW et al. Heterozygous germline mutations in BMPR2, encoding a TGF-beta receptor, cause familial primary pulmonary hypertension. The International PPH Consortium. Nat Genet 2000;26:81–4.

82. Yang X, Long L, Southwood M et al. Dysfunctional Smad signaling contributes to abnormal smooth muscle cell proliferation in familial pulmonary arterial hypertension. Circ Res 2005;96:1053–63.

83. Morrell NW, Yang X, Upton PD et al. Altered growth responses of pulmonary artery smooth muscle cells from patients with primary pulmonary hypertension to transforming growth factor-beta(1) and bone morphogenetic proteins. Circulation 2001;104:790–5.

84. West J, Fagan K, Steudel W et al. Pulmonary hypertension in transgenic mice expressing a dominant-negative BMPRII gene in smooth muscle. Circ Res 2004;94:1109–14.

85. Zaiman AL, Podowski M, Medicherla S et al. Role of the TGF-beta/Alk5 signaling pathway in monocrotaline-induced pulmonary hypertension. Am J Respir Crit Care Med 2008;177:896–905.

86. Inoue A, Yanagisawa M, Kimura S et al. The human endothelin family: three structurally and pharmacologically distinct isopeptides predicted by three separate genes. Proc Natl Acad Sci USA 1989;86:2863–7.

87. Yanagisawa M, Kurihara H, Kimura S et al. A novel potent vasoconstrictor peptide produced by vascular endothelial cells. Nature 1988;332:411–5.

88. Filep JG. Endothelin peptides: biological actions and pathophysiological significance in the lung. Life Sci 1993;52:119–33.

89. Opitz CF, Ewert R. Dual ET(A)/ET(B) vs. selective ET(A) endothelin receptor antagonism in patients with pulmonary hypertension. Eur J Clin Invest 2006; (36 Suppl 3):1–9.

90. Peacock AJ, Dawes KE, Shock A et al. Endothelin-1 and endothelin-3 induce chemotaxis and replication of pulmonary artery fibroblasts. Am J Respir Cell Mol Biol 1992;7:492–9.

91. Davie N, Haleen SJ, Upton PD et al. ET(A) and ET(B) receptors modulate the proliferation of human pulmonary artery smooth muscle cells. Am J Respir Crit Care Med 2002;165:398–405.

92. Hill NS, Warburton RR, Pietras L, Klinger JR. Nonspecific endothelin-receptor antagonist blunts monocrotaline-induced pulmonary hypertension in rats. J Appl Physiol 1997;83:1209–15.

93. Miyauchi T, Yorikane R, Sakai S et al. Contribution of endogenous endothelin-1 to the progression of cardiopulmonary alterations in rats with monocrotaline-induced pulmonary hypertension. Circ Res 1993;73:887–97.

94. Narumiya S, Sugimoto Y, Ushikubi F. Prostanoid receptors: structures, properties, and functions. Physiol Rev 1999; 79:1193–226.

95. Coleman RA, Smith WL, Narumiya S. International Union of Pharmacology classification of prostanoid receptors: properties, distribution, and structure of the receptors and their subtypes. Pharmacol Rev 1994;46:205–29.

96. Wharton J, Davie N, Upton PD et al. Prostacyclin analogues differentially inhibit growth of distal and proximal human pulmonary artery smooth muscle cells. Circulation 2000;102:3130–6.

97. Schermuly RT, Pullamsetti SS, Kwapiszewska G et al. Phosphodiesterase 1 upregulation in pulmonary arterial hypertension: target for reverse-remodeling therapy. Circulation 2007;115:2331–9.

98. Balabanian K, Foussat A, Dorfmuller P et al. CX(3)C chemokine fractalkine in pulmonary arterial hypertension. Am J Respir Crit Care Med 2002;165:1419–25.

99. Dorfmuller P, Zarka V, Durand-Gasselin I et al. Chemokine RANTES in severe pulmonary arterial hypertension. Am J Respir Crit Care Med 2002;165:534–9.

100. Perros F, Dorfmuller P, Souza R et al. Fractalkine-induced smooth muscle cell proliferation in pulmonary hypertension. Eur Respir J 2007;29:937–43.

101. Sanchez O, Marcos E, Perros F et al. Role of endothelium-derived CC chemokine ligand 2 in idiopathic pulmonary arterial hypertension. Am J Respir Crit Care Med 2007;176:1041–7.

102. Humbert M, Monti G, Brenot F et al. Increased interleukin-1 and interleukin-6 serum concentrations in severe primary pulmonary hypertension. Am J Respir Crit Care Med 1995;151:1628–31.

103. Hagen M, Fagan K, Steudel W et al. Interaction of interleukin-6 and the BMP pathway in pulmonary smooth muscle. Am J Physiol Lung Cell Mol Physiol 2007;292:L1473–9.

104. Bendeck MP, Zempo N, Clowes AW et al. Smooth muscle cell migration and matrix metalloproteinase expression after arterial injury in the rat. Circ Res 1994;75:539–45.

105. Strauss BH, Robinson R, Batchelor WB *et al.* In vivo collagen turnover following experimental balloon angioplasty injury and the role of matrix metalloproteinases. Circ Res 1996;79:541–50.

106. Cowan KN, Jones PL, Rabinovitch M. Elastase and matrix metalloproteinase inhibitors induce regression, and tenascin-C antisense prevents progression, of vascular disease. J Clin Invest 2000;105:21–34.

107. Jones PL, Chapados R, Baldwin HS *et al.* Altered hemodynamics controls matrix metalloproteinase activity and tenascin-C expression in neonatal pig lung. Am J Physiol Lung Cell Mol Physiol 2002;282:L26–35.

108. Cowan KN, Heilbut A, Humpl T *et al.* Complete reversal of fatal pulmonary hypertension in rats by a serine elastase inhibitor. Nat Med 2000;6:698–702.

109. Hagemann C, Rapp UR. Isotype-specific functions of Raf kinases. Exp Cell Res 1999;253:34–46.

110. Chong H, Vikis HG, Guan KL. Mechanisms of regulating the Raf kinase family. Cell Signal 2003;15:463–9.

111. Chang F, Steelman LS, Lee JT *et al.* Signal transduction mediated by the Ras/Raf/MEK/ERK pathway from cytokine receptors to transcription factors: potential targeting for therapeutic intervention. Leukemia 2003;17:1263–93.

112. Moreno-Vinasco L, Gomberg-Maitland M, Maitland ML *et al.* Genomic assessment of a multikinase inhibitor, sorafenib, in a rodent model of pulmonary hypertension. Physiol Genomics 2008;33:278–91.

113. Klein M, Schermuly RT, Ellinghaus P *et al.* Combined tyrosine and serine/threonine kinase inhibition by sorafenib prevents progression of experimental pulmonary hypertension and myocardial remodeling. Circulation 2008;118:2081–90.

114. Wilhelm SM, Carter C, Tang L *et al.* BAY 43-9006 exhibits broad spectrum oral antitumor activity and targets the RAF/MEK/ERK pathway and receptor tyrosine kinases involved in tumor progression and angiogenesis. Cancer Res 2004;64:7099–109.

115. Lugnier C. Cyclic nucleotide phosphodiesterase (PDE) superfamily: a new target for the development of specific therapeutic agents. Pharmacol Ther 2006;109:366–98.

116. Murray F, Patel HH, Suda RY *et al.* Expression and activity of cAMP phosphodiesterase isoforms in pulmonary artery smooth muscle cells from patients with pulmonary hypertension: role for PDE1. Am J Physiol Lung Cell Mol Physiol 2007;292:L294–303.

117. Schermuly RT, Kreisselmeier KP, Ghofrani HA *et al.* Antiremodeling effects of iloprost and the dual-selective phosphodiesterase 3/4 inhibitor tolafentrine in chronic experimental pulmonary hypertension. Circ Res 2004; 94:1101–8.

118. Wharton J, Strange JW, Moller GM *et al.* Antiproliferative effects of phosphodiesterase type 5 inhibition in human pulmonary artery cells. Am J Respir Crit Care Med 2005;172:105–13.

119. Rao A, Luo C, Hogan PG. Transcription factors of the NFAT family: regulation and function. Annu Rev Immunol 1997;15:707–47.

120. Hill-Eubanks DC, Gomez MF, Stevenson AS, Nelson MT. NFAT regulation in smooth muscle. Trends Cardiovasc Med 2003;13:56–62.

121. de Frutos S, Spangler R, Alo D, Bosc LV. NFATc3 mediates chronic hypoxia-induced pulmonary arterial remodeling with alpha-actin up-regulation. J Biol Chem 2007;282: 15081–9.

122. Bonnet S, Rochefort G, Sutendra G *et al.* The nuclear factor of activated T cells in pulmonary arterial hypertension can be therapeutically targeted. Proc Natl Acad Sci USA 2007;104:11418–23.

123. Duan SZ, Usher MG, Mortensen RM. Peroxisome proliferator-activated receptor-gamma-mediated effects in the vasculature. Circ Res 2008;102:283–94.

124. Gizard F, Bruemmer D. Transcriptional control of vascular smooth muscle cell proliferation by peroxisome proliferator-activated receptor-gamma: therapeutic implications for cardiovascular diseases. PPAR Res 2008;429123.

125. Hansmann G, de Jesus Perez VA, Alastalo TP *et al.* An antiproliferative BMP-2/PPARgamma/apoE axis in human and murine SMCs and its role in pulmonary hypertension. J Clin Invest 2008;118:1846–57.

PART 6

SURGICAL TREATMENT OF PULMONARY HYPERTENSION

Lung transplantation

PAUL A CORRIS

INTRODUCTION

Lung transplantation began in 1981 when Stanford University introduced combined transplantation of heart and lungs (HLT) in patients with pulmonary vascular disease (1). The indications for HLT were subsequently widened to include pulmonary parenchymal and airway diseases (2). Survival rates were good, and in marked contrast to the universal failures reported after single lung transplantation (SLT) in the preceding 25 years (3). It was realized, however, that many patients undergoing HLT received a new heart unnecessarily. After a period of research, clinical success with SLT in fibrosing lung disease was reported by the Toronto group in 1986 (4).

In 1988, double lung transplantation (DLT) with a tracheal anastomosis was introduced by Patterson and colleagues (5). However, this procedure was accompanied by more frequent problems with airway healing than HLT (6). In addition, the operation was more complex than HLT and the extensive mediastinal dissection led frequently to denervation of the recipient's native heart. Bleeding was at least as great a problem as for HLT, and by 1989 the procedure, as originally described, had been largely abandoned.

Noirclerc et al. (7) provided the solution to the problem of airway healing by performing two separate anastomoses, since, as in SLT, the donor bronchus is better vascularized initially if the anastomosis is close to the lung parenchyma. This concept was further developed by Pasque et al. (8) with the bilateral sequential single lung transplant (BLT). A previous study in hypoxic patients with idiopathic pulmonary fibrosis and pulmonary hypertension demonstrate sustained improvements in right ventricular function and falls in pulmonary artery pressure (PAP) following SLT (9).

This led to the successful application of isolated pulmonary transplantation in primary pulmonary hypertension in selected cases (Table 17.1.1) (10,11). Transplant centers, however, not only have a choice of transplant operations to offer patients with pulmonary vascular disease, but should also consider pulmonary thromboendarterectomy for patients presenting with severe pulmonary arterial hypertension (PAH) due to fibrotic organization of chronic massive thromboemboli in the proximal pulmonary arteries.

Investigations of all patients presenting with severe unexplained pulmonary hypertension should include radionuclide ventilation/perfusion imaging and/or CT angiography. Some patients will show evidence of multilobar or segmental non-matched perfusion defects. Such defects provide an indication for pulmonary angiography (including contrast CT) in order to define the anatomy of vascular obstruction with particular reference to the presence of chronic thromboembolic pulmonary hypertension (CTEPH). Many of these patients will benefit from thromboendarterectomy (12) rather than transplantation.

Table 17.1.1 Changes in hemodynamic data in seven patients undergoing single lung transplantation (SLT) for primary pulmonary hypertension

	Pre-SLT	Post-SLT	P
Mean PAP	64 ± 18 mmHg	18 ± 5 mmHg	0.001
Mean RAP	10 ± 6 mmHg	1 ± 2 mmHg	0.02
Cardiac index	2.54 ± 0.98 L/min m^{-2}	3.54 ± 0.7 L/min m^{-2}	0.065

PAP, pulmonary artery pressure; RAP, right atrial pressure. Adapted from ref 10.

CRITERIA AND INDICATIONS FOR TRANSPLANT ASSESSMENT

See Table 17.1.2 for guidelines on transplantation for pulmonary hypertension.

Choice of transplant operation

Historically there have been three operative procedures used in patients with PAH with each procedure having its own advocates (13), including single lung (14–18), bilateral lung (19) and heart/lung (21–23) transplantation.

Proponents of SLT have argued that it is technically an easier procedure to perform, has less morbidity and mortality when compared to BLT and HLT and allows more patients to receive lung transplants. Opponents have argued that patients transplanted with a single lung are more at risk not only for developing severe postoperative pulmonary edema (14,24), but also for severe ventilation/perfusion mismatches in case of acute or chronic rejection (25,26), both adversely affecting early and late survival and functional outcome. Any dysfunction that changes the compliance in the allograft can lead to rapid and sometimes marked hypoxemia in the recipient due to further shifting of ventilation from the allograft to the native lung. Early graft dysfunction due to reperfusion injury may be extremely difficult to manage, leading to severe hypoxemia

Table 17.1.2 Guidelines for transplant in pulmonary hypertension

Age limits
> Upper age limit 65 years (some countries and units have a lower cut-off)
> NYHA class III or IV despite trial of combination therapy including i.v. prostaglandin therapy for 3 months

Useful hemodynamic parameters
> Cardiac index $< 2\,L/min\,m^{-2}$
> Mean right atrial pressure $> 15\,mmHg$
> Mean pulmonary artery pressure $> 55\,mmHg$
> 6-Minute walk test $< 332\,m$
> Major hemoptysis

Contraindications
> Symptomatic osteoporosis
> Severe musculoskeletal disease of the thorax
> Current use of corticosteroids $> 20\,mg/day$
> Nutritional issues $< 70\%$ or $> 130\%$ of ideal body weight
> Tobacco and/or substance abuse
> Untreated/unresolved psychosocial problems
> Systemic diseases with multi-end-organ damage
> Creatinine clearance $< 50\,mg/mL\,min^{-1}$
> Active malignancy within 2 years with exceptions
> Hepatitis B and C with biopsy proven cirrhotic liver disease

and hemodynamic instability. Diffuse alveolar damage may result and is often associated with infection (14). Single lung transplantation is a very satisfactory procedure in patients with PAH secondary to pulmonary parenchymal diseases with no differences in outcome when compared to a same group of patients without PAH (27).

Proponents of BLT have argued that this procedure results in fewer ventilation/perfusion mismatches and as a result, patients are easier to look after in the immediate postoperative period. Moreover, this allows more marginal donor lungs to be utilized and hence makes best of the rare resource of donor lungs. Patients also have better pulmonary function and better long-term survival.

Heart/lung transplantation historically was the first and only procedure in these patients (1). Advocates of this procedure argue that this operation is not only technically more straightforward and thus associated with fewer postoperative complications (21). Opponents of this procedure argue that isolated lung transplantation alone will result in immediate and long-term normalization of pulmonary vascular resistance and right ventricular ejection fraction (16,17,28,29). The donor heart can be used for isolated cardiac transplantation. Patients subjected to HLT are also at risk for accelerated graft coronary disease, although the incidence in the series from Stanford University was only 8 percent at 5 years following the transplant (21). For all these reasons, many authors have pointed out that HLT should be reserved for special indications such as patients with Eisenmenger's syndrome caused by congenital heart disease and the results are better in patients with a VSD (20,30,31).

COMPARATIVE STUDIES

No prospective randomized studies are available to relieve the uncertainty as to the best lung transplant procedure for patients with pulmonary hypertension. In practice the majority of patients now receive bilateral lung transplantation with a smaller group receiving heart and lung transplantation.

Criteria and indications for transplant assessment

Four single centers have reported the outcomes between different transplant types for both primary and secondary hypertension. Chapelier and his colleagues reported on the results of HLT, BLT and SLT for PAH from the Paris-Sud University Lung Transplant Group (32). There was a similar improvement in early and late right-sided hemodynamic function, pulmonary function and 2-year and 4-year survival between HLT and BLT recipients. The sole patient who received a single lung developed severe pulmonary edema, left ventricular failure, persistent desaturation and an important ventilation/perfusion mismatch. They concluded that HLT and BLT are equally effective but single lung transplantation should be avoided.

The Pittsburgh group reported on their experience in two studies. In the first study published in 1994 by Bando et al. (33), pulmonary artery pressures decreased in all three allograft groups, but those in the single lung recipients remains significantly higher than in the two other groups. A significant ventilation/perfusion mismatch occurred in the SLT recipients but not in the others because of preferential blood flow to the allograft. Graft-related mortality was significantly higher and overall functional recovery was significantly lower at 1 year in the single compared to BLT and HLT recipients. The authors concluded that bilateral lung transplantation is a more satisfactory option for patients with pulmonary hypertension and that heart/lung transplantation should be preserved for recipients with complex congenital heart diseases or left ventricular dysfunction. In the second study from this group reported by Gammie et al. in 1998, SLT was compared to BLT with primary or secondary pulmonary hypertension (34). There was no difference in median duration of intubation, length of stay in the intensive care unit, hospital stay, 1-month, 1-year and 4-year survival and late functional status between both groups. During this study period, 58 patients with PAH died awaiting transplantation. The authors therefore concluded that SLT could be preferentially applied for patients on the waiting list. The group from Ann Arbor compared the outcome of SLT and simultaneous intracardiac repair versus HLT for patients with pulmonary hypertension secondary to congenital cardiac anomalies (30). One SLT recipient died perioperatively.

Three of the four remaining patients surviving the first year died during the second year. The two HLT recipients were doing well 15 and 18 months after the operation. The authors concluded that SLT and simultaneous repair of intracardiac defects may have good early results, but that long-term results are considerably less favorable.

Finally, the group at Johns Hopkins Hospital in Baltimore have reported their results in 57 recipients with primary and secondary pulmonary hypertension (35). The survival up to 4 years in patients with primary pulmonary hypertension was superior in BLT compared to SLT recipients (100 percent vs. 67 percent; $P = 0.02$). There was no clear advantage to SLT versus BLT for secondary pulmonary hypertension, although 4-year survival was better in single lung recipients if pulmonary artery pressure was ≤ 40 mmHg (91 percent vs. 75 percent; $P = 0.11$) and it was better in bilateral lung recipients if this value was ≥ 40 mmHg (88 percent vs. 62 percent; $P = 0.19$). The authors concluded that bilateral lung transplantation is the procedure of choice for patients with primary pulmonary hypertension and also with secondary hypertension with pulmonary artery pressures ≥ 40 mmHg.

The recent data from the Registry of The International Society for Heart and Lung Transplantation demonstrate that since 2008 virtually all isolated lung transplantations for pulmonary arterial hypertension worldwide are now carried out using bilateral lung transplantation and that single lung transplantation seems no longer to be considered as a suitable approach.

Transplant activity for patients with pulmonary arterial hypertension

The advent of effective combination disease targeted medical therapy for lung transplantation and the continued worldwide problem of donor lung shortage have led to significant reductions in the numbers of patients undergoing transplantation. Nevertheless the long-term outcomes of medically treated patients remain uncertain and transplantation will remain an important mode of therapy for those who fail on such therapy. Studies indicate up to 25 percent of patients with idiopathic PAH may fail to improve on disease targeted therapy and the prognosis of patients who remain in WHO-FC III or IV remains poor.

Numbers of patients transplanted for PAH have however progressively fallen worldwide and the Registry of the International Society for Heart and Lung Transplantation records only 41 such patients undergoing bilateral lung transplantation and 33 heart lung transplantations, including 16 with Eisenmenger's syndrome in 2006.

Timing of transplantation

The timing of referral for patients with pulmonary hypertension remains a difficult area, though there is true consensus in two specific diagnoses. Patients with pulmonary veno-occlusive disease and pulmonary capillary hemangiomyomatosis do not respond to medical therapy in the main and should be referred for transplantation consideration at diagnosis providing they appear suitable for consideration on general criteria.

There has, however, been considerable change in the approach to the assessment and listing of patients with severe PAH since the development of targeted medical therapy. Until the 1990s medical treatment had focused on non-disease-specific therapy based on calcium channel blockade, anticoagulation and use of diuretics, digoxin and oxygen. In the NIH Registry of 1991 (36), the median survival was 2.8 years and hence patients were generally referred for consideration of transplantation when they had reached New York Heart Association (NYHA) class III or class IV. A better comprehension of the pathogenesis of PAH has changed the focus of medical treatments to evaluate drugs that may reverse the vasoproliferative effects resulting in pulmonary vascular remodeling. The first drug shown to be effect was epoprostenol (PGI2) given by a continuous intravenous infusion. In a pivotal study by Barst and colleagues (37), 81 patients were randomized to receive epoprostenol or conventional therapy. The survival was significantly improved at 5 years from 27 percent to 54 percent in the epoprostenol-treated group. More recent studies suggest that median survival may be approaching 6 years and exercise performance and quality of life are also significantly improved. The development of combination medical therapy with prostaglandins, endothelin receptor antagonists and phosphodiesterase inhibitors has clearly impacted greatly on the timing of transplant listing. Moreover, two studies have demonstrated that 60–70 percent of patients who had previously been listed for transplantation on pre-epoprostenol criteria can be de-listed because of clinical improvement (38,39). The most recent survival data for the ISHLT Registry suggest a 5-year survival of approximately 40–50 percent following heart/lung or bilateral lung transplantation; however, PAH is one of the major risk factors for both early and late mortality with an odds ratio of 1.52 (40).

It is in this setting that pulmonary hypertension and transplant centers must decide whom to refer for listing and the timing of such a referral. One study (41) surveyed current practices in a wide variety of transplant centers throughout North America, Europe and Australia. Forty percent of centers felt all NYHA class III patients should be referred to transplant centers. By contrast, 57 percent of centers limited referral to those NYHA class III and IV patients who had failed to show benefit after an average of 3 months of epoprostenol therapy. A recent single-center report has demonstrated the value of assessment after 3 months of epoprostenol therapy. An improvement in NYHA to class II and a decrease in PVR of 30 percent or more is associated with a survival of 90 percent at 5 years.

Only 40 percent of centers use one or more hemodynamic criteria for listing. These include a mean right atrial pressure of more than 15 mmHg, PVR of 4–15 Wood units, a mixed venous oxygen saturation of less than 63 percent and a cardiac index of less than 2 L/min (42,43). The vast majority of centers use some form of exercise testing and echocardiography to help determine functional status referral and listing (44). No single measurement on echocardiogram has emerged as most useful. The evidence suggests, however, that exercise testing can be more helpful. A 6-minute walking test of more than 332 meters is associated with a good prognosis and this simple exercise test is both reproducible and correlates reasonably well with hemodynamics. It is also very sensitive in the detection of improvements related to therapy. A more formal exercise test with measurement of metabolic gas exchange is utilized by approximately 25 percent of centers with a mean oxygen consumption of less than 10 mL/kg min^{-1} used as an indicator for listing.

Overall, the results show that major pulmonary hypertension and transplant centers vary considerably regarding patterns of referral, listing and transplantation of patients and it is only with continued carefully collected registry data that guidelines for best practice will be refined. One important issue relates to the potential delay, for a NYHA class IV patient who fails to respond to intravenous epoprostenol over 3 months, in listing for transplantation and the effect this has on his or her overall chances of receiving a graft.

Patients who remain in a stable clinical state at NYHA class III will also prove a potentially difficult group and it is suggested that careful note is taken of the patients' informed views in this situation.

Patients who are experiencing problems with exertional syncope but who otherwise seem to have a good quality of life should be considered for atrial septostomy in addition to receiving prostenoid therapy.

Finally, potentially life-threatening hemoptysis should also be considered an indication for listing for transplant patients. A suggested guideline for transplant listing is shown in Table 17.1.2.

Bridging to transplantation

Patients who are failing on medical therapy may develop severe right heart failure whilst actively listed for transplantation.

Consideration should be given to atrial septostomy in such patients providing they conform to the guidelines for this procedure (see Chapter 17.2). Recently the use of a membrane oxygenator between pulmonary artery and left atrium has been described and in countries where there is a supra urgent lung transplant system full extracorporeal membrane oxygenator support has been used.

General issues

The International Society recommends an upper age limit for transplantation of 65 years though there are variations from unit to unit and country to country reflecting local views. The age criteria are influenced by data showing a progressive increase in mortality for procedures in patients over the age of 55 years. Patients who develop end-stage pulmonary vascular disease failing on medical therapy or may be considered for transplantation provided that they conform to other criteria below.

DISEASE IN OTHER ORGANS

The presence of uncontrolled systemic disease in addition in respiratory failure precludes lung transplantation. Good renal function is essential in view of cyclosporin toxicity and a creatinine clearance of more than 50 mL/min is required. Only minor abnormalities of liver function are acceptable with no abnormalities of coagulation. A raised hepatic alkaline phosphatase with minimal elevation of transaminases requires investigation, but does not preclude assessment. Pulmonary hypertension is seen occasionally in patients with cirrhosis (45) and hence it is important to exclude the presence of this in patients with pulmonary hypertension and abnormal liver function tests. Severe hepatic congestion may occur in patients with terminal pulmonary hypertension. Patients with severe pulmonary hypertension due to systemic disease, such as systemic sclerosis, may be suitable transplant recipients provided that there is no evidence of active vasculitis affecting other organs.

SEPSIS

The presence of localized sepsis may lead to severe systemic infection postoperatively because of the need for immunosuppressive therapy. Persistent extrapulmonary sepsis therefore reduces the chance of successful transplantation. Oral hygiene is important and all patients should have any dental sepsis eradicated preoperatively. The majority of patients with PAH who undergo transplantation will have an indwelling Hickman catheter preoperatively and it is important that there is no chronic low-grade infection associated with the line at the time of surgery leading to potential bacteremia.

PREVIOUS SURGERY

There is a risk of life-threatening hemorrhage when the native lungs are removed if there are extensive pleural adhesions. Clearly, there is a graduation of risk from scarring due to previous open lung biopsy via a limited thoracotomy to previous total pleurectomy though this scenario is very unlikely in patients with pulmonary hypertension. Lung biopsy is not recommended in such patients when the diagnosis is considered. There is the potential for patients with previous non-corrective surgery for complex congenital heart disease developing pulmonary vascular disease requiring consideration of transplantation. The use of the antifibrinolytic aprotinin during transplant surgery which reduced bleeding in patients who had undergone previous surgery (46) is no longer recommended. The development of single sequential lung transplantation (SSLT) via a transverse bilateral thoracotomy allows the surgeon much better access to the thorax than is afforded by a sternotomy. In this regard the SSLT has advantages over the original HLT.

PSYCHOLOGICAL FACTORS

Any potential recipient must be well motivated and want a lung transplant, be able to cope and have demonstrated a willingness to comply. A supportive family or circle of close friends is essential. Underlying psychiatric illness and abuse of alcohol or drugs including cigarettes are contraindications.

Matching donor to recipients

Donor matching is based on ABO compatibility alone. Size matching is achieved by calculating the predicted total lung capacity (TLC) of both donor and recipient using height, age and sex. No direct measurement of donor lung TLC is available. A screening lymphocytotoxic cross-match, using recipient serum and a banked pool of lymphocytes, is carried out in all potential recipients accepted for transplantation to exclude the presence of preformed antibodies. Direct cross-match with lymphocytes from a potential donor is only carried out prospectively when this screening test is positive. Wherever possible, donor and recipient are matched for cytomegalovirus (CMV) status. If active CMV infection occurs it can be ameliorated by giving valganciclovir and CMV hyperimmunoglobulin (47).

POSTOPERATIVE MANAGEMENT

Most patients can be extubated 12–24 hours after surgery and then begin an active program of mobilization. Fluid intake is restricted in the early postoperative period and diuresis encouraged to avoid accumulation of fluid in the lungs. The current methods of donor lung preservation all result in a degree of pulmonary vascular injury typified by the development of protein-rich edema fluid and neutrophil accumulation (48). Prophylactic antibiotics, such as flucloxacillin and metronidazole, are given for the first 5 days.

Routine immunosuppression

Initial immunosuppression comprises triple therapy comprising the cell cycle inhibitors azathioprine or mycophenolate mofetil, methylprednisolone and the calcineurine inhibitors cyclosporin or tacrolimus. There is no consensus on the role of induction therapy with either anti thymocyte globulin or the humanized IL-2 receptor blocking agents with approximately 50 percent of patients receiving these agents. Patients with PAH who have a low preoperative creatinine clearance may be considered for induction therapy in order to avoid initial use of calcineurine inhibitors and the potential for developing acute renal failure as a consequence. Methylprednisolone is substituted by oral prednisolone and is rapidly tailed via a reducing dose to a maintenance of 0.1 g/kg. Currently most patients remain on azathioprine or mycophenolate (MMF) cyclosporin or tacrolimus and oral steroids indefinitely. There is a growing use of the proliferation inhibitors sirolimus and everolimus though both agents must be avoided until there is clear evidence of either bronchial or tracheal healing. To date there is no convincing benefit of these agents improving outcomes in lung transplantation though they have been used in some patients with deteriorating renal function to allow either withdrawal or major reduction in calcineurine target levels. Cellular ejection episodes are generally treated with pulsed methylprednisolone 10 mg/kg i.v. for 3 days followed by increased oral prednisolone for 1 month. Rejection episodes refractory to increased steroids may be treated by photophoresis or total lymphoid irradiation. The role of non-cellular humeral rejection following lung transplantation remains a difficult area but patients with evidence of endothelitis on biopsy with capillary complement deposition and anti-HLA antibodies may benefit from intravenous immunoglobulin, plasmaphoresis and use of rituximab.

Acute pulmonary rejection

A diagnosis of rejection currently is based on trans-bronchial lung biopsy using alligator forceps under radiological screening (49). The principal morphological changes found in acute rejection are perivascular lymphocytic infiltrates which may extend into alveolar septa at the later stages of rejection. Additionally, airways may show a lymphocytic infiltrate. It is usual to carry out three or four biopsies from each lobe of one lung, since rejection may be patchy and multiple biopsies from different lobes afford a greater chance of positive diagnosis. There have been many studies trying to establish reliable, less invasive methods of diagnosing rejection on blood or bronchoalveolar lavage cells and fluid. To date, none has proven to be sufficiently sensitive and specific for routine clinical use, and though the Pittsburgh group reported some success using the donor-specific primed lymphocyte response of bronchoalveolar lavage cells in the diagnosis of lung allograft rejection (50) this has not stood the test of time.

Acute pulmonary rejection is now graded according to consensus guidelines reported by the International Society of Heart and Lung Transplantation (51). The classification is based on transbronchial lung biopsy specimens carried out during fiberoptic bronchoscopy and relates to the intensity of lymphocytic infiltrate (see Table 17.1.3). Many groups have encouraged home monitoring of FEV_1 by patients, using a hand-held spirometer, in an attempt to identify at an early stage those patients who are developing complications. Early studies have demonstrated that if routine surveillance biopsies are carried out at intervals during the first 6 months after transplantation, 20–25 percent show evidence of significant acute vascular rejection in the absence of clinical or functional deterioration. No study has shown that the use of protocol biopsies has improved the outcomes of lung transplantation.

Table 17.1.3 Histological grading system for acute vascular pulmonary rejection

Grade	Description
Normal (A0)	No significant abnormality
Minimal acute rejection (A1)	Infrequent perivascular infiltrates
Mild acute rejection (A2)	Frequent perivascular infiltrates around venules and arterioles
Moderate acute rejection (A3)	Dense perivascular infiltrates with extension into alveolar septa
Severe acute rejection (A4)	Diffuse perivascular, interstitial and air-space infiltrates; alveolar pneumocyte damage; possibly parenchymal necrosis, infarction or necrotizing vasculitis

Chronic allograft dysfunction

Obliterative bronchiolitis is the pathological feature of chronic allograft dysfunction which is the major limitation to long-term survival following lung transplantation affecting approximately 50 percent of patients by five years. It is defined physiologically by the presence of progressive airflow obstruction clinically termed bronchiolitis obliterans syndrome (BOS). It is associated with both an increased frequency and persistence of acute vascular rejection but there are numerous non-allogeneic associations now described including viral and bacterial infections and gastro-esophageal reflux.

Infection

The principal cause of early postoperative death is infection. Bacterial pneumonia is common in the early postoperative period, affecting up to 35 percent of patients, and is the major infectious complication in the intermediate and late postoperative periods (52). The factors that influence the development of pneumonia include both immunosuppression and alterations in the natural defense mechanisms, such as depressed cough reflex and reduced clearance due to depressed ciliary beat frequency (53). In the late postoperative period, the presence of obliterative bronchiolitis is often associated with colonization of the lungs by Gram-negative organisms.

CMV infection may cause problems, particularly 4–8 weeks post-surgery. It is a particular problem if CMV-negative recipients receive organs from CMV-positive donors. All centers now use prophylaxis with valganciclovir in this situation. Herpes pneumonia was reported in early series of lung transplants, but has been largely eliminated by the use of prophylactic aciclovir over the first 6 weeks after transplantation. Finally, fungal pneumonia should always be considered and Candida, in particular, may complicate the early postoperative period in part due to the high frequency of colonization in the airways of donor lungs. Aspergillus may also be a problem post-transplantation, and may present as fungal "bronchitis," invasive pneumonia or disseminated aspergillosis.

Prior to the application of prophylaxis, lung transplant recipients were also particularly prone to developing symptomatic infection with *Pneumocystis carinii*. Regular prophylactic oral treatment with trimethoprim/sulfamethoxazole provides extremely effective prophylaxis.

Results

The International Society for Heart and Lung Transplantation Registry shows a 1-year survival of 70 percent with a 5-year survival of approximately 50 percent following lung transplantation for PAH. The most important complications leading to death are opportunist infections and the development of obliterative bronchiolitis (OB). Functional results in survivors measured in terms of both FEV_1 and exercise performance are good with patients returning to NYHA class I from their preoperative level of class III or IV. Recipients can expect to attain their normal predicted FEV_1 and VC by 1 year in the absence of complications if they receive two new lungs, although the diffusing capacity usually remains reduced. All patients should expect restoration of normal lifestyle with little or no functional restriction during normal activities of daily living. Exercise data comparing the 6-minute walking distances and maximum oxygen consumption during an incremental symptom-limited exercise test show that recipients of successful transplants, irrespective of the operation, return to a normal 6-minute walking distance of 600 meters or greater by 1 year with no evidence of desaturation on exercise. The maximum oxygen consumption is significantly greater in HLT and BLT compared to SLT alone. However, maximum oxygen consumption during a symptom-limited test remains at around 50 percent predicted for a given subject in the first year, in part due to decompensation on account of the pre-transplant disability. Nevertheless, the functional results allow restoration of a comfortable lifestyle.

Lung function, computed tomographic scans and transbronchial lung biopsies have been normal in patients more than 5 years after transplantation, indicating the potential for prolonged survival in patients who do not develop OB. PAH, unfortunately, is one of the major risk factors for one-year mortality in lung transplant recipients with an odds ratio of 2.53 (95 percent CI: 1.87–3.42; $P < 0.0001$) (13).

OBLITERATIVE BRONCHIOLITIS

This process is defined functionally by the development of progressive airflow obstruction unresponsive to steroids, having excluded other causes such as anastomotic stricture (54). Functional evidence of OB leads to the clinical diagnosis of bronchiolitis obliterans syndrome (BOS). Pathology shows obliteration of bronchioles by organizing fibrin associated with myofibroblasts and mononuclear cells. Immunohistology shows that the walls of the bronchioles are infiltrated by CD8 lymphocytes (55). The small bronchioles are left as fibrous bands extending out to the pleura with associated dilatation and bronchiectasis of proximal airways. Vascular sclerosis affecting both pulmonary arteries and veins may be seen in conjunction with OB. Current evidence suggests that whilst OB is considered a feature of chronic rejection it may arise as a result of non-immune factors as described earlier. Moreover some recent uncontrolled studies have demonstrated that the macrolide antibiotic azithromycin may improve lung function in patients with BOS, particularly those who have a marked neutrophilia on bronchoalveolar lavage.

In non-responders BOS usually results in a progressive loss of function due to airflow obstruction over a period of 6–12 months, leading to respiratory failure and death (Figure 17.1.1). However, a few patients appear to "stabilize" with evidence of inactive OB on biopsy and an attenuation of the loss in FEV_1. Some patients with OB have demonstrated a clinical response to increased immunosuppression (56). Most transplant units switch patients from cyclosporine to tacrolimus-based immunosuppression when OB is diagnosed if they use the former calcineurine inhibitor as first line.

LYMPHOPROLIFERATIVE DISORDERS

An association between immunosuppression and lymphoproliferative disorders is well recognized. These lymphomas are usually associated with the Epstein–Barr virus and may involve any organ. Post-transplant lymphoproliferative

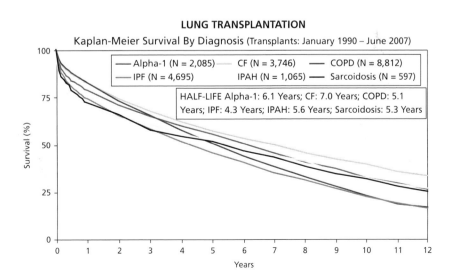

Figure 17.1.1 Kaplan-Meier survival curves for patients undergoing lung transplantation by underlying diagnosis.

disease often responds to a reduction in the level of immunosuppression alone. If disseminated, however, it may require use of the monoclonal antibody rituximab directed against the surface marker CD20. Lymphoma that has a less favorable histological appearance often requires more formal chemotherapy.

DISEASE RECURRENCE

There has been great interest in the study of lungs after successful lung transplantation to see if the acquired lung disease will recur in the allografts. To date, there is no evidence of idiopathic pulmonary hypertension returning in lung grafts. Vascular sclerosis of pulmonary vessels is seen in all patients who have obliterative bronchiolitis.

CONSEQUENCES OF DENERVATION

The surgery involved in lung transplantation severs all vagal supply to and from the lung. To date, there is no evidence of reinnervation with time after human lung transplantation. As a consequence of the denervation, the cough reflex is depressed, but the pattern of breathing during wakefulness and sleep remains normal. Most studies have demonstrated a normal ventilation response to hypercapnia. The pattern of increased ventilation on exercise has been reported as showing a faster rise in tidal volume and slower rise in rate compared to controls (57). Early reports suggest that the lungs of patients following HLT show evidence of denervation hypersensitivity to the muscarinic agonist methacholine (58). However, more recent *in vivo* studies have failed to confirm this convincingly, and *in vitro* studies of bronchial muscle from the lungs of transplant recipients have not demonstrated denervation hypersensitivity.

CONCLUSIONS

Lung transplantation now offers an effective therapy for patients with end-stage pulmonary vascular disease. Debate continues as to which transplant operation should be performed for such patients. The major practical problem facing lung transplantation at this time is a shortfall in suitable donor organs compared with the number of potential recipients. The shortfall in donor organs has led to the successful introduction of lungs from non-heart beating donors. There is much interest in the potential role of using *ex vivo* perfusion and ventilation of lungs which are not suitable for initial transplantation but may become viable organs after treatment. In the early postoperative period, opportunist infection and graft rejection remain major problems and, in the long term, obliterative bronchiolitis is the leading cause of graft failure. Much current research is aimed at understanding the pathophysiology of this condition. Patients who have received lung transplants and remain free of this complication enjoy an excellent standard of life with normal or near-normal restoration of activities and good prospects for prolonged survival.

KEY POINTS

- No prospective randomized studies are available to relieve the uncertainty as to the best lung transplant procedure for patients with PAH.
- There has been considerable change in the approach to the assessment and listing of patients with severe PAH since the development of targeted medical therapy.
- Overall the results show that major pulmonary hypertension and transplant centers vary considerably regarding patterns of referral, listing and transplantation of patients, and it is only with continued carefully collected registry data that guidelines for best practice will be refined.
- The International Society for Heart and Lung Transplantation Registry shows a 1-year survival of 70 percent with a 5-year survival of 50 percent following lung transplantation.

REFERENCES

• = Key primary paper

•1. Reitz BA, Wallwork J, Hunt SA *et al.* Heart-lung transplantation: a successful therapy for patients with pulmonary vascular disease. N Engl J Med 1982;306:557–63.
2. Penketh A, Higenbottam T, Hakim M *et al.* Heart and lung transplantation in patients with end stage lung disease. Br Med J 1987;295:311–14.
3. Wildevuuer CRH, Benfield JR. A review of 23 lung transplantations by 20 surgeons. Ann Thorac Surg 1979;9:489–515.
•4. Toronto Lung Transplant Group. Unilateral transplant for pulmonary fibrosis. N Engl J Med 1986;314:1140–5.
•5. Patterson GA, Cooper JD, Goldman B *et al.* Technique of successful clinical double lung transplantation. Ann Thorac Cardiovasc Surg 1988;45:626–33.
6. Patterson GA, Todd TR, Cooper JD *et al.* Airway complications after double lung transplantation. Toronto Lung Transplant Group. J Thorac Cardiovasc Surg 1990;99:14–20.
7. Noirclerc MJ, Metras D, Vaillant A *et al.* Bilateral bronchial anastomosis in double lung and heart lung transplantations. Eur J Cardiothorac Surg 1990;4:314–17.
8. Pasque ML, Cooper JD, Kaiser LR *et al.* Improved technique for bilateral lung transplantations: rationale and initial clinical experience. Ann Thorac Surg 1990;48:785–91.
9. Doig JC, Richens D, Corris PA *et al.* Resolution of pulmonary hypertension after single lung transplantation. Br Heart J 1991;66:431–4.

10. Pasque MK, Kaiser LR, Dresler CM *et al.* Single lung transplantation for pulmonary hypertension. J Thorac Cardiovasc Surg 1992;103:475–82.

• 11. Levine SM, Gibbons WJ, Dresler CM *et al.* Single lung transplantation for primary pulmonary hypertension. Chest 1990;98:1107–15.

12. Moser KM, Daily PA, Peterson K *et al.* Thromboendarterectomy for chronic major-vessel thromboembolic pulmonary hypertension. Immediate and long-term results in 42 patients. Ann Intern Med 1987;107:560–5.

13. Christie JD, Edwards LB, Aurora P *et al.* Registry of the International Society for Heart and Lung transplantation: Twenty fifth official adult lung and heart/lung transplant report 2008. J Heart Lung Transplant 2008;9:957-69.

14. Bando K, Keenan RJ, Paradis IL *et al.* Impact of pulmonary hypertension on outcome after single lung transplantation. Ann Thorac Surg 1994;58:1336–42.

15. McCarthy PM, Rosenkranz ER, White RD *et al.* Single lung transplantation with atrial septal defect repair for Eisenmenger's syndrome. Ann Thorac Surg 1991;52:300–3.

16. Pasque MK, Trulock EP, Kaiser LR *et al.* Single lung transplantation for pulmonary hypertension: three month haemodynamic follow up. Circulation 1991;84:2275–9.

17. Pasque MK, Trulock EP, Cooper JD *et al.* Single lung transplantation for pulmonary hypertension: single institution experience in 34 patients. Circulation 1995;92:2252–8.

18. Starnes VA, Stinson EB, Oyer PE *et al.* Single lung transplantation: a new therapeutic option for patients with pulmonary hypertension. Transplant Proc 1991;23:1209–10.

19. Ueno T, Smith JA, Snell GI *et al.* Bilateral sequential single lung transplantation for pulmonary hypertension and Eisenmenger's syndrome. Ann Thorac Surg 2000;69:381–7.

20. Birsan T, Zuckermann Z, Artemiou O *et al.* Bilateral lung transplantation for pulmonary hypertension. Transplant Proc 1997;29:2892–4.

21. White RI, Robbins RC, Altinger J *et al.* Heart-lung transplantation for primary pulmonary hypertension. Ann Thorac Surg 1999;67:937–42.

22. Mikhail G, Al-Kattan K, Banner N *et al.* Long term results of heart lung transplantation for pulmonary hypertension. Transplant Proc 1997;29:633.

23. Stoica SC, McNeil KD, Perreas K *et al.* Heart lung transplantation for Eisenmenger syndrome: early and long term results. Ann Thorac Surg 2001;72:1887–91.

24. Boujoukos AJ, Martich GD, Vega JD *et al.* Reperfusion injury in single lung transplant recipients with pulmonary hypertension and emphysema. J Heart Lung Transplant 1997;16:440–8.

25. Kramer MR, Marshall SE, McDougall IR *et al.* The distribution of ventilation and perfusion after single lung transplantation in patients with pulmonary fibrosis and pulmonary hypertension. Transplant Proc 1991;23:1215–16.

26. Levine SM, Jenkinson SG, Bryan CL *et al.* Ventilation-perfusion inequalities during graft rejection in patients undergoing single lung transplantation for primary pulmonary hypertension. Chest 1992;101:401–5.

27. Huerd SS, Hodges TN, Grover FL *et al.* Secondary pulmonary hypertension does not adversely affect outcome after single lung transplantation. J Thorac Cardiovasc Surg 2000; 19:458–65.

28. Kramer MR, Valantine HA, Marshall SE *et al.* Recovery of the right ventricle after single lung transplantation. Am J Cardiol 1994;73:494–500.

29. Shulman LR, Leibowitz DW, Anadarangam T *et al.* Variability of right ventricular functional recovery after lung transplantation. Transplantation 1996;62:622–5.

30. Lupinetti FM, Bolling SF, Bove EL *et al.* Selective lung or heart lung transplantation for pulmonary hypertension associated with congenital cardiac anomalies. Ann Thorac Surg 1994;57:1545–9.

31. Waddell TK, Bennett LW, Kennedy R *et al.* Lung or heart lung transplantation for Eisenmenger's syndrome: Analysis of the ISHLT/UNOS joint thoracic registry (abstract). J Heart Lung Transplant 2000;19:57.

32. Chapelier A, Vouhe P, Macchiarini P *et al.* Comparative outcome of heart lung and lung transplantation for pulmonary hypertension. J Thorac Cardiovasc Surg 1993;106:299–307.

• 33. Bando K, Armitage JM, Paradis IL *et al.* Indications for, and results of, single, bilateral and heart lung transplantation for pulmonary hypertension. J Thorac Cardiovasc Surg 1994;108:1056–65.

34. Gammie JS, Keenan RJ, Pham SM *et al.* Single versus double lung transplantation for pulmonary hypertension. J Thorac Cardiovasc Surg 1998;15:397–403.

35. Conte JV, Borja MJ, Patel CB *et al.* Lung transplantation for primary and secondary pulmonary hypertension. Ann Thorac Surg 2001;72:1673–80.

36. D'Alonzo GE, Barst RJ, Ayers SM *et al.* Survival in patients with primary pulmonary hypertension. Ann Intern Med 1991;15:343–9.

37. Barst RJ, Rubin LJ, Long WA *et al.* A comparison of continuous intravenous epoprostenol (prostacyclin) with conventional therapy for primary pulmonary hypertension. N Engl J Med 1996;334:296–301.

38. Robbins IM, Christman BW, Newman JH *et al.* A survey of diagnostic practices and the use of epoprostenol in patients with primary pulmonary hypertension. Chest 1998;14:1269–75.

39. Conte JV, Gaine SP, Orens JB *et al.* The influence of continuous intravenous prostacyclin therapy for primary pulmonary hypertension on the timing and outcome of transplantation. J Heart Lung Transplant 1998;17:679–85.

40. Hosenpud JD, Bennett LE, Keck BM *et al.* The registry of the International Society for Heart and Lung Transplantation: seventeenth official report. J Heart Lung Transplant 2000;19:909–31.

41. Pielsticker EJ, Martinex FJ, Rubenfire M. Lung and heart lung transplant practice patterns in pulmonary hypertension centres. J Heart Lung Transplant 2001;20:1297–304.

42. Rich S, Levy PS. Characteristics of surviving and non-surviving patients with primary pulmonary hypertension. Am J Med 1984;76:573–8.

43. Glanville AR, Burke CM, Theodore J *et al.* Primary pulmonary hypertension: length of survival of patients referred for heart and lung transplantation. Chest 1987;91:675–81.

44. Eysmann SB, Palevsky HI, Reichek N *et al.* Two dimensional echocardiography and cardiac catheterisation correlates of survival in primary pulmonary hypertension. Circulation 1989;79:353–60.

45. Morrison EB, Gaffrey FA, Eigenbrodt EH *et al.* Severe pulmonary hypertension associated with macronodular (post-necrotic) cirrhosis and auto-immune pneumonia. Am J Med 1980;69:513–19.

46. Bidstrup BP, Royston D, Supsfold RW *et al.* Reduction in blood loss and blood use after cardiopulmonary bypass with high dose aprotinin. J Thorac Cardiovasc Surg 1989;93:364–72.

47. Gould FK, Freeman R, Taylor CE *et al.* Prophylaxis and management of cytomegalovirus pneumonitis following pulmonary transplantation. J Heart Lung Transplant 1993;12:695–9.

48. Corris PA, Odom NJ, Jackson G *et al.* Reimplantation injury after lung transplantation in a rat model. J Heart Transplant 1987;6:234–7.

49. Higenbottam T, Stuart S, Penketh A *et al.* Transbronchial lung biopsy for the diagnosis of rejection in heart lung transplant recipients. Transplantation 1988;46:532–9.

50. Rabinowich H, Zeevi A, Paradis IL *et al.* Proliferative responses of bronchoalveolar lavage lymphocytes from heart lung transplant patients. Transplantation 1990;49:115–21.

51. Stewart S, Fishbein MC, Snell GS *et al.* Revision of the 1996 working formulation for the standardisation of nomenclature in the diagnosis of lung rejection. J Heart Lung Transplant 2007;26:1229–49.

52. Dauber JH, Paradis IL, Drummer JE *et al.* Allograft recipients. Clin Chest Med 1990;1:291–308.

53. Veale D, Glasper P, Gascoigne AD *et al.* Ciliary beat frequency in transplanted lungs. Thorax 1992;48:629–31.

54. Scott JP, Higenbottam TW, Sharples C *et al.* Risk factors for obliterative bronchiolitis in heart lung transplant recipients. Transplantation 1991;51:813–7.

55. Milne DS, Gascoigne AD, Wilkes J *et al.* The immunohistological features of obliterative bronchiolitis following lung transplantation. Transplantation 1992;54:748–50.

56. Glanville AR, Baldwin JC, Burke CM *et al.* Obliterative bronchiolitis after heart lung transplantation. Apparent arrest by augmented immunosuppression. Ann Intern Med 1987;107:300–4.

57. Sciurba FC, Owens GR, Sanders MH *et al.* Evidence of an altered pattern of breathing during exercise in recipients of heart lung transplants. N Engl J Med 1988;319:1186–92.

58. Glanville AR, Burke CM, Theodore J *et al.* Bronchial hyper-responsiveness after human cardiopulmonary transplantation. Clin Sci 1987;73:299–303.

Atrial septostomy and other interventional procedures

JULIO SANDOVAL AND JORGE GASPAR

INTRODUCTION

Right ventricular (RV) function is an important determinant of natural history in pulmonary arterial hypertension (PAH) (1): hemodynamic parameters that reflect RV dysfunction, such as an elevated mean right atrial pressure (RAP), a low cardiac output (CO), and low pulmonary arterial oxygen saturation are associated with poor prognosis (1). Right ventricular dysfunction and failure (RVF) from severe PAH is mainly the result of increased, long-standing, pressure overload (2–4). Other factors, such as RV ischemia, excessive sympathetic overdrive, RV volume overload, and altered RV gene expression (2–4), may contribute to modulate the response of the right ventricle and play a role in the pathogenesis of RVF (Figure 17.2.1). The mechanistic hypotheses for the development of RVF from severe chronic pressure overload were reviewed and discussed in the previous edition of this book (4).

This chapter reviews the role of atrial septostomy, an intervention specifically oriented to the relief of right ventricular failure (RVF), in the treatment scheme of PAH. The role of other interventional procedures including Stenting and Potts anastomosis is also discussed.

ATRIAL SEPTOSTOMY IN THE TREATMENT OF RIGHT VENTRICULAR FAILURE FROM PULMONARY ARTERIAL HYPERTENSION

Rationale

The use of AS in PAH is supported by the fact that survival in PAH is largely influenced by the functional status of the right ventricle; right ventricular failure and recurrent syncope are associated with poor short-term prognosis (1–4). Second, several experimental as well as clinical observations have suggested that an inter-atrial defect might be of benefit in severe pulmonary hypertension. Early animal studies by Austen et al. (5), showed that an inter-atrial communication allowed decompression of a hypertensive right ventricle and augmentation of systemic blood flow, particularly during exercise. In addition, clinical studies showed that patients with idiopathic PAH who had a patent foramen ovale lived longer than those without intracardiac shunting (6). Similarly, patients with Eisenmenger's syndrome appear to live longer and have heart failure less frequently than patients with idiopathic PAH (7,8). Taken together, these studies have suggested that deterioration in

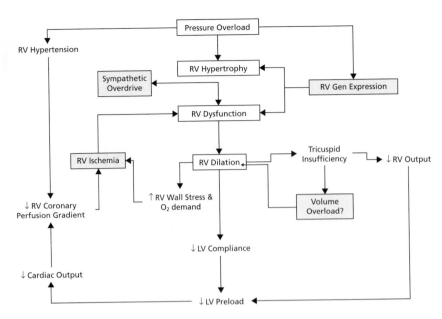

Figure 17.2.1 Mechanistic hypotheses for the development of right ventricular (RV) failure (RVF) from severe chronic pressure overload. RVF is mainly the result of pressure overload. Other factors, such as RV ischemia, excessive sympathetic overdrive, RV volume overload and altered RV gene expression, may contribute to modulate the response of the right ventricle and play a role in the pathogenesis of RVF. Changes in gene expression may dictate the response to either an appropriate RV hypertrophy or to RV dysfunction. RV dysfunction may elicit a sympathetic overdrive response, which in turn contributes to RV damage and dysfunction. RV dilation and dysfunction produces a reduction in left ventricular (LV) preload by both a reduction in LV compliance and a reduction in RV output due to tricuspid insufficiency and possibly to a deficit in RV systolic function. Tricuspid insufficiency might contribute to volume overload. As a result of low cardiac output and RV hypertension, the RV coronary perfusion gradient diminishes, which along with an increase in RV wall stress and oxygen demand produces RV ischemia, which contributes to RV dysfunction and failure. (From ref 4.)

symptoms; right heart failure and death in idiopathic PAH are associated with obstruction to systemic flow and failure of the right ventricle. The presence of an atrial septal defect in this setting would allow right-to-left shunting to increase systemic output that, in spite of the fall in systemic arterial oxygen saturation, will produce an increase in systemic oxygen transport (4,5). Furthermore, the shunt at the atrial level would allow decompression of the right atrium and right ventricle, alleviating signs and symptoms of right heart failure.

Historical background

In 1964, Austen *et al.* (5), based on their results in the canine model of hypertensive RV, had suggested that the surgical creation of interatrial communication should be considered in the treatment of patients with RVF from severe PAH. This operation was never conducted, in part, because two years later, Rashkind and Miller (9) described the catheter-balloon technique for the creation of an atrial defect without thoracotomy. The technique, indicated to increase pulmonary blood flow in children with transposition of the great vessels or with pulmonary atresia, had the problem of restenosis of the septostomy and, more important, it was difficult to do in older patients with thickened septum. To solve this problem, Park *et al.* in 1978 (10) reported the use of blade septostomy. Later, the septostomy

catheter was optimized and the safety and efficacy of this procedure were demonstrated in a multicenter trial reported in 1982 (11).

Blade balloon atrial septostomy (BBAS) as a palliative therapy for refractory idiopathic PAH was first reported by Rich and Lam in 1983 (12). Subsequent studies, particularly those of Nihill *et al.* (13) and Kerstein *et al.* (14) have shown that BBAS can be successfully performed in patients with advanced PAH and can bring about significant clinical and hemodynamic improvement. In addition to symptomatic improvement, there seems to be a trend toward improved survival in patients with severe PAH who have undergone successful BBAS (13–14). Similar results have been obtained with the use of graded balloon dilation atrial septostomy (BDAS) a variant of BBAS introduced by Hausknecht (15) and Rothman (16). BBAS is the technique most frequently used in recent series (17–29).

Worldwide experience with atrial septostomy in pulmonary hypertension

The precise role of AS in the treatment of PAH remains uncertain because most of the knowledge regarding its use comes from small series or case reports and there have been no randomized trials. The limitations of these studies include: (i) the series were all uncontrolled; (ii) the indication for performing the procedures varied between studies;

(iii) the etiology of the pulmonary vascular disease was not the same in all patients; and (iv) the medical treatment has changed over the past two decades (30). Despite these limitations, AS appears to have a place as therapeutic modality for advanced PAH, in fact, the performance of the procedure has steadily increased over the years (Figure 17.2.2).

The potential beneficial effects of atrial septostomy in the setting of PAH as well as the recommendations to reduce the risk for procedure-related mortality have been addressed in most recent guidelines (31–34). The knowledge has now expanded with the report of new cases in the last few years (17–29,35–40). Important issues derived from the analysis of the collective worldwide experience have been discussed and debated at the World Symposiums – Pulmonary Hypertension 2003 in Venice, Italy (33,34) and 2008 in Dana Point, California, USA (41). Information derived from this review regarding the role of AS in the setting of PAH is presented in this chapter.

Patients

There are 223 cases reported to date. Severe idiopathic PAH has been the main indication (81.4 percent) for AS. Other indications have included PAH associated to surgically corrected congenital heart disease (8.3 percent), PAH associated to collagen vascular disease (4.6 percent), peripheral (distal) chronic thromboembolic pulmonary hypertension not susceptible to surgical treatment in (2.8 percent), and other less frequent etiologies (2.8 percent). The procedure has been performed mainly in young women (70 percent).

Patients from the worldwide collective experience had a mean age of 27.7 ± 17 years. Congestive right heart failure (42.5 percent), syncope (38 percent), or both (19.4 percent) have been the main symptomatic indications for the

procedure. The mean NYHA functional class for the group is 3.56 ± 0.4.

Most patients who have undergone AS have had severe PAH unresponsive to conventional treatment, however, in the last few years, a significant proportion of patients (96/223) who had AS have been regarded as non-responsive to maximal medical treatment, including long-term intravenous prostacyclin infusion (n = 57), bosentan (n = 18), sildenafil (n = 8), beraprost (n = 6), subcutaneous treprostinil (n = 4), and inhaled Iloprost (n = 3). In 10 of these patients, different combinations of these drugs were used.

Procedure

Two types of atrial septostomy, BBAS (n = 71; 31.8 percent) and BDAS (n = 152; 68.2 percent), have been used in the treatment of PAH. The basic difference between the two procedures is that, in contrast to BBAS, in BDAS, the Park blade septostomy catheter is not used and the interatrial orifice is created by puncture with a Brockenbrough needle and use of progressively larger balloon catheters in a step-by-step fashion. Both procedures follow a similar protocol, that is, standard right and left heart catheterization performed under conscious sedation, and hemodynamic monitoring in the cardiac catheterization laboratory. A prospective evaluation of potential differences between the two procedures in regard to hemodynamic results and risk of complications has not been done.

The election to perform BBAS or BDAS should be a decision taken in each center based on institutional expertise. Regardless of the procedure, it is advisable to follow the recommendations to minimize the risk of death during the procedure (32) (Table 17.2.1) and the procedures should be performed only in centers experienced in both interventional cardiology and pulmonary hypertension (31,32).

EVALUATION AND PREPARATION FOR BDAS

To ensure preservation of systemic O_2 transport (SO_2T) once a right-to-left shunt is created, patients in whom BDAS is being considered should have a resting arterial O_2 saturation of at least 90 percent and a hematocrit level greater than 35 percent. In addition, in order to avoid the LV volume overload imposed by the shunt, LV function should be preserved (32), as evidenced by the absence of clinically apparent left heart failure and an ejection fraction by echocardiography greater than 0.45. If LV function is adequate, atrial septostomy can be attempted in the critically ill patient with the graded dilatation procedure.

BDAS TECHNIQUE

Whenever possible, the procedure is performed without supplementary oxygen in order to adequately gauge the

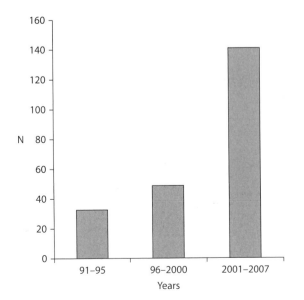

Figure 17.2.2 Worldwide performance of atrial septostomy over the years from reported cases and series.

Table 17.2.1 Recommendations to minimize the risk of procedure-related mortality of atrial septostomy

1. Atrial septostomy should be attempted only by those institutions with an established track record in the treatment of advanced pulmonary hypertension where atrial septostomy is performed with low morbidity.
2. Atrial septostomy should not be performed in the patient with impending death and severe right ventricular failure on maximal cardiorespiratory support. A mRAP > 20 mmHg, a PVRI > 55 U/m², and a predicted 1-year survival < 40% are all significant predictors of procedure-related death.
3. Before cardiac catheterization, it is important to confirm an acceptable baseline systemic oxygen saturation (> 90% in room air) as well as to optimize cardiac function (adequate right heart filling pressure, additional inotropic support if needed).
4. During cardiac catheterization is mandatory:
   a. Supplemental oxygen if needed.
   b. Mild and appropriate sedation to prevent anxiety.
   c. Careful monitoring of variables (LAP, SaO₂%, and mRAP).
   d. To attempt a step-by-step procedure.
5. After atrial septostomy, it is important to optimize oxygen delivery. Transfusion of packed red blood cells or erythropoietin (prior to and following the procedure if needed) may be necessary to increase oxygen content.

mRAP, mean right atrial pressure; PVRI, pulmonary vascular resistance index; LAP, left atrial pressure; SaO₂%, arterial oxygen saturation. (From ref 32.)

shunt-induced changes in arterial O_2 saturation which are of utmost importance to determine the final (optimal) size of the interatrial orifice. Mild conscious sedation may be used (i.e. midazolam 0.02–0.03 mg/kg), otherwise we prefer to avoid sedation in order to minimize its respiratory depressant effects.

A 6 F introducer is placed in the right femoral artery for left heart catheterization using a 6 F pigtail catheter. Two introducers are placed in the right femoral vein, with the punctures at least 2 cm apart. The most proximal puncture is for the trans-septal procedure and in the distal puncture a conventional introducer is placed for right heart catheterization using a balloon flow-directed catheter or a Cournand catheter. Anticoagulation is not initiated prior to the trans-septal puncture but frequent and thorough flushing of the catheters and sheaths, with heparinized saline (1000 U heparin in 1 L saline), is performed.

Right and left heart baseline pressures are recorded simultaneously and cardiac output is calculated through the indirect Fick principle using assumed oxygen consumption values. The finding of a large gradient between the right and left atria, which is considered a contraindication for blade atrial septostomy (31), is not considered a contraindication for the graded balloon technique. On the other hand, it is recommended that patients with a baseline LVEDP above 12 mmHg should not undergo atrial septostomy.

Trans-septal puncture is performed with the Mullins introducer (without the sheath) and Brockenbrough needle using standard techniques (42). We have always found the 2.5 cm Mullins catheter curve to be adequate but it should be kept in mind that in a large patient with a markedly dilated right atrium a 3.0 cm curve would allow an easier approach to the out-bulging inter-atrial septum. The adequacy of the intended puncture site can be mapped by a tiny contrast staining of the septum through the Mullins introducer before puncturing with the needle

(Figure 17.2.3A&B). As opposed to the situation where trans-septal puncture is done to perform percutaneous mitral commisurotomy (the most frequent current indication for trans-septal catheterization in adults), in the PPH population left atrial pressure is comparatively low and a brisk inspiration by the patient carries the theoretical risk of inadvertently allowing air to be suctioned into the left atrium. For this reason, once the correct and stable position of the Mullins introducer in the left atrium is confirmed, the needle is withdrawn and the catheter hub immediately occluded with a fingertip followed by a careful double flush. At this point heparin is administered (70 U/kg) and left atrial pressure is recorded. In our hospital we use the Inoue circular-end guidewire (Toray Industries, Inc., catalog number GMS-1) to maintain access in the left atrium because the rigidity of its shaft greatly facilitates balloon catheter trackability and the 4.5 cm diameter of its distal circled end, with a very soft tip, sits nicely and safely in the left atrium, providing great stability (Figure 17.2.3C). This guide wire has a diameter of 0.025 inch and the length of the straight segment is 150 cm (total length 175 cm) and therefore adequate for the majority of the current peripheral balloons. An alternative is to use a 0.035 inch extra support exchange guidewire which should be advanced deeply into the left inferior pulmonary vein for adequate tracking support.

Septostomy dilatation is then done in a graded step-by-step approach, beginning at 4 mm diameter with the Inoue septostomy dilator or at 3.7 mm with the dilator of a long 80 cm 11 F introducer (Super-Arrow-Flex, Arrow International, Inc.) (Figure 17.3.3D) and followed by successive balloon diameters of 8, 12 and 16 mm as shown in Figure 17.2.3E&F (if an 11 F dilator is used, its sheath can accommodate current low-profile peripheral balloons up to 18 mm diameter). After each step, a 3-minute waiting period is allowed to achieve steady state, followed by the careful measurement of LVEDP and arterial O_2 saturation.

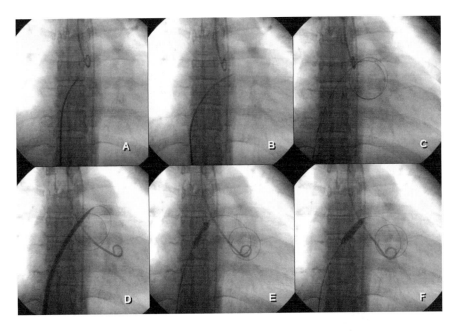

Figure 17.2.3 Balloon dilation atrial septostomy technique. The procedure involves a standard right and left heart catheterization. (A) AP view of the Mullins dilator with the Brockenbrough needle at its tip. A small contrast injection is done to map the intended puncture site, which can then be seen in different projections to determine its correct location. (B) Perforation of the septum with the Brockenbrough needle. (C) The Inoue circular-end guidewire is shown positioned in the left atrium. (D) A 4 mm initial dilation of the atrial septum is done with the Inoue dilator, and concluded with an 8 mm balloon. (E & F) Dilation of the atrial septum can occasionally offer moderate resistance but it has been always opened successfully with hand inflation, which has been measured to reach 4–6 ATM. Inflation is increased just enough to eliminate balloon waist (E) and is repeated at least twice to counter elastic recoil.

The final size of the defect is individualized for each patient and is determined when either of the following occurs:

- An LVEDP increase approaching 18 mmHg;
- An arterial oxygen saturation reduction near 80 percent; or
- When a 16 mm diameter dilatation has been achieved.

With the above criteria we have sought to decrease both the risk of excessive left ventricular volume overload that may lead to pulmonary edema and an excessive unwanted arterial oxygen desaturation, which have been identified as the causes of the high (25 percent) procedural-related death rate in earlier publications (31). Using this incremental dilation protocol, we have recently reported only one procedure related-death in a total of 50 procedures performed in 34 patients (43). Also, this approach allows performing atrial septostomy even in the setting of a high-pressure gradient between right and left atria, which should probably not be attempted with the blade septostomy technique as the size of the defect, and, therefore, the shunted volume cannot be adequately controlled with this approach (Figure 17.2.4). Using the described step-by-step approach some investigators have successfully dilated to 22 mm without complications (Naeije R, Personal communication).

After achieving the final septostomy dilatation, complete right and left heart pressure recording and cardiac output determination are repeated and the patient is started on supplementary oxygen. The sheaths are removed 2 hours after the procedure.

The patients are monitored in an intensive care setting during the first 48 hours after the procedure in a 30–45° upright position, with continuous supplementary oxygen administration. For the management of severe hypoxemia after septostomy, the use of inhaled iloprost has been recently suggested (28). Echocardiography is useful to monitor for evidence of LV volume overload and is also useful in determining the baseline inter-atrial orifice diameter, which should be approximately 20 percent smaller than the maximal balloon diameter used due to tissue recoil (Figure 17.2.5).

Immediate outcome after atrial septostomy

Atrial septostomy has been performed mostly in the setting of severe pulmonary hypertension and RVF. Accordingly, there is an inherent risk of complications and death during the procedure. In the current analysis of the 223 cases reported, mortality was 7.1 percent at 24 hours and 14.8 percent at 1 month. For the BDAS technique these figures are 4.2 percent and 10.3 percent, respectively.

Factors associated with procedure-related mortality (at one month) in the whole group are shown in Table 17.2.2. As in the prior analyses of the worldwide experience (32–34), a mean RAP > 20 mmHg remains as the most significant risk factor for procedure-related death (risk

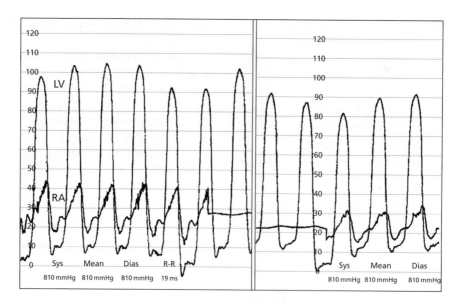

Figure 17.2.4 Pressure recordings before atrial septostomy show, on the left panel, a mean right atrial pressure (RA) of 28 mmHg and a left ventricular (LV) end-diastolic pressure (LVEDP) of 9 mmHg. Note the giant right atrial c–v waves peaking at 43 mmHg due to severe tricuspid regurgitation. After atrial septostomy (right panel), mean right atrial pressure falls to 21 mmHg and c–v waves to 30 mmHg, whilst LVEDP has increased to 15 mmHg. Modifications in the inter-atrial pressure gradient after septostomy are the result of both, a decrease in right atrial pressure and an increase in LVEDP. See text.

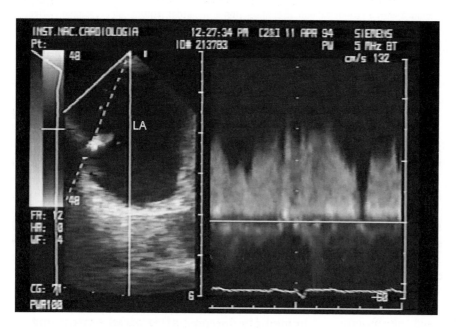

Figure 17.2.5 Multiplane trans-esophageal echocardiography to confirm and measure the diameter of the created inter-atrial defect. Note the right-to-left shunt at the level of atrial septum. LA, left atrium.

rate = 30.5; $P < 0.001$). A higher SaO_2 after the procedure, on the other hand, had a protective effect against the risk of death at one month.

Causes of death within one month in the 33 out of 223 cases reported were refractory hypoxemia (n = 20), progressive right heart failure (n = 6), procedural complications (n = 4), multiple organ failure (n = 1), hemoptysis (n = 1), and unrelated (voluntary dialysis withdrawal one case).

In most patients, symptoms and signs of RVF, including systemic venous congestion and syncope, are improved immediately after AS. In the current worldwide experience, (41) the clinical status after septostomy improved in 163 out of the 186 surviving patients (87.6 percent), was unchanged

in 23 (12.4 percent), and 31 (16.6 percent) patients were transplanted. NYHA functional class of the surviving patients decreased from 3.49 ± 0.58 to 2.1 ± 0.67 ($P < 0.001$) and, exercise endurance, as assessed by the six-minute walk, was also improved in most of the patients after septostomy in three studies evaluating this parameter (17,20,23) (Figure 17.2.6).

Immediate hemodynamic effects

Individual patient information regarding the hemodynamic parameters before and after AS has been reported

Table 17.2.2 Baseline variables associated with procedure-related mortality (one month)

Variable	HR (95% CI)	P<
Age (years)	0.99 (0.96–1.03)	0.966
Age > 18 years old	1.12 (0.29–4.34)	0.865
Gender, female	0.73 (0.18–2.8)	0.635
NYHA Functional Class	8.53 (0.89–81.2)	0.062
Diagnosis of CVD	3.18 (0.67–14.9)	0.143
Syncope	0.14 (0.03–0.66)	0.013
RHF	5.97 (0.75–47.2)	0.089
Septostomy type, blade	1.19 (0.30–4.6)	0.800
Mean RAP (mmHg)	1.19 (1.1–1.29)	**0.000**
RAP > 20 mmHg	30.5 (3.8–244)	**0.001**
Mean PAP (mmHg)	1.01 (0.98–1.05)	0.321
Mean LAP (mmHg)	1.11 (0.86–1.43)	0.420
Baseline CI (L/min m^{-2})	0.38 (0.09–1.6)	0.189
Baseline PVRI (U/m^2)	1.04 (0.98–1.09)	0.148
Baseline (SaO$_2$%)	0.97 (0.83–1.14)	0.773
SaO$_2$% after procedure	0.90 (0.84–0.96)	**0.001**
Mean SAP (mmHg)	0.96 (0.92–1.01)	0.148

CVD, collagen vascular disease; RHF, right heart failure; RAP, right atrial pressure; PAP, pulmonary artery pressure; LAP, left atrial pressure; CI, cardiac index; PVRI, pulmonary vascular resistance index; SaO$_2$%, arterial oxygen saturation; SAP, systemic artery pressure.

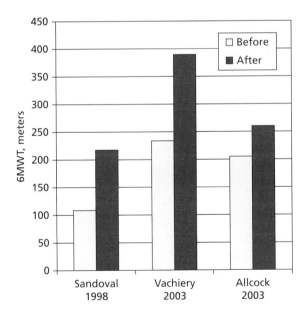

Figure 17.2.6 Effect of atrial septostomy on exercise endurance, as assessed by 6-minute walk test (6MWT), in three of the reported series.

only in 117 of the reported cases. In the group as a whole, there was a significant ($P < 0.000$) decrease in mRAP (from 14.6 ± 8 to 11.6 ± 6.3 mmHg), SaO$_2$ percent (from 93.3 ± 4.1 to 83 ± 8.5 percent); this was accompanied by an also significant ($P < 0.000$) increase in mLAP (from 5.7 ± 3.3 to 8.10 ± 3.98 mmHg) and CI (from 2.04 ± 0.69 to 2.62 ± 0.84 L/min/m^2). There were no significant

changes in mPAP or mean systemic artery pressure after the procedure.

The magnitude of hemodynamic changes is not the same for all patients and it depends on the level of baseline mRAP (4,31,32). As noted in Table 17.2.3, the hemodynamic changes after AS are progressively more important as the mRAP is higher. In patients with an mRAP less than 10 mmHg, the decrease in mRAP was not significant (10.6 percent from baseline) yet, there was a significant increase (22.5 percent) in CI. In patients with mRAP more than 20 mmHg, mRAP and SaO$_2$ percent decreased 25 percent and 14.5 percent respectively, whereas CI increased 38 percent from baseline. Patients with a baseline mRAP between 11 and 20 mmHg had an intermediate response; mRAP decreased by almost 20 percent and CI increased 30 percent.

It is important to stress the fact that it is in the group of patients with mRAP greater than 20 mmHg, in which the risk of procedure-related death is elevated. Likewise, it is important to note that although the decrease in mRAP was not significant in the group of patients with mRAP less than 10 mmHg (perhaps because it was already low), the changes in CI and NYHA functional class were significant and clinically relevant.

Although the hemodynamic changes after septostomy seem only moderate (particularly in the group with baseline mRAP less than 10 mmHg), these measurements represent only the resting state. The hemodynamic effects of atrial septostomy during exercise have not been established, however, the impact of septostomy is likely to manifest further during exercise, as shown in dogs with right ventricular hypertension (Figure 17.2.7) (5). Serial trans-esophageal echocardiograms performed in some of the patients at rest and during mild supine exercise support the concept that the decompression and shunting effects of atrial septostomy become more pronounced during exercise (17). A more significant hemodynamic effect of septostomy during exercise might also explain the increase in exercise endurance reported in humans after AS (17,20,23).

The effect of atrial septostomy on other hemodynamic variables such as pulmonary blood flow (PBF) and, therefore, on pulmonary vascular resistance are difficult to assess as in most of the studies reported so far, a direct measurement of PBF has not been done. In a recent work by Kurzyna and coworkers (28), a significant increase in PVR after septostomy was observed in some of the patients. This increase in PVR correlated with the level of mixed venous PO$_2$ after the procedure and it was though to be responsible in part for the presentation of refractory hypoxemia following septostomy. In their study, the authors were able to manage refractory hypoxemia with inhaled iloprost (28). This most interesting finding deserves future investigation.

Long-term hemodynamic effects

The long-term hemodynamic effects of atrial septostomy in PAH have been reported in two studies (14,35). Both

Table 17.2.3 Hemodynamic effects of atrial septostomy according to baseline mean right atrial pressure

Variable	RAP < 10 mmHg (n = 42)			RAP = 11–20 mmHg (n = 49)			RAP > 20 mmHg (n = 26)		
	Before	After	P<	Before	After	P<	Before	After	P<
mRAP (mmHg)	6.6 ± 2.4	5.9 ± 3.2	0.214	14.8 ± 2.8	11.9 ± 3.5	0.000	26.6 ± 4.4	19.9 ± 3.8	0.000
mPAP (mmHg)	62 ± 16	64 ± 19	0.329	66.4 ± 17	66.4 ± 16	1.000	63.4 ± 20	67.5 ± 20	0.102
mLAP (mmHg)	5.0 ± 2.7	6.8 ± 2.4	0.005	5.3 ± 3.6	7.8 ± 4.5	0.000	7.9 ± 3.0	10.9 ± 4.0	0.029
SaO₂ (%)	93.8 ± 4	85.8 ± 7	0.000	93.0 ± 4.0	82.8 ± 7.2	0.000	93.1 ± 4.3	78.6 ± 10.3	0.000
CI (L/min m⁻²)	2.36 ± 0.58	2.89 ± 0.72	0.000	2.04 ± 0.71	2.65 ± 0.96	0.000	1.55 ± 0.49	2.14 ± 0.56	0.000
mSAP (mmHg)	83 ± 15	83 ± 13	0.931	84.5 ± 14	88.8 ± 15	0.065	78 ± 20	81 ± 18	0.254
NYHA Class	3.25 ± 0.64	2.00 ± 0.65	0.000	3.63 ± 0.49	2.21 ± 0.78	0.000	3.71 ± 0.49	2.00 ± 0.0	0.000

mRAP, mean right atrial pressure; PAP, mean pulmonary artery pressure; mLAP, mean left atrial pressure; SaO₂, arterial oxygen saturation; CI, cardiac index; mSAP, mean systemic arterial pressure; NYHA, New York Heart Association.

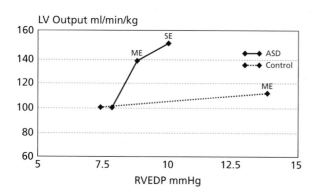

Figure 17.2.7 Effect of a surgically created atrial septal defect (ASD) on exercise performance in a canine model of right ventricular hypertension. Dogs with an ASD were able to significantly increase their cardiac output (CO) during both mild (ME) and severe exercise (SE) at the expense of only a modest increase in RVEDP. Dogs in the control group did not increase CO and had a marked increase in RVEDP at mild exercise. Four of these dogs died during or immediately after exercise. (Constructed with data from ref 5.)

studies found an improvement in right ventricular function over time, with a further decrease in mRAP and a further increase in CI in patients who had repeat catheterization after a mean of about 2 years after septostomy.

Effects on right heart structure and function

Echocardiography performed before and after septostomy in patients with PAH by our group (44) suggest that AS may also exert beneficial effects on right heart structure and function. We found significantly decreased right atrial and right ventricular systolic and diastolic areas after septostomy, reflecting less right heart dilation. RV systolic function, assessed by mean percentage change in area and the changes in global RV wall motion, also improved, particularly in patients with a severely depressed systolic function prior to the procedure. The easiest way to explain the beneficial effects of AS on RV function is that the simple decompression effect (decrease in radius) reduces wall

stress and improves performance via the La Place relationship (2–4); relief of RV wall tension and ischemia, mediated by decompression itself may also have contributed. Interestingly, neither RV wall thickness nor the bulging of atrial and ventricular septa toward the left chambers were affected by the procedure (44).

Compared with other therapeutic interventions such as calcium channel blockers, intravenous infusion of prostacyclin, pulmonary thromboendarterectomy, and lung transplantation (45–48), the effects of AS on RV structure and function are less dramatic. This is probably due to a more direct and pronounced effect of those interventions on RV afterload (i.e. decrease in PVR).

Long-term outcome and survival after atrial septostomy

Not all patients have clinical improvement after the procedure. Long-term clinical outcome after septostomy is dependent on the immediate hemodynamic response to the procedure, particularly the changes in CI and SO₂T (Table 17.2.4). Compared with patients with no clinical improvement, those with significant clinical benefit had a higher and significant increase in CI and SO₂T immediately after the procedure (4,18,32).

The true impact of AS on survival of patients with PAH has not been established in prospective and controlled studies. Most reported series, however, have suggested a short-term beneficial effect on the survival of these very sick patients (13,14,17,35,43). From the current worldwide experience, we have analyzed the survival characteristics of 106 patients in whom complete follow-up and outcome *after* septostomy (that is, excluding procedural deaths) were available. The mean survival time was 63.1 months (95 percent CI: 50 to 76.3 months). Kaplan–Meier survival curves after septostomy are shown in Figure 17.2.8. Long-term survival is limited by late deaths, primarily as a result of progression of the pulmonary vascular disease.

Factors associated with mortality after septostomy (including procedural deaths) are shown in Table 17.2.5. Mortality after septostomy (excluding procedure-related

Table 17.2.4 Comparison of selected hemodynamic variables before and after atrial septostomy as a function of clinical outcome

Variable	Improved clinically (n = 34)				Not improved clinically (n = 7)			
	Before	After	% Change	P<	Before	After	% Change	P<
mRAP (mmHg)	13.7 ± 7.9	10.1 ± 6.4	26.8	0.001	14.6 ± 9.4	12.3 ± 7.9	16	0.056
SaO$_2$ (%)	93.3 ± 4.4	84.1 ± 9.1	9.2	0.001	97 ± 1.4	90.1 ± 5.0	6.9	0.009
CI (L/min m^{-2})	2.0 ± 0.6	2.7 ± 0.7	35	0.001	2.2 ± 0.6	2.3 ± 0.4	4.5	0.3
SO$_2$T (mL/min m^{-2})	393 ± 126	457 ± 123	16.5	0.001	368 ± 125	370 ± 116	0.5	0.9

SO$_2$T, systemic oxygen transport. Rest of abbreviations as in Table 17.2.3. From ref 4.

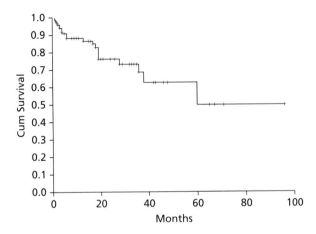

Figure 17.2.8 Kaplan–Meier survival curve in 106 patients from the current worldwide collective experience who had successful atrial septostomy. The mean survival time was 63.1 months (95% CI: 50 to 76.3 months). See text.

mortality) was dictated by older age (hazard ratio [HR]:1.04), scleroderma (HR:8.32), NYHA functional class (HR:4.71), NYHA class III and IV (HR:6.24), CI (HR:0.179), left atrial pressure (HR:0.737), and SOT (HR:0.99). The impact of baseline mRAP on long-term survival, which relevant at septostomy, disappears once the procedure has been performed.

Although there are undoubtedly many limitations in regard to the studied population, the impact of atrial septostomy on the survival of patients with severe pulmonary hypertension and right heart failure appears beneficial and at least comparable to that of other current pharmacologic therapeutic interventions. Three relatively large series have demonstrated this survival benefit to a similar extent (14,35,43) (Figure 17.2.9).

COMBINED THERAPY

As more experience has now accumulated, the initial concern that the administration of systemic vasodilators would be dangerous in patients with a right-to-left shunt is no longer present. A significant proportion of patients with AS in the worldwide experience were already receiving some of the current PAH-specific medications and in many cases continued to receive them after the procedure,

in fact, it is difficult to separate the potential beneficial effect that these medications could have had on the survival of the patients. Also, in the retrospective analysis of our own experience (43), there is a potential benefit of combining strategies (interventional plus pharmacological) in the management of PAH. In effect, we found that the benefit of AS alone on survival was significantly increased by the concomitant addition of PAH-specific drug therapies. As shown in Figure 17.2.10, the 3-, and 5-year survival of 100 percent and almost 90 percent, respectively for this combination, is impressive.

Although the concomitant use of drugs and AS has been used in many of the previously reported series, the sequence of combining these strategies is different from the one we have followed at our center. We have not waited until the failure of medical treatment was evident to perform AS, instead, the septostomy was performed first and then the specific drugs were added when they became available. In previous reports, AS septostomy has been used as the last or almost last resort in the management strategy, when the patients were most likely in an advanced stage of the disease. The performance of septostomy at a relatively earlier stage of the disease in our study may probably account for the encouraging results.

Possible mechanisms of improvement after atrial septostomy

Our understanding of the physiological changes occurring after septostomy is incomplete, but several mechanisms seem to be involved. In patients with PAH and right ventricular dysfunction (i.e. a marked increase in baseline mRAP), a decompression effect of the right heart chambers occurs (see above) (44). For those with less severe right ventricular dysfunction at baseline and only mild to moderate hemodynamic changes after septostomy, the benefit of the procedure may be more likely to manifest during exercise by preventing further right ventricular dilatation and dysfunction and by allowing right-to-left shunting to increase cardiac output (5). Finally, an increase in SO$_2$T also may produce beneficial effects on peripheral oxygen use (14) particularly during exercise, and be responsible for the improvement in functional class and exercise tolerance.

Table 17.2.5 Variables associated with long-term survival after atrial septostomy

Variable	HR (95% CI)	P<
Age (years)	1.03 (1.004–1.05)	0.021
Age > 18 years old	0.89 (0.399–2.01)	0.789
Gender, female	0.98 (0.439–2.2)	0.969
NYHA Functional Class	1.71 (0.78–3.72)	0.172
Diagnosis of CVD	5.56 (2.18–14.2)	**0.000**
Syncope	0.78 (0.38–1.60)	0.502
RHF	1.59 (0.73–3.46)	0.237
Septostomy type, blade	0.90 (0.40–1.98)	0.792
Mean RAP (mmHg)	1.08 (1.03–1.13)	**0.000**
RAP > 20 mmHg	3.58 (1.70–7.56)	**0.000**
Mean PAP (mmHg)	1.00 (0.97–1.03)	0.720
Mean LAP (mmHg)	0.84 (0.70–1.004)	0.055
Baseline CI (L/min m^{-2})	0.32 (0.14–0.70)	**0.004**
CI after procedure (L/min/m^{-2})	0.25 (0.12–0.51)	**0.000**
Baseline PVRI (U/m^2)	1.02 (0.98–1.06)	0.255
Baseline SaO$_2$%	0.94 (0.87–1.03)	0.213
SaO$_2$% after procedure	0.96 (0.92–1.007)	0.103
Mean SAP (mmHg)	0.98 (0.95–1.009)	0.212

Abbreviations as in Table 17.2.3.

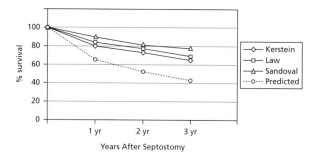

Figure 17.2.9 Effect of atrial septostomy on the survival of patients with pulmonary arterial hypertension in three of the reported series as compared with the estimated survival derived from the National Institutes of Health Study (1). The survival benefit achieved by the procedure is similar in these studies. (Data from refs 14, 35 and 43.)

Other mechanisms for improvement after AS are also likely. It has been shown that PAH patients have an increase in sympathetic nervous activity, as assessed by muscle sympathetic nerve activity (MSNA) (49), which may, in fact, be one of the pathophysiologic mechanisms leading to RVF (4). In a recent study, Ciarka et al. (29) demonstrated a significant decrease in MSNA after septostomy in patients with PAH. By decreasing sympathetic overdrive, atrial septostomy might also improve RV function. In the study of Ciarka et al. (29), the decrease in MSNA correlated with the decrease in RAP after septostomy, which is in support of the decompression phenomenon of the right heart after AS (44). In this regard, the

recent demonstration of a decrease in the levels of brain-type natriuretic peptide after septostomy is also in support of the decompression phenomenon (50).

Spontaneous closure of AS – the use of Amplatzer and Stenting

In most of the reported series, subsequent closure of the defect has been a relatively frequent (27/223 = 12.1 percent) and undesirable outcome of BDAS. The reason for this remains unknown. In our experience, there have not been significant differences in age, hemodynamic profile, or septostomy size between patients with spontaneous closure and those in whom the septostomy remained open. To solve the problem of closure, we have elected to repeat septostomy as many times as necessary, and achieved this without complications (43).

Recently, however, this problem has been approached differently by other investigators. Micheletti et al. (26), placed a custom-made fenestrated atrial septal device at the end of the procedure to maintain the septostomy open. By doing this in seven out of 20 children, the spontaneous closure of the defect was successfully avoided. This approach has been followed by other investigators with the use of Stents at the site of septostomy (38–40). These additional interventions may help in reducing the risk of the subsequent closure of the defect. At present, however, it is difficult to anticipate the long-term risk/benefit of this approach. In fact, in a recent communication, Lammers et al. (51) reported the occlusion of the fenestration in four out of nine patients, after a follow-up of 10 months, despite the concomitant use of aspirin or warfarin.

POTTS PROCEDURE

The Potts aorto-pulmonary anastomosis was originally introduced for the palliative treatment of tetralogy of Fallot and other congenital heart diseases characterized by a decreased pulmonary blood flow such as tricuspid and pulmonary atresia (52). Because of the difficulties encountered while attempting to close the shunt during subsequent corrective surgery, the Potts anastomosis has been largely replaced by alternative shunt procedures (53).

As is the case of atrial septostomy, the rationale for creating new right-to-left shunts is that patients with PAH associated to congenital heart disease and Eisenmenger physiology live longer and have less right ventricular failure than patients with idiopathic PAH (7,8). Thus, in an attempt to transform children with severe PAH to an Eisenmenger circulation type, avoiding supra-systemic pulmonary artery pressures, a direct side-to-side anastomosis between left pulmonary artery and descending aorta (Potts anastomosis) has been proposed (54).

In a recent communication, Serraf and coworkers (55), describe the use of this intervention in seven children

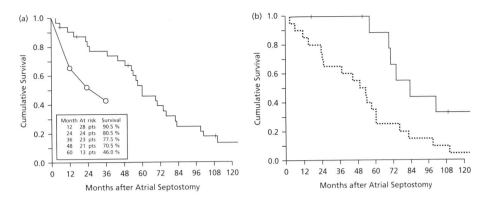

Figure 17.2.10   Impact of a combined management strategy (interventional plus PAH-specific drugs) on the survival of patients with PAH. (a) Kaplan–Meier survival estimates after atrial septostomy in the whole group of 32 patients with PAH. The median survival of the group was $60 \pm$ (SEM) 8 months (95% confidence interval (CI), 43 to 77 months). A predicted survival curve (open circles) is plotted for comparison. (b) The survival estimates for PAH patients with atrial septostomy plus PAH-specific pharmacologic treatment (n = 11; continuous line) are better than those in patients with atrial septostomy alone (n = 21; dotted line) [median survival 83 months (95% CI, 57 to 109) vs. 53 months (95% CI, 39 to 67) respectively; chi-square log-rank, 6.52; P = 0.01]. (From ref 43.)

(age 107 ± 50 months). All had supra-systemic PAH (systolic PAP = 134 ± 30 mmHg; PVR = 24 ± 0.9 UI/m^2). Six-minute walk distance was 170 ± 110 m and the NYHA class was 3 or 4. All patients were refractory to medical PAH therapy. The procedure was performed through left thoracotomy without cardio-pulmonary bypass. There was one procedure-related death which was attributed to a restrictive anastomosis. The postoperative course in the remaining patients was uneventful. After a mean follow-up of 26 ± 22 months all children improved by at least one NYHA functional class and 6-minute walk test increased to 502 ± 109 meters. As a result of the surgery, all patients showed a SaO$_2$ gradient between upper and lower limbs (97 ± 3 vs. 80 ± 9 percent).

Until now, the procedure has been performed exclusively in children with PAH where Potts anastomosis may be a life-saving procedure. There is an inherent risk for a surgical procedure of this magnitude in the PAH adult population. Although purely hypothetical, is the idea of creating a de-novo ductus arteriosus, through interventionism, with conduit, perhaps valved to prevent aortic back pressure surges into the pulmonary artery (56). Given the paucity of data it is difficult to draw a firm conclusion regarding the general application of this intervention. More experience and longer follow-up are necessary to confirm these initial and encouraging observations.

SUMMARY

Atrial septostomy stands as an additional, promising strategy in the treatment of severe PAH. Several reasons justify its use in this setting: (i) the deleterious impact of RVF on survival of patients; (ii) the unpredictable response to medical treatment; (iii) the limited access to lung transplantation; and (iv) the disparity in the availability of these treatments throughout the world.

Experience with this procedure is limited in part due to the relative availability and success of the new forms of pharmacological interventions. The definitive role of AS in the management of PAH is uncertain due to the lack of a prospective and controlled study. However, based on analyses of the worldwide experience, several general conclusions can be made: (i) atrial septostomy can be performed successfully in selected patients with advanced pulmonary vascular disease; (ii) in patients with PAH who have undergone successful AS, the procedure has resulted in a significant clinical improvement, beneficial and long-lasting hemodynamic effects at rest, and a trend toward improved survival. Although not prospectively assessed, the impact of AS on the survival of patients with severe PAH is beneficial and, in the mid-term, is at least comparable to that of other current pharmacological therapeutic interventions; (iii) the procedure-related mortality is still high but appears to be decreasing. Operator experience and strict adherence to WHO recommendations account for a low fatality rate. (iv) Because the disease process in PAH is unaffected by the procedure itself (late deaths), the long-term effects of an AS must be considered to be palliative.

Indications for the procedure include: (i) failure of maximal medical therapy (including oral CCB, prostacyclin analogues, bosentan, and phosphodiesterase-5 inhibitors, alone or combined) with persisting RV failure and/or recurrent syncope; (ii) as a bridge to transplantation; (iii) when no other therapeutic options exist (33,34).

KEY POINTS

Important issues derived from the analysis of the collective worldwide experience were discussed and debated at the World Symposiums – Pulmonary Hypertension 2008 in Dana Point, California, USA (41). General consensus and recommendations were as follows:

- The concept that atrial septostomy decompresses the RV in PAH is accepted.
- Uptake has been limited. Impediments to wider use of AS is related, in part, to the relative success of current medical treatment. Uptake may also be related to a lack of training pathway.
- Patients known to benefit have idiopathic PAH with syncope, persistent RV failure or have failed medical therapy.
- AS has a role in health care systems without drug access.
- AS has been used to bridge to lung transplant and might prolong survival on the waiting list. Its use in this setting should be delineated.
- Step-wise balloon dilation is the procedure of choice.
- The lack of data on exercise and long-term hemodynamics after AS needs to be addressed.
- Selection guidelines are unchanged from 2003 – do not undertake if baseline O_2 sat < 90 percent on room air or LVEDP > 18 mmHg.
- Procedural mortality is around 5 percent. Procedural deaths relate to inadvertent overly large defect, or fall in O_2 sat > 10 percent – more common if RAP > 20 mmHg. The defect created should be tailored to the end O_2 saturation.
- Closure of the defect may require repeat procedure. Data are sparse with Amplatzer devices, butterfly Stents, cutting edge balloons.
- Survival after AS is superior to NIH predicted survival. The benefit on survival differs from that of mono drug therapy in being immediately apparent.
- Current practice regarding the management of PAH is to consider atrial septostomy for treatment only after maximal medical (pharmacologic) therapy has failed. The advanced stage of PAH and RVF of the patients undergoing the procedure in the analysis of the current worldwide experience is in support of this. It is unknown how early in the course of PAH, AS may be beneficial.
- A combination approach of early AS (immediate results) with drug therapy seems attractive in Class IV patients.
- A trial of monotherapy patients (stable or deteriorating, Class III–IV) randomized to AS or no procedure is recommended.
- Use in children could be increased.

REFERENCES

- • = Key primary paper
- ◆ = Major review article
- ＊ = Management guideline

- •1. D'Alonso GE, Barst RJ, Ayres SM et al. Survival in patients with primary pulmonary hypertension. Results of a national prospective study. Ann Intern Med 1991;115:343–9.
- ◆2. Bristow MR, Zisman LS, Lances BD et al. The pressure-overloaded right ventricle in pulmonary hypertension. Chest 1998;114(Suppl):101S–106S.
- ◆3. Chin KM, Kim NHS, Rubin LJ. The right ventricle in pulmonary hypertension. Coron Art Dis 2005;16:13–8.
- ◆4. Sandoval J, Gaspar J. Atrial septostomy. In: Peacock AJ, Rubin LJ (eds). Pulmonary Circulation, 2nd edn. London: Edward Arnold, 2004:319–33.
- •5. Austen WG, Morrow AG, Berry WB. Experimental studies of the surgical treatment of primary pulmonary hypertension. J Thorac Cardiovasc Surg 1964;48:448–55.
- 6. Rozkovec A, Montanes P, Oakley CM. Factors that influence the outcome of primary pulmonary hypertension. Br Heart J 1986;55:449–58.
- •7. Hopkins WE, Ochoa LL, Richardson GW et al. Comparison of the hemodynamics and survival of adults with severe primary pulmonary hypertension or Eisenmenger syndrome. J Heart Lung Transplant 1996;15:100–5.
- 8. Hopkins WE. The remarkable right ventricle of patients with Eisenmenger syndrome. Coron Art Dis 2005;16:19–25.
- •9. Rashkind WJ, Miller WW. Creation of an atrial septal defect without thoracotomy. A palliative approach to complete transposition of the great arteries. JAMA 1966;196:173.
- 10. Park SC, Neches WH, Zuberbuhler JR et al. clinical use of blade atrial septostomy. Circulation 1978;58:600.
- 11. Park SC, Neches WH, Mullins CE et al. Blade Atrial Septostomy: Collaborative Study. Circulation 1982;66:258.
- •12. Rich S, Lam W. Atrial septostomy as palliative therapy for refractory primary pulmonary hypertension. Am J Cardiol 1983;51:1560–61.
- •13. Nihill MR, O'Laughlin MP, Mullins CE. Effects of atrial septostomy in patients with terminal cor pulmonale due to pulmonary vascular disease. Cathet Cardiovasc Diagn 1991;24:166–72.
- •14. Kerstein D, Levy PS, Hsu DT et al. Blade balloon atrial septostomy in patients with severe primary pulmonary hypertension. Circulation 1995;91:2028–35.
- •15. Hausknecht MJ, Sims RE, Nihill MR et al. Successful palliation of primary pulmonary hypertension by atrial septostomy. Am J Cardiol 1990;65:1045–6.
- •16. Rothman A, Beltran D, Kriett JM et al. Graded balloon dilation atrial septostomy as a bridge to transplantation in primary pulmonary hypertension. Am Heart J 1993;125:1763–6.
- •17. Sandoval J, Gaspar J, Pulido T et al. Graded balloon dilation atrial septostomy in severe primary pulmonary hypertension. A therapeutic alternative for patients

non-responsive to vasodilator treatment. J Am Coll Cardiol 1998;32:297–304.

•18. Rothman A, Slansky MS, Lucas VW et al. Atrial septostomy as a bridge to lung transplantation in patients with severe pulmonary hypertension. Am J Cardiol 1999;84:682–6.

•19. Reichenberger F, Pepke-Zaba J, McNeil K et al. Atrial septostomy in the treatment of severe pulmonary arterial hypertension. Thorax 2003;58:797–800.

20. Vachiery JL, Stoupel E, Boonstra A, Naeije R. Balloon atrial septostomy for pulmonary hypertension in the prostacyclin era. Am J Respir Crit Care Med 2003;167:A692.

21. Moscussi M, Dairywala IT, Chetcuti S et al. Balloon atrial septostomy in end-stage pulmonary hypertension guided a novel intracardiac echocardiographic transducer. Catheter Cardiovasc Interv 2001;52:530–4.

22. Kothari SS, Yusuf A, Juneja R et al. Graded balloon atrial septostomy in severe pulmonary hypertension. Indian Heart J 2002;54:164–9.

•23. Allcock RJ, O'Sullivan JJ, Corris PA. Atrial septostomy for pulmonary hypertension. Heart 2003;89:1344–7.

24. Kurzyna M, Dabrowsky M, Torbicki A et al. Atrial septostomy for severe primary pulmonary hypertension. Report of two cases. Kardiol Pol 2003;58:27–33.

25. Chau EMC, Fan KYY, Chow WH. Combined atrial septostomy and oral sildenafil for severe right ventricular failure due to primary pulmonary hypertension. Hong Kong Med J 2004;10:281–4.

•26. Micheletti A, Hislop A, Lammers A et al. Role of atrial septostomy in the treatment of children with pulmonary arterial hypertension. Heart 2006;92:969–72.

27. Hayden AM. Balloon atrial septostomy increases cardiac index and may reduce mortality among pulmonary hypertension patients awaiting lung transplantation. J Transpl Coord 1997;7:131–3.

•28. Kurzyna M, Dabrowski M, Bielecki D et al. Atrial septostomy in treatment of end-stage right heart failure in patients with pulmonary hypertension. Chest 2007;131:947–8.

•29. Ciarka A, Vachiery JL, Houssiere A et al. Atrial septostomy decreases sympathetic overactivity in pulmonary arterial hypertension. Chest 2007;131:1831–7.

◆30. Barst RJ. Role of atrial septostomy in the treatment of pulmonary vascular disease. Thorax 2000;55:95–6.

∗31. Rich S, Dodin E, McLaughlin VV. Usefulness of atrial septostomy as a treatment for primary pulmonary hypertension and guidelines for its application. Am J Cardiol 1997;80:369–71.

◆∗32. Sandoval J, Rothman A, Pulido T. Atrial septostomy for pulmonary hypertension. Clin Chest Med 2001; 22:547–60.

•33. Doyle RL, McCrory D, Channick RN, Simonneau G, Conte J. Surgical treatments/interventions for pulmonary arterial hypertension. ACCP Evidence-Based Clinical Practice Guidelines. Chest 2004;126:63S–71S

•34. Klepetko W, Mayer E, Sandoval J et al. Interventional and surgical modalities of treatment for pulmonary arterial hypertension. J Am Coll Cardiol 2004;43:73S–80S.

•35. Law MA, Grifka RG, Mullins CE, Nihill MR. Atrial septostomy improves survival in select patients with pulmonary hypertension. Am Heart J 2007;153:779–84.

36. Wawrzynska L, Remiszewski P, Kurzyna M et al. A case of a patient with idiopathic pulmonary arterial hypertension treated with lung transplantation: a bumpy road to success. Pol Arch Med Wewn 2006;115:565–71.

37. Rogan MP, Walsh KP, Gaine SP. Migraine with aura following atrial septostomy for pulmonary arterial hypertension. Nat Clin Pract Cardiovasc Med 2007; 4:55–8.

38. Fraisse A, Chetaille P, Amin Z et al. Use of Amplatzer fenestrated atrial septal defect device in a child with familial pulmonary hypertension. Pediatr Cardiol 2006;27:759–62.

•39. Prieto LR, Latson LA, Jennings C. Atrial septostomy using a butterfly stent in a patient with severe pulmonary arterial hypertension. Catheter Cardiovasc Interv 2006;68:642–7.

40. O'loughlin AJ, Keogh A, Muller DW. Insertion of a fenestrated Amplatzer atrial septostomy device for severe pulmonary hypertension. Heart Lung Circ 2006;15:275–7.

41. Keogh AM, Mayer E, Benza RL et al. Interventional and surgical modalities of treatment in pulmonary hypertension. J Am Coll Cardiol 2009;54:567–77.

•42. Baim DS. Percutaneous approach, including trans-septal and apical puncture. In: Baim DS, Grossman W (eds). Grossman's Cardiac Catheterization, Angiography, and Intervention, 6th edn. Philadelphia: Lippincott Williams and Wilkins, 2000;69–100.

43. Sandoval J, Gaspar J, Peña H et al. Effect of atrial septostomy on the survival of patients with severe pulmonary arterial hypertension. The benefit of combining strategies. Editorial Review.

•44. Espínola-Zavaleta N, Vargas-Barrón J, Tazar JI et al. Echocardiographic evaluation of patients with pulmonary hypertension before and after atrial septostomy. Echocardiography 1999;16:625.

45. Rich S, Brundage BH. High dose calcium channel blocking therapy for primary pulmonary hypertension: evidence for long-term reduction in pulmonary artery pressure and regression of right ventricular hypertrophy. Circulation 1987;76:135–41.

46. Hinderliter AL, Willis W, Barst RJ et al. Effects of long-term infusion of prostacyclin (Epoprostenol) on echocardiographic measures of right ventricular structure and function in primary pulmonary hypertension. Circulation 1997;95: 1479–86.

47. Dittrich HC, Nicod PH, Chow LC et al. Early changes of right heart geometry after pulmonary thromboendarterectomy. J Am Coll Cardiol 1998;11: 937–43.

48. Ritchie M, Waggoner A, Dávila-Roman VG et al. Echocardiographic characterization of the improvement in right ventricular failure in patients with severe pulmonary hypertension after single lung transplantation. J Am Coll Cardiol 1993;22:1170–4.

•49. Velez Roa S, Ciarka A, Najem B *et al.* Increased sympathetic nerve activity in pulmonary artery hypertension. Circulation 2004;110:1308–1312.

•50. O'Byrne ML, Berman-Rosenzweig ES, Barst RJ. The effect of atrial septostomy on the concentration of brain-type natriuretic peptide in patients with idiopathic pulmonary arterial hypertension. Cardiol Young 2007;17:557–9.

•51. Lammers AE, Derrick G, Haworth SG *et al.* Efficacy and long-term patency of fenestrated amplatzer devices in children. Catheter Cardiovasc Interv 2007;70:578–84.

•52. Potts WJ, Smith S, Gibson S. Anastomosis of the aorta to a pulmonary artery: Certain types in congenital heart disease. JAMA 1946;132:627–31.

53. Daniel FJ, Clarke CP, Richardson JP *et al.* An evaluation of Potts' aortopulmonary shunt for palliation of cyanotic heart disease. Thorax 1976;31:394–7.

•54. Blanc J, Vouhé P, Bonnet D. Potts shunt in patients with pulmonary hypertension. N Engl J Med 2004;350:623.

•55. Serraf A, Petit J, Belli E *et al.* Potts anastomosis for severe pulmonary arterial hypertension in children. Paper presented at the American Thoracic Society International Conference. San Diego, California, May 2007.

56. Keogh A. Novel shunts for PAH: Potts Anastomosis or 'de novo Ductus Arteriosus' – a hypothetical exercise. In: Keogh A, Mayers E (eds). Interventional and Surgical Modalities of Treatment in PAH (in press).

Pulmonary endarterectomy

ECKHARD MAYER

INTRODUCTION

Chronic thromboembolic pulmonary hypertension (CTEPH) is a frequently overlooked and underdiagnosed cause of pulmonary hypertension with a higher incidence than previously anticipated and a poor prognosis (1–7). Acute or recurrent pulmonary embolisms are considered to be the primary events followed by intraluminal thrombus organization and fibrous obstruction of pulmonary artery branches with consequent development of pulmonary hypertension and right heart dysfunction (8,9). Vascular remodeling occurs in patent areas of pulmonary microvasculature and further impairs pulmonary hemodynamics and exercise capacity (8,10). Therefore chronic thromboembolic pulmonary hypertension is a disease with a mechanical component judged amenable to surgery and a variable degree of small vessel arteriopathy (8,11).

The standard therapy for CTEPH is pulmonary endarterectomy (PEA; previous term: pulmonary thromboendarterectomy = PTE) (2). As the surgical treatment option for CTEPH is highly effective and potentially curative (4,12–17) and substantially differs from therapeutic concepts in pulmonary arterial hypertension (PAH), an exact diagnostic differentiation between CTEPH and PAH is mandatory for any particular patient with unexplained symptomatic pulmonary hypertension (2). Pulmonary endarterectomy is a complex surgical procedure and resembles a removal of fibrous obstructions of pulmonary artery branches by endarterectomy techniques using extracorporeal circulation and periods of deep hypothermic circulatory arrest. In experienced centers, the operative risk has been decreased to an acceptable level. Following successful surgery, long-term survival and quality of life are excellent.

ASSESSMENT OF OPERABILITY AND PATIENT SELECTION

Chronic thromboembolic pulmonary hypertension is defined as symptomatic pulmonary hypertension (mean pulmonary artery pressure $> 25 \, \text{mmHg}$) with persistent pulmonary perfusion defects. Diagnostic workup and algorithms for patients with chronic thromboembolic pulmonary hypertension are described in Part 10, Chapter 22.3. The detection of right ventricular dysfunction by transthoracic echocardiography and the presence of single or multiple perfusion defects in pulmonary perfusion scanning are suspicious findings for CTEPH (2). The degree of pulmonary hypertension and right ventricular impairment is determined by right heart catheterization providing an estimation of the spontaneous prognosis of the disease. Multiplanar pulmonary angiography (Figure 17.3.1) still remains the gold standard for the diagnosis of CTEPH and is recommended for the assessment of operability for each patient (14,18,19). High-resolution CT scanning (Figure 17.3.2) and MR imaging have become valuable complementary investigations in expert centers (20–23). However, as the evaluation with regard to operability vs. inoperability and the estimation of the operative risk and long-term benefit after surgery are crucial issues for any individual patient, a maximum of information on morphology of pulmonary artery branches, blood flow and lung parenchymal perfusion is mandatory, which can only be achieved by conventional multiplanar pulmonary angiography in the majority of patients. The combined results of ventilation perfusion scanning, high-resolution multi-slice computed tomography, magnetic resonance imaging and pulmonary angiography are sufficient to assess surgical accessibility and operability

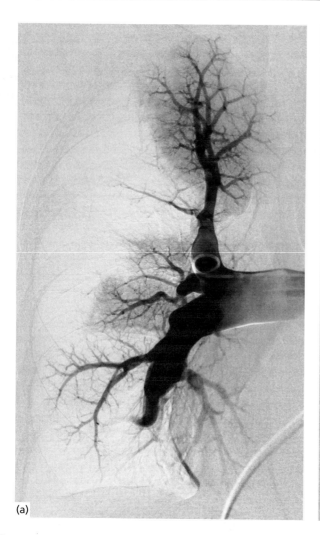
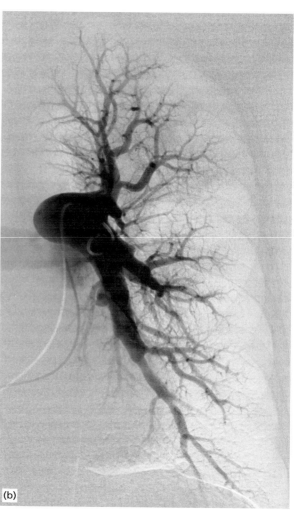

(a)

(b)

Figure 17.3.1 Pulmonary angiogram (a.p. view) showing significant obstructions and occlusions of right pulmonary artery branches and concomitant perfusion defects (a) and cut-offs of left lower lobe segmental arteries (b) in a 35-year-old female patient with severe CTEPH.

even in exclusively distal disease. In selected patients with unclear angiographic findings, pulmonary fiberoptic angioscopy can help to define operability and the risk of the surgical intervention (24,25).

Following careful assessment in a specialized multidisciplinary center and established diagnosis of CTEPH, patients should be referred for evaluation by a surgeon experienced in pulmonary endarterectomy operations. As there is a distinct learning curve with respect to diagnosis, evaluation of operability, surgical technique and perioperative management, team experience is the major prerequisite for a successful CTEPH treatment concept.

As there is inadequate evidence that medical therapy including PAH-specific therapy is an alternative to surgery, the operation should not be delayed in favor of medical therapy. The best outcomes after surgery at present are associated with concordance between PVR and anatomic disease depicted by angiography, preoperative PVR values < 1000–1200 dynes, absence of specific comorbidities (e.g. splenectomy, VA shunt, chronic infection, chronic bowel disease) and significant postoperative decrease in PVR

(4,13,14,26–29). Although pulmonary endarterectomy is the treatment of choice for CTEPH, surgery does not benefit all CTEPH patients either because of an increased operative risk or inadequate clinical and hemodynamic long-term improvement after surgery (2). There have been growing efforts to identify this high-risk group with a significant amount of distal arteriopathy preoperatively when the combination of high PVR and mild degree of angiographic pulmonary artery obstructions is present. In these patients who might present up to 40 percent of the CTEPH population PAH-specific therapy might be an alternative option (2,28,30–32). Therefore a preoperative classification system needs to be developed allowing a better stratification of surgical risk and long-term benefit for the particular patient. Variables other than PVR e.g. preoperative DLCO, upstream resistance and precise assessment of RV dysfunction may have a role in this future classification system (18,33,34). The San Diego classification (35) is based on operative findings of pulmonary artery obstruction and therefore not suitable for preoperative estimation of risk and long-term outcome of the operation. High quality imaging

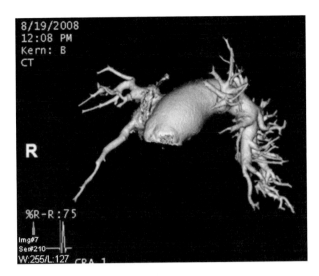

Figure 17.3.2 Computed tomography of pulmonary arteries (64-slice CT, 3-dimensional reconstruction of volumetric data set with retrospective electrocardiographic gating) detecting major occlusions of right pulmonary artery branches without proximal disease within left segmental arteries. Courtesy of Christopher Ahlers, MD, Department of Radiology, Johannes Gutenberg University Hospital, Mainz, Germany.

and a careful analysis of operability by an experienced multidisciplinary team are prerequisites for a recommendation of surgical treatment or alternative trial of medical therapy in CTEPH patients.

The decision for surgical treatment is made based on the severity of symptoms and the impairment of right ventricular function, pulmonary hemodynamics and gas exchange. Patients considered for surgery are usually severely incapacitated in their daily activities with dyspnea at low levels of exertion or at rest (New York Heart Association functional class III or IV). The preoperative pulmonary vascular resistance in surgical patients should be higher than 300 dyne/s cm^{-5} and average preoperative PVR values are approximately 800–1000 dynes in most larger patient cohorts (4,13,14). Patients with exertional dyspnea (NYHA functional class II), almost normal pulmonary vascular resistance at rest and a significant increase at exertion are also accepted for surgery to improve ventilation perfusion balance and avoid secondary microvascular arteriopathy of the patent pulmonary arteries. Patients with suprasystemic pulmonary artery pressures and excessive elevation of pulmonary vascular resistance (>1500 dyne/s cm^{-5}) are also accepted for surgery although the operative risk is significantly increased (13,36). Preoperative improvement of pulmonary hemodynamics by specific medical treatment might be an option to decrease the risk of surgery in this patient cohort (37,38).

Surgical accessibility of the thromboembolic lesions is an important prerequisite for a successful operation (24,25). It is heavily dependent on the surgeon's experience

and with growing experience, even patients with severe pulmonary hypertension and significant distal disease can be operated successfully. In order to achieve adequate early and late results, there should be no major discrepancy between the degree of pulmonary hypertension and the amount of surgically accessible thromboembolic material in the angiogram.

Right ventricular failure and concomitant hepatic and renal dysfunction are not considered as contraindications to surgery (4,39). However, patients with severe irreversible left ventricular dysfunction due to coronary artery, mitral or aortic valve disease or significant obstructive or restrictive lung disease are not accepted for surgery. All patients over 45 years undergo coronary angiography before surgery to rule out coronary disease. If necessary, coronary artery bypass grafting can be performed at the time of pulmonary endarterectomy.

PULMONARY ENDARTERECTOMY OPERATION

Although bilateral pulmonary endarterectomy has proved to be a potentially curative option for very sick patients with a poor prognosis, only approximately 4000 operations have been performed in a limited number of centers worldwide with the largest experience accumulated at the Division of Cardiothoracic Surgery at the University of California San Diego Medical Center (17,24,35,40–42).

The rationales of the operation are restoration of lung perfusion, ventilation perfusion balance and oxygenation, reduction of right ventricular afterload with consequent improvement of right heart function and concomitant recovery of multiorgan function and avoidance of secondary microvascular disease in patent areas of the pulmonary vasculature (Table 17.3.1). The surgical techniques and modifications necessary to reach these goals at a very acceptable operative risk have been well described by the San Diego group (40,41).

The operation is not an embolectomy or thrombectomy of fresh or old thromboembolic material from the central pulmonary artery and pulmonary artery branches, but a true endarterectomy removing the organized fibrous material with its neointima and parts of the medial layer (Figure 17.3.3). The operation is performed using extracorporeal circulation and periods of circulatory arrest under deep hypothermia (DHCA), as good visibility in a bloodless field is essential for a complete endarterectomy of the distal pulmonary artery branches and a maximal right ventricular afterload reduction. Circulatory arrest is necessary due to significant retrograde collateral blood flow from dilated bronchial arteries that would make an accurate distal endarterectomy procedure impossible. Different techniques avoiding circulatory arrest have been published (43–46) and intensely discussed (43,44).

Deep hypothermic circulatory arrest is believed to be a risk factor for neurological morbidity and mortality in aortic arch surgery although there are conflicting data in

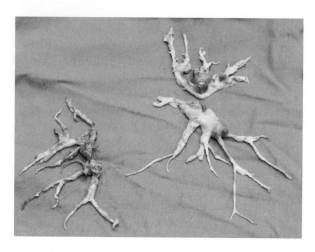

Figure 17.3.4 Surgical endarterectomy specimen of lobar, segmental and subsegmental PA branches.

Table 17.3.1 Rationales of PEA surgery

Rationales of PEA surgery
Restoration of lung perfusion
Reduction of right ventricular afterload
Improvement of right heart function
Restoration of ventilation perfusion balance and oxygenation
Recovery of multiorgan function
Avoidance of secondary microvascular pulmonary artery disease

this patient population with atherosclerotic aortic disease. However, operations on the aortic arch with circulatory arrest times greater than 25 minutes are very different procedures compared to endarterectomies of pulmonary arteries with maximum circulatory arrest times of less than 20 minutes in patients without significant atherosclerotic aortic disease. This is well demonstrated by the results of the San Diego Group reporting a 4.4 percent mortality and 0 percent neurological morbidity in a series of 500 consecutive PEA operations using deep hypothermic circulatory arrest. As long as early results in PEA programs avoiding circulatory events are significantly worse compared to published PEA outcomes including circulatory arrest (43,44), PEA operations without the use of hypothermia and/or circulatory arrest cannot be recommended. In addition, there are no long-term data on series without the use of DHCA and long-term outcomes are proven to be dependent on a complete endarterectomy and significant early reduction of PVR to less than 500 dynes (13). At present, PEA techniques described by the San Diego Group including deep hypothermic circulatory arrest are used by major centers in the world.

Following median sternotomy, cardiopulmonary bypass is instituted using ascending aortic and bicaval cannulation and cooling of the patient is initiated. When a 20°C core temperature is reached, the aorta is cross-clamped and cold cardioplegic solution is administered. The superior vena cava is mobilized and the right pulmonary artery is incised intrapericardially. Following removal of gross thrombus material, the correct endarterectomy plane is established. The endarterectomy is performed in 20-minute periods of circulatory arrest with exsanguination of the patient into the bypass reservoir. Developing the correct endarterectomy plane is difficult but crucial as incomplete endarterectomy with a plane that is too superficial will increase the surgical risk and lead to long-term residual pulmonary hypertension. If the endarterectomy plane is established too deeply within the vessel wall, intraoperative

perforation of a distal pulmonary artery branch might become a fatal complication by intrapulmonary hemorrhage. Using special blunt suction dissectors the endarterectomy specimen is circumferentially followed down to the segmental and subsegmental branches in each lobe, until a complete endarterectomy of the pulmonary vascular bed is achieved. Following reperfusion and closure of the right pulmonary artery incision, the left pulmonary artery is incised intrapericardially. Another period of circulatory arrest is necessary for the left pulmonary artery endarterectomy. Cardiopulmonary bypass is re-instituted and the left pulmonary artery incision is closed. Tricuspid valve repair is not necessary as tricuspid competence usually returns within days after successful pulmonary endarterectomy (47). In case of additional cardiac or coronary artery disease, valve or coronary bypass procedures can be performed in the rewarming period (48). Following rewarming, weaning from of cardiopulmonary bypass is cautiously performed. After achievement of hemostasis, wound closure is routine.

Jamieson and coworkers have proposed a surgical classification of pulmonary occlusive disease with regard to intraoperative findings (24,35). Type I and type II represent the typical condition of patients undergoing surgery. Peripheral type III occlusions on the segmental and subsegmental level require the most surgical experience and extremely careful exclusively distal dissection. Type IV disease represents secondary in-situ thrombosis in other forms of pulmonary hypertension, e.g. idiopathic pulmonary hypertension, and cannot be successfully treated by endarterectomy (4,49).

POSTOPERATIVE MANAGEMENT

In contrast to most other surgical procedures on the heart or proximal vessels using cardiopulmonary bypass the postoperative course of patients undergoing PEA is much more determined by right heart function and pulmonary circulation rather than left ventricular function and systemic circulation (50). Right heart dysfunction due to residual pulmonary hypertension and additional pulmonary vasoconstriction after extracorporeal circulation and a reperfusion edema within the endarterectomized segments of the lung are infrequent but significant problems after PEA

(14,25,50). Although the postoperative management after PEA surgery can be challenging with respect to ventilatory and hemodynamic treatment, the optimal postoperative care has not been defined and treatment protocols vary even amongst expert centers. Extensive ventilatory and circulatory monitoring including online measurement of cardiac output, mixed venous oxygen saturation and arterial blood gases have proved to be helpful for adequate evaluation of complications and instant therapeutic measures.

In most of the patients, right ventricular afterload reduction by removal of obstructive material from the pulmonary vasculature will result in an immediate and significant decrease of pulmonary artery pressures, a concomitant increase in cardiac index, good gas exchange and profound diuresis. In this group of patients, medical treatment consists of cautious fluid administration and application of vasoconstrictive drugs if systemic hypotension due to vasodilation is present. Reduction of cardiac index to preoperative levels may be necessary to avoid fluid overload of the lungs and relevant reperfusion edema. This problem is even more important in patients with a postoperative increase of cardiac index and an elevated but reversible degree of pulmonary hypertension. Aggressive diuretic therapy helps to reduce cardiac output and decreases the risk of pulmonary reperfusion edema (14,50).

In a small number of patients, postoperative right heart failure develops as a consequence of severe persistent pulmonary hypertension due to incomplete endarterectomy or small vessel disease and of the pulmonary vasoconstrictive effects of extracorporeal circulation, hypothermia and ischemia. As this group of patients is at a dramatically increased risk for death (25), all efforts should be made to optimize right heart function by administration of inotropic agents and by reducing right ventricular afterload. The role of treatment with specific pulmonary vasodilators in this challenging situation is unclear, although there is limited information that inhaled iloprost might be useful for the therapy of postoperative pulmonary hypertension (51).

Although the achievement of adequate gas exchange is a basic tenet of postoperative care after pulmonary endarterectomy and pulmonary reperfusion response can be a serious problem, there is no consensus with respect to ventilatory protocols even in specialized centers. It is uncertain whether mechanical ventilation with high tidal volumes and a limited degree of PEEP or a nonaggressive pressure-controlled ventilation with high PEEP provides better results with regard to gas exchange and hemodynamic effects. Nevertheless, early extubation on day 1 or 2 after surgery is possible with both protocols in more than 80 percent of the patients (14,50,52). Fifteen to 20 percent of the patients require prolonged ventilation mainly due to reperfusion edema and/or right ventricular dysfunction based on residual pulmonary hypertension or early pulmonary infections.

Early reocclusion prophylaxis using i.v. or s.c. heparin is essential for prevention of rethrombosis or embolism, although it might increase the degree of postoperative bleeding and rate of re-thoracotomy for bleeding. The routine preoperative insertion of an inferior vena cava filter to reduce the risk of perioperative or recurrent pulmonary embolism is a matter of debate, as the filter by itself might be a cause of thrombosis and source of recurrent embolism. Subsequent life-long anticoagulation is mandatory for all post PEA patients. A randomized trial to compare optimal surveillance anticoagulation with or without vena cava filters is warranted.

OUTCOME

Pulmonary endarterectomy in CTEPH has not been assessed in randomized controlled studies which are considered unethical in the absence of adequate alternative treatments. However, the outcome of pulmonary endarterectomy with respect to survival, functional status, hemodynamics, right ventricular function and pulmonary gas exchange is very favorable for most patients (14,25,53–55).

The concept of pulmonary endarterectomy has been transferred from the University of California, San Diego to an increasing number of centers around the world. The last surgical report from San Diego included a cohort of 965 patients operated between May 1998 and April 2006 and demonstrated a mortality of 4.9 percent in this group of severely ill patients (56). As early and late results are closely related to the experience of a surgeon and a multidisciplinary team, it is difficult for centers with a lower level of experience to reach similar results like the UC San Diego in the early phase of such a complex program treating a rare disease. Therefore it seems very important that PEA centers collaborate worldwide with regard to diagnostic procedures, patient selection, surgical techniques and postoperative management and the number of centers per country is limited in order to increase the number of annual pulmonary endarterectomies per center. Meanwhile it has been shown in several PEA programs worldwide that with increasing experience early mortality rates can be reduced to 5–10 percent in several hundred patients (14,43,57,58). However, as in the absence of adequate treatment alternatives the operation is also offered to patients with distal disease and very severe pulmonary hypertension, it is evident, that the operative risk for the individual patient in this group can be increased above the normal level. Lung transplantation for pulmonary hypertension is associated with a limited long-term survival (59) and therefore only a treatment option for highly selected patients with inoperable chronic thromboembolic pulmonary hypertension evaluated by an experienced interdisciplinary team.

Maximum benefits of surgery may not be immediate and take six months or more (60,61). In order to exclude residual or recurrent disease, patients must be systemically followed and ideally re-evaluated at 6–12 months after surgery with respect to exercise capacity and pulmonary hemodynamics including invasive evaluation with right heart catheterization. In case of residual or recurrent pulmonary hypertension specific pulmonary vasodilatory treatment might be beneficial (2,62,63), although further randomized controlled studies are necessary.

Late results

Compared to the reported survival without surgery (3,5) or with lung transplantation (59), long-term results after pulmonary endarterectomy are very favorable with a five-year survival rate of 75 to 80 percent (24,53,54). In 350 consecutive patients who underwent pulmonary endarterectomy at the Johannes Gutenberg-University hospital in Mainz in a 16-year period between 1989 and 2005, the five-year survival rate was 81 percent and the ten-year survival rate was 76 percent, respectively.

Quality of life

More than 90 percent of the patients report a significant improvement of the quality of life and exercise tolerance after surgery (53,54,60,61). Before surgery, most patients are in New York Heart Association functional class III or IV. In a survey of 306 patients after an average time since surgery of 3.3 years, 93 percent of them identified themselves as functional class I or II. And 96 percent considered their shortness of breath since surgery much improved or improved (54). The majority of post-PEA patients are enjoying a good functional status and quality of life with minimal utilization of health care services (54). These findings are supported by cardiopulmonary exercise tests in post-PEA patients. Peak oxygen uptake is significantly increasing over the first year after surgery and persistent for the second year whereas ventilatory response to carbon dioxide ($V(E)$-$V(CO_2)$) as a parameter of dead space ventilation is significantly decreasing within the first year after surgery and also persistently lowered in the second year (61).

Hemodynamic outcome and right ventricular function

In several studies, significant and persistent decreases of pulmonary artery pressures and pulmonary vascular resistance after PTE surgery are reported (25,53,54,60). More than five years after surgery, mean PAP and PVR are significantly lower compared to preoperative measurements with a normalization of right heart function evaluated by echocardiography in most of the patients (47,64,65). Restoration of pulmonary artery morphology and cardiac geometry and function can be impressively shown by magnetic imaging techniques (22).

It is estimated that in 10–15 percent of the patients residual or recurrent pulmonary hypertension and consequent right heart dysfunction occurs (2). If a reoperation is not feasible, these patients should be treated medically in a specialized center.

CONCLUSIONS

Pulmonary endarterectomy is an effective and potentially curative surgical treatment for patients with severe chronic thromboembolic pulmonary hypertension. Based on the experience of a multidisciplinary team, the operative risk has been reduced to an acceptable level. Long-term survival, NYHA functional status, exercise capacity, pulmonary hemodynamics and right ventricular function are significantly improved. Earlier referral to surgery might avoid the occurrence of a secondary vasculopathy and therefore further improve early and late results. Specific medical treatment might be an option for inoperable patients or patients with residual or recurrent pulmonary hypertension after pulmonary endarterectomy. Lung transplantation is not an option for the vast majority of CTEPH patients and should only be considered for selected patients who are not accepted for endarterectomy in a center with a large experience in this technically demanding surgical procedure.

KEY POINTS

- Pulmonary endarterectomy is the treatment of choice for chronic thromboembolic pulmonary hypertension.
- Once CTEPH is diagnosed, patients should be referred for surgical evaluation.
- Experience of a multidisciplinary team and surgeon is the prerequisite for successful treatment.
- The surgical technique is standardized but complex using extracorporeal circulation and deep hypothermic circulators arrest.
- Operative mortality should be < 10 percent, long-term benefits are very favorable for the majority of patients.
- PAH-specific medical treatment might be an option for inoperable patients or patients with residual or recurrent pulmonary hypertension after pulmonary endarterectomy.

REFERENCES

1. Pengo V *et al.* Incidence of chronic thromboembolic pulmonary hypertension after pulmonary embolism. N Engl J Med 2004;350(22):2257–64.
2. Hoeper MM *et al.* Chronic thromboembolic pulmonary hypertension. Circulation 2006;113(16):2011–20.
3. Riedel M, Widimsky J. (Prognosis of pulmonary hypertension in chronic thromboembolic disease). Vnitr Lek 1980;26(8):729–36.
4. Jamieson SW *et al.* Pulmonary endarterectomy: experience and lessons learned in 1,500 cases. Ann Thorac Surg 2003; 76(5):1457–62; discussion 1462–4.

5. Lewczuk J et al. Prognostic factors in medically treated patients with chronic pulmonary embolism. Chest 2001; 119(3):818–23.

6. Lang IM. Chronic thromboembolic pulmonary hypertension – not so rare after all. N Engl J Med 2004; 350(22):2236–8.

7. Tapson VF, Humbert M. Incidence and prevalence of chronic thromboembolic pulmonary hypertension:from acute to chronic pulmonary embolism. Proc Am Thorac Soc 2006;3(7):564–7.

8. Moser KM, Auger WR, Fedullo PF. Chronic major-vessel thromboembolic pulmonary hypertension. Circulation 1990; 81(6):1735–43.

9. Fedullo PF, Moser KM. Advances in acute pulmonary embolism and chronic pulmonary hypertension. Adv Intern Med 1997;42:67–104.

10. Moser KM, Bloor CM. Pulmonary vascular lesions occurring in patients with chronic major vessel thromboembolic pulmonary hypertension. Chest 1993;103(3):685–92.

11. Galie N, Kim NH. Pulmonary microvascular disease in chronic thromboembolic pulmonary hypertension. Proc Am Thorac Soc 2006;3(7):571–6.

12. Moser KM, Braunwald NS. Successful surgical intervention in severe chronic thromboembolic pulmonary hypertension. Chest 1973;64(1):29–35.

13. Dartevelle P et al. Chronic thromboembolic pulmonary hypertension. Eur Respir J 2004;23(4):637–48.

14. Mayer E. Surgical treatment of chronic thromboembolic pulmonary hypertension. Swiss Med Wkly 2006; 136(31–32):491–7.

15. Mayer E, Klepetko W. Techniques and outcomes of pulmonary endarterectomy for chronic thromboembolic pulmonary hypertension. Proc Am Thorac Soc 2006;3(7): 589–93.

16. Doyle RL et al. Surgical treatments/interventions for pulmonary arterial hypertension: ACCP evidence-based clinical practice guidelines. Chest 2004;126(1 Suppl): 63S–71S.

17. Daily PO et al. Surgical management of chronic pulmonary embolism: surgical treatment and late results. J Thorac Cardiovasc Surg 1980;79(4):523–31.

18. Kim NH. Assessment of operability in chronic thromboembolic pulmonary hypertension. Proc Am Thorac Soc 2006;3(7): 584–8.

19. Coulden R. State-of-the-art imaging techniques in chronic thromboembolic pulmonary hypertension. Proc Am Thorac Soc 2006;3(7):577–83.

20. Reichelt A et al. Chronic thromboembolic pulmonary hypertension: Evaluation with 64-detector row CT versus digital substraction angiography. Eur J Radiol 2008.

21. Kreitner KF et al. Chronic thromboembolic pulmonary hypertension – assessment by magnetic resonance imaging. Eur Radiol 2007;17(1):11–21.

22. Kreitner KF et al. Chronic thromboembolic pulmonary hypertension: pre- and postoperative assessment with breath-hold MR imaging techniques. Radiology 2004;232(2):535–43.

23. Ley S et al. Value of contrast-enhanced MR angiography and helical CT angiography in chronic thromboembolic pulmonary hypertension. Eur Radiol 2003;13(10):2365–71.

24. Jamieson SW, Kapelanski DP. Pulmonary endarterectomy. Curr Probl Surg 2000;37(3):165–252.

25. Fedull PF et al. Chronic thromboembolic pulmonary hypertension. N Engl J Med 2001;345(20):1465–72.

26. Bonderman D et al. Medical conditions increasing the risk of chronic thromboembolic pulmonary hypertension. Thromb Haemost 2005;93(3):512–6.

27. Bonderman D et al. Predictors of outcome in chronic thromboembolic pulmonary hypertension. Circulation 2007;115(16):2153–8.

28. Rubin LJ et al. Current and future management of chronic thromboembolic pulmonary hypertension: from diagnosis to treatment responses. Proc Am Thorac Soc 2006;3(7):601–7.

29. Tscholl D et al. Pulmonary thromboendarterectomy – risk factors for early survival and hemodynamic improvement. Eur J Cardiothorac Surg 2001;19(6):771–6.

30. Bresser P et al. Medical therapies for chronic thromboembolic pulmonary hypertension: an evolving treatment paradigm. Proc Am Thorac Soc 2006;3(7):594–600.

31. Ono F et al. Effect of orally active prostacyclin analogue on survival in patients with chronic thromboembolic pulmonary hypertension without major vessel obstruction. Chest 2003;123(5):1583–8.

32. Bonderman D et al. Bosentan therapy for inoperable chronic thromboembolic pulmonary hypertension. Chest 2005;128(4):2599–603.

33. Condliffe R et al. Prognostic and aetiological factors in chronic thromboembolic pulmonary hypertension. Eur Respir J 2008.

34. Kim NH et al. Preoperative partitioning of pulmonary vascular resistance correlates with early outcome after thromboendarterectomy for chronic thromboembolic pulmonary hypertension. Circulation 2004;109(1):18–22.

35. Thistlethwaite PA et al. Operative classification of thromboembolic disease determines outcome after pulmonary endarterectomy. J Thorac Cardiovasc Surg 2002;124(6):1203–11.

36. Thistlethwaite PA et al. Outcomes of pulmonary endarterectomy for treatment of extreme thromboembolic pulmonary hypertension. J Thorac Cardiovasc Surg 2006;131(2):307–13.

37. Nagaya N et al. Prostacyclin therapy before pulmonary thromboendarterectomy in patients with chronic thromboembolic pulmonary hypertension. Chest 2003;123(2):338–43.

38. Kerr KM, Rubin LJ. Epoprostenol therapy as a bridge to pulmonary thromboendarterectomy for chronic thromboembolic pulmonary hypertension. Chest 2003;123(2):319–20.

39. Klepetko W et al. Interventional and surgical modalities of treatment for pulmonary arterial hypertension. J Am Coll Cardiol 2004;43(12 Suppl S):73S–80S.

40. Daily PO et al. Modifications of techniques and early results of pulmonary thromboendarterectomy for chronic pulmonary embolism. J Thorac Cardiovasc Surg 1987;93(2):221–33.

41. Jamieson SW et al. Experience and results with 150 pulmonary thromboendarterectomy operations over a 29-month period. J Thorac Cardiovasc Surg 1993; 106(1):116–26; discussion 126–7.

42. Madani MM, Jamieson SW. Technical advances of pulmonary endarterectomy for chronic thromboembolic pulmonary hypertension. Semin Thorac Cardiovasc Surg 2006;18(3):243–9.

43. Thomson B et al. Pulmonary endarterectomy is possible and effective without the use of complete circulatory arrest – the UK experience in over 150 patients. Eur J Cardiothorac Surg 2008;33(2):157–63.

44. Macchiarini P et al. Pulmonary endarterectomy for chronic thromboembolic pulmonary hypertension: is deep hypothermia required? Eur J Cardiothorac Surg 2006;30(2):237–41; discussion 241–3.

45. Mikus PM et al. Pulmonary endarterectomy: is there an alternative to profound hypothermia with cardiocirculatory arrest? Eur J Cardiothorac Surg 2006;30(3):563–5.

46. Mikus PM et al. Pulmonary endarterectomy:an alternative to circulatory arrest and deep hypothermia: mid-term results. Eur J Cardiothorac Surg 2008;34(1):159–63.

47. Menzel T et al. Improvement of tricuspid regurgitation after pulmonary thromboendarterectomy. Ann Thorac Surg 2002;73(3):756–61.

48. Thistlethwaite PA et al. Pulmonary thromboendarterectomy combined with other cardiac operations: indications, surgical approach, and outcome. Ann Thorac Surg 2001;72(1):13–7; discussion 17–9.

49. Moser KM et al. Do patients with primary pulmonary hypertension develop extensive central thrombi? Circulation 1995;91(3):741–5.

50. Adams A, Fedullo PF. Postoperative management of the patient undergoing pulmonary endarterectomy. Semin Thorac Cardiovasc Surg 2006;18(3):250–6.

51. Kramm T et al. Inhaled iloprost to control residual pulmonary hypertension following pulmonary endarterectomy. Eur J Cardiothorac Surg 2005;28(6): 882–8.

52. Mares P et al. Pulmonary artery thromboendarterectomy: a comparison of two different postoperative treatment strategies. Anesth Analg 2000;90(2):267–73.

53. Kramm T et al. Long-term results after thromboendarterectomy for chronic pulmonary embolism. Eur J Cardiothorac Surg 1999;15(5):579–83; discussion 583–4.

54. Archibald CJ et al. Long-term outcome after pulmonary thromboendarterectomy. Am J Respir Crit Care Med 1999;160(2):523–8.

55. Corsico, A.G. et al. Long-term outcome after pulmonary endarterectomy. Am J Respir Crit Care Med 2008;178(4): 419–24.

56. Thistlethwaite PA, Madani M, Jamieson SW. Outcomes of pulmonary endarterectomy surgery. Semin Thorac Cardiovasc Surg 2006;18(3):257–64.

57. Lindner J et al. Implementation of a new programme for the surgical treatment of CTEPH in the Czech Republic – Pulmonary endarterectomy. Thorac Cardiovasc Surg 2006;54(8):528–31.

58. Rubens FD et al. Surgery for chronic thromboembolic pulmonary hypertension – inclusive experience from a national referral center. Ann Thorac Surg 2007;83(3): 1075–81.

59. Christie JD et al. Registry of the International Society for Heart and Lung Transplantation: twenty-fifth official adult lung and heart/lung transplantation report – 2008. J Heart Lung Transplant 2008;27(9):957–69.

60. Mayer E et al. Mid-term results of pulmonary thromboendarterectomy for chronic thromboembolic pulmonary hypertension. Ann Thorac Surg 1996; 61(6):1788–92.

61. Matsuda H et al. Long-term recovery of exercise ability after pulmonary endarterectomy for chronic thromboembolic pulmonary hypertension. Ann Thorac Surg 2006;82(4):1338–43; discussion 1343.

62. Hoeper MM et al. Bosentan therapy for inoperable chronic thromboembolic pulmonary hypertension. Chest 2005; 128(4):2363–7.

63. Reichenberger F et al. Long-term treatment with sildenafil in chronic thromboembolic pulmonary hypertension. Eur Respir J 2007;30(5):922–7.

64. Menzel T et al. Assessment of cardiac performance using Tei indices in patients undergoing pulmonary thromboendarterectomy. Ann Thorac Surg 2002;73(3): 762–6.

65. Menzel T et al. Pathophysiology of impaired right and left ventricular function in chronic embolic pulmonary hypertension: changes after pulmonary thromboendarterectomy. Chest 2000;118(4):897–903.

An integrated approach to the treatment of pulmonary arterial hypertension

MARIUS M HOEPER

INTRODUCTION

Until the turn of the century, the only treatments that were available for patients with pulmonary arterial hypertension (PAH) were calcium channel blockers (for patients fulfilling the responder criteria) (1) and intravenous epoprostenol (2). In the past few years this situation has changed considerably as now various intravenous, inhaled, subcutaneous and oral prostanoids are available as well as several endothelin receptor antagonists and phosphodiesterase-5 (PDE-5) inhibitors (3–5). Therefore, treatment of PAH is more rewarding now than it was before but it has also become more complex than ever. Physicians taking care of patients with PAH must decide when to start treatment, which drug(s) they use as initial therapy, when they switch medications and when they combine medications, whether they use different treatment strategies in different types of PAH, and when other options such as lung transplantation must be considered.

WHEN TO START THERAPY IN PAH?

The first randomized, controlled clinical trials in the PAH field enrolled predominantly patients in functional class WHO III and IV and thus, most of the PAH drugs were initially approved only for patients with advanced disease (2,6). It was unclear for some time whether treatment of PAH patients in functional class II would also be associated with beneficial clinical effects. Meanwhile, however, it has been shown that the PDE-5 inhibitor sildenafil as well as the endothelin receptor antagonist ambrisentan improve exercise capacity in patients presenting in functional class II (7,8). Perhaps more importantly, the EARLY study has demonstrated that the endothelin receptor antagonist bosentan slows disease progression in patients with mildly symptomatic PH, i.e. functional class II (9). As described in more detail in Chapter 16.4, the EARLY trial included 185 patients with PAH in functional class II who were randomized to receive either placebo or bosentan for 6 months. The study had two co-primary endpoints: change in pulmonary vascular resistance and change in 6-minute walk distance. While there was a significant decline in pulmonary vascular resistance after 6 months of bosentan therapy (-22.6 percent compared to placebo), the change in 6-minute walk distance ($+19.1$ m compared to placebo) did not reach statistical significance. Time to clinical worsening, however, a composite endpoint defined as death of any cause, hospitalization due to PAH complications, or symptomatic progression of PAH, significantly improved in the active treatment group. There were three events in the bosentan group compared to 13 events in the placebo group showing not only that PAH is a progressive disease, even in patients presenting with milder symptoms, but that disease progression can be slowed with modern therapy. One important observation of the EARLY trial was that medical therapy can slow disease progression even if exercise capacity does not improve. This observation may have therapeutic implications (see below).

Given the available data there is no longer any doubt that targeted therapy of PAH should start as early as possible. Sildenafil is currently approved in the US for all functional classes but in Europe only for functional class III. Ambrisentan has been approved for functional class II, III and IV in the US and for functional class II and III in Europe. Bosentan is approved for functional class III and IV in the US and for functional class II and III in Europe. Based on the available data and the approval status, these three drugs would currently be considered first choice therapy for PAH patients presenting in functional class II. However, as no head-to-head comparison studies are available, it is unknown if any of these substances is more efficacious than the other.

WHAT IS THE INITIAL THERAPY OF PAH?

Several factors influence the choice of the initial therapy of PAH patients: the severity of the disease, the underlying condition and concomitant diseases, the availability of drugs, local reimbursement regulations, physicians' and patients' preferences, and many more.

Patients presenting in functional class II

As outlined above, the recommended treatments for patients presenting in functional class II are PDE-5 inhibitors and/or endothelin receptor antagonists.

Patients presenting in functional class III

For patients presenting in functional class III, a broad spectrum of substances is available, including the endothelin receptor antagonists bosentan, sitaxentan*, and ambrisentan, the PDE-5 inhibitors sildenafil and tadalafil, intravenous epoprostenol, treprostinil and iloprost, inhaled iloprost, inhaled treprostinil, and subcutaneous treprostinil. Again, as there are no head-to-head comparisons between any of these treatments, the selection of the first-choice treatment remains difficult. Some experts argue that intravenous epoprostenol should be the treatment of choice for these patients as this remains the only therapy with a proven survival benefit. However, the survival advantage with epoprostenol treatment has been shown only in patients presenting in functional class IV (2). Of note, earlier studies by the Cambridge group showed that there was no survival benefit in PAH patients treated with intravenous prostanoids when the baseline mixed venous oxygen saturation was > 60 percent, i.e. when these patients had a normal or near-normal cardiac output (10,11). In addition, a study from France has provided data suggesting that the survival of patients in functional class III is the same with first-line bosentan therapy and with first-line epoprostenol therapy (12).

*Sitaxsentan was withdrawn in December 2010.

Based on these data, most expert centers now use oral drugs, i.e. endothelin receptor antagonists or PDE-5 inhibitors in the majority of their class III patients, and current international guidelines also recommend these drugs as first-choice therapy for class III patients.

Patients presenting in functional class IV

The recommended treatment for patients presenting in functional class IV is an intravenous prostacyclin derivative, such as epoprostenol, treprostinil or iloprost. Some centers also use subcutaneous treprostinil in these patients. In treatment-naïve patients who are hemodynamically stable, a treatment trial with PDE-5 inhibitors and/or endothelin receptor antagonists may also be justified but these patients need to be monitored closely and should proceed to parenteral prostanoid therapy once they don't improve rapidly and substantially. Patients who are hemodynamically unstable, i.e. presenting with right heart failure, should be treated with parenteral prostanoids as soon as possible. After stabilization, some of these patients may eventually be transitioned to less invasive therapies but this needs to be done with great caution. Some centers use upfront combination therapy with two or three classes of substances in this patient population, although there is a shortage of data to support this approach.

Today, lung transplantation is usually reserved for patients failing combination therapy including parenteral prostanoids. Atrioseptostomy is mostly performed in countries where disease-targeting medications are not available, apparently with some success (13). It also has been proposed that septostomy, especially when performed in the early stages of the disease, may be a useful adjunct to pharmacotherapy but there are no sufficient data that would demonstrate improved prognosis with this approach.

WHEN TO SWITCH AND WHEN TO COMBINE?

The vast majority of PAH patients are started on monotherapy with an endothelin receptor antagonist, a PDE-5 inhibitor, or a prostanoid. If a patient responds well to his or her current medication, therapy will usually be continued (14). However, it is unclear how to manage patients who fail to improve sufficiently, have no improvement at all, or even deteriorate while receiving active therapy. The EARLY trial, as mentioned above, has shown that active therapy can slow the progression of the disease even if patients have no improvement in their exercise capacity (9). This observation suggests that it might be useful to continue any active treatment even if it is not having a direct impact on the patient's performance. Thus, most experts tend to add new treatments to previous ones in cases of an unsatisfying response and consider withdrawing PAH-targeted therapy in situations where a patient would not tolerate a medication.

Therefore, whenever monotherapy is not sufficiently efficacious, treatments are not switched, but other classes of drugs are added to the therapeutic regimen. As outlined in detail in the combination therapy chapter elsewhere in this book (Chapter 16.6), there is preliminary evidence that various combinations improve hemodynamics, exercise capacity, and outcome in patients with PAH (14–18). The optimal time to institute combination therapy, however, is unknown, as is the optimal choice of drugs. Given the progressive nature and the poor prognosis of PAH, it is appealing to start combination therapy upfront, i.e. once the diagnosis has been made. This approach, however, has not yet been studied. For the present time, most pulmonary hypertension centers use a sequential approach starting with monotherapy and moving on to combination therapy once a treatment is not found to be sufficiently active (14). In order to decide whether or not combination therapy is necessary, the patient's status must be assessed and treatment goals need to be defined on an individual patient's basis to guide treatment decisions (see below).

Definition of patient status

As outlined in the recent guidelines on pulmonary hypertension published jointly by the *European Society of Cardiology* and the *European Respiratory Society*, the clinical condition of a patient can be defined as stable and satisfactory, stable but not satisfactory, unstable and deteriorating.

STABLE AND SATISFACTORY

These patients fulfill the characteristics listed in the "green zone" of Table 18.1. The most important criteria are absence of clinical signs of RV failure, stable WHO functional class I or II without syncope, a 6-minute walk distance greater

than 400–500 meters depending on the individual patient, a peak oxygen uptake $> 15\,mL/min\,kg^{-1}$, normal or near-normal BNP/NT-proBNP plasma levels, no pericardial effusion, tricuspid annular plane systolic excursion (TAPSE) determined by echocardiography $> 2.0\,cm$, right atrial pressure < 8 mmHg and a cardiac index greater than $2.5\,L/min\,m^{-2}$.

STABLE AND NOT SATISFACTORY

These patients are in a stable condition but have not achieved the status which patient and treating physician would consider desirable. Some of the limits described above for a stable and satisfactory condition and included in the "green zone" of Table 18.1 are not fulfilled. These patients require reevaluation and consideration for additional or different treatment.

UNSTABLE AND DETERIORATING

These patients fulfill some or all of the characteristics listed in the "red zone" of Table 18.1. In particular these patients present with right ventricular failure, progression of symptoms and signs, worsening in functional class, a 6-minute walk distance of less than 300–400 meters, a peak oxygen uptake $< 12\,mL/min\,kg^{-1}$, rising BNP/NT-proBNP plasma levels, evidence of pericardial effusion, TAPSE $< 1.5\,cm$, a right atrial pressure > 15 mmHg and rising, and a cardiac index below $2.0\,L/min\,m^{-2}$ and falling. Clinical warning signs are increasing edema and/or the need to escalate diuretic therapy, new onset or increasing frequency/severity of angina, and syncope, which is often an alarming sign and requires immediate attention as it is a common manifestation of a low cardiac output. Supraventricular arrhythmias, especially atrial flutter and atrial fibrillation, may contribute to the clinical deterioration.

Table 18.1 Risk determinants in pulmonary arterial hypertension

Low risk	Determinants of risk	High risk
No	Clinical evidence of RV failure	Yes
Gradual	Progression	Rapid
II, III	WHO class	IV
Longer (> 400–$500\,m$)	6-minute walk distance	Shorter ($< 300\,m$)
$\dot{V}O_2max > 14.5\,mL/min\,kg^{-1}$	Cardiopulmonary exercise testing	$\dot{V}O_2max < 12\,mL/min\,kg^{-1}$
Minimally elevated and stable	BNP/NT-proBNP	Very elevated and/or rising
$PaCO_2 > 34\,mmHg$	Blood gases	$PaCO_2 < 32\,mmHg$
Minimal RV dysfunction	Echocardiographic findings	Pericardial effusion
TAPSE $> 2.0\,cm$		RV dysfunction
		TAPSE $< 1.5\,cm$
Normal/near normal RAP and CI	Hemodynamics	High RAP, low CI

$\dot{V}O_2max$; maximum oxygen uptake; RV, right ventricle; TAPSE, tricuspid plane annular systolic excursion; RAP, right atrial pressure; CI, cardiac index; BNP, brain natriuretic peptide; NT-proBNP, N-terminal fragment of pro-brain natriuretic peptide.

COMPREHENSIVE PROGNOSTIC EVALUATION

A comprehensive and thorough prognostic evaluation is required to assure that patients are truly achieving the desired status, i.e. *stable and satisfactory*. Ideally these patients should be in functional class I or II without signs of disease progression. In elderly patients and those with co-morbidities, achieving functional class I or II is not always realistic and a good functional class III may be acceptable for the patient as well as the physician.

There are several elements of information that help to determine clinical status and stability which can be categorized into three different groups: (i) clinical signs and exercise capacity; (ii) biomarkers; and (iii) right ventricular function and hemodynamics.

Clinical signs and exercise capacity

Some important features of stability can be assessed by simple clinical means: clinical signs of right heart failure should be absent. The physical performance is a major determinant of quality of life in patients with PAH. Functional class assessment is based on a patient's self-reporting and it is a major treatment goal to bring or keep a patient in a good functional class, i.e. I or II. Nevertheless, patient self-reporting is often flawed and exercise capacity should be assessed by some objective measurements, too. The most commonly used tool is the 6-minute walk test. It has been demonstrated some years ago that it is not the improvement in 6-minute walk distance achieved with medical therapy that is of prognostic importance but the overall walking distance a patient is capable to cover (12,19). In several studies, a 6-minute walk distance of approximately 380 m while the patient was receiving therapy was the best prognostic discriminator, which has led to the suggestion that one treatment goal should be a 6-minute walk distance of at least 380–400 m. It was found later, however, that especially younger patients are often capable of walking more than 400 m despite the presence of severe pulmonary hypertension. For that reason, the 6-minute walk test treatment goal is now set between 400 and 500 m depending on the patient's age, height, physical condition and co-morbidities.

Cardiovascular exercise testing is another valuable tool to assess exercise capacity as well as cardiac performance during exercise. Although cardiopulmonary exercise testing can be performed safely in almost all disease stages, the prognostic information is most valuable in patients with mild-to-moderate symptoms and 6-minute walk distances above 400 m, as cardiopulmonary exercise testing may identify those patients who seem to do well but still have severely impaired right ventricular function and therefore a dubious prognosis. Several parameters obtained during cardiopulmonary exercise testing are of prognostic importance; the most widely used being the peak oxygen uptake. It has been shown that a peak oxygen uptake of less than 10.4 mL/min kg^{-1} is associated with a poor prognosis (20). Patients in functional class II usually have a peak oxygen uptake of 15.0 mL/min kg^{-1}, or higher (21). Thus, one important treatment goal is to achieve a peak oxygen uptake of more than 15.0 mL/min kg^{-1}.

Biomarkers

Biomarkers may also provide valuable information. BNP and NT-proBNP are most widely used as they correlate with right ventricular function and provide prognostic information (22,23). Cut-off levels associated with either a good or a poor outcome have not yet been sufficiently validated; however, markedly elevated BNP/NT-proBNP values that further increase despite targeted therapy are an indicator of a poor prognosis whereas normal or near-normal BNP and NT-proBNP values are usually associated with a well preserved right ventricular function and a good outcome.

Other biomarkers might also be useful: troponin is an indicator of myocardial injury and PAH patients with elevated troponin levels have a high risk of death (24).

A low arterial pCO_2 is a marker of disease severity in PAH as these patients with PAH tend to hyperventilate, which means that their pCO_2 is often lower than normal. The extent of hyperventilation worsens as cardiac output deteriorates and pCO_2 values < 32 mmHg indicate a poor prognosis (25).

Plasma levels of growth differentiation factor-15 (GDF-15) have recently been proposed as a marker of tissue injury and tissue hypoxia. GDF-15 appears to be a powerful prognostic marker in PAH, both alone and in addition to NT-proBNP (26). GDF-15 essays, however, are not yet commercially available.

Right ventricular function and hemodynamics

Regular assessment of right ventricular function and hemodynamics is critical in the management of PAH patients. The most widely used tools are echocardiography and right heart catheterization.

Echocardiography is used not only as an integral part of the diagnostic work-up of patients with PAH but also as a follow-up tool. One of the main problems with echocardiography as a follow-up tool is the interpretation of the right ventricular systolic pressure during the course of the disease. Physicians tend to use changes in the right ventricular systolic pressure as indicators of worsening or improvements of the disease. This interpretation, however, is often fundamentally wrong. There is no, or only a weak, correlation between the right ventricular or pulmonary arterial pressure and the severity of the disease, or the prognosis, respectively. This seems to be illogical on the first glance but it becomes clearer when one keeps in mind that the magnitude of pulmonary artery pressure elevation reflects not only the extent of pulmonary vascular obstruction but also the performance of the right ventricle and both factors tend to change the pulmonary artery pressure in opposite directions. This is exemplified by patients with Eisenmenger's disease who often have a well-preserved right ventricular function and therefore very high pulmonary artery pressures, but nevertheless often a relatively good long-term prognosis (27,28). On the other hand, a fall in the pulmonary arterial pressure can be a result of effective therapy as well as declining right ventricular function. It is for these reasons that the pulmonary artery pressure is not a useful marker of disease severity.

Thus, other echocardiographic parameters are being used to assess right ventricular function during the follow-up of patients with PAH, most importantly the right atrial area, the TEI-index, tricuspid annular plane systolic excursion (TAPSE) and the presence or absence of a pericardial effusion (see Chapter 7 for more details) (29–32). TAPSE has become one of the most widely used echocardiography indicators of right ventricular function and a value > 2.0 cm has been suggested as a threshold indicating well-preserved function (32).

Right heart catheterization is an invasive procedure but often provides invaluable information. The main rule for interpreting right heart catheterization data during follow-up of PAH patients is the same as for echocardiography: the pulmonary artery pressure is a poor determinant of disease severity and prognosis (19,33). The most important reason to conduct invasive reassessments during the course of the disease is to make sure that the determinants of right ventricular function, i.e. right atrial pressure, cardiac output and mixed-venous oxygen saturation are in the normal range.

Cardiac magnetic resonance imaging provides important information on the right ventricular dimensions and function but presently, this tool is mainly used for scientific purposes and usually not in clinical routine (34).

Timing of follow-up evaluations

The typical follow-up interval for PAH patients is 3 months but this may vary substantially from a few days in unstable patients to 6–12 months in patients who have been stable for several years. Not all of the abovementioned examinations need to be performed at each single visit, and follow-up strategies vary substantially among specialized centers. However, assessment of the disease status should never be based on a single variable alone. At least one objective parameter of exercise capacity should be measured at every visit, if possible together with at least one biomarker and either echocardiography or right heart catheterization to determine right ventricular function.

There are no generally accepted rules when and how often right heart catheterization should be repeated in PAH patients. Individual decisions are probably the best approach outside scientific programs. Follow-up right heart catheterizations make only sense when changes in

the therapeutic strategy are to be expected. Some centers find it useful to perform a right heart catheter whenever they consider changing the PAH medication, especially prior to starting combination therapy. However, in many cases the decision to change or adapt therapy can be based on the clinical presentation together with the abovementioned non-invasive assessments. Thus, other centers are more conservative and perform follow-up catheters mostly when the clinical presentation and the non-invasive findings are not concordant or when major treatment decisions such as the introduction of intravenous prostacyclin therapy or listing for lung transplantations are at issue. There are no data to show that the outcome of patients treated in centers who perform right heart catheterizations on a regular basis is different from the outcome of patients treated in centers where right heart catheterizations are performed less frequently.

GOAL-ORIENTED THERAPY

One of the current problems of modern management of PAH is that combination therapy is widely used in the absence of robust data in terms of the optimal timing and the best choice of drugs. As long as these data are not available, most centers will continue using a goal-directed treatment strategy (14). As treatment goals have also not been prospectively and comparatively assessed, they vary from center to center and from patient to patient. Table 18.1 shows several risk determinants and threshold for which there are data in the medical literature that allow linking these values to either a good or a poor outcome. These parameters have been discussed in some detail in the previous section of this chapter.

According to the concept of goal-oriented therapy, all indicated parameters, or at least the majority of them, should be in the "green zone" (Table 18.1). As long as this is the case, it is reasonable to continue the current therapeutic strategy. If treatment goals are not met and if the comprehensive assessment shows that this is due to the severity of pulmonary hypertension and not due to other concomitant conditions, treatment is usually intensified, which in the vast majority of the cases, means that new treatments are added to the existing regimen. The order of drugs and the choices of combination partners are currently left up to the discretion of the physician and the preferences of the patient as there are no data comparing long-term safety and efficacy of various combination strategies. Further details on combination therapy for PAH can be found in Chapter 16.6.

THERAPEUTIC ALGORITHM

Therapeutic algorithms have been published by various scientific communities in the past few years, the most recent one in August 2009 jointly by the *European Society of Cardiology* and the *European Respiratory Society.* The recommendations in this section are based on this algorithm. Of note, these recommendations apply only to patients with PAH and not to those with other forms of pulmonary hypertension.

The initial management of patients with newly diagnosed PAH consists of general measures, which may include the use of oxygen and/or diuretics, as needed. Infections and arrhythmias should be treated aggressively, especially in patients presenting with symptoms or signs of right heart failure (35). Excessive physical exertion must be avoided whereas supervised rehabilitation seems to be both safe and useful, although the best time to start a rehabilitation program is probably once medical therapy has been optimized (36).

Anticoagulation, usually with warfarin, is recommended for the majority of patients with PAH. The data to support this approach are limited, but all therapeutic guidelines recommend anticoagulation of PAH patients, unless there are contraindications.

The importance of referring patients with PAH to expert centers prior to invasive diagnostic procedures or initiation of targeted therapy cannot be overemphasized. Right heart catheterization should be performed at centers with a broad experience in managing patients with PAH, not only for safety reasons (37), but also to ensure complete hemodynamic assessment including pulmonary vasoreactivity testing, and pulmonary angiography, if appropriate (see the related chapters in this book).

Acute pulmonary vasoreactivity testing is part of the hemodynamic assessment during the first diagnostic right heart catheterization in patients with PAH. As described in another chapter of this book, vasoreactivity testing should be performed in experienced centers with selective and

short-acting pulmonary vasodilators, such as inhaled nitric oxide, inhaled iloprost, or intravenous epoprostenol. The only reason to perform acute pulmonary vasoreactivity testing outside clinical trials is to identify patients who may respond to treatment with calcium channel blockers. A positive response is defined as a fall in the mean pulmonary arterial pressure by $> 10\,\mathrm{mmHg}$ from baseline to less than $40\,\mathrm{mmHg}$ in the presence of a normal cardiac output (38,39). Only patients who fulfill these responder criteria should be exposed to calcium channel blockers with careful evaluation during the initial phase of therapy. Those patients who show a substantial clinical and hemodynamic response, ideally being in functional class I or II with normal or near-normal hemodynamics at rest should receive long-term therapy with calcium channel blockers. All other patients should move forward to treatment with PAH-targeted therapies, i.e. endothelin receptor antagonists, PDE-5 inhibitors or prostanoids. Of note, the presence or absence of an acute vasodilatory response has no predictive value for the response to treatments other than calcium channel blockers.

As mentioned above and shown in Figure 18.1, patients presenting in functional class I or II should be treated with endothelin receptor antagonists and/or phosphodiesterase-5 inhibitors. Prostanoids are currently not recommended for these patients. The various treatment options for patients presenting in functional class III or IV have been outlined above and are also shown in the treatment algorithm (Figure 18.1). Patients in any functional class who are not responding sufficiently to monotherapy, i.e. who do not meet the treatment goals outlined above, should be considered for combination therapy. Combination therapy may be induced as early as in functional class II since some of these patients have mild symptoms despite

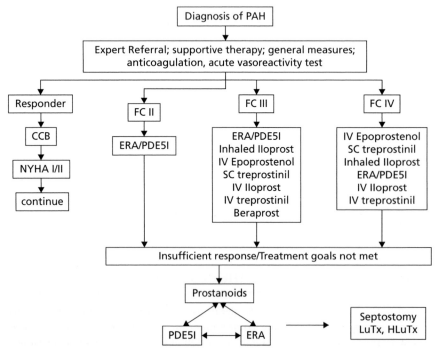

Figure 18.1 Algorithm for medical therapy of pulmonary arterial hypertension (PAH). CCB, calcium channel blockers; ERA, endothelin receptor antagonists; PDE5i, phosphodiesterase-5 inhibitors; IV, intravenous; SC, subcutaneous; LuTx, lung transplantation; HLuTx, heart and lung transplantation.

the presence of severe pulmonary hypertension. The rationale for using combination therapy in mildly symptomatic patients is not so much to improve exercise capacity but the hope that long-term prognosis is better when the disease is being treated aggressively early-on. For the present time, this approach is supported only by pathophysiological considerations as data from clinical trials addressing early combination therapy are not available.

PAH SUBPOPULATIONS

Most of the clinical trials that have been performed so far in the field of PAH have enrolled mainly patients with idiopathic disease and patients with systemic sclerosis. There are much less data on the other forms of PAH and there are some specific considerations for these subpopulations (the reader is also referred to the specific chapters dealing with these forms of PAH elsewhere in this book).

PAH associated with connective tissue disease (see also Chapter 15.3)

The vast majority of patients with PAH in association with connective tissue disease suffer from systemic sclerosis. As a general rule, these patients tend to respond less well to PAH-targeted therapy than patients with idiopathic PAH. The therapeutic principles, however, are similar and patients with systemic sclerosis and PAH usually do not respond to immunosuppressive therapy. The situation is different for patients with systemic lupus erythematosus who are also at increased risk of developing PAH, which, in contrast to PAH in the context of systemic sclerosis, may respond well to immunosuppressive therapy (40). In fact, milder forms of PAH in patients with lupus may initially be treated with immunosuppressants while PAH-targeted therapy is instituted only if PAH does not improve or resolve, respectively. If PAH is severe, the recommended approach is a combination of immunosuppressants and PAH-targeted therapy (with keeping in mind potentially dangerous drug–drug interactions, for example between endothelin receptor antagonists and calcineurin inhibitors). Patients with mixed connective tissue disease are somewhat in between patients with systemic sclerosis and patients with lupus erythematosus as PAH may also improve with immunosuppressive therapy but usually not as well as in patients with lupus, so that most of these patients require PAH-targeted medications (40).

PAH associated with congenital heart disease (see also Chapter 15.7)

The group *PAH associated with congenital heart disease* includes a broad and heterogeneous patient population

ranging from simple cardiac defects such as atrial and ventricular septal defects to complex abnormalities. Patients with simple or corrected defects often behave like patients with idiopathic PAH and are usually treated the same way and with similar treatment goals. Patients with complex abnormalities have not been included into clinical trials with PAH medications. The only exception was the BREATHE-5 study which assessed the safety and efficacy of the endothelin receptor antagonist bosentan in patients with Eisenmenger's syndrome (41). This study showed that bosentan is safe in this patient population and also demonstrated an improvement in exercise capacity with bosentan therapy. However, it is unknown if bosentan or any other PAH-targeted therapy does improve the long-term outcome of patients with Eisenmenger's disease or other complex cardiac abnormalities.

Patients with HIV infection (see also Chapter 15.6)

There are virtually no data from randomized controlled trials in patients with PAH and HIV infection. Open-label series, however, have suggested efficacy of PDE-5 inhibitors and endothelin receptor antagonists in this condition (42). Potential interactions of PAH drugs and antiretroviral therapy have to be kept in mind, especially between sildenafil and protease inhibitors. Other than that, treatment strategies and treatment goals are similar in patients with idiopathic PAH and HIV-associated PAH. It is still unclear if antiretroviral therapy has an effect on the course of PAH in these patients (43).

Portopulmonary hypertension (see also Chapter 15.5)

Treating patients with portopulmonary hypertension is often complex as both PAH as well as the underlying liver disease are life-threatening conditions (44). In general, patients with portopulmonary hypertension tend to respond well to PAH-targeted therapy (45,46). However, it has to be kept in mind that endothelin receptor antagonists are potentially hepatotoxic (47). Data from open-label series suggest that these drugs can be used safely in patients with mildly impaired liver function, i.e. with Child A disease. In fact, open-label case series have shown that patients with portopulmonary hypertension and Child A cirrhosis respond well to endothelin receptor antagonist therapy and one non-randomized study comparing bosentan and inhaled iloprost therapy in these patients suggested a survival benefit with bosentan (48). There are also a few case reports about the use of endothelin receptor antagonists in patients with more severe liver dysfunction, i.e. Child B or C disease. In the latter population, however, the pharmacokinetics of endothelin receptor antagonists are unknown and plasma concentrations of these compounds may be considerably higher in patients with liver dysfunction than in patients with normal liver function. The use of endothelin receptor antagonists in patients with Child B/C cirrhosis is not approved and must be discouraged until more data are available.

CONCLUSION

An integrated approach to PAH comprises optimized pharmacotherapy and non-pharmacological approaches such as rehabilitation programs. Pharmacotherapy follows an individual goal-oriented approach and combination of several PAH-targeted therapies is often required to achieve a satisfactory therapeutic result.

KEY POINTS

- Patients with PAH should receive disease-targeted therapy as early as possible in the course of their disease as early therapy can prevent clinical deterioration.
- Patients with PAH in functional class II are usually treated with endothelin receptor antagonists and/or PDE-5 inhibitors.
- For PAH patients presenting in functional class III and IV, a wide spectrum of drugs is now available. As none of these drugs cure the disease, combination therapy is widely used to achieve better long-term results.
- A goal-oriented strategy is widely used to guide treatment of PAH. Treatment is usually started as monotherapy and sequential combination therapy is used if pre-defined treatment goals are not met.
- The concept of goal-oriented therapy utilizes variables and thresholds of known prognostic importance, such as a achieving functional class II, a 6-minute walk test > 400–$500\,\mathrm{m}$ and a peak oxygen uptake $> 15.0\,\mathrm{mL/kg\,min^{-1}}$.
- Other parameters used to guide goal-oriented therapy are BNP/NT-pro BNP levels, echocardiographic determinants of right ventricular function such as the right atrial area, the TEI index and TAPSE, and hemodynamic parameters obtained during right heart catheterization.
- These parameters together are used for comprehensive prognostic evaluations which classify patients as *stable and satisfactory, stable but not satisfactory,* or *unstable and deteriorating.* The goal or therapy is to bring and keep patients in the first category.

REFERENCES

● = Key primary paper
◆ = Major review article

◆1. Rubin LJ. Primary pulmonary hypertension. N Engl J Med 1997;336(2):111–7.

●2. Barst RJ, Rubin LJ, Long WA, McGoon MD, Rich S, Badesch DB, Groves BM, Tapson VF, Bourge RC, Brundage BH et al. A comparison of continuous intravenous epoprostenol (prostacyclin) with conventional therapy for primary pulmonary hypertension. The Primary Pulmonary Hypertension Study Group. N Engl J Med 1996;334(5): 296–302.

◆3. Dupuis J, Hoeper MM. Endothelin receptor antagonists in pulmonary arterial hypertension. Eur Respir J 2008;31: 407–14.

◆4. Wilkins MR, Wharton J, Grimminger F, Ghofrani HA. Phosphodiesterase inhibitors for the treatment of pulmonary hypertension. Eur Respir J 2008;32(1):1 98–209.

◆5. Olschewski H, Gomberg-Maitland M. Prostacyclin therapies for the treatment of pulmonary arterial hypertension. Eur Respir J 2008;31:801–901.

●6. Rubin LJ, Badesch DB, Barst RJ, Galie N, Black CM, Keogh A, Pulido T, Frost A, Roux S, Leconte I, Landzberg M, Simonneau G. Bosentan therapy for pulmonary arterial hypertension. N Engl J Med 2002;346(12):896–903.

●7. Galie N, Olschewski H, Oudiz RJ et al. Ambrisentan for the treatment of pulmonary arterial hypertension: results of the ambrisentan in pulmonary arterial hypertension, randomized, double-blind, placebo–controlled, multicenter, efficacy (ARIES) study 1 and 2. Circulation 2008;117(23):3010–9.

●8. Galie N, Ghofrani HA, Torbicki A et al. Sildenafil Citrate therapy for pulmonary arterial hypertension. N Engl J Med 2005;353(20):2148–57.

●9. Galie N, Rubin L, Hoeper M, Jansa P, Al-Hiti H, Meyer G, Chiossi E, Kusic-Pajic A, Simonneau G. Treatment of patients with mildly symptomatic pulmonary arterial hypertension with bosentan (EARLY study): a double-blind, randomised controlled trial. Lancet 2008;371(9630): 2093–100.

10. Higenbottam T, Butt AY, McMahon A, Westerbeck R, Sharples L. Long-term intravenous prostaglandin (epoprostenol or iloprost) for treatment of severe pulmonary hypertension. Heart 1998;80(2):151–5.

11. Higenbottam TW, Butt AY, Dinh-Xaun AT, Takao M, Cremona G, Akamine S. Treatment of pulmonary hypertension with the continuous infusion of a prostacyclin analogue, iloprost. Heart 1998;79(2):175–9.

12. Provencher S, Sitbon O, Humbert M, Cabrol S, Jais X, Simonneau G. Long-term outcome with first-line bosentan therapy in idiopathic pulmonary arterial hypertension. Eur Heart J 2006;27(5):589–95.

13. Sandoval J, Gaspar J, Pulido T, Bautista E, Martinez-Guerra ML, Zeballos M, Palomar A, Gomez A. Graded balloon

dilation atrial septostomy in severe primary pulmonary hypertension. A therapeutic alternative for patients nonresponsive to vasodilator treatment. J Am Coll Cardiol 1998;32(2):297–304.

•14. Hoeper MM, Markevych I, Spiekerkoetter E, Welte T, Niedermeyer J. Goal-oriented treatment and combination therapy for pulmonary arterial hypertension. Eur Respir J 2005;26(5):858–63.

15. Ghofrani HA, Rose F, Schermuly RT et al. Oral sildenafil as long-term adjunct therapy to inhaled iloprost in severe pulmonary arterial hypertension. J Am Coll Cardiol 2003;42(1):158–64.

16. Mathai SC, Girgis RE, Fisher MR, Champion HC, Housten-Harris T, Zaiman A, Hassoun PM. Addition of sildenafil to bosentan monotherapy in pulmonary arterial hypertension. Eur Respir J 2007;29(3):469–75.

17. Hoeper MM, Faulenbach C, Golpon H, Winkler J, Welte T, Niedermeyer J. Combination therapy with bosentan and sildenafil in idiopathic pulmonary arterial hypertension. Eur Respir J 2004;24(6):1007–10.

18. Hoeper MM, Taha N, Bekjarova A, Gatzke R, Spiekerkoetter E. Bosentan treatment in patients with primary pulmonary hypertension receiving nonparenteral prostanoids. Eur Respir J 2003;22(2):330–4.

•19. Sitbon O, Humbert M, Nunes H, Parent F, Garcia G, Herve P, Rainisio M, Simonneau G. Long-term intravenous epoprostenol infusion in primary pulmonary hypertension: prognostic factors and survival. J Am Coll Cardiol 2002;40(4):780–8.

•20. Wensel R, Opitz CF, Anker SD et al. Assessment of survival in patients with primary pulmonary hypertension: importance of cardiopulmonary exercise testing. Circulation 2002;106(3):319–24.

21. Sun XG, Hansen JE, Oudiz RJ, Wasserman K. Exercise pathophysiology in patients with primary pulmonary hypertension. Circulation 2001;104(4):429–35.

22. Nagaya N, Nishikimi T, Uematsu M et al. Plasma brain natriuretic peptide as a prognostic indicator in patients with primary pulmonary hypertension. Circulation 2000;102(8):865–70.

23. Fijalkowska A, Kurzyna M, Torbicki A, Szewczyk G, Florczyk M, Pruszczyk P, Szturmowicz M. Serum N-terminal brain natriuretic peptide as a prognostic parameter in patients with pulmonary hypertension. Chest 2006;129(5): 1313–21.

24. Torbicki A, Kurzyna M, Kuca P et al. Detectable serum cardiac troponin T as a marker of poor prognosis among patients with chronic precapillary pulmonary hypertension. Circulation 2003;108(7):844–8.

25. Hoeper MM, Pletz MW, Golpon H, Welte T. Prognostic value of blood gas analyses in patients with idiopathic pulmonary arterial hypertension. Eur Respir J 2007;29(5): 944–50.

26. Nickel N, Kempf T, Tapken H et al. Growth differentiation factor-15 in idiopathic pulmonary arterial hypertension. Am J Respir Crit Care Med 2008;178(5):534–41.

27. Hopkins WE. The remarkable right ventricle of patients with Eisenmenger syndrome. Coron Artery Dis 2005;16(1): 19–25.

28. Hopkins WE, Ochoa LL, Richardson GW, Trulock EP. Comparison of the hemodynamics and survival of adults with severe primary pulmonary hypertension or Eisenmenger syndrome. J Heart Lung Transplant 1996; 15(1 Pt 1):100–105.

29. Hinderliter AL, Willis PWt, Long W et al. Frequency and prognostic significance of pericardial effusion in primary pulmonary hypertension. PPH Study Group. Primary pulmonary hypertension. Am J Cardiol 1999;84(4): 481–4, A410.

30. Raymond RJ, Hinderliter AL, Willis PW et al. Echocardiographic predictors of adverse outcomes in primary pulmonary hypertension. J Am Coll Cardiol 2002;39(7):1214–9.

31. Yeo TC, Dujardin KS, Tei C, Mahoney DW, McGoon MD, Seward JB. Value of a Doppler-derived index combining systolic and diastolic time intervals in predicting outcome in primary pulmonary hypertension. Am J Cardiol 1998;81(9):1157–61.

•32. Forfia PR, Fisher MR, Mathai SC et al. Tricuspid annular displacement predicts survival in pulmonary hypertension. Am J Respir Crit Care Med 2006;174(9):1034–41.

33. McLaughlin VV, Sitbon O, Badesch DB, Barst RJ, Black C, Galie N, Rainisio M, Simonneau G, Rubin LJ. Survival with first-line bosentan in patients with primary pulmonary hypertension. Eur Respir J 2005;25(2):244–9.

34. Hoeper MM, Tongers J, Leppert A, Baus S, Maier R, Lotz J. Evaluation of right ventricular performance with a right ventricular ejection fraction thermodilution catheter and MRI in patients with pulmonary hypertension. Chest 2001;120(2):502–7.

35. Tongers J, Schwerdtfeger B, Klein G, Kempf T, Schaefer A, Knapp JM, Niehaus M, Korte T, Hoeper MM. Incidence and clinical relevance of supraventricular tachyarrhythmias in pulmonary hypertension. Am Heart J 2007;153(1):127–32.

36. Mereles D, Ehlken N, Kreuscher S et al. Exercise and respiratory training improve exercise capacity and quality of life in patients with severe chronic pulmonary hypertension. Circulation 2006;114:1482–9.

37. Hoeper MM, Lee SH, Voswinckel R et al. Complications of right heart catheterization procedures in patients with pulmonary hypertension in experienced centers. J Am Coll Cardiol 2006;48(12):2546–52.

38. Sitbon O, Humbert M, Jais X et al. Long-term response to calcium channel blockers in idiopathic pulmonary arterial hypertension. Circulation 2005;111(23):3105–11.

◆39. Galie N, Torbicki A, Barst R et al. Guidelines on diagnosis and treatment of pulmonary arterial hypertension. The Task Force on Diagnosis and Treatment of Pulmonary Arterial Hypertension of the European Society of Cardiology. Eur Heart J 2004;25(24):2243–78.

40. Jais X, Launay D, Yaici A, Le Pavec J, Tcherakian C, Sitbon O, Simonneau G, Humbert M. Immunosuppressive therapy in

lupus- and mixed connective tissue disease-associated pulmonary arterial hypertension: a retrospective analysis of twenty-three cases. Arthritis Rheum 2008;58(2): 521–31.

•41. Galie N, Beghetti M, Gatzoulis MA, Granton J, Berger RM, Lauer A, Chiossi E, Landzberg M. Bosentan therapy in patients with Eisenmenger syndrome: a multicenter, double-blind, randomized, placebo-controlled study. Circulation 2006;114(1):48–54.

42. Sitbon O, Gressin V, Speich R et al. Bosentan for the treatment of human immunodeficiency virus-associated pulmonary arterial hypertension. Am J Respir Crit Care Med 2004;170(11):1212–7.

43. Sitbon O, Lascoux-Combe C, Delfraissy JF et al. Prevalence of HIV-related pulmonary arterial hypertension in the current antiretroviral therapy era. Am J Respir Crit Care Med 2008;177(1):108–13.

44. Hoeper MM, Krowka MJ, Strassburg CP. Portopulmonary hypertension and hepatopulmonary syndrome. Lancet 2004;363(9419):1461–8.

45. Reichenberger F, Voswinckel R, Steveling E et al. Sildenafil treatment for portopulmonary hypertension. Eur Respir J 2006;28(3):563–7.

46. Hoeper MM, Halank M, Marx C, Hoeffken G, Seyfarth HJ, Schauer J, Niedermeyer J, Winkler J. Bosentan therapy for portopulmonary hypertension. Eur Respir J 2005;25(3):502–8.

47. Humbert M, Segal ES, Kiely DG, Carlsen J, Schwierin B, Hoeper MM. Results of European post-marketing surveillance of bosentan in pulmonary hypertension. Eur Respir J 2007;30(2):338–44.

48. Hoeper MM, Seyfarth HJ, Hoeffken G, Wirtz H, Spiekerkoetter E, Pletz MW, Welte T, Halank M. Experience with inhaled iloprost and bosentan in portopulmonary hypertension. Eur Respir J 2007;30(6):1096–102.

PULMONARY HYPERTENSION DUE TO CAPILLARY OR POST CAPILLARY DISEASE

Pulmonary hypertension secondary to left heart failure

MARCO GUAZZI

INTRODUCTION

Pulmonary hypertension (PH) due to left-sided heart failure (HF) is perhaps the most common form of PH and its clinical manifestations are a continuous challenge for the bedside clinicians (1). According to the Dana Point (2008) PH nomenclature (2), left-sided PH is classified as a non-PH form due to diastolic or systolic dysfunction of the left ventricle or left-sided valvular disease. Definition and degree of severity of non-PH is the same as for other PH. With the exception of some valvular diseases, such as mitral valve stenosis, PH occurs in any setting where left ventricular filling pressure is elevated, with the degree of elevation usually proportional to the pulmonary wedge pressure (PCWP).

Although mitral stenosis was the most common cause of this entity decades ago, actual common cardiac causes of increased left ventricular filling pressures in referral practice are systemic hypertension and ischemic heart disease, conditions in which PH develops as the direct consequence of impaired LV diastolic relaxation and distensibility properties resulting in increase in LV diastolic, left atrial and pulmonary venous pressures. Pulmonary venous congestion is frequently associated with a reactive increase in pulmonary vascular resistance (PVR), that generates a higher transpulmonary pressure gradient superimposed on the pulmonary venous pressure. Cardiogenic pressure injury on the pulmonary capillary bed may develop as a consequence of acute, chronic or acute on chronic elevations of PH. In this continuum a wide spectrum of pathophysiological insights and clinical manifestations may well

be characterized. Notably, pathogenetic mechanisms that lead to anatomical and functional microvascular pulmonary abnormalities progressively develop in the time before the patient becomes symptomatic.

This chapter focuses on the pathogenetic mechanisms responsible for the development of acute left-sided PH and for its transition to chronic PH. The diagnosis, clinical assessment and treatment of this frequent disabling clinical disorder are also discussed.

PATHOGENETIC MECHANISMS INVOLVED IN ACUTE PH

Pressure-induced trauma and stress failure of alveolar capillaries

Any abnormal pressure elevation in the pulmonary capillary bed challenges the anatomical integrity and functional properties of lung capillaries and alveolar spaces (i.e. the blood–gas barrier). In the progressive modifications that the lung vasculature generates in response to hypertension, structural and functional abnormalities in lung capillaries may well anticipate those occurring at arteriolar and pulmonary artery level. However, PH development and its injury to the alveolar–capillary barrier have been classically regarded of pathophysiological importance merely for the acute clinical consequences (i.e. alveolar edema), mostly overlooking that a multistep "adaptive" process involves the microcirculation and the alveolar spaces carrying important clinical correlates of tissue organ damage (3).

From a physiological standpoint, the resistance opposed by lung capillaries to increased hydrostatic pressure has to deal with the thinness of the alveolar–capillary unit, a basic requirement for gas diffusion process. The anatomical configuration of the membrane is a three-layer structure with an epithelial layer with two differentiated types of cells (type I or epithelial cells, which provide mechanical support, and type II cells, which provide metabolic support), the interstitial space and the capillary endothelium. The pulmonary capillary endothelium is permeable to solutes, such as small molecules and ions, but has a low permeability to proteins (4), whereas the epithelium is quite resistant to the passive diffusion of small ions and solutes, and passively pumps water and solutes from the alveolar space to the interstitium (5). The ultrastructural appearance of the blood–gas barrier clearly shows one side of the membrane to be thinner than the other, and this difference is mainly related to the interstitial composition. On the thinner side, the interstitium is limited to the two fused basement membranes of the alveolar epithelium and the vascular endothelium; the thicker portion has a wider interstitial space with an increased concentration of fibroblasts and collagen. This double configuration allows the alveolar–capillary unit not only to promote gas diffusion, through the thinner portion, but also to protect the interstitium from fluid flux and electrolyte transition.

In a set of important experimental studies, West and coworkers (6) have described the anatomical consequences of abrupt increases of capillary pressure and have coined the term *stress failure* to refer to rupture of the alveolar capillary membrane components.

Specifically, in a rabbit model preparation, Tsukimoto *et al.* (7) reported the sequential morphological disruption of both the capillary endothelial and alveolar epithelial layers, during a stepwise increase in hydrostatic capillary pressure leading to a transition from a low-permeability form (leakage of protein into the interstitium) to a high-permeability form (leakage of proteins and red blood cells into the alveolar lumen) of pulmonary edema. After this evidence, a broad series of studies investigating the biology of alveolar stress failure have brought new insights into the cellular factors involved in the response to mechanical stress, suggesting that mechanisms additional to membrane thickness may determine the capillary stress. In a model of hydraulic overload, such as during controlled saline infusion to the capillary pulmonary circulation (180 min of saline infusion at 0.5 mL/min/kg in the rabbit lung), the morphometric analysis obtained in the very early postinfusion phase shows that 44 percent of the fluid leaks into the extravascular interstitial space; a process accompanied by significant ultrastructural changes and impairment in gas conductance (8). Changes occurring during hydraulic edema induce matrix proteoglycan fragmentation secondary to metalloproteases activation (9), as well as a marked change in plasma membrane composition with increase in endothelial membrane fluidity; a feature that may decrease the tensile strength in the membrane, contributing to endothelial stress failure (10).

Overall, these findings may well apply to the clinical condition of acute rise in PCWP and pulmonary edema, but human reports investigating the pathophysiological correlates of alveolar–capillary stress failure in cardiac patients are limited. In a study performed in patients with acute cardiogenic pulmonary edema, injury to the alveolar–capillary barrier was paralleled by increased levels in plasma surfactant protein A and B and tumor necrosis factor (TNF)-α (11). Persistence of elevated TNF-α levels until three days after edema resolution is suggestive of pulmonary parenchymal inflammation and may explain the potential recurrence of fluid accumulation despite hydrostatic stress failure resolution.

Molecular abnormalities in alveolar fluid clearance

Mechanical injury critically challenges alveolar fluid clearance, a process dependent on a series of complex cellular mechanisms. Primarily, Na^+ enters the apical membrane configuration of alveolar type II cells through the amiloride-sensitive epithelial Na^+ channels. Na^+ is then transported across the basolateral membrane into the interstitium through the ouabain-inhibitable Na^+/K^+ ATPase pump. This Na^+ transport generates an osmotic gradient that promotes removal of excessive intra-alveolar fluid. In several clinical conditions, such as heart failure (HF) an impairment in these mechanisms predisposes patients to pulmonary edema regardless of hydrostatic and oncotic pressures (Starling forces) and compensatory lymphatic drainage (12). In experimental preparations, with a progressive increase of left atrial pressure (LAP), a transient alveolar fluid reabsorption decrease by 50 percent was observed in lungs in which LAP was raised to 15 cm H_2O or further (13).

Interestingly, in rats overexpressing by adenovirus gene transfer the Na^+-K^+ ATPase β_1-subunit promotes an increase in fluid clearance (14). In the same model, Na^+ transport and alveolar fluid clearance during LAP elevation were comparable to those rats studied at normal LAP (15). Cellular growth factors and proinflammatory cytokines, particularly tumor necrosis factor α, also have been reported to alter the membrane permeability and to impair Na^+ and water transport (16,17). Hypoxia, another common association with chronic HF, is also capable to inhibit the alveolar Na^+-K^+ ATPase function and transalveolar fluid transport (18).

These findings support the intriguing hypothesis that an impaired Na^+ handling and a pathological Na^+-K^+ ATPase gene expression may occur during acute lung injury, and provide evidence that the result of a pressure overload on the lung microcirculation is an increase in capillary permeability to water and ions and disruption of local regulatory mechanisms for gas exchange.

PATHOGENETIC MECHANISMS INVOLVED IN CHRONIC PH

Alveolar–capillary remodeling

While there is evidence enough that stress failure is a reversible process (19), in the long term alveolar–capillary membrane becomes the target of a remodeling process and definitive evidence of reversibility is lacking. Studies performed in animals with pace-induced chronic HF, showed that alveolar–capillary membrane thickness was significantly increased compared to controls. This thickening process was mainly due to excessive deposition of collagen type IV (the major component of the alveolar–capillary membrane lamina densa) (20) and is similar to findings reported in patients with mitral stenosis and pulmonary venous hypertension (21), in whom the increased extracellular matrix thickness accounts for the more relevant structural changes.

An increased collagen content may be very likely triggered by local growth stimuli as angiotensin II, and has been interpreted to be protective against the increased amount of fluid leaking across the alveolar–capillary membrane (22). In this regard, an attractive hypothesis which is, however, based on isolated experimental evidence, suggests that during chronic capillary hydrostatic load, an increase in lung interstitial connective tissue would yield to an increase in extravascular fluid accumulation, given the high capability of the extracellular matrix components (mainly glycosaminoglycans) to absorb and hold fluid in the interstitial space. At least in conditions of subcritical, chronic LAP elevation, this mechanism could be protective in restraining the fluid in the extravascular interstitial spaces with no or little interference with gas diffusion between capillary blood and alveolar gas (23).

An additional factor that has been shown to specifically affect the extracellular matrix composition is the alveolar hypoxic stimulus that promotes alveolar–vascular remodeling by increasing the gene expression of extracellular matrix proteins (24). Overall, the anatomic changes that occur in the alveolar–capillary unit lead to an increased resistance across the membrane and impair gas transfer (3). On a clinical basis, the measure of lung gas diffusion may provide a correlate of the anatomic integrity and physiological properties of the alveolar–capillary membrane unit, and abnormalities in alveolar membrane conductance are of clinical and prognostic importance in patients with HF and left-sided PH (25). The continuum of the pathophysiological sequelae that lead to alveolar stress failure, capillary remodeling and prolonged path for gas diffusion is only partially known. A proposed sequence of events is reported in Figure 19.1.1 (26).

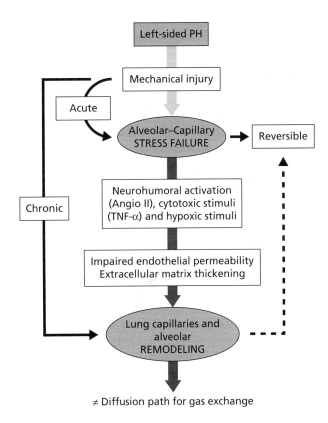

Figure 19.1.1 Elevation in pulmonary capillary pressure and proposed sequence of events that mediate capillary injury and alveolar membrane remodeling. Development of acute PH leads to alveolar stress failure, a process that has been shown to be reversible. In chronic PH a superimposition of additional factors other than mechanical, such as neurohumoral, citotoxic, hypoxic and genetic factors further injure lung capillaries and alveolar spaces leading to a remodeling alveolar process. (Adapted from ref 26.)

Structural vessel changes and histopathology of chronic pulmonary venous hypertension

Increase in venous pulmonary pressure promotes histological and functional changes of veins and arteries. Both intima and media of arterial vessels are affected. Media changes consist of hypertrophy and peripheral migration of smooth muscle into intra-acinar arterioles causing "muscolarization" of arterioles. A key step in the hypertrophic process is the induction of an endogenous vascular serine elastase (27) which releases growth factors and glycoproteins (tenascin-C and fibronectin). Pressure-induced endothelia disruption allows serum proteins into the vessel wall to activate endogenous vascular serine elastase and matrix metalloproteinases, which break up the elastic lamina in the wall and stimulate smooth muscle growth and collagen and elastin synthesis. Intima fibroproliferative changes derive from growth of smooth muscle cells and myofibroblast derived from the media. Pulmonary veins become dilated and develop medial hypertrophy as well. As medial hypertrophy becomes prominent, a process of vein "arterialization" takes place. Bronchial veins also become congested and dilated, because of increased flow through bronchopulmonary anastomoses. Plexiform lesions, which are complex, irreversible combined intimal and medial lesions located at the origin of small muscular pulmonary arteries, are generally not observed in patients with left-sided PH. There is a wide variability in the response of the pulmonary vascular structural changes to the elevated venous pressure, suggesting an important role of genetic factors. Clinically, regression of pulmonary vessels structural remodeling after normalization of pulmonary venous pressure by cardiac transplantation or mitral valve surgery are substantial, but usually not complete, and in patients evaluated for cardiac transplantation reversible hemodynamics following provocative vasodilator therapy carry a better prognosis (28).

Impaired vascular reactivity and endothelial dysfunction

PVR is elevated in left-sided PH as a result of abnormalities in smooth muscle tone and structural remodeling. The impairment in arterial smooth muscle tone relaxation is predominantly due to pulmonary vascular endothelial dysfunction and, as for other forms of PH, endothelial dysfunction seems to play an integral role in mediating the functional changes in the pulmonary vasculature. In the pulmonary circulation the central endothelium role in the local control of vessel tone is primarily based on the regulated release of nitric oxide (NO) and endothelin-1 (ET1). There is broad evidence that left-sided PH is critically influenced by an altered balance between these two opposing systems (29,30).

NO-DEPENDENT VASCULAR PULMONARY REGULATION

A series of studies investigating the effects of NO-blockade on pulmonary circulation have suggested that endothelium-derived NO is basically involved in determining both basal pulmonary vascular tone and dilation to endothelium-dependent stimuli.

In healthy humans, systemic infusion of NG-monomethil-L-arginine (L-NMMA), an analog of L-arginine with inhibitory activity on NO synthase, causes PH (31), aggravates hypoxia-induced pulmonary vasoconstriction (32) and impairs gas diffusion by inhibiting the alveolar-membrane gas conductance properties (33). In HF patients, direct L-NMMA infusion in the pulmonary artery causes a dose-dependent vasoconstriction which is partially attenuated by acetylcholine (34). Furthermore, experimental and human studies suggest that NO-dependent pulmonary vasodilation is impaired in left-sided PH. In humans, Porter et al. (35), by using intravascular ultrasounds to assess pulmonary artery diameter, found that intrapulmonary infusion of acetylcholine caused vasodilation in patients with HF and normal pulmonary artery pressure, but failed to cause dilation in those with PH.

Further observations in favor of a loss of a primary contribution of NO-dependent vasodilation to the development of PH were reported by measuring pulmonary blood flow velocity during intrapulmonary infusion of L-NMMA (36). In normal control subjects or patients with HF and a normal PVR, L-NMMA caused vasoconstriction, whereas in HF patients and PH, the vasoconstrictor response to L-NMMA was attenuated. The vasoconstrictor responses to phenylephrine were similar in the three groups.

ROLE OF ET1 IN THE REGULATION OF PULMONARY VASCULAR TONE

ET1, a 21-amino-acid vasoactive peptide with potent vasoconstrictor and platelet-aggregating properties, is widely distributed in the pulmonary endothelium. In mammals, two ET receptors have been described: ET_A, through which vasoconstriction and cellular growth is elicited, and ET_B, which can mediate either vasoconstriction by its effects on smooth muscle, or vasodilatation through action on endothelial cells (37). ET_B receptors also play an important role in ET-1 clearance (38). The ratio of ET_A to ET_B receptors on human resistance and conduit pulmonary arteries is approximately 9:1. The net effect of ET-1 in pulmonary arteries is constriction (39). ET1 may also contribute to pathological pulmonary vascular remodeling by causing proliferation and hypertrophy of vascular smooth muscle cells and increased collagen synthesis. ET1 immunoreactivity is abundant in pulmonary vascular endothelial cells from patients with left-sided PH (40) and increased plasma ET1 levels have been repeatedly reported in both experimental (41) and clinical HF (42). Interestingly, the extent of ET1 increase predicts mortality in chronic HF (43).

DIAGNOSIS AND ASSESSMENT OF LEFT-SIDED PH

Distinctive clinical signs and symptoms of left-sided PH are orthopnea and paroxysmal nocturnal dyspnea, which are not features of other forms of PH. Clinical tests often reveal findings suggestive of left-sided PH. The chest x-ray will often show pulmonary vascular congestion, pleural effusion and eventually pulmonary edema. The ECG may show LV hypertrophy rather than right ventricular (RV) hypertrophy. High resolution chest computed tomography can be helpful because it will often reveal a mosaic perfusion pattern and ground-glass opacities consistent with chronic pulmonary edema. Invasive measures of left ventricular end-diastolic, atrial and wedge pressures are required to definitively secure the diagnosis of elevated LV filling pressure and pulmonary venous hypertension.

In chronic conditions, when PH develops slowly, the RV can generate elevated peak systolic pressure due to an adaptive hypertrophy. Conversely, when RV failure develops, the pulmonary artery pressure may be relatively low despite marked elevation of the PVR. Recent years have brought increasing appreciation of the burden of diastolic heart failure (DHF) as a predominant cause of both acute (44) and chronic left-sided PH (45). However, the natural history and clinical follow-up of DHF patients with increased PH have not been systematically investigated in randomized clinical trials. DHF populations include predominantly elderly patients with systemic hypertension and left ventricular hypertrophy, coronary artery disease, diabetes mellitus and obesity.

Given the epidemic increase of this population, easily available non-invasive variables suggestive of increased LV filling pressure, abnormal LV relaxation and DHF have become of extreme importance, mainly in the presence of clinical suspicion of PH of cardiac origin (46,47). Essential in the evaluation of these patients is an echocardiogram, assumed that history, physical examination or chest x-ray are not sensitive for the differentiation between systolic and diastolic HF (48).

Several ultrasound findings may be suggestive of DHF such as the presence of a dilated left atrium, abnormal Doppler estimates of mitral and pulmonary venous velocity flows and mitral Tissue Doppler (TD) velocities. Standard Doppler flow indexes are equally determined by LA pressure and LV relaxation and may overestimate LV filling pressure since they cannot separate the effects of LV relaxation from preload as confounding variable. TD velocities are substantially related to LV relaxation and may be combined with standard Doppler flow indexes in order to separate the confounding factors. Accordingly, the most reliable correlate of LVEP and LAP has been found to be the combination of early mitral flow velocity (E) with early mitral TD velocity (E1) (48). The concept to use E/E1 ratio as a reliable estimate of LAP has been validated in heterogeneous groups of cardiac patients undergoing right heart catheterization (49). In patients with impaired relaxation and elevated LAP, E is elevated but E1 is reduced and an E/E1 ratio greater than 15 is almost invariably associated with a mean LA pressure greater than 15 mmHg (49).

Although echocardiography provides important and quite often definitive information to ascertain DHF diagnosis, invasive hemodynamics may still be required.

There is interesting evidence that along with diastolic impairment, an important determinant of PH in patients with LV dysfunction is the extent of functional mitral regurgitation, namely the mitral valve regurgitant orifice (46). The effective regurgitant mitral area is also a strong predictor of increased pulmonary pressure and acute pulmonary edema development in patients with functional mitral regurgitation due to ischemic heart disease (50).

Volume or exercise challenges can be used to unmask cases of left-sided PHs that may not be detectable at rest (i.e. normal LVEDP) due to unloading and diuretic therapies. Using a vasodilator challenge (51) or an inotropic challenge (52) during diagnostic cardiac catheterization is useful for evaluating changes in PCWP during cardiac output increase. A clinical example of exercise-induced increase in PCWP in patients with diastolic HF was reported by Kitzman *et al.* (53) in a group of selected patients with severe clinical HF, but with normal systolic function (LV preserved ejection fraction) and left ventricular concentric hypertrophy. These patients were compared to age- and gender-matched controls during symptom-limited upright

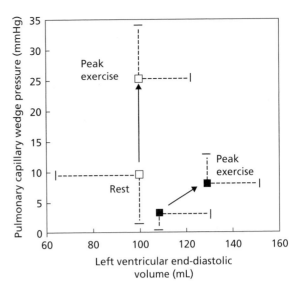

Figure 19.1.2   Changes in PCWP vs. LV end-diastolic volume from rest to peak exercise (arrows) in patients with diastolic HF (open squares) and controls (full squares). Patients had symptomatic HF but normal LV systolic function in the setting of hypertensive left ventricular hypertrophy. (Adapted from ref 53.)

bicycle exercise. Figure 19.1.2 shows that controls had more distensible left ventricles at rest as evidenced by a lower PCWP at larger LV end-diastolic volumes. During exercise, diastolic HF patients did not increase their LV end-diastolic volumes and the PCWP increased markedly to pulmonary edema levels. In a recent report, 406 unselected consecutive patients referred for unexplained dyspnea due to different causes of PH underwent invasive hemodynamic assessment. Interestingly, 48 percent of patients developed exercise PH due to left ventricular failure, and LV diastolic dysfunction represented one of the largest categories of unexplained exertional dyspnea (54). Assessment of functional mitral regurgitation may be very appropriate during effort also, given the very likely possibility that patients with no or minimal mitral regurgitation at rest develop severe insufficiency during exercise, which is another important clinical determinant of left-sided PH (55).

Clinical correlates of left-sided PH

Exertional dyspnea is the most frequent presenting symptom of left-sided PH that results from several pathophysiological impairments that may be unlocked by cardiopulmonary exercise testing (56,57). In HF patients with secondary PH, the pulmonary vasculature may importantly influence the exercise capacity. PVR may remain elevated throughout maximal exercise imposing an increased load to the RV and there is a positive correlation between right ventricular ejection fraction (RVEF) and peak VO$_2$ in patients referred for cardiac transplantation (58). Of note, patients with HF display a number of ventilatory abnormalities that are at least in part related to the development of left-sided PH. In stable HF patients an impaired exercise ventilation efficiency as assessed by the steepness of the relation between ventilation to CO_2 production rate (VE/VCO_2 slope) has been found to be related to pulmonary vasoconstriction, elevated pulmonary arterial pressure (PAP) (59) and right ventricular function (60). This has important implications considering the established strong predictivity of VE/VCO_2 slope for adverse clinical events in both systolic and diastolic HF (61,62). Moreover, a cyclic breathing pattern both at rest and during exercise correlates with PCWP and may disappear after correction of pulmonary vasoconstriction with nitroprusside infusion (63).

There is also an increasing recognized relationship between sleep disordered breathing and HF. In HF patients with elevated PCWP, incidence of central sleep apnea is more frequent and a highly significant relationship exists between PCWP, hypocapnia and central apnea severity (64).

Morbidity and mortality

The extent of left-sided PH is an important determinant of morbidity and mortality in patients with HF. An increased mortality and hospitalization rate is reported in HF patients with ecocardiographically determined PH (65) and PAP is an independent predictor of the need for cardiac transplant (66). At least two-thirds of patients with severe systolic LV dysfunction have PH with associated RV failure, and mortality associated with biventricular failure is twofold higher compared to isolated left ventricular failure (67) (Figure 19.1.3). Development of RV failure may also be an important concern for post-cardiac transplant patients, and data from the International Society of Heart Transplantation registry suggest that RV dysfunction accounts for 50 percent of all cardiac complications and 19 percent of early deaths (68).

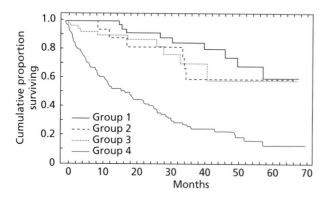

Figure 19.1.3 Survival rate among patients with chronic HF and different degrees of systolic dysfunction, PH and RVEF. Group 1: normal PAP and preserved RVEF (n = 73); Group 2: normal PAP and low RVEF (n = 68); Group 3: elevated PAP and preserved RVEF (n = 21); Group 4: high PAP/low RVEF (n = 215). (Adapted from ref. 67.)

TREATMENT OF LEFT-SIDED PH

Standard therapies for HF, including diuretics, RAS system inhibitors and nitrates may have a favorable effect on PVR. Only recently, however, the pulmonary circulation has been considered a therapeutic target in HF clinical evolution.

Recently, a number of so-called PH specific therapies have demonstrated clinical efficacy in randomized trials of idiopathic or other forms of PH. However, their role in the management of left-sided PH remains controversial and early experience evaluating specific treatments in the setting of left-sided PH was disappointing. The use of selective pulmonary vasodilators in patients with elevated PCWP was shown to confer a high risk of developing pulmonary edema and rapid clinical deterioration because of the important rise in cardiac output against a reduced PCWP and pulmonary venous pressure.

In the Floan International Randomized Survival Trial (FIRST), intravenous epoprostenol to treat advanced HF demonstrated a trend toward worse outcome and was terminated early for excess mortality (69). In a small study evaluating inhaled prostacyclin analog iloprost in patients undergoing assessment for cardiac transplantation, some improvement was observed in mPAP, PVR and PCWP during vasoreactivity testing with a positive effect on cardiac index and stroke volume (70).

ET1 receptor antagonists

Although the development of ET1 receptor antagonists has been viewed as an important means to define the pathogenetic role of ET1 antagonists in HF, positive results seem to be confined to experimental models. Both non-selective antagonists and ET1 selective antagonists have been shown to improve LV remodeling and survival in animal models of HF (71). In a pace-induced HF model with left-sided PH, PVR decreased after ET_A blockade, whereas an ET_B antagonist produced opposite effects (72). Despite initial promising results on pulmonary hemodynamics obtained in small studies of chronic HF patients with an acute administration of sitaxentan a selective ET_A antagonist (73), bosentan, a ET_A/ET_B antagonist, has been demonstrated to be ineffective in patients with systolic HF (74). No indication actually exists for use of both non-selective and selective ET1 antagonists in left-sided PH.

NO overexpression strategies

Based on the primary role of NO in the pathophysiology of pulmonary vascular function, strategies to increase NO availability in the lung have been developed. Use of inhaled NO has provided negative results. *NO inhalation has proven to be effective in reducing PVR, without changes in PAP and with some increase in PCWP due to the drop in transpulmonary gradient and to an increased preload of a poorly compliant LV (75,76). This untoward hemodynamic* effect has been shown to be associated with cases of acute pulmonary edema (77).

PHOSPHODIESTERASE 5 (PDE5)-INHIBITORS

PDE5-inhibition has recently been viewed and tested as an attractive therapeutic strategy to enhance the NO pathway pursued via cyclic 3′-5′-guanosine monophosphate (cGMP) signaling. PDE5 is the predominant isoenzyme that metabolizes cGMP, the second messenger of NO which is highly expressed in the smooth muscle cells in the medial layer of pulmonary arteries and veins of the normal lung. PDE5 activity has been shown to be increased in various experimental models of PH (78). Its inhibition by sildenafil has demonstrated efficacy in patients with various forms of PAH (idiopathic, repaired congenital systemic-to-pulmonary shunts and secondary to connective tissue disease). Sildenafil is an approved treatment for idiopathic PAH (79). At variance with other pulmonary selective vasodilators, there is increasing evidence that it may have a therapeutic key role in left-sided PH (80).

Studies performed by Guazzi et al. (81) and Lewis et al. (82) in patients with left-sided PH of different severity have provided evidence that acute oral sildenafil administration (50 mg) is well tolerated and rapidly lowers PAP and PVR, without significant effects on PCWP and systemic arterial pressure. The response of cardiac output is variable but the high pulmonary vascular resistances may prevent abrupt changes in PCWP. Of note, in addition to the acute pulmonary hemodynamic changes, an increase in capillary vascular bed NO concentration seems a basic mechanism for enhancing gas diffusion for carbon monoxide and alveolar–gas exchange conductance properties (81).

The same authors reported that favorable pulmonary hemodynamic effects observed after acute sildenafil administration are sustained over time in patients already receiving an optimal medical therapeutic regimen (83,84). Significant correlates of hemodynamic improvement were a higher peak VO$_2$ and a downward shift in the VE/VCO$_2$ slope. There is isolated evidence that the sildenafil and nitrate combination exerts a synergistic pulmonary vasodilatating activity without adverse systemic hemodynamic effects in advanced HF patients presenting with PH and systemic hypotension (85).

The clinical use of chronic sildenafil in left-sided PH has also been investigated in patients with severe HF who persistently exhibit PH despite LV unloading with left ventricular assist device (LVAD) implantation. Telford et al. recently demonstrated that after 2 to 4 weeks of oral PDE5 inhibitor therapy with sildenafil, mean PAP decreased by approximately one third, with an increase in cardiac output contributing to a decrease of PVR by approximately one half (86).

To date, there are no randomized clinical trials of pulmonary vasodilator therapy for patients with left-sided PH associated with normal systolic function, and no such treatment has yet been shown to favorably affect diastolic

HF patients with PH. There is an ongoing NIH sponsored large-scale trial examining the efficacy of long-term treatment with sildenafil in patients without LV dilatation and preserved systolic function, whose primary endpoints are gas exchange measured physical performance and LV remodeling and function. This trial will also provide robust information on the safety and tolerability of PDE5-inhibition in left-sided PH.

KEY POINTS

- Left-sided PH is classified as a non-PH form and includes left-sided ventricular or atrial disease and left-sided valvular disease, conditions associated with increased left ventricular filling pressure and/or pulmonary venous hypertension.
- Mitral stenosis was the most common cause of this entity decades ago; actual common cardiac causes of left-sided PH in referral practice are systemic hypertension and ischemic heart disease, conditions in which PH develops as consequence of impaired LV diastolic relaxation and distensibility properties yielding to increased LV diastolic, left atrial and pulmonary venous pressures.
- Diastolic HF is now regarded as the major cause of left-sided PH development.
- Cardiogenic pressure elevation leads to alveolar–capillary "stress failure" which consists of disruption of the alveolar anatomical configuration and impairment of cellular pathways involved in the fluid-flux regulation and gas exchange efficiency. These changes are reversible and may well anticipate a true remodeling process involving both the microcirculation and major pulmonary arterial vessels.
- In chronic left-sided PH, increase in pulmonary vascular resistance and pulmonary pressure occurs as a result of arterial abnormalities in smooth muscle tone and structural remodeling. The impairment in arterial smooth muscle tone relaxation is predominantly due to endothelial dysfunction and an imbalance between nitric oxide and endothelin-1 pathways endothelial control has been shown to play a key pathogenetic role.
- Distinctive clinical signs and symptoms of left-sided PH are orthopnea and paroxysmal nocturnal dyspnea. Echocardiography is essential in the evaluation of these patients, especially when assessing diastolic HF patients, assuming that history, physical examination and chest x-ray are non-sensitive for differentiating systolic from diastolic HF. Despite echocardiography providing important and quite often definitive information to ascertain left-sided PH, invasive measures of

432 Pulmonary hypertension secondary to left heart failure

LV end-diastolic, atrial and wedge pressure may be required to definitively secure the diagnosis.

- The extent of left-sided PH is an important determinant of morbidity and mortality, with a risk twofold higher for patients who develop right ventricular failure.
- Recently, greater attention has been suggested for targeting left-sided PH at earlier stages. The use of so-called PH-specific therapies, including epoprostenol and ET1 receptor antagonists, effective for other forms of PH, has provided disappointing results. Promising avenues seem to come from the use of PDE5-inhibitors, due to their specific selectivity for the lung circulation and nitric oxide pathway. At present, however, precise guidelines on the most beneficial and cost-effective therapeutic strategies for the cure of left-sided PH are still to be provided.

REFERENCES

1. Simonneau G, Robbins IM, Beghetti M, Channick RN, Delcroix M, Denton CP et al. Guidelines for the diagnosis and treatment of pulmonary hypertension: The Task Force for the Diagnosis and Treatment of Pulmonary Hypertension of the European Society of Cardiology (ESC) and the European Respiratory Society (ERS), endorsed by the International Society of Heart and Lung Transplantation (ISHLT). Eur Heart J 2009;30:2493-537.

2. Simonneau G, Robbins IM, Beghetti M, Channick RN, Delcroix M, Denton CP et al. Updated clinical classification of pulmonary hypertension. J Am Coll Cardiol 2009;54: 543-54.

3. Guazzi M. Alveolar gas diffusion abnormalities in heart failure. J Card Fail 2008;14:695-702.

4. Aird WC. Phenotypic heterogeneity of the endothelium: II. Representative vascular beds. Circ Res 2007;100:174-90.

5. Crone C, Saumon G, Basset G. News from the alveoli. News Physiol Sci 1990;5:50-3.

6. West JB, Mathieu-Costello O. Vulnerability of pulmonary capillaries in heart disease. Circulation 1995;92:622-31.

7. Tsukimoto K, Mathieu-Costello O, Prediletto R, Elliott AR, West JB. Ultrastructural appearances of pulmonary capillaries at high transmural pressures. J Appl Physiol 1991;71:573-82.

8. Conforti E, Fenoglio C, Bernocchi G, Bruschi O, Miserocchi GA. Morpho-functional analysis of lung tissue in mild interstitial edema. Am J Physiol 2002;282:L766-74.

9. Negrini D, Passi A, D Luca G, Miserocchi G. Pulmonary interstitial pressure and proteoglycans during development of pulmonary edema. Am J Physiol 1996:270:H2000-7.

10. Palestini P, Calvi E, Conforti L, Botto C, Fenoglio G, Miserocchi G. Composition, biophysical properties and morphometry of plasma membranes in pulmonary interstitial edema. Am J Physiol 2002;282:L1382-90.

11. De Pasquale CG, Arnolda LF, Doyle IR, Aylward PE, Chew DP, Bersten AD. Plasma surfactant protein-B: a novel biomarker in chronic heart failure. Circulation 2004;110:1091-6.

12. Matthay MA, Folkesson HG, Verkman AS. Salt and water transport across alveolar and distal airway epithelia in the adult lung. Am J Physiol 1996;270:L487-503.

13. Saldías FJ, Azzam ZS, Ridge KM, Yeldandi A, Rutschman DH, Schraufnagel D, Sznajder JI. Alveolar fluid reabsorption is impaired by increased left atrial pressures in rats. Am J Physiol Lung Cell Mol Physiol 2001;281(3):L591-7.

14. Factor P, Saldias F, Ridge K et al. Augmentation of lung liquid clearance via adenovirus-mediated transfer of a Na,K-ATPase beta1 subunit gene. J Clin Invest 1998;102:1421-30.

15. Azzam ZS, Dumasius V, Saldias FJ, Adir Y, Sznajder JI, Factor P. Na,K-ATPase overexpression improves alveolar fluid clearance in a rat model of elevated left atrial pressure. Circulation 2002;105(4):497-501.

16. Hocking DC, Phillips PG, Ferro TJ, Johnson A. Mechanisms of pulmonary edema induced by tumor necrosis factor-alpha. Circ Res 1990;67:68-77.

17. Dagenais A, Fréchette R, Yamagata Y et al. Downregulation of ENaC activity and expression by TNF-alpha in alveolar epithelial cells. Am J Physiol Lung Cell Mol Physiol. 2004;286:L301-11.

18. Suzuki S, Noda M, Sugita M, Ono S, Koike K, Fujimura S. Impairment of transalveolar fluid transport and lung Na(+)-K(+)-ATPase function by hypoxia in rats. J Appl Physiol 1999;87:962-8.

19. Elliott AR, Fu Z, Tsukimoto K, Prediletto R, Mathieu-Costello O, West JB. Short-term reversibility of ultrastructural changes in pulmonary capillaries caused by stress failure. J Appl Physiol 1992;73:1150-8.

20. Tomsley MI, Fu Z, Mathieu-Costello O et al Pulmonary microvascular permeability; responses to high vascular pressure after induction of pacing induced heart failure in dogs. Circ Res 1995;77:317-25.

21. Kay, JM, Edwards, FR Ultrastructure of the alveolar capillary wall in mitral stenosis. J Pathol 1973;111:239-45.

22. Lee, JS Electron microscopic studies on the alveolar-capillary barrier in patients with chronic pulmonary edema. Jpn Circ J 1979;43:945-54.

23. Drake, RE, Doursout, MF Pulmonary edema and elevated left atrial pressure: four hours and beyond. News Physiol Sci 2002;17:223-6.

24. Berg JT, Breen EC, Fu Z, Mathieu-Costello O, West JB. Alveolar hypoxia increases gene expression of extracellular matrix proteins and platelet-derived growth factor-B in lung parenchyma. Am J Respir Crit Care Med 1998; 158:1920-8.

25. Guazzi M, Pontone G, Brambilla R, Agostoni P, Rèina G. Alveolar-capillary membrane gas conductance: a novel prognostic indicator in chronic heart failure. Eur Heart J 2002;23:467-76.

26. Guazzi M. Alveolar-capillary membrane dysfunction in heart failure: evidence of a pathophysiologic role. Chest 2003;124:1090-2.

27. Rabinovitch M. EVE and beyond, retro and prospective insights. Am J Physiol 1999;277:L5-L12.

28. Stobierska B, Awad H, Michler RE. The evolving management of acute right-sided heart failure in cardiac transplant recipients. J Am Coll Cardiol 2001;38:923–31.

29. Ooi H, Colucci WS, Givertz MM. Endothelin mediates increased pulmonary vascular tone in patients with heart failure: demonstration by direct intrapulmonary infusion of sitaxentan. Circulation 2002;106:1618–21.

30. Cooper CJ, Jevnikar FW, Walsh T et al. The influence of basal nitric oxide activity on pulmonary vascular resistance in patients with congestive heart failure. Am J Cardiol 1998;82:609–14.

31. Stamler JS, Loh E, Roddy MA et al. Nitric oxide regulates basal systemic and pulmonary vascular resistance in healthy humans. Circulation 1994;89:2035–40.

32. Blitzer ML, Loh E, Roddy MA et al. Endothelium-derived nitric oxide regulates systemic and pulmonary vascular resistance during acute hypoxia in humans. J Am Coll Cardiol 1996;28:591–6.

33. Guazzi M, Arena R, Vicenzi M, Guazzi MD. Regulation of alveolar gas conductance by NO in man, as based on studies with NO donors and inhibitors of NO production. Acta Physiol 2009;196:267–77.

34. Cooper CJ, Jevnikar FW, Walsh T, Dickinson J, Mouhaffel A, Selwyn AP. The influence of basal nitric oxide activity on pulmonary vascular resistance in patients with congestive heart failure. Am J Cardiol 1998;82:609–14.

35. Porter TR, Taylor DO, Cycan A, Fields J, Bagley CW, Pandian NG, Mohanty PK. Endothelium-dependent pulmonary artery responses in chronic heart failure: influence of pulmonary hypertension J Am Coll Cardiol 1993;22:1418–24.

36. Cooper CJ, Jevnikar FW, Walsh T, Dickinson J, Mouhaffel A, Selwyn AP. The influence of basal nitric oxide activity on pulmonary vascular resistance in patients with congestive heart failure. Am J Cardiol 1998;82:609–14.

37. Yanagisawa M, Kurihara H, Kimura S, Tomobe Y, Kobayashi M, Mitsui Y, Yazaki Y, Goto K, Masaki T. A novel potent vasoconstrictor peptide produced by vascular endothelial cells. Nature 1988;332:411–5.

38. Dupuis J, Goresky CA, Fournier A. Pulmonary clearance of circulating endothelin-1 in dogs in vivo: exclusive role of ETB receptors. J Appl Physiol 1996;81:1510–5.

39. Fukuroda T, Kobayashi M, Ozaki S, Yano M, Miyauchi T, Onizuka M, Sugishita Y, Goto K, Nishikibe M. Endothelin receptor subtypes in human versus rabbit pulmonary arteries. J Appl Physiol 1994;76:1976–82.

40. Giaid A, Yanagisawa M, Langleben D et al. Expression of endothelin-1 in the lungs of patients with pulmonary hypertension. N Engl J Med 1993;328:1732–9.

41. Ray L, Mathieu M, Jespers P et al. Early increase in pulmonary vascular reactivity with overexpression of endothelin-1 and vascular endothelial growth factor in canine experimental heart failure. Exp Physiol 2008;93:434–42.

42. Cody RJ, Haas GJ, Binkley PF et al. Plasma endothelin correlates with the extent of pulmonary hypertension in patients with chronic congestive heart failure. Circulation 1992;85:504–9.

43. Hülsmann M, Stanek B, Frey B et al. Value of cardiopulmonary exercise testing and big endothelin plasma levels to predict short-term prognosis of patients with chronic heart failure. J Am Coll Cardiol 1998; 32:1695–700.

44. Gandhi SK, Powers JC, Nomeir AM, Fowle K, Kitzman DW, Rankin KM, Little WC. The pathogenesis of acute pulmonary edema associated with hypertension. N Engl J Med 2001;344:17–22.

45. Aurigemma GP, Gaasch WH: Diastolic heart failure. New Engl J Med 2004;351:1097–105.

46. Enriquez-Sarano M, Rossi A, Seward JB, Bailey KR, Tajik AJ. Determinants of pulmonary hypertension in left ventricular dysfunction. J Am Coll Cardiol 1997;29:153–9.

47. Lester SJ, Tajik AJ, Nishimura RA, Oh JK, Khandheria BK, Seward JB. Unlocking the mysteries of diastolic function: deciphering the Rosetta Stone 10 years later. J Am Coll Cardiol 2008;51:679–89.

48. Zile MR, Brutsaert DL. New concepts in diastolic dysfunction and diastolic heart failure: Part I: diagnosis, prognosis, and measurements of diastolic function. Circulation 2002;105:1387–93.

49. Nagueh SF, Middleton KJ, Kopelen HA, Zoghbi WA, Quiñones MA. Doppler tissue imaging: a noninvasive technique for evaluation of left ventricular relaxation and estimation of filling pressures. J Am Coll Cardiol 1997;30:1527–33.

50. Piérard LA, Lancellotti P. The role of ischemic mitral regurgitation in the pathogenesis of acute pulmonary edema. N Engl J Med 2004;351:1627–34.

51. Costard-Jäckle A, Fowler MB. Influence of preoperative pulmonary artery pressure on mortality after heart transplantation: testing of potential reversibility of pulmonary hypertension with nitroprusside is useful in defining a high risk group. J Am Coll Cardiol 1992; 19:48–54.

52. Givertz MM, Hare JM, Loh E, Gauthier DF, Colucci WS. Effect of bolus milrinone on hemodynamic variables and pulmonary vascular resistance in patients with severe left ventricular dysfunction: a rapid test for reversibility of pulmonary hypertension. J Am Coll Cardiol 1996;28:1775–80.

53. Kitzman DW, Higginbotham MB, Cobb FR, Sheikh KH, Sullivan MJ. Exercise intolerance in patients with heart failure and preserved left ventricular systolic function: failure of the Frank–Starling mechanism. J Am Coll Cardiol 1991;17:1065–72.

54. Tolle JJ, Waxman AB, Van Horn TL, Pappagianopoulos PP, Systrom DM. Exercise-induced pulmonary arterial hypertension. Circulation 2008;118:2183–9.

55. Tumminello G, Lancellotti P, Lempereur M, D'Orio V, Pierard LA. Determinants of pulmonary artery hypertension at rest and during exercise in patients with heart failure. Eur Heart J 2007;28:569–74.

56. Butler J, Chomsky DB, Wilson JR. Pulmonary hypertension and exercise intolerance in patients with heart failure. J Am Coll Cardiol 1999;34:1802–6.

57. McLaughlin VV, McGoon MD. Pulmonary arterial hypertension. Circulation 2006 26;114:1417–31.

58. Di Salvo TG, Mathier M, Semigran MJ, Dec GW. Preserved right ventricular ejection fraction predicts exercise

capacity and survival in advanced heart failure. J Am Coll Cardiol 1995;25:1143–53.

59. Reindl I, Wernecke KD, Opitz C, Wensel R, König D, Dengler T, Schimke I, Kleber FX. Impaired ventilatory efficiency in chronic heart failure: possible role of pulmonary vasoconstriction. Am Heart J 1998;136:778–85.

60. Lewis GD, Shah RV, Pappagianopolas PP, Systrom DM, Semigran MJ. Determinants of ventilatory efficiency in heart failure. The role of right ventricular performance and pulmonary vascular tone. Circ Heart Fail 2008;1:227–33.

61. Guazzi M, Myers J, Arena R. Cardiopulmonary exercise testing in the clinical and prognostic assessment of diastolic heart failure. J Am Coll Cardiol 2005;46:1883–90.

62. Arena R, Myers J, Abella J, Peberdy MA, Bensimhon D, Chase P, Guazzi M. Development of a ventilatory classification system in patients with heart failure. Circulation 2007;115:2410–17.

63. Olson TP, Frantz RP, Snyder EM, O'Malley KA, Beck KC, Johnson BD. Effects of acute changes in pulmonary wedge pressure on periodic breathing at rest in heart failure patients. Am Heart J 2007;153:104.e1–7.

64. Solin P, Bergin P, Richardson M, Kaye DM, Walters EH, Naughton MT. Influence of pulmonary capillary wedge pressure on central apnea in heart failure. Circulation 1999;99:1574–9.

65. Abramson SV, Burke JF, Kelly JJ Jr et al. Pulmonary hypertension predicts mortality and morbidity in patients with dilated cardiomyopathy. Ann Intern Med 1992;116:888–95.

66. Rickenbacher PR, Trindade PT, Haywood GA, Vagelos RH, Schroeder JS, Willson K, Prikazsky L, Fowler MB. Transplant candidates with severe left ventricular dysfunction managed with medical treatment: characteristics and survival. J Am Coll Cardiol 1996;27:1192–7.

67. Ghio S, Gavazzi A, Campana C et al. Independent and additive prognostic value of right ventricular systolic function and pulmonary artery pressure in patients with chronic heart failure. J Am Coll Cardiol 2001;37:183–8.

68. Hosenpud JD, Bennett LE, Keck BM, Boucek MM, Novick RJ.The Registry of the International Society for Heart and Lung Transplantation: seventeenth official report – 2000. J Heart Lung Transplant 2000;19:909–31.

69. Califf RM, Adams KF, McKenna WJ et al. A randomized trial of epoprostenol therapy for severe congestive heart failure: the Floan International Randomized Survival Trial (FIRST). Am Heart J 1997;134:44–54.

70. Sablotzki A, Czeslick E, Schubert S, Friedrich I, Mühling J, Dehne MG, Grond S, Hentschel T. Iloprost improves hemodynamics in patients with severe chronic cardiac failure and secondary pulmonary hypertension. Can J Anaesth 2002;49:1076–80.

71. Mulder P, Richard V, Derumeaux G et al. Role of endogenous endothelin in chronic heart failure: effect of long-term treatment with an endothelin antagonist on survival, hemodynamics, and cardiac remodeling. Circulation 1997;96:1976–82.

72. Wada A, Tsutamoto T, Fukai D et al. Comparison of the effects of selective endothelin ETA and ETB receptor antagonists in congestive heart failure. J Am Coll Cardiol 1997;30:1385–92.

73. Givertz MM, Colucci WS, LeJemtel TH et al. Acute endothelin A receptor blockade causes selective pulmonary vasodilation in patients with chronic heart failure. Circulation 2000;101:2922–27.

74. Packer M, McMurray J, Massie BM et al. Clinical effects of endothelin receptor antagonism with bosentan in patients with severe chronic heart failure: results of a pilot study. J Card Fail 2005;11:12–20.

75. Kieler-Jensen N, Ricksten SE, Stenqvist O et al. Inhaled nitric oxide in the evaluation of heart transplant candidates with elevated pulmonary vascular resistance. J Heart Lung Transplant 1994;13:366–75.

76. Hare JM, Shernan SK, Body SC, Graydon E, Colucci WS, Couper GS. Influence of inhaled nitric oxide on systemic flow and ventricular filling pressure in patients receiving mechanical circulatory assistance. Circulation 1997; 95:2250–53.

77. Bocchi EA, Bacal F, Auler Júnior JO, Carmone MJ, Bellotti G, Pileggi F. Inhaled nitric oxide leading to pulmonary edema in stable severe heart failure. Am J Cardiol 1994;74:70–2.

78. Murray F, MacLean MR, Pyne NJ Increased expression of the cGMP-inhibited cAMP-specific (PDE3) and cGMP binding cGMP-specific (PDE5) phosphodiesterases in models of pulmonary hypertension. Br J Pharmacol 2002;137:1187–94.

79. Galiè N, Ghofrani HA, Torbicki A et al. Sildenafil Use in Pulmonary Arterial Hypertension (SUPER) Study Group. N Engl J Med 2005;353:2148–57.

80. Guazzi M. Clinical use of phophodiesterase-5 inhibitors in chronic heart failure. Circ Heart Fail 2008;1:272–80.

81. Guazzi M, Tumminello G, Di Marco F, Fiorentini C, Guazzi MD. The effects of phosphodiesterase-5 inhibition with sildenafil on pulmonary hemodynamics and diffusion capacity, exercise ventilatory efficiency, and oxygen uptake kinetics in chronic heart failure. J Am Coll Cardiol 2004;44:2339–48.

82. Lewis GD, Lachmann J, Camuso J et al. Sildenafil improves exercise hemodynamics and oxygen uptake in patients with systolic heart failure. Circulation 2007;115:59–66.

83. Guazzi M, Samaja M, Arena R, Vicenzi M, Guazzi MD. Long-term use of sildenafil in the therapeutic management of heart failure. J Am Coll Cardiol 2007;50:2136–44.

84. Lewis GD, Shah R, Shahzad K et al. Sildenafil improves exercise capacity and quality of life in patients with systolic heart failure and secondary pulmonary hypertension. Circulation 2007;116:1555–62.

85. Stehlik J, Movesesian MA. Combined use of PDE5 inhibitors and nitrates in the treatment of pulmonary arterial hypertension in patients with heart failure. J Card Fail 2009;15:31–4.

86. Telford RJ, Hemnes AR, Russel SD et al. PDE5 inhibitor treatment of persistent pulmonary hypertension after mechanical circulatory support. Circ Heart Fail 2008;1:213–9.

Pulmonary veno-occlusive disease

BARBARA A COCKRILL AND CHARLES A HALES

INTRODUCTION

Pulmonary veno-occlusive disease (PVOD) is a rare disorder which causes pulmonary hypertension. The hallmark feature of PVOD is widespread microscopic obstruction of pulmonary venules due to intimal fibrosis and *in-situ* thrombus. According to the most recent World Health Organization classification, PVOD is considered a subset of pulmonary arterial hypertension (PAH) although it differs from other forms of PAH, including idiopathic PAH (IPAH) in that significant venous involvement is present in the pulmonary vasculature (1,2). This important distinction has been increasingly supported by differences in response to therapy when compared with other forms of PAH.

The first case to be recognized and reported was in 1934 by Hora (3). He described a 48-year-old baker who presented with progressive dyspnea and edema. The patient died within a year of presentation, and was found to have pulmonary vascular obstruction centered in the pulmonary veins. The term pulmonary veno-occlusive disease was not proposed until 1966 when in the case of a 37-year-old woman with iPAH clear division was made between the pathology of iPAH and PVOD (4).

INCIDENCE

Pulmonary veno-occlusive disease has been reported in all age groups from 8 weeks of age 5 into the seventh decade (6), although children and young adults appear to be most common. There may be a slight predilection for males, but this varies with series.

The actual incidence of PVOD is difficult to determine because, in the absence of lung biopsy, many cases may be misclassified as iPAH (7). As an example, in a review of the NHLBI registry biopsy specimens, seven of 58 patients thought to have IPAH were found to have PVOD (8). In a case series from the Mayo Clinic, five of 80 patients with IPAH were found to have PVOD on histopathological review (9). PVOD is clearly much less common than IPAH, probably accounting for about 10 percent of cases diagnosed as IPAH. Applying this figure to the incidence of IPAH yields an estimated incidence of 0.1 to 0.2 cases per million persons in the general population (1,7).

PATHOLOGY

Pathological findings in PVOD reflect a primary abnormality in the pulmonary venules and small veins, and the resulting "upstream" consequences in the pulmonary vessels and parenchyma. The characteristic finding on lung biopsy is narrowing of pulmonary venules and small veins by intimal fibrosis. The narrowing may be due to loose edematous connective tissue with variable cellularity or dense, sclerotic and acellular fibrotic tissue (10,11). This pattern of venous involvement is distinct from the histopathology found in other forms of pulmonary hypertension leading to the recent recommendation that the name be changed to pulmonary occlusive venopathy (11). The presence of both patterns in a single patient suggests progressive fibrosis. These lesions are usually distributed evenly throughout both lungs with no particular predilection for a specific lobe or region, although some patients with predominant upper lobe involvement have been described (10). Veins may be so abnormal with prominent medial muscularization that they resemble arteries, leading the pathologist on first pass to consider the pathology to be in the arteries (Figure 19.2.1).

Organizing thrombi are seen and appear to be formed *in situ* (9–11). The thrombi are usually limited to the pulmonary venules, and less commonly, are seen in the immediate precapillary circulation. The thrombi may be recannalized, most often with the formation of intraluminal fibrous septa (11,12). The portion of the vein proximal to the recannalized thrombus will frequently demonstrate medial hypertrophy and arterialization of the vein (11,13). The finding of organized and recannalized thrombi in the pulmonary venules is essentially universal being found in some percentage venules in all specimens (Figure 19.2.2). However, intimal thickening is more prevalent (Figure 19.2.3). For example, in a series of pathological specimens from five patients with PVOD, only 11–13 percent of small veins exhibited evidence of thrombosis and recanalization whereas increased intimal thickening was present in essentially all small veins. This suggests that intimal thickening

is the primary event that predisposes to subsequent *in situ* thrombosis (14).

Infiltration of the venular walls by inflammatory cells has been reported (15), but is a distinctly uncommon finding.

Parenchymal changes are less evident, and reflect capillary and lymphatic congestion due to downstream obstruction. A large amount of hemosiderin is present in the pulmonary interstitium and cytoplasm of alveolar macrophages. The interstitium typically shows significant edema located primarily in the lobular septa – which may progress to fibrosis (11). The findings of increased hemosiderin and interstitial edema are both consistent with the presence of venular obstruction, and resulting increased pulmonary capillary pressure. Characteristically, small nodular areas of congested and thickened alveolar walls often associated with hemorrhage and siderosis are demonstrated (10). These focal areas may represent sites of capillary disruption

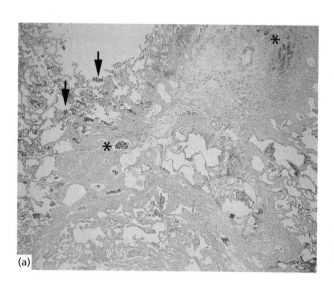
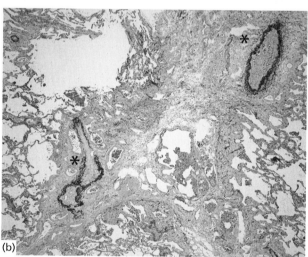

Figure 19.2.1 Photomicrograph of the lung in PVOD. Abnormal and occluded veins (asterisk) and areas of hemorrhage adjacent to the septum are seen (arrows). Left panel hematoxylin and eosin stained. Right panel elastic stain. Both images are original magnification (20×). (Images courtesy of Dr. Les Kopzik, Harvard Medical School.)

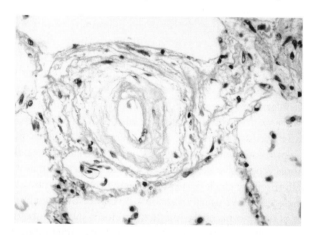
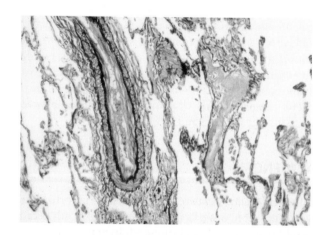

Figure 19.2.2 High power photomicrograph showing a small vein with both intimal and medial thickening resulting in marked luminal narrowing.

Figure 19.2.3 Medium power photomicrograph elastin tissue stain showing a sclerotic vein (right) and an arteriole with intimal hypertensive changes (left).

due to locally increased pressure with extravasation of blood, and subsequent healing. Dilated lymphatics and focal areas of congestion are frequent (11).

In approximately 50 percent of cases, remodeling of the pulmonary arteries and arterioles is present with moderate to severe medial hypertrophy and arterialization (11,13). Plexiform lesions are not present in PVOD. Pulmonary arterioles are variably involved, and when changes are present they are usually less striking than venular changes. The arterial findings tend to be patchy and crescent-shaped rather than being circumferential. However, at times, the obstruction may be equal to that seen in the pulmonary veins possibly reflecting the stage of the disease (13). As an example, in a case series of 26 patients, pulmonary arteries were narrowed or obliterated in approximately half of patients (13). In seven patients recent *in situ* thrombi were seen. However, fibrinoid necrosis, arteritis and plexiform lesions were absent. Interestingly, in this series lung biopsies with the most prominent arterial obstruction had the least severe parenchymal hemosiderosis – suggesting that the upstream occlusion protects that pulmonary capillary from stress disruption.

Chazova and colleagues compared venous and arterial changes in PVOD with two other forms of pulmonary venous hypertension: mitral stenosis and fibrosing mediastinitis. The venular abnormalities of intimal and adventitial thickening, while most striking in PVOD, were also clearly present in the other two diseases. The authors propose that the similarity of vascular changes in the three forms of pulmonary venous hypertension indicates that the increased pressure itself is one of the triggers to vascular remodeling (14). Increased cyclic cell stretch of the pulmonary vascular endothelium resulting from the higher intravascular pressures may play a role in both the venous and arterial remodeling (16).

In one case, examined at biopsy and then again 6 months later at the time of lung transplantation, progression of intimal venous changes and arterialization of veins was demonstrated. Medial thickening also progressed in the pulmonary arteries, but the total number of arteries with intimal and adventitial thickening was similar (14).

Lymphadenopathy is common both radiographically and pathologically. Lymph nodes resected during lung transplantations showed lymphatic congestion with vascular transformation of the sinuses and intra-sinusal hemorrhage. These findings are much more frequent in cases of PVOD compared with IPAH, and are probably primarily secondary to venous congestion (17).

ETIOLOGY AND PATHOGENESIS

Genetic predisposition

The cause of pulmonary veno-occlusive disease is unknown. It is likely that PVOD represents a syndrome of characteristic pathological responses to different insults in the setting of a permissive genetic predisposition.

Mutations in the BMPR2 gene have been identified in a number of patients with PVOD (18–20). BMPR2 encodes a type II receptor of the transforming growth factor-beta (TGF-β) superfamily of cell signaling receptors. As discussed in Chapter 15.2, Genetics of pulmonary arterial hypertension, mutations in this gene are identified in the majority of patients with familial PAH as well as a subset of sporadically occurring PAH. In a recent report, BMPR2 mutations were present in 2/24 patients with PVOD compared with 4/24 patients with sporadic PAH (21).

Further evidence that a genetic predisposition is present is suggested by a few case reports of disease occurring in siblings. As an example, a case of two siblings was reported in which a 14-year-old boy developed effort-induced dyspnea. He had a rapid course and died. Several months later, his 13-year-old sister died of the same process. At autopsy, severe veno-occlusive disease was found in both. No common exposure could be found (22).

PVOD has been reported in other sibling pairs, and in all of the reports, the disease onset in the siblings was within 1–2 years of each other (10,23,24). While these cases are suggestive of a genetic predisposition, the possibility of a common exposure cannot be discounted. Similar to the current theory on the pathogenesis of IPAH (25), it is our opinion that it is most likely that a permissive genetic milieu exists that allows a characteristic response to a toxic insult.

Infection

A preceding febrile illness resembling influenza has been described in many patients (4,10,26,27), but is not present in all. The relationship between the febrile illness and the subsequent development of PVOD is not certain.

A viral etiology is suggested in some cases. In one case examined at autopsy, a generalized lymphadenopathy with erythrophagocytosis was found and thought to indicate a viral origin. This patient had a preceding illness characterized by high spiking fevers (28). In the youngest patient thus far reported with PVOD, an intrauterine viral infection was suggested as the cause. The mother had a prolonged upper respiratory tract illness in the third trimester and the infant died at age 8 weeks. Autopsy showed PVOD associated with a subacute myocarditis and chronic interstitial pneumonia (5).

Two cases of PVOD associated with HIV have been reported, although both cases had confounding factors making the association with HIV uncertain. The first was in a 2-year-old child who was diagnosed with HIV at 8 months of age. Following a respiratory illness related to respiratory syncytial virus and influenza A, he developed signs and symptoms consistent with PVOD. At autopsy 9 months later, the child was found to have pathological findings consistent with lymphocytic interstitial pneumonia and PVOD. Thus, in this child, at least three viruses may be related to the development of PVOD: RSV, influenza A, and

HIV (29). The second report case was in a 27-year-old intravenous drug abuser. A preceding viral illness was not described. At open lung biopsy, occasional foreign bodies were found consistent with IV drug abuse, but the primary pathology was concentrated in the pulmonary venules (30). HIV disease is an accepted risk factor for the development of IPAH (31). It seems likely that more cases of PVOD in association with HIV have occurred, but have been attributed to IPAH.

Immune disorders

Autoimmune phenomena targeting the pulmonary venules with subsequent thrombosis, fibrosis and obstruction would be a logical explanation for the pathology seen in PVOD. Immune complexes are described in some patients (32), and it has been suggested that immune complex deposition in the basement membrane formation can lead to venular injury and intraluminal thrombosis. PVOD has been associated with collagen vascular diseases including systemic lupus erythematosis (33), progressive systemic sclerosis including the CREST (calcinosis cutis, Raynaud's phenomenon, esophageal dysfunction, sclerodactyly, and telangiectasia) variant (34–37), as well as in mixed connective tissue disease (38). However, PVOD is associated with autoimmune disorders in the minority of cases (7). PVOD may also rarely be associated with sarcoidosis (39).

PVOD has been described in a single patient as part of a generalized venulopathy. Liang and co-workers described a 39-year-old woman who presented with facial swelling, conjunctival and periorbital edema. She eventually died of severe pulmonary hypertension and cor pulmonale. Autopsy showed a generalized venulitis involving most organs. There was widespread phlebosclerosis of medium-sized venules with perivenular chronic inflammation. Pulmonary veins showed a similar pattern with marked obstruction. Thrombotic lesions within the pulmonary venules are not commented upon. Pulmonary arteries showed intimal hyperplasia and plexiform lesions – the latter is not usually described in PVOD (40).

Drug and chemical exposures

PVOD is a recognized but rare complication following hematopoietic stem cell transplantation and may be more common after bone-marrow transplantation, especially allogeneic transplantation, than after routine chemotherapy (7,41,42). Chemotherapeutic agents used in treatment of various malignancies have been reported in association with PVOD (43–45). Most patients were treated with a number of agents as well as total body irradiation in some reports. In the reported cases, bleomycin, BCNU, mitomycin-C appear the most commonly involved agents (41).

The possibility of a connection between hepatic veno-occlusive disease (HVOD) and PVOD is raised by the observations of Wingard and colleagues. In a large series,

154 patients who underwent intensive cytoreductive therapy were evaluated for HVOD. Thirty-nine patients were diagnosed with HVOD. Of 15 cases with HVOD who had an autopsy, 11 were found to have coexisting PVOD (46). In HVOD, endothelial cell damage and resulting inflammation and thrombosis are implicated in the pathogenesis, and it is hypothesized that the same process leads to PVOD in susceptible individuals (47).

There is a single reported case of PVOD developing in association with inhaled toxins. This involved a 14-year-old boy with a two-year history of inhaling a household cleaning product (48).

Case reports of PVOD in association with oral contraceptives (49) and pregnancy (50) raise the possibility that estrogens and hypercoaguable states may play a role in the development of PVOD. Thrombosis within the venules is a frequent, but not universal pathological finding. In a series of lung tissue taken from five patients with PVOD, Chazova *et al.* found thrombosis and recanalization in only 11–13 percent of venules examined despite striking intimal thickening in essentially all veins. This suggests that thickening of the intima is a primary event occurring in the absence of thrombosis (14). With currently available data, it cannot be concluded that *in situ* thrombosis or abnormalities in the clotting system are a primary factor (7). A more likely scenario is that a primary injury occurs in the venules which subsequently leads to *in-situ* thrombosis and recanalization.

There is no single factor that is consistently associated with the development of PVOD. As is the case with IPAH, it seems likely that the PVOD is a characteristic response to an injury in a susceptible, rather than due to a specific insult itself.

CLINICAL PRESENTATION AND DIAGNOSIS

Clinical findings

Clinically, it can be difficult to distinguish patients with PVOD from patients with IPAH or isolated pulmonary vascular disease of other causes. Patients with PVOD invariably present with progressive dyspnea on exertion. About half will have a dry cough. Both orthopnea and paroxysmal nocturnal dyspnea are described in a minority of patients, as is a preceding viral-like illness. As with primary pulmonary hypertension, atypical chest pain and near-syncope may be present, and probably represent more severe disease. In more advanced disease, patients may present with lower extremity edema. Hemoptysis is rare, although occult alveolar hemorrhage is common (51). Cyanosis may be more prominent in patients with PVOD than IPAH due to the underlying interstitial and alveolar edema which is present.

The physical findings of PVOD primarily reflect the presence of pulmonary hypertension. A prominent pulmonic heart sound and a murmur of tricuspid regurgitation are common. The majority of patients in the largest published series to describe physical exams findings had signs of overt right heart failure. Seven of 11 patients had elevated neck veins, a third heart sound, a right ventricular heave and lower extremity edema at the time of presentation (12). Clubbing was present in over 50 percent. A clue to the diagnosis is the presence of bibasilar crackles suggestive of pulmonary edema in a patient whose exam presentation is otherwise characteristic of IPAH. Physical findings of pulmonary edema are present in about half of patients (12,21).

Pulmonary function tests

Pulmonary function testing typically shows normal spirometry and lung volumes; however, both obstructive and restrictive patterns are also described (12). As noted above in the section on pathology, interstitial inflammation and fibrosis is not common and when present is mild. Thus, it is likely the restrictive pattern seen on pulmonary function testing is due to interstitial edema. In contrast to the spirometry and lung volumes, the diffusing capacity for carbon dioxide (D_LCO) is markedly reduced (52). Notably, the D_LCO is significantly low in patients with PVOD as compared to IPAH (21). This can provide a clue to diagnosis.

Blood gas analysis typically reveals a widened alveolar-arterial oxygen gradient, with varying degrees of hypoxemia, and a respiratory alkalosis (12). Similar to the D_LCO, the PaO_2 is lower in patients with PVOD than in IPAH. In cases which are not associated with a known collagen vascular disease, the anti-nuclear antibody titers are occasionally weakly elevated, but other markers of collagen vascular disease are negative.

Radiographic findings

Radiographic studies often suggest a patient with suspected IPAH actually has PVOD.

Plain films of the chest are usually nonspecific but may show enlarged pulmonary arteries and diffuse ground glass opacities may be seen. Kerley lines are often present as are pleural effusions (1). However, PVOD may be present in the absence of these findings as well (7).

Computed tomography frequently shows a distinguishing pattern (Figure 19.2.4): interlobular septal thickening, ground glass opacities and mediastinal adenopathy in the presence of pulmonary hypertension. Interlobular septal thickening – both smooth and nodular – is the most characteristic pattern (53). As an example, in one cases series of biopsy proven PVOD, 7/8 patients had smooth interlobular septal thickening (54). Diffuse ground glass opacities, especially with a centrilobular distribution are common (Figure 19.2.4), and probably represent some pulmonary interstitial edema. The finding of mediastinal lymphadenopathy is inconsistent being found in some cases (35) but not in others (12,53). However, when present, mediastinal

lymphadenopathy makes the diagnosis more likely. In our experience, chest CT scanning is the first study suggesting the diagnosis of PVOD – most often with findings of unexplained ground glass opacities, lymphadenopathy and pleural effusions (Figure 19.2.5). Holcomb and colleagues found that all eleven patients in their cases series had some radiological finding consistent with PVOD: 100 percent with an abnormal chest plain film, and 88 percent with an abnormal chest CT scan (12).

Results of pulmonary ventilation-perfusion scans are variable. The results have reported as normal (55), although more frequently there is some abnormal distribution of tracer material in the pulmonary vasculature (56). A segmental contour pattern of V/Q mismatch has been described (57). High-probability V/Q scans have been found in a subset of patients with PVOD in whom subsequent pulmonary angiography fails to demonstrate pulmonary emboli. The authors hypothesize that the downstream resistance to blood flow in PVOD could account for this finding. Tracer deposition during a V/Q scan is proportional to blood flow. Therefore the high downstream resistance would reduce the tracer deposition

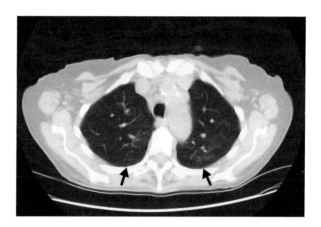

Figure 19.2.4 Computed tomography of the chest in a patient with PVOD. Note septal thickening and ground glass opacities (arrows) which probably represent pulmonary edema (see text).

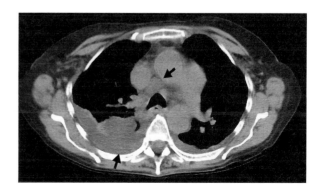

Figure 19.2.5 Computed tomography of the chest in a patient with PVOD. Note pleural effusion and mediastinal lymphadenopathy (arrow).

in the precapillary arterioles upstream from the venous resistance. Because the contrast material during a pulmonary arteriogram is performed with higher pressures, the downstream resistance may be overcome. Thus, the obstruction would not be apparent on angiogram. The authors further postulate that high probability scans may be found when larger pulmonary veins are involved in contrast to the more common finding of a diffuse patchy distribution of tracer material, when smaller pulmonary veins are most involved in the process.

Intravascular ultrasound (IVUS) is a developing technology in the diagnosis of pulmonary hypertension and more data are needed (59). To our knowledge, there is no published information regarding the use of IVUS in PVOD. As noted above, the thickening of the pulmonary arterial wall associated with PVOD is much less prominent than is present in the pulmonary venous circulation. We hypothesize that the finding of arterial wall thickness that is *less* than would be expected for the degree of pulmonary hypertension could be a clue that PVOD is present.

Hemodynamics

Pulmonary veno-occlusive disease is associated with severe pulmonary artery hypertension and as the process progresses, with right ventricular dysfunction.

The pulmonary artery occlusion pressure (PAOP) is characteristically normal. However, both elevated PAOP and measurements that vary in between sites in the lung are also reported. The mechanism of these findings is a source of some confusion (60). In order to understand how a PAOP can be normal or variable in the setting of a process which causes increased pulmonary capillary pressure and pulmonary edema, it is helpful to review the details of what a PAOP actually measures. As discussed in Chapter 10, the pulmonary artery catheter is a flow-directed catheter that therefore is carried by blood flow into the pulmonary artery. Balloon inflation encourages migration of the catheter tip from a main pulmonary artery into a smaller caliber vessel where it impacts and wedges. Blood flow distal to the site of impact is blocked, and a static column of blood is created beyond the inflated balloon. The pressure equilibrates between the site of balloon obstruction and the downstream junction with the next site of blood flow (the "j" point.). Therefore, the pressure measured at the catheter tip is equal to the pressure at the "j" point. The "j" point is usually in a pulmonary vein of equal caliber to the pulmonary artery in which the balloon is lodged – that is in a pulmonary vein *larger* than the venules that are most affected in PVOD. Thus, the PAOP measures a pressure that is distal to the site of increased resistance in the obstructed pulmonary venules in PVOD. For contrast, this is unlike the typical situation in fibrosing mediastinitis, another disease which affects the pulmonary veins and causes pulmonary edema. In fibrosing mediastinitis large pulmonary veins are narrowed when entering the left atrium, and the

small venules will join producing flow before reach the site of narrowing in the large veins. The PAOP in fibrosing mediastinitis will therefore be elevated. In both PVOD and fibrosing mediastinitis, when the balloon is deflated, and blood is again flowing past the site of resistance, increased pressure will be present in the pulmonary capillaries (Figure 19.2.6). In PVOD it is the increased pulmonary capillary pressure that leads to pulmonary edema.

Another finding that may be found on catheterization is when saline is injected through the distal port of the wedged catheter, the pressure rises disproportionately quickly and falls off very slowly. This is presumably due to the injected saline being trapped upstream from the site of increased venous resistance, and subsequent slow run-off (7). Some researchers have used this technique to assess the actual pulmonary capillary pressure when blood flow is present (61). The single arterial occlusion technique has also been used to attempt to partition the site of increase vascular

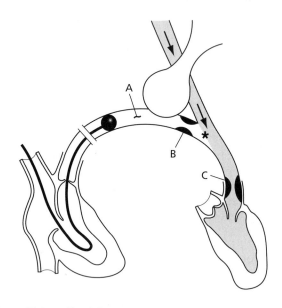

Figure 19.2.6 The definition of the pulmonary artery occlusion pressure (PAOP). Inflation of the catheter balloon, if properly done, stops blood flow through the segment of the pulmonary circulation distal to the catheter tip. The PAOP measured at point A equilibrates with the downstream pressure at the junction of static and flowing pulmonary venous blood (*). Point B, representing the pulmonary venules and small veins, is the site of increased resistance in PVOD. As shown in the diagram, point B is proximal to the junction point, and therefore is not reflected in the PAOP. However, when the balloon is deflated, blood flow past point B will result in increased upstream pressure in the pulmonary capillaries. Point C represents increased resistance in the large pulmonary veins, which is usually not present in PAOP. An elevated PAOP may be recorded in PVOD if larger veins are involved, or if the catheter has migrated into a very small caliber pulmonary artery and pressure at a more proximal junction point is measured (from Marini JJ, Wheeler AP (eds) Critical Care Medicine – The Essentials. Baltimore: Williams & Wilkins, 1989, with permission).

resistance. In the technique, after the catheter balloon is wedged in a pulmonary artery, the rate of fall in the pressure to the PAOP can be correlated with the site of increased resistance. If the obstruction is in the pulmonary arteries, after the balloon occludes the artery, the run pressure quickly falls. If the obstruction is in the pulmonary veins, the pressure falls off more gradually. Unfortunately, when this technique is applied to individual patients, there is too much overlap in values to be useful in making a diagnosis (62).

The issue of lung biopsy in patients with suspected PVOD is a difficult one. Patients with pulmonary hypertension are at increased risk for serious complications, including hemorrhage and death. However, the diagnosis can only be definitively made by examining lung tissue. It is our practice to consider lung biopsy in those patients deemed to be acceptable surgical risks.

TREATMENT

Because PVOD is so uncommon, it is difficult to make any general statements about treatment. Supplemental oxygen and careful diuresis should be considered in all patients. There have been no controlled trials and there is no confirmed treatment for PVOD, therefore the following discussion is based on case reports and small series.

Anticoagulants

The pathological observation of thrombosis within the venules in many cases of PVOD makes the use of anticoagulants as treatment for PVOD seem appropriate. Whether a primary or secondary event, progressive thrombus formation within the vessels would lead to clinical deterioration. There are observational data that patients with IPAH have improved survival – the thinking being that in-situ pulmonary arteriolar thrombosis contributes to progression of pulmonary hypertension. Particular caution is required when using anticoagulants in patients with PVOD given the frequency of occult alveolar hemorrhage, and the drugs should probably be withheld in any patient with a history of hemoptysis. There are no trials comparing the use of anticoagulants vs. withholding anticoagulants in PVOD. However, we and many others (7) routinely use long-term warfarin in these patients.

Immunosuppressive agents

A number of reports have described the use of immunosuppressive agents. The information is anecdotal, and patients who appear to respond frequently have PVOD in the setting of other signs of collagen vascular disease.

Corticosteroids have been used without consistent results (63,64). As an example, of 33 patients reported in the 1970s, seven were treated with corticosteroids. Only two of those seven patients survived more than three months after starting treatment (64). In contrast, Escamilla and colleagues reported a patient with biopsy proven HIV-associated PVOD who had a marked improvement in symptoms and pulmonary infiltrates after starting therapy with prednisone (30). A short-lived response to corticosteroids was seen in a patient with systemic sclerosis who improved within two months but died five months later of progressive disease (36). There may be a greater chance of response to corticosteroids if the PVOD follows bone-marrow transplant or is associated with chemotherapy (42,65).

In one case of PVOD associated with interstitial pneumonitis, there was fatal progression of pulmonary hypertension due to PVOD despite steroid-induced remission of the interstitial pneumonitis (63). In this case, transbronchial lung biopsies were performed initially, and revealed prominent chronic inflammatory cell infiltration, type II cell hyperplasia, and mild interstitial fibrosis as well as several small and medium-sized arteries which showed mild medial hypertrophy. Of note, PVOD was not documented on the initial biopsies. Symptoms were improved and infiltrates resolved within ten days of corticosteroid therapy. The patient remained stable for over two years without any recognizable change in her pulmonary artery pressures. However, 27 months after starting corticosteroids, she developed a rapidly progressive right heart failure and died. At autopsy, she had a mild interstitial pneumonitis. The pulmonary veins showed intimal proliferation and medial hypertrophy. Several small veins were thrombosed with occasional recanalization. There were some changes in the pulmonary arterioles as well (63). Despite the apparent safety in this case, we strongly advise against performing transbronchial biopsies in any patient with significant pulmonary hypertension due to the risk of uncontrolled and potentially fatal bleeding.

Azathioprine has been apparently successful in treating PVOD in the setting of severe collagen vascular disease. This patient had associated cutaneous vasculitis, myopathy and polyarteritis. She was initially treated with prednisone with some response, and subsequently treated with azathioprine and did well for at least 2 years (66).

Current knowledge is incomplete. We reserve the use of immunosuppressive agents for patients with either known or suspected collagen vascular disease. In this situation, we believe a therapeutic trial is indicated with careful and objective assessment for response.

PAH-specific therapy

Vasodilator agents have been used with mixed results. Unlike in the treatment of IPAH, the role of vasodilators is uncertain in PVOD at this time.

Great caution must be exercised, however, when use of these agents is attempted because of the potential for causing increased pulmonary edema. The capillary bed is the main exchange site for fluid between the intravascular and extravascular spaces in the lung. Increased capillary pressure and acute pulmonary edema will result when vasodilators cause a decrease in upstream pulmonary arteriolar resistance in the face of fixed disease in the pulmonary venous system. It is suggested that there may be some vasodilator tone in the pulmonary venules in patients with PVOD. We and others have found that pulmonary artery pressure and pulmonary vascular resistance decrease in response to inhaled nitric oxide in PVOD (21,67). Davis et al. calculated pulmonary capillary pressure in a single patient with PVOD, and suggest that post-capillary venules had vasomotor tone in this patient which required higher doses of prostacyclin to vasodilate than did the arteriolar tone (61). In this report, calculated pulmonary capillary pressure increased at prostacyclin doses < 6 ng/kg/min – the dose below which venular vasomotor tone was not affected. At doses 6–12 ng/kg/min, the calculated pulmonary capillary pressure was back at baseline. These findings must be confirmed by others, but if confirmed the issue for the clinician is whether the increase in pulmonary capillary pressure (and resultant pulmonary edema) at lower doses precludes further titration of the drug to higher doses.

Alpha–adrenergic blockers

Two patients have been described who did well initially when treated with the alpha-adrenergic blocker prasozin. Both had an acute vasodilator response to this agent. One did well initially, but had progressive right heart failure and died within two years, the other patient maintained clinical improvement for at least three years after starting therapy (68).

Calcium antagonists

Treatment with calcium channel antagonists has been attempted. Rich et al. report two patients who died within 48 hours of starting treatment with nifedipine apparently with pulmonary edema (69). The authors believed it due to an increase in cardiac output against a fixed pulmonary venous obstruction. Holcomb and colleagues report that six of 11 patients treated with calcium channel antagonists developed pulmonary edema. Only one of the episodes was during acute testing, the other episodes occurred between 3 days and 6 months after starting therapy (12).

Scattered reports of prolonged survival during treatment with calcium channel antagonists have also been reported. The first reported case of prolonged survival was in a patient with PVOD who had a significant reduction in pulmonary vascular resistance and pulmonary artery pressure when treated with long-term nifedipine. This patient survived for over 7 years. The authors speculate that the pulmonary artery vasodilating effect of the nifedipine allowed additional time for the PVOD to resolve before severe pulmonary arterial hypertensive changes occurred (41). Another patient was maintained on calcium channel antagonists with sustained clinical improvement for at least two years (69).

Caution must be taken when considering the use of calcium channel antagonists in any patient with poor right ventricular function as these agents are negative inotropes, and have been shown to adversely affect right ventricular contractility (67).

Prostacyclins

Fatal pulmonary edema during a low-dose prostacyclin infusion has been reported. A 42-year-old woman was treated with 2 ng/kg/min of prostacyclin. Within 15 minutes of starting the infusion the patient developed massive pulmonary edema. The infusion was stopped, but the patient died within two hours despite maximal support. Pulmonary veno-occlusive disease was confirmed at autopsy (70).

Two patients with PVOD were retrospectively identified at autopsy in a randomized trial designed to determine the effectiveness of prostacyclin in primary pulmonary hypertension. One patient initially responded with an improvement in symptoms, but died suddenly after two weeks of treatment. Pulmonary congestion was found at autopsy. The second patient developed acute pulmonary edema during dose-ranging treatment with prostacyclin. The drug was discontinued and the patient was not treated further with vasodilators. This patient died 1 month after the prostacyclin trial (71).

A recent study designed to identify radiographic predictors of epoprostenol therapy raises more concern about the use of epoprostenol in patients with PVOD (72). Of 73 consecutive patients, 12 died within 4 months of starting epoprostenol. Radiographic findings of PVOD or pulmonary capillary hemangiomatosis (PCH), including ground-glass opacities, septal lines, pleural effusion and adenopathy, were significantly more common in the patients who died. Six of 12 patients who had died had post-mortem examinations: in all six the pathology revealed PVOD or PCH. PCH is characterized by infiltration and compression of pulmonary veins by neocapillaries, and leads to "secondary" PVOD. Therefore, the authors did not distinguish these two entities in their data analysis. The authors suggest that patients with chest CT findings suggestive of either of these diagnoses have further evaluation before starting epoprostenol (72). Acute pulmonary edema and death has previously been described in a patient with PCH who was treated with epoprostenol (73).

In the largest reported experience to date since PAH specific treatment has been widely available, Montani and colleague describe eleven patients with PVOD who were treated with intravenous prostacyclin. Five of these patients (44 percent) developed pulmonary edema. Importantly, there were no clinical predictors that identified these patients, and none of the patients developed pulmonary edema with acute vasodilator testing. Centrilobular ground-glass opacities and septal lines were present in 100 percent of the pulmonary edema group (21).

Endothelin-1 antagonists

Endothelin-1 may have an important role in intimal hyperplasia in human saphenous vein grafts, and a potential therapeutic potential for the prevention of graft stenosis is suggested (74,75). There is little experience with the use of endothelin-1 antagonists in PVOD and it is unknown whether this therapy has any beneficial effects. In the report by Montani and colleagues, six patients with PVOD were treated with bosentan, and 2/6 (33.3 percent) developed pulmonary edema (21).

Sildenafil

The experience with sildenafil is similarly scant. One patient with familial PAH who was subsequently found on lung biopsy to have PVOD improved while on sildenafil therapy (76). In a different report, one patient who was deteriorating on intravenous epoprostenol improved with the addition of sildenafil (77).

In contrast to the treatment of IPAH, the role of PAH-specific therapy in treatment of PVOD is not certain. The mixture of apparently positive and negative results, combined with the certain risk of causing pulmonary edema in a significant number of patients should cause the clinician to be circumspect and very cautious with these agents. However, given the dismal prognosis, we generally give most patients a careful therapeutic trial with careful monitoring.

Imatinib

Recently, imatinib has been reported to improve hemodynamics both experimentally and in patients with IPAH (78–80). Imatinib is a platelet-derived growth receptor antagonist which has antiproliferative effects on pulmonary vascular smooth muscle cells. The drug is approved for the treatment of various malignancies. At the time of this writing, a single patient experience is reported: a 56-year-old woman with PVOD was treated with imatinib after deteriorating on high-dose epoprostenol. She demonstrated a rapid improvement in clinical status and ground glass opacities. The authors speculated that the rapid improvement may have been due to imatinib's effect on endothelial vascular integrity, and thus a decrease in pulmonary edema, in addition to antiproliferative effects on vascular smooth muscle (81).

Lung transplantation

It is clear from the previous discussion, the therapeutic options for patients with PVOD are unproven. Lung transplantation may be the only treatment that is consistently capable of prolonging survival in patients with PVOD (82). However, some patients may respond to medical therapy, and the optimal timing of transplantation is uncertain. In addition, PVOD has been reported to recur in the transplanted lungs within three months of transplantation (83). The success of transplantation is limited by the availability of organs resulting in a prolonged waiting time. Once the diagnosis is made and referral is made for lung transplantation evaluation, many patients with PVOD do not survive long enough to benefit.

The prognosis for patients with PVOD remains poor. In a case series of 11 patients, eight of 11 patients died within 1 year of diagnosis. Of the three surviving patients, one had a clinical response to oral nifedipine, one was treated with epoprostenol, and one underwent a successful lung transplantation (12). In the retrospective series by Montani and colleagues, by the time of the report, 22/24 patients with PVOD either died or underwent lung transplantation. The average time from diagnosis to one of these outcomes was 11.8 months (21). With currently available information, no conclusions can be made regarding the medical therapy of choice in patients with PVOD. Lung transplantation may to be the only treatment capable of significantly improving survival.

KEY POINTS

- PVOD is a rare cause of pulmonary hypertension.
- The disease is characterized by wide-spread pulmonary venular obstruction due to intimal hyperplasia, muscularization of venular walls and *in-situ* thrombosis. In some cases, retrograde histopathology is apparent in the pulmonary arterioles, but is much less prominent than the venous changes. These pathological findings are distinct from other forms of pulmonary hypertension such as IPAH.
- The pathogenesis of the disorder is uncertain, but it is likely that PVOD represents a characteristic response to venular injury. Documentation of mutations in the BMPR2 receptor, and reported familial cases raise the possibility of an underlying genetic predisposition.
- Clinically, PVOD is difficult to differentiate from IPAH. However, signs and symptoms of pulmonary hypertension and pulmonary edema in the absence of left ventricular dysfunction should raise the question of PVOD. Prognosis is poor, and treatment is largely supportive.

REFERENCES

• = Key primary paper

♦ = Major review article

♦1. Rubin LJ. Current concepts: primary pulmonary hypertension. N Engl J Med 1997;336:111–7.

2. Simonneau G et al. Updated clinical classification of pulmonary hypertension. J Am Coll Cardiol 2009;54:543-54.

3. Höra J. Zur Histologie der klinischen "primaren Pulmonalsklerose." Frankfurt Z Pathol 1934;47:100-8.

•4. Heath D, Segel N, Bishop J. Pulmonary veno-occlusive disease. Circulation 1966;34:242-8.

5. Wagenvoort CA, Losekoot G, Mulder E. Pulmonary veno-occlusive disease of presumably intrauterine origin. Thorax 1971;26:429-34.

6. Glassroth J, Woodford DW, Carrington CB, Gaensler EA. Pulmonary veno-occlusive disease in the middle-aged. Respiration 1985;47:309-21.

◆7. Mandel J, Mark EJ, Hales CA. State of the art: pulmonary veno-occlusive disease. Am J Respir Crit Care Med 2000;162:1964-73.

8. Pietra GG. The pathology of primary pulmonary hypertension. In: LJ Rubin, S Rich, eds. Primary pulmonary hypertension: lung biology in health and disease. New York: Marcel Dekker, 1997:19-63.

9. Bjornsson J, Edwards WD. Primary pulmonary hypertension: a histopathologic study of 80 cases. Mayo Clin Proc 1985;60:16-25.

•10. Wagenvoort CA, Wagenvoort N. The pathology of pulmonary veno-occlusive disease. Virchows Arch Pathol Anat Histol 1974;364:69-79.

11. Pietra GG, Capron F, Stewart S, Leone O, Humbert M, Robbins IM, Reid LM, Tuder RM. Pathologic assessment of vasculopathies in pulmonary hypertension. J Am Coll Cardiol 2004;43(Suppl 12):25S-32S.

12. Holcomb BW, Loyd JE, Ely EW, Johnson J, Robbins IM. Pulmonary veno-occlusive disease: a case series and new observations. Chest 2000;118:1671-9.

•13. Wagenvoort CA, Wagenvoort N, Takahashi T. Pulmonary veno-occlusive disease: involvement of pulmonary arteries and review of the literature. Hum Pathol 1985;16:1033-41.

14. Chazova I, Robbins I, Loyd J, Newman J, Tapson V, Zhdaov V, Meyrick B. Venous and arterial changes in pulmonary veno-occlusive disease, mitral stenosis and fibrosing mediastinitis. Eur Respir 2000;15(1):116-22.

15. Braun A, Greenberg SD, Malik S, Jenkins DE. Pulmonary veno-occlusive disease associated with pulmonary phlebitis. Arch Pathol 1973;95:67-70.

16. Matyal R, Hales CA, Quinn DA. Stretch-induced IL-8 production in human pulmonary artery endothelial cells. Am J Crit Respir Care Med 2000;161:A417.

17. de Montpreville VT, Dulmet E, Fadel E, Dartevelle P. Lymph node pathology in pulmonary veno-occlusive disease and pulmonary capillary hemangiomatosis. Virchows Arch 2008;453:171-6.

18. Runo JR, Vnencak-Jones CL, Prince M et al. Pulmonary veno-occlusive disease caused by an inherited mutation in bone morphogenetic protein receptor II. Am J Respir Crit Care Med 2003;167:889-94.

19. Machado RD, Aldred MA, James V et al. Mutations of the TGF-β type II receptor BMPR2 in pulmonary arterial hypertension. Human Mutation 2006;27(2):121-32.

20. Aldred MA, Vijayakrishnan J, James V et al. BMPR2 gene rearrangements account for a significant proportion of mutations in familial and idiopathic pulmonary arterial hypertension. Human Mutation: Mutation in Brief #869 (2006) Online. J Hum Mutat 2006;27:212-3.

21. Montani D, Achouh L, Dorfmuller P et al. Pulmonary veno-occlusive disease: clinical, functional, radiologic and hemodynamic characteristics and outcome of 24 cases confirmed by histology. Medicine 2008;87(4):220-33.

22. Davies P, Reid L. Pulmonary veno-occlusive disease in siblings: Case reports and morphometric study. Hum Pathol 1982;13:911-5.

23. Rosenthal A, Vawter G, Wagenvoort CA. Intra-pulmonary veno-occlusive disease. Virchow Arch [Pathol Anat] 1974;364:69.

24. Voordes CG, Kuipers JRG, Elema JD. Familial pulmonary veno-occlusive disease: a case report. Thorax 1977;32:763-6.

◆25. Archer S, Rich S. Primary pulmonary hypertension: A vascular biology and translational "work in progress." Circulation 2000;102:2871-91.

26. Carrington CB, Liebow AA. Pulmonary veno-occlusive disease. Hum Pathol 1970;1:322-4.

27. Tingelstad JB, Aterman K, Lambert EC. Pulmonary venous obstruction. Report of a case mimicking primary pulmonary artery hypertension, with a review of the literature. Am J Dis Child 1969;117:219-27.

28. McDonnell PJ, Summer WR, Hutchins GM. Pulmonary veno-occlusive disease: morphological changes suggesting a viral cause. JAMA 1981;246:667-71.

29. Ruchelli ED, Nojadera G, Rutstein RM, Rudy B. Pulmonary veno-occlusive disease: another vascular disorder associated with human immunodeficiency virus infection? Arch Pathol Lab Med 1994;118:664-6.

30. Escamilla R, Hermant C, Berjaud J, Mazerolles C, Daussy X. Pulmonary veno-occlusive disease in a HIV-infected intravenous drug abuser. Eur Respir J 1995;8:1982-4.

31. Mette SA, Palevsky HI, Pietra GG et al. Primary pulmonary hypertension in association with human immunodeficiency virus infection. A possible viral etiology for some forms of hypertensive pulmonary arteriopathy. Am Rev Respir Dis 1992;145:1196-200.

32. Corrin B, Spencer H, Turner-Warwick M, Beales SJ, Hamblin JJ. Pulmonary veno-occlusion - an immune complex disease? Virchows Arch A Pathol Anat Histol 1974;364:81-91.

33. Kishida Y, Kanai Y, Kuramochi S, Hosoda Y. Pulmonary veno-occlusive disease in a patient with systemic lupus erythematosus. J Rheumatol 1993;20:2161-2.

34. Morassut PA, Walley VM, Smith CD. Pulmonary veno-occlusive disease and the CREST variant of scleroderma. Can J Cardiol 1992;8:1055-8.

35. Scully RE, Mark EJ, McNeely WF, McNeely BU. Case records of the Massachusetts General Hospital: weekly clinicopathologic exercises. Case 48 - 1993: a 27-year-old woman with mediastinal lymphadenopathy and relentless cor pulmonale. N Engl J Med 1993;329:1720-8.

36. Saito A, Takizawa H, Ito K, Yamamoto K, Oka T. A case of pulmonary veno-occlusive disease associated with systemic sclerosis. Respirology 2003;8(3):383–5.

37. Johnson SR, Patsios D, Hwang DM, Granton JT. Pulmonary veno-occlusive disease and scleroderma associated pulmonary hypertension. J Rheumatol 2006;33(11):2347–50.

38. Zhang L, Visscher D, Rihal C, Aubry MC. Pulmonary veno-occlusive disease as a primary cause of pulmonary hypertension in a patient with mixed connective tissue disease. Rheumatol Int 2007;27(12):1163–5.

39. Nunes H, Humbert M, Capron F, Brauner M, Sitbon O, Battesti JP, Simonneau G, Valeyre D. Pulmonary hypertension associated with sarcoidosis:mechanisms, haemodynamics and prognosis. Thorax 2006;61(1):68–74.

40. Liang MH, Stern S, Fortinn PR, Louie DC, Marsh JD, Mudge GH, Murphy G. Fatal pulmonary venoocclusive disease secondary to a generalized venopathy: a new syndrome presenting with facial swelling and pericardial tamponade. Arthritis Rheum 1991;34:228–33.

41. Salzman D, Adkins DR, Craig F, Freytes C, LeMaistre CF. Malignancy-associated pulmonary veno-occlusive disease: report of a case following autologous bone marrow transplantation and review. Bone Marrow Transplant 1996;18:755–60.

42. Hackman RC, Madtes DK, Petersen FB, Clark JG. Pulmonary veno-occlusive disease following bone marrow transplantation. Transplantation 1989;47:989–92.

43. Joselson R, Warnock M. Pulmonary veno-occlusive disease after chemotherapy. Hum Pathol 1983;14:88–91.

44. Lombard CM, Churg A, Winokur S. Pulmonary veno-occlusive disease following therapy for malignant neoplasms. Chest 1987;92:871–6.

45. Swift GL, Gibbs A, Campbell IA, Wagenvoort CA, Tuthill D. Pulmonary veno-occlusive disease and Hodgkin's lymphoma. Eur Respir J 1993;6:596–8.

46. Wingard JR, Mellits ED, Jones RJ, Beschorner WE, Sostrin MB, Burns WH, Santos GW, Saral R. Association of hepatic veno-occlusive disease with interstitial pneumonitis in bone marrow transplant recipients. Bone Marrow Transplant 1989;4:685–9.

47. Bunte MC, Patnaik MM, Pritzker MR, Burns LJ. Pulmonary veno-occlusive disease following hematopoietic stem cell transplantation: a rare model of endothelial dysfunction. Bone Marrow Transplant 2008;41(8):677–86.

48. Liu L, Sackler JP. A case of pulmonary veno-occlusive disease: etiological and therapeutic appraisal. Angiology 1973;23:299–304.

49. Townend JN, Roberts DH, Jones EL, Davies MK. Fatal pulmonary venoocclusive disease after use of oral contraceptives. Am Heart J 1992;124:1643–4.

50. Tsou E, Waldhorn RE, Kerwin DM, Katz S, Patterson JA. Pulmonary venoocclusive disease in pregnancy. Obstet Gynecol 1984;64:281–4.

51. Rabiller A, Jais X, Hamid A et al. Occult alveolar hemorrhage in pulmonary veno-occlusive disease. Eur Respir J 2006; 27:108–13.

52. Elliott CG, Colby TV, Hill T, Crapo RO. Pulmonary veno-occlusive disease associated with severe reduction of single-breath carbon monoxide diffusing capacity. Respiration 1988;53:262–6.

53. Resten A, Maitre S, Humbert M, Rabiller A, Sitbon O, Capron F, Simonneau G, Musset D. Pulmonary hypertension: CT of the chest in pulmonary venoocclusive disease. AJR Am J Roentgenol 2004;183:65–70.

54. Swensen SJ, Tashjian JH, Myers JL, Engeler CE, Patz EF, Edwards WD, Douglas WW. Pulmonary venoocclusive disease: CT findings in eight patients. AJR Am J Roentgenol 1996;167:937–40.

55. Scheibel RL, Dedeker KL, Gleason DF, Pliego M, Kieffer SA. Radiographic and angiographic characteristics of pulmonary veno-occlusive disease. Radiology 1972;103:47–51.

56. Rich S, Pietra GG, Kieras K, Hart K, Brundage BH. Primary pulmonary hypertension: radiographic and scintigraphic patterns of histologic subtypes. Ann Intern Med 1986;105:499–502.

57. Sola M, Garcia A, Picado C, Ramirez J, Plaza V, Herranz R. Segmental contour pattern in a case of pulmonary venoocclusive disease. Clin Nucl Med 1993;18:679–81.

58. Bailey CL, Channick RN, Auger WR, Fedullo PF, Kerr KM, Yung GL, Rubin LJ. "High probability" perfusion lung scans in pulmonary venoocclusive disease. Am J Respir Crit Care Med 2000;162:1974–8.

59. Bressollette E, Dupuis J, Bonan R, Doucet S, Cernacek P, Tardif JC. Intravascular ultrasound assessment of pulmonary vascular disease in patients with pulmonary hypertension. Chest 2001;120:809–15.

60. Weed HG. Commentary: Pulmonary "capillary" wedge pressure not the pressure in the pulmonary capillaries. Chest 1991;100(4):1138–40.

61. Davis LL, deBoisblanc BP, Glynn CE, Ramirez C, Summer WR. Effect of prostacyclin on microvascular pressures in a patient with pulmonary veno-occlusive disease. Chest 1995;108:1754–6.

62. Fesler P, Pagnamenta A, Vachiery JL et al. Single arterial occlusion to locate resistance in patients with pulmonary hypertension. Eur Respir J 2003;21:31–6.

63. Gilroy RJ Jr, Teague MW, Lloyd JE. Pulmonary veno-occlusive disease: fatal progression of pulmonary hypertension despite steroid-induced remission of interstitial pneumonitis. Am Rev Respir Dis 1991;143:1130–3.

64. Chawla SK, Kittle CF, Faber LP, Jensik RJ. Pulmonary veno-occlusive disease. Ann Thorac Surg 1976;22:249–53.

65. Williams LM, Fussell S, Veith RW, Nelson S, Mason CM. Pulmonary veno-occlusive disease in an adult following bone marrow transplantation. Chest 1996;109:1388–91.

66. Sanderson JE, Spiro SG, Hendry AT, Turner-Warwick M. A case of pulmonary veno-occlusive disease responding to treatment with azathioprine. Thorax 1977;32:140–8.

67. Cockrill BA, Kacmarek RM, Fifer MA, Bigatello LM, Ginns LC, Zapol WM, Semigran MJ. Comparison of the effects of nitric oxide, nitroprusside, and nifedipine on hemodynamics

and right ventricular contractility in patients with chronic pulmonary hypertension. Chest 2001;119:128–36.

ψ68.   Palevsky HI, Pietra GG, Fishman AP. Pulmonary veno-occlusive disease and its response to vasodilator agents. Am Rev Respir Dis 1990;142:426–9.

ψ69.   Rich S, Kaufmann E, Levy PS. The effect of high doses of calcium-channel blockers on survival in primary pulmonary hypertension. N Engl J Med 1992;327:76–81.

70.   Palmer SM, Robinson LJ, Wang A, Gossage JR, Bashore T, Tapson VF. Massive pulmonary edema and death after prostacyclin infusion in a patient with pulmonary veno-occlusive disease. Chest 1998;113:237–40.

ψ71.   Rubin LJ, Mendoza J, Hood M, McGoon M, Barst R, Williams WB, Diehl JH, Crow J, Long W. Treatment of primary pulmonary hypertension with continuous intravenous prostacyclin (epoprostenol). Results of a randomized trial. Ann Intern Med 1990;112:485–91.

72.   Resten A, Maitre S, Humbert M, Sitbon O, Capron F, Simoneau G, Musset D. Pulmonary arterial hypertensioin: thin-section CT predictors of epoprostenol therapy failure. Radiology 2002;222:782–8.

73.   Humbert M, Maitre S, Capron F, Rain B, Musset D, Simonneau G. Pulmonary edema complicating continuous intravenous prostacyclin in pulmonary capillary hemangiomatosis. Am J Respir Crit Care Med 1998;157:1681–5.

74.   Porter KE, Olojugba DH, Masood I, Permberton M, Bell PR, London NJ. Endothelin-B receptors mediate intimal hyperplasia in an organ culture of human saphenous vein. J Vasc Surg 1998;28:695–701.

75.   Dumont AS, Lovren F, McNeill JH, Sutherlnad GR, Triggle CR, Anderson TJ, Verma S. Augmentation of endothelial function by endothelin antagonism in human saphenous vein conduits. J Neurosurg 2001;94:281–6.

76.   Barreto AC, Franchi SM, Castro CRP, Lopes AA. One-year follow-up of the effects of sildenafil on pulmonary artery hypertension and veno-occlusive disease. Brazil J Med Biol Res 2005;38:185–95.

77.   Kuroda T, Hirota H, Masaki M, Sugiyama S, Oshina Y, Terai K, Ito A, Yamauchi-Takihara K. Sildenafil as adjunct therapy to high-dose epoprostenol in a patient with pulmonary veno-occlusive disease. Heart Lung Circ 2006;15:139–42.

78.   Schermuly RT, Dony E, Ghofrani HA et al. Reversal of experimental pulmonary hypertension by PDGF inhibition. J Clin Invest 2005;115(10):2811–21.

79.   Ghofrani HA, Seeger W, Grimminger F. Imatinib for the treatment of pulmonary arterial hypertension. N Engl J Med 2005;353(13):1412–3.

80.   Souza R, Sitbon O, Parent F, Simmonneau G, Humbert M. Long term imatinib treatment in pulmonary arterial hypertension. Thorax 2006;61:736.

81.   Overbeek MJ, van Nieuw Amerongen GP, Boonstra A, Smit EF, Vonk-Noordegraaf A. Possible role of imatinib in clinical pulmonary veno-occlusive disease. Eur Respir J 2008;32:232–5.

82.   Cassart M, Gevenois PA, Kramer M, Jacobovitz D, de Francquen P, Yernault JC, Estenne M. Pulmonary venoocclusive disease: CT findings before and after single-lung transplantation. AJR Am J Roentgenol 1993; 160:759–60.

83.   Izbicki G, Shitrit D, Schechtman I, Bendayan D, Fink G, Sahar G, Saute M, Ben-Gal T, Kramer MR. Recurrence of pulmonary veno-occlusive disease after heart–lung transplantation. J Heart Lung Transplant 2005;24:635–7.

Pulmonary capillary hemangiomatosis

DAVID LANGLEBEN

INTRODUCTION

Pulmonary capillary hemangiomatosis (PCH) is a rare condition caused by an overabundance of thin-walled, capillary-like vessels in the lung. It can present as pulmonary hypertension. Little is known about its development and management, but recent advances in the understanding of vascular growth control provide hope for improved therapy in the future.

DEFINITION AND PATHOLOGY

Although clinical findings may offer clues to its presence, the definitive identification of PCH requires microscopic examination of the lung parenchyma. The classic finding is a diffuse excess of capillary-like vessels, which can infiltrate the walls of small arteries and veins, and also thicken and infiltrate the alveolar walls and space (1,2) (Figures 19.3.1 and 19.3.2). The major feature distinguishing PCH from other conditions causing capillary dilatation, such as left heart disease or veno-occlusive disease, is that the vessels in PCH truly infiltrate other pulmonary structures, including the walls of larger arteries and veins, intralobular fibrous septa, and bronchi (1). Furthermore, in PCH the proliferation of capillaries within the alveolar septa and interstitium is at least two cell layers thick (3). Secondary muscularization of proximal pulmonary arteries may also develop, as is seen with most other forms of pulmonary hypertension. The combination of pulmonary venous hypertension from infiltrated, narrowed and fibrosed pulmonary veins, and the thin-walled nature of the abnormal

infiltrating capillaries themselves, leads to extravasation of erythrocytes into the interstitium and airspaces, with subsequent macrophage engulfment and deposition of hemosiderin (1,2). On gross examination of the lungs, multiple hemorrhagic patches, with firmer nodular areas, may be found (4–6). Rarely, capillary proliferation has also been described in the pericardium (7), pleura (7), and mediastinal lymph nodes (8,9).

Several other disorders must be considered in the differential diagnosis. First, pulmonary atelectasis and congestion with capillary dilatation may be confused for PCH. However, in that condition, reticulin staining of lung sections will reveal only a single row of capillaries in the alveolar septa, and no infiltration of other structures (3). Pulmonary veno-occlusive disease presents with many similar clinical features, and may be indistinguishable from PCH except by histologic examination (10). With veno-occlusive disease, fibrosis or sclerosis of small intrapulmonary veins is found, with secondary capillary dilatation. There is no evidence of infiltration into other structures, and only a single layer of capillaries is found within the alveolar septa (4,11,12). Diffuse pulmonary hemangiomatosis has been described in childhood, and can present with a clinical picture of interstitial disease and pleural effusions, but the hemangiomas are larger and do not invade other structures (13). Pulmonary lymphangioleiomyomatosis, leiomyomatosis, tuberous sclerosis, and lymphangiomatosis may have some common clinical features with PCH, but are distinct histologically (14–16). Intravascular lymphomatosis, also termed malignant angioendotheliomatosis, is a rare lymphoma which can present with pulmonary hypertension, but with a different

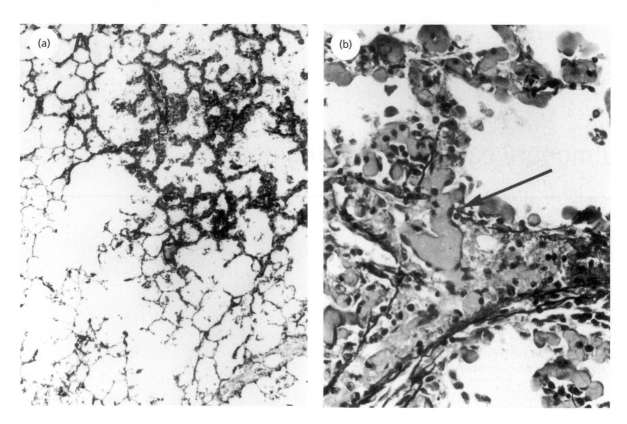

Figure 19.3.1 A low-power view (a) of a lung section showing the patchy and well-demarcated nature of the capillary proliferation within alveolar walls. Normal alveoli are present in the lower left. A higher power view (b) of an affected area. Capillaries of various sizes proliferate along the alveolar wall and bulge into the alveolar space. Some penetrate through the elastic lamina of a pulmonary venule (arrow) and proliferate inside the vessel. (Reproduced with permission from Annals Intern Med 1988;109:108.)

histology from PCH (17). Sclerosing hemangioma of the lung, originally attributed to proliferation of blood vessels with subsequent fibrosis, has been shown to be epithelial in origin, rather than endothelial (18). True isolated capillary hemangiomas of the lung may occur, and must be distinguished from PCH (19).

INCIDENCE/EPIDEMIOLOGY

PCH seems to be an exceedingly rare condition. Approximately 100 cases have been described in the literature (1–4,6–10,13,20–45). Its incidence is sporadic, although familial PCH has been described in three siblings, in a fashion suggesting autosomal recessive inheritance (20). PCH has been reported in patients ranging in age from neonates to late adulthood (13,31,32,43), with most patients presenting between the ages of 20 to 40 years. It appears that some individuals without any evidence of pulmonary hypertension may have PCH-like foci in their lungs at autopsy (3) or at incidental lung biopsy (41). In the autopsy series, eight (5.7 percent) of 140 patients had classic histologic findings of PCH (3). It is unknown whether they would have developed clinical symptoms with time. Survival after onset of symptoms ranges from one to five years.

ETIOLOGY, PATHOGENESIS AND CLASSIFICATION

There are no known causes of PCH. In the first case report of PCH in 1978, nuclear pleomorphism and hyperchromasia of the endothelial cells in the abnormal capillary-like vessels was described (1), suggesting a neoplastic process. After the recognition of a variety of disorders characterized by excessive blood vessel proliferation, termed angiogenic diseases (46), it was proposed that PCH represented an angiogenic disease of the lung (20). Abnormal monoclonal proliferation of endothelial cells has been described in idiopathic pulmonary arterial hypertension, consistent with neoplastic growth (47). Subsequently, mutations in the genes for receptors in the transforming growth factor-beta family, including bone morphogenic protein type II and activin like-kinase-I have been reported in heritable pulmonary arterial hypertension (48,49). These mutations may result in the proliferation of apoptosis-resistant endothelial clones (50,51). PCH may represent another form of unregulated endothelial growth. It might also be a *forme-fruste* of idiopathic pulmonary arterial hypertension. It is not known whether abnormalities of TGF-beta superfamily signal transduction cause PCH, but the possibility is intriguing. In support of the latter, there is one report of PCH in association with

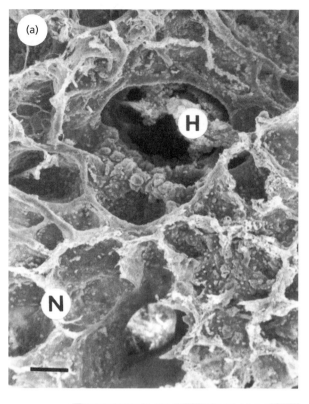

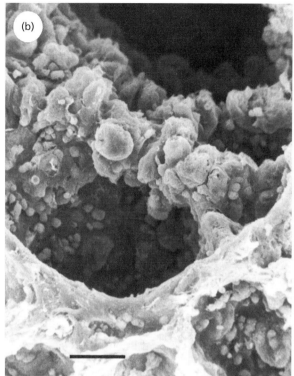

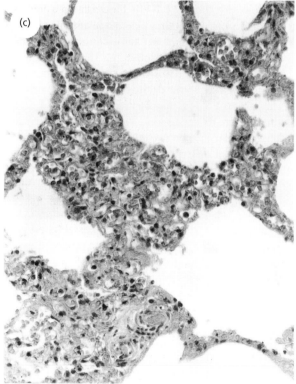

Figure 19.3.2 Scanning electron microscopy (a) of an affected lung. Capillaries are irregularly dilated and bulge into the alveolar space (H). The normal alveoli show a flat surface (N). A higher magnification (b) from area H of part A. Capillaries up to 30 m proliferate along the edge of, and also occasionally inside, the alveolus. Small round structures in the alveolus are mononuclear cells. A lung section (c) showing marked widening of alveolar walls by the capillary proliferation and thickening of the walls of small pulmonary blood vessels (bottom). (Reproduced with permission from Annals Intern Med 1988;109:108.)

hereditary hemorrhagic telangiectasia, a disorder that also causes heritable pulmonary arterial hypertension and is associated with mutations of receptors for the transforming growth factor beta family (52).

A variety of secondary disorders, including connective tissue disease or autoimmune disease, HIV infection, intracardiac shunts, and others, induce endothelial proliferation and plexiform lesion formation that is histologically similar to that of idiopathic pulmonary arterial hypertension (53). The mechanisms by which this process develops are not fully understood, but it has been suggested that chronic inflammation or shear stress injury to the pulmonary circulation can induce gene mutations that permit uncontrolled endothelial proliferation (54,55), similar to the phenomenon of chronic inflammatory bowel disease leading to colon cancer. PCH has been described in some patients with chronic illnesses (28–30,56–58), although it is not known if the occurrence is coincidental. The presence of fibrous long-spacing collagen, related to chronic inflammation or infection, has been associated with angiomatosis, and has been associated with one case of PCH (58).

As with idiopathic pulmonary arterial hypertension (59), endothelial nitric oxide synthase expression is decreased in PCH (36), but only in those patients who develop pulmonary hypertensive vascular remodeling. Similar to plexiform lesions, PCH lungs have increased expression of the proliferation and angiogenesis markers, vascular endothelial growth factor (VEGF) and MiB-1 (45). Unlike plexiform lesions, lungs affected by PCH retain some markers of cell growth suppression, such as peroxisome proliferator-activated receptor- and caveolin-1 (45). In another study, employing needle microdissection of proliferating capillaries from the explanted lungs of PCH patients, the genes for platelet-derived growth factor-B and platelet-derived growth factor receptor-ß, mast cell-related genes and type 2 pneumocyte genes were overexpressed (35). There were abundant mast cells in the lesions, as well as pericytes surrounding the proliferating capillaries. Urinary beta fibroblast growth factor levels have been described to be markedly increased, suggestive of pathologic angiogenesis (37). In that patient, levels of vascular endothelial growth factor and interleukin-8 were normal.

Despite many differences, there are many similarities of PCH and veno-occlusive disease to pulmonary arterial hypertension, and therefore both PCH and veno-occlusive disease are placed as category 1′, just beneath pulmonary arterial hypertension (category 1) in the recently revised pulmonary hypertension classification of the 4th World Symposium on Pulmonary Arterial Hypertension (60). There is still debate as to whether PCH and veno-occlusive disease represent separate entities (40).

CLINICAL PRESENTATION AND INVESTIGATIONS

There may be several distinct clinical presentations of PCH, depending on which pulmonary structures are infiltrated by the abnormal capillaries. Infiltration and narrowing of precapillary arterioles will cause the classic picture of idiopathic pulmonary arterial hypertension. Infiltration of pulmonary veins will cause a picture of pulmonary venous congestion, with secondary pulmonary hypertension. Infiltration of airspaces may affect gas transfer. Any and all of these patterns can be present in an individual patient.

The greatest diagnostic challenge is in patients who present with what seems to be classic idiopathic pulmonary

arterial hypertension, with clear lung fields on a chest x-ray, and a cardiac catheterization that detects pulmonary hypertension with a normal pulmonary artery wedge pressure (27). In those patients, the diagnosis is often missed, and PCH is only recognized when the patient deteriorates on vasodilator therapy. Any sign of pulmonary venous hypertension (Kerley-B lines, interstitial markings or pleural effusion on a chest x-ray or thoracic CT scan) in a patient with unexplained pulmonary hypertension should raise the possibility of PCH.

The initial case (1) and many subsequent cases have presented with signs of pulmonary venous dysfunction, and pulmonary congestion. Pulmonary hemorrhage with hemoptysis is present in over 30 percent of patients (8,26). Bronchoalveolar lavage may reveal erythrocyte extravasation into the bronchoalveolar fluid (9).The patients complain of dyspnea, orthopnea and cough. There may be a history of "asthma." Physical examination may reveal signs of increased pulmonary arterial pressure and right heart failure. Auscultation of the lungs may detect rales at the bases, and decreased air entry at the bases from pleural effusions.

On radiography of the chest, increased interstitial markings, patchy or diffuse reticulonodular infiltrates, cardiomegaly, enlarged central pulmonary vessels, and pleural effusions are found (6,7,23). Lung scintigraphy demonstrates a normal pattern of isotope distribution during inhalation of the isotope aerosol, or mildly decreased ventilation of the upper lobes, but the macroaggregated-albumin perfusion scans demonstrate nonhomogeneous perfusion, with some decreased perfusion to the upper lobes (26,61). There may be areas of enhanced perfusion, which seem to correspond to regions with particularly dense capillary proliferation (26). The lobar or segmental perfusion defects reported in chronic pulmonary thromboembolic disease have only been found in a few cases, and may correspond to areas of pulmonary hemorrhage or infarction (4,61). Thoracic CT scans reveal mediastinal and hilar adenopathy, enlargement of central pulmonary arteries, bilateral, diffuse intralobular septal thickening (smooth or nodular), centrilobular nodular opacities, focal areas of ground-glass opacification, and an absence of honeycombing (10,27,39,42). In the absence of histologic confirmation, the disorder may be confused for pulmonary veno-occlusive disease, even with the use of high-resolution CT scans (10).

Most patients develop signs of pulmonary hypertension with right failure. Cardiogenic shock, uncontrollable pulmonary edema, hemoptysis or pleural effusions are frequent causes of death.

PCH has been described in association with other diseases, including systemic lupus erythematosis, systemic sclerosis, hypertrophic cardiomyopathy, Takayasu's disease, sleep apnea, and AIDS (28–30,56–58). However, the rarity of the associations, and the finding of PCH-like foci in some clinically unaffected humans at routine autopsy, raises the possibility of coincidental occurrence (3).

TREATMENT/MANAGEMENT

A high index of suspicion of PCH must be present in patients with seeming idiopathic pulmonary arterial hypertension but who have signs of pulmonary venous congestion either before or during pulmonary vasodilator therapy. If any signs of pulmonary congestion are present, vasodilator therapy should be avoided, as the increased vascular flow in the presence of venous obstruction will result in alveolar capillary hydrostatic leakage. Catastrophic pulmonary congestion has been reported with either calcium blocker therapy or epoprostenol infusions (20,24,30).

Most cases of PCH have been diagnosed postmortem, but an increasing number are being diagnosed ante mortem, offering the opportunity for therapy (21,32). There are reports of successful treatment by orthotopic heart–lung transplantation in several (26,35), and by unilateral pneumonectomy in another case (21). However, *de novo* PCH in lungs from a previously healthy donor has been described 3 months after bilateral lung transplantation (38). Perhaps the most encouraging advance has been attempts at medical therapy. In one case, PCH was treated with the antiangiogenic agent, interferon alfa-2-a (32). The beneficial response was sustained at 14 months of therapy. However, another report described failure of interferon therapy (30). Another successful therapy in a single case involved oral doxycycline, a matrix metalloproteinase inhibitor which may reduce dysregulated angiogenesis (37). In that patient, after several weeks of therapy, pulmonary function test results and urinary beta-fibroblast growth factor levels had normalized, and there was sustained clinical benefit for greater than 18 months.

CONCLUSION

It has been proposed that PCH is not a new entity, but that it has only been recently been recognized (62). Reticulin staining of lung sections is particularly useful in the diagnosis as is CD 34 immunostaining to highlight the capillaries (40). There may be a wide spectrum of severity, and it is possible that many cases never become clinically relevant (3). However, with the appearance of symptoms, the course is usually fulminant and fatal. PCH may be neoplastic in origin, a congenital abnormality, or it may result from genetic mutations caused by chronic inflammation. At the present time, attacking the process with antiangiogenic agents may be the best option for medical therapy.

ACKNOWLEDGMENTS

Dr Langleben is a Chercheur-Boursier Clinicien National of the Fonds de la Recherche en Sante du Quebec, and is supported in part by the Bank of Montreal Center for the Study of Heart Disease in Women at the Jewish General Hospital.

REFERENCES

• = Key primary paper

•1. Wagenvoort CA, Beetstra A, Spijker J. Capillary hemangiomatosis of the lungs. Histopathology 1978; 2:401–6.
•2. Heath D, Reid R. Invasive pulmonary haemangiomatosis. Br J Diseases Chest 1985;79:284–94.
3. Havlik DM, Massie LW, Williams WL, Crooks LA. Pulmonary capillary hemangiomatosis-like foci. Am J Clin Pathol 2000; 113:655–62.
•4. Tron V, Magee F, Wright JL, Colby T, Churg A. Pulmonary capillary hemangiomatosis. Hum Pathol 1986;17:1144–50.
5. al-Fawaz IM, al-Mobaireek KF, al-Suhaibani M, Ashour M. Pulmonary capillary hemangiomatosis: a case report and review of the literature. Pediatr Pulmonol 1995;19:243–8.
6. Frazier AA, Franks TJ, Mohammed TL, Ozbudak IH, Galvin JR. From the archives of the AFIP: Pulmonary veno-occlusive disease and pulmonary capillary hemangiomatosis. RadioGraphics 2007;27:867–82.
7. Vevaina JR, Mark EJ. Thoracic hemangiomatosis masquerading as interstitial lung disease. Chest 1988; 93:657–9.
8. Whittaker JS, Pickering CAC, Heath D, Smith P. Pulmonary capillary haemangiomatosis. Diagnostic Histopathol 1983;6:77–84.
9. Domingo C, Encabo B, Roig J, Lopez D, Morera J. Pulmonary capillary hemangiomatosis: Report of a case and review of the literature. Respiration 1992;59:178–80.
10. Dufour B, Maitre S, Humbert M, Capron F, Simonneau G, Musset D. High-resolution CT of the chest in four patients with pulmonary capillary hemangiomatosis or pulmonary venoocclusive disease. Am J Roentgenol 1998;171:1321–4.
11. Wagenvoort CA, Wagenvoort N. The pathology of pulmonary veno-occlusive disease. Virchows Arch Pathol Anat 1974;364:69–79.

12. Daroca PJ, Mansfield RE, Ichinose H. Pulmonary veno-occlusive disease: report of a case with pseudoangiomatous features. Am J Surg Pathol 1977;1:349–55.

13. Rowen M, Thompson JR, Williamson RA, Wood BJ. Diffuse pulmonary hemangiomatosis. Radiology 1978;127:445–51.

14. Sherrier RH, Chiles C, Roggli V. Pulmonary lymphangioleiomyomatosis: CT findings. Am J Roentgenol 1989;153:937–40.

15. Wagener OE, Roncoroni AJ, Barcat JA. Severe pulmonary hypertension with diffuse smooth muscle proliferation of the lungs. Chest 1989;95:234–7.

16. Tazelaar HD, Kerr D, Yousem SA, Saldana MJ, Langston C, Colby TV. Diffuse pulmonary lymphangiomatosis. Hum Pathol 1993;24:1313–22.

17. Snyder LS, Harmon KR, Estensen RD. Intravascular lymphomatosis malignant angioendotheliomatosis presenting as pulmonary hypertension. Chest 1989;96:1199–200.

18. Alvarez-Fernandez E, Carretero-Albinana L, Menarguez-Palanaca J. Sclerosing hemangioma of the lung. Arch Pathol Lab Med 1989;113:121–4.

19. Fugo K, Matsuno Y, Okamoto K et al. Solitary capillary hemangioma of the lung: report of two resected cases detected by high-resolution CT. Am J Surg Pathol 2006; 30:750–3.

20. Langleben D, Heneghan JM, Batten AP, Wang NS, Fitch N, Schlesinger RD, Guerraty A, Rouleau JL. Familial pulmonary capillary hemangiomatosis resulting in primary pulmonary hypertension. Ann Intern Med 1988;109:106–9.

21. Wagenaar SJSC, Mulder JJS, Wagenvoort CA, Van Den Bosch JMM. Pulmonary capillary hemangiomatosis diagnosed during life. Histopathology 1989;14:212–4.

22. Masur Y, Remberger K, Hoefer M. Pulmonary capillary hemangiomatosis as a rare cause of pulmonary hypertension. Path Res Pract 1996;192:290–5.

23. Lippert JL, White CS, Cameron EW, Sun CC, Liang X, Rubin LJ. Pulmonary capilary hemangiomatosis: radiographic appearance. J Thoracic Imaging 1998;13:49–51.

24. Humbert M, Maitre S, Capron F, Rain B, Musset D, Simonneau G. Pulmonary edema complicating continuous intravenous prostacyclin in pulmonary capillary hemangiomatosis. Am J Resp Crit Care Med 1998;157:1681–5.

25. Magee F, Wright JL, Kay JM, Peretz D, Donevan R, Churg A. Pulmonary capillary hemangiomatosis. Am Rev Respir Dis 1985;132:922–5.

26. Faber CN, Yousem SA, Dauber JH, Griffith BP, Hardesty RL, Paradis IL. Pulmonary capillary hemangiomatosis. Am Rev Respir Dis 1989;140:808–13.

27. Eltorky MA, Headley AS, Winer-Muram H, Garrett HE, Griffin JP. Pulmonary capillary hemangiomatosis: a clinicopathologic review. Ann Thoracic Surg 1994;57:772–6.

28. Jing X, Yokoi T, Nakamura Y, Nakamura M, Shan L, Tomimoto S, Hano T, Kakudo K. Pulmonary capillary hemangiomatosis. A unique feature of congestive vasculopathy associated with hypertrophic cardiomyopathy. Arch Pathol Lab Med 1998;122:94–6.

29. Fernandez-Alonso J, Zulueta T, Reyes-Ramirez JR, Castillo-Palma MJ, Sanchez-Roman J. Pulmonary capillary hemangiomatosis as a cause of pulmonary hypertension in a young woman with systemic lupus erythematosus. J Rheumatology 1999;26:231–3.

30. Gugnani MK, Pierson C, Vanderheide R, Girgis RE. Pulmonary edema complicating prostacyclin therapy in pulmonary hypertension associated with scleroderma. Arthritis Rheum 2000;43:699–703.

31. Cioffi U, De Simone M, Pavoni G, Poggi L, Pisani D, Ferrero S, Santambrogio L. Pulmonary capillary hemangiomatosis in an asymptomatic elderly patient. Int Surg 1999;84:168–70.

•32. White CW, Sondheimer HM, Crouch EC, Wilson H, Fan LL. Treatment of pulmonary hemangiomatosis with recombinant interferon alfa-2-a. N Engl J Med 1989;320:1197–200.

33. Unterborn J, Mark EJ. Case records of the Massachusetts General Hospital: weekly clinicopathological exercises. New Engl J Med 2000;343:1788–96.

34. Channick RN, Olschewski H, Seeger W, Staub T, Voswinckel R, Rubin LJ. Safety and efficacy of inhaled treprostinil as add-on therapy to bosentan in pulmonary arterial hypertension. J Am Coll Cardiol 2006;48:1433–7.

35. Assaad AM, Kawut SM, Arcasoy SM, Rosenzweig EB, Wilt JS, Sonett JR, Borczuk AC. Platelet-derived growth factor is increased in pulmonary capillary hemangiomatosis. Chest 2007;131:850–5.

36. Kradin R, Matsubara O, Mark EJ. Endothelial nitric oxide synthase expression in pulmonary capillary hemangiomatosis. Exp Mol Pathol 2005;79:194–7.

•37. Ginns LC, Roberts DH, Mark EJ, Brusch JL, Marler JJ. Pulmonary capillary hemangiomatosis with atypical endotheliomatosis: successful antiangiogenic therapy with doxycycline. Chest 2003;124:2017–22.

38. de Perrot M, Waddell TK, Chamberlain D, Hutcheon M, Keshavjee S. De novo pulmonary capillary hemangiomatosis occurring rapidly after bilateral lung transplantation. J Heart Lung Transplant 2003;22:698–700.

39. El-Gabaly M, Farver CF, Budev MA, Mohammed TL. Pulmonary capillary hemangiomatosis imaging findings and literature update. (Review) (17 refs). J Computer Assisted Tomogr 2007;31:608–10.

40. Lantuejoul S, Sheppard MN, Corrin B, Burke MM, Nicholson AG. Pulmonary veno-occlusive disease and pulmonary capillary hemangiomatosis: a clinicopathologic study of 35 cases. Am J Surg Pathol 2006;30:850–7.

41. Moritani S, Ichihara S, Seki Y, Kataoka M, Yokoi T. Pulmonary capillary hemangiomatosis incidentally detected in a lobectomy specimen for a metastatic colon cancer. Pathol Internat 2006;56:350–7.

42. Lawler LP, Askin FB. Pulmonary capillary hemangiomatosis: multidetector row CT findings and clinico-pathologic correlation. J Thoracic Imag 2005;20:61–3.

43. Oviedo A, Abramson LP, Worthington R, Dainauskas JR, Crawford SE. Congenital pulmonary capillary hemangiomatosis: Report of two cases and review of the literature. Pediatr Pulmonol 2003;36:253–6.

44. Oviedo A, Abramson LP, Worthington R, Dainauskas JR, Crawford SE. Congenital pulmonary capillary

hemangiomatosis: Report of two cases and review of the literature. Pediatr Pulmonol 2003;36:253–6.

45. Sullivan A, Chmura K, Cool CD, Keith R, Schwartz GG, Chan ED. Pulmonary capillary hemangiomatosis: an immunohistochemical analysis of vascular remodeling. Eur J Med Res 2006;11:187–93.

46. Folkman J, Klagsbrun M. Angiogenic factors. Science 1987;235:442–7.

47. Lee SD, Shroyer KR, Markham NE, Cool CD, Voelkel NF, Tuder RM. Monoclonal endothelial cell proliferation is present in primary but not secondary pulmonary hypertension. J Clin Invest 1998;101:927–34.

48. Deng Z, Morse JH, Slager SL et al. Familial primary pulmonary hypertension gene PPH1 is caused by mutations in the bone morphogenic protein receptor-II gene. Am J Hum Genet 2000;67:737–44.

49. Lane KB, Machado RD, Pauciulo MW, Thompson JR, Phillips JA, Loyd JE, Nichols WC, Trembath RC. Heterozygous germline mutations in BMPR2, encoding a TGF-beta receptor, cause familial primary pulmonary hypertension. The International PPH Consortium. Nature Genet 2000;26:81–4.

50. Teichert-Kuliszewska K, Kutryk MJB, Kuliszewski MA et al. Bone morphogenic protein receptor-2 signalling promotes pulmonary arterial endothelial cell survival: implications for loss-of-function mutations in the pathogenesis of pulmonary hypertension. Circ Res 2006;98:209–17.

51. Michelakis ED. Spatio-temporal diversity of apoptosis within the vascular wall in pulmonary hypertension: heterogeneous BMP signalling may have therapeutic implications. Circ Res 2006;98:172–5.

•52. Varnholt H, Kradin R. Pulmonary capillary hemangiomatosis arising in hereditary hemorrhagic telangiectasia. Hum Pathol 2004;35:266–8.

53. Rich S. Executive summary from the World Symposium – Primary Pulmonary Hypertension. Available at: http://www.who.int/ncd/cvd/pph.html. 1998.

54. Yeager ME, Halley GR, Galphon HA, Voelkel NF, Tuder RM. Microsatellite instability of endothelial cell growth and apoptosis genes within plexiform lesions in primary pulmonary hypertension. Circ Res 2001;88:E2–E11.

55. Voelkel NF, Cool CD, Lee SD, Wright L, Geraci MW, Tuder RM. Primary pulmonary hypertension between inflammation and cancer. Chest 1998;114:225S–30S.

56. Kakkar N, Vasishta RK, Banerjee AK, Singh S, Kumar L. Pulmonary capillary hemangiomatosis as a cause of pulmonary hypertension in Takayasu's aortoarteritis. Respiration 1997;64:381–3.

57. Ahemd Q, Chung-Park M, Tomashefski JF. Cardiopulmonary pathology in patients with sleep apnea/obesity hypoventilation syndrome. Hum Pathol 1997;28:264–9.

58. Borczuk AC, Niedt G, Sablay LB, Kress Y, Mannion CM, Factor SM, Tanaka KE. Fibrous long-spacing collagen in bacillary angiomatosis. Ultrastructural Pathol 1998;22:127–33.

59. Giaid A, Saleh D. Reduced expression of endothelial nitric oxide synthase in the lungs of patients with primary pulmonary hypertension. N Engl J Med 1995;333:214–21.

60. Simonneau G et al. Updated clinical classification of pulmonary hypertension. J Am Coll Cardiol 2009;54:543–54.

61. Rush C, Langleben D, Schlesinger RD, Stern J, Wang NS, Lamoureux E. Lung scintigraphy in pulmonary capillary hemangiomatosis. Clin Nucl Med 1991;16:913–7.

62. Thurlbeck WM. Pulmonary capillary hemangiomatosis as a rare cause of pulmonary hypertension. Pathol Res Pract 1996;192:298–9.

PULMONARY HYPERTENSION ASSOCIATED WITH DISORDERS OF THE RESPIRATORY SYSTEM AND/OR HYPOXEMIA

PART 8

Pulmonary hypertension due to chronic hypoxic lung disease: Chronic obstructive pulmonary disease and interstitial lung disease

JOAN ALBERT BARBERÀ, ISABEL BLANCO AND SANDRA PIZARRO

INTRODUCTION

Pulmonary hypertension (PH) is an important complication in the natural history of chronic respiratory diseases, particularly in chronic obstructive pulmonary disease (COPD) and interstitial lung diseases (ILD). In these conditions, the presence of PH is associated with reduced survival and worse clinical course. The prevalence of PH in respiratory diseases is not negligible. It can be close to 50 percent or even greater in patients with advanced disease. In respiratory diseases PH is usually of moderate severity and progresses slowly, without altering right ventricular function in the majority of cases. Nevertheless, a reduced subgroup of patients may present disproportionate PH, with pulmonary artery pressure (PAP) largely exceeding the severity of respiratory impairment. These patients may depict a clinical picture similar to more severe forms of PH and have greater mortality. Recent studies providing evidence on the important role of the endothelial cell and its derived mediators in the pathogenesis of PH associated with respiratory diseases have provided the rationale for the potential use of agents that modulate endothelial function in the treatment of this condition.

In the present chapter we will review the clinical relevance of PH, its pathogenesis, diagnosis and management, in the setting of the two most common respiratory disorders presenting this complication, COPD and ILD.

PULMONARY HYPERTENSION IN COPD

Chronic obstructive pulmonary disease is defined in terms of airflow obstruction that results from an inflammatory process affecting the airways and lung parenchyma. Despite major abnormalities in the airways and lung parenchyma, changes in pulmonary vessels represent an important component of the disease. Alterations in vessel structure are highly prevalent and abnormalities in their function impair gas exchange and result in PH, one of the principal factors associated with reduced survival in COPD. Studies revealing endothelial dysfunction at early disease stages have contributed to a better understanding of the pathogenesis of PH in this disease (1,2) and opened a potential new approach for its treatment.

Prevalence

The actual prevalence of PH in COPD is unknown, because it has not been screened systematically using right heart catheterization in the wide clinical spectrum of the disease. Furthermore, the criteria used to define PH in COPD vary among different studies. Whereas some authors have used the conventional criteria used to define pulmonary arterial hypertension (PAH), that is mean PAP ≥ 25 mmHg, others have used a value greater than 20 mmHg, the upper limit of PAP in healthy subjects (3) (Table 20.1.1).

Table 20.1.1 Hemodynamic characteristics and prevalence of pulmonary hypertension in COPD

Author	N	Design	FEV$_1$	PaO$_2$ (mmHg)	DLCO (percent pred.)	mPAP (mmHg)	CI (L/min/m²)	PVR (dyn s cm^{-5})	Defining PH criteria[a] (mPAP)	Prevalence of PH[b] (percent)
Burrows (14)	50	Prospective	37 percent FVC	NR	81	26	2.5	468	>25 mmHg	20
Weitzenblum (11)	175	Prospective	40 percent FVC	63	NR	20	3.2	NR	>20 mmHg	35
Weitzenblum (37)	93	Prospective	41 percent FVC	66	NR	19	3.6	NR	>20 mmHg	34
Oswald-Mammosser (13)	84	Prospective. Patients undergoing LTOT	36 percent FVC	52	NR	27	NR	NR	>20 mmHg	77
Scharf (38)	120	Retrospective. patients included in NETT	27 percent pred.	66	27	26	2.9	193	>20 mmHg	91
Thabut (7)	215	Retrospective. candidates for LVRS or LT	24 percent pred.	62	NR	27	3.0	376[c]	>25 mmHg	50

[a]Value of mean pulmonary artery pressure (mPAP) used to define pulmonary hypertension (PH). [b]According to the defining PH criteria. [c]Pulmonary vascular resistance (PVR) index.

Abbreviations: FEV$_1$: forced expiratory volume in the first second; PaO$_2$: partial pressure of arterial oxygen; DLCO: diffusion capacity for carbon monoxide; CI: cardiac index; NR: not reported; FVC: forced vital capacity; LTOT: long-term oxygen therapy; NETT: national emphysema treatment trial; LT: lung transplantation; LVRS: lung volume reduction surgery.

Hemodynamic studies involving a large number of subjects have been performed in patients with advanced COPD (stage IV of the GOLD classification) (4). In this subgroup the prevalence of PH is very high, ranging between 50 percent and 91 percent, depending on the criteria used to define it (Table 20.1.1). Nevertheless, in the majority of patients PH is of mild-to-moderate severity (<30 mmHg). Severe PH is rarely seen in COPD. In a retrospective study conducted in 998 COPD patients, Chaouat *et al.* (5) identified only 27 patients with PAP >40 mmHg. Whereas 16 of them had another disease capable of causing PH, in 11 (1.1 percent of the whole group), COPD was the only cause. The latter group of patients had moderate airway obstruction (FEV$_1$ 50 percent pred.), severe hypoxemia, hypercapnia and very low CO diffusing capacity (DLCO). These findings indicate that there is a reduced subset of COPD patients with *out-of-proportion* PH that share some clinical features with idiopathic PAH (6). Similar results have been obtained by Thabut *et al.* (7) who identified in a cluster analysis a subgroup of COPD patients characterized by moderate impairment of airway function and high levels of PAP, along with severe arterial hypoxemia (Figure 20.1.1).

In patients with mild-to-moderate disease, the prevalence of PH is considered to be low. However, in these patients PH might not be present at rest, but develops during exercise (8). The exact prevalence of exercise-induced PH in patients with moderate COPD is unknown, but might be high based on histological analyses revealing significant pulmonary vascular changes in the majority of patients with mild COPD (2,9,10).

Prognostic significance

Patients with COPD and PH have shorter survival than patients with normal PAP (11) and the presence of PH or *cor pulmonale* is one of the best predictors of mortality (12,13). Survival is inversely related to PH severity (14) and mortality is significantly increased in patients with out-of-proportion PH (5) (Figure 20.1.2). Furthermore, echocardiographic signs of right ventricular dysfunction (15) and electrocardiographic signs of right ventricular hypertrophy or right atrial overload (16) are also predictive of survival in COPD.

In addition to the prognostic significance in relation to survival, the presence of PH in COPD is associated with poor clinical evolution and more frequent use of health care resources (17). A PAP >18 mmHg is one of the best predictors of increased risk of hospitalization for COPD exacerbation, likely suggesting that patients with an abnormal pulmonary vascular bed might have lesser functional reserve to overcome the changes that occur during exacerbation episodes.

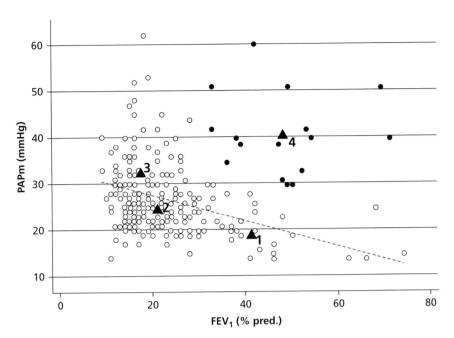

Figure 20.1.1 Relationship between pulmonary artery pressure (PAP) and FEV$_1$ in 215 patients with severe COPD. A cluster analysis identified four groups of patients. Groups 1, 2 and 3 (open symbols) followed the expected inverse relationship between PAP and FEV$_1$. Group 4 consists of a group of patients characterized by moderate airflow obstruction that contrast with high (out-of-proportion) pulmonary hypertension (closed symbols). Triangles indicate the average values in each group. (From Thabut et al. (7).)

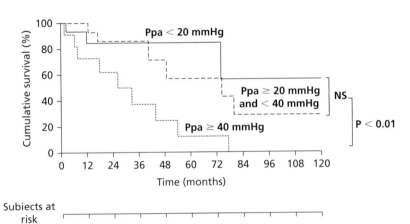

Figure 20.1.2 Survival of patients with COPD and no other detectable cause of pulmonary hypertension divided according to the value of mean pulmonary artery pressure (Ppa). The probability of survival, estimated using the Kaplan–Meier method, was significantly reduced in the subgroup of patients with out-of-proportion pulmonary hypertension (Ppa > 40 mmHg). NS = not significant. (From Chaouat et al. (5).)

Pulmonary vascular remodeling

Remodeling of pulmonary vessels is the major cause of PH in COPD. It affects small and precapillary arteries and has been identified at different degrees of disease severity. The most prominent feature of pulmonary vascular remodeling is the enlargement of the intimal layer in muscular arteries (2,9,18). Intimal hyperplasia is produced by the proliferation of smooth muscle cells (SMC), which in advanced stages conform bundles of longitudinal muscle that differs from the normal circumferential disposition (19), and deposition of elastic and collagen fibers (19–21) (Figure 20.1.3). In the arterioles there is development of a medial coat of circular smooth muscle bounded by a new elastic lamina (19,22).

Intimal hyperpalasia of pulmonary muscular arteries is apparent at all disease stages. In mild-to-moderate COPD the majority of SMC proliferating in hyperplasic intimas have a poorly differentiated phenotype, as shown by the

lack of expression of contractile filaments that are characteristic of mature cells (23) (Figure 20.1.3).

Changes in the tunica media are less conspicuous and the majority of morphometric studies have failed to demonstrate differences in the thickness of the muscular layer when comparing COPD patients with control subjects (2,9,18).

Remodeling of pulmonary arteries is not restricted to patients with an established diagnosis of COPD. Indeed, intimal thickening, the magnitude of which does not differ from that seen in patients with mild-to-moderate COPD, is also present in heavy smokers with normal lung function (23).

COPD is an inflammatory disease, hence inflammatory cells might contribute to the alterations of pulmonary vessels. Patients with COPD have an increased number of inflammatory cells infiltrating the adventitia of pulmonary muscular arteries, as compared with nonsmokers (10). This inflammatory infiltrate is largely constituted by activated

T-lymphocytes with a predominance of the CD8[+] subset (10,24) (Figure 20.1.3). By contrast, the number of neutrophils, macrophages and B-lymphocytes are minimal and do not differ from control subjects.

Interestingly, smokers with normal lung function also show an increased number of CD8[+] T-cells in the arterial adventitia, with a reduction of the CD4[+]/CD8[+] ratio, as compared with nonsmokers, which does not differ from patients with mild-to-moderate COPD (10).

Pathogenesis

As in other pulmonary hypertensive states, endothelial dysfunction of pulmonary arteries plays a crucial role in the pathogenesis of PH in COPD. It has been shown in patients with end-stage COPD (25) and also in patients with mild-to-moderate disease (2). Impairment of endothelial function is associated with or results from changes in the expression or balanced release of endothelium-derived vasoactive agents. The expression of endothelial nitric oxide synthase (eNOS) and prostacyclin synthase (PGI_2-S) are significantly reduced in pulmonary arteries of COPD patients (26,27) (Figure 20.1.3). Furthermore, the expression of some growth factors (vascular endothelial growth factor, VEGF) (21) or their receptors (transforming growth factor-β type II receptor) (28) is upregulated in pulmonary arteries of COPD patients.

Hypoxia has been classically considered the main pathogenic mechanism of PH in COPD. However, its role is currently being reconsidered because pulmonary vascular remodeling and endothelial dysfunction can be observed in patients with mild COPD who do not have hypoxemia and in smokers with normal lung function (9,10,23), and because long-term oxygen therapy does not fully reverse PH (29). Furthermore, the relationship between arterial PO_2 and PAP is very weak (Figure 20.1.4).

Recent observations indicate that cigarette smoke products might cause pulmonary vascular impairment in COPD (1). This suggestion arises from the observation that smokers with normal lung function show remodeling in pulmonary arteries (23), impairment of endothelial function (2), reduced expression of eNOS (26), increased VEGF expression (21) and inflammatory cell infiltrate (10), that are indistinguishable from those seen in patients with mild-to-moderate COPD, and clearly differ from nonsmokers. Furthermore, guinea pigs chronically exposed to cigarette smoke develop PH and vessel remodeling (30), changes that antecede the development of emphysema (31). In this animal model, cigarette smoke exposure induces rapid changes in gene expression of VEGF, VEGF receptor-1, endothelin-1 (ET-1) and inducible NOS (32), mediators that regulate vascular cell growth and vessel contraction, and are likely involved in the pathogenesis of pulmonary vascular changes of COPD. In addition, exposure of pulmonary artery endothelial cells to cigarette smoke extract causes an irreversible inhibition of eNOS activity, which is

due to diminished protein content and mRNA (33). Cigarette smoke contains a number of products that have the potential to produce endothelial injury; among these the aldehyde acrolein seems to play a prominent role (27).

Accordingly, the initial event in the natural history of PH in COPD appears to be the injury of pulmonary endothelium by cigarette-smoke products. Indeed, lesions of endothelial cells in pulmonary arteries from COPD patients can be identified on microscopic observation as areas of denuded endothelium (34) (Figure 20.1.5). Endothelial damage results in the abnormal synthesis and release of vasoactive mediators that impair endothelium-dependent vasodilation (2,26) and favors the action of factors that promote the proliferation of SMC and extracellular matrix deposition. All these changes may contribute to intimal hyperplasia with the ensuing reduction of arterial lumen and increase of pulmonary vascular resistance (PVR). Arteries with endothelial dysfunction are more susceptible to the action of additional factors. Among these, sustained arterial hypoxemia and alveolar hypoxia in poorly ventilated lung units play a crucial role, since they may induce further endothelial impairment and vessel remodeling, either directly or through VEGF-dependent mechanisms, thus amplifying the initial effects of cigarette smoke products. Similar effects might be produced by cytokines released by inflammatory cells.

Pathophysiology and natural history

Pulmonary hypertension in COPD is usually of low to moderate severity and mean PAP rarely exceeds 35–40 mmHg. Cases exceeding these values are considered out-of-proportion PH and represent only 1–3 percent of patients (5,7). Both right atrial pressure and pulmonary artery occlusion pressure tend to be normal, as well as the cardiac output (14,35,36).

At their initial stage, PH in COPD may not be apparent at rest, but might develop during exercise (8). Patients with exercise-induced PH are more prone to develop resting PH in subsequent years (8).

Pulmonary hypertension in COPD progresses over time and its severity correlates with the degree of airflow obstruction and the impairment of pulmonary gas exchange (37,38). The rate of progression of PH is slow, with an average PAP increase of 0.6 mmHg per year (37). Since PAP is only moderately elevated and its rate of progression is slow, the right ventricle (RV) has time to adapt to such a modest increase in afterload. When PAP is chronically elevated the RV dilates and both end-diastolic and end-systolic volumes increase. The stroke volume of the RV is usually maintained, whereas its ejection fraction decreases. Yet, in clinically stable patients RV contractility lies within normal limits irrespective of the PAP value (39,40). Decreased RV contractility in COPD has been observed only during exacerbation episodes in patients presenting marked peripheral edema (41,42).

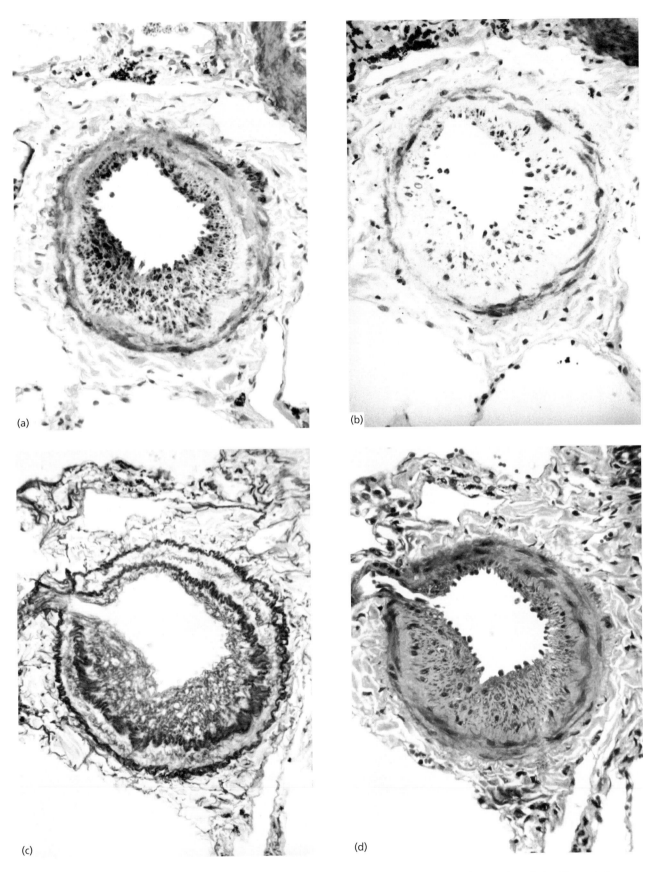

Figure 20.1.3 Pulmonary vascular remodeling in COPD. Sections of pulmonary muscular arteries showing prominent intimal hyperplasia. Immunostaining for α-smooth muscle actin (a) reveals intimal proliferation of smooth muscle cells, although not all them show immunoreactivity to desmin (b) a contractile filament expressed in mature smooth muscle cells, thus indicating a poorly differentiated state. Staining for elastic (c) and collagen (d) fibers shows marked elastosis and fibrosis of the intima. Immunostaining with monoclonal antibody against CD8.

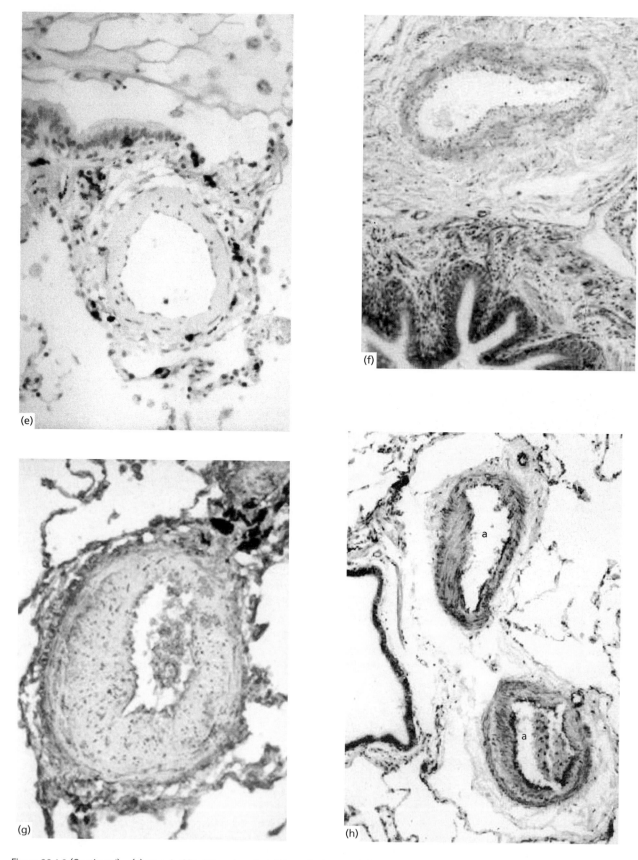

Figure 20.1.3 (Continued)   (e) reveals CD8 T-lymphocyte infiltrate in the arterial adventitia. Pulmonary arteries of patients with mild-to-moderate COPD show reduced expression of endothelial nitric oxide synthase (eNOS) in endothelial cells (f) with no increase in the expression of endothelin-1 (g). In contrast, the expression of vascular endothelial growth factor (VEGF) is augmented in the arterial wall in moderate COPD (h) [*a* denotes pulmonary muscular artery].

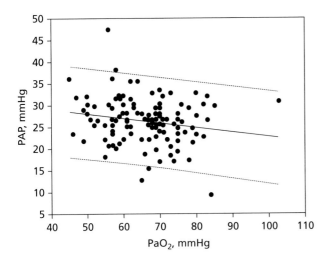

Figure 20.1.4 Relationship between partial pressure of arterial oxygen (PaO_2) and pulmonary artery pressure (PAP) in 120 patients with severe emphysema. Despite a significant correlation between both measurements ($r = -0.11$, $P = 0.03$), the plot of the data reveals substantial scatter in the relationship (data obtained from Scharf *et al.* (38).)

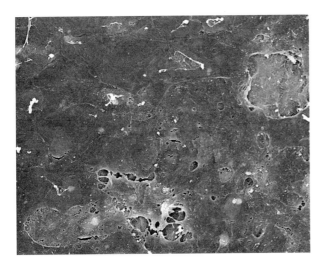

Figure 20.1.5 Scanning electron microscopy of the endothelial surface of pulmonary arteries in COPD. The endothelial surface shows denuded areas where endothelial cells have detached from the subendothelial tissue and gaps between endothelial junctions.

In clinically stable COPD, peripheral edema is not a sign of RV failure since it might be present in patients without evidence of reduced cardiac output (41,43). In COPD, peripheral edema results from a complex interaction between the hemodynamic changes and the balance between edema-promoting and edema-protective mechanisms (44,45). In patients with PH associated with chronic respiratory failure, both hypoxemia and hypercapnia aggravate venous congestion by further activating the sympathetic nervous system, already stimulated by right atrial distension. Sympathetic activation decreases renal plasma flow, stimulates the renin-angiotensin-aldosterone system,

and promotes tubular absorption of bicarbonate, sodium and water. Vasopressin also contributes to edema formation. It is released when patients become hyponatremic and its plasma levels rise in patients with hypoxemia and hypercapnia (44).

Evaluation and diagnosis

Recognition of PH in COPD is difficult, especially in its mildest form, because symptoms due to PH, such as dyspnea or fatigue, are difficult to differentiate from the clinical picture of COPD. Furthermore, the identification of some clinical signs may be obscured by chest hyperinflation or the large swings in intrathoracic pressure. Usually, the main suspicion is based in the presence of peripheral edema, but, as discussed above, in COPD this may not be a sign of right ventricular failure. Cardiac sounds may be disturbed by the presence of bronchial rales or overinflated lungs and the typical auscultatory findings of PH are uncommon in COPD patients.

Evaluation may include:

- Routine examinations (4,5,16,46,47)
- Echocardiography (Table 20.1.2 and 48–54)
- Right heart catheterization (55, not routinely recommended)

In summary, clinical suspicion of PH in patients with COPD should be high if clinical deterioration is not matched to the decline in pulmonary function. Profound hypoxemia, hyperventilation and low DLCO are indicators of possible PH. Once PH is suspected patients should be evaluated by Doppler echocardiography and, if confirmed, undergo right heart catheterization in those circumstances where the result of the procedure will determine its clinical management.

Treatment

In patients with associated PH, COPD should be optimally treated according to existing guidelines (4). Treatment addressed to ameliorate PH in COPD includes long-term oxygen therapy (LTOT) (40,56–63); vasodilators (Figure 20.1.6; 64–82) and, eventually, new specific PAH therapy (see below).

NEW SPECIFIC THERAPY FOR PULMONARY ARTERIAL HYPERTENSION

Specific PAH therapy (prostanoids, ET-1 receptor antagonists and phosphodiesterase-5 inhibitors), addressed to revert or compensate the unbalanced release of endothelium-derived vascular mediators, improves symptoms, exercise performance, pulmonary hemodynamics and survival in some forms of PAH. Considering that the pathogenesis of PH in COPD shares some common pathways with that of

Table 20.1.2 Doppler echocardiography in the diagnosis of pulmonary hypertension in COPD

Author	N	Defining PH criteria[a] (mmHg)	Sensitivity (95 percent CI)	Specificity (95 percent CI)	PPV (95 percent CI)	NPV (95 percent CI)
Arcasoy (51)	96	>45	76 (50–93 percent)	65 (54–75 percent)	32 (18–48 percent)	93 (83–98 percent)
Fisher (52)	63	>40	60 percent (42–76 percent)	74 percent (58–87 percent)	68 percent (49–83 percent)	67 percent (51–81 percent)

[a]Value of systolic pulmonary artery pressure estimated by Doppler echocardiography used to define pulmonary hypertension (PH).
Abbreviations: CI: confidence interval; PPV: positive predictive value; NPV: negative predictive value.

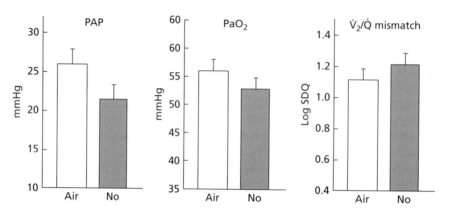

Figure 20.1.6 Effect of the inhibition of hypoxic pulmonary vasoconstriction in COPD. The administration of inhaled nitric oxide (NO) to 13 patients with COPD produced a significant decrease of pulmonary artery pressure (PAP), but at the same time worsened arterial hypoxemia. The latter resulted from the increase in ventilation-perfusion (V_A/Q) mismatching due to the inhibition of hypoxic pulmonary vasoconstriction by NO (Data obtained from Barberà et al. (56).)

PAH, it is conceivable that drugs that may correct the endothelial vasoconstrictor-dilator imbalance could be of clinical benefit in COPD (83,84). See also Table 20.1.3 and refs 85–92.

In summary, the treatment of choice in patients with PH associated with COPD who are hypoxemic is LTOT. In the subgroup of patients with out-of-proportion PH, specific PAH therapy might be considered, although ideally this should be done in the setting of clinical trials. The use of specific PAH therapy in patients with COPD and moderate PH is currently discouraged because there are no systematic data regarding its efficacy and there is compelling evidence indicating that these drugs might worsen pulmonary gas exchange.

PULMONARY HYPERTENSION IN INTERSTITIAL LUNG DISEASES

Interstitial lung diseases (ILD) are a group of diffuse parenchymal lung diseases that share similar clinical, radiologic and pulmonary function characteristics, resulting from the damage of lung parenchyma by varying patterns of inflammation and fibrosis (93). Interstitial lung diseases consist of disorders of known causes (collagen vascular disease, environmental or drug related) and disorders

of unknown etiology. The latter group includes idiopathic interstitial pneumonias (IIPs), granulomatous lung disorders (e.g. sarcoidosis) and other forms of ILD (lymphangioleiomyomatosis (LAM), pulmonary Langerhans' cell histiocytosis and eosinophilic pneumonia). The most important distinction among IIPs is between idiopathic pulmonary fibrosis (IPF) and the other interstitial pneumonias (nonspecific interstitial pneumonia, desquamative interstitial pneumonia, respiratory bronchiolitis-associated interstitial lung disease, acute interstitial pneumonia, cryptogenic organizing pneumonia and lymphocytic interstitial pneumonia) (93).

The majority of ILD have been associated with PH, although its prevalence varies greatly depending on the underlying disease. The most extensive available data refers to IPF associated PH.

Epidemiology

The prevalence of PH, assessed by right heart catheterization, in patients with severe IPF ranges between 32 percent and 46 percent (94–97) (Table 20.1.4). Pulmonary hypertension is more prevalent in patients with worse lung function, although other factors including age, duration of the disease, need for supplemental oxygen and reduced exercise tolerance are also associated with the presence of PH

Table 20.1.3 New specific therapy for pulmonary arterial hypertension in COPD

Author	Drug	Design	N	Dose (mg)	Time (months)	6MWD (m)		PAP (mmHg)		PaO$_2$ (mmHg)	
						Pre	Post	Pre	Post	Pre	Post
Alp (90)	Sildenafil	Uncontrolled	6	50 b.i.d.	3	351 ± 49	433 ± 52*	30 ± 6	25 ± 4*	NR	NR
Madden[a] (89)	Sildenafil	Uncontrolled	7	50 t.i.d.	2	107 ± 76	145 ± 96*	39 ± 10	35 ± 9	NR	NR
Rietema (91)	Sildenafil	Uncontrolled	14	20 t.i.d.	3	385 ± 135	394 ± 116	20 ± 9	NR	NR	NR
Stolz (88)	Bosentan	Double-blind, placebo-controlled	30	125 b.i.d.	3	331 ± 123	329 ± 94	32 (29–38)[b]	30 (26–34)[b]	65 ± 11	61 ± 8*

[a]Four patients had COPD and three idiopathic pulmonary fibrosis. [b]Measured by Doppler echocardiography; values are median (interquartile range).
*$P < 0.05$ compared with pre-treatment value.
Definition of abbreviations: 6MWD: distance covered in the 6 min walk test; PAP: pulmonary artery pressure; PaO$_2$: partial pressure of arterial oxygen; NR: not reported.

in IPF. The combination of lung fibrosis with emphysema is associated with a higher prevalence of PH (98).

In sarcoidosis, the presence of PH is often associated with advanced fibrotic disease and the development of hypoxemia. One study reported a 28 percent prevalence of PH in patients with sarcoidosis (94). The prevalence of PH in other ILD is unknown. It has been rarely reported in LAM and in Langerhans' cell hystiocitosis.

The presence of PH has prognostic importance in IPF. Nadrous *et al.* (99) reported shorter survival in patients with IPF and systolic PAP > 50 mmHg, assessed by echocardiography, than patients below this value. Furthermore, Lettieri *et al.* (94) showed that in patients with IPF listed for lung transplantation, the presence of PH was associated with greater mortality (Figure 20.1.7). Considering that mean survival after the diagnosis in IPF is only 2.5–3.5 years (100), the presence of associated PH represents a sign of very poor prognosis in this condition.

Pathology and pathogenesis

There is probably no single pathologic mechanism that links ILD to PH. The vasculopathy of IPF consists of medial and intimal enlargement of pulmonary arteries. In addition, intimal lesions can progress to fibrosis with the consequent luminal obliteration. Presumably, the most important mechanism involved in the pathogenesis of PH in IPF is the destruction of lung tissue, with the consequent loss of vasculature, and vessel fibrosis in the affected regions. Fibrotic areas have markedly reduced vascular density, as shown by the absence of endothelial cell markers in fibroblastic foci (101).

A weak correlation between PAP and PaO$_2$ suggests a potential role of hypoxemia in the development of PH in IPF (102). However, the pattern of vascular remodeling, the lack of reversibility with oxygen and the presence of PH in patients with mild hypoxemia suggests that hypoxemia *per se* is not the only cause of this complication.

Alterations in the synthesis and release of certain endothelium-derived vasoactive mediators may be involved in the pathogenesis of IPF-associated PH. Among those, ET-1 appears to play a prominent role. Endothelin-1 is prominently expressed in lung tissue of patients with IPF, specially in airway epithelium and type II pneumocytes, particularly those lining areas of young granulation tissue (103). Interestingly, ET-1 immunoreactivity and mRNA are present in pulmonary vascular endothelial cells in patients with associated PH (103). Furthermore, patients with IPF have increased plasma levels of ET-1 and its concentration correlates with disease progression and the presence of PH (104).

Pathophysiology

In general, in IPF PH is of mild-to-moderate severity, with only few subjects developing severe PH, usually at the end-stage of the disease.

Pulmonary vascular involvement in ILD affects the efficiency of gas exchange. Agustí *et al.* (105) showed that the increase in mean PAP, along with the decline in arterial PO$_2$, and the impairment of V$_A$/Q distributions during exercise were related to the severity of structural vascular changes.

Evaluation and diagnosis

Similarly to that which occurs in COPD, in ILD clinical symptoms of PH appear late in the course of the disease and may be masked by the underlying pulmonary disorder. Suspicion of the disease might be raised by conventional examinations like ECG, usually showing right ventricular hypertrophy and right atrial dilatation, and chest x-ray that may show proximal pulmonary artery and/or right ventricular enlargement.

In patients with ILD the DLCO falls due to the enlargement of the interstitial space and the vascular disease (106).

Table 20.1.4 Prevalence of pulmonary hypertension in idiopathic pulmonary fibrosis

Author	N	Design	FVC (percent pred.)	DLCO (percent pred.)	PaO$_2$ (mmHg)	mPAP (mmHg)	CI (L min m^{-2})	Defining PH criteria[a]	Prevalence of PH[b] (percent)
Lettieri (94)	79	Retrospective. patients undergoing LT	49	31	NR	30	3.2	RHC mPAP >25 mmHg	32
Shorr (95)	2525	Retrospective. LT registry	48	NR	41	NR	2.8	RHC mPAP >25 mmHg	46
Zisman (96)	61	Retrospective	54	30	58	34	NR	RHC mPAP >25 mmHg	39
Nadrous (99)[c]	88	Retrospective	64	54	74	43[d]	2.7	DE sPAP >35 mmHg	84
Nathan (97)	60	Retrospective	51	30	NR	25	NR	RHC mPAP >25 mmHg	35

[a]Value of mean pulmonary artery pressure (PAP) used to define pulmonary hypertension (PH). [b]According to the defining PH criteria. [c]Patients who underwent Doppler echocardiography at initial evaluation. [d] Estimated by Doppler echocardiography.

Abbreviations: FVC: forced vital capacity; percent pred.: percentage of predicted value; DLCO: diffusion capacity for carbon monoxide; PaO$_2$: partial pressure of arterial oxygen; mPAP: mean pulmonary artery pressure; CI: cardiac index; RHC: right heart catheterization, LT: lung transplantation; NR: not reported; DE: Doppler echocardiography; sPAP: estimated systolic PAP.

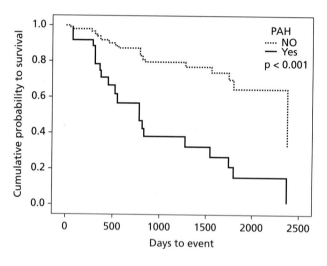

Figure 20.1.7 Prognostic significance of pulmonary hypertension in idiopathic pulmonary fibrosis (IPF). Kaplan–Meier estimates of survival in 79 patients with IPF divided according to the presence of pulmonary hypertension (mean pulmonary artery pressure >25 mmHg). Survival was significantly reduced in patients presenting pulmonary hypertension (from Lettieri *et al.* (94).)

In these patients, a reduction in DLCO disproportionate to the reduction in lung volumes might suggest underlying pulmonary vascular disease. Indeed, in IPF the prevalence of PH is higher in subjects with DLCO values below 40 percent predicted (93).

As in other conditions, Doppler echocardiography is the essential tool for the detection of PH. Nevertheless, its accuracy in ILD is low. In IPF, Nathan *et al.* (97) have recently reported that only 40 percent of echocardiographic measurements accurately reflected the value of systolic PAP,

as compared with right heart catheter measurements (97). In general, echocardiography tends to overestimate the true PAP value. The sensitivity of echocardiography in detecting catheter-proven PH was 73 percent and the specificity 45 percent, considering a cut-off value of systolic PAP >40 mmHg (97). The diagnostic performance of Doppler echocardiography improved slightly when it was considered together with the results of the 6 min walk test and pulmonary function testing (97).

Accordingly, right heart catheterization is mandatory to confirm the diagnosis of PH in ILD. The procedure should be reserved to those patients in whom the result of the hemodynamic assessment will determine treatment options (e.g. listing or prioritization for lung transplant) or cases potentially suitable for specific PAH therapy.

Treatment

There is no specific information on the hemodynamic effects of LTOT in patients with ILD and associated PH. Conceivably, LTOT might be of clinical benefit, especially in patients experiencing oxygen desaturation during exercise or nocturnal hypoxemia.

A number of trials have evaluated the effects of vasodilators (hydralazine, calcium channel blockers) for the treatment of PH in ILD, all of them with negative results (107). Furthermore, there are some theoretical risks to vasodilation in patients with ILD since these drugs inhibit HPV and might contribute to worsening gas exchange, since in IPF HPV contributes to V$_A$/Q matching (105).

Few studies have evaluated the efficacy of specific PAH therapy in patients with ILD and associated PH. See refs 108–112 for more details.

Based on the pathogenic role that some mediators may have in both the development of PH and the progression of pulmonary fibrosis, clinical trials are currently conducted addressed to assess the effects of specific PAH therapy in ILD associated PH. Results of these trials will provide evidence on the potential usefulness of that therapy in ILD. In the meantime, it seems reasonable to consider the use of specific PAH therapy only in those cases with disproportionally elevated PH in the setting of clinical trials or registries and in PH expert units.

KEY POINTS

- Pulmonary hypertension (PH) is a common complication of chronic obstructive pulmonary disease (COPD) and idiopathic pulmonary fibrosis (IPF) that, when present, is associated with greater mortality and worse clinical course.
- In advanced COPD, PH is highly prevalent, affecting more than 50 percent of patients. In end-stage IPF, the prevalence of PH ranges between 32 percent and 46 percent.
- In chronic respiratory diseases, PH is usually of mild-to-moderate severity and progresses slowly, with preserved right ventricular function. Only a reduced subgroup of patients (1–3 percent in COPD) may present severe PH, with PAP exceeding 40–45 mmHg, disproportionately high to the degree of respiratory impairment. These patients have shorter survival and share some clinical features similar to idiopathic PAH.
- Echocardiography is the best screening tool for the assessment of PH in respiratory diseases, although its diagnostic performance is lower than in other forms of PH. The diagnosis of PH relies on right heart catheterization. The procedure is indicated in candidates to surgical treatments; suspected out-of-proportion PH potentially amenable with targeted therapy; and, in general, those conditions where the result of the hemodynamic assessment will determine treatment options.
- The treatment of choice for patients with chronic respiratory diseases and associated PH who are hypoxemic is long-term oxygen therapy.
- Conventional vasodilators are not recommended because they may impair gas exchange due to the inhibition of hypoxic pulmonary vasoconstriction, and their lack of efficacy after long-term use.
- In the subgroup of patients with out-of-proportion PH, targeted PH therapy could be considered, preferably in expert centers and in the context of clinical trials. The use of targeted therapy in patients with respiratory diseases and moderate PH is currently discouraged because there are no systematic data regarding its safety or efficacy.

REFERENCES

1. Barberà JA, Peinado VI, Santos S. Pulmonary hypertension in chronic obstructive pulmonary disease. Eur Respir J 2003;21:892–905.
2. Peinado VI, Barberà JA, Ramirez J, Gomez FP, Roca J, Jover L, Gimferrer JM, Rodriguez-Roisin R. Endothelial dysfunction in pulmonary arteries of patients with mild COPD. Am J Physiol 1998;274:L908–13.
3. Kovacs G, Scheidl S, Olschewski H. Pulmonary arterial pressure at rest and during exercise in normal controls. Eur Respir J 2008;32:261s.
4. Rabe KF, Hurd S, Anzueto A, Barnes PJ, Buist SA, Calverley P et al. Global strategy for the diagnosis, management, and prevention of chronic obstructive pulmonary disease: GOLD executive summary. Am J Respir Crit Care Med 2007;176:532–55.
5. Chaouat A, Bugnet AS, Kadaoui N, Schott R, Enache I, Ducolone A et al. Severe pulmonary hypertension and chronic obstructive pulmonary disease. Am J Respir Crit Care Med 2005;172:189–94.
6. Chaouat A, Naeije R, Weitzenblum E. Pulmonary hypertension in COPD. Eur Respir J 2008;32:1371–85.
7. Thabut G, Dauriat G, Stern JB, Logeart D, Levy A, Marrash-Chahla R, Mal H. Pulmonary hemodynamics in advanced COPD candidates for lung volume reduction surgery or lung transplantation. Chest 2005;127:1531–6.
8. Kessler R, Faller M, Weitzenblum E, Chaouat A, Aykut A, Ducolone A, Ehrhart M, Oswald-Mammosser M. "Natural history" of pulmonary hypertension in a series of 131 patients with chronic obstructive lung disease. Am J Respir Crit Care Med 2001;164:219–24.
9. Barberà JA, Riverola A, Roca J, Ramirez J, Wagner PD, Ros D, Wiggs BR, Rodriguez-Roisin R. Pulmonary vascular abnormalities and ventilation-perfusion relationships in mild chronic obstructive pulmonary disease. Am J Respir Crit Care Med 1994;149:423–9.
10. Peinado VI, Barberà JA, Abate P, Ramirez J, Roca J, Santos S, Rodriguez-Roisin R. Inflammatory reaction in pulmonary muscular arteries of patients with mild chronic obstructive pulmonary disease. Am J Respir Crit Care Med 1999;159:1605–11.
11. Weitzenblum E, Hirth C, Ducolone A, Mirhom R, Rasaholinjanahary J, Ehrhart M. Prognostic value of pulmonary artery pressure in chronic obstructive pulmonary disease. Thorax 1981;36:752–8.
12. Traver GA, Cline MG, Burrows B. Predictors of mortality in chronic obstructive pulmonary disease. A 15-year follow-up study. Am Rev Respir Dis 1979;119:895–902.
13. Oswald-Mammosser M, Weitzenblum E, Quoix E, Moser G, Chaouat A, Charpentier C, Kessler R. Prognostic factors in COPD patients receiving long-term oxygen therapy. Importance of pulmonary artery pressure. Chest 1995;107:1193–8.
14. Burrows B, Kettel LJ, Niden AH, Rabinowitz M, Diener CF. Patterns of cardiovascular dysfunction in chronic obstructive lung disease. N Engl J Med 1972;286:912–8.

15. Burgess MI, Mogulkoc N, Bright-Thomas RJ, Bishop P, Egan JJ, Ray SG. Comparison of echocardiographic markers of right ventricular function in determining prognosis in chronic pulmonary disease. J Am Soc Echocardiogr 2002;15:633–9.

16. Incalzi RA, Fuso L, De Rosa M, Di Napoli A, Basso S, Pagliari G, Pistelli R. Electrocardiographic signs of chronic cor pulmonale: a negative prognostic finding in chronic obstructive pulmonary disease. Circulation 1999;99:1600–5.

17. Kessler R, Faller M, Fourgaut G, Mennecier B, Weitzenblum E. Predictive factors of hospitalization for acute exacerbation in a series of 64 patients with chronic obstructive pulmonary disease. Am J Respir Crit Care Med 1999;159:158–64.

18. Magee F, Wright JL, Wiggs BR, Paré PD, Hogg JC. Pulmonary vascular structure and function in chronic obstructive pulmonary disease. Thorax 1988;43:183–9.

19. Wilkinson M, Langhorne CA, Heath D, Barer GR, Howard P. A pathophysiological study of 10 cases of hypoxic cor pulmonale. Q J Med 1988;249:65–85.

20. Wright JL, Petty T, Thurlbeck WM. Analysis of the structure of the muscular pulmonary arteries in patients with pulmonary hypertension and COPD: National Institutes of Health nocturnal oxygen therapy trial. Lung 1992;170:109–24.

21. Santos S, Peinado VI, Ramirez J, Morales-Blanhir J, Bastos R, Roca J, Rodriguez-Roisin R, Barbera JA. Enhanced expression of vascular endothelial growth factor in pulmonary arteries of smokers and patients with moderate chronic obstructive pulmonary disease. Am J Respir Crit Care Med 2003;167:1250–6.

22. Hale KA, Ewing SL, Gosnell BA, Niewoehner DE. Lung disease in long-term cigarette smokers with and without chronic airflow obstruction. Am Rev Respir Dis 1984;130:716–21.

23. Santos S, Peinado VI, Ramirez J, Melgosa T, Roca J, Rodriguez-Roisin R, Barberà JA. Characterization of pulmonary vascular remodelling in smokers and patients with mild COPD. Eur Respir J 2002;19:632–8.

24. Saetta M, Baraldo S, Corbino L, Turato G, Braccioni F, Rea F et al. CD8+ve cells in the lungs of smokers with chronic obstructive pulmonary disease. Am J Respir Crit Care Med 1999;160:711–7.

25. Dinh-Xuan AT, Higenbottam T, Clelland C, Pepke-Zaba J, Cremona G, Butt AY et al. Impairment of endothelium-dependent pulmonary-artery relaxation in chronic obstructive pulmonary disease. N Engl J Med 1991;324:1539–47.

26. Barberà JA, Peinado VI, Santos S, Ramirez J, Roca J, Rodriguez-Roisin R. Reduced expression of endothelial nitric oxide synthase in pulmonary arteries of smokers. Am J Respir Crit Care Med 2001;164:709–13.

27. Nana-Sinkam SP, Lee JD, Sotto-Santiago S, Stearman RS, Keith RL, Choudhury Q et al. Prostacyclin prevents pulmonary endothelial cell apoptosis induced by cigarette smoke. Am J Respir Crit Care Med 2007;175:676–85.

28. Beghe B, Bazzan E, Baraldo S, Calabrese F, Rea F, Loy M et al. Transforming growth factor-β type II receptor in pulmonary arteries of patients with very severe COPD. Eur Respir J 2006;28:556–62.

29. Weitzenblum E, Sautegeau A, Ehrhart M, Mammosser M, Pelletier A. Long-term oxygen therapy can reverse the progression of pulmonary hypertension in patients with chronic obstructive pulmonary disease. Am Rev Respir Dis 1985;131:493–8.

30. Wright JL, Churg A. Effect of long-term cigarette smoke exposure on pulmonary vascular structure and function in the guinea pig. Exp Lung Res 1991;17:997–1009.

31. Yamato H, Churg A, Wright JL. Guinea pig pulmonary hypertension caused by cigarette smoke cannot be explained by capillary bed destruction. J Appl Physiol 1997;82:1644–53.

32. Wright JL, Tai H, Dai J, Churg A. Cigarette smoke induces rapid changes in gene expression in pulmonary arteries. Lab Invest 2002;82:1391–8.

33. Su Y, Han W, Giraldo C, Li YD, Block ER. Effect of cigarette smoke extract on nitric oxide synthase in pulmonary artery endothelial cells. Am J Respir Cell Mol Biol 1998;19:819–25.

34. Peinado VI, Ramirez J, Roca J, Rodriguez-Roisin R, Barbera JA. Identification of vascular progenitor cells in pulmonary arteries of patients with chronic obstructive pulmonary disease. Am J Respir Cell Mol Biol 2006;34:257–63.

35. Fishman AP. State of the art: chronic cor pulmonale. Am Rev Respir Dis 1976;114:775–94.

36. Naeije R. Should pulmonary hypertension be treated in chronic obstructive pulmonary disease? In: Weir EK, Archer SL, Reeves JT (eds). The diagnosis and treatment of pulmonary hypertension. Mount Kisco, Futura Publishing, 1992;209–39.

37. Weitzenblum E, Sautegeau A, Ehrhart M, Mammosser M, Hirth C, Roegel E. Long-term course of pulmonary arterial pressure in chronic obstructive pulmonary disease. Am Rev Respir Dis 1984;130:993–8.

38. Scharf SM, Iqbal M, Keller C, Criner G, Lee S, Fessler HE. Hemodynamic characterization of patients with severe emphysema. Am J Respir Crit Care Med 2002;166:314–22.

39. Crottogini AJ, Willshaw P. Calculating the end-systolic pressure–volume relation. Circulation 1991;83:1121–3.

40. Biernacki W, Flenley DC, Muir AL, MacNee W. Pulmonary hypertension and right ventricular function in patients with COPD. Chest 1988;94:1169–75.

41. MacNee W, Wathen CG, Flenley DC, Muir AD. The effects of controlled oxygen therapy on ventricular function in patients with stable and decompensated cor pulmonale. Am Rev Respir Dis 1988;137:1289–95.

42. Weitzenblum E, Apprill M, Oswald M, Chaouat A, Imbs JL. Pulmonary hemodynamics in patients with chronic obstructive pulmonary disease before and during an episode of peripheral edema. Chest 1994;105:1377–82.

43. MacNee W, Wathen CG, Hannan WJ, Flenley DC, Muir AL. Effects of pirbuterol and sodium nitroprusside on pulmonary haemodynamics in hypoxic cor pulmonale. Br Med J (Clin Res Ed) 1983;287:1169–72.

44. Lee-Chiong TL, Matthay RA. The heart in the stable COPD patient. In: Similowski T, Whitelaw WA, Derenne JP (eds). Clinical management of chronic obstructive pulmonary disease. New York: Marcel Dekker, Inc., 2002:475–532.

45. Palange P. Renal and hormonal abnormalities in chronic obstructive pulmonary disease (COPD). Thorax 1998;53: 989–91.

46. Oswald-Mammosser M, Oswald T, Nyankiye E, Dickele MC, Grange D, Weitzenblum E. Non-invasive diagnosis of pulmonary hypertension in chronic obstructive pulmonary disease. Comparison of ECG, radiological measurements, echocardiography and myocardial scintigraphy. Eur J Respir Dis 1987;71:419–29.

47. Wiedemann HP, Matthay RA. Heart Disease. A Textbook of Cardiovascular Medicine. Philadelphia: WB Saunders Company, 1997.

48. Torbicki A, Skwarski K, Hawrylkiewicz I, Pasierski T, Miskiewicz Z, Zielinski J. Attempts at measuring pulmonary arterial pressure by means of Doppler echocardiography in patients with chronic lung disease. Eur Respir J 1989;2: 856–60.

49. Laaban JP, Diebold B, Zelinski R, Lafay M, Raffoul H, Rochemaure J. Noninvasive estimation of systolic pulmonary artery pressure using Doppler echocardiography in patients with chronic obstructive pulmonary disease. Chest 1989;96:1258–62.

50. Naeije R, Torbicki A. More on the noninvasive diagnosis of pulmonary hypertension: Doppler echocardiography revisited. Eur Respir J 1995;8:1445–9.

51. Arcasoy SM, Christie JD, Ferrari VA, Sutton MS, Zisman DA, Blumenthal NP, Pochettino A, Kotloff RM. Echocardiographic assessment of pulmonary hypertension in patients with advanced lung disease. Am J Respir Crit Care Med 2003; 167:735–40.

52. Fisher MR, Criner GJ, Fishman AP, Hassoun PM, Minai OA, Scharf SM, Fessler AH. Estimating pulmonary artery pressures by echocardiography in patients with emphysema. Eur Respir J 2007;30:914–21.

53. Turhan S, Dincer I, Ozdol C, Rahimov U, Kilickap M, Altin T et al. Value of tissue Doppler myocardial velocities of tricuspid lateral annulus for the diagnosis of right heart failure in patients with COPD. Echocardiography 2007; 24:126–33.

54. Takakura M, Harada T, Fukuno H, Okushi H, Taniguchi T, Sawada S et al. Echocardiographic detection of occult cor pulmonale during exercise in patients with chronic obstructive pulmonary disease. Echocardiography 1999; 16:127–34.

55. Yusen RD, Lefrak SS, Trulock EP. Evaluation and preoperative management of lung volume reduction surgery candidates. Clin Chest Med 1997;18:199–224.

56. Barberà JA, Roger N, Roca J, Rovira I, Higenbottam TW, Rodriguez-Roisin R. Worsening of pulmonary gas exchange with nitric oxide inhalation in chronic obstructive pulmonary disease. Lancet 1996;347:436–40.

57. DeGaute JP, Domenighetti G, Naeije R, Vincent JL, Treyvaud D, Perret C. Oxygen delivery in acute exacerbation of chronic obstructive pulmonary disease. Effects of controlled oxygen therapy. Am Rev Respir Dis 1981;124:26–30.

58. MacNee W. Pathophysiology of cor pulmonale in chronic obstructive pulmonary disease. Part Two. Am J Respir Crit Care Med 1994;150:1158–68.

59. Lejeune P, Mols P, Naeije R, Hallemans R, Melot C. Acute hemodynamic effects of controlled oxygen therapy in decompensated chronic obstructive pulmonary disease. Crit Care Med 1984;12:1032–5.

60. Olvey SK, Reduto LA, Stevens PM, Deaton WJ, Miller RR. First pass radionuclide assessment of right and left ventricular ejection fraction in chronic pulmonary disease. Effect of oxygen upon exercise response. Chest 1980;78:4–9.

61. Report of the Medical Research Council Working Party. Long term domiciliary oxygen therapy in chronic hypoxic cor pulmonale complicating chronic bronchitis and emphysema. Lancet 1981;i:681–5.

62. Nocturnal oxygen therapy trial group. Continuous or nocturnal oxygen therapy in hypoxemic chronic obstructive lung disease. A clinical trial. Ann Intern Med 1980;93: 391–8.

63. Ashutosh K, Mead G, Dunsky M. Early effects of oxygen administration and prognosis in chronic obstructive pulmonary disease and cor pulmonale. Am Rev Respir Dis 1983;127:399–404.

64. Simonneau G, Escourrou P, Duroux P, Lockhart A. Inhibition of hypoxic pulmonary vasoconstriction by nifedipine. N Engl J Med 1981;304:1582–5.

65. Muramoto A, Caldwell J, Albert RK, Lakshminarayan S, Butler J. Nifedipine dilates the pulmonary vasculature without producing symptomatic systemic hypotension in upright resting and exercising patients with pulmonary hypertension secondary to chronic obstructive pulmonary disease. Am Rev Respir Dis 1985;132:963–6.

66. Agustí AGN, Barberà JA, Roca J, Wagner PD, Guitart R, Rodriguez-Roisin R. Hypoxic pulmonary vasoconstriction and gas exchange during exercise in chronic obstructive pulmonary disease. Chest 1990;97:268–75.

67. Naeije R, Melot C, Mols P, Hallemans R. Effects of vasodilators on hypoxic pulmonary vasoconstriction in normal man. Chest 1982;82:404–10.

68. Barberà JA. Chronic obstructive pulmonary disease. In: Roca J, Rodriguez-Roisin R, Wagner PD (eds). Pulmonary and peripheral gas exchange in health and disease. New York: Marcel Dekker, Inc., 2000:229–61.

69. Mélot C, Hallemans R, Naeije R, Mols P, Lejeune P. Deleterious effect of nifedipine on pulmonary gas exchange in chronic obstructive pulmonary disease. Am Rev Respir Dis 1984;130:612–6.

70. Bratel T, Hedenstierna G, Nyquist O, Ripe E. The use of a vasodilator, felodipine, as an adjuvant to long-term oxygen treatment in COLD patients. Eur Respir J 1990;3:46–54.

71. Andrivet P, Chabrier PE, Defouilloy C, Brun-Buisson C, Adnot S. Intravenously administered atrial natriuretic factor in patients with COPD. Effects on ventilation-perfusion relationships and pulmonary hemodynamics. Chest 1994;106:118–24.

72. Adnot S, Kouyoumdjian C, Defouilloy C, Andrivet P, Sediame S, Herigault R, Fratacci MD. Hemodynamic and gas exchange responses to infusion of acetylcholine and inhalation of nitric oxide in patients with chronic obstructive lung disease and pulmonary hypertension. Am Rev Respir Dis 1993;148:310–6.

73. Sturani C, Bassein L, Schiavina M, Gunella G. Oral nifedipine in chronic cor pulmonale secondary to severe chronic obstructive pulmonary disease (COPD). Chest 1983;84:135–42.

74. Agostoni P, Doria E, Galli C, Tamborini G, Guazzi MD. Nifedipine reduces pulmonary pressure and vascular tone during short- but not long-term treatment of pulmonary hypertension in patients with chronic obstructive pulmonary disease. Am Rev Respir Dis 1989;139:120–5.

75. Saadjian AY, Philip-Joet FF, Vestri R, Arnaud AG. Long-term treatment of chronic obstructive lung disease by Nifedipine: an 18-month haemodynamic study. Eur Respir J 1988;1:716–20.

76. Morrell NW, Higham MA, Phillips PG, Shakur BH, Robinson PJ, Beddoes RJ. Pilot study of losartan for pulmonary hypertension in chronic obstructive pulmonary disease. Respir Res 2005;6:88.

77. Roger N, Barberà JA, Roca J, Rovira I, Gomez FP, Rodriguez-Roisin R. Nitric oxide inhalation during exercise in chronic obstructive pulmonary disease. Am J Respir Crit Care Med 1997;156:800–6.

78. Katayama Y, Higenbottam TW, Diaz de Atauri MJ, Cremona G, Akamine S, Barberà JA, Rodriguez-Roisin R. Inhaled nitric oxide and arterial oxygen tension in patients with chronic obstructive pulmonary disease and severe pulmonary hypertension. Thorax 1997;52:120–4.

79. Frostell C, Blomqvist H, Hedenstierna G, Lundberg J, Zapol WM. Inhaled nitric oxide selectively reverses human hypoxic pulmonary vasoconstriction without causing systemic vasodilation. Anesthesiology 1993;78:427–35.

80. Yoshida M, Taguchi O, Gabazza EC, Kobayashi T, Yamakami T, Kobayashi H, Maruyama K, Shima T. Combined inhalation of nitric oxide and oxygen in chronic obstructive pulmonary disease. Am J Respir Crit Care Med 1997;155:526–29.

81. Germann P, Ziesche R, Leitner C, Roeder G, Urak G, Zimpfer M, Sladen R. Addition of nitric oxide to oxygen improves cardiopulmonary function in patients with severe COPD. Chest 1998;114:29–35.

82. Vonbank K, Ziesche R, Higenbottam TW, Stiebellehner L, Petkov V, Schenk P, Germann P, Block LH. Controlled prospective randomised trial on the effects on pulmonary haemodynamics of the ambulatory long term use of nitric oxide and oxygen in patients with severe COPD. Thorax 2003;58:289–93.

83. Naeije R, Barberà JA. Pulmonary hypertension associated with COPD. Crit Care 2001;5:286–9.

84. Higenbottam T. Pulmonary hypertension and chronic obstructive pulmonary disease: a case for treatment. Proc Am Thorac Soc 2005;2:12–9.

85. Stevens D, Sharma K, Szidon P, Rich S, McLaughlin V, Kesten S. Severe pulmonary hypertension associated with COPD. Ann Transplant 2000;5:8–12.

86. Archer SL, Mike D, Crow J, Long W, Weir EK. A placebo-controlled trial of prostacyclin in acute respiratory failure in COPD. Chest 1996;109:750–5.

87. Dernaika TA, Beavin ML, Kinasewitz GT. Iloprost improves gas exchange in COPD patients with pulmonary arterial hypertension (PAH). Am J Respir Crit Care Med 2008;177:A443.

88. Stolz D, Rasch H, Linka A, Di VM, Meyer A, Brutsche M, Tamm M. A randomised, controlled trial of bosentan in severe COPD. Eur Respir J 2008;32:619–28.

89. Madden BP, Allenby M, Loke TK, Sheth A. A potential role for sildenafil in the management of pulmonary hypertension in patients with parenchymal lung disease. Vascul Pharmacol 2006;44:372–6.

90. Alp S, Skrygan M, Schmidt WE, Bastian A. Sildenafil improves hemodynamic parameters in COPD – an investigation of six patients. Pulm Pharmacol Ther 2006;19:386–90.

91. Rietema H, Holverda S, Bogaard HJ, Marcus JT, Smit HJ, Westerhof N et al. Sildenafil treatment in COPD does not affect stroke volume or exercise capacity. Eur Respir J 2008;31:759–64.

92. Zhao L, Mason NA, Morrell NW, Kojonazarov B, Sadykov A, Maripov A et al. Sildenafil inhibits hypoxia-induced pulmonary hypertension. Circulation 2001;104:424–8.

93. American Thoracic Society and European Respiratory Society. International Multidisciplinary Consensus Classification of the Idiopathic Interstitial Pneumonias. Joint statement of the American Thoracic Society (ATS) and the European Respiratory Society (ERS). Am J Respir Crit Care Med 2002;165:277–304.

94. Lettieri CJ, Nathan SD, Barnett SD, Ahmad S, Shorr AF. Prevalence and outcomes of pulmonary arterial hypertension in advanced idiopathic pulmonary fibrosis. Chest 2006;129:746–52.

95. Shorr AF, Wainright JL, Cors CS, Lettieri CJ, Nathan SD. Pulmonary hypertension in patients with pulmonary fibrosis awaiting lung transplant. Eur Respir J 2007;30:715–21.

96. Zisman DA, Ross DJ, Belperio JA, Saggar R, Lynch JP, III, Ardehali A, Karlamangla AS. Prediction of pulmonary hypertension in idiopathic pulmonary fibrosis. Respir Med 2007;101:2153–9.

97. Nathan SD, Shlobin OA, Barnett SD, Saggar R, Belperio JA, Ross DJ et al. Right ventricular systolic pressure by echocardiography as a predictor of pulmonary hypertension in idiopathic pulmonary fibrosis. Respir Med 2008;102:1305–10.

98. Cottin V, Nunes H, Brillet PY, Delaval P, Devouassoux G, Tillie-Leblond I et al. Combined pulmonary fibrosis and emphysema: a distinct underrecognised entity. Eur Respir J 2005;26:586–93.

99. Nadrous HF, Pellikka PA, Krowka MJ, Swanson KL, Chaowalit N, Decker PA, Ryu JH. Pulmonary hypertension in patients with idiopathic pulmonary fibrosis. Chest 2005;128:2393–9.

100. Martinez FJ, Safrin S, Weycker D, Starko KM, Bradford WZ, King TE, Jr. et al. The clinical course of patients with

idiopathic pulmonary fibrosis. Ann Intern Med 2005;
142:963–97.

101. Ebina M, Shimizukawa M, Shibata N, Kimura Y, Suzuki T,
Endo M et al. Heterogeneous increase in CD34-positive
alveolar capillaries in idiopathic pulmonary fibrosis.
Am J Respir Crit Care Med 2004;169:1203–8.

102. Weitzenblum E, Ehrhart M, Rasaholinjanahary J, Hirth C.
Pulmonary hemodynamics in idiopathic pulmonary fibrosis
and other interstitial pulmonary diseases. Respiration
1983;44:118–27.

103. Giaid A, Michel RP, Stewart DJ, Sheppard M, Corrin B,
Hamid Q. Expression of endothelin-1 in lungs of patients
with cryptogenic fibrosing alveolitis. Lancet 1993;341:
1550–54.

104. Simler NR, Brenchley PE, Horrocks AW, Greaves SM,
Hasleton PS, Egan JJ. Angiogenic cytokines in patients with
idiopathic interstitial pneumonia. Thorax 2004;59:581–5.

105. Agustí AGN, Roca J, Gea J, Wagner PD, Xaubet A, Rodriguez-
Roisin R. Mechanisms of gas-exchange impairment in
idiopathic pulmonary fibrosis. Am Rev Respir Dis 1991;
143:219–25.

106. Bonay M, Bancal C, de ZD, Arnoult F, Saumon G, Camus F.
Normal pulmonary capillary blood volume in patients with
chronic infiltrative lung disease and high pulmonary artery
pressure. Chest 2004;126:1460–6.

107. Kennedy JI, Fulmer JD. Pulmonary hypertension in the
interstitial lung diseases. Chest 1985;87:558–60.

108. Ghofrani HA, Wiedemann R, Rose F, Schermuly RT,
Olschewski H, Weissmann N et al. Sildenafil for treatment
of lung fibrosis and pulmonary hypertension: a randomised
controlled trial. Lancet 2002;360:895–900.

109. Olschewski H, Ghofrani HA, Walmrath D, Schermuly R,
Temmesfeld-Wollbruck B, Grimminger F, Seeger W. Inhaled
prostacyclin and iloprost in severe pulmonary hypertension
secondary to lung fibrosis. Am J Respir Crit Care Med
1999;160:600–7.

110. Collard HR, Anstrom KJ, Schwarz MI, Zisman DA. Sildenafil
improves walk distance in idiopathic pulmonary fibrosis.
Chest 2007;131:897–9.

111. Gunther A, Enke B, Markart P, Hammerl P, Morr H, Behr J et al.
Safety and tolerability of bosentan in idiopathic pulmonary
fibrosis: an open label study. Eur Respir J 2007;29:713–9.

112. King TE, Jr., Behr J, Brown KK, du Bois RM, Lancaster L,
de Andrade JA et al. BUILD-1: a randomized placebo-
controlled trial of bosentan in idiopathic pulmonary
fibrosis. Am J Respir Crit Care Med 2008;177:75–81.

20.2

Pulmonary hypertension in obstructive sleep apnea

KATHLEEN SARMIENTO AND STEVEN M SCHARF

INTRODUCTION

Obstructive sleep apnea (OSA) is a common disorder, affecting 4 percent of men, 2 percent of women, with higher prevalence in the elderly and overweight (1). OSA patients develop periodic obstruction of the upper airway at night while respiratory efforts continue. Hypoxemia ensues, and the apneic period is terminated by an arousal and return of patency to the upper airway (Figure 20.2.1). Many patients with OSA demonstrate a smaller number of "central" apneas as well, in which both airflow and respiratory effort cease. Apneas may also be "mixed" in which the initial part is central, and the latter part is obstructive. There has been a rapid accumulation of evidence linking OSA and cardiovascular morbidity and mortality. For example, OSA patients have an increased prevalence of hypertension (2,3) and coronary artery disease, independent of other known risk factors (4,5). Disordered breathing is a robust predictor of acute myocardial infarction in humans and animals (6). It has become clear that even in patients without overt cardiovascular disease endothelial function is impaired, leading to abnormalities in endothelial dependent activities such as vasodilation and production of pro-inflammatory cytokines (7–9).

In 1956, Burwell *et al.* described a patient with obesity, severe sleepiness, hypoxia, hypoventilation, and cor pulmonale (10). He coined the term "Pickwickian" syndrome because of the resemblance of the patient to a character in the 1837 Dickens novel "The Posthumous Papers of the Pickwick Club." Later, Gastaut *et al.* raised the possibility that many patients with Pickwickian syndrome actually suffer from upper airway obstruction during sleep (11), or, as called today, sleep apnea syndrome. As the patient described by Burwell demonstrated clinical signs of right

heart failure, the question naturally arises as to whether the clinical presentation, including pulmonary hypertension (PH) and cor pulmonale, are typical in patients with this common disorder.

This chapter focuses on the link between OSA and PH. We will focus on the prevalence and potential mechanisms for development of PH, emphasizing the effects of OSA on the pulmonary vasculature and the RV. We will review what we have learned from animal models as well as human studies. Finally, we will attempt to draw some conclusions and consider directions for future studies.

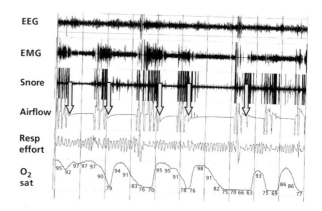

Figure 20.2.1 Example of sleep study in a patient with severe OSA. Obstructive apneas are identified as cessations of airflow associated with continued respiratory effort (arrows). Note the burst of EEG and EMG activity (arousals) and intermittent decreases in oxygen levels associated with each apnea. EEG, electroencephalogram; EMG, electromyogram (submentalis muscle); airflow, through the nose; Resp effort, recorded from an abdominal pneumobel; O_2 sat, recorded from a pulse oximeter.

There is some disagreement as to the true prevalence of PH in patients with OSA. Different estimates are likely due to differing definitions of PH, techniques for estimating PH, and patient populations. Two series have estimated the prevalence of PH among patients with OSA to be approximately 20 percent (12,13). This estimate originated from studies done on patients identified with severe OSA, though many of them also suffered from underlying obstructive lung disease or alveolar hypoventilation associated with chronic hypoxemia (12–15). This led to the conclusion that daytime hypoxemia was necessary for the development of sustained PH in OSA, and that nocturnal changes associated with OSA were themselves not sufficient to cause PH and cor pulmonale (15). Subsequently, studies reported PH in the absence of daytime hypoxemia in patients with OSA (16,17). Six studies (18–23) evaluating patients with OSA without underlying pulmonary disease have reported a prevalence of PH and/or cor pulmonale between 10 and 47 percent.

Recently, O'Hearn *et al.* studied patients with OSA and pretibial edema (24), a common finding in patients with OSA (25) as well as patients with right heart failure (26). None of the subjects with or without edema showed any clinical signs of heart failure. Among the 70 subjects enrolled in the study, 29 had edema and 41 did not. PH was assessed during daytime catheterization in edematous subjects only. An elevated RAP (mean RAP > 5 mmHg) was found in 26 (93 percent) patients with lower extremity edema. An elevation in mean pulmonary artery pressure (PAM $\geq$ 20 mmHg) was found in 24 patients (86 percent) and an elevated pulmonary artery systolic pressure ($\geq$ 30 mmHg) was found in 23 patients (82 percent). Severe PH (PAM $\geq$ 30 mmHg) was found in seven (25 percent). Increased pulmonary artery wedge pressure (> 12 mmHg) was seen in 20 patients (71 percent), suggesting a large contribution of LV dysfunction to PH in these patients. Cardiac index was normal. Patients without edema were not studied at cardiac catheterization. However, RV function using first pass radionuclide ventriculography showed dysfunction (RVD = ejection fraction < 40 percent) in 77 percent of the edematous and 61 percent of the non-edematous subjects (NS). Thus, at the very least, pretibial edema in OSA patients signals a high likelihood of PH with RVD. There is also a high incidence of RVD in non-edematous subjects as well.

MECHANISMS

The cardiovascular effects of OSA are generally thought to be related to one or more of the following mechanisms: (i) exaggerated inspiratory swings in intrathoracic pressure; (ii) intermittent hypoxia; (iii) post-apneic arousals. A complete review of the hemodynamic effects of exaggerated inspiratory swings in intrathoracic pressure is available elsewhere (27,28), but includes inspiratory increased in venous return, leading to increased RV and decreased left

ventricular (LV) diastolic filling, and increased LV afterload. As there are few data addressing the role of postapneic arousals in PH, we will concentrate on the first two factors. However, it should be noted that these arousals contribute to an increase in sympathoadrenal tone, a factor that could influence pulmonary hemodynamics.

To determine the effects of chronically exaggerated inspiratory swings in intrathoracic pressure, Salejee *et al.* performed tracheal banding on rats (29). This caused exaggerated inspiratory swings in intrathoracic pressure (approximately 30 mmHg), mild chronic hypercapnia, but no hypoxemia. Rats were studied at 7 weeks and 1 year following tracheal banding. There was no evidence of pulmonary congestion, LV hypertrophy or hepatic congestion. However, there were increases in RV to total body weight ratio by 50 percent compared to sham operated animals in both groups of obstructed animals. The extent of RV hypertrophy was directly correlated with inspiratory swing in intrathoracic pressure. These authors postulated that large increases in venous return during inspiration could have led to RV hypertrophy. Tarasiuk and Scharf assessed the effects of intermittent upper airway obstruction on venous return in a large animal model simulating the periodic airway obstruction seen in OSA (Figure 20.2.2) (30,31). They demonstrated that inspiratory venous return was approximately fivefold that of expiratory venous return during obstructed inspirations.

The animal findings likely explain the echocardiographic findings of Shiomi *et al.* in humans with OSA showing RV enlargement associated with leftward septal shift and decreased LV preload (32). The large increase in right-sided pressures engendered by increased venous return dilates the

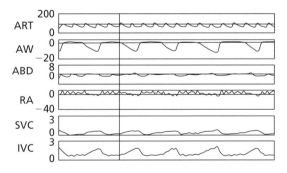

Figure 20.2.2 Effects of obstructive apneas on venous return in intubated anesthetized dogs. Periodic occlusions of the endotracheal tube were done for one minute, interspersed with one minute of normal breathing. This illustration is from an occluded phase (15 sec). Respiratory efforts are indicated by decreasing airway pressure (AW) and increasing respiratory effort. The vertical line indicates the start of one respiratory effort. ART, arterial pressure; AW, airway pressure; ABD, abdominal pressure; RA, right atrial pressure; SVC, superior vena cava flow; IVC, inferior vena cava flow. Note the large inspiratory increase in both SVC and IVC. Pressures in mmHg; flow in liters/min. (Redrawn from ref 31 with permission.)

RV and compresses the LV by the mechanisms of ventricular interdependence. Podzus *et al.* studied patients with OSA at night (27,33). These workers used pulmonary arterial transmural pressure (PATM) as an index of PH. They found that during central apneas, or the central part of mixed apneas, there were no or only mild increases in PATM, in spite of the fact that oxygen saturation fell. On the other hand, during obstructive apneas, when intrathoracic pressure fell, there were increases in PATM, unrelated to the fall in oxygen saturation. Schafer *et al.* also demonstrated the independent effects of hypoxemia and mechanical factors (increased negative intrathoracic pressure) on elevating PATM (34) (Figure 20.2.3). Thus, it must be concluded that during obstructive apneas, exaggerated decreases in intrathoracic pressure increase PATM and thus impose a load on the RV.

Patients with OSA often develop hypoxemia during and immediately following their apneic episodes (Figure 20.2.1). The severity of hypoxia varies depending on the duration of the disordered breathing event, lung volumes and the presence or absence of concomitant lung disease. Hypoxia in OSA is intermittent since with resumption of breathing, oxygen saturation usually returns to normal or near normal levels. Since hypoxia occurs nightly, it is called chronic intermittent hypoxemia (CIH). As is well known, chronic continuous hypoxia leads to PH, pulmonary vascular remodeling and RV failure in patients with chronic hypoxemia. Recently the effects of CIH in animal models have been extensively studied. In one model, rats are placed in chambers in which the ambient oxygen concentration is lowered from room air to 4–6 percent approximately once per minute, followed by return to room air (Figure 20.2.4). This is done for varying periods of time ranging up to 7 weeks. This model thus isolates one aspect of OSA, the CIH, from the mechanical swings in intrathoracic pressure related to upper airway obstruction. Since the pioneering work of Fletcher *et al.* demonstrated the occurrence of systemic hypertension in animals exposed to CIH37, this model has been used to study cardiovascular effects of CIH, and by implication, OSA. It is clear that CIH is a potent stimulus for sympathetic activation (37) both peripherally and centrally. In addition, Chen *et al.* demonstrated LV hypertrophy and dysfunction at both the whole organ and cellular level (38,39). This was independent of the development of systemic hypertension, but was associated with oxidant stress and myocardial apoptosis. While RV hypertrophy was not demonstrated by these authors, it has been demonstrated by others using similar models in rats (40–43) and mice (44–46).

The demonstration of oxidant stress as a result of CIH provides one plausible mechanism contributing to the development of PH in OSA, as it is known that oxidant stress can lead to PH with hypoxia (41,42). There are several detailed reviews available discussing the relationship between OSA and oxidative stress (43,44). In addition, mechanisms associated with the development of PH in continuous hypoxia could contribute to PH with CIH.

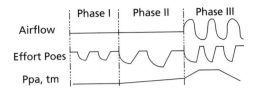

Figure 20.2.3 Obstructive apnea in three phases. Poes, esophageal pressure; Ppa, tm, transmural pulmonary artery pressure. (Reproduced from ref 34 with permission.)

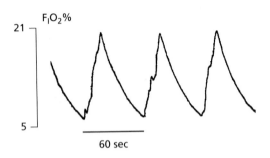

Figure 20.2.4 Changes in fraction of oxygen in a chamber of a rat exposed to chronic intermittent hypoxia.

Recently, Snow *et al.* compared the effects of continuous and intermittent hypoxia on pulmonary vasoreactivity (45). Both continuous and hypocapnic intermittently hypoxic animals developed PH, vascular remodeling and RV hypertrophy, and increased vascular eNOS expression, although the responses were less in CIH than in continuous hypoxia. However, the lungs from the hypocapnic CIH animals did not show increased ionomycin dependent vasodilation characteristic of continuous hypoxia. Further, maintenance of eucapnia by addition of exogenous CO_2 attenuated the responses compared to hypocapnic animals. These findings suggest that CIH can produce pulmonary vascular and RV effects similar to those seen in continuous hypoxia, and further that there is an adjunct role for elevated arterial CO_2 tensions.

It is known that hypercapnia with acidosis can lead to PH (47). The amount by which arterial PCO_2 increases with nocturnal disordered breathing events will depend on a number of factors including extent of the hypoventilation engendered by upper airway occlusion (apnea, hypopnea), the duration of the event, baseline arterial PCO_2, and respiratory drive. In an animal model of periodic apneas in pigs, in which the extent and duration of obstruction were standardized, Chen and Scharf showed that arterial PCO_2 increased from approximately 40 to approximately 60 mmHg during 30-second simulated obstructive apneas (48). However, these authors showed that the pressor responses to hypercapnia were far less important than those to hypoxia in the genesis of acute systemic hypertension. In patients who develop chronic (daytime) hypercapnia with OSA, this factor could conceivably have a greater contributing effect to PH. In a recent study, Kawata *et al.*

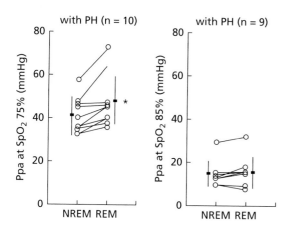

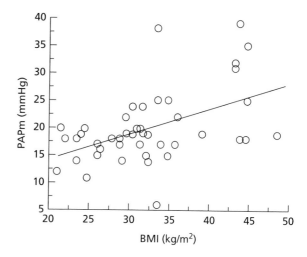

Figure 20.2.5 Pulmonary artery pressure (Ppa) evaluated at the same level of SpO_2 during NREM and REM sleep with and without daytime PH. Note greater sensitivity to hypoxia in REM sleep in patients with PH. *$P < 0.01$. (Redrawn from ref 50 with permission.)

Figure 20.2.6 Correlation between mean pulmonary artery pressure (PAPm) and BMI; $r = 0.50$; $P = 0.0006$. (Redrawn from ref 19 with permission.)

found that 14 percent of a large group of patients with OSA showed daytime hypercapnia (49). This was predicted by higher body mass index (BMI), and greater severity of OSA.

It is known that alpha sympathetic stimulation can lead to pulmonary vasoconstriction. However, the role of sympathoadrenal stimulation in the genesis of PH is unclear. In rats with CIH Huang *et al.* demonstrated downregulation of nNOS mRNA expression and decreased post-transcriptional nNOS protein centrally, suggesting a central effect of NO in sympathoexitation (51). In addition, there is evidence suggesting a neural component to oxidative stress and a heightened pulmonary vasoconstriction (50). Increased pulmonary artery pressures occur during REM sleep in patients with daytime PH compared to those without (51) (Figure 20.2.5). While the mechanism is not known, REM sleep is often associated with large fluctuations in autonomic tone, and increased sympathetic tone and/or sensitivity to sympathetic tone may be the mechanism.

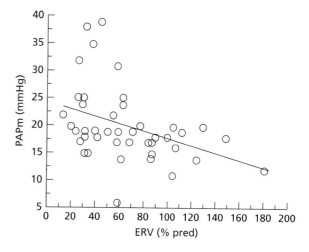

Figure 20.2.7 Correlation between PAPm and expiratory reserve volume (ERV); $r = -0.40$; $P = 0.007$. (Redrawn from ref 19 with permission.)

PREDICTIVE FACTORS AND TREATMENT

Many potential predictive factors for the development of PH in sleep-disordered breathing have been studied. The most consistently cited include lower daytime arterial oxygen content, elevated BMI, and lower minimum nocturnal saturation (MinSPO$_2$ percent). Bady *et al.* showed a clear linear correlation between PAPm and BMI, a negative linear correlation between mean pulmonary artery pressure (PAPm) and expiratory reserve volume, and additional significant correlations between PAPm and indices of hypoxemia and hypercapnia (19) (Figures 20.2.6 and 20.2.7). Sajkov *et al.* studied pulmonary hemodynamics and lung function in OSA patients with and without PH (52). PH patients did not differ from normals in lung function,

severity of OSA, age or BMI. However, PH patients had increased small airways closure during tidal breathing, greater V/Q inequality and greater pulmonary artery pressor response to hypoxia and a marked rise in pulmonary artery pressure with increased blood flow. These findings suggest that there may be patients with a greater tendency to develop PH in the presence of certain stimuli that could occur with OSA.

By contrast, RVD appears to be predicted by AHI and extent of nocturnal oxyhemoglobin saturation, but not by age, BMI, gender, blood gas analysis, pulmonary function, pulmonary artery pressure, or LV ejection fraction (18,53). It is possible that the presence of RVD is not directly the result of nor does it predict the presence PH (e.g. oxidant stress could cause direct myocardial damage). It is clear that both PH and RVD should be simultaneously studied to clarify these issues in OSA.

The most common treatment for OSA is continuous positive airway pressure (CPAP). CPAP maintains airway patency and eliminates apneic episodes. Thus, there is relief of the mechanical stress of respiration against an occluded airway, sympathetic surge during arousals, and intermittent hypoxia. Additionally, CPAP reduces markers of inflammation and oxidative stress to within normal ranges and enhances release of nitric oxide by the pulmonary microvasculature (8,54). Finally, reversal of persistent daytime hypercapnia, PH, and RV remodeling have been reported with CPAP (55–58).

FUTURE DIRECTIONS

While it appears that PH and cor pulmonale may be one of the common manifestations of OSA, it is not clear whether the clinical course, presentation or prognosis of OSA is affected by the changes in pulmonary hemodynamics. For example, are there effects on degree of daytime sleepiness, mortality, or quality of life in patients with PH as opposed to those without PH? If pulmonary hemodynamics have major prognostic significance, then building in an evaluation of these factors as part of the routine evaluation of OSA should be considered. Additional studies are also indicated for exploring mechanisms leading to PH and cor pulmonale. These could include proliferation of pulmonary vascular growth mediators due to CIH or large inspiratory increases in blood flow. There are also potential therapeutic implications for elucidating these mechanisms. For example, if the primary mechanisms leading to pulmonary vascular remodeling center around the hypoxemic component of OSA (CIH), it is potentially feasible to treat OSA patients with oxygen alone. This could improve compliance with therapy, which is often suboptimal with CPAP masks. While there has been a great deal of emphasis on systemic vascular and left heart function, there has been less emphasis on changes in pulmonary vasculature and right-sided cardiac function. We would urge that more attention be paid to this part of the OSA syndrome in future clinical and basic studies.

KEY POINTS

- OSA is a disease characterized by chronic intermittent hypoxemia, oxidative stress, exaggerated intrathoracic pressure swings, and increased sympathoadrenal tone.
- These derangements all contribute to the development of PH and RV remodeling.
- Treatment with CPAP alleviates the metabolic and structural changes induced by OSA.

REFERENCES

● = Key primary paper

●1. Young T, Peppard PE. Epidemiological evidence for and association of sleep disordered breathing with hypertension and cardiovascular disease. In: Bradley TD, Floras JS. Sleep Apnea. Implications in Cardiovascular and Cerebrovascular Disease. New York: Marcel Dekker, 2000:261–84.

●2. Lavie P, Here P, Hoffstein V. Obstructive sleep apnoea syndrome as a risk factor for hypertension: population study. BMJ 2000;320:479–82.

●3. Grote L, Hedner J, Peter JH. Sleep-related breathing disorder is an independent factor for uncontrolled hypertension. J Hypertens 2000;18:679–85.

●4. Shahar E, Whitney CW, Redline S et al. for the Sleep Heart Health Study Research group. Sleep-disordered breathing and cardiovascular disease cross-sectional results of the Sleep Heart Health Study. Am J Respir Crit Care Med 2001;163:19–25.

●5. Mooe T, Rabben T, Wiklund U et al. Sleep-disordered breathing in men with coronary artery disease. Chest 1996;109:659–63.

●6. Podszus TE, Greenberg H, Scharf SM. Influence of sleep state and sleep-disordered breathing on cardiovascular function. In: Sullivan CE, and Saunders NA (eds). Sleep and Breathing II. New York: Marcel Dekker, 1993:257–310.

●7. Drager LF, Bortolotto LA, Lorenzi MC et al. Early signs of atherosclerosis in obstructive sleep apnea. Am J Respir Crit Care Med 2005;172:613–8.

●8. Jelic S, Margherita P, Kawut SM et al. Inflammation, oxidative stress, and repair capacity of the vascular endothelium in obstructive sleep apnea. Circulation 2008;117:2270–8.

●9. Williams A, Scharf SM. Obstructive sleep apnea, cardiovascular disease, and inflammation – is NF-kB the key? Sleep and Breathing 2007;11:69–76.

●10. Burwell CS, Robin ED, Whaley RD, Bicklemann AG. Extreme obesity associated with alveolar hypoventilation: a Pickwickian syndrome. Am J Med 1956;21:811–8.

●11. Gastaut H, Tassinari CA, Duron B. Polygraphic study of the episodic diurnal and nocturnal (hypnic and respiratory) manifestations of the Pickwick syndrome. Br Res 1966;1:167–86.

●12. Chaouat A, Weitzenblum E, Krieger J et al. Pulmonary hemodynamics in the obstructive sleep apnea syndrome. Chest 1996;109:380–6.

●13. Sanner BM, Doberaurer C, Konermann M et al. Pulmonary hypertension in patients with obstructive sleep apnea syndrome. Arch Intern Med 1997;157:2483–7.

●14. Weitzenblum E, Krieger J, Apprill M et al. Daytime pulmonary hypertension in patients with obstructive sleep apnea syndrome. Am Rev Respir Dis 1988;138:345–9.

●15. Bradley TD, Rutherford R, Grossman RF et al. Role of daytime hypoxemia in the pathogenesis of right heart failure in the obstructive sleep apnea syndrome. Am Rev Respir Dis 1985;131:835–9.

•16. Podszus T, Bauer W, Mayer J et al. Sleep apnea and pulmonary hypertension. Klin Wochenschr 1986;64:131–4.

•17. Laks L, Lehrhaft B, Grunstein RR, Sullivan CE. Pulmonary hypertension in obstructive sleep apnea. Eur Respir J 1995;8:537–41.

•18. Sanner BM, Konermann M, Sturm A et al. Right ventricular dysfunction in patients with obstructive sleep apnea syndrome. Eur Respir J 1997;10:2079–83.

•19. Bady E, Achkar A, Pascal S et al. Pulmonary arterial hypertension in patients with sleep apnea syndrome. Thorax 2000;55:934–9.

•20. Weber K, Podszus T, Krupp O et al. Prevalence of pulmonary hypertension in patients with obstructive sleep apnea. Sleep Res 1990;19:308. (abstract)

•21. Sajkov D, Cowie RJ, Thornton AT et al. Pulmonary hypertension and hypoxemia in obstructive sleep apnea syndrome. Am J Respir Crit Care Med 1994;149:416–22.

•22. Yamakawa H, Shiomi T, Sasanabe R et al. Pulmonary hypertension in patients with severe obstructive sleep apnea. Psych and Clin Neurosci 2002;56:311–2.

•23. Hetzel M, Kochs M, Marx N et al. Pulmonary hemodynamics in obstructive sleep apnea: frequency and causes of pulmonary hypertension. Lung 2003;181:157–66.

•24. O'Hearn DJ, Gold AR, Gold MS et al. Lower extremity edema and pulmonary hypertension in morbidly obese patients with obstructive sleep apnea. Sleep Breathing 2009;13:25–34.

•25. Iftikhar I, Ahmed M, Tarr S et al. Comparison of obstructive sleep apnea patients with and without leg edema. Sleep Med 2008;8:890–93.

•26. Schoen FJ. The heart. In: Vinay K, Abbas AK, Fausto N (eds). Pathologic basis of disease. Philadelphia: Saunders, 2005.

•27. Podszus TE, Feddersen CO, Scharf SM. Sleep apnea and right ventricular function. In: Scharf SM, Pinsky MR, Magder S (eds). Respiratory-Circulatory Interactions in Health and Disease. New York: Marcel Dekker, 2001:641–50.

•28. Scharf SM, Sica AS, Heart-lung interactions. In: Haddad GG, Abman SH, Chernick V (eds). Basic Mechanisms of Pediatric Respiratory Disease, 2nd edn. Hamilton: BC Dekker, 2002:234–49.

•29. Salejee I, Tarasiuk A, Reder I, Scharf SM. Chronic upper airways obstruction produces right but not left ventricular hypertrophy in rats. Am Rev Resp Dis 1993;148:1346–50.

•30. Tarasiuk A, Scharf SM. Effects of periodic obstructive apneas on venous return in closed chest dogs. Am Rev Resp Dis 1993;148:323–9.

•31. Tarasiuk A, Chen L, Scharf SM. Effects of periodic obstructive apnoeas on superior and inferior venous return in dogs. Acta Physiol Scand 1997;161:187–94.

•32. Shiomi T, Guilleminault C, Stoohs R, Schnittger I. Leftward shift of the interventricular septum and pulsus paradoxus in obstructive sleep apnea syndrome. Chest 1991;100: 894–902.

•33. Podzus T, Peter JH, Guilleminault C, von Wichert F. Pulmonary artery pressure during sleep apnea. Chest 1990;(Suppl);97:81S.

•34. Schafer H, Hasper E, Ewig S et al. Pulmonary hemodynamics in obstructive sleep apnoea: time course and associated factors. Eur Respir J 1998;12:679–84.

•35. Sica AL, Greenberg HE, Ruggiero DA, Scharf SM. Chronic intermittent hypoxia: a model of sympathetic activation in the rat. Resp Physiol 2000;121:173–84.

•36 Campden MJ, Shimoda LA, O'Donnell CP. Acute and chronic cardiovascular effects of intermittent hypoxia in C57BL/6J mice. J Appl Physiol 2005;99:2028–35.

•37. Fletcher EC, Lesske J, Qian W et al. Repetitive episodic hypoxia causes diurnal elevations of systemic blood pressure in rats. Hypertension 1992;19:555–61.

•38. Chen L, Einbinder E, Zhang Q et al. Oxidative stress and left ventricular function with chronic intermittent hypoxia in rats. Am J Resp Crit Care Med 2005;172:915–20.

•39. Chen L, Zhang J, Gan TX et al. Left ventricular dysfunction and associated cellular injury in rats exposed to chronic intermittent hypoxia. J Appl Physiol 2008;104:218–23.

•40. McGuire M, Bradford A. Chronic intermittent hypoxia increases haematocrit and causes right ventricular hypertrophy in the rat. Respir Physiol 1999;117:53–8.

•41. Hoshikawa Y, Ono S, Suzuki S et al. Generation of oxidative stress contributes to the development of pulmonary hypertension induced by hypoxia. J Appl Physiol 2001;90:1299–306.

•42. DeMarco VG, Habibi J, Whaley-Connell AT et al. Oxidative stress contributes to pulmonary hypertension in the transgenic (mRen2) 27 rat. Am J Physiol Heart Circ Physiol 2008;294:H2659–68.

•43. Lavie L. Obstructive sleep apnea syndrome – an oxidative stress disorder. Sleep Med Rev 2003;7:35–51.

•44. Budhiraja R, Parthasarathy S, Quan S. Endothelial dysfunction in obstructive sleep apnea. J Clin Sleep Med 2007;3:409–15.

•45. Snow JR, Kitzis V, Norton CE et al. Differential effects of chronic hypoxia and intermittent hypocapnic and eucapnic hypoxia on pulmonary vasoreactivity. J Appl Physiol 2008;104:110–8.

•46. Fagan KA. Physiological and genomic consequences of intermittent hypoxia selected contribution: pulmonary hypertension in mice following intermittent hypoxia. J Appl Physiol 2001;90:2502–7.

•47. Enson Y, Giuntii C, Lewis ML et al. The influence of hydrogen ion concentration and hypoxia on the pulmonary circulation. J Clin Invest 1964;43:1146–62.

•48. Chen L, Sica AL,Greenberg H, Scharf SM. Role of hypoxemia and hypercapnia in acute cardiovascular response to simulated central apneas in sedated pigs. Resp Phys 1998;111:257–69.

•49. Kawata N, Tatsumi K, Terada J et al. Daytime hypercapnia in obstructive sleep apnea syndrome. Chest 2007;132:1832–8.

•50. Niijima M, Kimura H, Edo H et al. Manifestation of pulmonary hypertension during REM sleep in obstructive sleep apnea syndrome. Am J Respir Crit Care Med 1999;159:1766–72.

•51. Huang J, Tamisier R, Ji E *et al.* Chronic intermittent hypoxia modulates nNOS mRNA and protein expression in the rat hypothalamus. Respir Physio Neurobiol 2007;158:30–8.

•52. Sajkov D, Wang T, Saunders N *et al.* Daytime pulmonary hemodynamics in patients with obstructive sleep apnea without lung disease. Am J Respir Crit Care Med 1999;159:1518–26.

•53. Dursunoglu N, Dursunoglu D, Kilic M. Impact of obstructive sleep apnea on right ventricular global function: sleep apnea and myocardial performance index. Respir 2005; 72:278–84.

•54. Lattimore J, Wilcox I, Adams M *et al.* Treatment of obstructive sleep apnea leads to enhanced pulmonary vascular nitric oxide release. Int J Cardiol 2008;126:229–33.

•55. Alchanatis M, Tourkohoriti G, Kakouros S *et al.* Daytime pulmonary hypertension in patients with obstructive sleep apnea: the effect of continuous positive airway pressure on pulmonary hemodynamics. Respir 2001;68:566–72.

•56. Chaouat A, Weitzenblum E, Krieger J *et al.* Prognostic value of lung function and pulmonary haemodynamics in OSA patients treated with CPAP. Eur Respir J 1999;13:1091–6.

•57. Sajkov D, Wang T, Saunders N *et al.* Continuous positive airway pressure treatment improves pulmonary hemodynamics in patients with obstructive sleep apnea. Am J Respir Crit Care Med 2002;165:152–8.

•58. Arias M, Garcia-Rio F, Alonso-Fernandez A *et al.* Pulmonary hypertension in obstructive sleep apnea: effects of continuous positive airway pressure. Eur Heart J 2006;27:1106–13.

•59. Zielinski J. Effects of intermittent hypoxia on pulmonary haemodynamics: animal models versus studies in humans. Eur Respir J 2005;25:173–80.

An integrated approach to the treatment of pulmonary hypertension related to hypoxic lung diseases*,†

ARI CHAOUAT, EMMANUEL GOMEZ, MATTHIEU CANUET, CHRISTINE SELTON-SUTY, FRANÇOIS CHABOT AND EMMANUEL WEITZENBLUM

INTRODUCTION

Pulmonary hypertension (PH) complicates the course of most advanced chronic lung diseases (1). Chronic alveolar hypoxia is the predominant cause of PH in this category (2). However, it would be inappropriate to consider all these PH as similar since it is a very heterogeneous group of PH (3). Table 20.3.1 shows most types of chronic lung diseases that can be complicated by PH. The usual mean to categorize these diseases is to separate them as obstructive, restrictive, mixed (obstructive and restrictive) and those without significant impairment of the mechanical properties of the respiratory system as of central origin.

The current definition of PH is a resting mean pulmonary artery pressure (PAP) ≥ 25 mmHg (4,5). The same group of experts, which proposed this definition, mentioned that a normal mean PAP is comprised between 8 and 20 mmHg (4,5). In chronic lung diseases most studies have set the definition of PH as a mean PAP > 20 mmHg since it appears that a mean PAP above this threshold is associated with worse outcomes (6). In this category of PH,

cor pulmonale is a frequently used term (1,7,8). It is defined as right ventricle (RV) hypertrophy, dilatation or both secondary to PH caused by respiratory disorders.

This chapter will underline current knowledge on treatment of PH in stable hypoxic lung diseases. It must be emphasized that COPD is the most frequent and studied cause.

In order to determine the efficacy of treatment of PH which could be expected in patients with chronic lung diseases, some knowledge of the pathophysiology of PH will be considered in the first part of this chapter. The second part will be dedicated to the therapeutic strategy.

CAUSES OF PH IN PATIENTS WITH CHRONIC LUNG DISEASES

Alveolar hypoxia

Alveolar hypoxia is the consequence of ventilation – perfusion inequality and/or alveolar hypoventilation that

---

*The authors have no conflicts of interest to disclose.

†Abbreviations: Arterial oxygen partial pressure, PaO₂; Arterial oxygen saturation, SaO₂; Chronic obstructive pulmonary disease, COPD; Long-term oxygen therapy, LTOT; Lung volume reduction surgery, LVRS; Non-invasive intermittent positive-pressure ventilation, NIPPV; Pulmonary arterial hypertension, PAH; Pulmonary artery pressure, PAP; Pulmonary artery wedge pressure, PWP; Pulmonary hypertension, PH; Pulmonary vascular resistance, PVR; Right ventricle, RV.

Table 20.3.1 Chronic lung diseases associated with pulmonary hypertension: group 3 of the current clinical classification

Obstructive lung diseases
COPD*
Asthma (with irreversible airway obstruction)
Cystic fibrosis#
Bronchiectasis
Bronchiolitis obliterans

Restrictive lung diseases
Neuromuscular diseases
Kyphoscoliosis#
Sequelae of pulmonary tuberculosis
Sarcoidosis#
Pneumoconiosis
Drug-related lung diseases
Extrinsic allergic alveolitis
Connective tissue diseases#
Idiopathic interstitial pulmonary fibrosis#
Interstitial pulmonary fibrosis of known origin#
Combined pulmonary fibrosis and emphysema#

Respiratory insufficiency of central origin
Central alveolar hypoventilation
Obesity-hypoventilation syndrome#
Sleep apnea syndrome

COPD, chronic obstructive pulmonary disease.
*Very frequent cause of pulmonary hypertension.
#Frequent cause of pulmonary hypertension.

complicate the course of many lung diseases (2). Acute alveolar hypoxia induces a rise of PAP and pulmonary vascular resistance (PVR) that is accounted for by hypoxic pulmonary vasoconstriction (9). Although hypoxic pulmonary vasoconstriction is less active in patients with significant structural changes of small pulmonary arteries as observed in patients with advanced chronic lung diseases (10), this response of pulmonary vascular bed to alveolar hypoxia can have important clinical consequences. Indeed, exacerbation, sleep-related oxygen desaturations and exercise are clearly the origin of repetitive gas exchange impairment and peaks of PH in many chronic lung diseases.

Chronic effects of hypoxia on the pulmonary circulation are known from clinical and pathological studies performed in subjects living at high altitude (11) and from animal models of PH (12). Hypoxia induces changes in structure and function of all cells of the pulmonary vasculature as well as important change in extracellular matrix of the vascular wall.

Alveolar hypoxia – other than in states of severe hypoxia – has been considered as a minor factor in recent reviews (13,14) since only weak correlations were found between PAP, PVR on the one hand and arterial oxygen partial pressure (PaO_2) and arterial oxygen saturation (SaO_2) on the other hand. However, as developed below, alveolar hypoxia may have important effects in genetically predisposed patients.

Loss and remodeling of the pulmonary vascular bed

In COPD patients, diffuse pulmonary emphysema induces a loss of pulmonary vessels. This phenomenon is correlated with an increase in mean PAP during exercise and at rest in advanced forms of pulmonary emphysema (15). It has also been shown that the pulmonary vascular remodeling is related to inflammatory process in the vascular wall (16–18). Peinado et al. have reported a relationship between the number of inflammatory cells infiltrating the wall of pulmonary arteries on the one hand, and the enlargement of the intimal layer and the endothelial dysfunction on the other (16). Circulating pro-inflammatory cytokines, interleukin 6 levels were correlated with PAP values in a large series of COPD patients (19). It has also been shown that functional polymorphisms of pro-inflammatory cytokines or related to the proliferation of smooth muscle cells were accountable for a higher risk for the development of PH in chronic lung diseases (20). These data show how the pathological process of the underlying disease may favor the development of PH probably in combination with alveolar hypoxia. These phenomena may explain why mean PAP and PVR do not return to normal under long-term oxygen therapy (LTOT).

Similar processes of loss and remodeling of the pulmonary vascular bed are observed in interstitial lung diseases and particularly in patients with severe idiopathic lung fibrosis (21). It has also been observed in granulomas in the pulmonary vascular wall of patients with sarcoidosis (22) and muscle proliferation around vessels in patients with lymphangio-leiomyomatosis (23). These observations suggest that it is of paramount importance to treat and control the underlying disease otherwise the improvement of pulmonary hemodynamics will not be possible.

Associated left ventricular dysfunction

The increase in PAP is mainly due to an increase in PVR in chronic lung diseases; however an elevation of pulmonary artery wedge pressure (PWP) can also contribute to the development of PH particularly in patients with COPD (15,24). Knowing that most COPD patients are elderly and are smokers or ex-smokers it is not surprising to find in such a population some patients with a post-capillary component (PWP > 15 mmHg) in the development of PH. Epidemiological studies and large pharmaceutical trials (25) have found frequent association with left heart disease and an important proportion of death due to cardiovascular events. These data might be extrapolated to other chronic lung diseases such as interstitial lung diseases as illustrated in the study case of Table 20.3.2 and Figure 20.3.1. It is important to emphasize that the post-capillary component of PH may be covered up by chronic lung disease whereas a treatment of these associated cardiac diseases may improve the functional status and the life expectancy.

Table 20.3.2   Study case: 67-year-old man

Six-minute walk distance: 220 meters

Severe hypoxemia (ambient air pH 7.43, $PaCO_2$ 34 mmHg and
  PaO_2 46 mmHg)

FVC 70% of pred., FEV_1 72% of pred., FEV_1/FVC 78% and TLC 71%
  of pred.

History of left heart disease

High-resolution computed tomography (Figure 20.3.1)

  Ground glass opacities

  Interlobular interstitial thickening

  Traction bronchiectasis

  Thin-walled cysts

  Dilated left atrium

Echocardiography: left ventricular ejection fraction 45% and
  systolic PAP 75 mmHg

Diagnosis

Idiopathic nonspecific interstitial pneumonia

Ischemic cardiomyopathy

Pre and post-capillary pulmonary hypertension

Treatments

LTOT

Systemic corticosteroid

Angiotensin receptor blocker

Follow-up (6 months)

Clinical improvement

Six-minutes walk distance: 410 metres

pH 7.41, $PaCO_2$ 37 mmHg and PaO_2 58 mmHg (ambient air)

Systolic PAP 40 mmHg

FVC, forced vital capacity; % pred., percentage of the predicted value;
FEV_1, forced expiratory volume in 1 second; TLC, total lung capacity;
PAP, pulmonary artery pressure.

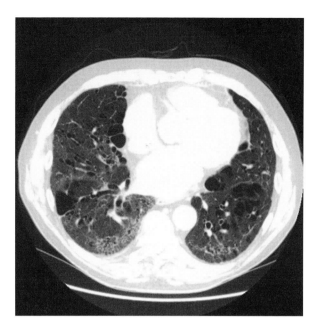

Figure 20.3.1   A computed tomography scan, through the lower zones, of a patient with idiopathic nonspecific interstitial pneumonia (study case, Table 20.3.2). There are ground glass opacities, interlobular interstitial thickening, traction bronchiectasis, thin-walled cyst and a dilated left atrium.

hyperviscosity caused by polycythemia and compression of arterioles and capillaries during expiration increase PAP and PVR in chronic lung diseases (1). However, their role seems small compared to alveolar hypoxia and anatomical factors due to the underlying disease.

PHYSIOLOGICAL CONSEQUENCES OF PH

Worsening of oxygenation

Patients with PH tend to have greater hypoxemia and exercise desaturation compared to patients with similar lung mechanics impairment but without PH (29). Several pathophysiological mechanisms explain why gas exchange worsens when PH complicates the course of chronic lung diseases. It has been shown that pulmonary artery endothelial dysfunction frequently encountered in severe chronic lung diseases modifies pulmonary vascular response to hypoxia and therefore worsens gas exchange. It is likely that the more PAP increases the more ventilation – perfusion distribution worsens. Additionally, patients who have patent *foramen ovale* and PH develop severe hypoxemia as soon as right atrial pressure increases above the level of left atrial pressure.

Right ventricular dysfunction

The RV is a flow generator. It adapts well to changes of preload but has limited adjustment to increase in afterload (30). It has been shown in COPD (this is also probably true

Some studies have also reported left diastolic dysfunction in patients with chronic lung disease without any associated disorder of the heart (26,27). These studies suggest that several mechanisms are involved in the elevation of PWP. First, chronic hypoxia can lead to an imbalance between left ventricular oxygen supply and demand and induce an abnormal myocardial relaxation. Second, the so-called ventricular interdependence may compromise left ventricular filling even when PAP is mildly elevated. Third, it has been observed in patients with severe distention (severe emphysema and to less extent in other obstructive diseases) that the increase in PWP particularly during exercise is in part due to hyperinflation (28).

These observations show that there are complex interactions between PAP and the left heart preload. These interactions should be taken into account for therapeutic approach.

Other factors

Other functional factors must be considered. Indeed, several studies have shown that hypercapnic acidosis, for most chronic lung diseases) that PAP is not severely increased in stable state and its rate of progression is slow. Therefore, the RV usually hypertrophies to reduce the wall stress due to the increased pressure and its dilatation (31). Patients with mild or moderate chronic lung disease usually have preserved right systolic function at rest (32). We might speculate that RV function is also preserved in most other chronic lung diseases but our knowledge concerning the role of the RV dysfunction in the natural history of most chronic lung diseases is limited. More studies are required in this area. For instance, the fast progression of PH in patients with end-stage idiopathic lung fibrosis may induce a loss in RV contractility. Indeed, an increase in RV wall stress in a circumstance of severe hypoxemia may favor RV failure. It is likely that such a worsening of RV function would impact on the clinical status.

Peripheral edema

Patients with severe chronic lung disease frequently develop peripheral edema. Mechanisms leading to peripheral edema are numerous. For instance in patients with COPD, edemas are observed in patients with normal cardiac output and normal right atrial pressure (33). It has been shown that they are linked with the level of hypercapnia. Carbon dioxide induces vasodilatation therefore there is a reduction of the effective circulating volume in the arterial systemic system. These changes may induce a decrease in the renal blood flow without fall of the glomerular filtration. Compensating neurohumoral factors are also involved. Elevated levels of rennin, aldosterone and atrial natriuretic peptide have been observed in patients with edema (34).

It is noteworthy that during acute exacerbation of COPD some patients develop true right heart failure (33,35). These patients exhibit important peripheral edema impossible to differentiate clinically between edema due to salt–water imbalance described above.

It is obvious that the mechanisms of peripheral edema in COPD are intricate and not completely understood. In addition, we must admit that less is known in that field concerning other chronic lung diseases.

CLINICAL CONSEQUENCES OF PH

Dyspnea and exercise limitation

It is a well-known fact that most chronic lung diseases and pulmonary vasculopathies such as pulmonary arterial hypertension (PAH) cause dyspnea on exertion and exercise limitation. The main mechanisms of dyspnea in COPD are dynamic hyperinflation, increase in ventilatory demand, respiratory muscle weakness and in the most severe patients hypoxemia and hypercapnia (36). Less is known about the mechanisms of exertional dyspnea in restrictive lung diseases. In interstitial lung diseases, it appears that

increased chemoreceptor activation secondary to hypoxia, altered vagal afferent activity and increased muscle respiratory effort are involved in the development of dyspnea and exercise limitation (37).

In PAH, it has been shown that elevated functional NYHA classes are linked with a high right atrial pressure and a low cardiac output mainly reflecting the right ventricular dysfunction (38). Furthermore, an increased ratio of dead space volume to tidal volume that is due to the pulmonary vascular bed loss leads to an increase in ventilatory requirement and participates to the feeling of dyspnea. The excess of ion hydrogen due to low aerobic threshold and oxygen desaturation during exercise secondary to cardiovascular abnormalities also contribute to dyspnea on exertion (39). These findings suggest that the severity of dyspnea on exertion is mainly a reflection of right ventricular abnormalities and the loss of the pulmonary vascular bed in PAH.

On the other hand, as mentioned above patients with PH related to hypoxic lung diseases usually have preserved right heart function. Thus, cardiac consequences of PH in chronic lung diseases may not be the main cause of exertional dyspnea and exercise limitation. Therefore, it is likely that solely lowering PAP may not improve dyspnea or exercise capacity in chronic lung diseases.

Survival and PH related to hypoxic lung diseases

Numerous studies have emphasized the prognostic value of PH complicating chronic lung diseases. It has been shown that an elevated PAP impacts significantly on life expectancy in patients with COPD even under LTOT (6,40). In idiopathic pulmonary fibrosis an elevated systolic PAP (> 50 mmHg) estimated with echocardiography is associated to a lower survival (41). In the same disease, the level of mean PAP measured with right heart catheterization before listing patients for lung transplantation is a good predictor of mortality (42).

In summary, it is often difficult to differentiate the clinical consequences of PH and those of the airflow limitation and parenchymal lesions in chronic lung disease. Nevertheless, it is important to detect an associated condition (Figure 20.3.2) which could impact on the pulmonary circulation such as a left heart disease in order to apply any recommended treatment. Furthermore, the control of the underlying disease appears necessary in the purpose to treat PH related to chronic lung diseases.

DISTINCT CHARACTERISTICS OF SEVERE AND OUT-OF-PROPORTION PH

Due to the high prevalence of chronic lung diseases, it is frequent to observe two chronic lung diseases or an associated left heart disease in an individual. It is also not unexpected to find co-morbidities such as thromboembolic

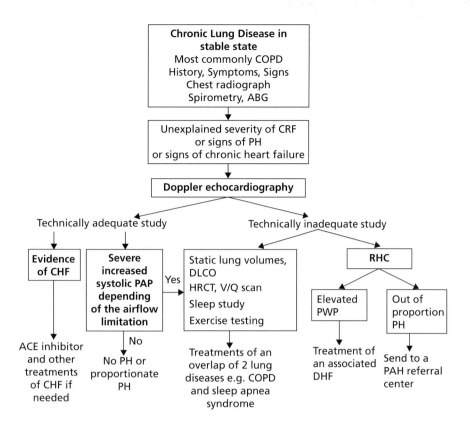

Figure 20.3.2 Proposal for a diagnosis strategy of an integrated approach to the treatment of pulmonary hypertension related to hypoxic lung diseases. COPD, chronic obstructive pulmonary disease; ABG, arterial blood gases; CRF, chronic respiratory failure; PH, pulmonary hypertension; CHF, chronic heart failure; ACE, angiotensin-converting enzyme; PAP, pulmonary artery pressure; DLCO, diffusion capacity for carbon monoxide; HRCT, high-resolution computed tomography; V/Q scan, ventilation/perfusion lung scan; RHC, right heart catheterization; PWP, pulmonary artery wedge pressure; DHF, diastolic heart failure.

disease, connective tissue diseases, portal hypertension or the use of appetite suppressant (43). All these associated conditions may act in tandem to increase the PAP and may explain in some patients the severity of PH. These co-morbid conditions are often difficult to identify. It is of paramount importance to well characterize these patients since some associated co-morbidities are treatable (Figure 20.3.2).

A subset of patients exhibit severe PH and mild to moderate impairment of lung mechanics. Two recent studies (43,44) have found that few patients with COPD without severe airflow limitation have severe PH also termed disproportionate PH. In this latter condition, it is not known whether some patients with COPD present genetic predisposition to develop severe PH when exposed to tobacco or an association of idiopathic PAH and COPD. Recent publications from Cottin *et al.* (45) have also shown that patients with combined pulmonary fibrosis and emphysema develop severe PH. In this latter condition, it is conceivable that fibrosis and emphysema act concomitantly to reduce the pulmonary vascular bed and explain the severity of PH.

Patients with severe PH or disproportionate PH have severe dyspnea on exertion (43) and less exercise capacity compared with patients without severe PH. Whether severe PH is the main cause of exercise limitation in these patients with chronic lung diseases is unknown. It has been hypothesized that PH in such a condition as disproportionate PH in COPD patients deserves to be specifically treated.

TREATMENT STRATEGIES

The objectives of treatment of PH in chronic lung diseases are to improve pulmonary hemodynamics and as an expected result to improve the functional status and survival of these patients. As mentioned above due to the important interplay between lung mechanisms, gas exchange, pulmonary hemodynamics and cardiac function treatment acting only on the post-load of the RV may have limited efficiency. The goals of treatments could be reached (i) by acting on the etiology of chronic lung disease; (ii) by correcting alveolar hypoxia with oxygen therapy or mechanical ventilation; (iii) by treating an associated left heart dysfunction; (iv) by improving pulmonary hemodynamics with vasodilators and/or drugs devoted to PAH; and (v) finally in case of right heart failure by improving RV contractility.

Treatment of the underlying disease

To stop or slow down the progression of the underlying disease may have a positive impact on the pulmonary circulation. Since it is beyond the scope of this chapter to review all treatments of chronic lung diseases, only few examples of interaction with the pulmonary circulation will be considered.

Animal models have shown that exposure to cigarette smoke induces pulmonary artery remodeling (46). Systemic inflammation was observed in smokers and was shown as an associated factor in the development of PH in COPD (19). Therefore, smoking cessation, among other positive effects, may help to lower the risk to develop PH in COPD.

Exercise and respiratory training, designated as pulmonary rehabilitation, in COPD have a positive impact. It improves exercise capacity and quality of life and reduces dyspnea on exertion with a high level of evidence. Conversely, in severe PH it is believed that physical activities have a negative impact and may favor a worsening of the disease. Pulmonary rehabilitation has been performed in patients with PAH or severe chronic thromboembolic PH and showed beneficial results (47). Thus, exercise and respiratory training can be accomplished in COPD patients or other chronic lung diseases with PH. It is probably wise to refer patients with severe PH to an expert center in order to start and monitor pulmonary rehabilitation.

Lung volume reduction surgery (LVRS) is a treatment of severe emphysema (48). Few studies have been performed on pulmonary hemodynamics before and after LVRS (49,50). It has been suspected that LVRS may have adverse effects on pulmonary hemodynamics due to the reduction of the vascular bed after the resection of lung tissue. A recent study as part of the National Emphysema Treatment Trial has shown no significant increases in terms of mean PAP and PVR, 6 months after medical treatment or LVRS (50).

In interstitial lung diseases, corticosteroids and immunosuppressive drugs are recommended (51). The goal of the treatment is to avoid the progression and occasionally to reverse the course of the disease. The effect of these drugs on PH has never been studied in idiopathic pulmonary fibrosis. Knowing the lack of efficacy on the course of the disease it is likely that corticosteroids are ineffective to treat PH in these patients. Concerning sarcoidosis, which does not belong to group 3 of the current clinical classification of PH but nevertheless is a chronic lung disease, few studies have shown that corticosteroids may improve pulmonary hemodynamics (22,52).

It is important to emphasize that lung and heart–lung transplantations are the ultimate therapeutic option in selected patients with chronic lung diseases and severe PH. One of the most frequent indications of transplantation in chronic lung diseases is COPD and idiopathic lung fibrosis. As expected when there is no graft dysfunction, PAP significantly improves after lung transplantation (53).

Remedy to alveolar hypoxia with oxygen therapy or mechanical ventilation

Alveolar hypoxia is considered to be the major determinant of the elevation of PVR and PAP in COPD patients and in other chronic lung diseases (1,8,12). One of the aims of LTOT is the improvement of PH induced by chronic alveolar hypoxia. Experimental data have raised the hope that pulmonary vascular changes could be reversed in chronic lung diseases under LTOT. In fact, we know that the structural changes of the small pulmonary vessels, which are observed in advanced chronic lung diseases are not completely reversible under LTOT (54) and we do not know whether these changes are fully accounted for by chronic alveolar hypoxia. The well-known NOTT (55) and MRC (56) studies were not mainly devoted to the pulmonary hemodynamics evolution under LTOT in COPD patients, but pulmonary hemodynamics data were available at the onset in all patients and follow-up right heart catheterization was performed in a relatively high number of patients. These studies showed that (i) PAP increased in patients who were not treated with oxygen therapy; (ii) remained stable in patients who received LTOT from 12 to 15 hours per day; and (iii) slightly decreased in patients treated with continuous LTOT (>18 h/day).

Nocturnal hypoxemia is frequently encountered in patients with chronic lung disease particularly in REM sleep and in patients who experience obstructive sleep apneas (57). These nocturnal desaturations provoke nocturnal peaks of PH (58). These episodes of severe hypoxemia have probably a deleterious effect on the pulmonary circulation. It is believed that the correction of nocturnal hypoxemia in these patients improves their pulmonary hemodynamics. To correct nocturnal hypoxemia in these patients on nocturnal oxygen therapy, continuous positive airway pressure support plus oxygen therapy or noninvasive intermittent positive-pressure ventilation (NIPPV) associated or not with oxygen therapy are usually necessary. Only few studies have been performed on that subject. Patients with obesity hypoventilation syndrome and severe kyphoscoliosis develop chronic hypercapnic respiratory failure frequently complicated with pulmonary hypertension. In these patients peripheral edema is a relatively good sign of chronic cor pulmonale. In one study including a small number of patients, Masa *et al.* (59) have shown that 4 months of NIPPV lead to an improvement of peripheral edema and of arterial blood gases. This study suggests that long-term mechanical ventilation can improve pulmonary hypertension due to chronic hypercapnic respiratory failure.

Treatment of an associated left heart dysfunction

The most frequent co-morbidity that can worsen PH in patients with chronic lung disease is an associated left heart dysfunction. There is no trial assessing the effect of angiotensin-converting enzyme inhibitors, angiotensin receptor blockers, beta-blockers on pulmonary hemodynamics in patients with chronic lung diseases and coexisting chronic left heart failure. In COPD several trials indicate that the benefits of selective beta-1-blockers in cardiac patients with COPD outweigh the risks (60). Accordingly, beta-blockers should not be denied to patients with post-capillary HP due to a left heart disease and an associated chronic lung disease. The effect and tolerance of all these drugs remain to be assessed in patients with pre- and post-capillary HP. However, we currently know that angiotensin-converting inhibitors failed to improve functional status and pulmonary hemodynamics in COPD patients with pre-capillary PH (61,62).

Due to the pleiotropic effect of HMG-CoA reductase inhibitors, these drugs improve left ventricular ejection fraction and functional status in patients with chronic heart failure (63) and reduce pulmonary remodeling in a rat model of PH (64). Thus, HMG-CoA reductase inhibitors are promising in the treatment of PH in chronic lung disease particularly in patients with an associated left heart dysfunction.

All treatments currently indicated in chronic left heart disease need to be rigorously studied to assess their efficacy and safety in patients with chronic lung disease and mixed (pre- and post-capillary) PH.

Medical treatments acting on the remodeling and tone of pulmonary arteries

Experience with vasodilators has come from the treatment of idiopathic PAH. It is based on the belief that pulmonary vasoconstriction is an important component of PH, which may not be true in most patients. The acute effects of some drugs, such as calcium channel blockers and urapidil (65) have been somewhat favorable, but there have been very few long-term studies, all were performed in patients with COPD and their results were disappointing (66). Two studies on angiotensin inhibitors to test the long-term effect (>30 days) showed no significant difference in term of pulmonary hemodynamic variables (61,62).

Inhaled nitric oxide is a selective and potent pulmonary vasodilator. Acutely it may improve pulmonary hemodynamics in chronic lung disease. However, some studies performed in COPD have shown that it worsens ventilation-perfusion mismatch and hypoxemia (67). There has been one long-term study (68), again also carried out in patients with COPD showing that the addition of NO to LTOT allowed a significant improvement in PAP, PVR and cardiac output. These results are promising but the technological and toxicological problems related to the prolonged use of inhaled NO are far from being solved, and clearly we need further studies in this field.

Treatments of PAH have shown a dramatic change in the past few years (5). Synthetic prostacyclin (epoprostenol), prostacyclin analogs, endothelin-1 receptor antagonists and phosphodiesterase-5 inhibitors were tested in randomized controlled trials, leading to the approval of several drugs in each class. It is tempting to use these drugs in PH complicating chronic lung disease. Unfortunately, only few studies were published in this field (long-term effect) (69–71).

These studies were performed in stable patients with COPD. In an uncontrolled trial, including six patients with advanced COPD an acute administration of sildenafil produced a pulmonary hemodynamics improvement (70). In the same study, after 3 months of oral treatment with sildenafil, mean PAP and PVR decreased significantly. Exercise capacity was also significantly improved. No side effect of sildenafil is reported in this study. A recent report has shown that one endothelin-1 receptor antagonist had deleterious effect on gas exchange in patients with COPD (71).

Therefore, it is recommended to not treat PH due to chronic lung diseases with these drugs outside trials. In patients with severe or out-of-proportion PH when the pulmonary vascular consequences are in the forefront, it may be legitimate to use a prostacyclin analogue, an endothelin-1 receptor antagonist or a phosphodiesterase-5 inhibitor.

Treatment of right heart failure

As mentioned above, RV function is usually preserved in PH complicating chronic lung disease. However, in some conditions, such as severe idiopathic lung fibrosis, out-of-proportion PH in COPD and combined pulmonary fibrosis and emphysema syndrome RV function may be significantly altered. In these conditions the improvement of RV contractility may improve cardiac output and the functional status of these patients (31). Unfortunately, only a recent experimental study has confirmed this hypothesis (72). Indeed, sildenafil a phosphodiesterase-5 inhibitor in a rat model of PH produced an improvement of cardiac contractility.

A recent review suggests that a treatment of neurohormonal consequences of right heart failure and the reduction of inflammation and reactive oxygen species/reactive nitrogen species imbalance acting on cardiomyocytes may deserve to be treated (31).

In fact, the current treatment of RV failure in chronic lung diseases is based on treating respiratory failure and diuretics. However, diuretics should be used with caution as it may induce metabolic alkalosis that could aggravate arterial hypercapnia.

SUMMARY

In order to treat pulmonary hypertension related to hypoxic lung diseases the first stage is to well characterize which hypoxic lung disease(s) is or are accountable (Figure 20.3.2). When PH is unusually high (mean PAP above 35–40 mmHg), it is of paramount importance to exclude PH due to left heart disease or venous thromboembolic disease. All these associated conditions must be taken into account for treatment choice. All chronic lung diseases and associated conditions should be treated according to the current guidelines to avoid a worsening of PH. Rectifying hypoxemia with LTOT, and hypercapnia with NIPPV when alveolar hypoventilation is the main cause of chronic respiratory

Table 20.3.3 Current methods of treatment of pulmonary hypertension in chronic lung disease

Methods	References	At least one randomized trial?
LTOT	55, 56	Yes
Nocturnal oxygen therapy	8	Yes
NIPPV	59	No
Ca^{2+} channel blockers	66	No
Urapidil	65	No
Angiotensin inhibitors	62	Yes
Inhaled nitric oxide	68	Yes
Medical treatment dedicated to PAH	69, 70, 71	Yes
Lung transplantation	53	No

LTOT, long-term oxygen therapy; NIPPV, non-invasive intermittent positive-pressure ventilation; PAH, pulmonary arterial hypertension.

failure, avoids the progress of PH in hypoxic lung diseases. Whether this latter effect improves functional status and survival is controversial. Nonspecific pulmonary vasodilators have never been demonstrated efficiently in long-term clinical trials. Drugs approved for idiopathic PAH are not recommended for use in PH related to hypoxic lung diseases. Table 20.3.3 summarizes current methods of treatment of PH in chronic lung diseases. Ideal future drugs should lower the RV post-load and improve RV function without worsening of gas exchange.

KEY POINTS

- The development of pulmonary hypertension in patients with COPD and probably in other chronic lung diseases is associated with a short life expectancy.
- When pulmonary hypertension is unusually high (mean pulmonary artery pressure above 35–40 mmHg), it is of paramount importance to exclude pulmonary hypertension due to left heart disease, venous thromboembolic disease or an association of two chronic lung diseases.
- Few patients with mild to moderate impairment of lung mechanics develop severe pulmonary hypertension termed out of proportion pulmonary hypertension.
- All chronic lung diseases and associated conditions should be treated according to the current guidelines.
- Rectifying hypoxemia with long-term oxygen therapy, and hypercapnia with mechanical ventilation

when alveolar hypoventilation is the main cause of chronic respiratory failure, avoids the progress of PH.
- Drugs approved for idiopathic pulmonary arterial hypertension are not recommended for use in pulmonary hypertension related to hypoxic lung diseases.

REFERENCES

1. Weitzenblum E. Chronic cor pulmonale. Heart 2003;89: 225–30.
2. Fishman AP. Hypoxia on the pulmonary circulation. How and where it acts. Circ Res 1976;38:221–31.
3. Simonneau G, Robbins IM, Beghetti M, Channick RN et al. Updated clinical classification of pulmonary hypertension. J Am Coll Cardiol 2009;54:S43–54.
4. Badesch DB, Champion HC, Sanchez MA, Hoeper MM et al. Diagnosis and assessment of pulmonary arterial hypertension. J Am Coll Cardiol 2009;54:S55–66.
5. Galie N, Hoeper MM, Humbert M, Torbicki A et al. Guidelines for the diagnosis and treatment of pulmonary hypertension: The Task Force for the Diagnosis and Treatment of Pulmonary Hypertension of the European Society of Cardiology (ESC) and the European Respiratory Society (ERS), endorsed by the International Society of Heart and Lung Transplantation (ISHLT). Eur Heart J 2009;30:2493–537.
6. Weitzenblum E, Hirth C, Ducolone A, Mirhom R et al. Prognostic value of pulmonary artery pressure in chronic obstructive pulmonary disease. Thorax 1981;36:752–8.
7. Han MK, McLaughlin VV, Criner GJ, Martinez FJ. Pulmonary diseases and the heart. Circulation 2007;116:2992–3005.
8. Chaouat A, Naeije R, Weitzenblum E. Pulmonary hypertension in COPD. Eur Respir J 2008;32:1371–85.
9. Archer S, Michelakis E. The mechanism(s) of hypoxic pulmonary vasoconstriction: potassium channels, redox O(2) sensors, and controversies. News Physiol Sci 2002;17:131–7.
10. Barbera JA, Riverola A, Roca J, Ramirez J et al. Pulmonary vascular abnormalities and ventilation–perfusion relationships in mild chronic obstructive pulmonary disease. Am J Respir Crit Care Med 1994;149:423–9.
11. Heath D, Smith P, Rios Dalenz J, Williams D et al. Small pulmonary arteries in some natives of La Paz, Bolivia. Thorax 1981;36:599–604.
12. Stenmark KR, Fagan KA, Frid MG. Hypoxia-induced pulmonary vascular remodeling: cellular and molecular mechanisms. Circ Res 2006;99:675–91.
13. Wright JL, Levy RD, Churg A. Pulmonary hypertension in chronic obstructive pulmonary disease: current theories of pathogenesis and their implications for treatment. Thorax 2005;60:605–9.
14. Peinado VI, Pizarro S, Barbera JA. Pulmonary vascular involvement in COPD. Chest 2008;134:808–14.

15. Scharf SM, Iqbal M, Keller C, Criner G *et al.* Hemodynamic characterization of patients with severe emphysema. Am J Respir Crit Care Med 2002;166:314–22.

16. Peinado VI, Barbera JA, Abate P, Ramirez J *et al.* Inflammatory reaction in pulmonary muscular arteries of patients with mild chronic obstructive pulmonary disease. Am J Respir Crit Care Med 1999;159:1605–11.

17. Saetta M, Baraldo S, Corbino L, Turato G *et al.* CD8 +ve cells in the lungs of smokers with chronic obstructive pulmonary disease. Am J Respir Crit Care Med 1999;160:711–7.

18. Santos S, Peinado VI, Ramirez J, Melgosa T *et al.* Characterization of pulmonary vascular remodelling in smokers and patients with mild COPD. Eur Respir J 2002;19:632–8.

19. Chaouat A, Savale L, Chouaid C, Tu L *et al.* Role for interleukin-6 in COPD-related pulmonary hypertension. Chest 2009;136:678–87.

20. Eddahibi S, Chaouat A, Morrell N, Fadel E *et al.* Polymorphism of the serotonin transporter gene and pulmonary hypertension in chronic obstructive pulmonary disease. Circulation 2003;108:1839–44.

21. Nathan SD, Noble PW, Tuder RM. Idiopathic pulmonary fibrosis and pulmonary hypertension: connecting the dots. Am J Respir Crit Care Med 2007;175:875–80.

22. Nunes H, Humbert M, Capron F, Brauner M *et al.* Pulmonary hypertension associated with sarcoidosis: mechanisms, haemodynamics and prognosis. Thorax 2006;61:68–74.

23. McCormack FX. Lymphangioleiomyomatosis: a clinical update. Chest 2008;133:507–16.

24. Chabot F, Schrijen F, Poincelot F, Polu JM. Interpretation of high wedge pressure on exercise in patients with chronic obstructive pulmonary disease. Cardiology 2001;95:139–45.

25. Calverley PM, Anderson JA, Celli B, Ferguson GT *et al.* Salmeterol and fluticasone propionate and survival in chronic obstructive pulmonary disease. N Engl J Med 2007;356:775–89.

26. Funk GC, Lang I, Schenk P, Valipour A *et al.* Left ventricular diastolic dysfunction in patients with COPD in the presence and absence of elevated pulmonary arterial pressure. Chest 2008;133:1354–9.

27. Lamia B, Molano LC, Mouton D, Muir JF *et al.* Echocardiographic diagnosis of left ventricular diastolic dysfunction in COPD patients with pulmonary arterial hypertension. Am J Respir Crit Care Med 2009;179:A1484.

28. Butler J, Schrijen F, Henriquez A, Polu JM *et al.* Cause of the raised wedge pressure on exercise in chronic obstructive pulmonary disease. Am Rev Respir Dis 1988;138:350–4.

29. Vodoz JF, Cottin V, Glerant JC, Derumeaux G *et al.* Right-to-left shunt with hypoxemia in pulmonary hypertension. BMC Cardiovasc Disord 2009;9:15.

30. MacNee W. Pathophysiology of cor pulmonale in chronic obstructive pulmonary disease. Part two. Am J Respir Crit Care Med 1994;150:1158–68.

31. Bogaard HJ, Abe K, Vonk Noordegraaf A, Voelkel NF. The right ventricle under pressure: cellular and molecular mechanisms of right-heart failure in pulmonary hypertension. Chest 2009;135:794–804.

32. Vonk-Noordegraaf A, Marcus JT, Holverda S, Roseboom B *et al.* Early changes of cardiac structure and function in COPD patients with mild hypoxemia. Chest 2005;127: 1898–903.

33. Weitzenblum E, Apprill M, Oswald M, Chaouat A *et al.* Pulmonary hemodynamics in patients with chronic obstructive pulmonary disease before and during an episode of peripheral edema. Chest 1994;105:1377–82.

34. de Leeuw PW, Dees A. Fluid homeostasis in chronic obstructive lung disease. Eur Respir J Suppl 2003;46:33s–40s.

35. MacNee W, Wathen CG, Flenley DC, Muir AD. The effects of controlled oxygen therapy on ventricular function in patients with stable and decompensated cor pulmonale. Am Rev Respir Dis 1988;137:1289–95.

36. O'Donnell DE. Hyperinflation, dyspnea, and exercise intolerance in chronic obstructive pulmonary disease. Proc Am Thorac Soc 2006;3:180–4.

37. O'Donnell DE, Voduc N. Mechanisms of dyspnea in restrictive lung disease. In: Malher DA, O'Donnell DE, eds. Dyspnea: mechanisms, measurement and management. Boca Raton: Taylor & Francis Group 2005:87–113.

38. Rich S, Dantzker DR, Ayres SM, Bergofsky EH *et al.* Primary pulmonary hypertension. A national prospective study. Ann Intern Med 1987;107:216–23.

39. Sun XG, Hansen JE, Oudiz RJ, Wasserman K. Exercise pathophysiology in patients with primary pulmonary hypertension. Circulation 2001;104:429–35.

40. Oswald-Mammosser M, Weitzenblum E, Quoix E, Moser G *et al.* Prognostic factors in COPD patients receiving long-term oxygen therapy. Importance of pulmonary artery pressure. Chest 1995;107:1193–8.

41. Nathan SD, Shlobin OA, Ahmad S, Urbanek S *et al.* Pulmonary hypertension and pulmonary function testing in idiopathic pulmonary fibrosis. Chest 2007;131:657–63.

42. Shorr AF, Wainright JL, Cors CS, Lettieri CJ *et al.* Pulmonary hypertension in patients with pulmonary fibrosis awaiting lung transplant. Eur Respir J 2007;30:715–21.

43. Chaouat A, Bugnet AS, Kadaoui N, Schott R *et al.* Severe pulmonary hypertension and chronic obstructive pulmonary disease. Am J Respir Crit Care Med 2005;172:189–94.

44. Thabut G, Dauriat G, Stern JB, Logeart D *et al.* Pulmonary hemodynamics in advanced COPD candidates for lung volume reduction surgery or lung transplantation. Chest 2005;127:1531–6.

45. Cottin V, Le Pavec J, Prevot G, Mal H *et al.* Pulmonary hypertension in patients with combined pulmonary fibrosis and emphysema syndrome. Eur Respir J 2010;35:105–11.

46. Wright JL, Sun JP, Churg A. Cigarette smoke exposure causes constriction of rat lung. Eur Respir J 1999;14:1095–9.

47. Mereles D, Ehlken N, Kreuscher S, Ghofrani S *et al.* Exercise and respiratory training improve exercise capacity and quality of life in patients with severe chronic pulmonary hypertension. Circulation 2006;114:1482–9.

48. Fishman A, Martinez F, Naunheim K, Piantadosi S et al. A randomized trial comparing lung-volume-reduction surgery with medical therapy for severe emphysema. N Engl J Med 2003;348:2059–73.

49. Oswald-Mammosser M, Kessler R, Massard G, Wihlm JM et al. Effect of lung volume reduction surgery on gas exchange and pulmonary hemodynamics at rest and during exercise. Am J Respir Crit Care Med 1998;158:1020–5.

50. Criner GJ, Scharf SM, Falk JA, Gaughan JP et al. Effect of lung volume reduction surgery on resting pulmonary hemodynamics in severe emphysema. Am J Respir Crit Care Med 2007;176:253–60.

51. Bradley B, Branley HM, Egan JJ, Greaves MS et al. Interstitial lung disease guideline: the British Thoracic Society in collaboration with the Thoracic Society of Australia and New Zealand and the Irish Thoracic Society. Thorax 2008;(63 Suppl 5):v1–58.

52. Rodman DM, Lindenfeld J. Successful treatment of sarcoidosis-associated pulmonary hypertension with corticosteroids. Chest 1990;97:500–2.

53. Bjortuft O, Simonsen S, Geiran OR, Fjeld JG et al. Pulmonary haemodynamics after single-lung transplantation for end-stage pulmonary parenchymal disease. Eur Respir J 1996;9:2007–11.

54. Wright JL, Petty T, Thurlbeck WM. Analysis of the structure of the muscular pulmonary arteries in patients with pulmonary hypertension and COPD: National Institutes of Health nocturnal oxygen therapy trial. Lung 1992;170:109–24.

55. Nocturnal Oxygen Therapy Trial Group. Continuous or nocturnal oxygen therapy in hypoxemic chronic obstructive lung disease: a clinical trial. Ann Intern Med 1980;93:391–8.

56. Long term domiciliary oxygen therapy in chronic hypoxic cor pulmonale complicating chronic bronchitis and emphysema. Report of the Medical Research Council Working Party. Lancet 1981;1:681–6.

57. Chaouat A, Weitzenblum E, Krieger J, Ifoundza T et al. Association of chronic obstructive pulmonary disease and sleep apnea syndrome. Am J Respir Crit Care Med 1995;151:82–6.

58. Fletcher EC, Levin DC. Cardiopulmonary hemodynamics during sleep in subjects with chronic obstructive pulmonary disease. The effect of short- and long-term oxygen. Chest 1984;85:6–14.

59. Masa JF, Celli BR, Riesco JA, Hernandez M et al. The obesity hypoventilation syndrome can be treated with noninvasive mechanical ventilation. Chest 2001;119:1102–7.

60. Chen J, Radford MJ, Wang Y, Marciniak TA et al. Effectiveness of beta-blocker therapy after acute myocardial infarction in elderly patients with chronic obstructive pulmonary disease or asthma. J Am Coll Cardiol 2001;37:1950–6.

61. Bertoli L, Fusco M, Lo Cicero S, Micallef E et al. Influence of ACE inhibition on pulmonary haemodynamics and function in patients in whom beta-blockers are contraindicated. Postgrad Med J 1986;(62 Suppl 1):47–51.

62. Morrell NW, Higham MA, Phillips PG, Shakur BH et al. Pilot study of losartan for pulmonary hypertension in chronic obstructive pulmonary disease. Respir Res 2005;6:88.

63. Node K, Fujita M, Kitakaze M, Hori M et al. Short-term statin therapy improves cardiac function and symptoms in patients with idiopathic dilated cardiomyopathy. Circulation 2003;108:839–43.

64. Lee JH, Lee DS, Kim EK, Choe KH et al. Simvastatin inhibits cigarette smoking-induced emphysema and pulmonary hypertension in rat lungs. Am J Respir Crit Care Med 2005;172:987–93.

65. Adnot S, Defouilloy C, Brun-Buisson C, Abrouk F et al. Hemodynamic effects of urapidil in patients with pulmonary hypertension. A comparative study with hydralazine. Am Rev Respir Dis 1987;135:288–93.

66. Saadjian AY, Philip-Joet FF, Vestri R, Arnaud AG. Long-term treatment of chronic obstructive lung disease by Nifedipine: an 18-month haemodynamic study. Eur Respir J 1988;1:716–20.

67. Roger N, Barbera JA, Roca J, Rovira I et al. Nitric oxide inhalation during exercise in chronic obstructive pulmonary disease. Am J Respir Crit Care Med 1997;156:800–6.

68. Vonbank K, Ziesche R, Higenbottam TW, Stiebellehner L et al. Controlled prospective randomised trial on the effects on pulmonary haemodynamics of the ambulatory long term use of nitric oxide and oxygen in patients with severe COPD. Thorax 2003;58:289–93.

69. Rietema H, Holverda S, Bogaard HJ, Marcus JT et al. Sildenafil treatment in COPD does not affect stroke volume or exercise capacity. Eur Respir J 2008;31:759–64.

70. Alp S, Skrygan M, Schmidt WE, Bastian A. Sildenafil improves hemodynamic parameters in COPD – an investigation of six patients. Pulm Pharmacol Ther 2006;19:386–90.

71. Stolz D, Rasch H, Linka A, Di Valentino M et al. A randomized, controlled trial of bosentan in severe COPD. Eur Respir J 2008;32:619–28.

72. Nagendran J, Archer SL, Soliman D, Gurtu V et al. Phosphodiesterase type 5 is highly expressed in the hypertrophied human right ventricle, and acute inhibition of phosphodiesterase type 5 improves contractility. Circulation 2007;116:238–48.

PART 9

OTHER IMPORTANT CAUSES OF PULMONARY HYPERTENSION

Schistosomiasis and others in group 5

ROGÉRIO SOUZA, ANDRÉ HOVNANIAN, CAIO JÚLIO CÉSAR DOS SANTOS FERNANDES AND CARLOS VIANA POYARES JARDIM

SCHISTOSOMIASIS

Schistosomiasis is a tropical disease, first described in 1851 by a German physician, Theodor Bilharz, while working in Cairo, Egypt (1). By that time, Bilharz not only described the worms but also their eggs with spines in different positions (apical or lateral) that later would be recognized as features of different species of the trematode responsible for the disease (schistosoma) (2). Nowadays, schistosomiasis is still considered as one of the most prevalent infectious diseases, with around 200 million people infected in 74 countries (85 percent living in sub-Saharan Africa) (3,4). Many different species of schistosoma exist, with different geographic distribution worldwide (Figure 21.1), but three of them (*Schistosoma mansoni, Schistosoma haematobium* and *Schistosoma japonicum*) represent the vast majority of cases (5,6).

Schistosoma infections are closely related to direct contact with fresh water contaminated with the larval forms of the parasite known as cercariae, which have the ability to penetrate human skin. After this, the cercariae shed their tails and enter capillaries and lymphatic vessels towards the

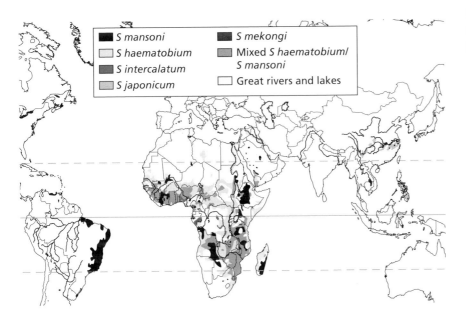

Figure 21.1 Global distribution of schistosomiasis according to the different species of schistosoma.

■ S mansoni
□ S haematobium
■ S intercalatum
▨ S japonicum
■ S mekongi
▨ Mixed S haematobium/ S mansoni
□ Great rivers and lakes

lungs and after several days, the portal venous system, where they mature. The adult forms then migrate to the mesenteric circulation and start egg production. The eggs will then be liberated in the circulation (impacting then on other tissues) or eliminated in feces or urine (depending on the schistosoma species). The life cycle ends after another form of the parasite (miracidium) is released from the egg and infects freshwater snails, from which cercariae are released after two generations (4,7).

Up to one-third of the eggs produced by *S. mansoni* and *S. japonicum* species are deposited in the small veins of the liver, via the portal flow (7). Most of the lesions associated with chronic schistosomiasis are not related to the worms but to the released eggs (5). At the pre-sinusoidal stage, the eggs induce a granulomatous inflammatory response and periportal fibrosis with subsequent portal hypertension, which, in turn, can be responsible for portacaval shunts, generating pulmonary blood overflow and enabling the eggs to be carried to the lung capillaries, where they may lodge (7). Due to attempt of the pre-sinusoidal territory, the development of cirrhosis is not a feature of schistosomiasis, even in the presence of advanced hepatosplenic disease (8).

Different cytokines have been implicated in the immunological processes that modulate chronic host response to schistosoma infection (mainly in the setting of hepatosplenic disease), as IL13, interferon gamma, TNF and IL5; nevertheless, their specific role in each phase of human schistosomiasis is still to be determined (9). Chronic schistosomiasis may be present in up to 20 percent of infected patients and its most common manifestations are hepatosplenic disease with portal hypertension (*S. mansoni* and *S. japonicum*) (10). About 4 to 8 percent of patients with schistosomiasis develop hepatosplenic disease (4,11).

There is a clear association between the development of peri-portal fibrosis and the impairment of the pulmonary circulation, more specifically the development of pulmonary hypertension. An autopsy evaluation of 313 cases of mansoni schistosomiasis evidenced a 7.7 percent prevalence of hepatosplenic disease with findings of pulmonary hypertension (12). Initial studies considering this association emphasized the mechanical role of the ova in causing vascular obstruction and focal arteritis (13). Later, some authors suggested that inflammation also had a significant role in the genesis of the vasculopathy (14–18) as recently recognized for other forms of pulmonary hypertension (19). These early works already acknowledged the presence of plexiform lesions unrelated to the angiomatoid lesions characteristically described as the main pathological feature of schistosomiasis (15,20). Preliminary results of an ongoing study, comparing the lung specimens from patients with idiopathic PAH and schistosomiasis PH also support the spectrum of vascular lesions not related to the presence of eggs or granuloma (21) (Figure 21.2).

From the pulmonary hypertension standpoint, schistosomiasis-associated pulmonary hypertension may represent up to 30 percent of all pulmonary hypertension patients studied at reference centers in Brazil (22). These

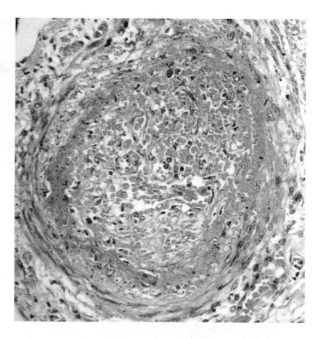

Figure 21.2 Plexiform lesion from a patient with schistosomiasis-associated pulmonary hypertension. (Courtesy of Prof. Thais Mauad, Pathology Department, University of São Paulo Medical School, with permission.)

data emphasize the importance of such a clinical condition in developing countries, suggesting that an unrecognized burden of pulmonary hypertension may exist (23). Recently, the results of a screening program for pulmonary hypertension in patients with hepatosplenic schistosomiasis mansoni found a 7.6 percent prevalence of pulmonary hypertension. Interestingly, about 4.6 percent were further diagnosed (through right heart catheterization) as having pulmonary arterial hypertension (with normal pulmonary artery occlusion pressure) whilst 3.0 percent presented post-capillary pulmonary hypertension, reinforcing the belief that multiple pathophysiological mechanisms might be implicated in the development of pulmonary hypertension in schistosomiasis mansoni. This result also underlines the importance of invasive hemodynamic measurements for the appropriate diagnosis (24). Taken together, the prevalence of both hepatosplenic disease and pulmonary arterial hypertension in this subgroup, may indicate that schistosomiasis-associated pulmonary arterial hypertension might represent the most prevalent form of pulmonary arterial hypertension worldwide.

The recognition of the potential pathways related to the genesis of pulmonary hypertension-associated schistosomiasis led to several changes in its classification in the setting of all other causes of pulmonary hypertension. In the Evian classification, schistosomiasis was classified in the inflammatory group; in the Venice classification, schistosomiasis was in the non-thrombotic embolic group, thus emphasizing the mechanical effect of egg obstruction in the lung vasa (25); recently it has been suggested that schistosomiasis should be relocated in the pulmonary arterial hypertension

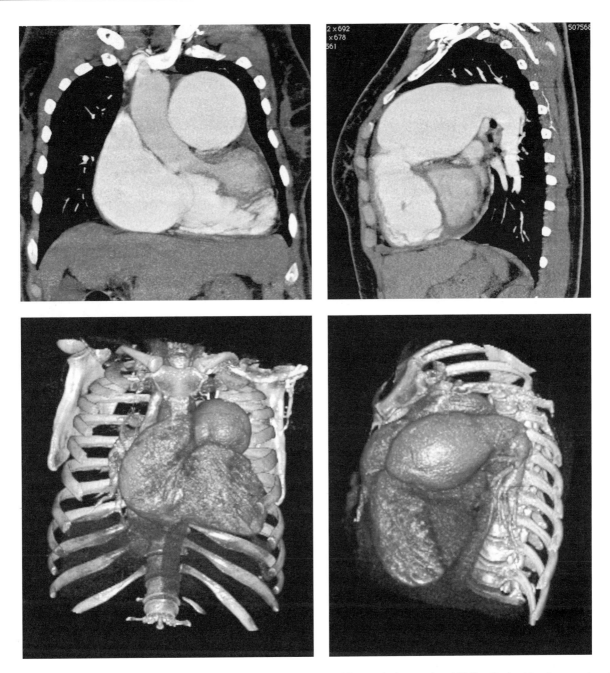

Figure 21.3   Chest CT scan and three-dimensional reconstruction from a schistosomiasis-associated PAH patient evidencing prominent enlargement of pulmonary artery. (Courtesy of Dr Dany Jasinowodolinsk and Dr Claudia Figueiredo, Radiology Department, Fleury Research Institute, with permission.)

group, as a result of the recent findings regarding pathology and hemodynamic presentation. Nevertheless, it is important to re-emphasize that schistosomiasis is a multifactorial disease and that the proper diagnosis of pulmonary arterial hypertension associated with its hepatosplenic form is highly dependent on right heart catheterization to exclude the post-capillary presentation, also common in this clinical setting.

Clinical presentation of schistosomiasis-associated pulmonary hypertension is indistinguishable from other forms of PAH, especially idiopathic PAH (22). Symptoms include

dyspnea, chest pain, peripheral edema and syncope, usually in a progressive pattern over years. Some radiological features are compatible with an insidious process with significant vascular dilatations (26). Compared to idiopathic pulmonary arterial hypertension, the main pulmonary artery enlargement of patients with schistosomiasis-associated PAH is significantly more evident, regardless of the hemodynamic severity (Figure 21.3).

Environmental exposure is a key feature for the diagnosis of schistosomiasis, as important as the identification of the parasite's eggs in stool exam or in rectal biopsy (7). Abdominal ultrasonographic findings such as liver left lobe enlargement or periportal fibrosis raise the suspicion of schistosomiasis and in prevalent areas have a high positive predictive value, even in the absence of viable eggs in stool (27). In fact, the presence of hepatosplenic abnormalities may be considered mandatory to establish the association of schistosomiasis with the development of pulmonary hypertension, not because the disease may not be a cause of pulmonary hypertension in the absence of portal abnormalities, but because it is currently not feasible to distinguish it from the idiopathic form of pulmonary arterial hypertension; even lung biopsies might be inconclusive. Serology tests, by means of the ELISA technique, are also available for the identification of previous contact with various forms of *Schistosoma*, but its usefulness may be confined to patients from non-endemic areas of the disease, since the massive population exposure lowers its value as a disease marker (28).

The cardiovascular investigation of schistosomiasis-associated pulmonary hypertension follows the same algorithm established for other forms of pulmonary hypertension (29). After clinical suspicion or at a screening program, an echocardiogram is performed and in the presence of signs of pulmonary hypertension, right heart catheterization is mandatory to confirm the elevated pulmonary artery pressure levels and also to assess which is the main vascular territory implicated (pre- or post-capillary), since both forms of pulmonary hypertension are common in patients with hepatosplenic schistosomiasis (24). A recent study comparing consecutive newly diagnosed patients with schistosomiasis-related PAH and idiopathic PAH showed that schistosomiasis patients presented a more favorable hemodynamic profile at diagnosis and no acute response at the vasodilator test, compared with nearly 15 percent of response found in the idiopathic group (personal communication, presented at ERS 2007 (E3281)). The clinical course of schistosomiasis-associated pulmonary arterial hypertension also seems to be better than expected compared with idiopathic pulmonary arterial hypertension; unpublished data from our group showed that regardless of hemodynamic severity at baseline, patients with schistosomiasis-associated pulmonary arterial hypertension presented a better 3-year survival than would be expected for patients with idiopathic pulmonary arterial hypertension (to be presented at ATS 2009).

The effect of specific treatment in this particular setting of PAH remains to be determined as well as the role of antiparasitic treatment. Preliminary reports have shown improvement in right ventricular function with sildenafil (30). No data are available regarding the role of other drugs, such as endothelin receptor antagonists or prostanoids. Also, the use of high-dosage calcium-channel blockers is not advised, due to the virtual presence of portal hypertension in all cases. Conventional pulmonary hypertension therapy such as diuretics and oxygen should be implemented as needed. Caution is necessary in the use of oral anticoagulation, because of the high risk of life-threatening bleeding due to the presence of esophageal varices. In schistosomiasis-associated hepatosplenic disease, the effect of antiparasitic treatment is greatly variable, from resolution of periportal fibrosis to absence of response (31). A single case report has described improvement in hemodynamics after antiparasitic treatment (32). Nevertheless, as the treatment of the parasite usually requires one-day treatment with praziquantel, a drug with few side effects, it may be reasonable to treat all the diagnosed patients who have not been treated yet, even in the absence of viable worms or eggs.

The currently ongoing programs to control schistosomiasis in the developing world are of major importance to decrease the morbidity and mortality associated with schistosomiasis, even considering that patients with schistosomiasis-associated pulmonary hypertension will still be seen after decades of schistosomiasis control. This fact, along with the recently acquired knowledge about potential pathophysiological features and its current prevalence, invite us to design appropriate trials addressing the role of different therapeutic approaches for the management of this particular clinical condition that may represent the most prevalent form of PAH worldwide.

SARCOIDOSIS–ASSOCIATED PULMONARY HYPERTENSION

Sarcoidosis is a disease of unknown etiology with a myriad of presentations. Any organ system may be involved, but the lungs and intrathoracic lymph nodes are those most affected. Pulmonary hypertension (PH) is a well-defined complication of sarcoidosis that can result in significant morbidity and mortality (33). Due to the diversity of pathophysiological mechanisms that might be implicated in the genesis of PH in sarcoidosis, together with the paucity of robust data related to this particular association, sarcoidosis-associated PH is currently under the miscellaneous category within the pulmonary hypertension classification (25).

The prevalence rates of PH in sarcoidosis remain unclear. Literature results are widely heterogeneous, ranging from 1 to 74 percent, depending on how PH is defined and on the technique used for diagnosis (34–37). In spite of the higher prevalence rates of PH in more advanced stages of the disease (36,38), some data suggest that the severity of PH does not correlate well with the degree of pulmonary fibrosis or hypoxemia (39) as depicted in a follow-up French study showing an incidence of 32 percent of PH in 22 sarcoidosis patients without pulmonary fibrosis (40). Furthermore, some observations examining the degree of PH in other types of advanced lung disease (e.g. DPOC, cystic fibrosis and interstitial lung diseases) have found systolic pulmonary arterial pressure (sPAP) levels much lower than those observed in sarcoidosis patients (41–44).

All these findings support the rationale that the development of PH is not exclusively attributed to the septal and capillary destruction due to fibrosis and/or to chronic hypoxemia as it occurs in other forms of interstitial lung disease. Other mechanisms might play role in the linkage between PH and sarcoidosis.

There is continuous evidence in favor of multiple and variable mechanisms participating in the development of sarcoidosis-associated PH (40,45–49):

1. compression of pulmonary arteries by hilar or mediastinal nodes;
2. pulmonary vasoconstriction due to an imbalance between vasodilator and vasoconstrictor factors, as evidenced by the increased urinary, plasma and BAL levels of endothelin-1 in sarcoidosis patients;
3. pulmonary vessel adventitia, intimal and media infiltration by noncaseating granulomas;
4. hypoxic pulmonary vasoconstriction;
5. scarring and occlusion of pulmonary veins by granulomas and/or giant cells, mimicking pulmonary veno-occlusive disease;
6. left ventricular systolic and/or diastolic dysfunction due to direct myocardial involvement;
7. porto-pulmonary syndrome related to liver disease.

Diagnosis is difficult, owing to the nonspecific and quite variable clinical presentation. Essentially, symptoms and signs depend on the presence or absence of lung fibrosis and right ventricular function compromise. However, other conditions such as myopathy, anemia, airway obstruction and occult cardiac disease may also impair exercise capacity or result in dyspnea on exertion, thus making the diagnosis even more complicated (50–52).

The only way to perform an accurate diagnosis of PH is by means of right heart catheterization (RHC). This is even more relevant in the presence of advanced lung parenchymal disease when the estimation of systolic right ventricular pressure by transthoracic echocardiogram becomes challenging (53). In this particular presentation, the poor correlation between RVSP and invasive sPAP leads to an underestimation of peak right ventricular pressure (54). In addition, invasive hemodynamic measurements allow the identification of left heart disease in a significant proportion of patients (55). Despite the unequivocal role of RHC, investigation is necessary also in the field of noninvasive studies. A recent study depicted the presence of desaturation of < 90 percent in a 6-min walk test and a diffusion capacity of the lung for carbon monoxide levels < 60 percent as potential predictors of PH in sarcoidosis patients (38). The combination of echocardiogram and these other noninvasive markers may be used as a better indication for the RHC, providing an earlier and more accurate diagnosis of PH in sarcoidosis patients.

It is well known that the presence of PH identifies a subgroup of sarcoidosis patients with poor prognosis (40,56) and probably could serve as a surrogate marker of survival. Thus, it seems well justified to treat PH in this population, but the appropriate management of such a complication is not as well defined as it is for other forms of PH such as idiopathic or scleroderma-associated pulmonary arterial hypertension. Furthermore, there is no evidence that the reversal is true, i.e., if standard treatments for sarcoidosis could positively affect the progression of PH.

Data referring to specific PH treatments are scarce and based on small non-randomized uncontrolled studies. Trials on hemodynamic response to treatment with vasodilators are controversial. Nunes et al. reported that none of their patients had acute vasodilator response with either inhaled nitric oxide (iNO) or intravenous (IV) epoprostenol (40). Others studies revealed clinical and functional improvement to iNO43 and IV prostacyclin (57) in selected patients. Epoprostenol IV therapy was also tested in short- (43) and long-term settings (44) both demonstrating reduction on pulmonary vascular resistance. In a long-term study of epoprostenol use in sarcosis-associated PH, with a mean follow-up time of 29 months, four of seven patients improved in terms of functional status and remained transplant-free during the follow-up (44). The use of bosentan was reported to be useful in case reports or small case series (55,58). Lastly, sildenafil demonstrated a hemodynamic benefit in 12 patients with end-stage sarcoidosis-associated PH (59). Even with these relatively optimistic results, the evidence for recommendation of PAH-specific therapy in the spectrum of sarcoidosis-associated PH is poor and caution should be taken, particularly in patients with parenchymal disease and in those with radiological features that might suggest the presence of predominant venous disease.

In the same way, data about specific therapies for sarcoidosis are even more controversial. The use of corticosteroids is the mainstay of treatment for sarcoidosis. However, its impact on the progression of PH is quite confusing and its benefit difficult to predict. While some reports describe regression or resolution of PH with corticosteroid treatment in selected patients (40,60,61), others show no benefit or even PH worsening (45,46,55,62). In relation to other immunosuppressive agents commonly used in sarcoidosis, there are no systematic studies regarding patients with PH.

The multiple mechanisms related to the pathophysiology of PH in sarcoidosis are quite intriguing, varying from inflammatory and granulomatous processes to mechanical compression of the pulmonary vessels, passing through known pathways related to vascular remodeling, common to other forms of PAH. This feature makes the approach to sarcoidosis-associated PH much more complex, but also opens a diversity of fields of study that could result in specific therapeutic approaches taking into account these particular characteristics of sarcoidosis-associated PH.

HISTIOCYTOSIS AND PULMONARY HYPERTENSION

Pulmonary Langerhans'-cell histiocytosis (HX) is an uncommon smoking-related interstitial lung disease of unknown etiology and unpredictable clinical course that affects young adults (63). Histiocytosis X is characterized by proliferation of specific histiocytic cells (Langerhans' cells) infiltrating different organs (64–66); lung parenchyma involvement is particularly common as an isolated presentation. The disease characteristically affects young smokers (between 20 and 40 years old) although it has also been described in other ages (67).

Clinical presentation is widely variable. Symptoms might be perceived as related only to smoking and may not be significant even in the presence of diffuse lung involvement (68). Pneumothorax with chest pain is not an uncommon presentation and may make the diagnosis difficult (69). The clinical course of the disease is unpredictable. It may regress spontaneously or after steroid therapy and/or smoking cessation. In a minority of cases, it may progress to lung fibrosis leading to important clinical and functional impairment. Chest CT scan is of major importance for the diagnosis, usually presenting small limited/cavitated nodules and thick- and thin-walled cysts; as the disease progresses cysts become the predominant abnormality (68).

From a histopathological standpoint, the classical findings are the formation of bronchiolocentric inflammation with aggregates of large numbers of Langherhans' cells and interstitial fibrosis with cyst formation (70). These findings explain the development of obstructive and/or restrictive lung mechanics and their corresponding clinical aspects.

Pulmonary hypertension is a frequent complication of advanced pulmonary histiocytosis. In contrast to other forms of lung fibrosis, in advanced disease, the diminished exercise capacity and reduction on DLCO both seem to be related to a prominent pulmonary vascular dysfunction (71), which seems to be out of proportion with the alterations seen on pulmonary function tests (72). This is in agreement with histopathological findings of association between both conditions, demonstrating prominent pulmonary vascular involvement in advanced histiocytosis. In addition to the bronchiolocentric inflammation with aggregation of Langerhans' cells and fibrosis, widespread vascular abnormalities were observed in a high proportion of HX cases, characterized by granuloma infiltration of small and medium-sized arteries primarily in the regions of HX nodules, but medial and subintimal thickening were also described in unaffected areas (65,66). The consequence is a proliferative vasculopathy, including venular involvement with aspects of veno-occlusive disease, independent of small airway and parenchymal disease (72). Also, as in other forms of PAH (19), inflammation might play a role in the development of PH in histiocytosis patients (73). All these remodeling processes result in loss of vascular compliance and reduction of cross-sectional area, increasing right ventricle afterload and having PH as a direct consequence.

Data on hemodynamics in HX patients are scarce. In a study including 21 consecutive advanced HX patients, invasive hemodynamic measurements revealed PH in all of them. In comparison with other forms of chronic lung disease, HX patients displayed significant higher levels of mean pulmonary arterial pressure (mPAP) and pulmonary vascular resistance (PVR) as well as lower cardiac index (CI) even in the presence of less severe lung function test abnormalities. The proportion of patients that acutely responded

at the vasodilator challenge was similar to that obtained in patients with idiopathic PAH (72), although the clinical relevance of such a finding is not clear.

With respect to prognosis, in a large retrospective analysis of 102 patients, five and ten-year survival rates were 74 and 64 percent, respectively (63). Nevertheless, these values did not account for the presence of PH; its impact on survival is still to be determined.

Treating PH in HX is unknown. A single case report has shown clinical and hemodynamic improvement with a prolonged corticosteroid regimen (74). There are no robust data on the use of specific PH therapies for the treatment of histiocytosis-associated PH, even considering that isolated successful cases are now being reported (75). It is particularly important to consider the prominent venous involvement and even the veno-occlusive pattern described in histiocytosis patients (72,76). Arterial vasodilation, in this setting, may be hazardous to this population due to the pulmonary edema that may result from it. While there is no evidence for adequate disease management, lung transplantation remains the standard of care for selected advanced cases.

Vascular involvement might be interpreted as a pivotal process in advanced pulmonary histiocytosis. Given all the available clinical and histopathological evidence, it must be stressed that addressing the vascular component of the disease can potentially modify its clinical course. Further studies are still necessary to properly investigate the role of vascular impairment in the progression of this intriguing disease.

KEY POINTS

- Schistosomiasis associated PH might represent one of the most prevalent forms of PH worldwide. There is a clear need to address the impact of specific treatment in the different forms of PH associated with schistosomiasis.
- Multiple mechanisms are associated with the development of PH in sarcoidosis. A comprehensive evaluation is mandatory to identify the predominant one before any treatment attempt is considered.
- PH is a frequent complication of advanced pulmonary hystiocytosis, although its impact on prognosis is still to be proplerly determined.

REFERENCES

1. Bilharz T. Further observations concerning Distonum Haematobium, from a letter to C. T. von Siebald. Z Wissensch Zool 1853;4:454–6.
2. Sandbach FR. The history of schistosomiasis research and policy for its control. Med Hist 1976;20:259–75.

3. Taylor M. Global trends in schistosomiasis control. Bull World Health Organ 2008;86:738.

4. Ross AG, Bartley PB, Sleigh AC, Olds GR, Li Y, Williams GM, McManus DP. Schistosomiasis. N Engl J Med 2002;346: 1212–20.

5. Gryseels B, Polman K, Clerinx J, Kestens L. Human schistosomiasis. Lancet 2006;368:1106–18.

6. Chitsulo L, Engels D, Montresor A, Savioli L. The global status of schistosomiasis and its control. Acta Trop 2000;77:41–51.

7. Prata A. Mansonic Schistosomiasis, 8th edn. Doenças Infecciosas e Parasitárias, ed. R. Veronesi, R. Foccacia, and R. Dietze. São Paulo: Guanabara Koogan, 1991:838–55.

8. Schwartz E. Pulmonary schistosomiasis. Clin Chest Med 2002;23:433–43.

9. Pearce EJ, MacDonald AS. The immunobiology of schistosomiasis. Nat Rev Immunol 2002;2:499–511.

10. Pedroso ER. [Lung changes associated with schistosomiasis mansoni]. Mem Inst Oswaldo Cruz 1989;84 Suppl 1:46–57.

11. Conceicao MJ, Borges-Pereira J, Coura JR. A thirty years follow-up study on *Schistosomiasis mansoni* in a community of Minas Gerais, Brazil. Mem Inst Oswaldo Cruz 2007;102:1007–9.

12. Goncalves EC, Fonseca AP, Pittella JE. Frequency of schistosomiasis mansoni, of its clinicopathological forms and of the ectopic locations of the parasite in autopsies in Belo Horizonte, Brazil. J Trop Med Hyg 1995;98:289–95.

13. Shaw AP, Ghareeb A. The pathogenesis of pulmonary schistosomiasis in Egypt with special reference to Ayerza's disease. J Pathol Bacteriol 1938;46:401–24.

14. Chaves E. [Pulmonary schistosomiasis arteritis; morphological study of 54 cases with special reference to hypersensitivity reactions]. Hospital (Rio J) 1964;66: 1335–46.

15. Chaves E. [Plexiform lesions in chronic cor pulmonale in schistosomiasis]. Hospital (Rio J) 1965;68:635–45.

16. Chaves E. [Pathology of pulmonary endarteritis obliterans in Manson's schistosomiasis]. An Inst Med Trop (Lisb) 1965;22:171–7.

17. Chaves E. The pathology of the arterial pulmonary vasculature in Manson's schistosomiasis. Dis Chest 1966;50:72–7.

18. Magalhaes Filho A. Pulmonary lesions in mice experimentally infected with Schistosoma mansoni. Am J Trop Med Hyg 1959;8:527–35.

19. Dorfmuller P, Perros F, Balabanian K, Humbert M. Inflammation in pulmonary arterial hypertension. Eur Respir J 2003;22:358–63.

20. de Cl, Tompson G, de S, Barbosa FS. Pulmonary hypertension in schistosomiasis. Br Heart J 1962;24:363–71.

21. Pozzan G, Souza R, Jardim C, Dolhnikoff M, Mello G, Canzian M, Bernardi F, Mauad T, Grunberg K. Histopathological features of pulmonary vascular disease in chronic *Schistosomia mansoni* infection are not different from those in idiopathic pulmonary hypertension. Am J Respir Crit Care Med 2008;177:A443.

22. Lapa MS, Ferreira EV, Jardim C, Martins Bdo C, Arakaki JS, Souza R. [Clinical characteristics of pulmonary hypertension patients in two reference centers in the city of Sao Paulo.] Rev Assoc Med Bras 2006;52: 139–43.

23. Humbert M, Khaltaev N, Bousquet J, Souza R. Pulmonary hypertension: from an orphan disease to a public health problem. Chest 2007;132:365–7.

24. Lapa M, Dias B, Jardim C, Fernandes CJ, Dourado PM, Figueiredo M, Farias A, Tsutsui J, Terra-Filho M, Humbert M, Souza R. Cardiopulmonary manifestations of hepatosplenic schistosomiasis. Circulation 2009;119:1518–23.

25. Simonneau G, Galie N, Rubin LJ et al. Clinical classification of pulmonary hypertension. J Am Coll Cardiol 2004;43: 5S–12S.

26. Figueiredo C, Souza R, Ota JS, Moises V, Barone R, Rocha M. Pulmonary hypertension in schistosomiasis: a chest CT study. Am J Respir Crit Care Med 2004;169:A174.

27. Hatz C, Jenkins JM, Ali QM, Abdel-Wahab MF, Cerri GG, Tanner M. A review of the literature on the use of ultrasonography in schistosomiasis with special reference to its use in field studies. 2. *Schistosoma mansoni.* Acta Trop 1992;51:15–28.

28. Igreja RP, Matos JA, Goncalves MM, Barreto MM, Peralta JM. Schistosoma mansoni-related morbidity in a low-prevalence area of Brazil: a comparison between egg excretors and seropositive non-excretors. Ann Trop Med Parasitol 2007;101:575–84.

29. Galie N, Manes A, Branzi A. Evaluation of pulmonary arterial hypertension. Curr Opin Cardiol 2004;19:575–81.

30. Loureiro R, Mendes A, Bandeira A, Cartaxo H, Sa D. Oral sildenafil improves functional status and cardiopulmonary hemodynamics in patients with severe pulmonary hypertension secondary to chronic pulmonary schistosomiasis: a cardiac magnetic resonance study. American Heart Association International Meeting 2004:2569.

31. Richter J. Evolution of schistosomiasis-induced pathology after therapy and interruption of exposure to schistosomes: a review of ultrasonographic studies. Acta Trop 2000; 77:111–31.

32. Bouree P, Piveteau J, Gerbal JL, Halpen G. [Pulmonary arterial hypertension due to bilharziasis. Apropos of a case due to *Schistosoma haematobium* having been cured by praziquantel]. Bull Soc Pathol Exot 1990;83:66–71.

33. Diaz-Guzman E, Farver C, Parambil J, Culver DA. Pulmonary hypertension caused by sarcoidosis. Clin Chest Med 2008;29:549–63, x.

34. Mayock RL, Bertrand P, Morrison CE, Scott JH. Manifestations of Sarcoidosis. Analysis of 145 Patients, with a Review of Nine Series Selected from the Literature. Am J Med 1963;35:67–89.

35. Battesti JP, Georges R, Basset F, Saumon G. Chronic cor pulmonale in pulmonary sarcoidosis. Thorax 1978;33: 76–84.

36. Gluskowski J, Hawrylkiewicz I, Zych D, Wojtczak A, Zielinski J. Pulmonary haemodynamics at rest and during

exercise in patients with sarcoidosis. Respiration 1984;46:26–32.

37. Shorr AF, Helman DL, Davies DB, Nathan SD. Pulmonary hypertension in advanced sarcoidosis: epidemiology and clinical characteristics. Eur Respir J 2005;25:783–8.

38. Bourbonnais JM, Samavati L. Clinical predictors of pulmonary hypertension in sarcoidosis. Eur Respir J 2008;32:296–302.

39. Emirgil C, Sobol BJ, Herbert WH, Trout K. The lesser circulation in pulmonary fibrosis secondary to sarcoidosis and its relationship to respiratory function. Chest 1971;60:371–8.

40. Nunes H, Humbert M, Capron F, Brauner M, Sitbon O, Battesti JP, Simonneau G, Valeyre D. Pulmonary hypertension associated with sarcoidosis: mechanisms, haemodynamics and prognosis. Thorax 2006;61:68–74.

41. Scharf SM, Iqbal M, Keller C, Criner G, Lee S, Fessler HE. Hemodynamic characterization of patients with severe emphysema. Am J Respir Crit Care Med 2002;166:314–22.

42. Arcasoy SM, Christie JD, Ferrari VA, Sutton MS, Zisman DA, Blumenthal NP, Pochettino A, Kotloff RM. Echocardiographic assessment of pulmonary hypertension in patients with advanced lung disease. Am J Respir Crit Care Med 2003; 167:735–40.

43. Preston IR, Klinger JR, Landzberg MJ, Houtchens J, Nelson D, Hill NS. Vasoresponsiveness of sarcoidosis-associated pulmonary hypertension. Chest 2001;120:866–72.

44. Fisher KA, Serlin DM, Wilson KC, Walter RE, Berman JS, Farber HW. Sarcoidosis-associated pulmonary hypertension: outcome with longterm epoprostenol treatment. Chest 2006;130:1481–8.

45. Barst RJ, Ratner SJ. Sarcoidosis and reactive pulmonary hypertension. Arch Intern Med 1985;145:2112–4.

46. Damuth TE, Bower JS, Cho K, Dantzker DR. Major pulmonary artery stenosis causing pulmonary hypertension in sarcoidosis. Chest 1980;78:888–91.

47. Levine BW, Saldana M, Hutter AM. Pulmonary hypertension in sarcoidosis. A case report of a rare but potentially treatable cause. Am Rev Respir Dis 1971;103:413–7.

48. Portier F, Lerebours-Pigeonniere G, Thiberville L, Dominique S, Tayot J, Muir JF, Nouvet G. [Sarcoidosis simulating a pulmonary veno-occlusive disease]. Rev Mal Respir 1991;8:101–2.

49. Salazar A, Mana J, Sala J, Landoni BR, Manresa F. Combined portal and pulmonary hypertension in sarcoidosis. Respiration 1994;61:117–9.

50. Spruit MA, Thomeer MJ, Gosselink R, Troosters T, Kasran A, Debrock AJ, Demedts MG, Decramer M. Skeletal muscle weakness in patients with sarcoidosis and its relationship with exercise intolerance and reduced health status. Thorax 2005;60:32–8.

51. Kabitz HJ, Lang F, Walterspacher S, Sorichter S, Muller-Quernheim J, Windisch W. Impact of impaired inspiratory muscle strength on dyspnea and walking capacity in sarcoidosis. Chest 2006;130:1496–502.

52. Chambellan A, Turbie P, Nunes H, Brauner M, Battesti JP, Valeyre D. Endoluminal stenosis of proximal bronchi in

sarcoidosis: bronchoscopy, function, and evolution. Chest 2005;127:472–81.

53. Homma A, Anzueto A, Peters JI, Susanto I, Sako E, Zabalgoitia M, Bryan CL, Levine SM. Pulmonary artery systolic pressures estimated by echocardiogram vs. cardiac catheterization in patients awaiting lung transplantation. J Heart Lung Transplant 2001;20:833–9.

54. Brecker SJ, Gibbs JS, Fox KM, Yacoub MH, Gibson DG. Comparison of Doppler derived haemodynamic variables and simultaneous high fidelity pressure measurements in severe pulmonary hypertension. Br Heart J 1994; 72:384–9.

55. Baughman RP, Engel PJ, Meyer CA, Barrett AB, Lower EE. Pulmonary hypertension in sarcoidosis. Sarcoidosis Vasc Diffuse Lung Dis 2006;23:108–16.

56. Arcasoy SM, Christie JD, Pochettino A, Rosengard BR, Blumenthal NP, Bavaria JE, Kotloff RM. Characteristics and outcomes of patients with sarcoidosis listed for lung transplantation. Chest 2001;120:873–80.

57. Jones K, Higenbottam T, Wallwork J. Pulmonary vasodilation with prostacyclin in primary and secondary pulmonary hypertension. Chest 1989;96:784–9.

58. Foley RJ, Metersky ML. Successful treatment of sarcoidosis-associated pulmonary hypertension with bosentan. Respiration 2008;75:211–4.

59. Milman N, Burton CM, Iversen M, Videbaek R, Jensen CV, Carlsen J. Pulmonary hypertension in end-stage pulmonary sarcoidosis: therapeutic effect of sildenafil? J Heart Lung Transplant 2008;27:329–34.

60. Davies J, Nellen M, Goodwin JF. Reversible pulmonary hypertension in sarcoidosis. Postgrad Med J 1982;58: 282–5.

61. Rodman DM, Lindenfeld J. Successful treatment of sarcoidosis-associated pulmonary hypertension with corticosteroids. Chest 1990;97:500–2.

62. Gluskowski J, Hawrylkiewicz I, Zych D, Zielinski J. Effects of corticosteroid treatment on pulmonary haemodynamics in patients with sarcoidosis. Eur Respir J 1990;3:403–7.

63. Vassallo R, Ryu JH, Schroeder DR, Decker PA, Limper AH. Clinical outcomes of pulmonary Langerhans'-cell histiocytosis in adults. N Engl J Med 2002;346:484–90.

64. Vassallo R, Ryu JH, Colby TV, Hartman T, Limper AH. Pulmonary Langerhans'-cell histiocytosis. N Engl J Med 2000;342:1969–78.

65. Colby TV, Lombard C. Histiocytosis X in the lung. Hum Pathol 1983;14:847–56.

66. Travis WD, Borok Z, Roum JH, Zhang J, Feuerstein I, Ferrans VJ, Crystal RG. Pulmonary Langerhans cell granulomatosis (histiocytosis X). A clinicopathologic study of 48 cases. Am J Surg Pathol 1993;17:971–86.

67. Kulwiec EL, Lynch DA, Aguayo SM, Schwarz MI, King TE Jr. Imaging of pulmonary histiocytosis X. Radiographics 1992;12:515–26.

68. Tazi A. Adult pulmonary Langerhans' cell histiocytosis. Eur Respir J 2006;27:1272–85.

69. Howarth DM, Gilchrist GS, Mullan BP, Wiseman GA, Edmonson JH, Schomberg PJ. Langerhans cell

histiocytosis: diagnosis, natural history, management, and outcome. Cancer 1999;85:2278–90.

70. Kambouchner M, Basset F, Marchal J, Uhl JF, Hance AJ, Soler P. Three-dimensional characterization of pathologic lesions in pulmonary Langerhans cell histiocytosis. Am J Respir Crit Care Med 2002;166:1483–90.

71. Crausman RS, Jennings CA, Tuder RM, Ackerson LM, Irvin CG, King TE Jr. Pulmonary histiocytosis X: pulmonary function and exercise pathophysiology. Am J Respir Crit Care Med 1996;153:426–35.

72. Fartoukh M, Humbert M, Capron F, Maitre S, Parent F, Le Gall C, Sitbon O, Herve P, Duroux P, Simonneau G. Severe pulmonary hypertension in histiocytosis X. Am J Respir Crit Care Med 2000;161:216–23.

73. Kannourakis G, Abbas A. The role of cytokines in the pathogenesis of Langerhans cell histiocytosis. Br J Cancer Suppl 1994;23:S37–40.

74. Benyounes B, Crestani B, Couvelard A, Vissuzaine C, Aubier M. Steroid-responsive pulmonary hypertension in a patient with Langerhans' cell granulomatosis (histiocytosis X). Chest 1996;110:284–6.

75. Bendayan D, Shitrit D, Kramer MR. Combination therapy with prostacyclin and tadalafil for severe pulmonary arterial hypertension: a pilot study. Respirology 2008;13:916–8.

76. Hamada K, Teramoto S, Narita N, Yamada E, Teramoto K, Kobzik L. Pulmonary veno-occlusive disease in pulmonary Langerhans' cell granulomatosis. Eur Respir J. 2000;15:421–3.

PART 10

ACUTE AND CHRONIC PULMONARY THROMBOEMBOLISM, PULMONARY VASCULAR TUMORS AND PULMONARY VASCULITIS

Diagnosis of acute pulmonary thromboembolism

ARNAUD PERRIER AND HENRI BOUNAMEAUX

INTRODUCTION

Pulmonary embolism is the third cause of mortality by cardiovascular disease after coronary artery disease and stroke. In Western countries, it remains the leading cause of death in the puerperium and the postoperative period. It has been estimated that over one million venous thromboembolic (VTE) events or deaths occur each year in six large European countries, with three quarters of the VTE-related deaths being from hospital-acquired VTE, which is, therefore, a major health concern (1). Nonetheless, pulmonary embolism is difficult to diagnose because of protean clinical manifestations and poor sensitivity and specificity of symptoms and signs. Therefore, it is still underdiagnosed and up to 80 percent of pulmonary emboli found at autopsy have not been suspected ante mortem, a proportion which has not decreased in the last 40 years (2). However, considerable progress has been made in the workup of patients with clinically suspected pulmonary embolism with the advent of novel diagnostic instruments such as plasma D-dimer measurement (3), lower limb venous compression ultrasonography to detect deep vein thrombosis (4) and helical CT scan (5) and of rational and cost-effective diagnostic strategies (6–10). Finally, deep venous thrombosis and pulmonary embolism are now considered as a single disease, venous thromboembolism, with common risk factors and treatment. Indeed, more than 90 percent of pulmonary emboli originate from a deep venous thrombosis of the lower limbs and approximately 50 percent of patients with a proximal deep venous thrombosis have a silent concomitant pulmonary embolism (11,12).

DEFINITIONS

Traditionally, pulmonary embolism was classified as massive or non-massive. However, that definition was ambiguous, because the term massive could refer either to the clinical presentation of pulmonary embolism accompanied by shock, or to the radiological description of a more than 50 percent amputation of the pulmonary vasculature. Moreover, that classification did not account for those patients who despite absence of overt shock have repercussions of pulmonary embolism on right ventricular function. Hence, pulmonary embolism is usually classified into three categories:

- Massive pulmonary embolism: pulmonary embolism provoking shock or cardiorespiratory arrest.
- Submassive pulmonary embolism: pulmonary embolism provoking right ventricular strain (dilatation and hypokinesis) despite normal systemic blood pressure.
- Non-massive pulmonary embolism: pulmonary embolism associated with normal systemic blood pressure and normal right ventricular function.

More recently, the guidelines of the European Society of Cardiology have proposed a new terminology that emphasizes the mortality associated with increasing severity of pulmonary embolism (Table 22.1.1) (7).

Table 22.1.1   Classification of pulmonary embolism according to early (in-hospital) mortality risk

	PE-related early mortality	Risk markers		
		Shock or hypotension	RV dysfunction[†]	RV injury[¶]
High-risk PE	> 15%	Yes	Yes*	Yes*
Intermediate-risk PE	4 to 10%	No	Yes	Yes or no
Low-risk PE	< 1%	No	No	No

PE: pulmonary embolism. RV: right ventricle.
*Usually present, but not required to define high-risk PE.
[†]As assessed by echocardiography.
[¶]Elevated biomarkers of myocardial injury (troponin).
Adapted from ref 7.

EPIDEMIOLOGY

Several recent population-based studies have established that the incidence of venous thromboembolism is around 1 per 1000 subjects per year, with an incidence of pulmonary embolism approximately half that of deep venous thrombosis (13,14). Venous thromboembolic recurrences account for one-third of those events. Age is an important determinant of the incidence of venous thromboembolism. Above 40 years, the incidence of venous thromboembolism doubles for every ten additional years. Finally, the disease is slightly more common in male than in female subjects.

The case-fatality rate of treated pulmonary embolism has been a matter of debate. In the large multicenter Prospective Investigation on Pulmonary Embolism Diagnosis (PIOPED) study (15), despite a high 15 percent mortality in the three months following the acute event, only 10 percent of those deaths were attributed to pulmonary embolism. In contrast, in the large International Cooperative Pulmonary Embolism Registry (ICOPER) (16), pulmonary embolism recurrence was the main cause of death in the 17.5 percent of patients who died during the 3-month follow-up period. In a Geneva series (17), 3-month mortality was 8.4 percent and more than half of the deaths that occurred during the first 15 days were due to pulmonary embolism recurrence. The much lower recurrence and case-fatality rates observed in a recent meta-analysis of randomized controlled trials on treatment of venous thromboembolism (18) are probably due to selection bias and exclusion of the sicker patients. Hence, the true recurrence rate in patients with pulmonary embolism is probably around 4 percent in the first three months, and approximately half of those events are fatal (19) Finally, cancer, heart failure and presence of concomitant deep vein thrombosis are significant risk factors for recurrent pulmonary embolism (19).

ETIOLOGY

Venous thromboembolism is a multigenic disease with a strong influence of environmental factors. The basic pathophysiological hypothesis formulated by Virchow at the end of the 19th century is still valid (20). Virchow's triad consists of venous stasis in the lower limbs, an imbalance of the haemostatic system towards thrombosis (hypercoagulable state), and direct lesions of the venous endothelium. Although the relative importance of those factors varies according to the clinical situation, venous thrombosis usually results from an interaction of those mechanisms. For instance, venous stasis and clotting activation predominate in thrombosis after surgery, but patients with more severe hypercoagulability due to cancer or a genetic thrombophilic mutation are more prone to thrombotic complications in that setting.

Genetic determinants

In recent years, several molecular markers of an increased thrombotic risk have been identified, of which the two most prevalent are the Leiden mutation of factor V which confers a resistance to activated protein C, and the G20210A mutation of prothrombin (Table 22.1.2) (21). Deficiency in protein S, protein C or antithrombin are much less prevalent (21). Patients who are heterozygous for two of these anomalies present a much greater thrombotic risk. Conversely, certain genetic factors seem to protect from thrombosis despite the existence of a thrombophilic mutation. For instance, the O blood group appears to reduce the risk of venous thrombosis in carriers of factor V Leiden (22). Protective factors are yet largely non-investigated. Factor V Leiden and prothrombin mutation are stronger risk factors for deep vein thrombosis than for pulmonary embolism, raising the question whether clot composition might be different when those anomalies are present and, therefore more adherent (23). Finally, elevated levels of homocysteine, factor VIII, IX and XI have been identified as risk factors for venous thromboembolism, but the underlying genetic defects are yet unidentified (24). Gender seems to also play an important role, and the risk of recurrent VTE in patients with a first idiopathic event appears to be higher in men than in women (25).

Table 22.1.2 Prevalence of genetic risk factors for pulmonary embolism

Anomaly	General population (%)	Subjects with pulmonary embolism (%)	Relative risk
Antithrombin deficiency	0.02	1	50
Protein C deficiency	0.2	3	15
Protein S deficiency	0.1	1–2	10–20
Factor V Leiden*	4	12	3
G20210A prothrombin mutation	4	10	2.5

*Frequency of the anomaly is very different according to the country of origin (15% in the South of Sweden vs. 5% overall in Europe).

Environmental determinants

The main environmental risk factors for pulmonary embolism are detailed in Table 22.1.3. Recent data from the Nurses' Health Study (26) and a French epidemiological study (27) have identified heavy smoking and arterial hypertension as additional risk factors. Hormone replacement therapy increases the thromboembolic risk threefold, similar to oral contraception (28). However, the absolute incidence of venous thromboembolism is 10-fold higher in women over 50 compared to women in their third decade and hormone replacement therapy may hence be responsible for a higher number of cases. Raloxifene, a new selective modulator of the estrogen receptor, is also associated with an increased risk of venous thromboembolism (29).

Searching for specific etiologies

TESTING FOR THROMBOPHILIA

The opportunity of searching for a genetic thrombophilia depends on the probability of finding an anomaly in a given individual, on the feasibility of biological diagnosis and most of all on the existence of consequences on patient management (24). Recent trials failed to report an increased recurrence rate after a first venous thromboembolic event in patients with the most frequent anomalies (heterozygous factor V Leiden or prothrombin mutation) (30). Hence, prolonged anticoagulation treatment after a first episode is not justified. In contrast, detection of thrombophilic defects may be important in particular situations. For instance, thrombotic risk is greatly increased during pregnancy in some thrombophilias such as antithrombin deficiency, justifying prophylactic anticoagulation throughout. Common recommendations are to investigate patients with a positive family history of venous thromboembolism, recurrent idiopathic venous thrombosis or thrombosis after a trivial triggering event (travel, pregnancy, estrogen therapy), first thrombotic episode before 50 years of age, association of arterial and venous thrombosis, superficial thrombosis in a nonvaricose vein, thrombosis in unusual sites, and association of thrombosis and fetal loss (24).

Table 22.1.3 Environmental and acquired risk factors for venous thromboembolism

Acquired thrombophilia
  Lupus anticoagulant
  Antiphospholipid syndrome
  Acquired deficiency in coagulation inhibitors
  Hyperhomocysteinemia
Hormonal treatment
  Oral contraceptives
  Hormone replacement therapy
  Tamoxifen, raloxifen
  Pregnancy
Cancer
Surgery
Trauma
Immobilization
  Hemiplegia, paraplegia
Congestive heart failure
Myocardial infarction
Chronic inflammatory bowel disease
Nephrotic syndrome

Nevertheless, screening decisions should be individualized according to the family and individual history, the type of suspected anomaly, patient age and consequences of a positive finding. Finally, any patient with one of the above cited characteristics should be considered as having a clinical thrombophilia, even if the laboratory tests do not disclose a known anomaly, and given appropriate prophylaxis in at-risk situations. Specialized counseling and performance of tests in a reference laboratory should be preferred to routine testing.

SEARCHING FOR CANCER

Neoplastic cells are able to activate the clotting cascade either directly through activation of thromboplastin or indirectly by stimulating monocytes and macrophages to synthesize a variety of procoagulant molecules. Hence, cancer is a significant risk factor for venous thromboembolism and the risk of discovering a cancer during the first 6 months to one year after an acute episode venous thromboembolism is increased approximately three- to fourfold (31–33). The prevalence of cancer may be higher in patients with idiopathic venous thromboembolism (34), and in the rare patients with bilateral deep vein thrombosis (35). In a recent series most cancers were detected by clinical examination and simple tests such a complete blood count, sedimentation rate and chest radiography (36), and the 34-month cancer-free survival was similar in patients with a negative initial workup and a control group without deep vein thrombosis. The only randomized trial on this issue compared extensive screening to usual care (37). The proportion of occult cancer identified by extensive screening was higher (13.1 percent versus 1.0 percent), but the 2-year cancer-related mortality was again similar. Therefore, an extensive diagnostic workup for cancer does not appear warranted in patients with acute venous thromboembolism.

CLINICAL PRESENTATION

Clinical syndromes

Symptoms of pulmonary embolism are very non-specific. In 65 percent of patients, pulmonary embolism is evoked because of pleuritic pain accompanied or not by dyspnea. Isolated dyspnea, usually acute but sometimes slowly progressive and without an obvious alternative cause, points towards pulmonary embolism in 20 percent of patients. Syncope or shock are a rare clinical presentation of pulmonary embolism (less than 10 percent). Last, pulmonary embolism is exceptionally discovered in the absence of a clinical suspicion during the investigation of a radiologic infiltrate. Those clinical presentations correspond to three syndromes of different pathology and variable severity (38).

ALVEOLAR HEMORRHAGE

The clinical hallmark of this syndrome is pleuritic pain due to irritation of the visceral pleura, and more rarely hemoptysis. It is due to peripheral emboli. Although it is often incorrectly referred to as "pulmonary infarction," the histopathological correlate is in fact an alveolar hemorrhage probably provoked by the afflux of blood from the high-pressure bronchial circulation in the segment obstructed by the embolus (39). The classic radiologic picture is a wedge-shaped pleural-based infiltrate that affects around 20 percent of patients (40). Other common chest X-ray anomalies include platelike atelectasis and pleural effusion. Tachycardia and dyspnea are less frequent than in this clinical syndrome reflecting the peripheral character and lesser hemodynamic repercussions of such pulmonary emboli (38).

ISOLATED DYSPNEA

The absence of pleuritic pain in this syndrome is probably due to more proximal embolization of the pulmonary vasculature. Patients may complain of retrosternal chest pain

oppressive in character evoking the differential diagnosis of angina. In fact, such pain probably reflects true myocardial ischemia due to increased right ventricular wall tension and reduced right coronary artery flow. Tachycardia, although more frequent, is still present in only 45 percent of patients (38). Electrocardiogram is rarely normal, but its anomalies are often non-specific. Although dyspnea is usually of abrupt or rapid onset, in some patients it may progress over several days.

SHOCK

Syncope and/or shock are the clinical manifestations of massive pulmonary embolism causing acute severe pulmonary hypertension and right ventricular failure. It is usually due to large central clots. Although suggestive of pulmonary embolism in patients with obvious risk factors such as recent surgery, syncope may be a misleading presentation (41). Suspected massive pulmonary embolism with shock is a distinct situation requiring a specific diagnostic approach detailed in an appropriate section.

Laboratory tests

CHEST RADIOGRAPH

The most frequent anomalies of the chest radiograph are cardiomegaly, pleural effusion, band atelectasis and elevated hemidiaphragm (40,42). Their presence raises the probability of pulmonary embolism, albeit modestly. Pulmonary artery enlargement and oligemia are rare and non-specific. The typical infiltrate of so-called pulmonary infarction has already been discussed. Nevertheless, the chest radiograph remains extremely useful in a patient with suspected pulmonary embolism for differential diagnosis with conditions such as left ventricular failure, pneumonia or pneumothorax.

ELECTROCARDIOGRAM

The electrocardiogram is usually normal in small peripheral pulmonary embolism. Larger pulmonary embolism may induce modifications such as large P waves in derivations DII, DIII and AVF, the S1Q3 pattern or ST segment depression in derivations V1 to V4. A right bundle branch block or right axial deviation are also possible (43). When all present in a patient with a suggestive clinical presentation and risk factors for venous thromboembolism, those anomalies may be useful.

BLOOD GASES

Hypocapnia and hypoxemia are frequent in pulmonary embolism. However, approximately 20 percent of patients with proven pulmonary embolism have a normal arterial oxygen pressure and alveoloarterial oxygen gradient (44,45).

Clinical probability of pulmonary embolism

Sensitivity and specificity of clinical symptoms, signs and abnormalities of blood gases, chest radiograph and electrocardiogram in suspected pulmonary embolism are low when considered singly. Nevertheless, these findings can be combined effectively by clinicians, either implicitly (15,46) or by prediction rules (47,48). Both means of assessing clinical likelihood of pulmonary embolism allow a fairly accurate stratification of patients into three categories corresponding to a prevalence of pulmonary embolism of around 10 percent (low clinical probability), 30 percent (intermediate clinical probability) and 65 percent (high clinical probability), respectively (49,50). The majority of patients (80 to 90 percent) have a low or intermediate clinical probability of pulmonary embolism. Clinical assessment is necessary to correctly interpret test results, as the posttest probability of pulmonary embolism depends not only on test characteristics (sensitivity and specificity) but also on pretest probability. Table 22.1.4 shows two recently developed prediction rules. The Wells rule (48) has been widely validated and can be applied to both out- and inpatients, but it requires a subjective judgment on the probability of an alternative diagnosis, which reduces its interobserver reliability. The revised Geneva score (47) has only been validated in outpatients (49), but it is entirely standardized. In summary, clinical evaluation allows classifying patients in probability categories corresponding to an increasing prevalence of PE, whether assessed by implicit clinical judgment or by a validated prediction rule.

INVESTIGATIONS

The individual characteristics of the main diagnostic tests for pulmonary embolism are summarized in Table 22.1.5. Likelihood ratios are adapted from a recent meta-analysis (51).

D-dimer

Plasma D-dimer, a degradation product of crosslinked fibrin, has been extensively investigated in recent years (52). D-dimer levels are elevated in plasma in the presence of an acute clot, because of simultaneous activation of coagulation and fibrinolysis. Hence, a normal D-dimer level renders acute pulmonary embolism unlikely. On the other hand, although D-dimer is very specific for fibrin, the specificity of fibrin for venous thromboembolism is poor, because

Table 22.1.4 Clinical prediction rules for pulmonary embolism

Revised Geneva score (47)		Wells score (48)	
Variables	**Points**	**Variables**	**Points**
Risk factors		**Risk factors**	
Age >65 years	+1	Previous PE or DVT	+1.5
Previous DVT or PE	+3	Recent surgery or immobilization	+1.5
Surgery or fracture within one month	+2	Cancer	+1
Active malignancy	+2		
Symptoms		**Symptoms**	
Unilateral lower limb pain	+3	Hemoptysis	+1
Hemoptysis	+2		
Clinical signs		**Clinical signs**	
Heart rate		Heart rate >100/min	+1.5
75 to 94 beats per minute	+3	Clinical signs of DVT	+3
≥95 beats per minute	+5		
Pain on lower limb deep vein palpation and unilateral edema	+4		
		Clinical judgment	
		Alternative diagnosis less likely than PE	+3
Clinical probability	**Total**	**Clinical probability**	**Total**
Low	0–3	Low	0–1
Intermediate	4–10	Intermediate	2–6
High	≥11	High	≥7
		PE unlikely	0 to 4
		PE likely	>4 points

DVT, deep vein thrombosis; PE, pulmonary embolism.

Table 22.1.5   Performances of diagnostic tests for non-massive pulmonary embolism

Test	Sensitivity (%)	Specificity (%)	Likelihood ratio	
			Positive result	Negative result
V/Q lung scan				
Normal	99	–	–	0.05
Nondiagnostic	–	–	0.9	–
High probability	–	91	18	–
Plasma D–dimer				
Rapid ELISA	97	40	1.6	0.08
Immunoturbidimetric	95	50	1.9	0.1
Whole blood agglutination	85	65	2.4	0.2
Lower limb venous ultrasonography	30	97	10	0.7
Helical CT scan				
Single-detector	70	90	7	0.3
Multidetector	83	96	20.8	0.2
Echocardiography	60	90	6	0.4

V/Q: ventilation-perfusion.
Adapted from ref 51.

fibrin is produced in a wide variety of conditions, such as cancer, inflammation, infection, or necrosis. Therefore, D-dimer is not useful for confirming pulmonary embolism. There are a number of available assays with different characteristics (52). The quantitative ELISA or ELISA-derived assays have a sensitivity over 95 percent and a specificity around 40 percent (Table 22.1.5) (52,53). They can therefore be used to exclude pulmonary embolism in patients with either a low or a moderate probability of pulmonary embolism. In the emergency department, a negative ELISA D-dimer can exclude pulmonary embolism without further testing in approximately 30 percent of patients (49,50, 54–56). Outcome studies using the Vidas D-dimer assay have shown that the three-month thromboembolic risk in patients was below 1 percent in patients left untreated based on a negative test result (Table 22.1.6). Quantitative latex-derived assays and a whole-blood agglutination assay have lower sensitivity in the range of 85 to 90 percent (Table 22.1.5) and are often referred to as moderately sensitive assays (53,57). The most extensively studied to date in outcome studies are the Tinaquant and the SimpliRED assays, which yield a less than 1 percent 3-month thromboembolic risk in patients with a low clinical probability left untreated (Table 22.1.6) (50,58–62). However, their safety for ruling out pulmonary embolism has not been established in the moderate clinical probability category when using a three-level probability scheme. When using the dichotomous Wells rule which classifies patients as "pulmonary embolism unlikely" and "pulmonary embolism likely" (Table 22.1.4), moderately sensitive assays are safe to exclude pulmonary embolism in patients categorized as "pulmonary embolism unlikely," i.e. with a score of 4 points or less (50).

The diagnostic yield of D-dimer relies on its specificity, which varies according to patient characteristics. The specificity of D-dimer in suspected pulmonary embolism decreases steadily with age and may reach 10 percent or less in patients above 80 years (63). D-dimer is also more frequently elevated in patients with cancer (57,64), in hospitalized patients and during pregnancy (65,66). Therefore, the number of suspected patients in whom D-dimer must be measured to exclude one pulmonary embolism (also referred to as the number needed to test or NNT) varies between 3 in the emergency department and 10 or above in the specific situations listed above. Deciding whether measuring D-dimer is worthwhile in a given situation remains a matter of clinical judgment. In summary, a normal D-dimer level by a highly sensitive assay safely excludes pulmonary embolism in patients with a low or moderate clinical probability, while a moderately sensitive assay excludes pulmonary embolism only in patients with a low clinical probability. When using a recently introduced two-level clinical probability assessment scheme, a normal D-dimer level excludes pulmonary embolism safely in "pulmonary embolism less likely" patients either by a highly or moderately sensitive assay.

Lower limb venous compression ultrasonography and CT venography

Lower limb venous compression ultrasonography has become the diagnostic criterion standard for proximal deep venous thrombosis (67). Finding a deep vein thrombosis by ultrasonography in a patient with clinically suspected pulmonary embolism is sufficient evidence to

Table 22.1.6 Three-month thromboembolic risk in patients left untreated according to various diagnostic criteria for ruling out pulmonary embolism

Diagnostic criterion	Patients (n)	3-month thromboembolic risk (%) (95% CI)	Reference
Normal pulmonary angiogram	1050	1.7 (1.0 to 2.7)	94
Normal lung scan	1278	0.7 (0.4 to 1.3)	73–77
Plasma ELISA D-dimer level $< 500\,\mu g/L$ and low to intermediate clinical probability of PE	5060	0.1 (0 to 0.4)	49, 50, 54–56, 60
Negative immunoturbidimetric D-dimer and low clinical probability or PE unlikely	2071	0.6 (0.3 to 1.5)	50, 61, 62
Negative whole blood D-dimer assay and low clinical probability	1175	0.4 (0.1 to 1.4)	58, 59
Non-diagnostic lung scan and negative proximal US and low clinical probability of PE	864	2.3 (1.5 to 3.5)	46, 76
Negative single-detector CT scan angiography and negative proximal US and low or intermediate clinical probability of PE	975	1.6 (1.0 to 2.6)	55, 81
Negative multidetector CT scan angiography and low/intermediate clinical probability or PE unlikely	6449	0.8 (0.6 to 1.2)	49, 50, 56, 73

IPE, pulmonary embolism; US, lower limb venous compression ultrasonography.

warrant anticoagulant treatment without further testing. However, compression ultrasonography shows a deep vein thrombosis in only approximately 30 to 50 percent of patients with proven pulmonary embolism (Table 22.1.5) (4,49). In a recent randomized trial comparing two strategies for diagnosing pulmonary embolism, with and without venous ultrasonography, ultrasound performed in patients with an elevated D-dimer allowed avoiding a CT in only 9 percent of patients and the strategy including ultrasound was not cost-effective. The diagnostic yield of venous ultrasound in suspected pulmonary embolism might be raised by performing a complete ultrasonography including the distal veins, but a modest increase in sensitivity appears to be offset by a decrease in specificity (68). Finally, the probability of a positive proximal CUS in suspected pulmonary embolism is higher in patients with leg symptoms and signs than in asymptomatic patients (4).

More recently, CT venography has been advocated as a simple way to diagnose DVT in patients with suspected pulmonary embolism as it can be combined with chest CT angiography as a single procedure using only one intravenous injection of contrast dye. In the recent PIOPED II study, combining CT venography with CT angiography increased sensitivity for pulmonary embolism from 83 percent to 90 percent and had a similar specificity (around 95 percent) (69). However, the corresponding increase in negative predictive value was not clinically significant. Therefore, CT venography increases the overall detection rate only marginally in patients with suspected pulmonary embolism and adds a significant amount of irradiation, which may be a concern especially in younger women (70).

Ventilation–perfusion lung scintigraphy

Perfusion lung scintigraphy is a non-invasive technique allowing the visualization of pulmonary perfusion through intravenous injection of albumin macroaggregates labeled by Technetium 99m. The macroaggregates are trapped in approximately 0.1 percent of the pulmonary capillary vessels and may be imaged by a gamma-camera. Pulmonary hypoperfusion is not highly specific for an embolus, since any disease which narrows the airways or fills the alveoli with fluid will result in hypoxic pulmonary vasoconstriction, a protective mechanism designed to minimize the shunt effect due to poorly ventilated alveolar units. A perfusion defect corresponding to a segment or a large part of a segment is more specific for pulmonary embolism. The addition of ventilation scintigraphy (by Xenon 133, Krypton 81m or aerosolized Technetium 99m) further increases specificity, a so-called mismatched defect (perfusion defect with normal ventilation) usually representing pulmonary embolism (71). The interpretation of lung scan has long been based on criteria validated in the landmark Prospective Investigation On Pulmonary Embolism Diagnosis (PIOPED) study (15), and their subsequent revision (72). More recently, it has been greatly simplified and lung scan results are now classified into three categories: normal, high probability and non-diagnostic (73). Attribution of a lung scintigram to the high probability category requires two or more mismatched segmental defects or, if only one is present, the addition of two large mismatched subsegmental defects according to the revised PIOPED criteria (72). The presence of one or more mismatched segmental defects or two or more large mismatched subsegmental defects suffices for the Canadian classification (73), but these differences of interpretation appear to be of little clinical consequence (Figure 22.1.1). The high negative predictive value of a normal lung scan has been confirmed by several studies, including a large outcome study (73–77) and is recognized as a valid criterion for excluding pulmonary embolism (Table 22.1.5). The positive predictive value of a high probability scan is approximately 90 percent (15) and most clinicians consider such a result to rule in pulmonary embolism (Table 22.1.5). Recent evidence suggests that the ventilation scan may be validly replaced by chest X-ray with an overall agreement of 88 percent and a positive predictive value of 86 percent for a scintigraphic mismatch (78). The main weakness of ventilation-perfusion scintigraphy is the high proportion of non-diagnostic results (around 50 percent in recent series) (63,73,76). However, further testing can be safely withheld in patients with a low clinical probability of pulmonary embolism, a non-diagnostic lung scan result and no proximal deep venous thrombosis on proximal compression ultrasonography (46,76).

Helical computed tomography

The value of CT angiography for the decision making in suspected pulmonary embolism has changed with recent improvements in available technology. Single-detector CT angiography (Figures 22.1.2 and 22.1.3) had a high specificity but a low sensitivity (around 70 percent) for

pulmonary embolism (79,80). Therefore, a negative single-detector CT was not safe for ruling out pulmonary embolism, and venous compression ultrasonography was required to ensure the absence of a proximal DVT. Indeed, around 10 to 15 percent of patients finally classified as having pulmonary embolism had a proximal DVT despite a negative chest single-detector spiral CT. Conversely, non-high-probability patients left untreated because of a negative single-detector CT and absence of proximal DVT had only a 1 percent 3-month thromboembolic risk in two large-scale outcome studies (55,81). Since the introduction of multidetector-row computed tomography (MDCT) with high spatial and temporal resolution and quality of arterial opacification, CT angiography has become the method of choice for imaging the pulmonary vasculature for suspected pulmonary embolism in routine clinical practice. It allows an adequate visualization of the pulmonary arteries up to at least the segmental level (Figure 22.1.4) (82). The large recent PIOPED II series observed a sensitivity of 83 percent and a specificity of 96 percent of multidetector (mainly 4-detector) CT (69). That sensitivity, although higher than that of single-detector CT, may appear disappointing. However, most false-negative CT results occurred in patients with a high clinical probability, again highlighting the importance of clinical assessment. Indeed, in patients with a low or intermediate clinical probability of pulmonary embolism as assessed by the Wells score, a negative CT had a high negative predictive value for pulmonary embolism (96 percent and 89 percent, respectively), while it was only 60 percent in those with

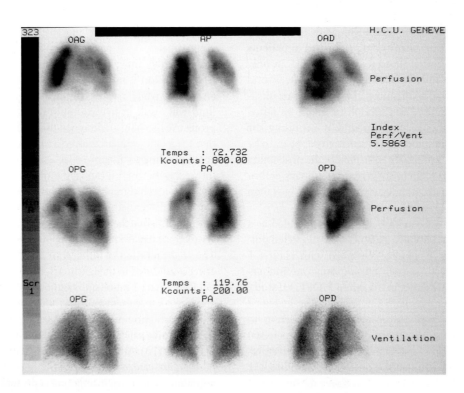

Figure 22.1.1   High probability lung scan. The six perfusion views (upper part of figure) show multiple segmental defects, mismatched compared to the three ventilation views (lower part). Such a lung scan result is highly specific for pulmonary embolism.

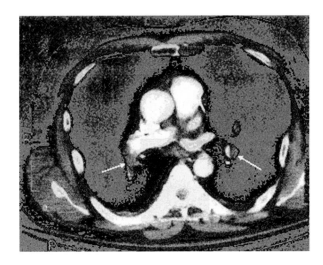

Figure 22.1.2 Single-detector helical computed tomography showing a pulmonary embolism. This CT image was taken in the same patient as the lung scan in Figure 22.1.1. Bilateral thrombi in the main and lobar pulmonary artery are clearly visible (arrows).

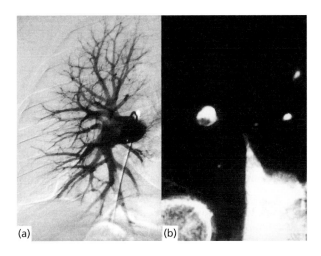

(a)   (b)

Figure 22.1.3 Helical computed tomography and corresponding pulmonary angiogram. The CT shows an isolated segmental thrombus, confirmed by a vascular filling defect in the same segmental artery on pulmonary angiography (arrows).

a high pretest probability. Conversely, the positive predictive value of a positive CT was high (92 to 96 percent) in patients with an intermediate or high clinical probability but much lower (58 percent) in patients with a low pretest likelihood of pulmonary embolism. Nevertheless, four recent outcome studies in which MDCT was used for clinical decision-making, among which two randomized studies, provide evidence in favor of CT as a stand-alone test to exclude pulmonary embolism (49,50,56,73). Table 22.1.7 summarizes the findings of those studies. Whether patients with a negative CT and a high clinical probability should be further investigated by venous compression ultrasonography and/or ventilation-perfusion scintigraphy or pulmonary angiography is controversial, but this is a

rare occurrence. Another controversial area is the clinical significance of isolated subsegmental pulmonary embolism, i.e. the presence of a single subsegmental clot on MDCT, which is found in 1 percent to 5 percent in patients with suspected pulmonary embolism undergoing MDCT (56,83). Indeed, the positive predictive value of such a finding is low, and results from outcome studies suggest that such patients left untreated by anticoagulants may have an uneventful course (84). In summary, a single-detector or MDCT showing a thrombus up to the segmental level can be taken as adequate evidence of pulmonary embolism in most instances, whereas the necessity to treat isolated subsegmental thrombi in a patient without a deep vein thrombosis is unclear. In patients with a non high clinical probability, a negative single-detector CT must be combined to a negative venous compression ultrasonography to safely exclude pulmonary embolism, whereas MDCT may be used as a stand-alone test. Whether further testing is mandatory in the rare patients who have a negative MDCT despite a high clinical probability is not settled.

Pulmonary angiography

Although formerly considered the criterion standard for diagnosing pulmonary embolism, pulmonary angiography (Figure 22.1.3) is difficult to interpret, frequent disagreement occurring even between expert readers, more often on the absence (17 percent of angiograms) than on the presence of pulmonary embolism (8 percent of angiograms) (15). It is also costly and invasive. The mortality due to pulmonary angiography is around 0.2 percent (85). The rare deaths attributable to pulmonary angiography occur in very sick patients with hemodynamic compromise or acute respiratory failure. This should be kept in mind when discussing diagnostic strategies for suspected massive pulmonary embolism. On the other hand, complications do not appear to be more frequent in patients with preexisting pulmonary hypertension in recent series (86).

Echocardiography

Doppler echocardiography has several uses in suspected pulmonary embolism and it may play a role in risk stratification. In a small subset of patients with pulmonary embolism, transthoracic echocardiography allows a direct visualization of the clot in the right heart chambers or in the right main pulmonary artery (87). However, the most frequent echocardiographic manifestations of pulmonary embolism are indirect and reflect the hemodynamic changes caused by an acute increase in pulmonary arterial resistance and pulmonary hypertension. Pulmonary arterial pressure may be estimated in most patients by the tricuspid regurgitation velocity. A cutoff value of 2.7 m/sec for the presence of pulmonary arterial hypertension was adopted in several series. Signs of right ventricular dysfunction include dilation of the right ventricle, right ventricular hypokinesis, and in

Table 22.1.7   Safety of a negative multidetector CT for ruling out pulmonary embolism in recent large-scale outcome studies

	Setting	Patients (n)	PE (%)	Negative CT, not treated	Clinical probability	3-month thromboembolic risk, (%) (95% CI)
CTEP3 study (56)	Outpatient	756	26	318	Non-high	1.6 (0.7 to 3.9)
Christopher study (50)	Out- and inpatient	3306	21	1505	Any	1.3 (0.9 to 2.0)
PEDS study (73)	Out- and inpatient	694	19	561	Any	0.4 (0.1 to 1.3)
CTEP4 study (49)	Outpatient	1693	22	1359	Non-high	0.3 (0.1 to 0.8)
Pooled results		6449	21	3743		0.8 (0.6 to 1.2)

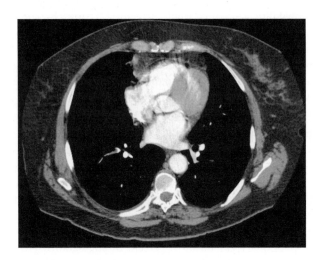

Figure 22.1.4   Multidetector computed tomography showing a segmental clot extending in a subsegmental branch (arrow). Note the higher definition compared with Figure 22.1.2 (single-detector CT).

severe cases, paradoxical motion of the interventricular septum. Several echocardiographic measurements have been proposed to quantify right ventricular dilation, of which the most standardized is the right ventricle over left ventricle diameter ratio. However, a visual estimate appears to be as accurate in the eyes of an experienced observer (88). A particular pattern of right ventricular hypokinesis characterized by akinesia of the mid-free wall and preservation of apex motion (McConnell's sign) appears to be quite specific for acute as opposed to chronic pulmonary hypertension (89). Conversely, right ventricular hypertrophy and pulmonary artery pressures above 60 mmHg suggest chronic pulmonary hypertension. The sensitivity of these signs which are often combined, lies between 40 and 70 percent in clinically suspected pulmonary embolism, and their specificity is approximately 90 percent, provided the patient does not have another disease causing chronic pulmonary hypertension (Table 22.1.5) (90).

Echocardiography is the first-line test in suspected massive pulmonary embolism. Indeed, in patients with shock, it is extremely effective for differential diagnosis with tamponade and cardiogenic shock. Moreover, absence of pulmonary hypertension and/or right ventricular dilation and hypokinesis in that situation renders pulmonary embolism as the cause of shock unlikely.

DIAGNOSTIC STRATEGIES

Suspected non–massive pulmonary embolism

Computed tomography angiography (CT) has become the main thoracic imaging test for investigating suspected pulmonary embolism (7,10). Ventilation-perfusion scintigraphy remains a valid option but it is increasingly abandoned because of a high proportion of inconclusive results. However, since most patients with suspected pulmonary embolism do not have the disease, CT should not be the first-line test. In patients admitted to the emergency department, plasma D-dimer measurement combined with clinical probability assessment is the logical first step and allows ruling out pulmonary embolism in around 30 percent of patients, with a 3-month thromboembolic risk in patients left untreated below 1 percent (Table 22.1.6). D-dimer should not be measured in patients with a high clinical probability because of a low negative predictive value in that population (91), nor in hospitalized patients due to a high number needed to test to obtain a clinically relevant negative result. In most centers, MDCT is the second-line test in patients with an elevated D-dimer level and the first-line test in patients with a high clinical probability (Figure 22.1.5). MDCT is considered diagnostic of pulmonary embolism when it shows a clot at least at the segmental level or the pulmonary arterial tree. A negative MDCT has been shown to safely exclude pulmonary embolism in several large-scale outcome studies (49,50,56,73). False-negative results of MDCT have been reported in patients with a high clinical probability of

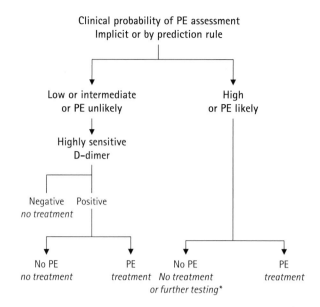

Figure 22.1.5 Algorithm for diagnostic workup of suspected non-massive pulmonary embolism. PE, pulmonary embolism. Note that this scheme is appropriate when using a highly sensitive D-dimer assay.

pulmonary embolism (69). Whether further tests should be performed in such patients is controversial (92).

Suspected massive pulmonary embolism

Patients with suspected massive pulmonary embolism have a very high mortality rate and require emergent thrombolytic treatment, in the event pulmonary embolism is confirmed. The clinical presentation evokes a differential diagnosis with other causes of shock such as pericardial tamponade or myocardial infarction and cardiogenic shock. The clot burden is usually high in that situation, and the diagnostic yield of any imaging study, whether ventilation-perfusion lung scan or helical CT, is likely to be high. Therefore, the logical initial test in such patients is transthoracic echocardiography. An echocardiogram showing signs of acute pulmonary hypertension and right ventricular strain in a shocked patient with a normal left ventricular contractility is a very strong argument in favor of massive pulmonary embolism. In fact, most clinicians would readily begin thrombolytic treatment in such a patient without awaiting further diagnostic information, if the patient were highly unstable. On the other hand, in a patient temporarily stabilized by vasopressive drugs (dopamine or noradrenaline), confirmation may be sought by either lung scan or helical CT, whichever is the most rapidly available. Angiography should be avoided whenever possible since it carries the highest risk in this patient population (85) and increases the risk of a major bleed at the puncture site due to thrombolytic treatment (93).

KEY POINTS

- The incidence of pulmonary embolism is around 1/1000 per year. It is the third cardiovascular cause of death in Western countries.
- Pulmonary embolism is a potentially fatal complication of deep vein thrombosis. Both disorders belong to a single disease entity, venous thromboembolism.
- Venous thromboembolism is a multigenic disease with a strong environmental influence. The indication to search for genetic thrombophilic defects should be individualized.
- Clinical assessment either implicit or by a prediction rule allows an accurate stratification of patients in categories of increasing prevalence of pulmonary embolism (low, intermediate and high clinical probability, or pulmonary embolism unlikely or likely).
- For most patients, the diagnosis of pulmonary embolism rests on clinical assessment, D-dimer measurement in outpatients and multidetector CT. In patients with a contraindication to CT, lower limb venous ultrasonography and ventilation-perfusion scintigraphy remain valid options.
- The validation of diagnostic strategies for pulmonary embolism requires outcome or management studies to identify patients who can be safely left untreated by antoicoagulants.
- Massive pulmonary embolism is a distinct clinical entity with a specific diagnostic approach. Echocardiography should be the initial test in a shocked patient with suspected pulmonary embolism.

REFERENCES

● = Key primary paper
◆ = Major review article

1. Cohen AT, Agnelli G, Anderson FA, Arcelus JI, Bergqvist D, Brecht JG *et al.* Venous thromboembolism (VTE) in Europe. The number of VTE events and associated morbidity and mortality. Thromb Haemost 2007;98:756–64.
2. Stein PD, Henry JW. Prevalence of acute pulmonary embolism among patients in a general hospital and at autopsy. Chest 1995;108:978–81.
3. Righini M, Perrier A, De Moerloose P, Bounameaux H. D-Dimer for venous thromboembolism diagnosis: 20 years later. J Thromb Haemost 2008;6:1059–71.
4. Kearon C, Ginsberg JS, Hirsh J. The role of venous ultrasonography in the diagnosis of suspected deep venous thrombosis and pulmonary embolism. Ann Intern Med 1998;129:1044–9.

5. Quiroz R, Kucher N, Zou KH, Kipfmueller F, Costello P, Goldhaber SZ et al. Clinical validity of a negative computed tomography scan in patients with suspected pulmonary embolism: a systematic review. JAMA 2005;293:2012–7.

•6. Wells PS. Integrated strategies for the diagnosis of venous thromboembolism. J Thromb Haemost 2007;5 Suppl 1:41–50.

•7. Torbicki A, Perrier A, Konstantinides S, Agnelli G, Galie N, Pruszczyk P et al. Guidelines on the diagnosis and management of acute pulmonary embolism: the Task Force for the Diagnosis and Management of Acute Pulmonary Embolism of the European Society of Cardiology (ESC). Eur Heart J 2008;29:2276–315.

8. Stein PD, Sostman HD, Bounameaux H, Buller HR, Chenevert TL, Dalen JE et al. Challenges in the diagnosis of acute pulmonary embolism. Am J Med 2008;121:565–71.

•9. Le Gal G, Perrier A. Contemporary approach to the diagnosis of non-massive pulmonary embolism. Curr Opin Pulm Med 2006;12:291–8.

10. British Thoracic Society guidelines for the management of suspected acute pulmonary embolism. Thorax 2003; 58:470–83.

11. Meignan M, Rosso J, Gauthier H, Brunengo F, Claudel S, Sagnard L et al. Systematic lung scans reveal a high frequency of silent pulmonary embolism in patients with proximal deep venous thrombosis. Arch Intern Med 2000;160:159–64.

12. Moser KM, Fedullo PF, LitteJohn JK, Crawford R. Frequent asymptomatic pulmonary embolism in patients with deep venous thrombosis. JAMA 1994;271:223–5.

13. Spencer FA, Emery C, Lessard D, Anderson F, Emani S, Aragam J et al. The Worcester Venous Thromboembolism study: a population-based study of the clinical epidemiology of venous thromboembolism. J Gen Intern Med 2006;21:722–7.

◆14. Heit JA. Venous thromboembolism: disease burden, outcomes and risk factors. J Thromb Haemost 2005;3:1611–7.

◆15. The PIOPED Investigators. Value of the ventilation-perfusion scan in acute pulmonary embolism. JAMA 1990;263:2753–9.

16. Goldhaber SZ, Visani L, De Rosa M. Acute pulmonary embolism: clinical outcomes in the International Cooperative Pulmonary Embolism Registry (ICOPER). Lancet 1999;353: 1386–9.

17. Wicki J, Perrier A, Perneger TV, Bounameaux H, Junod AF. Predicting adverse outcome in patients with acute pulmonary embolism: a risk score. Thromb Haemost 2000;84:548–52.

18. Douketis JD, Kearon C, Bates S, Duku EK, Ginsberg JS. Risk of fatal pulmonary embolism in patients with treated venous thromboembolism. JAMA 1998;279:458–62.

19. Douketis JD, Foster GA, Crowther MA, Prins MH, Ginsberg JS. Clinical risk factors and timing of recurrent venous thromboembolism during the initial 3 months of anticoagulant therapy. Arch Intern Med 2000;160: 3431–6.

20. von Virchow R. Weitere Untersuchungen ueber die Verstopfung der Lungenarterien und ihre Folge. Traube's Beitraege exp Path u Physiol. Berlin, 1846, p. 21–31.

•21. Rosendaal FR. Venous thrombosis: a multicausal disease. Lancet 1999;353:1167–73.

22. Gonzalez Ordonez AJ, Medina Rodriguez JM, Martin L, Alvarez V, Coto E. The O blood group protects against venous thromboembolism in individuals with the factor V Leiden but not the prothrombin (factor II G20210A) mutation. Blood Coagul Fibrinolysis 1999;10:303–7.

•23. Perrier A. Deep vein thrombosis and pulmonary embolism: A single disease entity with different risk factors? Chest 2000;118:1234–6.

•24. de Moerloose P, Alhenc-Gelas M, Boehlen F, Bounameaux H, Aiach M. Deep venous thrombosis and thrombophilia: indications for testing and clinical implications. Sem Vasc Med 2001;1:89–95.

25. Kyrle PA, Minar E, Bialonczyk C, Hirschl M, Weltermann A, Eichinger S. The risk of recurrent venous thromboembolism in men and women. N Engl J Med 2004;350:2558–63.

26. Goldhaber SZ, Grodstein F, Stampfer MJ, Manson JE, Colditz GA, Speizer FE et al. A prospective study of risk factors for pulmonary embolism in women. JAMA 1997;277:642–5.

27. Samama MM. An epidemiologic study of risk factors for deep vein thrombosis in medical outpatients: the Sirius study. Arch Intern Med 2000;160:3415–20.

◆28. Grady D, Wenger NK, Herrington D, Khan S, Furberg C, Hunninghake D et al. Postmenopausal hormone therapy increases risk for venous thromboembolic disease. The Heart and Estrogen/progestin Replacement Study. Ann Intern Med 2000;132:689–96.

29. Cummings SR, Eckert S, Krueger KA, Grady D, Powles TJ, Cauley JA et al. The effect of raloxifene on risk of breast cancer in postmenopausal women: results from the MORE randomized trial. Multiple Outcomes of Raloxifene Evaluation. JAMA 1999;281:2189–97.

◆30. De Stefano V, Martinelli I, Mannucci PM, Paciaroni K, Chiusolo P, Casorelli I et al. The risk of recurrent deep venous thrombosis among heterozygous carriers of both factor V Leiden and the G20210A prothrombin mutation. N Engl J Med 1999;341:801–6.

◆31. Baron JA, Gridley G, Weiderpass E, Nyren O, Linet M. Venous thromboembolism and cancer. Lancet 1998;351:1077–80.

32. Sorensen HT, Mellemkjaer L, Steffensen FH, Olsen JH, Nielsen GL. The risk of a diagnosis of cancer after primary deep venous thrombosis or pulmonary embolism. N Engl J Med 1998;338:1169–73.

33. Carrier M, Le Gal G, Wells PS, Fergusson D, Ramsay T, Rodger MA. Systematic review: the Trousseau syndrome revisited: should we screen extensively for cancer in patients with venous thromboembolism? Ann Intern Med 2008;149:323–33.

34. Prandoni P, Lensing AW, Buller HR, Cogo A, Prins MH, Cattelan AM et al. Deep-vein thrombosis and the incidence of subsequent symptomatic cancer. N Engl J Med 1992;327:1128–33.

35. Rance A, Emmerich J, Guedj C, Fiessinger JN. Occult cancer in patients with bilateral deep-vein thrombosis. Lancet 1997;350:1448–9.

36. Cornuz J, Pearson SD, Creager MA, Cook EF, Goldman L. Importance of findings on the initial evaluation for cancer

in patients with symptomatic idiopathic deep venous thrombosis. Ann Intern Med 1996;125:785–93.

♦37. Piccioli A, Lensing AW, Prins MH, Falanga A, Scannapieco GL, Ieran M et al. Extensive screening for occult malignant disease in idiopathic venous thromboembolism: a prospective randomized clinical trial. J Thromb Haemost 2004;2:884–9.

38. Stein PD, Henry JW. Clinical characteristics of patients with acute pulmonary embolism stratified according to their presenting syndromes. Chest 1997;112:974–9.

39. Dalen JE, Haffajee CI, Alpert JS, Howe JP, Ockens IS, Paraskos JA. Pulmonary embolism, pulmonary hemorrhage, pulmonary infarction. N Engl J Med 1977;296:1431–5.

40. Elliott CG, Goldhaber SZ, Visani L, DeRosa M. Chest radiographs in acute pulmonary embolism. Results from the International Cooperative Pulmonary Embolism Registry. Chest 2000;118:33–8.

41. Thames MD, Alpert JS, Dalen JE. Syncope in patients with pulmonary embolism. JAMA 1977;238:2509–11.

42. Stein PD, Terrin ML, Hales CA, Palevsky HI, Saltzman HA, Thompson T et al. Clinical, laboratory, roentgenographic, and electrocardiographic findings in patients with acute pulmonary embolism and no pre-existing cardiac or pulmonary disease. Chest 1991;100:598–603.

43. Rodger M, Makropoulos D, Turek M, Quevillon J, Raymond F, Rasuli P et al. Diagnostic value of the electrocardiogram in suspected pulmonary embolism. Am J Cardiol 2000;86:807–9.

44. Rodger MA, Carrier M, Jones GN, Rasuli P, Raymond F, Djunaedi H et al. Diagnostic value of arterial blood gas measurement in suspected pulmonary embolism. Am J Respir Crit Care Med 2000;162:2105–8.

45. Stein PD, Goldhaber SZ, Henry JW. Alveolar–arterial oxygen gradient in the assessment of acute pulmonary embolism. Chest 1995;107:139–43.

♦46. Perrier A, Miron MJ, Desmarais S, de Moerloose P, Slosman D, Didier D et al. Using clinical evaluation and lung scan to rule out suspected pulmonary embolism: Is it a valid option in patients with normal results of lower-limb venous compression ultrasonography? Arch Intern Med 2000;160:512–6.

♦47. Le Gal G, Righini M, Roy PM, Sanchez O, Aujesky D, Bounameaux H et al. Prediction of pulmonary embolism in the emergency department: the revised Geneva score. Ann Intern Med 2006;144:165–71.

♦48. Wells PS, Anderson DR, Rodger M, Ginsberg JS, Kearon C, Gent M et al. Derivation of a simple clinical model to categorize patients' probability of pulmonary embolism: increasing the models utility with the SimpliRED D-dimer. Thromb Haemost 2000;83:416–20.

♦49. Righini M, Le Gal G, Aujesky D, Roy PM, Sanchez O, Verschuren F et al. Diagnosis of pulmonary embolism by multidetector CT alone or combined with venous ultrasonography of the leg: a randomised non-inferiority trial. Lancet 2008;371:1343–52.

♦50. van Belle A, Buller HR, Huisman MV, Huisman PM, Kaasjager K, Kamphuisen PW et al. Effectiveness of managing suspected pulmonary embolism using an algorithm combining clinical probability, D-dimer testing, and computed tomography. JAMA 2006;295:172–9.

•51. Roy PM, Colombet I, Durieux P, Chatellier G, Sors H, Meyer G. Systematic review and meta-analysis of strategies for the diagnosis of suspected pulmonary embolism. BMJ 2005;331:259.

•52. Di Nisio M, Squizzato A, Rutjes AW, Buller HR, Zwinderman AH, Bossuyt PM. Diagnostic accuracy of D-dimer test for exclusion of venous thromboembolism: a systematic review. J Thromb Haemost 2007;5:296–304.

53. Stein PD, Hull RD, Patel KC, Olson RE, Ghali WA, Brant R et al. D-Dimer for the exclusion of acute venous thrombosis and pulmonary embolism: a systematic review. Ann Intern Med 2004;140:589–602.

54. Perrier A, Desmarais S, Miron MJ, de Moerloose P, Lepage R, Slosman D et al. Non-invasive diagnosis of venous thromboembolism in outpatients. Lancet 1999;353:190–5.

55. Perrier A, Roy PM, Aujesky D, Chagnon I, Howarth N, Gourdier AL et al. Diagnosing pulmonary embolism in outpatients with clinical assessment, D-dimer measurement, venous ultrasound, and helical computed tomography: a multicenter management study. Am J Med 2004;116:291–9.

♦56. Perrier A, Roy PM, Sanchez O, Le Gal G, Meyer G, Gourdier AL et al. Multidetector-row computed tomography in suspected pulmonary embolism. N Engl J Med 2005;352:1760–8.

57. Di Nisio M, Sohne M, Kamphuisen PW, Buller HR. D-Dimer test in cancer patients with suspected acute pulmonary embolism. J Thromb Haemost 2005;3:1239–42.

♦58. Wells PS, Anderson DR, Rodger M, Stiell I, Dreyer JF, Barnes D et al. Excluding pulmonary embolism at the bedside without diagnostic imaging: management of patients with suspected pulmonary embolism presenting to the emergency department by using a simple clinical model and D-dimer. Ann Intern Med 2001;135:98–107.

59. de Groot MR, van Marwijk Kooy M, Pouwels JG, Engelage AH, Kuipers BF, Buller HR. The use of a rapid D-dimer blood test in the diagnostic work-up for pulmonary embolism: a management study. Thromb Haemost 1999; 82:1588–92.

60. Kruip MJ, Slob MJ, Schijen JH, van der Heul C, Buller HR. Use of a clinical decision rule in combination with D-dimer concentration in diagnostic workup of patients with suspected pulmonary embolism: a prospective management study. Arch Intern Med 2002;162:1631–5.

61. Leclercq MG, Lutisan JG, van Marwijk Kooy M, Kuipers BF, Oostdijk AH, van der Leur JJ et al. Ruling out clinically suspected pulmonary embolism by assessment of clinical probability and D-dimer levels: a management study. Thromb Haemost 2003;89:97–103.

62. Ten Wolde M, Hagen PJ, MacGillavry MR, Pollen IJ, Mairuhu AT, Koopman MM et al. Non-invasive diagnostic work-up of patients with clinically suspected pulmonary embolism; results of a management study. J Thromb Haemost 2004;2:1110–7.

♦63. Righini M, Goehring C, Bounameaux H, Perrier A. Effects of age on the performance of common diagnostic tests for pulmonary embolism. Am J Med 2000;109:357–61.

64. Righini M, Le Gal G, De Lucia S, Roy PM, Meyer G, Aujesky D et al. Clinical usefulness of D-dimer testing in cancer

patients with suspected pulmonary embolism. Thromb Haemost 2006;95:715–9.

65. Chabloz P, Reber G, Boehlen F, Hohlfeld P, de Moerloose P. TAFI antigen and D-dimer levels during normal pregnancy and at delivery. Br J Haematol 2001;115:150–2.

66. Francalanci I, Comeglio P, Liotta AA, Cellai AP, Fedi S, Parretti E et al. D-dimer concentrations during normal pregnancy, as measured by ELISA. Thromb Res 1995;78:399–405.

67. Kearon C, Julian JA, Math M, Newman TE, Ginsberg JS. Noninvasive diagnosis of deep venous thrombosis. Ann Intern Med 1998;128:663–77.

68. Elias A, Colombier D, Victor G, Elias M, Arnaud C, Juchet H et al. Diagnostic performance of complete lower limb venous ultrasound in patients with clinically suspected acute pulmonary embolism. Thromb Haemost 2004;91:187–95.

69. Stein PD, Fowler SE, Goodman LR, Gottschalk A, Hales CA, Hull RD et al. Multidetector computed tomography for acute pulmonary embolism. N Engl J Med 2006;354:2317–27.

•70. Brenner DJ, Hall EJ. Computed tomography – an increasing source of radiation exposure. N Engl J Med 2007;357: 2277–84.

71. Alderson PO, Martin EC. Pulmonary embolism: diagnosis with multiple imaging modalities. Radiology 1987;164:297–312.

72. Gottschalk A, Sostman HD, Coleman RE, Juni JE, Thrall J, McKusick KA et al. Ventilation-perfusion scintigraphy in the PIOPED study. Part II. Evaluation of scintigraphic criteria and interpretations. J Nucl Med 1993;34:1119–26.

◆73. Anderson DR, Kahn SR, Rodger MA, Kovacs MJ, Morris T, Hirsch A et al. Computed tomographic pulmonary angiography vs ventilation-perfusion lung scanning in patients with suspected pulmonary embolism: a randomized controlled trial. JAMA 2007;298:2743–53.

74. Hull RD, Raskob GE, Coates G, Panju AA. Clinical validity of a normal perfusion lung scan in patients with suspected pulmonary embolism. Chest 1990;97:23–6.

75. Kipper MS, Moser KM, Kortman KE, Ashburn WL. Longterm follow-up of patients with suspected pulmonary embolism and a normal lung scan. Chest 1982;82:411–5.

◆76. Wells PS, Ginsberg JS, Anderson DR, Kearon C, Gent M, Turpie AG et al. Use of a clinical model for safe management of patients with suspected pulmonary embolism. Ann Intern Med 1998;129:997–1005.

77. van Beek EJ, Kuyer PM, Schenk BE, Brandjes DP, ten Cate JW, Buller HR. A normal perfusion lung scan in patients with clinically suspected pulmonary embolism. Frequency and clinical validity. Chest 1995;108:170–3.

78. Sostman HD, Miniati M, Gottschalk A, Matta F, Stein PD, Pistolesi M. Sensitivity and specificity of perfusion scintigraphy combined with chest radiography for acute pulmonary embolism in PIOPED II. J Nucl Med 2008;49:1741–8.

◆79. Perrier A, Howarth N, Didier D, Loubeyre P, Unger PF, de Moerloose P et al. Performance of helical computed tomography in unselected outpatients with suspected pulmonary embolism. Ann Intern Med 2001;135:88–97.

80. Rathbun SW, Raskob GE, Whitsett TL. Sensitivity and specificity of helical computed tomography in the diagnosis of pulmonary embolism: a systematic review. Ann Intern Med 2000;132:227–32.

◆81. Musset D, Parent F, Meyer G, Maitre S, Girard P, Leroyer C et al. Diagnostic strategy for patients with suspected pulmonary embolism: a prospective multicentre outcome study. Lancet 2002;360:1914–20.

82. Ghaye B, Szapiro D, Mastora I, Delannoy V, Duhamel A, Remy J et al. Peripheral pulmonary arteries: how far in the lung does multi-detector row spiral CT allow analysis? Radiology 2001;219:629–36.

83. Eyer BA, Goodman LR, Washington L. Clinicians' response to radiologists' reports of isolated subsegmental pulmonary embolism or inconclusive interpretation of pulmonary embolism using MDCT. AJR Am J Roentgenol 2005;184:623–8.

84. Le Gal G, Righini M, Parent F, van Strijen M, Couturaud F. Diagnosis and management of subsegmental pulmonary embolism. J Thromb Haemost 2006;4:724–31.

85. Stein PD, Athanasoulis C, Alavi A, Greenspan RH, Hales CA, Saltzman HA et al. Complications and validity of pulmonary angiography in acute pulmonary embolism. Circulation 1992;85:462–8.

86. Hudson ER, Smith TP, McDermott VG, Newman GE, Suhocki PV, Payne CS et al. Pulmonary angiography performed with iopamidol: complications in 1434 patients. Radiology 1996;198:61–5.

87. Come PC. Echocardiographic evaluation of pulmonary embolism and its response to therapeutic interventions. Chest 1992;101:151S–62S.

88. Jardin F, Dubourg O, Bourdarias JP. Echocardiographic pattern of acute cor pulmonale. Chest 1997;111:209–17.

89. McConnell MV, Solomon SD, Rayan ME, Come PC, Goldhaber SZ, Lee RT. Regional right ventricular dysfunction detected by echocardiography in acute pulmonary embolism. Am J Cardiol 1996;78:469–73.

90. Jackson RE, Rudoni RR, Hauser AM, Pascual RG, Hussey ME. Prospective evaluation of two-dimensional transthoracic echocardiography in emergency department patients with suspected pulmonary embolism. Acad Emerg Med 2000;7: 994–8.

91. Righini M, Aujesky D, Roy PM, Cornuz J, de Moerloose P, Bounameaux H et al. Clinical usefulness of D-dimer depending on clinical probability and cutoff value in outpatients with suspected pulmonary embolism. Arch Intern Med 2004;164:2483–7.

92. Douma RA, Kamphuisen PW, Huisman MV, Buller HR. False normal results on multidetector-row spiral computed tomography in patients with high clinical probability of pulmonary embolism. J Thromb Haemost 2008;6:1978–9.

•93. Kearon C, Kahn SR, Agnelli G, Goldhaber S, Raskob GE, Comerota AJ. Antithrombotic therapy for venous thromboembolic disease: American College of Chest Physicians Evidence-Based Clinical Practice Guidelines, 8th edn. Chest 2008;133:454S–545S.

94. van Beek EJ, Brouwerst EM, Song B, Stein PD, Oudkerk M. Clinical validity of a normal pulmonary angiogram in patients with suspected pulmonary embolism – a critical review. Clin Radiol 2001;56:838–42.

Treatment of acute pulmonary embolism

VICTOR F TAPSON

INTRODUCTION

Venous thromboembolism (VTE) includes the spectrum of deep vein thrombosis (DVT) and pulmonary embolism (PE). The vast majority of acute PE cases arise from the deep veins of the legs, and the therapeutic approach for it is generally the same for DVT and PE. However, in certain settings, the treatment of PE becomes more complex. When it manifests with hemodynamic compromise (massive PE), more aggressive therapy including thrombolytic therapy or pulmonary embolectomy requires consideration. Therapy for acute VTE generally consists of two phases – initial parenteral anticoagulation treatment with heparin, low molecular weight heparin (LMWH) or fondaparinux and long-term treatment with oral anticoagulants. The development of new oral agents for both initial and long-term treatment is likely to ultimately simplify therapy. This chapter will focus on the approach to proven acute PE including scenarios involving more aggressive therapy. While long-term therapy will be discussed, the primary focus will be the initial phase of treatment.

RISK STRATIFICATION FOR ACUTE PULMONARY EMBOLISM

The clinical presentation of acute VTE may vary from incidental discovery of asymptomatic DVT or PE to massive embolism causing immediate death. Treatment can reduce the risk of death, and appropriate primary prophylaxis is usually effective. If PE is suspected, a careful assessment based on the history, physical examination, and known risk factors is necessary. If PE is confirmed by radiographic imaging, treatment is initiated.

For most patients presenting with acute PE, initial therapy consists of parenteral anticoagulation. In fact, anticoagulation should be considered even prior to the diagnosis of PE if the clinical suspicion is high and the risk of bleeding deemed low (1). Risk stratification is important when PE is diagnosed so that when appropriate, more aggressive therapy than anticoagulation can be considered (1).

Hemodynamics and echocardiography

The anatomic extent of PE correlates with pulmonary hemodynamics, and pulmonary vascular resistance increases dramatically when vascular obstruction exceeds 50–60 percent (2). However, PE-related mortality appears to be more closely associated with clinical findings at the time of diagnosis than it is to the actual degree of vascular obstruction. In the International Cooperative Pulmonary Embolism Registry (ICOPER) which included more than 2000 patients, the mortality rate was 58 percent in patients with unstable hemodynamics but was only 15 percent in clinically stable individuals (3). Furthermore, a systolic blood pressure below 90 mmHg was independently associated with a greater risk of death with an odds ratio (OR) of 2.9 and 95 percent confidence interval (CI) of 1.7 to 5.0. Another large, multicenter registry included 1001 patients with major PE, defined as right heart failure or pulmonary hypertension (4). Four groups of patients were prospectively defined: (i) patients with right ventricular (RV) pressure overload or pulmonary hypertension, but with normal blood pressure; (ii) patients with systemic arterial hypotension (systolic blood pressure < 90 mmHg or a drop of at least 40 mmHg for more than 15 minutes), but without cardiogenic shock or need for catecholamine support; (iii) patients with systemic hypotension and cardiogenic shock and/or need for catecholamine administration to maintain adequate tissue perfusion; (iv) patients with circulatory collapse who underwent cardiopulmonary resuscitation. The hospital mortality rate was 8.1 percent in group 1, 15.2 percent in group 2, 25 percent in group 3 and 62.5 percent in group 4 (4). Other studies have confirmed that the early mortality rate in patients with shock exceeds 25 percent (5–7). Based upon these data, the definition of massive PE is now based on clinical rather than radiographic parameters and, more specifically, on the presence of hemodynamic instability (persistent arterial hypotension and/or cardiogenic shock) at presentation (1,8).

PE patients with stable hemodynamics at presentation have a low death rate when anticoagulated, provided that they have no major underlying disease. A meta-analysis comparing unfractionated heparin (UFH) with LMWH for the initial treatment of PE found in-hospital mortality rates of 1.4 percent for UFH and 1.2 percent for LMWH, however, most of these patients had symptomatic DVT with asymptomatic PE (9). In a multicenter randomized clinical trial of 1017 clinically stable patients with symptomatic PE who received LMWH or UFH followed by 6 months of oral anticoagulation, the mortality rate was shown to be 4.4 percent (10). Thus, stable patients with acute PE are treated with either LMWH or UFH (1).

While more aggressive therapy is recommended when hemodynamics are unstable, and while prognosis is quite good in non-massive PE patients enrolled in clinical trials, clinical researchers have attempted to identify a subgroup of apparently stable patients with "submassive PE" who may have a higher mortality rate than those with normal blood pressure. In a nonrandomized study by Ribeiro and colleagues, the mortality rate in patients with RV dysfunction was 14 percent (10 deaths among 70 patients) compared with no deaths among 56 patients in those with normal findings by echocardiography ($P = 0.002$) (11). In ICOPER, the in-hospital mortality of patients with RV dysfunction on echocardiography was 18 percent although, again, patients with shock were not analyzed separately (12). Several recent studies have investigated the outcome of patients without hypotension but with RV dysfunction on echocardiography (6,7,13–15). In these studies, the mortality rate varied between 3 percent and 16 percent in patients with RV dysfunction and between 0 percent and 8 percent in patients with normal RV function. Although most studies have reported higher mortality rates in patients with RV dysfunction (12,16), this has not been a universal finding (7,18). Right ventricular dysfunction by echocardiography was not defined consistently in these studies and use of thrombolytic therapy was not controlled.

These study limitations may account for the inconsistent findings.

Biomarkers and clinical scoring

High levels of brain natriuretic peptide (BNP), pro-BNP, and cardiac troponins (T and I) have been associated with a greater risk of death in patients with PE. In a Polish series, the in-hospital mortality of patients with normal blood pressure, high troponin levels and RV enlargement was 25 percent (19). A study by the same investigators demonstrated that clinically stable patients with high pro-BNP levels had a mortality rate of 17 percent (20). In another series of 141 patients with PE, an overall 30 day mortality rate of 19.9 percent was observed. In the subset of patients with both RV enlargement and a high troponin I concentration (32 percent), the mortality rate was 38 percent (16). However, lack of randomization and differing definitions for significant elevation of biomarkers, prevent firm conclusions.

A clinical score for predicting early mortality in patients with PE has recently been described by Aujesky, and associates (21). The score was derived from a large hospital database and has been prospectively validated in several independent cohorts (21,22). Higher scores were associated with advanced age, male sex, number of comorbid conditions and certain clinical abnormalities. Patients could be assigned to one of five groups based on this score. Mortality rates 3 months after diagnosis are as follows: 2.5 percent for groups I and II, 7 percent for group III, 11 percent for group IV and 24 percent for group V (21–24). If such a scoring system could be linked with reduced mortality with thrombolytic therapy, it would represent a significant advance. A summary of factors to be considered when risk stratifying a patient with acute PE is shown in Box 22.2.1.

INITIAL ANTICOAGULATION

If risk stratification suggests that more aggressive measures are not needed, then anticoagulation alone is continued.

BOX 22.2.1: Factors to Consider when Risk Stratifying a Patient with Acute Pulmonary Embolism

- Vital signs (excessive tachycardia/tachypnea, hypotension)*
- Echocardiography (RV enlargement/hypokinesis).
- Biomarkers (troponin/BNP).
- Oxygenation.
- Comorbid disease/cardiopulmonary reserve.
- Bleeding risk.
- Extensive residual DVT.

*Unstable hemodynamics is the clearest indication for thrombolytic therapy.

The majority of studies on initial anticoagulation therapy of VTE have included primarily patients with acute DVT; patients with PE have comprised a smaller number of patients studied and their outcome has generally not been given separately. However, patients treated for PE are more likely to die of recurrent PE than patients with DVT. The risk of fatal recurrent PE appears to be four times higher in patients with PE than in patients with DVT during 3 months of anticoagulant treatment (1.5 vs. 0.4 percent) (25). As a result, more recent studies have specifically evaluated patients with PE (10,26). Because most patients who die from PE appear to do so within the first few hours of admission to the hospital (27), and because the observed mortality rate is high in untreated patients, early initiation of anticoagulation while awaiting objective confirmation, if PE is strongly suspected, and if the bleeding risk is deemed low appears justified (1).

Unfractionated heparin

Barritt and Jordan (28), carried out the only randomized controlled trial comparing UFH with no treatment in a small group of patients with PE diagnosed on clinical grounds. In this study, heparin was associated with a significantly lower rate of recurrent PE and death due to PE. Based on these data and the results of additional studies in patients with DVT, the experts of the last consensus conference of the American College of Chest Physicians (ACCP) strongly recommended the use of UFH or LMWH for the initial treatment of PE, with LMWH being favored when possible, based upon certain specific advantages (1).

The largest study to date examining UFH in patients with acute PE reported to date is the Matisse PE trial, a randomized controlled trial comparing fondaparinux with UFH for the initial treatment of PE (see fondaparinux below) (26). The results of this trial strongly support in a large cohort of patients, that treatment with IV UFH followed by warfarin is a safe and effective therapeutic option for patients with PE.

In spite of the demonstrated efficacy of UFH, its use is limited by the need for a continuous IV infusion, and frequent dose adjustment with aPTT monitoring. However, subcutaneous (SC) UFH without monitoring has also proven effective. In the recent Fixed-Dose heparin (FIDO) study (29), patients with VTE, including 134 with PE, were randomized to receive either SC LMWH twice daily or SC UFH at an initial dose of 330 IU followed by 250 IU, twice daily, without aPTT monitoring or dose adjustment. Both therapies overlapped with warfarin, which was continued for 3 months. While the PE patients were not analyzed separately, recurrence and bleeding rates were similar and low in both groups (29). Nonetheless, the substantially greater number of patients effectively treated with LMWH without monitoring as well as the balance of data supporting a lower risk of heparin-induced thrombocytopenia

(HIT) in patients receiving LMWH compared with UFH supports the use of LMWH for VTE rather than SC unmonitored UFH (30). While no HIT was reported in patients receiving UFH in the Matisse PE (26) and FIDO (29) studies, platelet counts were not routinely monitored in the FIDO study. In patients with severe renal insufficiency, UFH is the most appropriate option for initial PE therapy (1). Due to its short half-life, and complete reversibility with protamine, UFH is also advantageous for patients with a high risk of bleeding, such as patients who have recently suffered bleeding or undergone surgery. The use of LMWH together with thrombolytic treatment has not been evaluated in PE. Thus, UFH is favored in patients in whom thrombolytic therapy is planned or has recently been administered, although this has not been studied in randomized trials.

Low molecular weight heparin

A number of clinical trials have compared LMWH with UFH for the treatment of acute VTE. Simonneau and associates (31) conducted and published the THESEE study, more than a decade ago. In this study, the largest of the randomized trials comparing a LMWH (tinzaparin) with UFH for initial PE therapy, 612 patients with symptomatic PE were randomized to receive SC tinzaparin at a fixed dose of 175 IU/kg once daily or IV UFH with aPTT monitoring. Warfarin was overlapped and continued for at least 3 months, with the international normalized ratio (INR) maintained between 2 to 3. By day 8, three of the 304 patients given tinzaparin had experienced recurrent VTE, three had suffered major bleeding and four had died. Two of the 308 patients given UFH had experienced recurrences, five had suffered major bleeding and three had died. The combined endpoint of recurrent VTE, major bleeding or death was reached by nine patients (3 percent) in the tinzaparin group and nine in the UFH group (2.9 percent). At the end of the 3-month follow-up period for this landmark study, no difference was observed between the groups (31). A number of meta-analyses have examined LMWH with UFH for treatment of acute VTE. Quinlan and colleagues carried out a meta-analysis of 12 trials comparing LMWH and UFH as initial therapy in 1951 patients with either symptomatic PE or asymptomatic PE and symptomatic DVT (8). They found a nonsignificant trend in favor of LMWH for recurrent VTE, with a relative risk (RR) of 0.68 (95 percent CI 0.42 to 1.09). For major bleeding, the RR was 0.67 (95 percent CI 0.36 to 1.27) and for death, 0.77 (95 percent CI 0.52 to 1.55) (9).

The largest group of patients with PE receiving LMWH followed by oral anticoagulation reported to date is that studied in the recent van Gogh trial (10). In this study, 1120 clinically stable patients with symptomatic PE received standard therapy with UFH (n = 119; 10.9 percent), LMWH (tinzaparin or enoxaparin) (n = 914; 83.7 percent) or both LMWH and UFH (n = 59; 5.4 percent), followed by oral anticoagulation for either 3 or 6 months. Recurrence rates and bleeding rates were very low and the mortality was only 4.4 percent at 6 months (10). Thus, the use of a fixed dose of LMWH is a safe and effective treatment for patients with symptomatic PE.

Studies assessing LMWH for the initial treatment of PE have used a fixed dose adjusted for body weight, without monitoring, as there is no convincing evidence to suggest that the risk of recurrent VTE or bleeding depends on anti-Xa levels in patients receiving LMWH. Low molecular weight heparin may accumulate in renal failure, increasing the risk of bleeding (32). It is generally recommended to use UFH with monitoring in this setting rather than LMWH with anti-Xa measurement (1). Heparin-induced thrombocytopenia is a rare complication in medical patients and has been most commonly associated with therapeutic doses of LMWH. In a series of 728 patients receiving therapeutic doses of LMWH for various indications, HIT was observed in 0.8 percent of patients and was more frequent in patients who had (1.7 percent) previously been exposed to UFH or LMWH, than in those who had not (0.3 percent) (33). Medical patients treated with therapeutic doses of LMWH for periods of only 5–7 days are thought to have a low risk of heparin-induced thrombocytopenia and routine platelet count monitoring is therefore not required in these patients (34). Advantages of LMWH over UFH are outlined in Box 22.2.2.

Fondaparinux

Fondaparinux, a long-acting inhibitor of factor X, was evaluated for the initial treatment of PE in the Matisse PE study (26). In this study, 2213 patients with PE were randomized to groups receiving SC fondaparinux once daily at a fixed dose adapted to body weight (5.0, 7.5 and 10.0 mg in patients weighing less than 50 kg, 50–100 kg and more than 100 kg, respectively) or heparin, given as a constant IV infusion with aPTT monitoring, and oral anticoagulation followed. Forty-two of the 1103 patients assigned to the fondaparinux group (3.8 percent) developed symptomatic and objectively confirmed recurrent VTE by 3 months, compared with 56 of the 1110 patients assigned to the UFH group (5.0 percent), giving an absolute difference of −1.2 percent in favor of fondaparinux (95 percent CI −3.0 to 0.5); thus, fondaparinux was not inferior to heparin (26). Major bleeding was observed during initial therapy in 14 patients (1.2 percent) on fondaparinux and 12 patients (1.1 percent) on heparin. At the end of the 3-month treatment period, 57 deaths (5.2 percent) were recorded in patients initially treated with fondaparinux and 48 (4.4 percent) deaths were recorded in patients initially treated with heparin (26). Thus, once-daily, subcutaneous administration of fondaparinux without monitoring was at least as effective and as safe as IV UFH in the initial treatment of patients with stable acute PE (26).

BOX 22.2.2: Advantages of Low Molecular Weight Heparin Over Standard, Unfractionated Heparin

- LMWH is at least as effective as UFH.
- In certain *prophylactic* settings, it is *more* effective.*
- No intravenous line needed with LMWH.†
- More bioavailable than UFH; thus, generally no monitoring with LMWH.†
- LMWH facilitates outpatient therapy.
- Better quality of life, fewer nosocomial complications with LMWH.
- Less HIT with LMWH.

*Examples include, total hip replacement, total knee replacement, acute stroke with hemiplegia, spinal cord injury.
†One clinical trial supports therapy of acute DVT with subcutaneous, unmonitored standard, unfractionated heparin (29), but the vast majority are intravenous studies. Monitoring anti-Xa levels while on LMWH can be considered if renal function is changing, with long-term use in pregnancy, in extremes of body weight, or anytime absorption or therapeutic levels are questioned.
Abbreviations: LMWH = low molecular weight heparin; UFH = standard, unfractionated heparin

---

OTHER APPROVED ANTICOAGULANTS

Heparin-induced thrombocytopenia

The setting of HIT requires special consideration. More than 90 percent of patients with clinical HIT have a platelet count fall of 50 percent or more during treatment with heparin. The decision to treat should not wait for laboratory confirmation because of the time delay in obtaining results. There is a high risk of thrombosis in HIT despite cessation of heparin therapy. Among patients with HIT associated thrombocytopenia, the initial rate of thrombosis is about 5–10 percent per day over the first 1–2 days after discontinuation of heparin and the cumulative 30-day risk is about 50 percent (34). Anticoagulation with a direct thrombin inhibitor (e.g., argatroban or lepirudin) should be considered for HIT. Warfarin should not be initiated until the disease process has been controlled and the platelet count has returned to the normal range because of the potential for worsening thrombotic complications, including venous limb gangrene and warfarin-induced skin necrosis. Hepatic and renal function must be considered when HIT is present; Lepirudin is excreted by the kidneys, and argatroban is metabolized in the liver. While a detailed discussion of HIT is beyond the scope of this chapter, guidelines have been formulated to assist in clinical decisions in this setting (34).

MASSIVE AND SUBMASSIVE PULMONARY EMBOLISM

Patients with PE may present with circulatory collapse or respiratory failure. In large registries, these patients account for less than 5 percent of all patients admitted with PE (3), although this may represent an inaccurate depiction of "real life" since unidentified patients in whom the presentation is fatal PE are not included. The treatment of these patients combines symptomatic interventions to reverse hemodynamic instability and respiratory failure and treatments designed to decrease pulmonary vascular obstruction rapidly. Transfer to the intensive care unit should be considered in any PE patient with unstable vital signs, significant hypoxemia, or evidence of unstable hemodynamics.

Oxygen and respiratory support

Oxygen and intubation with mechanical ventilation are instituted as clinically indicated is administered as based upon oxygen saturation/arterial blood gas assessment. The potential detrimental effects of mechanical ventilation on right heart function must be realized.

Fluid loading

The traditional first-line treatment for hypotension is volume expansion. Evidence from animal experiments suggests that in cases of pulmonary hypertension, this may increase myocardial oxygen consumption, resulting in RV ischemia and worsening RV function. Nonetheless, certain clinical data suggest that fluid loading may improve the hemodynamic status of patients with massive PE (35). In an uncontrolled series of 13 normotensive patients with acute PE and a low cardiac index, a 500 mL infusion of dextran over 20 minutes was shown to be associated with a significant increase in cardiac index, from 1.6 ± 0.1 to $2.0 \pm 0.1 \, L/min/m^2$ (36). The effect of fluid loading on cardiac index was inversely correlated with baseline RV end-diastolic volume index.

Inotropes and vasopressors

In experimental animal models with massive PE and severe hypotension, isoproterenol has not proven beneficial and may be detrimental (35,37). In contrast, norepinephrine improved RV function in animal experiments, increasing systemic arterial pressure over a wide range of blood pressure and RV afterload, suggesting that its effects were not limited to the subset of animals with profound hypotension (35). Evidence relating to the effects of norepinephrine in patients with massive PE and shock arises from small case series or single case reports in which patients also received thrombolytic therapy and other vasopressors,

making conclusions difficult (38–40). Epinephrine appears to combine the beneficial vasoconstrictive effects of norepinephrine with the positive inotropic effect of dobutamine and may be the drug of choice in PE patients with marked hypotension. However, clinical data are sparse (38,41). Both dopamine and dobutamine have been shown to increase cardiac output in experimental PE. The effect of dopamine on cardiac output is often limited by tachycardia (42). The effects of dobutamine on hemodynamics and gas exchange in patients with PE have been described in two small case series (43,44). In these studies, dobutamine increased cardiac output and improved oxygen transport, although hypoxemia worsened in some patients (44).

Nitric oxide

Inhaled nitric oxide induces selective pulmonary arterial vasodilation, inducing an increase in cardiac output in patients with increased right ventricular afterload. Clinical experience with inhaled nitric oxide in patients with PE is limited to a small case series and a few case reports, but may be beneficial. In four patients with massive PE, inhaled nitric oxide, at concentrations of 5–20 ppm, induced a dose-dependent decrease in pulmonary artery pressure and an increase in cardiac output and blood oxygen saturation in all patients (45). While all patients improved initially, two ultimately died. It has also been shown that inhaled nitric oxide can correct the profound hypoxemia associated with right-to-left shunt through a patent foramen ovale in patients with massive PE (46).

In summary, in acute massive PE, hemodynamic instability may improve with fluid administration. If shock persists after a 500 mL fluid challenge, inotropic support is indicated. Dobutamine appears reasonable in cases of moderate systemic hypotension or norepinephrine in cases of more profound systemic hypotension (35). Inhaled nitric oxide may also prove beneficial. Clearly, more clinical trial data would be useful, but these patients are extremely difficult to randomize, and require individualized care.

Thrombolytic therapy

In isolated clinical studies, thrombolytic agents are associated with rapid and statistically significant improvement in hemodynamic parameters (47). Various studies have shown that, when compared to heparin alone for the treatment of PE, thrombolytics result in significantly reduced mean pulmonary arterial pressures, total pulmonary resistance, and RV end diastolic pressure as well as a significant increase in cardiac index (47–49). While the use of thrombolytic therapy in patients with hemodynamic compromise is fairly well accepted in clinical practice, the crux of the debate lies with the patient with "submassive PE." One early randomized trial evaluating recombinant tissue-type plasminogen activator (tPA) used echocardiography to evaluate RV wall motion and tricuspid regurgitation in patients with confirmed PE who then received either tPA in addition to heparin or heparin alone. The study revealed a rapid, statistically significant improvement in RV wall movement and tricuspid regurgitation at 3 and 24 hours after thrombolytic therapy (50).

To date, only a limited number of randomized controlled trials have compared thrombolytic therapy to conventional unfractionated heparin in the treatment of acute PE (50–56). Together, these studies account for fewer than 800 patients. Unfortunately, only ten of these studies include mortality data (47–50,52–56) and only one was designed and powered to detect clinical endpoints (56). Since the latter study, a meta-analysis has combined data from the randomized trials, and concluded that administration of thrombolytics to an unselected patient population has not demonstrated a mortality benefit (57) in part due to low event rates. A future trial would likely need at least 1000 patients in order to have sufficient power to detect clinical endpoints (58).

Thus far, only one randomized trial of thrombolytic therapy versus heparin alone included *only* patients with hemodynamic instability (55). In this study, eight patients were randomized to a bolus of streptokinase followed by heparin, or heparin alone. The four patients who received streptokinase all survived to two years of follow-up while all four patients who received heparin alone died within a few hours of presentation, however, patients in this study did not have proven PE, but were only considered to have a high clinical suspicion (55). A subgroup analysis of five randomized trials that included, but were not limited to, patients presenting with cardiogenic shock reported a 6.2 percent death rate in the thrombolytic group compared to 12.7 percent in the group that received heparin alone (OR 0.47, 95 percent CI 0.20 to 1.10) (57). Although there was a trend towards decreased mortality in the thrombolytic group, this did not reach statistical significance (57). The ACCP currently carries a Grade 1B level of evidence recommendation in support of thrombolytic administration to hemodynamically unstable patients with acute PE (1), and most clinicians accept this criterion, in the absence of absolute contraindications (59). A summary of the ACCP recommendations for administration of thrombolytic therapy is outlined in Box 22.2.3.

In hemodynamically stable patients with RV dysfunction, Konstantinides and associates (56), demonstrated that patients who received tPA were significantly less likely to clinically deteriorate than those who received placebo, i.e., 11 percent versus 25 percent, with a relative risk reduction of 55 percent (95 percent CI 21 percent to 75 percent) and number needed to treat of 8. However, there was no difference in all-cause mortality. An important study limitation involves the fact that treating physicians were allowed to break protocol and administer thrombolysis if they believed that a patient was doing poorly. The high rate of rescue thrombolysis may have driven the composite end point to statistical significance. Thus, the potential

---

BOX 22.2.3: A Synopsis of Key Thrombolytic Therapy Recommendations from the 8th ACCP Consensus (1)*

- All PE patients should undergo rapid risk stratification (Grade 1C).†
- With hemodynamic compromise, thrombolytic therapy is recommended, unless there are major contraindications due to bleeding risk (Grade 1B).‡
- In selected high-risk patients without hypotension, and with a low risk of bleeding, administration of thrombolytic therapy is suggested (Grade 2B).
- In acute PE, when a thrombolytic agent is used, peripheral vein administration rather than direct pulmonary artery infusion is recommended (Grade 1B).
- In patients with acute PE, we recommend use of thrombolytic regimens with short infusion times (e.g. a 2-h infusion) over those with prolonged infusion times (e.g., a 24-h infusion) (Grade 1B).

*The decision to use thrombolytics depends on the clinician's assessment of PE severity, prognosis, and bleeding risk.
†Grade 1 denotes a strong recommendation, and grade 2 a weak recommendation ("suggestion"). Level A would be based upon high-quality randomized trial data, while B indicates moderate-quality evidence, and C low or very low-quality evidence.
‡Unstable hemodynamics is the clearest indication for thrombolytic therapy. It is controversial as to whether hypotension caused by PE, in the absence of the need for pressors constitutes a clear indication for thrombolysis. The need for pressors mandates strong consideration for thrombolytics.

---

mortality benefit of thrombolytics in PE patients with RV dysfunction but preserved systemic arterial blood pressure, remains unproven.

As described, biomarkers, including cardiac troponins and brain natriuretic peptide (BNP) have been used to risk stratify (19,20). While a firm evidence-based recommendation cannot be made in this regard, it appears appropriate to consider them in the risk stratification armamentarium. Another potential avenue to explore, would be better delineation of *degrees* of RV enlargement and dysfunction. A significant proportion (73 percent) of pulmonologists surveyed indicated they would strongly consider thrombolytics in PE associated with severe hypoxemia (59). The presence of extensive residual thrombus in the lower extremities could be a risk for higher mortality in acute PE, particularly in those patients who already have RV dysfunction, and perhaps thrombolytic therapy would be beneficial in this setting. However, this also remains unstudied and unproven. Future investigations should address these issues.

Thrombolytics naturally possess the ability to lyse clots anywhere within the vasculature and thus, complications from bleeding, including fatal intracranial hemorrhage must be considered. A number of absolute and relative contraindications to thrombolytic therapy have been proposed in order to minimize the bleeding risk (Box 22.2.4). However, in dire clinical circumstances even absolute contraindications may not preclude the use of thrombolytics in the view of some clinicians. Pooled data from randomized trials of thrombolytics for acute PE have shown a trend toward increased major hemorrhagic events in the thrombolytic group versus the group that received heparin alone, although at 9.1 percent for thrombolytic therapy, versus 6.1 percent for UFH the difference (OR 0.67; 95 percent CI 0.40 to 1.12) did not reach statistical significance (57). Not surprisingly, minor bleeding events were significantly increased in the thrombolytic group. Previous intracranial hemorrhage active significant bleeding, and recent major surgery (previous 1 to 2 weeks depending on the specific procedure and patient) would be of significant concern regarding thrombolytic administration.

Generalizing the significance of bleeding data beyond the confines of the clinical research setting is limited, as clinical trials frequently have strict exclusion criteria, and investigators may be more reluctant to enroll patients with

relative contraindications or with significant comorbid illness. Registry data from the International Cooperative Pulmonary Embolism Registry (ICOPER), reported that 21.9 percent of patients who received thrombolytics for the treatment of PE had a major bleeding complication, with 3 percent demonstrating intracranial hemorrhage, compared with 0.3 percent in the heparin-treated group (2). However, the baseline characteristics were not similar between these patient groups.

Thrombolytic therapy is generally administered by peripheral IV infusion. While animal and clinical trials have suggested the potential benefit of central and even direct intraembolic infusion, the inadequate evidence base suggests that systemic delivery is favored except in exceptional circumstances (1).

EMBOLECTOMY AND VENA CAVA FILTER PLACEMENT

No clear guidelines can be offered for pulmonary embolectomy. It is reasonable to consider in patients with proven massive PE and hemodynamic instability, particularly when thrombolytic therapy has failed or is contraindicated (1,60,61). Because the condition of these patients is very compromised, the risk of death may be high with this approach. A surgical approach is sometimes considered when there are right heart thrombi, with or without paradoxical embolism, but no data from randomized trials are available; thrombolysis is also commonly considered in such cases.

The main indications for inferior vena caval filter (IVCF) placement include contraindications to anticoagulation, major bleeding complications during anticoagulation, and recurrent embolism while on therapeutic anticoagulation (1). Filters are sometimes placed in the case of massive PE, when it is believed that additional emboli might be lethal, either with or without thrombolytic therapy. However, this latter indication is not based on solid clinical trial data. While filters are effective in reducing the incidence of PE, they have not been shown to increase overall survival (62). Retrieval is feasible after many months, and removal approximately 1 year after placement has been reported (63,64). Recommendations for the use of vena caval filters have recently been published (63).

BOX 22.2.4: Absolute and Relative Contraindications to Thrombolytic Therapy

Absolute contraindications*

Previous intracranial hemorrhage
Known intracranial malignancy, arteriovenous malformation or aneurysm
Significant head trauma
Active internal bleeding
Known bleeding diathesis
Intracranial or intraspinal surgery within 3 months
Cerebrovascular accident within 2 months

Relative contraindications

Recent internal bleeding
Recent surgery or organ biopsy
Recent trauma, including cardiopulmonary resuscitation
Venipuncture at non-compressible site
Uncontrolled hypertension
Pregnancy
Diabetic retinopathy

Age > 75 years

*These absolute contraindications should be carefully assessed, but some (except concurrent intracranial hemorrhage) may not be "absolute" in extreme circumstances of massive PE. These settings are best individualized; risk/benefit must be considered.

HOME THERAPY/EARLY DISCHARGE FOR ACUTE PULMONARY EMBOLISM

Because bed rest is not recommended for acute DVT unless there is substantial pain and swelling (1), outpatient management in selected patients has become common, with LMWH simplifying the initial management of DVT. However, patients treated for PE appear to be almost four times as likely (1.5 percent vs. 0.4 percent) to die of a recurrence in the next year than are patients treated for DVT (25). While for certain experienced physicians, outpatient care for carefully selected acute PE patients may already be a reality (65), most practitioners are not secure with this approach.

Kovacs and colleagues (66) published results from a non-randomized but prospective cohort of PE patients managed in the outpatient setting, clearly outlining inclusion and exclusion criteria. In these carefully selected patients, the recurrence rates demonstrated were about the same as in large randomized trials examining predominantly for only DVT in the outpatient setting (67–69) and the major bleeding rates as low or lower. While non-randomized, this study set the stage for a closer look. Additional prospective data also suggest that carefully scrutinized patients can be managed after very brief hospitalization or observation (70). If outpatient PE therapy is considered, careful triage of patients is crucial; clinical judgment together with scoring systems described above which take into account severity of the event may prove effective in facilitating patient selection (23,24). A means by which the approach to outpatient therapy can be more standardized is crucial. While a reduction in iatrogenic problems and nosocomial disease are potential benefits, more data are needed.

LONG-TERM TREATMENT OF ACUTE PULMONARY EMBOLISM

While the focus of this review is on the initial therapy of acute PE, some fundamental data regarding long-term therapy are offered. Patients with acute VTE require long-term anticoagulation to prevent symptomatic extension and recurrent VTE. Documented VTE in patients with transient risk factors should be treated for 3 to 6 months, but more extended treatment is appropriate when significant risk factors persist, when thromboembolism is idiopathic, or when previous episodes of VTE have been documented (1,71). Recent data suggest that D-dimer levels may help guide decisions about the duration of therapy; persistently elevated levels appear to be associated with an increased recurrence rate (72). In patients with active cancer, long-term treatment of DVT with the LMWH dalteparin, as compared with warfarin has been shown to be associated with fewer VTE recurrences (73).

NEW AGENTS

A number of parenteral and oral anticoagulants are being studied in Phase III clinical trials. Idraparinux is a very long-acting parenteral synthetic antithrombin inhibitor administered weekly by the SC route, and its biotinylated form is reversible. This compound was developed for both the initial and long-term treatment of VTE (10). Oral direct thrombin inhibitors, such as dabigatran, and oral anti-factor Xa inhibitors, such as rivaroxaban and apixaban, are being

evaluated for both prophylaxis and therapy. Aptamers, derived from nucleic acid templates, act as reversible antagonists of coagulation factors, have the potential to be developed together with a specific antidote, and are in early phase clinical trials. While none of these agents are approved for commercial use for therapy of acute VTE, preliminary data are very promising.

KEY POINTS

- Therapy for acute PE should be initiated if the clinical suspicion is high and the perceived bleeding risk is low.
- As anticoagulation is initiated and PE is diagnosed, risk stratification should be considered.
- Depending on the scenario, more aggressive treatment with thrombolytic therapy or embolectomy can be considered.
- There is now a large body of evidence from large randomized comparisons that UFH, LMWH and fondaparinux are all safe and effective approaches to initial anticoagulation.
- Low molecular weight heparin and fondaparinux are easier to administer, do not require monitoring, and are backed by a substantial evidence base in the modern era.
- Documented VTE in patients with transient risk factors should be treated for 3 to 6 months, but more extended treatment is appropriate when significant risk factors persist, when VTE is idiopathic, or when VTE is recurrent.
- Bleeding risk should also be considered.
- IVC filter placement should be undertaken if anticoagulation is contraindicated due to bleeding.
- Evidence-based guidelines continue to be refined based upon new clinical trial data. New anticoagulants are on the horizon.

REFERENCES

1. Kearon C, Kahn SR, Agnelli G *et al.* Antithrombotic therapy for venous thromboembolic disease. Chest 2008;133:454S–545.
2. Azarian R, Wartski M, Collignon MA *et al.* Lung perfusion scans and hemodynamics in acute and chronic pulmonary embolism. J Nucl Med 1997;38:980–3.
3. Goldhaber SZ, Visani L, De Rosa M. Acute pulmonary embolism: clinical outcomes in the International Cooperative Pulmonary Embolism Registry (ICOPER). Lancet 1999;353:1386–9.
4. Kasper W, Konstantinides S, Geibel A *et al.* Management strategies and determinants of outcome in acute major

pulmonary embolism: results of a multicenter registry. J Am Coll Cardiol 1997;30:1165–71.

5. Alpert JS, Smith R, Carlson J et al. Mortality in patients treated for pulmonary embolism. JAMA 1976;236:1477–80.

6. Grifoni S, Olivotto I, Cecchini P et al. Short-term clinical outcome of patients with acute pulmonary embolism, normal blood pressure and echocardiographic right ventricular dysfunction. Circulation 2000;101:2817–22.

7. Vieillard-Baron A, Page B, Augarde R et al. Acute cor pulmonale in massive pulmonary embolism: incidence, echocardiographic pattern, clinical implications and recovery rate. Intensive Care Med 2001;27:1481–6.

8. Task Force on Pulmonary Embolism, European Society of Cardiology. Guidelines on diagnosis and management of acute pulmonary embolism. Eur Heart J 2000;21:1301–36.

9. Quinlan DJ, McQuillan A, Eikelboom JW. Low-molecular-weight heparin compared with intravenous unfractionated heparin for treatment of pulmonary embolism: a meta-analysis of randomized, controlled trials. Ann Intern Med 2004;140:175–83.

10. Büller HR, Cohen AT, Davidson B et al. Idraparinux versus standard therapy for venous thromboembolic disease. N Engl J Med 2007;357:1094–104.

11. Ribeiro A, Lindmarker P, Juhlin-Dannfelt A et al. Echocardiography Doppler in pulmonary embolism: right ventricular dysfunction as a predictor of mortality rate. Am Heart J 1997;134:479–87.

12. Kucher N, Rossi E, De Rosa M, Goldhaber SZ. Prognostic role of echocardiography among patients with acute pulmonary embolism and a systolic arterial pressure of 90 mmHg or higher. Arch Intern Med 2005;165:1777–81.

13. Kostrubiec M, Pruszczyk P, Bochowicz A et al. Biomarker-based risk assessment model in acute pulmonary embolism. Eur Heart J 2005;26:2166–72.

14. Kucher N, Printzen G, Goldhaber SZ. Prognostic role of brain natriuretic peptide in acute pulmonary embolism. Circulation 2003;107:2545–7.

15. Pieralli F, Olivotto I, Vanni S et al. Usefulness of bedside testing for brain natriuretic peptide to identify right ventricular dysfunction and outcome in normotensive patients with acute pulmonary embolism. Am J Cardiol 2006;97:1386–90.

16. Konstantinides S, Geibel A, Olschewski M et al. Association between thrombolytic treatment and the prognosis of hemodynamically stable patients with major pulmonary embolism: results of a multicenter registry. Circulation 1997;96:882–8.

17. Scridon T, Scridon C, Skali H et al. Prognostic significance of troponin elevation and right ventricular enlargement in acute pulmonary embolism. Am J Cardiol 2005;96:303–5.

18. Hamel E, Pacouret G, Vincentelli D et al. Thrombolysis or heparin therapy in massive pulmonary embolism with right ventricular dilation: results from a 128-patient monocenter registry. Chest 2001;120:120–5.

19. Pruszczyk P, Bochowicz A, Torbicki A et al. Cardiac troponin T monitoring identifies high-risk group of normotensive patients with acute pulmonary embolism. Chest 2003;123:1947–52.

20. Pruszczyk P, Kostrubiec M, Bochowicz A et al. N-terminal pro-brain natriuretic peptide in patients with acute pulmonary embolism. Eur Respir J 2003;22:649–53.

21. Aujesky D, Perrier A, Roy PM et al. Validation of a clinical prognostic model to identify low-risk patients with pulmonary embolism. J Intern Med 2007;261:597–604.

22. Aujesky D, Obrosky DS, Stone RA et al. Derivation and validation of a prognostic model for pulmonary embolism. Am J Respir Crit Care Med 2005;172:1041–6.

23. Aujesky D, Obrosky DS, Stone RA et al. A prediction rule to identify low-risk patients with pulmonary embolism. Arch Intern Med 2006;166:169–75.

24. Aujesky D, Roy PM, Le Manach CP et al. Validation of a model to predict adverse outcomes in patients with pulmonary embolism. Eur Heart J 2006;27:476–81.

25. Douketis JD, Kearon C, Bates S et al. Risk of fatal pulmonary embolism in patients with treated venous thromboembolism. JAMA 1998;279:458–62.

26. Büller HR, Davidson BL, Decousus H et al. Subcutaneous fondaparinux versus intravenous unfractionated heparin in the initial treatment of pulmonary embolism. N Engl J Med 2003;349:1695–702.

27. Heit JA, Silverstein MD, Mohr DN et al. Predictors of survival after deep vein thrombosis and pulmonary embolism: a population-based, cohort study. Arch Intern Med 1999;159:445–53.

28. Barritt DW, Jordan SC. Anticoagulant drugs in the treatment of pulmonary embolism: a controlled trial. Lancet 1960;i:1309–12.

29. Kearon C, Ginsberg JS, Julian JA et al. Comparison of fixed-dose weight-adjusted unfractionated heparin and low molecular-weight heparin for acute treatment of venous thromboembolism. JAMA 2006;296:935–42.

30. Martel N, Lee J, Wells PS. Risk for heparin-induced thrombocytopenia with unfractionated and low molecular-weight heparin thromboprophylaxis: a meta-analysis. Blood 2005;106:2710–5.

31. Simonneau G, Sors H, Charbonnier B et al. A comparison of low molecular-weight heparin with unfractionated heparin for acute pulmonary embolism. The THESEE Study Group. Tinzaparine ou Heparine Standard: Evaluations dans l'Embolie Pulmonaire. N Engl J Med 1997;337:663–9.

32. Gouin-Thibault I, Pautas E, Siguret V. Safety profile of different low molecular weight heparins used at therapeutic dose. Drug Saf 2005;28:333–49.

33. Prandoni P, Siragusa S, Girolami B, Fabris F. The incidence of heparin-induced thrombocytopenia in medical patients treated with low molecular-weight heparin: a prospective cohort study. Blood 2005;106:3049–54.

34. Warkentin TE, Greinacher A, Koster A, Lincoff AM. Treatment and prevention of heparin-induced thrombocytopenia. Chest 2008;133:340S–380S.

35. Layish DT, Tapson VF. Pharmacologic hemodynamic support in massive pulmonary embolism. Chest 1997;111:218–24.

36. Mercat A, Diehl JL, Meyer G, Teboul JL, Sors H. Hemodynamic effects of fluid loading in acute massive pulmonary embolism. Crit Care Med 1999;27:540–4.

37. McDonald IG, Hirsh J, Hale GS, Cade JF, McCarthy RA. Isoproterenol in massive pulmonary embolism: haemodynamic and clinical effects. Med J Aust 1968;2:201–5.

38. Boulain T, Lanotte R, Legras A, Perrotin D. Efficacy of epinephrine therapy in shock complicating pulmonary embolism. Chest 1993;104:300–2.

39. Hopf HB, Flossdorf T, Breulmann M. Recombinant tissue-type plasminogen activator for the emergency treatment of perioperative life-threatening pulmonary embolism (stage IV). Results in 7 patients. Anaesthesist 1991;40:309–14.

40. Scheeren TW, Hopf HB, Peters J. Intraoperative thrombolysis with rt-PA in massive pulmonary embolism during venous thrombectomy. Anasthesiol Intensivmed Notfallmed Schmerzther 1994;29:440–5.

41. Igarashi A, Amagasa S, Yokoo N. Case of postoperative pulmonary embolism after tonsillectomy in a healthy young woman. Masui 2007;56:1085–7.

42. Mathru M, Venus B, Smith RA, Shirakawa Y, Sugiura A. Treatment of low cardiac output complicating acute pulmonary hypertension in normovolemic goats. Crit Care Med 1986;14:120–4.

43. Jardin F, Genevray B, Brun-Ney D, Margairaz A. Dobutamine: a hemodynamic evaluation in pulmonary embolism shock. Crit Care Med 1985;13:1009–12.

44. Manier G, Castaing Y. Influence of cardiac output on oxygen exchange in acute pulmonary embolism. Am Rev Respir Dis 1992;145:130–6.

45. Capellier G, Jacques T, Balvay P et al. Inhaled nitric oxide in patients with pulmonary embolism. Intensive Care Med 1997;23:1089–92.

46. Estagnasie PG, Le Bourdelles L, Mier F, Coste D, Dreyfuss. Use of inhaled nitric oxide to reverse flow through a patent foramen ovale during pulmonary embolism. Ann Intern Med 1994;120:757–9.

47. The Urokinase Pulmonary Embolism Trial: a national cooperative study. Circulation 1973;47 Suppl II:II1–108.

48. Tibbutt DA, Davies JA, Anderson JA et al. Comparison by controlled clinical trial of streptokinase and heparin in the treatment of life-threatening pulmonary embolism. Br Med J 1974;1:343–7.

49. Ly B, Arnesen H, Eie H et al. A controlled clinical trial of streptokinase and heparin in the treatment of major pulmonary embolism. Acta Med Scand 1978;203:465–70.

50. Goldhaber SZ, Haire WD, Feldstein ML et al. Alteplase versus heparin in acute pulmonary embolism: randomised trial assessing right-ventricular function and pulmonary perfusion. Lancet 1993;341:507–11.

51. Dotter CT, Seamon AJ, Rosch J et al. Streptokinase and heparin in the treatment of pulmonary embolism: a randomized clinical trial. Vasc Surg 1979;13:42–52.

52. Marini C, Di Ricco G, Rossi G et al. Fibrinolytic effects of urokinase and heparin in acute pulmonary embolism: a randomized clinical trial. Respiration 1988;54:162–73.

53. Levine M, Hirsh J, Weitz J et al. A randomized trial of a single bolus dosage regimen of recombinant tissue plasminogen activator in patients with acute pulmonary embolism. Chest 1990;98:1473–9.

54. Dalla-Volta S, Palla A, Santolicandro A et al. PAIMS 2: alteplase combined with heparin versus heparin in the treatment of acute pulmonary embolism. Plasminogen Activator Italian Multicenter Study 2. J Am Coll Cardiol 1992;20:520–6.

55. Jerjes-Sanchez C, Ramiez-Rivera A, de Lourdes Garcia M et al. Streptokinase and heparin versus heparin alone in massive pulmonary embolism: a randomized controlled trial. J Thromb Thrombolysis 1995;2:227–9.

56. Konstantanides S, Geibel A, Heusel G et al. Heparin plus alteplase compared with heparin alone in patients with submassive pulmonary embolism. NEJM 2002;347:1143–50.

57. Wan S, Quinlan DJ, Agnelli G et al. Thrombolysis compared with heparin for the initial treatment of pulmonary embolism: a meta-analysis of the randomized controlled trials. Circulation 2004;110:744–9.

58. Goldhaber SZ. Thrombolytic therapy for patients with pulmonary embolism who are hemodynamically stable but have right ventricular dysfunction: pro. Arch Intern Med 2005;165:2197–9.

59. Witty LA, Krichman A, Tapson VF. Thrombolytic therapy for venous thromboembolism: Utilization by practicing pulmonologists. Arch Intern Med 1994;154:1601–4.

60. Leacche M, Unic D, Goldhaber SZ et al. Modern surgical treatment of massive pulmonary embolism: results in 47 consecutive patients after rapid diagnosis and aggressive surgical approach. J Thorac Cardiovasc Surg 2005;129:1018–23.

61. Meyer G, Tamisier D, Sors H et al. Pulmonary embolectomy: a 20-year experience at one center. Ann Thorac Surg 1991;51:232–6.

62. Decousus H, Leizorovicz A, Parent F et al. A clinical trial of vena caval filters in the prevention of pulmonary embolism in patients with proximal deep-vein thrombosis. N Engl J Med 1998;338:409–15.

63. Mismetti P, Rivron-Guillot K, Quenet S et al. A prospective long-term study of 220 patients with a retrievable vena cava filter for secondary prevention of venous thromboembolism. Chest 2007;131:223–9.

64. Kaufman JA, Kinney TB, Streiff MB et al. Guidelines for the use of retrievable and convertible vena cava filters: report from the Society of Interventional Radiology multidisciplinary consensus conference. J Vasc Interv Radiol 2006;17:449–59.

65. Wells PS, Anderson DR, Rodger MA et al. A randomized trial comparing 2 low-molecular-weight heparins for the outpatient treatment of deep vein thrombosis and pulmonary embolism. Arch Intern Med 2005;165:733–8.

66. Kovacs MJ, Anderson D, Morrow B et al. Outpatient treatment of pulmonary embolism with dalteparin. Thromb Haemost 2000;83:209–11.

67. Columbus Investigators. Low-molecular-weight heparin in the treatment of patients with venous thromboembolism. N Engl J Med 1997;337:657–62.

68. Levine M, Gent M, Hirsh J *et al.* A comparison of low-molecular-weight heparin administered primarily at home with unfractionated heparin administered in the hospital for proximal deep-vein thrombosis. N Engl J Med 1996;334:677–81.

69. Koopman MM, Prandoni P, Piovella F *et al.* Tasman Study Group. Treatment of venous thrombosis with intravenous unfractionated heparin administered in the hospital as compared with subcutaneous LMWH administered at home. N Engl J Med 1996;334:682–7.

70. Davies CWH, Wimperis J, Green ES *et al.* Early discharge of patients with pulmonary embolism: a two-phase observational study. Eur Respir J 2007;30:708–14.

71. Campbell IA, Bentley DP, Prescott RJ *et al.* Anticoagulation for three versus six months in patients with deep vein thrombosis or pulmonary embolism, or both: randomised trial. BMJ 2007;334:674.

72. Palareti G, Cosmi B, Legnani C *et al.* D-dimer testing to determine the duration of anticoagulation therapy. N Engl J Med 2006;355:1780–9.

73. Lee AYY, Levine MN, Baker RI *et al.* Low-molecular-weight heparin versus a coumarin for the prevention of recurrent venous thromboembolism in patients with cancer. N Engl J Med 2003;349:146–53.

74. Bauer K. New anticoagulants. Hematology Am Soc Hematol Educ Program 2006:450–6.

75. Rusconi CP, Scardino E, Layzer J *et al.* RNA aptamers as reversible antagonists of coagulation factor IXa. Nature 2002;419:90–4.

Chronic thromboembolic pulmonary hypertension

DIANA BONDERMAN AND IRENE M LANG

INTRODUCTION

Recent advances in the understanding and treatment of pulmonary vascular disease have contributed to a growing interest in chronic thromboembolic pulmonary hypertension (CTEPH), and have enhanced this relatively young research area in many aspects.

Traditionally, a line was drawn between the pathobiological processes underlying CTEPH versus non-thromboembolic precapillary pulmonary hypertension (PAH). While CTEPH was classified as a variant of pulmonary hypertension (PH) driven by simple mechanical obstruction of the pulmonary arteries, non-thromboembolic PH was attributed to remodeling and proliferation of the vascular wall as the consequence of complex molecular mechanisms that attracted attention and grant support.

For years, the scientific debate of CTEPH was mainly focused around its thromboembolic nature because of striking dissimilarities to classical venous thromboembolism, for example the lack of risk factors for venous thrombosis (1,2), the lack of clinically apparent pulmonary embolism in a majority of patients (3), the difficulty to reproduce the disease in animal models of thrombosis (4), and the nature of the pulmonary vascular obstructions that are dissociated from hemodynamic compromise (5,6). However, recent epidemiologic studies have demonstrated a clear association between venous thromboembolism and the evolution of CTEPH (7,8), and have largely resolved this debate.

Because no correlations could be found between the extent of thrombotic pulmonary arterial obstructions and pulmonary vascular resistance (5), recent research has concluded that CTEPH is a dual vascular disorder, comprised of major vessel vascular remodeling of thrombus resolution and a small-vessel arteriopathy that is indistinguishable from classical PAH (9). The identification of other than thrombotic disease-modifying conditions (8,10,11) has shed new light on disease pathobiology. The perception of CTEPH as an exceptional prothrombotic state with frequently recurring thromboembolic events has been abandoned. It seems that in affected patients, minor or major thromboembolic events in combination with infection, inflammation, autoimmunity or malignancy trigger an intravascular remodeling process that involves the thrombus itself as well as the vascular wall of small resistance vessels.

The new view on CTEPH pathogenesis has impacted clinical routine. The primary treatment remains surgical pulmonary endarterectomy (PEA). However, experiences from CTEPH centers worldwide suggest that up to 50 percent of patients are not suitable for surgical removal of pulmonary obstructions. Based on the concept of a disorder that involves the small pulmonary arterioles, vasodilator therapy has been proposed for those patients. Although the BENEFIT study (12), the first multi-center randomized controlled trial of the dual endothelin receptor antagonist bosentan in inoperable CTEPH patients failed to achieve the second component of the co-primary endpoint, the availability of novel vasodilator substances and adaptive study designs permit hope for medical treatments of inoperable CTEPH patients.

DEFINITION

CTEPH is defined by the following observations that are made after at least 3 months of effective anticoagulation (13):

1. a mean pulmonary arterial pressure > 25 mmHg with a pulmonary capillary wedge pressure $\geqslant 25$ mmHg, and

2. one or more mismatched segmental or larger
   perfusion defects detected by ventilation-perfusion
   lung scanning/multi-detector computed
   tomographic angiography/pulmonary angiography
   (Figure 22.3.1).

EPIDEMIOLOGY

The incidence and prevalence of CTEPH are unknown.
Classical estimates of disease frequency refer to the number
of CTEPH cases per survived pulmonary thromboembolic
events (7,13–15), and reported cumulative incidences range
between 0.1 percent and 3.8 percent of survived pulmonary thromboemboli. However, more than 30 percent of
affected patients deny previous symptoms or a diagnosis of
previous acute venous thromboembolism (8).

Over recent years, a number of apparently unrelated
conditions have been identified as risk factors for CTEPH.
Populations at risk are those with a history of splenectomy
(10,11,16), carriers of ventriculo-atrial (VA) shunts for the
treatment of hydrocephalus, or carriers of pacemakers with
a history of device infection (8,10), patients with inflammatory bowel disease (10), thyroid hormone replacement (8),
circulating antiphospholipid antibodies (2,8,17), survived
cancer (8), individuals with blood groups non-0 (8,18) and
elevated plasma coagulation factor VIII (18), as well as carriers of the fibrinogen Aα Thr312Ala polymorphism (19).
Table 22.3.1 summarizes currently known CTEPH risk factors according to the strength of the statistical relationship
compared with a control cohort. Evidence on reported risk
factors mainly originates from observational case-control
analyses of CTEPH patients, as no long-term longitudinal
prospective analyses are available on risk populations. A
multi-center prospective CTEPH registry is under way and
will elucidate incidence, diagnosis, treatments and outcomes
of contemporary CTEPH patients in Europe.

ETIOLOGY

CTEPH results from single of recurrent pulmonary emboli
arising from sites of venous or, not of-norm thrombosis.
The current concept is that failing thrombus resolution,
fibrous obstruction and secondary remodeling processes
of the pulmonary vascular bed lead to an increase in pulmonary vascular resistance, progressive right heart failure
and death.

Although CTEPH is understood as a thromboembolic
disorder, neither classical plasmatic risk factors for venous
thromboembolism nor defects in fibrinolysis are associated
with CTEPH. Compared with the general population no
increased prevalence of the factor V Leiden mutation was
found (1,2). Other hereditary thrombotic risk factors, such
as deficiencies in antithrombin, protein C, protein S or the
prothrombin gene mutation (2,17) lack an association with
CTEPH. Efforts to identify functional defects (20,21) or

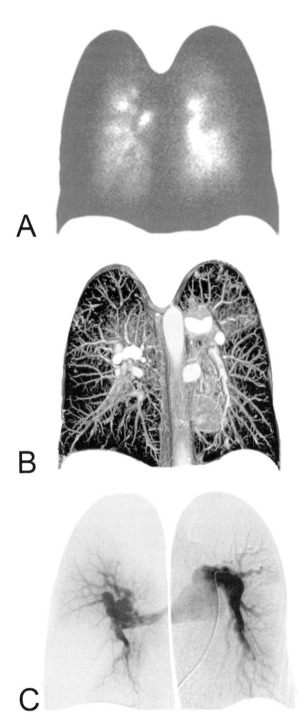

Figure 22.3.1 Imaging in CTEPH. Parallel investigations of a
single representative CTEPH case are shown. (A) Planar images of
99mTc-albumin lung scintigraphy show multiple segmental
defects. In the absence of pulmonary parenchymal abnormalities,
perfusion scintigraphy is diagnostic. (B) Three-dimensional
visualization of the pulmonary arterial tree with multiple
detector-row spiral computed tomography. In this patient,
thrombotic occlusions (shown in red) are found in the main
pulmonary trunk, and in the right lobar arteries. (C) Pulmonary
angiography illustrates low perfusion of the right lower lobe, with
an irregular appearance of the pulmonary trunk representing the
contours of major vessel thrombus.

Table 22.3.1 Risk factors for CTEPH listed in the order of the magnitude of published odds ratios

Risk factor (Ref)	Odds ratio [confidence interval]
Infected VA-shunt/pacemaker (8,10)	13.00 [2.5–129] and 76.40 [7.67–10350.62]
Splenectomy (8,10)	13.00 [2.7–127] and 17.87 [1.56–2438]
Recurrent VTE (8)	14.49 [5.40–43.08]
Thyroid disease (8)	6.10 [2.73–15.05]
Previous VTE (8)	4.52 [2.35–9.12]
Antiphospholipid antibodies (8)	4.20 [1.56–12.21]
Survived cancer (8)	3.76 [1.47–10.43]
Inflammatory bowel disease (8)	3.19 [0.74–16.03]
Blood groups non-O (8)	2.09 [1.12–3.94]
Fibrinogen Aα Thr312Ala polymorphism (19)	1.68 [1.13–2.49]
HLA-B*5201 (Japan) (78)	2.14 [1.29–3.55]
HLA-DPB1*0202 (Japan) (78)	3.41 [1.71–6.74]

VTE, venous thromboembolism.

gene polymorphisms (19) in the pulmonary vascular fibrinolytic system of affected individuals have failed. Neither alterations in plasma levels of type 1 plasminogen activator inhibitor nor tissue-type plasminogen activator could be linked with CTEPH (22).

The identification of clinical risk factors for CTEPH has shed new light on molecular mechanisms underlying thrombus persistence and its fibrous transformation. The observation that carriers of VA-shunts represent a CTEPH risk population (8,10) has stimulated experimental research. Shunt infection is common in patients with VA-shunts, and *Staphylococcus aureus* or *S. epidermidis* is responsible for up to one-half of these infections (23), leading to thrombosis and device failure (24). We observed that the majority of our CTEPH patients carrying either VA-shunt or pacemaker had a history of device infection. Indeed, staphylococcal DNA was present in six out of seven PEA specimens from VA-shunt/pacemaker carriers. In a murine model of stagnant-flow venous thrombosis, staphylococcal infection delayed thrombus resolution in parallel with an up-regulation of profibrotic molecules, such as transforming growth factor beta and connective tissue growth factor (25). Based on the available data it cannot be said whether the risk to develop CTEPH is to be attributed to hypothyroidism or thyroid hormone replacement therapy, or both. In tumor survivors, the interaction of tissue factor, thrombin and other coagulation factors with protease activated receptor proteins expressed by tumor cells and host vascular cells may have led to the induction of genes related to angiogenesis, cell survival and cell adhesion and migration. Of note, time delays between the occurrence of a CTEPH-associated medical condition and manifestation of CTEPH is in the order of 2–40 years (10).

Pulmonary vascular remodeling is believed to occur in areas free of thrombosis, and is histologically indistinguishable from other forms of PH (9,26–28). There is a broad individual variation with respect to the degree of pulmonary arteriopathy, that has been labeled as "secondary vascular changes" by Kenneth Moser (13). Although concomitant pulmonary vascular disease predicts adverse outcome (6,29), biological mechanisms that predict the degree of vascular involvement have not been identified. Mutations in the type-2 bone morphogenetic protein receptor gene that have been linked to the development of pulmonary vascular disease in familial and idiopathic PH cases (30,31) could not be related to CTEPH (32). Interestingly, CTEPH patients with a medical history of splenectomy, infected VA-shunt, inflammatory bowel disease or osteomyelitis face an adverse outcome as compared to affected patients without a clinical risk factor (33). This finding has been attributed to more severe small vessel pathology, although the exact mechanisms remain unclear.

CLINICAL PRESENTATION

Symptoms and physical signs

Similar to patients with other PH entities, CTEPH patients suffer from symptoms of progressive right heart failure. In earlier stages of disease typical patient complaints are dyspnea on exertion, fatigue and rapid exhaustion. Symptoms of overt right heart failure in advanced stages of disease are resting dyspnea and fluid retention. Physical findings are often subtle and may include a prominent pulmonary component of S2, left parasternal heave, and a systolic murmur, if tricuspid regurgitation is present. Typical clinical signs of right heart failure are extended neck veins, leg edema, ascites, hepatomegaly, and acrocyanosis. A rare but typical clinical finding is bruits over peripheral lung fields (34). This acoustic phenomenon is thought to occur in approximately 10 percent of CTEPH patients and has been attributed to turbulent blood flow in partially occluded pulmonary vessels (35).

Clinical course

Despite similarities in symptoms and physical signs, the course of CTEPH is clearly different from non-thromboembolic PH. A major difference is encountered in the age of disease onset. On average, CTEPH patients are 7 years older at the time of diagnosis, with the majority of patients presenting between the sixth and seventh life decade (8). In contrast to a progressive course of non-thromboembolic PH, CTEPH progresses episodically with months-to-years-lasting "honeymoon periods" between episodes of severe desaturation and deterioration. If left untreated, a mean survival of 6.8 years after diagnosis has been reported in CTEPH patients from Japan (36). For comparison, patients with idiopathic PAH face an untreated median survival of less than 3 years after diagnosis (37).

INVESTIGATIONS

CTEPH is a curable PH subset. CTEPH that is successfully (38) subjected to bilateral surgical PEA regains near-normal functional capacity (39). Thus, a major goal in the diagnostic work-up of patients presenting with PH is to test for the presence of CTEPH. If CTEPH is suspected, patients ought to be referred to specialized PEA centers, where further diagnostic testing is undertaken with the goal to explore operability. Imaging has become central to the diagnosis of CTEPH, and in the assessment of operability. Although visualization of thrombus site and extent may serve as surgical "road map," the operability statement is complex and hardly standardized. It is determined by thrombus location, underlying disease modifying factors, general comorbidities, the status of the lung parenchyma, hemodynamics in absolute numbers, i.e. pulmonary vascular resistance above $1000\,\mathrm{dyn/s\,cm^{-5}}$ confers increased risk, the relation of hemodynamic compromise and thrombus extension, previous cardiothoracic surgeries, hemodynamics after a previous PEA, personal experience of the surgeon, unilateral versus bilateral disease, the response to nitric oxide during acute testing (6), upstream resistance (29), and plasma levels of biomarkers, i.e., ADMA (40) and FABP (41). Because the degree of concomitant small vessel arteriopathy has a major impact on PEA outcome, a series of techniques have been developed that may help to assess the functional status of the distal pulmonary vascular bed (6,29).

In experienced PEA centers in Europe and the United States, available imaging techniques are used complementary. Traditionally, ventilation-perfusion scanning and pulmonary angiography have been key diagnostic tools for CTEPH. In light of the technical evolution, multi-detector computed tomographic angiography and magnetic resonance angiography may supersede traditional imaging techniques. Emerging non-invasive imaging modalities are described in dedicated chapters of this textbook.

Ventilation–perfusion scanning

Ventilation-perfusion lung scanning represents a mainstay in the diagnostic work-up of PH patients. A normal ventilation-perfusion scintigram virtually rules out CTEPH (42–46), while in the presence of PH, one or more mismatched segmental or larger defects generally indicate CTEPH (45). In clinical routine, an abnormal perfusion scan alone is diagnostic in the absence of severe pulmonary parenchymatous disease.

Pulmonary angiography

Pulmonary angiography has been a cornerstone in the management of patients with CTEPH. Allowing for the visualization of thromboembolic occlusions to the distality of the pulmonary vascular tree, pulmonary angiography is the established gold standard in CTEPH diagnosis, and key data source for the assessment of operability (47–49). Major draw-backs of this technique are its invasiveness and limited access, which results in limited expertise, especially in low-volume centers.

Right heart catheterization

Concomitant pulmonary vascular disease is a predictor of adverse surgical outcome in patients with CTEPH (6,29). Kim and co-workers (29) invasively analyzed pulmonary arterial occlusion pressure waveforms, a technique that has been used for partitioning pulmonary vascular resistance. Preoperative assessment of upstream resistance in 26 CTEPH patients correlated with both postoperative total pulmonary resistance index and postoperative mean pulmonary artery pressure. More recently, Skoro-Sajer et al. (6) demonstrated that acute vasoreactivity testing with nitric oxide may disclose the functional status of pulmonary microvasculature and predict surgical outcome. A total of 62 patients were followed for a median of 70.9 months after PEA. Those who experienced a reduction in mPAP > 10.4 percent with nitric oxide inhalation had lower postoperative pulmonary pressures and a clear long-term survival benefit as opposed to patients with acute vasoreactivity below this threshold.

TREATMENT

PEA is the treatment of choice in patients with confirmed CTEPH. It can be considered curative, as a majority of patients nearly normalize their hemodynamics and experience substantial relief from symptoms (50–52). However, surgical success largely depends on patient suitability. Beyond established standards and parameters that predict surgical success (51), operability is dependent on the expertise of the surgical team and on the resources available. Thus, the proportion of CTEPH patients not suitable for PEA varies from center to center, and may be as high as 50 percent.

Current criteria for the PEA include: confirmed diagnosis of CTEPH in NYHA functional classes II, III or IV, a preoperative pulmonary vascular resistance $> 300 \, dyn/s \, cm^{-5}$, surgical accessibility of thrombi in the main, lobar or segmental pulmonary arteries, absence of severe co-morbidities, and patient consent (53).

A crucial issue in the preoperative assessment of CTEPH patients is the definition of the degree of secondary arteriopathy and its contribution to overall pulmonary vascular resistance. Patients with thromboembolic defects in the main, lobar, or proximal segmental level are characterized as having proximal disease and represent the main target population for PEA. In contrast, patients with significant PH but little or no visible evidence of thromboembolic pathology are considered poor candidates for surgery (54). This latter group is usually characterized by severe pulmonary arteriopathy. Operability remains a center-specific assessment, and may vary largely.

In fact, patients who do not undergo surgery or suffer from persistent or residual PH after PEA face a poor prognosis. Particularly, in patients with a mean pulmonary artery pressure $> 50 \, mmHg$, 5-year survival rates are as low as 10 percent (55–58). Medical therapies currently used in the management of CTEPH come from a number of drug classes, such as anticoagulants, diuretics, or digitalis. Supportive treatment with anticoagulants reduces the risk of recurrent pulmonary thromboembolic events, and maintenance of lifelong anticoagulation is recommended (35). Diuretics may be used in conditions of fluid overload, and chronic oxygen supplementation is used for the treatment of hypoxemia.

The evidence for pathogenic mechanisms held in common between non-thromboembolic PH and CTEPH provides a strong rationale for the usefulness of vasodilator drugs in CTEPH patients. Pharmacotherapy is currently not approved but justified for "compassionate use" in inoperable patients, or as a "therapeutic bridge" to PEA in patients considered at high risk due to poor hemodynamics, or in patients with persistent or residual PH after PEA, or when surgery is contraindicated due to significant comorbidity.

Current knowledge on the effects of vasodilator treatment in patients with CTEPH primarily originates from uncontrolled single-center experiences, retrospective evaluations, and trials primarily assessing non-thromboembolic PH that included, but did not exclusively evaluate, patients with CTEPH. Prostacyclin and -analogs, endothelin receptor antagonists and phosphodiesterase-5 inhibitors were employed.

Prostacyclin and prostacyclin analogs

BERAPROST SODIUM

Ono and co-workers (59) studied the efficacy of oral beraprost sodium in inoperable patients with CTEPH. Patients were classified into two groups, one receiving oral beraprost sodium (n = 20), the other conventional therapy (n = 23). In contrast to the control group, treated patients experienced improvements in NYHA functional class. In a subgroup of patients undergoing hemodynamic evaluation after 2 ± 1 months, oral beraprost sodium treatment resulted in significant improvements in mean pulmonary arterial pressure and total pulmonary resistance, but not cardiac output. Overall, the study suggested that vasodilator treatment on top of conventional therapy improves 1- and 5-year survival. Vizza and co-workers (60) compared the effects of 6 months of beraprost treatment in eight patients with distal CTEPH and matched individuals with idiopathic pulmonary arterial hypertension. The authors concluded that in patients with CTEPH beraprost led to similar mid-term clinical and hemodynamic improvements as in patients with non-thromboembolic PH.

EPOPROSTENOL

Beneficial effects were also observed when patients were treated with epoprostenol. Nagaya and colleagues (61) administered intravenous epoprostenol in 12 CTEPH patients scheduled for PEA. Because of severe PH with pulmonary vascular resistance values exceeding $1200 \, dyn/s \, cm^{-5}$, these patients were considered high-risk surgical candidates. During a mean follow-up period of 46 ± 12 days, the intravenous administration of prostacyclin resulted in a 28 percent decrease in pulmonary vascular resistance before surgery. Moreover, plasma brain natriuretic peptide levels markedly decreased, suggesting improvement in right ventricular function. In another retrospective series (62), nine patients with moderate to severe CTEPH were treated with intravenous epoprostenol for 2 to 26 months before PEA. Six patients experienced either clinical stability or improvement that was associated with a mean reduction in pulmonary vascular resistance of 28 percent (range 0–46 percent). Three patients experienced clinical deterioration during epoprostenol administration, with a significant increase in pulmonary vascular resistance in two patients. Data from an Italian patient cohort (63) comprising 16 patients with non-thromboembolic PH and 11 with surgically untreatable CTEPH suggested that epoprostenol therapy over a median period of 12.4 months improves clinical status, exercise capacity, and NYHA functional class. In a more recent analysis conducted by Cabrol and colleagues (64), 27 consecutive patients with inoperable distal CTEPH were treated with long-term intravenous epoprostenol. After 20 ± 8 months of treatment, there was sustained improvement of exercise capacity and hemodynamic parameters in those who survived.

TREPROSTINIL

At our institution, subcutaneous treprostinil was administered in 25 patients with severe inoperable thromboembolic disease (65). A historical control group of 31 conventionally treated inoperable CTEPH patients were analyzed in parallel. We found a beneficial treatment effect on exercise capacity, hemodynamics and survival.

ILOPROST

A subgroup of patients enrolled in the AIR (Aerosolized Iloprost Randomized) study, a prospective randomized placebo-controlled trial, suffered from CTEPH. The study failed to demonstrate significant beneficial effects of inhaled iloprost in this subpopulation (66). Kramm et al. (67) studied the effect of inhaled iloprost administered immediately before PEA, after intensive care unit admission, and 12 hours after surgery (n = 10). Preoperative treatment had no significant effect on hemodynamic parameters, but led to detrimental systemic vasodilation and hypotension. Postoperative treatment, however, showed beneficial effects on pulmonary vascular resistance and mean pulmonary arterial pressure on top of the relief of hemodynamics by PEA. The same investigators administered aerosolized iloprost in a randomized placebo-controlled fashion in the setting of persistent PH in the postoperative period (68). Iloprost significantly enhanced cardiac index and reduced mean pulmonary arterial pressure and pulmonary vascular resistance in contrast to placebo.

Endothelin receptor antagonists

BOSENTAN

We assessed the effects of the dual endothelin receptor antagonist bosentan in 16 inoperable patients with CTEPH (69). After 6 months of treatment, NYHA functional class improved in 11 patients. In addition, a significant improvement was encountered in the 6-minute walking distance, paralleled by a reduction in serum levels of N-terminal brain natriuretic peptide. In the same issue of Chest, Hoeper et al. (70) published results from a prospective, multi-center, open-label trial evaluating bosentan treatment in CTEPH patients. At the 3-month follow-up visit, the 6-minute walking distance as well as hemodynamic parameters and serum levels of N-terminal brain natriuretic peptide had significantly improved in the treatment groups as compared to controls. Another retrospective, open-label study assessed bosentan treatment in 20 patients with CTEPH (71). After at least 3 months of treatment, Hughes and colleagues found significant improvement in the 6-minute walking distance as well as in hemodynamic parameters, such as pulmonary vascular resistance and cardiac index. Mean pulmonary artery pressure was also reduced but did not reach statistical significance as compared to the baseline value. Moreover, Hughes and co-investigators reported findings from a retrospective, open-label study evaluating long-term efficacy and safety of bosentan in CTEPH patients from three European centers (n = 47) (72). A clear improvement was observed in

6-minute walking distance at 1-year follow-up. A total of 28 patients had undergone right heart catheter after one year, and demonstrated significant improvement in cardiac index and a decrease in total pulmonary resistance. Seyfarth and co-authors (73) investigated the effect of long-term bosentan treatment on exercise tolerance and right ventricular function, as measured by the Tei index. Twelve consecutive patients with CTEPH not eligible for PEA or following partial or complete failure of PEA were included in a non-randomized, open-label prospective study. After 24 months of therapy, a beneficial effect on both outcome measures was achieved. The Swiss BOCTEPH study (74) was a national open-label trial assessing the effect of bosentan on hemodynamics, exercise capacity, quality of life, safety and tolerability in patients with CTEPH. Fifteen patients not eligible or waiting for surgery were enrolled. Similar to previous results, positive effects on all study endpoints could be achieved after 6 months of treatment.

Phosphodiesterase-5 inhibitors

SILDENAFIL

Ghofrani and co-workers (75) assessed sildenafil treatment in 12 patients with inoperable distal CTEPH. In this open-label study, acute vasodilator testing with sildenafil showed considerable vasoreactivity, and clear hemodynamic improvement and an increase in 6-minute walking distance were achieved after a mean treatment duration of 6.5 ± 1.1 months. Sheth and colleagues (76) investigated six patients with inoperable CTEPH and left ventricular dysfunction. After 6 weeks of sildenafil therapy, beneficial effects on mean pulmonary artery pressure, pulmonary capillary wedge pressure, and NYHA functional class were shown. In a double-blind, placebo-controlled pilot study performed by Suntharalingam et al. (77), 19 subjects with inoperable CTEPH were randomly assigned to sildenafil or placebo for 12 weeks. The primary endpoint was change in 6-minute walking distance. Secondary endpoints included changes in World Health Organization (WHO) class, cardiopulmonary hemodynamics, quality of life scores, and N-terminal brain natriuretic peptide. All subjects were transferred to open-label sildenafil at the end of the study and offered repeat assessment at 12 months. Although the study was not sufficiently powered to test the primary endpoint, it did suggest beneficial effects in favor of sildenafil in several secondary endpoints at both 3 months and 12 months.

The mainly positive experience gained from small observational series supported the concept of vasodilator treatment in inoperable CTEPH patients and led to the first double-blind, randomized, placebo-controlled trial in inoperable CTEPH. The BENEFIT study investigated Bosentan Effects in inoperable Forms of chronic Thromboembolic pulmonary hypertension (12). A total of 157 patients were enrolled and randomized in a 1:1 fashion to receive bosentan or placebo for 16 weeks. The study population consisted of symptomatic patients in WHO functional classes II, III, or IV with a 6-minute walking distance <450 m. A diagnosis of CTEPH had to be demonstrated by ventilation-perfusion lung scanning and pulmonary angiography. Patients could only be included if CTEPH had been judged inoperable because of peripheral localization of thrombotic material, or persistent/recurrent PH after PEA, without evidence of recurrent thromboembolism. To select a homogenous population of truly inoperable subjects, an Operability Evaluation Committee consisting of two specialized pulmonologists and two PEA surgeons was asked for re-evaluation of the inoperability status. Patients who were unanimously judged operable were excluded from the primary analysis.

Pulmonary vascular resistance that directly reflects disease pathobiology, and the 6-minute walk test as a measure of exercise capacity were chosen as co-primary endpoints. Although a statistically significant treatment effect of bosentan over placebo on pulmonary vascular resistance could be demonstrated (-24.1 percent of baseline [95 percent CI: -31.5 percent to -16.0 percent]), the effect on 6-minute walking distance was as low as $+2.2$ m ([95 percent CI: -22.5 m to $+28.8$ m]). The reasons for these discrepant results remain unclear. One explanation was the age difference between the patient population enrolled in the BENEFIT trial and the typical patient with idiopathic PAH studied in vasodilator trials. Because CTEPH patients were significantly older, comorbid conditions or skeletal muscle deconditioning could prevent or delay recovery of exercise capacity. Another hypothesis was that the duration of the study was not long enough to demonstrate improvement in the 6-minute walking distance.

The finding of a significant hemodynamic benefit without improvement in exercise capacity fueled a debate over the usefulness of the 6-minute walk test in this particular patient population. Tailoring trial designs to this unique form of PH will be one of the challenges in the near future. Currently, the effect of other vasodilator compounds, e.g. riociguat (CHEST) or treprostinil (CETREPH), are tested in multi-national placebo-controlled trials.

Future directions of therapy

Successful PEA represents the only curative therapy for patients with CTEPH, and will remain the treatment of choice. However, the assessment and definition of concomitant pulmonary vascular disease that may preclude an adequate relief from PH after PEA and increases perioperative mortality remains a black box in the preoperative diagnostic work-up of CTEPH patients. Promising techniques for the evaluation of the functional status of the distal pulmonary vascular bed have been introduced. One of the future efforts to be undertaken by the scientific community are standardized approaches. Preoperative quantification of small-vessel disease together with a precise estimate of thrombus load may set the stage for a clear-cut

differentiation between surgical candidates and those who are not. At present, none of the vasodilator compounds established in the treatment of non-thromboembolic PH are approved for the treatment of inoperable CTEPH patients. Despite its outcome the BENEFIT trial reinforced the principle of vasodilator use as a future direction in CTEPH research.

KEY POINTS

- CTEPH is a dual vascular disorder comprising major vessel vascular remodeling of thrombus resolution and a classical small-vessel arteriopathy.
- In general, only a small minority of patients who have survived an acute thromboembolic event continue to develop CTEPH.
- Traditional plasmatic prothrombotic risk factors are not risk factors for CTEPH.
- By contrast, splenectomy, infected ventriculo-atrial shunt, inflammatory bowel disease, thyroid hormone replacement therapy, or survived cancer have been identified as CTEPH-associated conditions.
- Because of potential surgical curability of the disorder, a diagnosis of pulmonary hypertension should always be followed by the search for underlying thromboembolism.
- Pulmonary endarterectomy is the treatment of choice in patients with confirmed CTEPH. However, the proportion of patients not suitable for surgery varies from center to center, and may be as high as 50 percent.
- Vasodilator trials in patients with inoperable CTEPH will clarify whether medical therapy for CTEPH is effective.

REFERENCES

1. Lang IM, Klepetko W, Pabinger I. No increased prevalence of the factor V Leiden mutation in chronic major vessel thromboembolic pulmonary hypertension (CTEPH). Thromb Haemost 1996;76:476–7.
2. Wolf M, Boyer-Neumann C, Parent F, Eschwege V, Jaillet H, Meyer D, Simonneau G. Thrombotic risk factors in pulmonary hypertension. Eur Respir J 2000;15:395–9.
3. Lang IM. Chronic thromboembolic pulmonary hypertension – not so rare after all. N Engl J Med 2004;350:2236–8.
4. Marsh JJ, Konopka RG, Lang IM, Wang HY, Pedersen C, Chiles P, Reilly CF, Moser KM. Suppression of thrombolysis in a canine model of pulmonary embolism. Circulation 1994;90:3091–97.
5. Azarian R, Wartski M, Collignon MA, Parent F, Herve P, Sors H, Simonneau G. Lung perfusion scans and hemodynamics

in acute and chronic pulmonary embolism. J Nucl Med 1997;38:980–3.

6. Skoro-Sajer N, Hack N, Sadushi-Kolici R et al. Pulmonary vascular reactivity and prognosis in patients with chronic thromboembolic pulmonary hypertension: a pilot study. Circulation 2009;119:298–305.

7. Pengo V, Lensing AW, Prins MH et al. Incidence of chronic thromboembolic pulmonary hypertension after pulmonary embolism. N Engl J Med 2004;350:2257–64.

8. Bonderman D, Wilkens H, Wakounig S et al. Risk factors for chronic thromboembolic pulmonary hypertension. Eur Respir J 2009;33:325–51.

9. Moser KM, Bloor CM. Pulmonary vascular lesions occurring in patients with chronic major vessel thromboembolic pulmonary hypertension. Chest 1993;103:685–92.

10. Bonderman D, Jakowitsch J, Adlbrecht C et al. Medical conditions increasing the risk of chronic thromboembolic pulmonary hypertension. Thromb Haemost 2005;93:512–6.

11. Jais X, Ioos V, Jardim C, Sitbon O, Parent F, Hamid A, Fadel E, Dartevelle P, Simonneau G, Humbert M. Splenectomy and chronic thromboembolic pulmonary hypertension. Thorax 2005;60:1031–4.

12. Jais X, D'Armini AM, Jansa P et al. Bosentan for treatment of inoperable chronic thromboembolic pulmonary hypertension: BENEFiT (Bosentan Effects in iNopErable Forms of chronIc Thromboembolic pulmonary hypertension), a randomized, placebo-controlled trial. J Am Coll Cardiol 2008;52:2127–34.

13. Moser KM, Auger WR, Fedullo PF. Chronic major-vessel thromboembolic pulmonary hypertension. Circulation 1990;81:1735–43.

14. Ribeiro A, Lindmarker P, Johnsson H, Juhlin-Dannfelt A, Jorfeldt L. Pulmonary embolism: one-year follow-up with echocardiography Doppler and five-year survival analysis. Circulation 1999;99:1325–30.

15. Becattini C, Agnelli G, Pesavento R, Silingardi M, Poggio R, Taliani MR, Ageno W. Incidence of chronic thromboembolic pulmonary hypertension after a first episode of pulmonary embolism. Chest 2006;130:172–5.

16. Condliffe R, Kiely DG, Gibbs JS et al. Prognostic and aetiological factors in chronic thromboembolic pulmonary hypertension. Eur Respir J 2009;33:332–8.

17. Auger WR, Permpikul P, Moser KM. Lupus anticoagulant, heparin use, and thrombocytopenia in patients with chronic thromboembolic pulmonary hypertension: a preliminary report. Am J Med 1995;99:392–6.

18. Bonderman D, Turecek PL, Jakowitsch J et al. High prevalence of elevated clotting factor VIII in chronic thromboembolic pulmonary hypertension. Thromb Haemost 2003;90:372–6.

19. Suntharalingam J, Goldsmith K, van Marion V et al. Fibrinogen alpha Thr312Ala polymorphism is associated with chronic thromboembolic pulmonary hypertension. Eur Respir J 2008;31:736–41.

20. Lang IM, Marsh JJ, Olman MA, Moser KM, Loskutoff DJ, Schleef RR. Expression of type 1 plasminogen activator inhibitor in chronic pulmonary thromboemboli. Circulation 1994;89:2715–21.

21. Lang IM, Marsh JJ, Olman MA, Moser KM, Schleef RR. Parallel analysis of tissue-type plasminogen activator and type 1 plasminogen activator inhibitor in plasma and endothelial cells derived from patients with chronic pulmonary thromboemboli. Circulation 1994;90:706–12.

22. Olman MA, Marsh JJ, Lang IM, Moser KM, Binder BR, Schleef RR. Endogenous fibrinolytic system in chronic large-vessel thromboembolic pulmonary hypertension. Circulation 1992;86:1241–8.

23. Schoenbaum SC, Gardner P, Shillito J. Infections of cerebrospinal fluid shunts: epidemiology, clinical manifestations, and therapy. J Infect Dis 1975;131:543–52.

24. Colli BO, Starr EM, Martelli N. [Surgical treatment of hydrocephalus in children. II. Complications]. Arq Neuropsiquiatr 1981;39:408–19.

25. Bonderman D, Jakowitsch J, Redwan B et al. Role for staphylococci in misguided thrombus resolution of chronic thromboembolic pulmonary hypertension. Arterioscler Thromb Vasc Biol 2008;28:678–84.

26. Moser KM, Braunwald NS. Successful surgical intervention in severe chronic thromboembolic pulmonary hypertension. Chest 1973;64:29–35.

27. Arbustini E, Morbini P, D'Armini AM, Repetto A, Minzioni G, Piovella F, Vigano M, Tavazzi L. Plaque composition in plexogenic and thromboembolic pulmonary hypertension: the critical role of thrombotic material in pultaceous core formation. Heart 2002;88:177–82.

28. Blauwet LA, Edwards WD, Tazelaar HD, McGregor CG. Surgical pathology of pulmonary thromboendarterectomy: a study of 54 cases from 1990 to 2001. Hum Pathol 2003;34:1290–8.

29. Kim NH, Fesler P, Channick RN, Knowlton KU, Ben-Yehuda O, Lee SH, Naeije R, Rubin LJ. Preoperative partitioning of pulmonary vascular resistance correlates with early outcome after thromboendarterectomy for chronic thromboembolic pulmonary hypertension. Circulation 2004;109:18–22.

30. Deng Z, Morse JH, Slager SL et al. Familial primary pulmonary hypertension (gene PPH1) is caused by mutations in the bone morphogenetic protein receptor-II gene. Am J Hum Genet 2000;67:737–44.

31. Thomson JR, Machado RD, Pauciulo MW et al. Sporadic primary pulmonary hypertension is associated with germline mutations of the gene encoding BMPR-II, a receptor member of the TGF-beta family. J Med Genet 2000;37:741–5.

32. Du L, Sullivan CC, Chu D, Cho AJ, Kido M, Wolf PL, Yuan JX, Deutsch R, Jamieson SW, Thistlethwaite PA. Signaling molecules in nonfamilial pulmonary hypertension. N Engl J Med 2003;348:500–9.

33. Bonderman D, Skoro-Sajer N, Jakowitsch J et al. Predictors of outcome in chronic thromboembolic pulmonary hypertension. Circulation 2007;115:2153–8.

34. ZuWallack RL, Liss JP, Lahiri B. Acquired continuous murmur associated with acute pulmonary thromboembolism. Chest 1976;70:557–9.

35. Hoeper MM, Mayer E, Simonneau G, Rubin LJ. Chronic thromboembolic pulmonary hypertension. Circulation 2006;113:2011–20.

36. Kunieda T, Nakanishi N, Satoh T, Kyotani S, Okano Y, Nagaya N. Prognoses of primary pulmonary hypertension and chronic major vessel thromboembolic pulmonary hypertension determined from cumulative survival curves. Intern Med 1999;38:543–6.

37. D'Alonzo GE, Barst RJ, Ayres SM, Bergofsky EH, Brundage BH, Detre KM, Fishman AP, Goldring RM, Groves BM, Kernis JT et al. Survival in patients with primary pulmonary hypertension. Results from a national prospective registry. Ann Intern Med 1991;115:343–9.

38. Bonderman D, Martischnig AM, Vonbank K et al. Right ventricular load at exercise is a cause of persistent exercise limitation in patients with normal resting pulmonary vascular resistance after pulmonary endarterectomy. Chest 2011.

39. Mayer E, Klepetko W. Techniques and outcomes of pulmonary endarterectomy for chronic thromboembolic pulmonary hypertension. Proc Am Thorac Soc 2006;3:589–93.

40. Skoro-Sajer N, Mittermayer F, Panzenboeck A et al. Asymmetric dimethylarginine is increased in chronic thromboembolic pulmonary hypertension. Am J Respir Crit Care Med 2007;176:1154–60.

41. Lankeit M, Dellas C, Panzenbock A et al. Heart-type fatty acid-binding protein for risk assessment of chronic thromboembolic pulmonary hypertension. Eur Respir J 2008;31:1024–9.

42. Fedullo PF, Auger WR, Kerr KM, Rubin LJ. Chronic thromboembolic pulmonary hypertension. N Engl J Med 2001;345:1465–72.

43. Fishman AJ, Moser KM, Fedullo PF. Perfusion lung scans vs. pulmonary angiography in evaluation of suspected primary pulmonary hypertension. Chest 1983;84:679–83.

44. Moser KM, Page GT, Ashburn WL, Fedullo PF. Perfusion lung scans provide a guide to which patients with apparent primary pulmonary hypertension merit angiography. West J Med 1988;148:167–70.

45. Lisbona R, Kreisman H, Novales-Diaz J, Derbekyan V. Perfusion lung scanning: differentiation of primary from thromboembolic pulmonary hypertension. AJR Am J Roentgenol 1985;144:27–30.

46. Powe JE, Palevsky HI, McCarthy KE, Alavi A. Pulmonary arterial hypertension: value of perfusion scintigraphy. Radiology 1987;164:727–30.

47. Pitton MB, Duber C, Mayer E, Thelen M. Hemodynamic effects of nonionic contrast bolus injection and oxygen inhalation during pulmonary angiography in patients with chronic major-vessel thromboembolic pulmonary hypertension. Circulation 1996;94:2485–91.

48. Auger WR, Fedullo PF, Moser KM, Buchbinder M, Peterson KL. Chronic major-vessel thromboembolic pulmonary artery obstruction: appearance at angiography. Radiology 1992;182:393–8.

49. Nicod P, Peterson K, Levine M, Dittrich H, Buchbinder M, Chappuis F, Moser K. Pulmonary angiography in severe chronic pulmonary hypertension. Ann Intern Med 1987;107:565–8.

50. Jamieson SW, Kapelanski DP, Sakakibara N et al. Pulmonary endarterectomy: experience and lessons learned in 1500 cases. Ann Thorac Surg 2003;76:1457–62; discussion 1462–54.

51. Klepetko W, Mayer E, Sandoval J et al. Interventional and surgical modalities of treatment for pulmonary arterial hypertension. J Am Coll Cardiol 2004;43:73S–80S.

52. Dartevelle P, Fadel E, Mussot S et al. Chronic thromboembolic pulmonary hypertension. Eur Respir J 2004;23:637–48.

53. Doyle RL, McCrory D, Channick RN, Simonneau G, Conte J. Surgical treatments/interventions for pulmonary arterial hypertension: ACCP evidence-based clinical practice guidelines. Chest 2004;126:63S–71S.

54. Kim NH. Assessment of operability in chronic thromboembolic pulmonary hypertension. Proc Am Thorac Soc 2006;3:584–8.

55. Riedel M, Stanek V, Widimsky J, Prerovsky I. Long-term follow-up of patients with pulmonary thromboembolism. Late prognosis and evolution of hemodynamic and respiratory data. Chest 1982;81:151–8.

56. Hartz RS, Byrne JG, Levitsky S, Park J, Rich S. Predictors of mortality in pulmonary thromboendarterectomy. Ann Thorac Surg 1996;62:1255–9; discussion 1259–60.

57. Archibald CJ, Auger WR, Fedullo PF et al. Long-term outcome after pulmonary thromboendarterectomy. Am J Respir Crit Care Med 1999;160:523–8.

58. Lewczuk J, Piszko P, Jagas J, Porada A, Wojciak S, Sobkowicz B, Wrabec K. Prognostic factors in medically treated patients with chronic pulmonary embolism. Chest 2001;119:818–23.

59. Ono F, Nagaya N, Okumura H, Shimizu Y, Kyotani S, Nakanishi N, Miyatake K. Effect of orally active prostacyclin analogue on survival in patients with chronic thromboembolic pulmonary hypertension without major vessel obstruction. Chest 2003;123:1583–8.

60. Vizza CD, Badagliacca R, Sciomer S et al. Mid-term efficacy of beraprost, an oral prostacyclin analog, in the treatment of distal CTEPH: a case control study. Cardiology 2006;106:168–73.

61. Nagaya N, Sasaki N, Ando M, Ogino H, Sakamaki F, Kyotani S, Nakanishi N. Prostacyclin therapy before pulmonary thromboendarterectomy in patients with chronic thromboembolic pulmonary hypertension. Chest 2003;123:338–43.

62. Bresser P, Fedullo PF, Auger WR, Channick RN, Robbins IM, Kerr KM, Jamieson SW, Rubin LJ. Continuous intravenous epoprostenol for chronic thromboembolic pulmonary hypertension. Eur Respir J 2004;23:595–600.

63. Scelsi L, Ghio S, Campana C, D'Armini AM, Serio A, Klersy C, Piovella F, Vigano M, Tavazzi L. Epoprostenol in chronic thromboembolic pulmonary hypertension with distal lesions. Ital Heart J 2004;5:618–23.

64. Cabrol S, Souza R, Jais X et al. Intravenous epoprostenol in inoperable chronic thromboembolic pulmonary hypertension. J Heart Lung Transplant 2007;26:357–62.

65. Skoro-Sajer N, Bonderman D, Wiesbauer F, Harja E, Jakowitsch J, Klepetko W, Kneussl MP, Lang IM. Treprostinil

for severe inoperable chronic thromboembolic pulmonary hypertension. J Thromb Haemost 2007;5:483–9.

66. Olschewski H, Simonneau G, Galie N *et al.* Inhaled iloprost for severe pulmonary hypertension. N Engl J Med 2002;347:322–9.

67. Kramm T, Eberle B, Krummenauer F, Guth S, Oelert H, Mayer E. Inhaled iloprost in patients with chronic thromboembolic pulmonary hypertension: effects before and after pulmonary thromboendarterectomy. Ann Thorac Surg 2003;76:711–8.

68. Kramm T, Eberle B, Guth S, Mayer E. Inhaled iloprost to control residual pulmonary hypertension following pulmonary endarterectomy. Eur J Cardiothorac Surg 2005;28:882–8.

69. Bonderman D, Nowotny R, Skoro-Sajer N, Jakowitsch J, Adlbrecht C, Klepetko W, Lang IM. Bosentan therapy for inoperable chronic thromboembolic pulmonary hypertension. Chest 2005;128:2599–603.

70. Hoeper MM, Kramm T, Wilkens H, Schulze C, Schafers HJ, Welte T, Mayer E. Bosentan therapy for inoperable chronic thromboembolic pulmonary hypertension. Chest 2005;128:2363–7.

71. Hughes R, George P, Parameshwar J, Cafferty F, Dunning J, Morrell NW, Pepke-Zaba J. Bosentan in inoperable chronic thromboembolic pulmonary hypertension. Thorax 2005;60:707.

72. Hughes RJ, Jais X, Bonderman D *et al.* The efficacy of bosentan in inoperable chronic thromboembolic pulmonary

hypertension: a 1-year follow-up study. Eur Respir J 2006;28:138–43.

73. Seyfarth HJ, Hammerschmidt S, Pankau H, Winkler J, Wirtz H. Long-term bosentan in chronic thromboembolic pulmonary hypertension. Respiration 2007;74:287–92.

74. Ulrich S, Speich R, Domenighetti G *et al.* Bosentan therapy for chronic thromboembolic pulmonary hypertension. A national open label study assessing the effect of Bosentan on haemodynamics, exercise capacity, quality of life, safety and tolerability in patients with chronic thromboembolic pulmonary hypertension (BOCTEPH-Study). Swiss Med Wkly 2007;137:573–80.

75. Ghofrani HA, Schermuly RT, Rose F *et al.* Sildenafil for long-term treatment of nonoperable chronic thromboembolic pulmonary hypertension. Am J Respir Crit Care Med 2003;167:1139–41.

76. Sheth A, Park JE, Ong YE, Ho TB, Madden BP. Early haemodynamic benefit of sildenafil in patients with coexisting chronic thromboembolic pulmonary hypertension and left ventricular dysfunction. Vascul Pharmacol 2005;42:41–5.

77. Suntharalingam J, Treacy CM, Doughty NJ *et al.* Long-term use of sildenafil in inoperable chronic thromboembolic pulmonary hypertension. Chest 2008; 134:229–36.

78. Tanabe N, Kimura A, Amano S *et al.* Association of clinical features with HLA in chronic pulmonary thromboembolism. Eur Respir J 2005;25:131–8.

Pulmonary vascular tumors

KIM M KERR

INTRODUCTION

Primary tumors of the pulmonary artery are extremely rare (1). The majority of these tumors are malignant, sarcomatous neoplasms (2), yet primary sarcomas of the lung represent only one in every 500 primary lung cancers. Primary soft tissue sarcomas of the lung are divided into three categories based on site of origin: parenchymal sarcomas, small-vessel sarcomas, and large-vessel sarcomas (3). This chapter will focus on large-vessel sarcomas.

Large-vessel sarcomas are primarily intravascular tumors that arise from within the pulmonary artery. They arise proximally and spread within the lumen with multiple sites of attachment making the origin difficult to define (4). Symptoms result from obstruction of the pulmonary vascular bed and right ventricular failure. Patients are most likely to be incorrectly diagnosed with pulmonary embolism with most patients not receiving the correct diagnosis until the time of autopsy (4,5). Distant metastases are uncommon (5). It has been postulated that the low incidence of distant metastases may be due to the vital location of the primary tumor preventing most patients from surviving long enough to develop disseminated disease (6). Surgery has the potential to palliate symptoms (2), improve survival (5) and potentially cure this disease (7–9). Hence, it is important that physicians be aware of this disease entity so that the correct diagnosis can be made and appropriate therapy instituted.

EPIDEMIOLOGY

Mandelstamm first described pulmonary artery sarcoma in 1923 (10). Because of its rarity, what is known about pulmonary artery sarcoma is based upon individual case reports and small series with approximately 200 cases reported to date in the literature. A slight female predominance has been identified (1:1.3) (4). The vast majority of cases occur in adults, with an average age of 50 years (5); however, several cases have been diagnosed in adolescents (11,12) as well as in an infant (13). The etiology remains obscure and no risk factors for the development of these tumors have been identified. On average, patients are symptomatic for 8 months before an aggressive search for an etiology is instituted (5).

CLINICAL PRESENTATION

Patients present with symptoms related to pulmonary artery obstruction, pulmonary hypertension and right ventricular dysfunction as well as nonspecific symptoms secondary to the presence of malignancy. Based upon 110 cases reported in the literature, Nomura et al found that the most common symptom is dyspnea (67 percent), followed by chest/back pain (54 percent), cough (43 percent), and hemoptysis (22 percent). Systemic symptoms include malaise (13 percent), weight loss (12 percent), and fever (10 percent) (4).

Findings on physical exam in patients with pulmonary artery sarcoma include jugular venous distension, a bruit over the pulmonary artery, a systolic flow murmur, hepatomegaly, edema, cyanosis, and clubbing (4).

Given this constellation of symptoms, it is not surprising that the most common clinical diagnosis given these patients is pulmonary thromboembolism (4,5). However, an alternative diagnosis should be sought in patients who present with symptoms of systemic disease such as fever or weight loss. Clubbing is also not a feature of thromboembolic disease and should stimulate a search for another etiology (14). Other preoperative or *ante mortem* diagnoses included mediastinal tumor, lung cancer and cardiac tumor of the right ventricle (4).

EVALUATION

Right ventricular hypertrophy is the most common electrocardiographic abnormality, occurring in up to one half of patients. The chest radiograph may be normal or demonstrate a hilar mass, prominent pulmonary artery(ies), hilar infiltrate, decreased pulmonary vascular markings, nodules, or cavities (4,5,15). The perfusion scan demonstrates areas of decreased or absent perfusion (4,5) indistinguishable from thromboembolic disease. Perfusion defects that do not improve or that increase in size with anticoagulation suggest a diagnosis other than acute pulmonary embolism. In addition, unilateral perfusion abnormalities on scintigraphy are rare in chronic thromboembolic disease and should prompt a search for other causes of large-vessel pulmonary artery obstruction including tumor (bronchogenic carcinoma, pulmonary artery sarcoma) as well as fibrosing mediastinitis, pulmonary arteritis and congenital anomoly (16).

Two-dimensional echocardiography may demonstrate evidence of pulmonary hypertension and may also allow for direct visualization of the tumor. A pedunculated mass arising from the RV outflow tract, pulmonary valve or pulmonary trunk would suggest the diagnosis of sarcoma (8).

While bronchoscopy is frequently performed to evaluate patients who present with hemoptysis or lung mass, it is likely to be non-diagnostic in pulmonary artery sarcoma cases. However, there are rare case reports of tumor eroding through the airway allowing the diagnosis of neoplasm to be made (17).

Pulmonary angiography typically demonstrates a proximal mass partially or totally obstructing the pulmonary artery (Figure 22.4.1). Sarcomas are often lobulated and polypoid (18), but smooth gradual tapering of the pulmonary artery, indistinguishable from chronic thromboembolic disease, has also been described (19). The mass may be fixed or pedunculated and mobile with a "to-and-fro" movement with each cardiac cycle. Demonstration of a pressure gradient across the mass is especially helpful since such gradients are not typically seen in chronic thromboembolic disease (20). As with scintography, vascular obstruction that increases in size on serial angiography is also very suggestive of a neoplastic process. Pulmonary angioscopy may allow for direct visualization of the tumor (2).

CT scanning and magnetic resonance imaging are very useful modalities for evaluating pulmonary artery sarcomas (Figure 22.4.2). Both allow exclusion of some competing diagnoses such as extravascular obstruction from bronchogenic carcinoma or mediastinal fibrosis. CT and

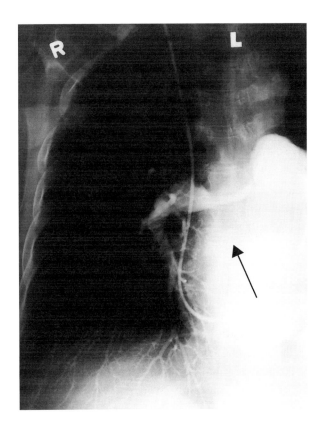

Figure 22.4.1 Angiographic image of a sarcoma causing a large filling defect in the right main pulmonary artery (arrow).

MRI are useful in assessing tumor size, degree of vascular obstruction, and the presence of extravascular invasion as well as to look for evidence of metastases. Yi *et al.* compared the CT findings of seven patients with pulmonary artery sarcoma to 40 patients with pulmonary emboli. They found a low attenuation filling defect occupying the entire luminal diameter of the main or proximal pulmonary artery to be present in all with pulmonary artery sarcoma and none of the patients with pulmonary embolism (21). Other CT findings suggestive of pulmonary artery sarcoma include inhomogeneous attenuation (possibly due to hemorrhage or necrosis of tumor), contiguously soft tissue filled pulmonary arteries, vascular distension, and extravascular spread. These finding are more likely to occur in advanced disease (21,22). Heterogenous enhancement with gadolinium-diethylene-triamine-pentaacetic acid (Gd-DTPA) demonstrated by MRI is characteristic of a vascularized tumor and allows the elimination of thromboembolic disease as a diagnosis since thrombus does not enhance on T1 weighted images after the administration of gadolinium (8,22,23). Tumor emboli, vasculitis (23), and septic emboli (24) may also enhance with Gd-DTPA. MRI may be especially helpful in the diagnosis of recurrent or residual disease (24).

The role of positron emission tomography in the evaluation of patients with pulmonary sarcoma remains to be defined. FDG-PET tumor imaging has been reported

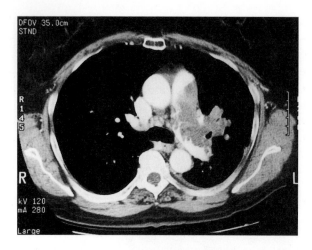

Figure 22.4.2 Angiosarcoma in a 74-year-old female. Transverse CT angiogram demonstrates a large lobulated mass in the left main pulmonary artery which extends into the left upper lobe and left descending pulmonary arteries.

to distinguish sarcoma from thromboembolism when the appropriate diagnosis could not be obtained from CT scanning alone (25). However, acute pulmonary emboli and large-vessel arteritis can also cause an increase in FDG uptake in the region of the pulmonary artery on PET scan (26).

Ultimately, tissue must be obtained for a definitive diagnosis. Biopsies may be obtained via intravascular forceps during angiography (23), transvenous catheter suction biopsy (27), CT-guided transthoracic needle aspiration (15), or surgical exploration. Often, patients undergo surgery for presumed thromboembolism which leads to the correct diagnosis of sarcoma. The majority of patients, however, are diagnosed at autopsy (4,5).

PATHOLOGY

At surgery or autopsy the pulmonary trunk is distended by a multinodular mucoid or gelatinous tumor which is often mixed with thrombus and may contain foci of more firm, fibrotic as well as bony hard material depending upon the histologic composition of the tumor. The tumor extends distally along the pulmonary arteries and may also extend proximally or arise from the right ventricle (28,29). Frequently, the sites of attachment to the pulmonary artery are multiple and the apparent origin is difficult to define (4). The pulmonary trunk is most commonly involved (80 percent of cases) with equal likelihood of involvement of the left (58 percent) and the right pulmonary arteries (57 percent). Both pulmonary arteries are involved in 37 percent of cases, the pulmonary valve is affected in 28 percent, and the right ventricle in 8 percent (4). Some tumors remain localized to the artery, but direct extension

into the lung parenchyma or mediastinum is frequently present (29). Intrapulmonary metastases are common, occurring in 40 percent of cases and are presumably embolic (4). Nodules of metastatic tumor are usually small, but may be as large as 3 cm and may be either confined to the pulmonary vasculature or be associated with bronchial or parenchymal invasion. Pulmonary infarction may also be seen as a consequence of extensive tumor growth, tumor emboli, or thromboemboli occluding pulmonary vessels (29). While distant metastases are less common (19 percent), they have been reported to involve the pericardium, heart, pleura, adrenal gland, pancreas, stomach, jejunum, brain, bone, liver, retroperitoneum, diaphragm, skin and tongue (4,30).

The majority of pulmonary artery sarcomas are thought to originate from pluripotent intimal cells, hence generating the term *intimal sarcoma*. These sarcomas are typically poorly differentiated malignant mesenchymal tumors, but some carry distinct histologic features permitting subclassification such as osteogenic sarcoma, chondrosarcoma, etc. Leiomyosarcomas are thought to be distinctly different from intimal sarcomas, arising from the media of the vessel and are referred to as *mural sarcomas*. The distinction between intimal and mural sarcomas is at the microscopic level as both tumors grossly appear the same (30,31). McGlennan *et al.* summarized the pathology of 100 cases of pulmonary artery sarcoma from the literature. They found the histopathology to be heterogenous with the sarcomatous elements most commonly described as undifferentiated (34 percent), consisting of cells with variations in cytologic attributes. Other pathologic types included myogenous (26 percent), fibrocytic (17 percent), mesenchymoma (6 percent), chondrosarcoma (4 percent), vascular (4 percent), osteogenic sarcoma (3 percent) and two were classified as malignant fibrous histiocytoma (2 percent) (12). With the current classifications of soft tissue sarcomas, more cases are now being diagnosed as malignant fibrous histiocytoma (32). Tavora *et al.* reported on 43 cases of sarcomas arising in the pulmonary artery that were seen in consultation at the Armed Forces Institute of Pathology. Twenty-eight of the 43 cases were classified as pleomorphic-fascicular sarcomas, the majority of which were malignant fibrous histiocytoma-like (9).

TREATMENT/MANAGEMENT

Surgical resection is the treatment of choice for pulmonary artery sarcoma offering palliation (2,8) and increased length of survival (5). Aggressive surgical resection is potentially curative in patients with localized lesions (33). Surgical therapy depends upon tumor location, distal extension, and the presence of pulmonary metastases. Techniques include tumor and pulmonary artery resection and reconstruction, endarterectomy techniques, and pneumonectomy (2,8).

Kruger reviewed 93 cases of primary sarcoma of the pulmonary artery reported in the literature up to 1990. The tumor was resected in 27 patients; 13 underwent tumor excision from the vascular bed and 14 underwent pneumonectomy. Median survival for the 93 patients was 1.5 months from diagnosis with most patients dying from the consequences of decompensated right heart failure due to right ventricular outflow obstruction by the tumor. However, despite a 22 percent early mortality after resection, median survival was prolonged to 10 months in those patients who underwent surgery. It is notable that 58 percent of patients had evidence of lung metastases at the time of diagnosis, yet no survival benefit was demonstrated for those who underwent pneumonectomy and presumed simultaneous resection of metastases versus simple tumor excision. In addition, survival was similar for both those with and without identified metastases. It appears that prognosis following successful surgery depends upon recurrence of tumor in the pulmonary artery rather than progression of metastatic disease (5). Devendra reported 16 cases of pulmonary artery sarcoma undergoing surgery at a single institution. There was no surgical mortality and the average length of hospital stay was 14 days. Hemodynamic improvement was noted following surgery with an increase in cardiac output and a decrease in mean pulmonary artery pressure. The postoperative average length of survival was 17 months and one patient remained alive 54 months following surgery (7). Others have also reported an improvement in functional status with surgery (2,8). Huo reported a series of 12 patients who underwent surgery for pulmonary artery sarcoma and provided follow-up on eight of those patients. Mean survival was 13.2 months, but an interesting observation was that prolonged survival was associated with the diagnosis of leiomyosarcoma with one patient lost to follow-up (alive) at 40 months and another alive with disease at 68 months (30). Tavora provided follow-up on 32 patients included in their series of 43 pulmonary artery sarcomas. Only two cases were alive without disease at 10 years, both were low-grade myofibroblastic sarcomas. Only four other patients survived longer than 3 years, all died with disease. Diagnosis at age 60 years and above was associated with a poorer prognosis (9).

The rarity of pulmonary artery sarcomas and the histologic heterogeneity of the tumors make it difficult to comment on the role of adjuvant treatment modalities. Chemotherapeutic agents such as ifosfomide, doxorubicin, cyclophosphamide, vincristine and postoperative radiotherapy have been employed alone and in combination in the treatment of pulmonary artery sarcomas (2,5,6,8,13,15,34). Unfortunately, there are no clinical trials to define the role of adjuvant therapy in this disease. Heart–lung transplant has been utilized in the treatment of pulmonary artery sarcoma, but the appearance of metastatic disease following transplant limits the utility of this aggressive approach, especially given the limited availability of donor organs (34–36).

PULMONARY TUMOR EMBOLISM

Tumor emboli to the lungs may also present with progressive dyspnea, chest pain and evidence of pulmonary hypertension with right ventricular failure. Most patients will have an established diagnosis of malignancy, usually metastatic. The malignancies most commonly associated with tumor embolism include breast, lung, prostate, stomach and liver (37) and tend to involve smaller pulmonary arteries (38,39). The chest radiograph is usually unremarkable. Radionuclide perfusion scanning commonly demonstrates numerous small, peripheral, subsegmental perfusion defects in the presence of normal ventilation, but findings can range from normal (40) to large perfusion defects (41). Pulmonary angiography is typically normal or demonstrates small vessel abnormalities and is usually performed to establish or exclude the competing diagnosis of venous thromboembolic disease. Right heart catheterization in symptomatic patients will confirm the presence of pulmonary hypertension (37). Pulmonary wedge aspiration cytology can be examined for the presence of tumor cells (42,43), but lung biopsy is usually required to make the diagnosis of tumor embolism. It is not yet known if early diagnosis of tumor embolism changes prognosis, but it may avoid unnecessary anticoagulation (37).

Rarely, tumor emboli may present with more proximal pulmonary artery obstruction, typically arising from tumors that invade the inferior vena cava or larger veins. Distinguishing tumor emboli from venous thromboembolic disease can be difficult, but progression of disease despite adequate anticoagulation would suggest the former diagnosis. Survival following surgical resection has been reported in atrial myxoma (44), renal cell carcinoma (45–47), Wilms' tumor (48) and choriocarcinoma (49), testicular cancer (50), and intravenous leiomyoma (51).

KEY POINTS

- Primary pulmonary artery sarcomas are extremely rare.
- The diagnosis is often difficult and delayed due to symptoms which mimic more common causes of pulmonary vascular obstruction such as pulmonary embolism.
- The diagnosis should be entertained in patients who also present with systemic symptoms (weight loss, fever) or in patients who fail to improve with anticoagulation.
- CT and MRI scanning may be helpful in distinguishing sarcoma from competing diagnoses.
- The prognosis is grim without surgical intervention with most patients dying quickly from right ventricular failure.

- Early surgical resection palliates symptoms, lengthens survival, and provides the only potential for cure.
- The role of adjuvant therapy (chemotherapy or radiotherapy) has yet to be defined.

REFERENCES

• = Key primary paper

1. Colby TV. Malignancies in the lung and pleura mimicking benign processes. Sem Diagnost Pathol 1995;12:30–44.
2. Anderson MB, Kriett JM, Kapelanski DP, Tarazi R, Jamieson SW. Primary pulmonary artery sarcoma: a report of six cases. Ann Thorac Surg 1995;59:1487–90.
3. Miller DL, Allen MS. Rare pulmonary neoplasms. Mayo Clin Proc 1993;68:492–8.
4. Nonomura A, Kurumaya H, Kono N et al. Primary pulmonary artery sarcoma. Report of two autopsy cases studied by immunohistochemistry and electron microscopy, and review of 110 cases reported in the literature. Acta Pathol Jpn 1988;38:883–96.
•5. Kruger I, Borowski A, Horst M, de Vivie ER, Theissen P, Gross-Fengel W. Symptoms, diagnosis, and therapy of primary sarcomas of the pulmonary artery. Thorac Cardiovasc Surg 1990;38:91–5.
6. Fer MF, Greco A, Haile KL, Rosenblatt PA, Johnson RL, Glick AD, Oldham RK. Unusual survival after pulmonary sarcoma. South Med J 1981;74:624–6.
7. Devendra G, Mo M, Kerr KM, Fedullo PF, Yi J, Kapelanski DP, Jamieson S, Auger WR. Pulmonary artery sarcomas: the UCSD experience. Am J Respir Crit Care Med 2002; 165:A24.
8. Mayer E, Kriegsmann J, Gaumann A et al. Surgical treatment of pulmonary artery sarcoma. J Thorac Cardiovasc Surg 2001;121:77–82.
9. Tavora F, Miettinen M, Fanburg-Smith J, Franks TJ, Burke A. Pulmonary artery sarcoma: a histologic and follow-up study with emphasis on a subset of low-grade myofibroblastic sarcomas with a good long-term follow-up. Am J Surg Pathol 2008; 32(12):1751-61.
•10. Mandelstamm M. ̇yber primäre neubildungen des herzens. Virchows Arch (Pathol Anat) 1923;245:43–54.
11. Farooki ZQ, Chang CH, Jackson WL, Clapp SK, Hakimi M, Arcieniegas E, Pinsky WW. Primary pulmonary artery sarcoma in two children. Pediatr Cardiol 1988;9:243–51.
12. McGlennan RC, Manivel JC, Stanley SJ, Slater DL, Wick MR, Dehner LP. Pulmonary artery trunk sarcoma: a clinicopathologic, ultrastructural, and immunohistochemical study of four cases. Mod Pathol 1989;2:486–94.
13. Chappell T, Creech CB, Parra D, Strauss A, Scholl F, Whitney G. Presentation of pulmonary artery intimal sarcoma in an infant with a history of neonatal valvular pulmonic stenosis. Ann Thorac Surg 2008;85:1092–4.
14. Loredo JS, Fedullo PF, Piovella F, Moser KM. Digital clubbing associated with pulmonary artery sarcoma. Chest 1996;109:1651–3.
15. Parish JM, Rosenow EC, Swensen SJ, Crotty TB. Pulmonary artery sarcoma; clinical features. Chest 1996;110:1480–8.
16. Bergin CJ, Hauschildt JP, Brown MA, Channick RN, Fedullo PF. Identifying the cause of unilateral hypoperfusion in patients suspected to have chronic thromboembolism: diagnostic accuracy of helical CT and conventional angiography. Radiology 1999;213:743–9.
17. Nguyen GK. Exfoliative cytology of angiosarcoma of the pulmonary artery. Acta Cytologica 1985;29:624–7.
18. Rafal RB, Nichols JN, Markisz J. Pulmonary artery sarcoma: diagnosis and postoperative follow-up with gadolinium-diethylenetriamine pentaacetic acid-enhanced magnetic resonance imaging. Mayo Clin Proc 1995;70:173–6.
19. Schermoly M, Overman J, Pingleton SK. Pulmonary artery sarcoma – unusual pulmonary angiographic finding – a case report. Angiology 1987;38:617–21.
20. Hynes JK, Smith HC, Holmes DR, Edwards WD, Evans TC, Orszulak TA. Preoperative angiographic diagnosis of primary sarcoma of the pulmonary artery. Circulation 1982;66:672–4.
21. Yi Ca, Lee KS, Choe YH, Han D, Kwon OJ, Kim S. Computed tomography in pulmonary artery sarcoma; distinguishing features from pulmonary embolic disease. J Comput Assist Tomogr 2004;28:34–9.
22. Kauczor HU, Schwickert HC, Mayer E, Kersjes W, Moll R, Schwede F. Pulmonary artery sarcoma mimicking chronic thromboembolic disease: computed tomography and magnetic resonance imaging findings. Cardiovasc Intervent Radiol 1994;17:185–9.
23. Scully RE, Mark EJ, Ebeling SH, Ellenders SM, Peters, CC. Case Records of the Massachusetts General Hospital. N Engl J Med 2000;343:493–500.
24. Kacl GM, Bruder E, Pfammatter T, Follath F, Salomon F, Debatin JF. Primary angiosarcoma of the pulmonary arteries: dynamic contrast-enhanced MRI. J Comput Assist Tomogr 1998;22:687–91.
25. Thurer RL, Thorsen A, Parker JA, Karp DD. FDG Imaging of a pulmonary artery sarcoma. Ann Thorac Surg 2000; 70:1414–5.
26. Wittram C, Scott JA. 18F-FDG PET of pulmonary embolism. AJR 2007;189:171–5.
27. Yamada N, Kamei S, Yasuda F, Isaka N, Yada I, Nakano T. Primary leiomyosarcoma of the pulmonary artery confirmed by catheter suction biopsy. Chest 1998;113:555–6.
28. Yi ES. Tumors of the pulmonary vasculature. Cardiol Clin 2004;22:431–40.
29. Dail DH. Uncommon tumors. In: Dail DH, Hammar SP, eds. Pulmonary Pathology. New York, Spring-Verlag, 1994:1279–461.
30. Huo L, Moran CA, Fuller GN, Gladish G, Suster S. Pulmonary artery sarcoma; a clinicopathologic and immunohistochemical study of 12 cases. Am J Clin Pathol 2006;125:419–24.

31. Burke AP, Virmani R. Sarcomas of the great vessels; a clinicopathologic study. Cancer 1993;71:1761–73.

32. Virmani R, Burke A, Farb A. Tumors of great vessels. In: Virmani R, Burke A, Farb A, eds. Atlas of Cardiovascular Pathology. Philadelphia: W.B. Saunders, 1996:154–8.

33. Mattoo A, Fedullo PF, Kapelanski D, Illowite JS. Pulmonary artery sarcoma; a case report of surgical cure and 5-year follow-up. Chest 2002;122:745–7.

34. Talbot SM, Taub RN, Keohan ML, Edwards N, Galantowicz ML, Schulman LL. Combined heart and lung transplantation for unresectable primary cardiac sarcoma. J Thorac Cardiovasc Surg 2002;124:1145–8.

35. Chhaya NC, Goodwin AT, Jenkins DP et al. Surgical treatment of pulmonary artery sarcoma. J Thorac Cardiovasc Surg 2006;131:1410–1.

36. Britton PD. Primary pulmonary artery sarcoma – a report of two cases with a special emphasis on the diagnostic problems. Clin Radiol 1990;41:92–4.

37. Bassiri AG, Haghighi B, Doyle RL, Berry GJ, Rizk NW. Pulmonary tumor embolism. Am J Respir Crit Care Med 1997;155:2089–95.

38. Soares FA, Pinto APFE, Landell GA, Mello de Oliveira JA. Pulmonary tumor embolism to arterial vessels and carcinomatous lymphangitis. Arch Pathol Lab Med 1993;117:827–31.

•39. Goldhaber SZ, Dricker E, Buring JE, Eberlein K, Godleski JJ, Mayer RJ, Hennekens CH. Clinical suspicion of autopsy-proven thrombotic and tumor pulmonary embolism in cancer patients. Am Heart J 1987;114:1432–5.

40. Domanski MJ, Cunnion RE, Fernicola DJ, Roberts WC. Fatal cor pulmonale caused by extensive tumor emboli in the small pulmonary arteries without emboli in the major pulmonary arteries or metastasis in the pulmonary parenchyma. Am J Cardiol 1993;72:233–4.

41. Moores LK, Burrell LM, Morse RW, Belgrave CH, Balingit AG. Diffuse tumor microembolism. A rare cause of a high-probability perfusion scan. Chest 1997; 111:1122–3.

42. Babar SI, Sobonya RE, Snyder LS. Pulmonary microvascular cytology for the diagnosis of pulmonary tumor embolism. WJM 1998;168:47–50.

43. Bhuvaneswaran JS, Venkitachalam CG, Sandhyamani S. Pulmonary wedge aspiration cytology in the diagnosis of recurrent tumor embolism causing pulmonary arterial hypertension. Int J Cardiol 1993;39:209–12.

44. Keenan DJM, Morton P, O'Kane HO. Right atrial myxoma and pulmonary embolism: rational basis for investigation and treatment. Br Heart J 1982;48:510–21.

45. Daughtry JD, Stewart BH, Golding LAR, Groves LK. Pulmonary embolus presenting as the initial manifestation of renal cell carcinoma. Ann Thorac Surg 1977;24:178–81.

46. Isringhaus H, Naber M, Kopper B. Successful treatment of tumor embolism of an hypernephroma with complete occlusion of the left pulmonary artery. Thorac Cardiovasc Surg 1987;35:65–6.

47. Kubota H, Furuse A, Kotsuka Y, Yagyu K, Kawauchi M, Saito H. Successful management of massive pulmonary tumor embolism from renal cell carcinoma. Ann Thorac Surg 1996;61:708–10.

48. Bulas DI, Thompson R, Reaman G. Pulmonary emboli as a primary manifestation of Wilms' tumor. AJR 1991; 156:155–6.

49. Watanabe S, Shimokawa S, Sakasegawa K, Masuda H, Sakata R, Higashi M. Choriocarcinoma in the pulmonary artery treated with emergency pulmonary embolectomy. Chest 2002;121:654–6.

50. Haab F, Cour F, Boutan Laroze A, Squara P, Lucas G. Testicular neoplasm presenting as a major pulmonary embolism. Eur Urol 1996;29:494–6.

51. Marcus SG, Krauss T, Freedberg RS, Culliford AT, Weinreich DJ, Kronzon I. Pulmonary embolectomy for intravenous uterine leiomyomatosis. Am Heart J 1994;127:1642–5.

Pulmonary vasculitis

KARINA KEOGH AND SEAN P GAINE

INTRODUCTION

Vasculitis is inflammation involving the walls of blood vessels. It may be localized to a single organ or can affect multiple different organs (1–3). The primary vasculitic disorders may be categorized based on size of the vessel involved, into small-, medium- and large-vessel vasculitides, as proposed at the Chapel Hill Consensus Conference in 1994 (4) (Table 22.5.1 and Figure 22.5.1). The large-vessel diseases affect the aorta and its major branches. The medium-vessel diseases predominantly, if not exclusively, affect the main visceral arteries including renal, hepatic, mesenteric and coronary arteries and their major branches. The small-vessel vasculitides are distinguished by their involvement of arterioles, venules, and capillaries, however they may also affect larger vessels (1). Other forms of vasculitis not covered by this classification include vasculitis due to infection (e.g. *R. rickettsi*), medications (e.g. hydralazine), serum sickness and paraneoplastic syndromes (1). Pulmonary involvement in vasculitis is most commonly associated with the small-vessel vasculitides: Wegener's granulomatosis, microscopic polyangiitis, and Churg–Strauss syndrome (5,6) (Table 22.5.2). Pulmonary involvement may rarely occur in the large-vessel vasculitides and thoracic aneurysms have been found in up to 17 percent of patients with temporal arteritis (7,8). Pulmonary vasculitis may also be prominent in connective tissue diseases, such as systemic lupus erythematosus and rheumatoid arthritis (6,9,10). One of the causes of pulmonary hypertension associated with HIV infection is pulmonary vasculitis (11). Pulmonary hypertension may also be seen in conjunction with Takayasu's vasculitis (12), and there are also case

Table 22.5.1 Classification of the primary systemic vasculitides based on the size of the blood vessel involvement (1)

Large vessel
Takayasu's arteritis
Giant cell (temporal) arteritis

Medium-sized vessel
Kawasaki syndrome
Polyarteritis nodosa (PAN)

Small vessel
Churg–Strauss syndrome (CSS)
Cutaneous leukocytoclastic vasculitis
Essential cryoglobulinemic vasculitis
Henoch–Schönlein purpura (HSP)
Microscopic polyangiitis (MPA)
Wegener's granulomatosis (WG)

reports of pulmonary arterial hypertension in the setting of ANCA-associated vasculitis (13).

EPIDEMIOLOGY

Primary vasculitides are rare, and therefore epidemiologic data are limited. They are typically first diagnosed in middle life, although all ages may be affected. The average annual incidence of primary vasculitides has been estimated at 42–115 cases per million (14–16). The incidence of individual vasculitic disorders may also vary with ethnicity. For example, Takayasu's arteritis is more common in Asians, whereas giant cell arteritis has a higher prevalence among

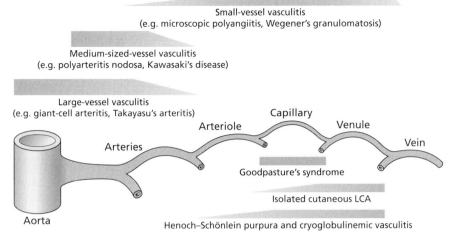

Figure 22.5.1 Preferred sites of vascular involvement by selected vasculitides. The widths of the trapezoids indicate the frequencies of involvement of various portions of the vasculature. LCA denotes leukocytoclastic angiitis. (From Jennette JC, Falk RJ. Small-vessel vasculitis. N Engl J Med 1997;**337**:1512–23, Figure 1, with permission.)

Table 22.5.2   Vasculitis involving the lung

Large vessel

Takayasu's arteritis

Giant cell (temporal) arteritis

Small vessel

ANCA-related

    Wegener's granulomatosis (WG)

    Microscopic polyangiitis (MPA)

    Churg–Strauss syndrome (CSS)

    Isolated pauci-immune

Collagen vascular disorders

    Systemic lupus erythematosus

    Rheumatoid arthritis

    Polymyositis

    Scleroderma

    Mixed connective tissue disease

Pulmonary allograft rejection

Goodpasture's disease

Henoch–Schönlein purpura (HSP)

IgA nephropathy

Idiopathic pauci-immune glomerulonephritis

Behçet's disease

Antiphospholipid syndrome

Essential cryoglobulinemia

Drug-related hypersensitivity vasculitis

Infection-related vasculitis

Paraneoplastic vasculitis

Sarcoid vasculitis

Myasthenia gravis

Ulcerative colitis

Autologous bone marrow transplantation

northern Europeans (17,18). Over the last decade a trend towards an increased incidence of vasculitis has been reported (19), though whether this is due to more accurate diagnosis rather than a true increase in the incidence rate is unclear. Many of the vasculitides were once uniformly fatal, but with the advent of corticosteroid therapy, and the development of other immunosuppressive agents, significant improvements have been made (20–27). However, particularly in the case of Wegener's and microscopic polyangiitis many patients experience one or more relapse, and there is still significant morbidity from both the disease itself and from the immunosuppressant drugs used to treat it (28).

PATHOLOGY

The hallmark of vasculitis is inflammation and necrosis involving the blood vessel wall. This can lead to two typical anatomical patterns; either there is sufficient inflammation to cause luminal narrowing and occlusion or alternatively, the extent of inflammation may cause sufficient weakening of the wall to cause aneurysm formation or vessel rupture. Vasculitic lesions are often both focal and segmental, meaning that the pathology will not be seen in all vessels of a similar size and even in those vessels that are affected, the lesions are generally not present in a uniform manner throughout. Parts of the vessel may be spared entirely. Inflammation may or may not extend through all vessel layers. Moreover, histologically there are only a limited number of patterns seen despite the many different etiologies and diffuse manifestations. Therefore pathologic findings are not generally diagnostic for a specific syndrome, though they may be suggestive such as IgA and C3 deposition in Henoch–Schönlein purpura (29).

In the lung, small-vessel vasculitis affects the arterioles, venules and capillaries within the interstitial compartment. The interstitial inflammation, as denoted by a neutrophilic infiltrate, edema and fibrin deposition, with fibrinoid necrosis of the capillary walls is termed necrotizing pulmonary capillaritis. Damage to capillaries in the interstitium, may cause leakage of blood into the alveolar spaces, and diffuse alveolar hemorrhage. Arteriolar and capillary thrombosis can also be seen. Chronically there may be evidence of pulmonary fibrosis and/or changes consistent with emphysema (6,30).

ETIOLOGY

A variety of pathophysiological processes have been implicated in the development of vasculitis, including immune-complex deposition, clonal lymphocyte expansion, cytokine production, autoantibody formation against neutrophilic granules and antigens presented by endothelial cells to circulating lymphocytes, thereby generating a localized immune response (29,31–34). Within individual syndromes, it is felt that various different processes may lead to a final common pathway and therefore, similar histological pictures. The small-vessel vasculitides that affect the lung are generally associated with antineutrophil cytoplasmic antibodies (ANCA) (33,35–53).

Antineutrophil cytoplasmic antibodies (ANCA)

See Figures 22.5.2, 22.5.3 and refs 38–53.

CLINICAL PRESENTATION

Common pulmonary manifestations of vasculitis include dyspnea and cough with infiltrates (both localized and diffuse), or inflammatory nodules (often cavitary) demonstrated radiologically. Hemoptysis may be seen, secondary to alveolar hemorrhage and may be fatal (6,54). Significant alveolar hemorrhage may occur in the absence of overt hemoptysis. In these patients a diagnosis of diffuse alveolar hemorrhage may be made on the basis of bilateral alveolar infiltrates, a falling hematocrit, and a bronchoalveolar lavage showing aliquots that are sequentially more bloody and/or have hemosiderin-laden macrophages (54). Pulmonary hypertension is rarely a feature in patients with pulmonary vasculitis, but may be a feature in patients with more severe disease, or those with a history of thromboembolism. ANCA-associated vasculitis is associated with a high incidence of venous thromboembolic disease (55).

Granulomatous inflammation of the upper airways is frequently seen. Upper airway symptoms can include sinus pain, nasal discharge and epistaxis. Nasal erosions and crusting are frequently seen in patients with Wegener's or lymphomatoid granulomatosis. Destruction of the nasal cartilage may lead to septal perforation or saddle nose deformity. Oral ulcerations are characteristic of Behçet's disease. In patients with tracheobronchial involvement, necrotizing granulomatous inflammation may cause ulcerative lesions, or inflammatory pseudotumors – "cobblestoning." Ultimately this may lead to bronchial stenosis and or bronchiomalacia. This inflammation has a predilection for the subglottic area. Tracheal stenosis preferentially affects younger patients.

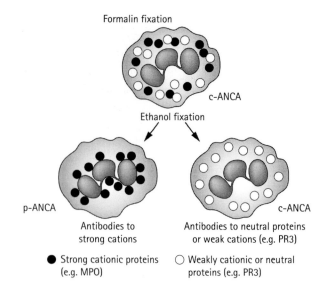

Figure 22.5.2 Antinuclear cytoplasmic antibodies (ANCA). The use of cross-linking fixatives (e.g. formalin) during the preparation of the neutrophil substrate results in ANCA-relevant antigens remaining in the cytoplasm. The pANCA fluorescent pattern represents an artifact of ethanol fixation. Ethanol fixation leads to alterations in granule membranes, allowing positively charged constituents to migrate to the negatively charged nuclear membrane. Because this does not occur with formalin fixation, use of both types of fixation allows the distinction of a true pANCA from an antinuclear antibody (ANA). With formalin-fixed neutrophils, antibodies that would cause pANCA patterns (on ethanol-fixed cells) will display diffuse granular cytoplasmic staining, whereas nuclear staining would indicate the presence of an ANA. MPO, myeloperoxidase; PR3, proteinase 3. (From Hoffman GS, Specks U. Antineutrophil cytoplasmic antibodies. Arthritis Rheum 1998;41(9):1521–37. Reprinted with permission from Wiley-Liss Inc., a subsidiary of John Wiley & Sons, Inc.)

Pulmonary vasculitis generally occurs in the setting of systemic manifestations. These may include nonspecific symptoms of fever, malaise, arthralgias or specific organ involvement (1).

- **The skin** typically may reveal purpura, bullae or ulceration, livido reticularis and Raynaud's phenomenon (56,57).
- **Renal** involvement is frequently found in the systemic vasculitic disorders. Wegener's granulomatosis commonly manifests with significant glomerulonephritis and may present with acute renal failure (26,58). Renal disease less commonly occurs with Churg–Strauss syndrome and is rarely associated with significant loss of renal function (36,59,60).
- **Central nervous system** involvement commonly occurs in giant cell arteritis and Takayasu's and to a lesser extent in Churg–Strauss syndrome and Wegner's granulomatosis (62).
- **Peripheral nerve** lesions, such as mononeuritis multiplex are common in polyarteritis nodosa and Churg–Strauss syndrome (62,63).

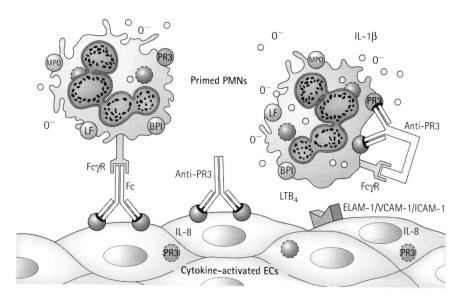

Figure 22.5.3 Hypothetical scheme for ANCA enhancement of vascular injury. In vitro activation of neutrophils and apoptosis is associated with translocation of numerous cytoplasmic proteins to the cell surface. Antibodies (e.g. anti-PR3) bound to appropriately displayed target antigens enhance neutrophil oxidative burst and degranulation. The magnitude of effect may be influenced by antibody specificity for different PR3 epitopes, IgG subclass, and the Fc(gamma) receptor [Fc(gamma)R] phenotype engaged. PR3 [and other proteins, e.g. elastase, lactoferrin (LF)] from degranulated neutrophils become bound to endothelial cells (ECs) and may cause enhanced expression of adhesion molecules and increased endothelial production of interleukin (IL)-8. ANCA have also been shown to enhance monocyte production of monocyte chemoattractant protein 1 and IL-8. Augmented chemotaxis and endothelial cell adhesion of leukocytes may follow, setting the stage for vascular injury. BPI, bactericidal/permeability-increasing protein; ELAM-1, endothelial leukocyte adhesion molecule 1; ICAM-1, intercellular adhesion molecule 1; LTB4, leukotriene B4; MPO, myeloperoxidase; PMN, polymorphonuclear cells; PR3, proteinase 3; VCAM-1, vascular cell adhesion molecule 1. (From Hoffman GS, Specks U. Antineutrophil cytoplasmic antibodies. Arthritis Rheum 1998;41(9):1521–37. Reprinted with permission from Wiley-Liss, Inc., a subsidiary of John Wiley & Sons, Inc.)

- **Gastrointestinal disease** may also occur (58,60,64). Clinical manifestations range from abdominal pain (likely related to ischemia), bowel perforation, pancreatitis and bleeding.
- **Eye disease** is also frequently seen in Wegener's (scleritis, iritis, orbital pseudotumor) and Behçet's (iritis).

DIAGNOSTIC EVALUATION

Diagnostic evaluation involves:

- Pulmonary function testing (26,65).
- Radiological evaluation (5,26,67–69 and Figure 22.5.4).
- Laboratory testing and biopsy (4,26,70–74).

TREATMENT

The treatment of pulmonary vasculitis requires individualization. Different treatment protocols are followed for induction of remission and then for remission maintenance. Treatment of Wegener's granulomatosis also depends on whether the patient has limited or severe disease. Limited disease is characterized by necrotizing granulomatous pathology, with no affected organ at risk for irreversible damage. In contrast, generalized or severe disease includes all patients with life-threatening or organ threatening disease. Manifestations of severe/generalized disease include alveolar hemorrhage, glomerulonephritis, nervous system, or cardiac involvement. Rarely localized necrotizing granulomatous lesions may be in life-threatening locations, and require treatment as for generalized disease. In order to prevent *Pneumocystis jirovecii* pneumonia, prophylaxis with trimethoprim/sulfamethoxazole or alternate agents is recommended.

Remission induction

The standard regimen for remission induction of severe/generalized disease is corticosteroids (often 1 g methylprednisolone iv for 3 days then prednisone 1 mg/kg/day, not to exceed 80 mg/day), in conjunction with oral cyclophosphamide (2 mg/kg/day, adjusted for renal function) (75). For more details, see refs 28, 58, 75–82.

Induction therapy for limited disease

In limited disease, methotrexate (target dose 25 mg once a week) is used in conjunction with prednisone (1 mg/kg/day, not to exceed 80 mg/day). It is less toxic and appears to have similar efficacy to cyclphosphamide, with regards to inducing remission in these patients (85). However, methotrexate use has been associated with higher relapse rates,

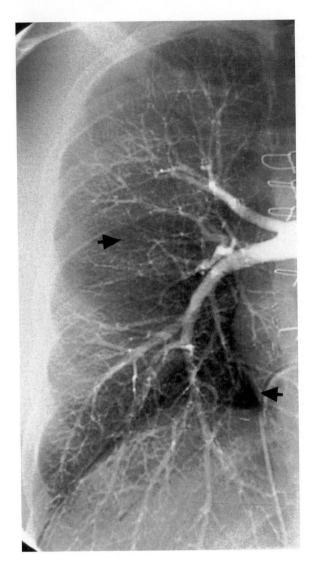

Figure 22.5.4 Radiology of Takayasu's arteritis. Pulmonary angiogram demonstrating diffusely narrowed vessels with areas of occlusion. (Image provided courtesy of the Mayo Foundation.)

particularly renal relapses (86). Methotrexate is contraindicated in patients with significant renal dysfunction. Patients on methotrexate should also receive folic acid 1 mg per day to minimize toxicity. Liver function and white cell count need to be monitored while on this drug.

Remission maintenance

After disease remission has been achieved patients need to remain on immunosuppressive therapy for another 18 months. Some clinicians would continue immunosuppressant therapy indefinitely (2). Methotrexate was the first drug demonstrated to be an efficacious alternative to cyclophosphamide for remission maintenance, without comparable side effects (78,79). The methotrexate dose used for remission maintenance is the same as that used for remission induction. Azathioprine appears to be as effective as methotrexate for remission maintenance (76),

and may be the preferred agent as it can be used in patients with diminished and renal function, and has less hepatotoxicity. Prior to its administration patients should be tested for thiopurine-methyltransferase deficiency. Those with a significant deficiency of this enzyme should not receive the drug as their difficulty in metabolizing the azathioprine puts them at high risk for profound and prolonged pancytopenia. Azathioprine is usually given at a dose of 2 mg/kg/day. Both white cell counts and liver function tests need to be monitored. Mycophenolate mofetil is a second-line agent for remission maintenance, used when the above two agents are contraindicated. It is dosed at 2 mg/kg orally. Initial reports suggest that it can be used successfully to maintain remission after standard induction therapy. The drug is generally well tolerated (87). Leflunomide is another option for a second-line agent (88).

Refractory disease

In patients whose disease is refractory to maximal standard therapy (i.e. cyclophosphamide and corticosteroids), treatment choices are very limited. There is growing evidence to support the use of the monoclonal antibody rituximab. It appears to be well tolerated and effective for the induction and maintenance of stable remission in Wegener's. The short-term safety profile is encouraging (89). The efficacy and safety of rituximab in comparison with cyclophosphamide for remission induction in patients with newly diagnosed or acutely relapsing ANCA-associated vasculitis (WG or microscopic polyangiitis) has been studied formally in a double-masked, double placebo-controlled multicenter trial (90). Plasma exchange may also be considered (91). The TNF alpha antagonist, etanercept does not appear to be effective (92).

Relapase

Relapse of Wegener's granulomatosis has been associated with infection of the upper respiratory tract (93) and there is some evidence that trimethoprim-sulfamethoxazole reduces the rate of relapse (93). Relapses off treatment require a return to induction therapy as above. When they occur on treatment they require an increase in immunosuppression. Minor flares may require an increase in prednisone alone. More serious flares require cyclophosphamide. Flares occurring on cyclophosphamide require treatment as outlined in the refractory disease section above.

Prophylaxis

Patients receiving long-term steroids should also receive prophylaxis against osteoporosis including: calcium, vitamin D, and bisphosphonates. Prophylaxis against *Pneumocystis jirovecii* should be considered in any patient on chronic immunosuppressive therapy or corticosteroids in excess of 20 mg per day (94,95).

SPECIFIC DISORDERS

Wegener's granulomatosis

Wegener's granulomatosis is the most common of the vasculitides that typically affect the lung, with an estimated prevalence of 3 per 100 000 (24). Moreover, the lung is the most frequently involved organ in Wegener's, with up to 90 percent of patients having pulmonary symptoms (24,96).

The blood vessels involved in Wegener's granulomatosis are predominantly the small arteries and veins. Classically, the pathology shows a triad of (1) necrotizing vasculitis; (2) necrotizing granulomatous upper and lower respiratory tract inflammation; and (3) necrotizing glomerulonephritis (97). However, limited forms may also occur (98). The American College of Rheumatology criteria for the diagnosis of Wegener's granulomatosis are highlighted in Table 22.5.3. Two out of four criteria must be met (99). For more details on symptoms, see refs 24 and 100.

Patient survival has improved dramatically from the original case series by Wegener, where all patients died within 7 months, to a 5-year mortality of less than 20 percent (24,58). A significant proportion of the morbidity and mortality is now related to treatment. Treatment of Wegener's granulomatosis is outlined below:

- Generalized Wegener's granulomatosis
  Induction: corticosteroids and cyclophosphamide (rituximab is under investigation as a potential alternative agent to cyclophosphamide).
  Maintenance: azathioprin, methotrexate.
  Mycophenolate mofetil (second line).
- Localized Wegener's granulomatosis
  Induction: corticosteroids and methotrexate.
  Maintenance: methotrexate, azathioprine.
  Mycophenolate mofetil (second line).

Subglottic stenosis may require mechanical dilatations and corticosteroid injections. Tracheostomy is now less commonly necessary. Direct involvement of the main pulmonary artery with stenosis and right heart failure has also been described (101) (Figure 22.5.5).

Microscopic polyangiitis

Microscopic polyangiitis (MPA) is a non-granulomatous necrotizing vasculitis involving small and medium vessels that shares many features with Wegener's granulomatosis. The kidneys are invariably affected, and as in Wegener's the renal disease may deteriorate rapidly. Pulmonary hemorrhage may occur in 10–30 percent and may be fatal. Rashes and mononeuritis multiplex are less common, as is gastrointestinal involvement. Ocular and ENT symptoms are much less common than in Wegener's (42,102–104). MPA was not widely accepted as an entity distinct from

Table 22.5.3 The American College of Rheumatology criterion for the diagnosis of Wegener's granulomatosis (2 of 4 criteria are necessary) (99)

Wegener's granulomatosis
1. Nasal or oral inflammation.
2. Abnormal chest x-ray (nodules, fixed infiltrates or cavities).
3. Abnormal urinary sediment.
4. Granulomatous inflammation on biopsy.

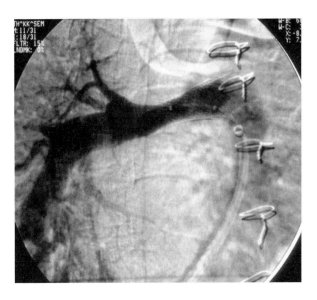

Figure 22.5.5 Radiology of pulmonary artery stenosis and stent. Stenosis of the right pulmonary artery in a patient with Wegener's granulomatosis corrected by the placement of an endovascular stent.

polyarteritis nodosa in the United States until the early 1990s, and is not included in the American College of Rheumatology classification scheme. It is defined as: "necrotizing vasculitis with few or no immune deposits affecting small vessels" (4). It is generally diagnosed on the basis of renal biopsy showing focal pauci-immune segmental glomerulonephritis, with extracapillary proliferation forming crescents. ANCA is present in 40–80 percent of patients with MPA and while in most studies the majority of patients are pANCA positive, cANCA positivity is reported at 10–50 percent. Skin biopsy generally shows leukocytoclastic vasculitis. There may be infiltrates on chest x-ray. Visceral angiogram is generally unhelpful even in the setting of abdominal symptoms as the involved vessels are too small to be visualized (104).

Churg–Strauss syndrome

Churg–Strauss syndrome (CSS) is a necrotizing vasculitis of small- and medium-sized vessels also commonly affecting the lung, but unlike Wegener's granulomatosis and

Table 22.5.4 The American College of Rheumatology criterion for the diagnosis of Churg–Strauss syndrome (4 of 6 criteria are necessary) (108)

Churg–Strauss syndrome
1. Asthma.
2. Peripheral eosinophilia greater than 10 percent of the total white cell count.
3. Peripheral neuropathy attributable to a systemic vasculitis.
4. Transient pulmonary infiltrates on chest x-ray.
5. Paranasal sinus disease.
6. Biopsy containing a blood vessel with extravascular eosinophils.

microscopic polyangiitis, it is typically associated with asthma and peripheral eosinophilia (105,106). There may be three distinct phases of Churg–Strauss. The first being a prodromal asthmatic/allergic phase which tends to precede the other features, often by many years. It is maybe associated with allergic rhinitis and nasal polyposis. The second is an eosinophilic phase with peripheral eosinophilia measured in excess of 1.5×10^9/liter. This phase may be associated with eosinophilic infiltrations of the lung (Loeffler's syndrome or eosinophilic pneumonia) or gastrointestinal tract (eosinophilic gastroenteritis). Finally there is a vasculitic phase of Churg–Strauss. It has been recognized however that all three phases are often not seen simultaneously in the same patient. Disease expression may also be modified by drug therapy, and increasingly "formes frustes" of CSS have been recognized (107). The American College of Rheumatology criteria suggest the diagnosis of Churg–Strauss if four of six criteria are present (Table 22.5.4) (108). Renal involvement in CSS is less prominent than in Wegener's and microscopic polyangiitis, and rarely leads to renal failure (36,59,60). However, peripheral nerve involvement with mononeuritis multiplex is more common. Organs that may be involved include the skin, heart, peripheral and central nervous system and abdominal viscera. Churg–Strauss is typically pANCA positive, and ANCA status appears to correlate with disease activity, though not with organ manifestation (33,36).

Recently it has been suggested that the use of leukotriene receptor antagonists in the treatment of asthma may play a causative role in the development of CSS, however, generally these agents allow for corticosteroid dose reduction and therefore may unmask pre-existing Churg–Strauss rather than play a primary "vasculitogenic" role (109–111). The mainstay of treatment is corticosteroids while the cytotoxic agent most commonly used is cyclophosphamide. If there are life-threatening or organ threatening manifestations, treatment is the same as that outlined above for severe Wegener's granulomatosis (36). Other drugs that have been used include azathioprine, methotrexate, and alpha interferon (112).

Giant cell arteritis

Giant cell or temporal arteritis is a large-vessel vasculitic disorder. It generally effects patients over the age of 50 and is more common in women and in those of Northern European origin (14,113). A subacute onset may include early symptoms of malaise, fatigue, weight loss and fever associated with a very high erythrocyte sedimentation rate. Alternatively an abrupt, painless visual loss may occur (in 15 percent of patients) due to vasculitic involvement of the ophthalmic or posterior ciliary's artery (113). Permanent blindness may be preceded by amaurosis fugax. Other common symptoms include headaches, tenderness over the temporal arteries and jaw claudication. Giant cell arteritis is frequently seen in association with polymyalgia rheumatica. Biopsy of the temporal arteries is diagnostic with pathology showing giant cells and lymphocytes, with intimal proliferation and destruction of the elastic membranes. Bilateral biopsies of the temporal arteries are generally obtained, as there may be skip lesions (114). The aortic arch and its branches are clinically involved in 10–15 percent of patients (115) and may lead to cough and aortic arch syndrome. There are several reports of pulmonary involvement (116).

Isolated pauci-immune pulmonary capillaritis

There have been several reports of an isolated pauci-immune pulmonary capillaritis causing diffuse alveolar hemorrhage (117,118). These patients have had variable pANCA positivity. In a series of 29 patients with mean follow-up of 43 months, there was no evidence for a systemic disease (118).

Takayasu's arteritis

Takayasu's arteritis affects vessels with abundant elastic tissue such as the aorta and its major branches. The pulmonary vasculature has an elastic component to the peripheral lobular branches and these may be affected in up to 50 percent of patients with the disease with up to 70 percent having moderate pulmonary hypertension (66,67,69,119). Takayasu's arteritis is most common in Asian women and almost universally occurs in those less than 50 years of age. Early symptoms include malaise and arthralgia. Later symptoms of vascular obstruction become apparent such as headaches, dizziness and visual disturbances. If the coronary ostia are involved the patient may develop angina. There may be claudication in the arms or the legs due to involvement to the subclavian, or the distal aorta and the iliac vessels. Cerebral and intra abdominal ischemia may also develop. On examination almost all patients have an asymmetrical reduction in peripheral pulses, with blood pressure differences of > 10 mmHg. They may also have bruits over the large vessels or a murmur of aortic insufficiency due to aortic root dilatation. Tests show normocytic anemia, a raised erythrocyte sedimentation rate and thrombocytosis. The electrocardiogram may show ischemia and the chest x-ray may show a dilated aortic arch. The diagnosis is generally confirmed on angiography that shows aneurysms with smooth tapered narrowings and occlusions of involved vessels (Figure 22.5.4). CT and MRA are most commonly used in follow-up, rather than to make the initial diagnosis. Biopsy is rarely pursued because of the size of the vessels involved. These patients generally follow a chronic course, with a 15-year survival of greater than 80 percent with immunosuppressant therapy (120).

Polyarteritis nodosa

Polyarteritis nodosa was the first form of vasculitis described in 1866 by Kussmaul and Maier (121,122). It affects small- and medium-sized muscular arteries, but not arterioles, venules or capillaries. Classically polyarteritis nodosa affects the joints, gastrointestinal tract, including liver and the peripheral and central nervous systems. While in the past pulmonary involvement has been reported, most if not all of these patients would now be classified as having Churg–Strauss syndrome, or microscopic polyangiitis.

Miscellaneous causes of pulmonary vasculitis

Pulmonary vasculitis may also occur in a number of other diseases including Goodpasture's disease, Henoch–Schönlein purpura, Beçhet's disease and connective tissue diseases including rheumatoid arthritis and systemic lupus erythematosus (123–127). It may also be seen in sarcoidosis and infectious processes such as HIV and CMV (11, 128–130).

KEY POINTS

- Vasculitis is inflammation and necrosis of blood vessel walls.
- Primary vasculitic disorders may be categorized based on size of vessel (small, medium, large).
- Pulmonary involvement in vasculitis is most commonly associated with small-vessel vasculitides.
- Most common diseases are Wegener's granulomatosis, microscopic polyangiitis, Churg–Strauss syndrome.
- Pulmonary vasculitides commonly associated with antineutrophilic cytoplasmic antibodies.
- Treatment involves steroids +/− other immunosuppressants.

REFERENCES

- • = Key primary paper
- ◆ = Major review article

◆1. Jennette JC, Falk RJ. Small-vessel vasculitis. N Engl J Med 1997;337(21):1512–23.

2. Savage CO, Harper L, Adu D. Primary systemic vasculitis. Lancet 1997;349(9051):553–8.

3. Savage CO, Harper L, Cockwell P, Adu D, Howie AJ. ABC of arterial and vascular disease: vasculitis. BMJ 2000; 320(7245):1325–8.

•4. Jennette JC, Falk RJ. Nomenclature of systemic vasculitides. Arthrit Rheumat 1994;37:187–92.

5. Burns A. Pulmonary vasculitis. Thorax 1998;53(3):220–7.

◆6. Schwarz MI, Brown KK. Small vessel vasculitis of the lung. Thorax 2000;55(6):502–10.

7. Larson TS, Hall S, Hepper NG, Hunder GG. Respiratory tract symptoms as a clue to giant cell arteritis. Ann Intern Med 1984;101(5):594–7.

8. Evans J, Hunder GG. The implications of recognizing large-vessel involvement in elderly patients with giant cell arteritis. Curr Opin Rheumatol 1997;9(1):37–40.

9. Zamora MR, Warner ML, Tuder R, Schwarz MI. Diffuse alveolar hemorrhage and systemic lupus erythematosus. Clinical presentation, histology, survival, and outcome. Medicine (Baltimore) 1997;76(3):192–202.

10. Schwarz MI, Zamora MR, Hodges TN, Chan ED, Bowler RP, Tuder RM. Isolated pulmonary capillaritis and diffuse alveolar hemorrhage in rheumatoid arthritis and mixed connective tissue disease. Chest 1998;113(6):1609–15.

11. Khunnawat C, Mukerji S, Havlichek D Jr, Touma R, Abela GS. Cardiovascular manifestations in human immunodeficiency virus-infected patients. Am J Cardiol 2008;102(5):635–42.

12. Caverio MA, Maicas C, Silva L, Ortigosa J, Yebra M, Camacho C, de Artaza M. Takayasu's disease causing pulmonary hypertension and right heart failure. Am Heart J 1994;127(2):450–1.

13. Launay D, Souza R, Guillevin L, Hachulla E, Pouchot J, Simonneau G, Humbert M.Pulmonary arterial hypertension in ANCA-associated vasculitis. Sarcoid Vasc Diffuse Lung Dis 2006;23(3):223–8.

14. Scott DG, Watts RA. Classification and epidemiology of systemic vasculitis. Br J Rheumatol 1994;33(10):897–9.

15. Haugeberg G, Bie R, Bendvold A, Larsen AS, Johnsen V. Primary vasculitis in a Norwegian community hospital: a retrospective study. Clin Rheumatol 1998;17(5):364–8.

◆16. Gonzalez-Gay MA, Garcia-Porrua C. Epidemiology of the vasculitides. Rheum Dis Clin North Am 2001;27(4):729–49.

17. Kerr GS, Hallahan CW, Giordano J, Leavitt RY, Fauci AS, Rottem M et al. Takayasu arteritis. Ann Intern Med 1994;120(11):919–29.

18. Nordborg E, Nordborg C. Giant cell arteritis: epidemiological clues to its pathogenesis and an update on its treatment. Rheumatology 2003;42(3):413–21.

19. Watts RA, Gonzalez-Gay MA, Lane SE, Garcia-Porrua C, Bentham G, Scott DG. Geoepidemiology of systemic vasculitis: comparison of the incidence in two regions of Europe. Ann Rheumat Dis 2001;60(2):170–2.

20. Walton EW. Giant cell granuloma of the respiratory tract (Wegener's granulomatosis). BMJ 1958(2):265–70.

21. Hollander D, Manning RT. The use of alkylating agents in the treatment of Wegener's granulomatosis. Ann Intern Med 1967;67(2):393–8.

•22. Fauci AS, Wolff SM. Wegener's granulomatosis: studies in eighteen patients and a review of the literature. Medicine (Baltimore) 1973;52(6):535–61.

23. Reza MJ, Dornfeld L, Goldberg LS, Bluestone R, Pearson CM. Wegener's granulomatosis. Long-term follow-up of patients treated with cyclophosphamide. Arthritis Rheum 1975;18(5):501–6.

•24. Fauci AS, Haynes BF, Katz P, Wolff SM. Wegener's granulomatosis: prospective clinical and therapeutic experience with 85 patients for 21 years. Ann Intern Med 1983;98(1):76–85.

25. Savage CO, Winearls CG, Evans DJ, Rees AJ, Lockwood CM. Microscopic polyarteritis: presentation, pathology and prognosis. Q J Med 1985;56(220):467–83.

•26. Hoffman GS, Kerr GS, Leavitt RY, Hallahan CW, Lebovics RS, Travis WD et al. Wegener granulomatosis: an analysis of 158 patients. Ann Intern Med 1992;116(6):488–98.

27. Cotch M, Hoffman G, Yerg D, Kauffman G, Targonski P. The epidemiology of Wegener's granulomatosis: estimates of the five-year period prevalence, annual mortality, and geographic disease distribution from population-based data sources. Arthritis Rheum 1996;39:87–92.

•28. Seo P, Min YI, Holbrook JT, Hoffman GS, Merkel PA, Spiera R, Davis JC, Ytterberg SR, St Clair EW, McCune WJ, Specks U, Allen NB, Luqmani RA, Stone JH; WGET Research Group. Damage caused by Wegener's granulomatosis and its treatment: prospective data from the Wegener's Granulomatosis Etanercept Trial (WGET). Arthritis Rheum 2005;52(7):2168–78.

29. Faille-Kuyber EH, Kater L, Kooiker CJ, Dorhout Mees EJ. IgA-deposits in cutaneous blood-vessel walls and mesangium in Henoch–Schonlein syndrome. Lancet 1973;1(7808):892–3.

30. Mark EJ, Ramirez JF. Pulmonary capillaritis and hemorrhage in patients with systemic vasculitis. Arch Pathol Lab Med 1985;109(5):413–8.

31. Weyand CM, Schonberger J, Oppitz U, Hunder NN, Hicok KC, Goronzy JJ. Distinct vascular lesions in giant cell arteritis share identical T cell clonotypes. J Exp Med 1994;179(3):951–60.

32. Weyand CM, Hicok KC, Hunder GG, Goronzy JJ. Tissue cytokine patterns in patients with polymyalgia rheumatica and giant cell arteritis. Ann Intern Med 1994;121(7):484–91.

♦33. Hoffman GS, Specks U. Antineutrophil cytoplasmic antibodies. Arthritis Rheum 1998;41(9):1521–37.

34. Hughes CC, Savage CO, Pober JS. The endothelial cell as a regulator of T-cell function. Immunol Rev 1990;117:85–102.

35. Cohen Tervaert JW, Limburg PC, Elema JD, Huitema MG, Horst G, The TH et al. Detection of autoantibodies against myeloid lysosomal enzymes: a useful adjunct to classification of patients with biopsy-proven necrotizing arteritis. Am J Med 1991;91(1):59–66.

•36. Gayraud M, Guillevin L, le Toumelin P, Cohen P, Lhote F, Casassus P et al. Long-term follow-up of polyarteritis nodosa, microscopic polyangiitis, and Churg–Strauss syndrome: analysis of four prospective trials including 278 patients. Arthrit Rheum 2001;44(3):666–75.

37. Solans R, Bosch JA, Perez-Bocznegra C, Selva A, Huguet P, Alijotas J et al. Churg–Strauss syndrome: outcome and long-term follow-up of 32 patients. Rheumatology (Oxford) 2001;40:763–771.

38. Davies D, Moran J, Niall J. Segmental necrotizing glomerulonephritis with antineutrophil antibody: possible arbovirus aetiology. BMJ 1982;285:606.

39. Specks U, Wiegert EM, Homburger HA. Human mast cells expressing recombinant proteinase 3 (PR3) as substrate for clinical testing for antineutrophil cytoplasmic antibodies (ANCA). Clin Exp Immunol 1997;109:286–95.

40. Cohen Tervaert JW, Goldschmeding R, Elema JD, von dem Borne AE, Kallenberg CG. Antimyeloperoxidase antibodies in the Churg–Strauss syndrome. Thorax 1991;46(1):70–1.

41. Lauque D, Cadranel J, Lazor R, Pourrat J, Ronco P, Guillevin L et al. Microscopic polyangiitis with alveolar hemorrhage. A study of 29 cases and review of the literature. Groupe d'Etudes et de Recherche sur les Maladies "Orphelines" Pulmonaires (GERM "O"P). Medicine (Baltimore) 2000;79(4):222–33.

•42. Guillevin L, Durand-Gasselin B, Cevallos R, Gayraud M, Lhote F, Callard P et al. Microscopic polyangiitis: clinical and laboratory findings in eighty-five patients. Arthritis Rheum 1999;42(3):421–30.

43. Savige JA, Gallicchio MC, Stockman A, Cunningham TJ, Rowley MJ, Georgiou T et al. Anti-neutrophil cytoplasm antibodies in rheumatoid arthritis. Clin Exp Immunol 1991;86(1):92–8.

44. Saxon A, Shanahan F, Landers C, Ganz T, Targan S. A distinct subset of antineutrophil cytoplasmic antibodies is associated with inflammatory bowel disease. J Allergy Clin Immunol 1990;86(2):202–10.

45. Merkel PA, Polisson RP, Chang Y, Skates SJ, Niles JL. Prevalence of antineutrophil cytoplasmic antibodies in a large inception cohort of patients with connective tissue disease. Ann Intern Med 1997;126(11):866–73.

46. Short AK, Lockwood CM. Antigen specificity in hydralazine associated ANCA positive systemic vasculitis. QJM 1995; 88(11):775–83.

47. Aebi C, Theiler F, Aebischer CC, Schoeni MH. Autoantibodies directed against bactericidal/permeability-increasing protein in patients with cystic fibrosis: association with microbial respiratory tract colonization. Pediatr Infect Dis J 2000;19(3):207–12.

48. Russell KA, Specks U. Are antineutrophil cytoplasmic antibodies pathogenic? Experimental approaches to understand the antineutrophil cytoplasmic antibody phenomenon. Rheum Dis Clin North Am 2001;27(4): 815–32, vii.

49. Harper JM, Thiru S, Lockwood CM, Cooke A. Myeloperoxidase autoantibodies distinguish vasculitis mediated by anti-neutrophil cytoplasm antibodies from immune complex disease in MRL/Mp-lpr/lpr mice: a spontaneous model for human microscopic angiitis. Eur J Immunol 1998;28(7):2217–26.

50. Harbeck RJ, Launder T, Staszak C. Mononuclear cell pulmonary vasculitis in NZB/W mice. II. Immunohistochemical characterization of the infiltrating cells. Am J Pathol 1986;123(2):204–11.

51. Foucher P, Heeringa P, Petersen AH, Huitema MG, Brouwer E, Cohen Tervaert JW et al. Antimyeloperoxidase-associated lung disease. An experimental model. Am J Respir Crit Care Med 1999;160(3):987–94.

52. Brouwer E, Huitema MG, Klok PA, de Weerd H, Tervaert JW, Weening JJ et al. Antimyeloperoxidase-associated proliferative glomerulonephritis: an animal model. J Exp Med 1993;177(4):905–14.

53. Pall AA, Savage CO. Mechanisms of endothelial cell injury in vasculitis. Springer Semin Immunopathol 1994; 16(1):23–37.

54. Green RJ, Ruoss SJ, Kraft SA, Duncan SR, Berry GJ, Raffin TA. Pulmonary capillaritis and alveolar hemorrhage. Update on diagnosis and management. Chest 1996;110(5):1305–16.

•55. Merkel PA, Lo GH, Holbrook JT, Tibbs AK, Allen NB, Davis JC Jr, Hoffman GS, McCune WJ, St Clair EW, Specks U, Spiera R, Petri M, Stone JH; Wegener's Granulomatosis Etanercept Trial Research Group. Brief communication: high incidence of venous thrombotic events among patients with Wegener granulomatosis: the Wegener's Clinical Occurrence of Thrombosis (WeCLOT) Study. Ann Intern Med 2005; 142(8):620–6.

56. Blanco R, Martinez-Taboada VM, Rodriguez-Valverde V, Garcia-Fuentes M. Cutaneous vasculitis in children and adults. Associated diseases and etiologic factors in 303 patients. Medicine (Baltimore) 1998;77(6):403–18.

57. Gibson LE. Cutaneous vasculitis update. Dermatol Clin 2001;19(4):603–15, vii.

•58. Reinhold-Keller E, Beuge N, Latza U, de Groot K, Rudert H, Nolle B et al. An interdisciplinary approach to the care of patients with Wegener's granulomatosis: long-term outcome in 155 patients. Arthritis Rheum 2000; 43(5):1021–32.

•59. Chumbley LC, Harrison RG, DeRemee RA. Allergic granulomatosis and angiitis (Churg–Strauss syndrome). Mayo Clin Proc 1977;52:477–84.

•60. Guillevin L, Cohen P, Gayraud M, Lhote F, Jarrousse B, Casassus P. Churg–Strauss syndrome. Clinical study and long-term follow-up of 96 patients. Medicine 1999;78(1):26–37.

61. Ferro JM. Vasculitis of the central nervous system. J Neurol 1998;245(12):766–76.

62. Lhote F, Guillevin L. Polyarteritis nodosa, microscopic polyangiitis, and Churg–Strauss syndrome. Clinical aspects and treatment. Rheum Dis Clin North Am 1995;21(4):911–47.

63. Sehgal M, Swanson JW, DeRemee RA, Colby TV. Neurologic manifestations of Churg–Strauss syndrome. Mayo Clin Proc 1995;70(4):337–41.

64. Levine SM, Hellmann DB, Stone JH. Gastrointestinal involvement in polyarteritis nodosa (1986–2000): presentation and outcomes in 24 patients. Am J Med 2002;112(5):386–91.

65. Rosenberg DM, Weinberger SE, Fulmer JD, Flye MW, Fauci AS, Crystal RG. Functional correlates of lung involvement in Wegener's granulomatosis. Use of pulmonary function tests in staging and follow-up. Am J Med 1980;69(3):387–94.

66. Lie JT. Isolated pulmonary Takayasu arteritis: clinicopathologic characteristics. Mod Pathol 1996; 9(5):469–74.

67. Tanigawa K, Eguchi K, Kitamura Y, Kawakami A, Ida H, Yamashita S et al. Magnetic resonance imaging detection of aortic and pulmonary artery wall thickening in the acute stage of Takayasu arteritis. Improvement of clinical and radiologic findings after steroid therapy. Arthritis Rheum 1992;35(4):476–80.

68. Takahashi K, Honda M, Furuse M, Yanagisawa M, Saitoh K. CT findings of pulmonary parenchyma in Takayasu arteritis. J Comput Assist Tomogr 1996;20(5):742–8.

69. Hara M, Sobue R, Ohba S, Kitase M, Sasaki S, Ogino H et al. Diffuse pulmonary lesions in early phase Takayasu arteritis predominantly involving pulmonary artery. J Comput Assist Tomogr 1998;22(5):801–3.

70. Hunder GG, Arend WP, Bloch DA, Calabrese LH, Fauci AS, Fries JF et al. The American College of Rheumatology 1990 criteria for the classification of vasculitis. Introduction. Arthritis Rheum 1990;33(8):1065–7.

71. Rao JK, Allen NB, Pincus T. Limitations of the 1990 American College of Rheumatology classification criteria in the diagnosis of vasculitis. Ann Intern Med 1998;129(5): 345–52.

72. Hunder GG. The use and misuse of classification and diagnostic criteria for complex diseases. Ann Intern Med 1998;129(5):417–8.

73. Savige J, Gillis D, Benson E, Davies D, Esnault V, Falk RJ et al. International Consensus Statement on Testing and Reporting of Antineutrophil Cytoplasmic Antibodies (ANCA). Am J Clin Pathol 1999;111(4):507–13.

74. Schnabel A, Holl-Ulrich K, Dalhoff K, Reuter M, Gross WL. Efficacy of transbronchial biopsy in pulmonary vaculitides. Eur Resp J 1997;10(12):2738–43.

75. Langford CA, Talar-Williams C, Barron KS, Sneller MC. A staged approach to the treatment of Wegener's granulomatosis: induction of remission with glucocorticoids and daily cyclophosphamide switching to methotrexate for remission maintenance. Arthritis Rheum 1999;42:2666–73.

•76. PagnouxC, Mahr A, Hamidou MA, Boffa JJ, Ruivard M, Ducroix JP, Kyndt X, Lifermann F, Papo T, Lambert M, Le Noach J, Khellaf M, Merrien D, Puechal X, Vinzio S, Cohen P, Mouthon L, Cordier JF, Guillevin L; French Vasculitis Study Group. Azathioprine or methotrexate maintenance for ANCA associated vasculitis. N Engl J Med 2008;25;359(26):2790–803.

•77. Fauci AS, Wolff SM, Johnson JS. Effect of cyclophosphamide upon the immune response in Wegener's granulomatosis. N Engl J Med 1971;285(27):1493–6.

•78. Jayne D, Rasmussen N, Andrassy K, Bacon P, Tervaert JW, Dardoniene J, Ekstrand A, Gaskin G, Gregorini G, de Groot K, Gross W, Hagen EC, Mirapeix E, Pettersson E, Siegert C, Sinico A, Tesar V, Westman K, Pusey C; European Vasculitis Study Group. A randomized trial of maintenance therapy for vasculitis associated with antineutrophil cytoplasmic autoantibodies. N Engl J Med 2003;349(1):36–44.

79. Langford CA, Talar-Williams C, Barron KS, Sneller MC. Use of a cyclophosphamide-induction methotrexate – maintenance regimen for the treatment of Wegener's granulomatosis: extended follow-up and rate of relapse. Am J Med 2003;114(6):463–9.

80. Hoffman GS. Treatment of Wegener's granulomatosis: time to change the standard of care? Arthritis Rheum 1997; 40(12):2099–104.

81. Hoffman GS, Leavitt RY, Fleisher TA, Minor JR, Fauci AS. Treatment of Wegener's granulomatosis with intermittent high-dose intravenous cyclophosphamide. Am J Med 1990;89(4):403–10.

82. Guillevin L, Cordier JF, Lhote F, Cohen P, Jarrousse B, Royer I et al. A prospective, multicenter, randomized trial comparing steroids and pulse cyclophosphamide versus steroids and oral cyclophosphamide in the treatment of generalized Wegener's granulomatosis. Arthritis Rheum 1997;40(12):2187–98.

83. Regan MJ, Hellmann DB, Stone JH. Treatment of Wegener's granulomatosis. Rheum Dis Clin North Am 2001;27(4): 863–86, viii.

•84. de Groot K, Adu D, Savage CO. The value of pulse cyclophosphamide in ANCA-associated vasculitis: meta-analysis and critical review. Nephrol Dialysis Transplant 2001;16:2018–27.

85. Specks U. Methotrexate for Wegener's granulomatosis: what is the evidence? Arthritis Rheum. 2005;52(8):2237–42.

86. Reinhold-Keller E, Fink CO, Herlyn K. High rate of renal relapse in 71 patients with Wegener's granulomatosis under maintenance of remission with low-dose methotrexate. Arthritis Rheum 2002;47:326–32.

87. Langford CA, Talar-Williams C, Sneller MC. Mycophenolate mofetil for remission maintenance in the treatment of Wegener's granulomatosis. Arthritis Rheum 2004; 51(2):278–83.

88. Metzler C, Fink C, Lamprecht P, Gross WL, Reinhold-Keller E. Maintenance of remission with leflunomide in Wegener's granulomatosis. Rheumatology 2004;43(3):315–20.

89. Keogh KA, Ytterberg SR, Fervenza FC, Carlson KA, Schroeder DR, Specks U. Rituximab for refractory Wegener's granulomatosis: report of a prospective, open label pilot trial. Am J Resp Crit Care Med 2006:173(2): 180–87.

•90. Stone JH, Merkel PA, Spiera R, Seo P, Langford CA, Hoffman GS, Kallenserg CG, St Clair FW, Turkiewicz A, Tchao NK, Webber L, Ding L, Sejismundo LP, Mieras K, Weitzenkamp D, Ikle D, Seyfert-Margolis V, Mueller M, Brunetta P, Allen NB, Fervenza FC, Geetha D, Keogh KA, Kissin EY, Monach PA, Peikert T, Stegeman C, Ytterberg SR, Specus U, RAVE-ITN Research Group. Rituximab versus Cyclophosphanide for ANCA-associated vasculitis. N Engl J Med 2010;363: 221–32.

♦91. Mukhtyar C, Guillevin L, Cid MC, Dasgupta B, de Groot K, Gross W, Hauser T, Hellmich B, Jayne D, Kallenberg CG, Merkel PA, Raspe H, Salvarani C, Scott DG, Stegeman C, Watts R, Westman K, Witter J, Yazici H, Luqmani R. European Vasculitis Study Group. EULAR recommendations for the management of primary small and medium vessel vasculitis. Ann Rheum Dis 2009;68(3):310–7.

92. Stone JH, Uhlfelder ML, Hellmann DB, Crook S, Bedocs NM, Hoffman GS. Etanercept combined with conventional treatment in Wegener's granulomatosis: a six-month open-label trial to evaluate safety. Arthritis Rheum 2001;44(5):1149–54.

93. Stegeman CA, Cohen Tervaert JW, Sluiter WJ, Manson WL, de Jong PE, Kallenberg CG. Association of chronic nasal carriage of Staphyloccus aureus and higher relapse rates in Wegener's granulomatosis. Ann Intern Med 1994; 1994(120):12–7.

•94. Stegeman CA, Tervaert JW, de Jong PE, Kallenberg CG. Trimethoprim-sulfamethoxazole (co-trimoxazole) for the prevention of relapses of Wegener's granulomatosis. New Engl J Med 1996;335:16–20.

95. Ognibene FP, Shelhamer JH, Hoffman GS, Kerr GS, Reda D, Fauci AS et al. Pneumocystis carinii pneumonia: a major complication of immunosuppressive therapy in patients with Wegener's granulomatosis. Am J Respir Crit Care Med 1995;151(3 Pt 1):795–9.

96. Cordier JF, Valeyre D, Guillevin L, Loire R, Brechot JM. Pulmonary Wegener's granulomatosis. A clinical and imaging study of 77 cases. Chest 1990;97(4):906–12.

97. Godman GC, Churg J. Wegener's granulomatosis: pathology and review of the literature. Arch Pathol 1954;58:533–53.

98. Carrington CB, Liebow A. Limited forms of angiitis and granulomatosis of Wegener's type. Am J Med 1966; 41(4):497–527.

•99. Leavitt RY, Fauci AS, Bloch DA, Michel BA, Hunder GG, Arend WP et al. The American College of Rheumatology 1990 criteria for the classification of Wegener's granulomatosis. Arthritis Rheum 1990;33(8):1101–7.

100. Daum TE, Specks U, Colby TV, Edell ES, Brutinel MW, Prakash UB et al. Tracheobronchial involvement in Wegener's granulomatosis. Am J Respir Crit Care Med 1995;151(2 Pt 1):522–6.

101. Case records of the Massachusetts General Hospital. Weekly clinicopathological exercises. Case 31–1986. A 39-year-old woman with stenosis of the subglottic area and pulmonary artery. N Engl J Med 1986;315(6): 378–87.

102. Bosch X, Font J, Mirapeix E, Revert L, Ingelmo M, Urbano-Marquez A. Antimyeloperoxidase autoantibody-associated necrotizing alveolar capillaritis. Am Rev Resp Dis 1992; 146(5 Pt 1):1326–9.

103. Niles JL, Bottinger EP, Saurina GR, Kelly KJ, Pan G, Collins AB et al. The syndrome of lung hemorrhage and nephritis is usually an ANCA-associated condition. Arch Intern Med 1996;156(4):440–5.

104. Guillevin L, Lhote F. Distinguishing polyarteritis nodosa from microscopic polyangiitis and implications for treatment. Curr Opin Rheumatol 1995;7(1):20–4.

•105. Churg J, Strauss L. Allergic granulomatosis, allergic angiitis and periarteritis nodosa. Am J Pathol 1951;27:277–94.

•106. Lanham JG, Elkon KB, Pusey CD, Hughes GR. Systemic vasculitis with asthma and eosinophilia: a clinical approach to the Churg–Strauss syndrome. Medicine 1984; 63(2):65–81.

107. Churg A, Brallas M, Cronin SR, Churg J. Formes frustes of Churg–Strauss syndrome. Chest 1995;108(2):320–3.

•108. Masi AT, Hunder GG, Lie JT, Michel BA, Bloch DA, Arend WP et al. The American College of Rheumatology 1990 criteria for the classification of Churg–Strauss syndrome (allergic granulomatosis and angiitis). Arthritis Rheum 1990;33(8): 1094–100.

109. Knoell DL, Lucas J, Allen JN. Churg–Strauss syndrome associated with zafirlukast. Chest 1998;114(1):332–4.

110. Wechsler ME, Pauwels R, Drazen JM. Leukotriene modifiers and Churg–Strauss syndrome: adverse effect or response to corticosteroid withdrawal? Drug Safety 1999;21(4): 241–51.

•111. Weller PF, Plaut M, Taggart V, Trontell A. The relationship of asthma therapy and Churg–Strauss syndrome: NIH workshop summary report. J Allergy Clin Immunol 2001; 108(2):175–83.

112. Tatsis E, Schnabel A, Gross WL. Interferon-alpha treatment of four patients with the Churg–Strauss syndrome. Ann Intern Med 1998;129(5):370–4.

113. Machado EB, Michet CJ, Ballard DJ, Hunder GG, Beard CM, Chu CP et al. Trends in incidence and clinical presentation of temporal arteritis in Olmsted County, Minnesota, 1950–1985. Arthritis Rheum 1988;31(6):745–9.

114. Klein RG, Campbell RJ, Hunder GG, Carney JA. Skip lesions in temporal arteritis. Mayo Clin Proc 1976;51(8):504–10.

115. Lie JT. Aortic and extracranial large vessel giant cell arteritis: a review of 72 cases with histopathological documentation. Sem Arthritis Rheum 1995;24:422–31.

116. Glover MU, Muniz J, Bessone L, Carta M, Casellas J, Maniscalco BS. Pulmonary artery obstruction due to giant cell arteritis. Chest 1987;91(6):924–5.

117. Nierman DM, Kalb TH, Ornstein MH, Gil J. A patient with antineutrophil cytoplasmic antibody-negative pulmonary capillaritis and circulating primed neutrophils. Arthritis Rheum 1995;38(12):1855–8.

118. Jennings CA, King TE, Jr., Tuder R, Cherniack RM, Schwarz MI. Diffuse alveolar hemorrhage with underlying isolated, pauci-immune pulmonary capillaritis. Am J Respir Crit Care Med 1997;155(3):1101–9.

119. Lupi E, Sanchez G, Horwitz S, Gutierrez E. Pulmonary artery involvement in Takayasu's arteritis. Chest 1975;67(1):69–74.

120. Ishikawa K, Maetani S. Long-term outcome for 120 Japanese patients with Takayasu's disease. Clinical and statistical analyses of related prognostic factors. Circulation 1994;90(4):1855–60.

•121. Kussmaul A, Maier R. On a previously undescribed peculiar arterial disease (periarteritis nodosa), accompanied by Bright's disease and rapidly progressive general muscle weakness. Deutsches Arch Klin Med 1866(1):484–518.

122. Matteson EL. Commemorative Translation of the 130-year anniversary of the original article by Adolf Kussmaul and Rudolf Maier. Rochester, Minnesota: Mayo Foundation; 1996.

123. Salama AD, Levy JB, Lightstone L, Pusey CD. Goodpasture's disease. Lancet 2001;358(9285):917–20.

124. Wright WK, Krous HF, Griswold WR, Billman GF, Eichenfield LF, Lemire JM et al. Pulmonary vasculitis with hemorrhage in anaphylactoid purpura. Pediatr Pulmonol 1994;17(4): 269–71.

125. Erkan F, Cavdar T. Pulmonary vasculitis in Behçet's disease. Am Rev Resp Dis 1992;146(1):232–9.

126. Anaya JM, Diethelm L, Ortiz LA, Gutierrez M, Citera G, Welsh RA et al. Pulmonary involvement in rheumatoid arthritis. Semin Arthritis Rheum 1995;24(4):242–54.

127. Matthay RA, Schwarz MI, Petty TL, Stanford RE, Gupta RC, Sahn SA et al. Pulmonary manifestations of systemic lupus erythematosus: review of twelve cases of acute lupus pneumonitis. Medicine (Baltimore) 1975;54(5):397–409.

128. Fernandes SR, Singsen BH, Hoffman GS. Sarcoidosis and systemic vasculitis. Semin Arthrit Rheum 2000;30(1): 33–46.

129. Chetty R. Vasculitides associated with HIV infection. J Clin Pathol 2001;54(4):275–8.

130. Golden MP, Hammer SM, Wanke CA, Albrecht MA. Cytomegalovirus vasculitis. Case reports and review of the literature. Medicine 1994;73(5):246–55.

PART **11**

PULMONARY HYPERTENSION IN PEDIATRICS

Idiopathic pulmonary arterial hypertension in children

DUNBAR IVY

INTRODUCTION

Untreated, idiopathic pulmonary arterial hypertension (IPAH) in children carries a poor prognosis. Data from 1965 revealed that 22 of 35 children diagnosed with IPAH died within one year of diagnosis (1). This poor prognosis without targeted therapy was confirmed prior to the current treatment era (2). In the NIH registry, the median untreated survival for children after diagnosis was reported to be 10 months as opposed to 2.8 years for adults (3). As recently as 1999, further studies by Barst *et al.* showed that survival for children with idiopathic pulmonary arterial hypertension who were candidates for intravenous prostacyclin but were unable to be treated with this therapy was poor with a survival of 45 percent, 34 percent, 29 percent, and 29 percent, respectively, at 1, 2, 3, and 4 years (4). Recent advances in the understanding of the pathobiology of idiopathic pulmonary arterial hypertension and new treatment therapies have resulted in marked improvement in the prognosis for children with IPAH (5,6). Similarities and differences persist in comparison of children with IPAH and adults. In both groups, disease progression is rapid, perhaps more rapid in children than in adults, and left untreated elevation of pulmonary arterial pressure and resistance leads to right ventricular failure, clinical deterioration and death (7,8). Prevalence of pediatric PH in a French study was estimated at 3.7 cases/million with IPAH in 60 percent and familial PAH in 10 percent (9). A cure for IPAH has not been found and the aim of treatment is to improve quality of life, hemodynamics, exercise capacity, and survival. As will be discussed in this chapter, medical management of children follows a similar algorhythm to that of adults treated with idiopathic pulmonary vascular disease (10). In contrast, many aspects of pulmonary vascular disease of children are distinct from adult pulmonary hypertension. Pediatric pulmonary hypertension is intrinsically linked to lung growth and development in the younger child. Furthermore, the onset of pulmonary vascular injury in the younger child may determine the possibility of greater reversal of pulmonary vascular disease. Children appear to be more reactive to acute vasodilator testing compared with adults (11). However, children with IPAH and PAH associated with other diseases may have a better long-term outcome to pulmonary arterial hypertension specific therapies than adults (Figure 23.1.1) (12). Unfortunately, the therapeutic strategy studied for adult pulmonary hypertension has not been sufficiently studied in children with regard to optimal dosing and endpoints for clinical trials.

DEFINITION

Similar to adults, pulmonary arterial hypertension is defined as a mean pulmonary arterial pressure greater than 25 mmHg at rest with a normal pulmonary artery wedge

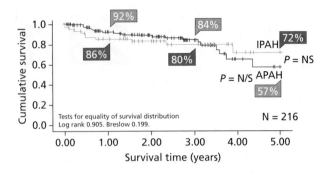

Figure 23.1.1   Kaplan–Meier survival curve of children with IPAH and APAH from the UK Pulmonary Hypertension service from 2001–2007. Haworth *et al.* Heart 2009;95:312–7.

pressure less than 15 mmHg and an increased pulmonary vascular resistance greater than 3 Wood units $\times$ m^2 (13). The Venice classification is appropriate for adults and children. This classification has recently been updated at the Dana Point, California WHO meeting with modifications of the Venice classification (14). In younger children, the pulmonary arterial pressure is frequently referenced as a ratio to systemic arterial pressure with a significant difference being greater than 0.5. In adults and children, the diagnosis of IPAH is one of exclusion and therefore requires a complete evaluation of all possible etiologies of associated pulmonary arterial hypertension, left heart disease, and respiratory disease (15).

HERITABILITY

Bone morphogenetic protein receptor type 2 (BMPR2) mutations have been identified in children and adults with IPAH and familial PAH (16–20). This genetic mutation in the TGF-beta receptor has been found in patients with familial PAH (50–70 percent) (19) and sporadic PAH (15–26 percent) (20). The pattern of inheritance in children with BMPR2 mutations is the same as adults with an autosomal dominant pattern with reduced penetrance and genetic anticipation. In many families, it is the child who presents first with severe disease, and then further evaluation of first degree relatives reveals milder disease in the parents or grandparents (21). BMPR2 mutations have been evaluated in several pediatric series with inconsistent results. Grunig found no BMPR2 mutations or deletions in 13 children with IPAH (18). However, in a study by Harrison *et al.*, 22 percent of children with IPAH or pulmonary hypertension associated with congenital heart disease had activin-like kinase type-1 (ALK-1) or BMPR2 mutations (17). More recently, a study by Rosenzweig *et al.* evaluated whether children and adults with pulmonary arterial hypertension had a positive response to acute vasodilator testing. In this study, the authors found BMPR2 mutation positive children appeared less likely to respond

to acute vasodilator testing than mutation negative children (22). Furthermore, these children had lower mixed venous saturation and cardiac index than BMPR2 mutation negative patients. A limitation of this study was that there were very few children who were positive for the BMPR2 mutation. These findings are similar to those by Elliott *et al.* who reported that IPAH and FPAH adult patients with BMPR2 mutations are less likely to respond to acute vasodilator testing than BMPR2 mutation negative patients (23).

Other genetic loci may also play important roles. Studies have suggested an important role of the serotonin transporter gene in some adults with PAH (24), and a study in children found that homozygosity for the long variant of the serotonin transporter gene was highly associated with idiopathic pulmonary hypertension in children (25).

EVALUATION

A complete evaluation for all possible causes of PAH is required before the diagnosis of IPAH is made. Certain diseases, such as connective tissue disease or chronic thromboembolic pulmonary hypertension, are less likely to be discovered in children, but still should be excluded. As discussed below, cardiac catheterization is required to rule out subtle congenital heart disease, such as pulmonary vein disease, to determine right atrial pressure, pulmonary arterial pressure, pulmonary vascular resistance, and to determine vasoreactivity to acute vasodilator testing. Lung biopsy is rarely performed but may be helpful to exclude certain diseases, such as pulmonary veno-occlusive disease, pulmonary capillary hemangiomatosis or alveolar capillary dysplasia. Furthermore, in certain forms of interstitial lung disease, such as pulmonary capillaritis or hypersensitivity pneumonitis, lung biopsy may be beneficial as treatment of these disorders varies markedly from the approach used in IPAH. Several additional tests may help quantitate exercise capacity and response to therapy.

As in adults, the 6-minute walk (6MW) test is feasible and has been used to measure sub maximal exercise. Unfortunately, the 6MW test has not been validated in children with PAH. In general, children with PAH tend to walk further than their adult counterparts with the same WHO functional class, and therefore, have "walked out" of many PAH trials. This may be partially explained by the infrequent prevalence of right heart failure in children. Another concern is that younger children may have difficulty focusing during the examination. Recently several studies have begun to evaluate the 6MW test in children. Lammers studied healthy children aged 4 to 11 years (26). The mean distance walked in 6 minutes was 470 ± 59 m. Distance walked correlated with age ($r = 0.64$, $P < 0.0001$), weight ($r = 0.51$, $P < 0.0001$) and height ($r = 0.65$, $P < 0.0001$) with no significant difference between boys and girls. The distance walked increased significantly from 4 to 7 years of age

(4 years 383 ± 41 m; 5 years 420 ± 39 m, 6 years 463 ± 40 m; 7 years 488 ± 35 m; $P < 0.05$ between each) with further modest increases beyond 7 years of age (26) (Figure 23.1.2).

Cardiopulmonary exercise testing in children over 7 years of age is useful to determine peak oxygen consumption, VE/VCO_2, and anaerobic threshold (27,28). Children with pulmonary hypertension have significant impairment in aerobic capacity, with a peak oxygen consumption of 20.7 ± 6.9 versus 35.5 ± 7.4 mL/kg/min in healthy controls ($P < 0.0001$). Peak oxygen consumption was strongly correlated with invasive measures of disease severity, including pulmonary vascular resistance index ($r = -0.6$, $P = 0.006$). Furthermore, children with adverse events had a lower peak VO_2 and higher VE/VCO_2 (27) (Table 23.1.1).

In adults, brain natriuretic peptide (BNP) is a useful tool to assess mortality risk, progression of the disease and response to therapy (29,30). Recent studies in children have begun to identify usefulness of BNP or N-terminal pro brain natriuretic peptide (NT-proBNP) (31–33). BNP correlates positively with functional status in children with PAH and values above 130 pg/mL are associated with increased risk of death or need for transplantation (32). Furthermore, change in BNP measurements over time

correlates with the change in the hemodynamic and echocardiographic parameters of children with PAH; with a BNP value > 180 pg/mL predicting a decreased survival rate (Figure 23.1.3). The change in BNP level in a specific patient over time was shown to be more helpful in determining risk or hemodynamic response to therapy than the average value in a pediatric PAH population (31). NT-proBNP, uric acid, or norepinephrine levels have also been shown to correlate with outcome in children with PAH (33). After initiation of treatment, NT-proBNP appears to decrease, which correlates with an increase in exercise capacity as documented by the 6MW test (33). An NT-proBNP greater than 605 pg/mL was predictive of mortality (33).

Newer techniques have begun to evaluate right ventricular function by cardiac MRI, 3-dimensional echocardiography or by determination of total right ventricular afterload by measuring impedance. Normal values for tricuspid annular plane systolic excursion (TAPSE) have been published (34). TAPSE ranged from a mean of 0.91 cm (z score ± 3, 0.56–1.26 cm) in neonates to 2.47 cm (z score ± 3, 1.84–3.10 cm) in 18-year-olds. TAPSE values showed positive correlations with age and body surface area. Pulmonary vascular resistance (PVR) is the current standard for evaluating reactivity in children with pulmonary arterial hypertension (PAH). However, PVR measures only the mean component of right ventricular afterload and neglects pulsatile effects. Total right ventricular afterload can be measured as pulmonary vascular input impedance and consists of a dynamic component (compliance/stiffness) and a static component (resistance) (Figure 23.1.4) (35–37). In the normal pulmonary circulation, resistance contributes 90 percent of total RV afterload, whereas in significant PAH, 30 percent of RV afterload may be contributed by compliance and 70 percent by resistance. Increases in PVR and decreases in compliance of the larger pulmonary arteries will increase right ventricular afterload, and can lead to right ventricular dysfunction (35,38,39).

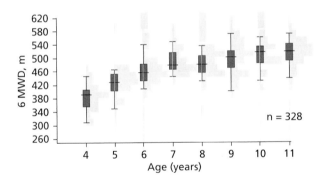

Figure 23.1.2 The distance walked in 6 minutes in healthy children. Data are shown as histograms and box-and-whisker-plots illustrating the median, 25th, and 75th percentile (grey box) and 5th and 95th percentile. Lammers AE *et al.* Arch Dis Child 2008;93:464–8.

Table 23.1.1 Cardiopulmonary exercise testing in pediatric pulmonary hypertension

Variable	Adverse outcome	No adverse outcome	P
Age	11.5 ± 0.7	11.5 ± 3.5	NS
Peak VO_2	14.6 ± 3.9	26.8 ± 7.2	< 0.0001
% peak VO_2	33 ± 8	60 ± 14	< 0.0001
VE/VCO_2	55 ± 11	39 ± 8	< 0.0001
% VE/VCO_2	170 ± 32	126 ± 20	< 0.0001
% O_2 pulse	40%	66%	0.04

Yetman AT *et al.* Am J Cardiol 2005;95(5):697–9.

CONVENTIONAL THERAPY

Conventional therapy in patients used to treat right ventricular failure is frequently used in pulmonary arterial hypertension in children. Digoxin is used in the presence of right ventricular failure, although there are no clear-cut data in children (40). Furthermore, warfarin and other antithrombotic agents are generally recommended to prevent thrombosis *in situ*, although data specific to the pediatric population are lacking. In adults and children who receive anticoagulation, low-dose warfarin is frequently used to target an INR of 1.5 to 2 (41). However, in younger children, maintenance of an adequate level is frequently difficult and toddlers may be treated with aspirin or very low-dose warfarin when benefit outweighs risk. Anticoagulation is more often used in children with IPAH

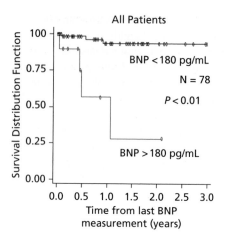

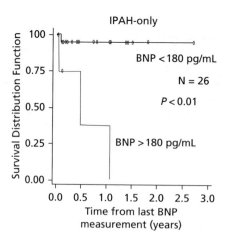

Figure 23.1.3 Kaplan–Meier survival curves for children with IPAH and PAH associated with a congenital left-to-right shunt. Survival curves are shown for (A) all patients (left) and for the subgroup of IPAH patients (right) categorized with either BNP > 180 pg/mL or < 180 pg/mL. Bernus A *et al*. Chest 2009;135: 745–51.

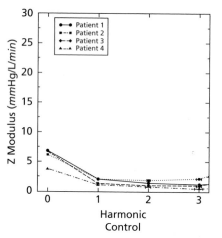

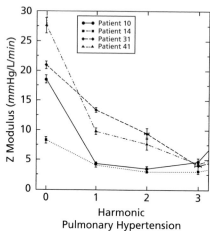

Figure 23.1.4 Typical impedance curves from children with normal pulmonary artery pressure (left) and with pulmonary arterial hypertension (right). Impedance is the sum of $Z_0 + Z_1 + Z_2 + Z_3$. Z_0 correlates with pulmonary vascular resistance index whereas $Z_1 + Z_2 + Z_3$ correlates with body surface area $\times$ pulse pressure/ stroke volume. Hunter KS *et al*. Am Heart J 2008;155:166–74.

and especially in those with a central venous line for intra-venous prostanoid therapy. Studies of aspirin and clopidog-rel in IPAH in adults have suggested a favorable effect of aspirin on the ratio of thromboxane to prostacyclin meta-bolites, but studies in children are lacking (42). Diuretics are used to treat peripheral edema or ascites in the pres-ence of right heart failure, however, excessive diuresis should be avoided. Careful attention to respiratory tract infections is required as this may worsen alveolar hypoxia. Routine influenza vaccination as well as pneumococcal vaccination is recommended. We recommend against the use of decongestants with pseudoephedrine or other stimulant-type medications as these have been associated with PAH (43). In children who require the use of oral contraceptive agents either for prevention of pregnancy or for regulation of menses, we recommend agents that have no estrogen content. Pulse oximetry and polysom-nography is indicated and chronic hypoxemia or nighttime desaturation is aggressively treated. However, oxygen therapy is not used as a mainstay of therapy in children with normal daytime saturations. In the presence of resting hypoxemia, chronic supplemental oxygen may be used.

CO-MORBIDITY

As in adults, children with idiopathic pulmonary arterial hypertension may have associated co-morbidities. Approxi-mately 5 percent of children with idiopathic disease may have an elevation of antinuclear antibodies as well as evi-dence of hypothyroidism or hyperthyroidism suggesting an autoimmune association (44,45). Furthermore, chil-dren should be screened for evidence of a hypercoagulable state as some may have an underlying coagulopathy such as antiphospholipid antibody syndrome. Reversible lower airways obstruction is the most common lung function abnormality among pediatric patients with IPAH. Whether airway reactivity is a cause of or the result of IPAH remains to be determined (46).

VASOREACTIVITY TESTING

As in adults, cardiac catheterization with acute vasodilator testing is essential prior to selecting targeted therapy in children. Cardiac catheterization carries a greater risk in those children with baseline suprasystemic pulmonary arterial pressure (Odds Ratio = 8.1, $P = 0.02$) (47,48). As in adults, a short-acting vasodilator is used, such as inhaled nitric oxide (15). Previously, patients were considered responsive to acute vasodilator testing if there was a 20 percent fall in mean pulmonary artery pressure and pulmonary vascular resistance to a vasodilator agent with no change or an increase in cardiac output (4). Based on studies by Sitbon, more stringent criteria for acute vasoreactivity in adults have been established, with the fall in mean pulmonary artery pressure greater than 10 mmHg to less than 40 mmHg (49). Although the more strict criteria are currently used in children, this has not been adequately studied in this population. In recent studies by Yung et al., either criteria predicted long-term response to calcium channel blockade.

PHARMACOLOGICAL THERAPY OF PAH

Based on known mechanisms of action, three classes of drugs have been extensively studied for the treatment of IPAH in adults: prostanoids (epoprostenol, treprostinil, iloprost, beraprost), endothelin receptor antagonists (bosentan, sitaxsentan*, ambrisentan), and phosphodiesterase inhibitors (sildenafil, tadalafil).

Before commencing vasodilator therapy for chronic PAH, vasodilator responsiveness should be assessed in a controlled situation, ideally in the cardiac catheterization unit (see above). A positive response is defined by assessing the change of cardiac and pulmonary catheter data to acute acting vasodilators (50). The younger the child at the time of testing, the greater the likelihood of acute pulmonary vasodilation in response to vasoreactivity testing (11). Many oral and inhaled vasodilators have been used for testing of vasodilator responsiveness (51–54).

Nitric oxide

The use of newer vasodilator agents, particularly inhaled nitric oxide, has been an important advance in safely determining vasoreactivity. Inhaled nitric oxide therapy improves gas exchange and selectively lowers pulmonary vascular resistance in several clinical diseases, including idiopathic pulmonary hypertension and congenital heart disease (51,52). Inhaled nitric oxide diffuses to the adjacent smooth muscle cell, where it activates soluble guanylate cyclase, resulting in an increase in cGMP and vasodilation. Currently, inhaled nitric oxide with oxygen is recommended by many centers as the agent of choice for evaluating pulmonary vasoreactivity (55).

The role of chronic inhaled nitric oxide (iNO) in the treatment of pulmonary hypertensive disorders has been studied. Although iNO therapy causes sustained decreases in pulmonary vascular resistance, adverse hemodynamic

*Sitaxsentan was withdrawn in December 2010.

effects may complicate iNO therapy after abrupt withdrawal (56,57). Inhibition of phosphodiesterase type 5 (see below), which degrades cGMP within vascular smooth muscle, causes vasodilation and may attenuate this rebound effect (57–59). Alterations in endogenous endothelial activity during NO inhaled therapy may mediate the rebound effect. ET-1 signaling pathways have been implicated in the rebound phenomena. Reactive oxygen species (ROS) may mediate these alterations and superoxide scavenging to stop the tissue increases in superoxide and peroxynitrite, preserves NOS activity, decreasing eNOS nitration, and prevents the rebound phenomena (60). Currently few patients are treated with inhaled NO at home as other therapies are available, but advancements in the use of NO in the non-intubated patient have led to greater use in the pre- and postoperative setting (61,62).

Calcium channel blockers

The use of calcium channel antagonists to evaluate vasoreactivity is dangerous, as these drugs can cause a decrease in cardiac output or a marked drop in systemic blood pressure (8). Such deleterious effects may be prolonged due to the relatively long half-life of calcium channel blockers. Consequently, elevated right atrial pressure and low cardiac output are contraindications to acute or chronic calcium channel blockade. The number of patients treated with calcium channel blockers is steadily decreasing. Recent data have shown that 7.4 percent of children with IPAH and 6 percent of those with APAH are responders to acute vasodilator testing (12).

Our preference is to perform an acute trial of calcium channel blocker therapy only in those patients who are acutely responsive to either nitric oxide or prostacyclin. Likewise, patients who do not have an acute vasodilatory response to short acting agents and who are then placed on calcium channel blocker therapy are unlikely to benefit from this form of therapy (4). A recent study examined a previously identified cohort of 77 children diagnosed between 1982 and 1995 with idiopathic pulmonary arterial hypertension and followed up through 2002. For acute responders treated with CCB (n = 31), survival at 1, 5, and 10 years was 97 percent, 97 percent, and 81 percent, respectively; treatment success was 84 percent, 68 percent, and 47 percent, respectively (63). A total of 60–80 percent of children with severe pulmonary hypertension are non-responsive to acute vasodilator testing, and therefore requires therapy other than calcium channel antagonists. Children and adults treated with calcium channel blockers may lose this response over time and must be monitored carefully for sustained efficacy (4,63).

Prostacyclins

Adults with IPAH and children with congenital heart disease demonstrate an imbalance in the biosynthesis of thromboxane A_2 and prostacyclin (64,65). Likewise, adults and children with severe pulmonary hypertension show diminished prostacyclin synthase expression in the lung vasculature (66). Prostacyclin administered over the long term, utilizing intravenous epoprostenol, has shown to improve survival and quality of life in adults and children with idiopathic pulmonary arterial hypertension (4,63,67–69).

The choice of therapy for children with PAH is impacted by severity of disease, pharmacologic adverse effects, and the patients' and families' willingness to use invasive therapy. Children who demonstrate a positive response to acute vasodilator challenge in the cardiac catheterization laboratory with inhaled nitric oxide are candidates for calcium channel blocker therapy. Only 20–40 percent of children are candidates for calcium channel blocker therapy as compared to only 10–25 percent of adults, which suggests an age-dependent response (4).

Prostacyclin and prostacyclin analogs impact the cyclic-AMP pathway to increase pulmonary vasodilation. Intravenous epoprostenol-prostacyclin was first used in the 1980s and continues to be the gold standard for treatment of severe disease. The treatment of patients with prostacyclin is promising, however the therapy is cumbersome. The prostacyclin must be infused 24 hours/day via a central venous catheter and kept cold with ice packs; the half-life of the drug is 2–5 minutes placing the patient at risk for an acute pulmonary hypertensive crisis if there is an accidental discontinuation of the medication. In addition, the side effects of the drug include nausea, diarrhea, jaw pain, bone pain and headaches Epoprostenol was FDA approved in 1995. In a recent study, 77 children diagnosed between 1982 and 1995 with IPAH were followed up through 2002. Survival for all children treated with epoprostenol (n = 35) at 1, 5, and 10 years was 94 percent, 81 percent, and 61 percent, respectively, while treatment success was 83 percent, 57 percent, and 37 percent, respectively (Figure 23.1.5) (63). Due to the development of tolerance, the dose of intravenous prostacyclin is incrementally increased and is usually higher in children than adults. The mean dose in young children is usually 50–90 ng/kg/min but may be higher. Some children with IPAH or HPAH may be weaned off intravenous epoprostenol successfully if strict weaning criteria are used (70).

The prostacyclin analog, treprostinil was approved by the FDA, initially for subcutaneous use (2002), and more recently for intravenous administration (2004) and by inhalation (2009). While subcutaneous treprostinil allows patients to remain free of central venous catheters, it can cause severe pain at the infusion site. Recent data have shown long-term efficacy in adults with PAH (71), but it has not been well studied in children. Treprostinil has also been given in the intravenous form (72,73). Intravenous treprostinil requires central line access and continuous infusion, but is easier for families to mix, may be used at room temperature, and has a half-life of four hours. Intravenous treprostinil has fewer side effects than intravenous epoprostenol, but there are no studies comparing

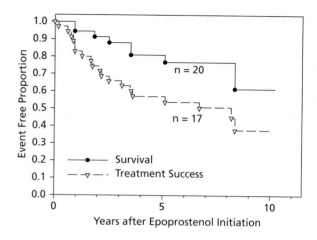

Figure 23.1.5 Kaplan–Meier curves for survival and treatment success in all patients with IPAH who received epoprostenol (n = 37). Survival rates at 1, 3, 5, and 10 years were 94%, 88%, 81%, and 61%, respectively; treatment success rates at 1, 3, 5, and 10 years were 83%, 65%, 57%, and 37%, respectively. Yung D *et al.* Circulation 2004;110:660–665.

efficacy (73). Some studies have suggested a higher rate of bacteremia in children and adults treated with intravenous treprostinil (74), but this may be decreased by protecting catheter connections and avoiding water on any connection (75). Treprostinil is also being used in an inhaled form (76), but data are lacking in children.

An inhaled prostacyclin analog, iloprost, received approval for the treatment of PAH in the United States in December 2004. This medication is administered by nebulization 6–9 times a day. Iloprost has been shown to improve hemodynamics and exercise capacity. Iloprost requires patient cooperation with the treatment administration lasting 10–15 minutes (77–79), which is difficult for young children (54). The advantage of an inhaled prostacyclin is that it can cause selective pulmonary vasodilation without affecting systemic blood pressure. In the acute setting, inhaled iloprost lowers mean pulmonary artery pressure and improves systemic oxygen saturation (80). In a select patient population, inhaled iloprost may benefit children as add-on therapy or to replace intravenous therapy in children with repeated central line infections. However, some children may develop reactive airways obstruction limiting usefulness of this therapy. Inhaled iloprost has also been studied in combination with bosentan and sildenafil, among others (78). In some cases, intravenous iloprost has been studied with beneficial effects but this form has not received authority approval (81–83).

Beraprost is an orally active prostacyclin analog with a half-life of 35–40 minutes. While beneficial effects have been noted in short-term trials (84), these may be attenuated with prolonged treatment (85,86). Long-acting beroprost has been approved in Japan (87).

Endothelin receptor antagonists

Another target for treatment of pulmonary hypertension is the vasoconstrictor peptide endothelin (ET) (88,89). The endothelins are a family of isopeptides consisting of ET-1, ET-2, and ET-3. ET-1 is a potent vasoactive peptide produced primarily in the vascular endothelial cell, but also may be produced by smooth muscle cells. Two receptor subtypes, ET_A and ET_B, mediate the activity of ET-1. ET_A and ET_B receptors on vascular smooth muscle mediate vasoconstriction, whereas ET_B receptors on endothelial cells cause release of nitric oxide (NO) and prostacyclin (PGI2), and act as clearance receptors for circulating ET-1. ET-1 expression is increased in the pulmonary arteries of patients with pulmonary hypertension.

Bosentan, a dual ET receptor antagonist, lowers pulmonary artery pressure and resistance, and improves exercise tolerance in adults with pulmonary arterial hypertension (88). Bosentan has been approved since 2001 for the treatment of WHO functional Class III and IV patients over 12 years of age, and has recently shown beneficial effects in Class II patients (90). These results have been extrapolated to children (68,91–95). In BREATHE-3, treatment with bosentan resulted in an increase in cardiac index of $0.5 \, L/min/m^2$, a decrease in mean pulmonary artery pressure of 8 mmHg and a decrease in pulmonary vascular resistance index of 3.8 Wood units/m^2 after 12 weeks (92). In this study, the dosing regimen of 31.25 mg bid was used for patients weighing 10–20 kg, 62.5 mg bid for those weighing 20–40 kg and 125 mg bid for those weighing > 40 kg. Risks associated with endothelin receptor antagonist therapy include dose-related hepatotoxicity, teratogenicity and perhaps male infertility (92). Bosentan therapy added on to epoprostenol in children allowed for a decrease in epoprostenol dose and its associated side effects (68). A more recent retrospective study of 86 children on bosentan for a median exposure of 14 months with and without concomitant therapy found that bosentan as part of an overall treatment strategy provided a sustained clinical and hemodynamic improvement was overall well tolerated, and two-year survival estimates were 88 percent in IPAH. In this study, 90 percent improved or remained unchanged in WHO FC after median treatment duration of 14 months (93). Comparable results were reported by Maiya et al., except that in IPAH stabilization was achieved in 95 percent but combined therapy with epoprostenol was necessary in 60 percent (94). Elevated hepatic aminotransferase levels occur in approximately 12 percent of adults treated with bosentan but were only 3.5 percent in children (93). Recently, a European, prospective, non-interventional, Internet-based postmarketing surveillance database was evaluated. Pediatric patients (aged 2–11 years) were compared with patients over 12 years of age. Over a 30-month period, 4994 patients, including 146 bosentan-naive pediatric patients, were captured in the database. PAH was idiopathic in 40 percent and related to congenital heart disease in 45 percent. The median exposure to bosentan

was 29.1 weeks, and elevated aminotransferases were reported in 2.7 percent of children under 12 years of age versus 7.8 percent in older patients. The discontinuation rate was 14.4 percent in children versus 28.1 percent in patients over 12 years (95). A specific pediatric formulation has been recently approved in Europe (96).

Selective ET_A receptor blockade has also been studied using ambrisentan or sitaxsentan, ET receptor antagonists with high oral bioavailability and a long duration of action, and high specificity for the ET_A receptor. Selective ET_A receptor blockade may benefit patients with pulmonary arterial hypertension by blocking the vasoconstrictor effects of ET_A receptors while maintaining the vasodilator/clearance functions of ET_B receptors. Sitaxsentan given orally for 12 weeks improved exercise capacity and cardiopulmonary hemodynamics in patients with pulmonary arterial hypertension that was idiopathic, or related to connective tissue or congenital heart disease (97,98). Ambrisentan, an endothelin receptor antagonist that is selective for the endothelin type-A (ET_A) receptor was approved by the U.S. FDA in June 2007. Adults showed significant improvements in 6-minute walk distance and significant delay in clinical worsening on ambrisentan. The incidence of elevated hepatic aminotransferase levels was 2.8 percent (99). There is no data on use of selective ET_A receptor blockade in children.

Phosphodiesterase-5 inhibitors

In models of PAH, phosphodiesterase-5 activity is increased and protein is localized to vascular smooth muscle (100). Specific phosphodiesterase-5 inhibitors, such as sildenafil, (12,90,101–107) promote an increase in cGMP levels and thus promote pulmonary vasodilation and remodeling. Sildenafil is as effective a pulmonary vasodilator as inhaled NO (104) and may potentiate the effects of inhaled NO (108–111). In certain settings, intravenous sildenafil may worsen oxygenation (111,112). However, sildenafil has been shown to prevent rebound PAH on withdrawal from inhaled NO (58,59). Addition of sildenafil to long-term intravenous epoprostenol therapy in adults with PAH has been shown to be beneficial (90).

Sildenafil has been approved for the treatment of WHO functional class II–IV PAH adult patients (103); the data in children remain limited. In a pilot study of 14 children with PAH, oral sildenafil decreased significantly PAP and PVR and improved the mean 6-MWD but a plateau was reached between 6 and 12 months (101) (Figure 23.1.6). In a small study of children with IPAH and PH associated with congenital heart disease, sildenafil has been shown to improve oxyhemoglobin saturation and exercise capacity without significant side effects (102). Moreover, phosphodiesterase type 5 appears to be highly expressed in the hypertrophied human right ventricle and acute inhibition with oral sildenafil has been shown to improve right ventricular contractility (113). Side effects include headache, flushing, exacerbation of nosebleeds, and rare systemic

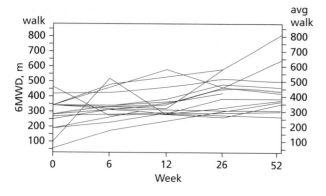

Figure 23.1.6 Six-minute walk distance in children treated with sildenafil for 12 months. Humpl T *et al. Circulation* 2005;111: 3274–80.

hypotension or erections. A randomized placebo controlled trial of oral sildenafil has been competed in pediatric patients with the initial results presented in abstract form (114).

Although no formal dose-response study has been performed, the doses generally used are 0.5–1 mg/kg/dose given three to four times a day with some children requiring even higher doses.

Intravenous sildenafil has been shown to potentiate the increase in cGMP in response to NO in children with increased PVR related to CHD or to postoperative state. Nevertheless, sildenafil infusion was associated with increased intrapulmonary shunting and augmentation of hypoxemia related to V/Q mismatch in the postoperative CHD patient (111,112). However, a recent study of intravenous sildenafil has shown improvement in oxygenation index in persistent pulmonary hypertension of the newborn in patients treated with or without inhaled nitric oxide (115).

Tadalafil, another selective phosphodiesterase type 5 inhibitor, has a longer duration of action (116). In adults with severe PAH, tadalafil has been used in addition to prostacyclin with some improvement (117,118). Little data are available in children.

ATRIAL SEPTOSTOMY AND POHS SHUNT FOR REFRACTORY PAH

The general indications for atrial septostomy include pulmonary hypertension, syncope and intractable heart failure refractory to chronic vasodilator treatment (119–122) and symptomatic low cardiac output states. Risks associated with this procedure include worsening of hypoxemia with resultant right ventricular ischemia, worsening right ventricular failure, increased left atrial pressure, and pulmonary edema. We favor a graded balloon dilation approach utilizing intracardiac echo and saturation monitoring to determine adequacy of shunt. We have frequently used a cutting balloon with the initial inflation followed by static

balloon dilations. Recently, a Potts anastamosis with connection of the left pulmonary artery to descending aorta, has been attempted to allow a direct shunt allowing an immediate reduction in right ventricular afterload, but this has rarely been performed (123).

TRANSPLANTATION

For patients who do not respond to prolonged vasodilator treatment, lung transplantation should be considered (124–129). Cystic fibrosis accounts for the majority of pediatric lung transplants. IPAH as an indication for transplantation is seen in approximately 8–16 percent of patients. Unconditional half-life for all children receiving lung transplantation for the era 1995–2005 was 4.5 years. The number of living related donor lung transplantations has decreased in recent years (129). A recent study of lung transplantation in adults with IPAH quoted survival as high as 86 percent at 1 year, 75 percent at 5 years, and 66 percent at 10 years (128). The most common causes of post-transplant death include graft failure, technical issues and infection, whereas infection and bronchiolitis obliterans syndrome are the most common causes of late death. Calculation of mean right atrial pressure × pulmonary vascular resistance may help determine timing of intervention in these patients (130).

KEY POINTS

- Children with IPAH often present with syncope.
- The pathology, pathobiology, diagnostic and treatment strategies used in adults are appropriate for most children.
- Treatment of children with IPAH is based more on experience (expert opinion) than evidence (randomized trials).
- Abnormalities of lung development, such as bronchopulmonary dysplasia, alveolar capillary dysplasia or pulmonary vein disease, are many times more common than IPAH in the infant under 6 months of age.
- CT scan is important to rule out interstitial lung disease in the evaluation of children with suspected IPAH.
- Current survival of IPAH at several centers is greater than 70% at 5 years.
- Children with IPAH generally have preserved cardiac output and right atrial pressure and thus do not have right heart failure until the late stages of the disease.
- Children with IPAH routinely walk further than adults with the same degree of hemodynamic abnormality.

REFERENCES

1. Thilenius OG, Nadas AS, Jockin H. Primary pulmonary vascular obstruction in children. Pediatrics 1965;36:75–87.
2. Sandoval J, Bauerle O, Gomez A, Palomar A, Martinez Guerra ML, Furuya ME. Primary pulmonary hypertension in children: clinical characterization and survival. J Am Coll Cardiol 1995;25(2):466–74.
3. D'Alonzo GE, Barst RJ, Ayres SM, Bergofsky EH, Brundage BH, Detre KM et al. Survival in patients with primary pulmonary hypertension. Results from a national prospective registry. Ann Intern Med 1991;115(5):343–9.
4. Barst RJ, Maislin G, Fishman AP. Vasodilator therapy for primary pulmonary hypertension in children. Circulation 1999;99(9):1197–208.
5. Rashid A, Ivy D. Severe paediatric pulmonary hypertension: new management strategies. Arch Dis Child 2005;90(1):92–8.
6. Ivy DD, Feinstein JA, Humpl T, Rosenzweig EB. Non-congenital heart disease associated pediatric pulmonary arterial hypertension. Progr Pediatr Cardiol 2009;27:13–23.
7. Haworth SG. The management of pulmonary hypertension in children. Arch Dis Child 2008;93(7):620–5.
8. Rosenzweig EB, Barst RJ. Pulmonary arterial hypertension in children: a medical update. Curr Opin Pediatr 2008; 20(3):288–93.
9. Fraisse A, Jais X, Schleich JM, di Filippo S, Maragnes P, Beghetti M et al. Characteristics and prospective 2-year follow-up of children with pulmonary arterial hypertension in France. Arch Cardiovasc Dis 2010;103(2):66–74.
10. Barst RJ, Gibbs JS, Ghofrani HA, Hoeper MM, McLaughlin VV, Rubin LJ et al. Updated evidence-based treatment algorithm in pulmonary arterial hypertension. J Am Coll Cardiol 2009;54(1 Suppl):S78–84.
11. Barst RJ. Pharmacologically induced pulmonary vasodilatation in children and young adults with primary pulmonary hypertension. Chest 1986;89(4):497–503.
12. Haworth SG, Hislop AA. Treatment and survival in children with pulmonary arterial hypertension: the UK Pulmonary Hypertension Service for Children 2001–2006. Heart 2009; 95(4):312–7.
13. Rich S, ed. Primary Pulmonary hypertension. Executive Summary from the World Symposium. Primary Pulmonary Hypertension World Health Orgnization, 1998.
14. Simonneau G, Robbins IM, Beghetti M, Channick RN, Delcroix M, Denton CP et al. Updated clinical classification of pulmonary hypertension. J Am Coll Cardiol 2009;54 (1 Suppl):S43–54.
15. Rosenzweig EB, Feinstein JA, Humpl T, Ivy DD. Pulmonary arterial hypertension in children: Diagnostic work up and challenges. Progr Pediatr Cardiol 2009;27:7–11.
16. Trembath RC, Harrison R. Insights into the genetic and molecular basis of primary pulmonary hypertension. Pediatr Res 2003;53(6):883–8.
17. Harrison RE, Berger R, Haworth SG, Tulloh R, Mache CJ, Morrell NW et al. Transforming growth factor-beta receptor mutations and pulmonary arterial hypertension in childhood. Circulation 2005;111(4):435–41.
18. Grunig E, Koehler R, Miltenberger-Miltenyi G, Zimmermann R, Gorenflo M, Mereles D et al. Primary pulmonary hypertension in children may have a different genetic background than in adults. Pediatr Res 2004;56(4): 571–8.
19. Newman JH, Wheeler L, Lane KB, Loyd E, Gaddipati R, Phillips JA, 3rd et al. Mutation in the gene for bone morphogenetic protein receptor II as a cause of primary pulmonary hypertension in a large kindred. N Engl J Med 2001;345(5):319–24.
20. Thomson JR, Machado RD, Pauciulo MW, Morgan NV, Humbert M, Elliott GC et al. Sporadic primary pulmonary hypertension is associated with germline mutations of the gene encoding BMPR-II, a receptor member of the TGF-beta family. J Med Genet 2000;37(10):741–5.
21. Loyd JE, Slovis B, Phillips JA, 3rd, Butler MG, Foroud TM, Conneally PM et al. The presence of genetic anticipation suggests that the molecular basis of familial primary pulmonary hypertension may be trinucleotide repeat expansion. Chest 1997;111(6 Suppl):82S–3S.
22. Rosenzweig EB, Morse JH, Knowles JA, Chada KK, Khan AM, Roberts KE et al. Clinical implications of determining BMPR2 mutation status in a large cohort of children and adults with pulmonary arterial hypertension. J Heart Lung Transplant 2008;27(6):668–74.
23. Elliott CG, Glissmeyer EW, Havlena GT, Carlquist J, McKinney JT, Rich S et al. Relationship of BMPR2 mutations to vasoreactivity in pulmonary arterial hypertension. Circulation 2006;113(21):2509–15.
24. Eddahibi S, Adnot S. The serotonin pathway in pulmonary hypertension. Arch Mal Coeur Vaiss 2006;99(6): 621–5.
25. Willers ED, Newman JH, Loyd JE, Robbins IM, Wheeler LA, Prince MA et al. Serotonin transporter polymorphisms in familial and idiopathic pulmonary arterial hypertension. Am J Respir Crit Care Med 2006;173(7):798–802.
26. Lammers AE, Hislop AA, Flynn Y, Haworth SG. The 6-minute walk test: normal values for children of 4–11 years of age. Arch Dis Child 2008;93(6):464–8.
27. Yetman AT, Taylor AL, Doran A, Ivy DD. Utility of cardiopulmonary stress testing in assessing disease severity in children with pulmonary arterial hypertension. Am J Cardiol 2005;95(5):697–9.
28. Garofano RP, Barst RJ. Exercise testing in children with primary pulmonary hypertension. Pediatr Cardiol 1999;20(1):61–4; discussion 5.
29. Nagaya N, Nishikimi T, Okano Y, Uematsu M, Satoh T, Kyotani S et al. Plasma brain natriuretic peptide levels increase in proportion to the extent of right ventricular dysfunction in pulmonary hypertension. J Am Coll Cardiol 1998;31(1):202–8.
30. Nagaya N, Nishikimi T, Uematsu M, Satoh T, Kyotani S, Sakamaki F et al. Plasma brain natriuretic peptide as a prognostic indicator in patients with primary pulmonary hypertension. Circulation 2000;102(8):865–70.
31. Bernus A, Wagner BD, Accurso F, Doran A, Kaess H, Ivy DD. Brain natriuretic peptide levels in managing pediatric

patients with pulmonary arterial hypertension. Chest 2009;135(3):745–51.

32. Lammers AE, Hislop AA, Haworth SG. Prognostic value of B-type natriuretic peptide in children with pulmonary hypertension. Int J Cardiol 2009;135(1):21–6.

33. Van Albada ME, Loot FG, Fokkema R, Roofthooft MT, Berger RM. Biological serum markers in the management of pediatric pulmonary arterial hypertension. Pediatr Res 2008;63(3):321–7.

34. Koestenberger M, Ravekes W, Everett AD, Stueger HP, Heinzl B, Gamillscheg A et al. Right ventricular function in infants, children and adolescents: reference values of the tricuspid annular plane systolic excursion (TAPSE) in 640 healthy patients and calculation of z score values. J Am Soc Echocardiogr 2009;22(6):715–9.

35. Weinberg CE, Hertzberg JR, Ivy DD, Kirby KS, Chan KC, Valdes-Cruz L et al. Extraction of pulmonary vascular compliance, pulmonary vascular resistance, and right ventricular work from single-pressure and Doppler flow measurements in children with pulmonary hypertension: a new method for evaluating reactivity: in vitro and clinical studies. Circulation 2004;110(17):2609–17.

36. Hunter KS, Gross JK, Lanning CJ, Kirby KS, Dyer KL, Ivy DD et al. Noninvasive methods for determining pulmonary vascular function in children with pulmonary arterial hypertension: application of a mechanical oscillator model. Congenit Heart Dis 2008;3(2):106–16.

37. Hunter KS, Lee PF, Lanning CJ, Ivy DD, Kirby KS, Claussen LR et al. Pulmonary vascular input impedance is a combined measure of pulmonary vascular resistance and stiffness and predicts clinical outcomes better than pulmonary vascular resistance alone in pediatric patients with pulmonary hypertension. Am Heart J 2008;155(1):166–74.

38. Mahapatra S, Nishimura RA, Oh JK, McGoon MD. The prognostic value of pulmonary vascular capacitance determined by Doppler echocardiography in patients with pulmonary arterial hypertension. J Am Soc Echocardiogr 2006;19(8):1045–50.

39. Mahapatra S, Nishimura RA, Sorajja P, Cha S, McGoon MD. Relationship of pulmonary arterial capacitance and mortality in idiopathic pulmonary arterial hypertension. J Am Coll Cardiol 2006;47(4):799–803.

40. Rich S SM, Dodin E et al. The short-term effects of digoxin in patients with right ventricular dysfunction from pulmonary hypertension. Chest 1998;114:787–92.

41. Rich S, Kaufmann E, Levy PS. The effect of high doses of calcium-channel blockers on survival in primary pulmonary hypertension. N Engl J Med 1992;327(2):76–81.

42. Robbins IM, Kawut SM, Yung D, Reilly MP, Lloyd W, Cunningham G et al. A study of aspirin and clopidogrel in idiopathic pulmonary arterial hypertension. Eur Respir J 2006;27(3):578–84.

43. Barst RJ, Abenhaim L. Fatal pulmonary arterial hypertension associated with phenylpropanolamine exposure. Heart 2004;90(7):e42.

44. Barst RJ, Flaster ER, Menon A, Fotino M, Morse JH. Evidence for the association of unexplained pulmonary hypertension in children with the major histocompatibility complex. Circulation 1992;85(1):249–58.

45. Roberts KE, Barst RJ, McElroy JJ, Widlitz A, Chada K, Knowles JA et al. Bone morphogenetic protein receptor 2 mutations in adults and children with idiopathic pulmonary arterial hypertension: association with thyroid disease. Chest 2005;128(6 Suppl):618S.

46. Rastogi D, Ngai P, Barst RJ, Koumbourlis AC. Lower airway obstruction, bronchial hyperresponsiveness, and primary pulmonary hypertension in children. Pediatr Pulmonol 2004;37(1):50–5.

47. Carmosino MJ, Friesen RH, Doran A, Ivy DD. Perioperative complications in children with pulmonary hypertension undergoing noncardiac surgery or cardiac catheterization. Anesth Analg 2007;104(3):521–7.

48. Friesen RH, Williams GD. Anesthetic management of children with pulmonary arterial hypertension. Paediatr Anaesth 2008;18(3):208–16.

49. Sitbon O, Humbert M, Jais X, Ioos V, Hamid AM, Provencher S et al. Long-term response to calcium channel blockers in idiopathic pulmonary arterial hypertension. Circulation 2005;111(23):3105–11.

50. Rosenzweig EB, Barst RJ. Idiopathic pulmonary arterial hypertension in children. Curr Opin Pediatr 2005;17(3):372–80.

51. Balzer DT, Kort HW, Day RW, Corneli HM, Kovalchin JP, Cannon BC et al. Inhaled Nitric Oxide as a Preoperative Test (INOP Test I): the INOP Test Study Group. Circulation 2002;106(12 Suppl 1):I76–81.

52. Berner M, Beghetti M, Spahr-Schopfer I, Oberhansli I, Friedli B. Inhaled nitric oxide to test the vasodilator capacity of the pulmonary vascular bed in children with long-standing pulmonary hypertension and congenital heart disease. Am J Cardiol 1996;77(7):532–5.

53. Rimensberger PC, Spahr-Schopfer I, Berner M, Jaeggi E, Kalangos A, Friedli B et al. Inhaled nitric oxide versus aerosolized iloprost in secondary pulmonary hypertension in children with congenital heart disease: vasodilator capacity and cellular mechanisms. Circulation 2001;103(4):544–8.

54. Ivy DD, Doran AK, Smith KJ, Mallory GB, Jr., Beghetti M, Barst RJ et al. Short- and long-term effects of inhaled iloprost therapy in children with pulmonary arterial hypertension. J Am Coll Cardiol 2008;51(2):161–9.

55. Atz AM AI, Lock JE et al. Combined effects of nitric oxide and oxygen during acute pulmonary vasodilator testing. J Am Coll Cardiol 1999;33(3):813–9.

56. Atz AM AI, Wessel DL. Rebound pulmonary hypertension after inhalation of nitric oxide. Ann Thorac Surg 1996;62(6):1759–64.

57. Ivy DD, Kinsella JP, Ziegler JW, Abman SH. Dipyridamole attenuates rebound pulmonary hypertension after inhaled nitric oxide withdrawal in postoperative congenital heart disease. J Thorac Cardiovasc Surg 1998;115(4):875–82.

58. Atz AM, Wessel DL. Sildenafil ameliorates effects of inhaled nitric oxide withdrawal. Anesthesiology 1999;91:307–10.

59. Namachivayam P, Theilen U, Butt WW, Cooper SM, Penny DJ, Shekerdemian LS. Sildenafil prevents rebound pulmonary hypertension after withdrawal of nitric oxide in children. Am J Respir Crit Care Med 2006;174(9):1042-7.

60. Oishi P, Grobe A, Benavidez E, Ovadia B, Harmon C, Ross GA et al. Inhaled nitric oxide induced NOS inhibition and rebound pulmonary hypertension: a role for superoxide and peroxynitrite in the intact lamb. Am J Physiol Lung Cell Mol Physiol 2006;290(2):L359-66.

61. Ivy DD, Griebel JL, Kinsella JP, Abman SH. Acute hemodynamic effects of pulsed delivery of low flow nasal nitric oxide in children with pulmonary hypertension. J Pediatr 1998;133(3):453-6.

62. Ivy DD, Parker D, Doran A, Kinsella JP, Abman SH. Acute hemodynamic effects and home therapy using a novel pulsed nasal nitric oxide delivery system in children and young adults with pulmonary hypertension. Am J Cardiol 2003;92(7):886-90.

63. Yung D, Widlitz AC, Rosenzweig EB, Kerstein D, Maislin G, Barst RJ. Outcomes in children with idiopathic pulmonary arterial hypertension. Circulation 2004;110(6):660-5.

64. Christman BW, McPherson CD, Newman JH, King GA, Bernard GR, Groves BM et al. An imbalance between the excretion of thromboxane and prostacyclin metabolites in pulmonary hypertension. New Engl J Med 1992;327(2): 70-5.

65. Adatia I, Barrow SE, Stratton PD, Miall-Allen VM, Ritter JM, Haworth SG. Thromboxane A2 and prostacyclin biosynthesis in children and adolescents with pulmonary vascular disease. Circulation 1993;88(5 Pt 1):2117-22.

66. Tuder RM, Cool CD, Geraci MW, Wang J, Abman SH, Wright L et al. Prostacyclin synthase expression is decreased in lungs from patients with severe pulmonary hypertension. Am J Respir Crit Care Med 1999;159(6):1925-32.

67. Lammers AE, Hislop AA, Flynn Y, Haworth SG. Epoprostenol treatment in children with severe pulmonary hypertension. Heart 2007;93(6):739-43.

68. Ivy DD, Doran A, Claussen L, Bingaman D, Yetman A. Weaning and discontinuation of epoprostenol in children with idiopathic pulmonary arterial hypertension receiving concomitant bosentan. Am J Cardiol 2004;93(7):943-6.

69. Barst RJ. A comparison of continuous intravenous epoprostenol (prostacyclin) with conventional therapy for primary pulmonary hypertension. N Engl J Med 1996: 296-302.

70. Melnick L, Barst RJ, Rowan CA, Kerstein D, Rosenzweig EB. Effectiveness of transition from intravenous epoprostenol to oral/inhaled targeted pulmonary arterial hypertension therapy in pediatric idiopathic and familial pulmonary arterial hypertension. Am J Cardiol 2010;105(10): 1485-9.

71. Barst RJ, Galie N, Naeije R, Simonneau G, Jeffs R, Arneson C et al. Long-term outcome in pulmonary arterial hypertension patients treated with subcutaneous treprostinil. Eur Respir J 2006;28(6):1195-203.

72. Tapson VF, Gomberg-Maitland M, McLaughlin VV, Benza RL, Widlitz AC, Krichman A et al. Safety and efficacy of IV treprostinil for pulmonary arterial hypertension: a prospective, multicenter, open-label, 12-week trial. Chest 2006;129(3):683-8.

73. Ivy DD, Claussen L, Doran A. Transition of stable pediatric patients with pulmonary arterial hypertension from intravenous epoprostenol to intravenous treprostinil. Am J Cardiol 2007;99(5):696-8.

74. Bloodstream infections among patients treated with intravenous epoprostenol or intravenous treprostinil for pulmonary arterial hypertension – seven sites, United States, 2003-2006. MMWR Morb Mortal Wkly Rep 2007;56(8):170-2.

75. Doran AK, Ivy DD, Barst RJ, Hill N, Murali S, Benza RL. Guidelines for the prevention of central venous catheter-related blood stream infections with prostanoid therapy for pulmonary arterial hypertension. Int J Clin Pract Suppl 2008;160:5-9.

76. Channick RN, Olschewski H, Seeger W, Staub T, Voswinckel R, Rubin LJ. Safety and efficacy of inhaled treprostinil as add-on therapy to bosentan in pulmonary arterial hypertension. J Am Coll Cardiol 2006;48(7):1433-7.

77. Hoeper MM, Schwarze M, Ehlerding S, Adler-Schuermeyer A, Spiekerkoetter E, Niedermeyer J et al. Long-term treatment of primary pulmonary hypertension with aerosolized iloprost, a prostacyclin analogue. N Engl J Med 2000;342(25): 1866-70.

78. McLaughlin VV, Oudiz RJ, Frost A, Tapson VF, Murali S, Channick RN et al. Randomized study of adding inhaled iloprost to existing bosentan in pulmonary arterial hypertension. Am J Respir Crit Care Med 2006;174(11): 1257-63.

79. Olschewski H, Simonneau G, Galie N, Higenbottam T, Naeije R, Rubin LJ et al. Inhaled iloprost for severe pulmonary hypertension. N Engl J Med 2002;347(5): 322-9.

80. Limsuwan A, Wanitkul S, Khosithset A, Attanavanich S, Samankatiwat P. Aerosolized iloprost for postoperative pulmonary hypertensive crisis in children with congenital heart disease. Int J Cardiol 2007;129(3):333-8.

81. Ewert R, Opitz CF, Wensel R, Winkler J, Halank M, Felix SB. Continuous intravenous iloprost to revert treatment failure of first-line inhaled iloprost therapy in patients with idiopathic pulmonary arterial hypertension. Clin Res Cardiol 2007;96(4):211-7.

82. Hallioglu O, Dilber E, Celiker A. Comparison of acute hemodynamic effects of aerosolized and intravenous iloprost in secondary pulmonary hypertension in children with congenital heart disease. Am J Cardiol 2003;92(8): 1007-9.

83. Hoeper MM, Spiekerkoetter E, Westerkamp V, Gatzke R, Fabel H. Intravenous iloprost for treatment failure of aerosolised iloprost in pulmonary arterial hypertension. Eur Respir J 2002;20(2):339-43.

84. Galie N, Humbert M, Vachiery JL, Vizza CD, Kneussl M, Manes A et al. Effects of beraprost sodium, an oral prostacyclin analogue, in patients with pulmonary arterial hypertension: a randomized, double-blind,

placebo-controlled trial. J Am Coll Cardiol 2002;39(9): 1496–502.

85. Badesch DB, Abman SH, Ahearn GS, Barst RJ, McCrory DC, Simonneau G et al. Medical therapy for pulmonary arterial hypertension: ACCP evidence-based clinical practice guidelines. Chest 2004;126(1 Suppl):35S–62S.

86. Barst RJ, McGoon M, McLaughlin V, Tapson V, Rich S, Rubin L et al. Beraprost therapy for pulmonary arterial hypertension. J Am Coll Cardiol 2003;41(12):2119–25.

87. Kunieda T, Nakanishi N, Matsubara H, Ohe T, Okano Y, Kondo H et al. Effects of long-acting beraprost sodium (TRK-100STP) in Japanese patients with pulmonary arterial hypertension. Int Heart J 2009;50(4):513–29.

88. Rubin LJ, Badesch DB, Barst RJ, Galie N, Black CM, Keogh A et al. Bosentan therapy for pulmonary arterial hypertension. N Engl J Med 2002;346(12):896–903.

89. Abman SH. Role of endothelin receptor antagonists in the treatment of pulmonary arterial hypertension. Annu Rev Med 2009;60:13–23.

90. Simonneau G, Rubin LJ, Galie N, Barst RJ, Fleming TR, Frost AE et al. Addition of sildenafil to long-term intravenous epoprostenol therapy in patients with pulmonary arterial hypertension: a randomized trial. Ann Intern Med 2008; 149(8):521–30.

91. Carter NJ, Keating GM. Bosentan: in pediatric patients with pulmonary arterial hypertension. Paediatr Drugs 2010;12(1):63–73.

92. Barst RJ, Ivy D, Dingemanse J, Widlitz A, Schmitt K, Doran A et al. Pharmacokinetics, safety, and efficacy of bosentan in pediatric patients with pulmonary arterial hypertension. Clin Pharmacol Ther 2003;73(4):372–82.

93. Rosenzweig EB, Ivy DD, Widlitz A, Doran A, Claussen LR, Yung D et al. Effects of long-term bosentan in children with pulmonary arterial hypertension. J Am Coll Cardiol 2005;46(4):697–704.

94. Maiya S, Hislop AA, Flynn Y, Haworth SG. Response to bosentan in children with pulmonary hypertension. Heart 2006;92(5):664–70.

95. Beghetti M, Hoeper MM, Kiely DG, Carlsen J, Schwierin B, Segal ES et al. Safety experience with bosentan in 146 children 2–11 years old with pulmonary arterial hypertension: results from the European Postmarketing Surveillance program. Pediatr Res 2008;64(2):200–4.

96. Beghetti M, Haworth SG, Bonnet D, Barst RJ, Acar P, Fraisse A et al. Pharmacokinetic and clinical profile of a novel formulation of bosentan in children with pulmonary arterial hypertension: the FUTURE-1 study. Br J Clin Pharmacol 2009;68(6):948–55.

97. Barst RJ, Langleben D, Badesch D, Frost A, Lawrence EC, Shapiro S et al. Treatment of pulmonary arterial hypertension with the selective endothelin-A receptor antagonist sitaxsentan. J Am Coll Cardiol 2006;47(10):2049–56.

98. Barst RJ, Langleben D, Frost A, Horn EM, Oudiz R, Shapiro S et al. Sitaxsentan therapy for pulmonary arterial hypertension. Am J Respir Crit Care Med 2004;169(4): 441–7.

99. Galie N, Olschewski H, Oudiz RJ, Torres F, Frost A, Ghofrani HA et al. Ambrisentan for the treatment of pulmonary arterial hypertension: results of the ambrisentan in pulmonary arterial hypertension, randomized, doubleblind, placebo-controlled, multicenter, efficacy (ARIES) study 1 and 2. Circulation 2008;117(23):3010–9.

100. Hanson KA, Ziegler JW, Rybalkin SD, Miller JW, Abman SH, Clarke WR. Chronic pulmonary hypertension increases fetal lung cGMP phosphodiesterase activity. Am J Physiol 1998;275(5 Pt 1):L931–41.

101. Humpl T, Reyes JT, Holtby H, Stephens D, Adatia I. Beneficial effect of oral sildenafil therapy on childhood pulmonary arterial hypertension: twelve-month clinical trial of a single-drug, open-label, pilot study. Circulation 2005; 111(24):3274–80.

102. Karatza AA, Bush A, Magee AG. Safety and efficacy of sildenafil therapy in children with pulmonary hypertension. Int J Cardiol 2005;100(2):267–73.

103. Galie N, Ghofrani HA, Torbicki A, Barst RJ, Rubin LJ, Badesch D et al. Sildenafil citrate therapy for pulmonary arterial hypertension. N Engl J Med 2005;353(20):2148–57.

104. Michelakis E TW, Lien D, Webster L, Hasimoto K, Archer S. Oral sildenafil is an effective and specific pulmonary vasodilator in patients with pulmonary arterial hypertension: comparison with inhaled nitric oxide. Circulation 2002;105: 2398–403.

105. Michelakis ED, Tymchak W, Noga M, Webster L, Wu XC, Lien D et al. Long-term treatment with oral sildenafil is safe and improves functional capacity and hemodynamics in patients with pulmonary arterial hypertension. Circulation 2003;108(17):2066–9.

106. Sastry BK, Narasimhan C, Reddy NK, Raju BS. Clinical efficacy of sildenafil in primary pulmonary hypertension: a randomized, placebo-controlled, double-blind, crossover study. J Am Coll Cardiol 2004;43(7):1149–53.

107. Wilkins MR, Paul GA, Strange JW, Tunariu N, Gin-Sing W, Banya W et al. Sildenafil versus Endothelin Receptor Antagonist for Pulmonary Hypertension (SERAPH) Study. Am J Respir Crit Care Med 2005;171.

108. Abrams D, Schulze-Neick I, Magee AG. Sildenafil as a selective pulmonary vasodilator in childhood primary pulmonary hypertension. Heart 2000;84(2):E4.

109. Prasad S, Wilkinson J, Gatzoulis MA. Sildenafil in primary pulmonary hypertension. N Engl J Med 2000;343(18):1342.

110. Atz Am LA, Fairbrother DL, Uber WE, Bradley SM. Sildenafil augments the effect of inhaled nitric oxide for postoperative pulmonary hypertensive crisis. J Thorac Cardiovasc Surg 2002;124:628–9.

111. Schulze-Neick I, Hartenstein P, Li J, Stiller B, Nagdyman N, Hubler M et al. Intravenous sildenafil is a potent pulmonary vasodilator in children with congenital heart disease. Circulation 2003;108 (Suppl 1):II167–73.

112. Stocker C, Penny DJ, Brizard CP, Cochrane AD, Soto R, Shekerdemian LS. Intravenous sildenafil and inhaled nitric oxide: a randomised trial in infants after cardiac surgery. Intensive Care Med 2003;29(11):1996–2003.

113. Nagendran J, Archer SL, Soliman D, Gurtu V, Moudgil R, Haromy A *et al*. Phosphodiesterase type 5 is highly expressed in the hypertrophied human right ventricle, and acute inhibition of phosphodiesterase type 5 improves contractility. Circulation 2007;116(3):238–48.

114. Barst RJ, Richardson H, Konourina I, Group S. Oral sildenafil treatment in children with pulmonary arterial hypertension(PAH): results of a double-blind, placebo-controlled, dose-ranging study. ERJ 2009; 34(Suppl 53):S3–S4.

115. Steinhorn RH, Kinsella JP, Pierce C, Butrous G, Dilleen M, Oakes M *et al*. Intravenous sildenafil in the treatment of neonates with persistent pulmonary hypertension. J Pediatr 2009;155(6):841–7 e1.

116. Galie N, Brundage BH, Ghofrani HA, Oudiz RJ, Simonneau G, Safdar Z *et al*. Tadalafil therapy for pulmonary arterial hypertension. Circulation 2009;119(22):2894–903.

117. Bendayan D, Shitrit D, Kramer MR. Combination therapy with prostacyclin and tadalafil for severe pulmonary arterial hypertension: a pilot study. Respirology 2008; 13(6):916–8.

118. Wrishko RE, Dingemanse J, Yu A, Darstein C, Phillips DL, Mitchell MI. Pharmacokinetic interaction between tadalafil and bosentan in healthy male subjects. J Clin Pharmacol 2008;48(5):610–8.

119. Barst RJ. Role of atrial septostomy in the treatment of pulmonary vascular disease. Thorax 2000;55(2):95–6.

120. Kerstein D, Levy PS, Hsu DT, Hordof AJ, Gersony WM, Barst RJ. Blade balloon atrial septostomy in patients with severe primary pulmonary hypertension. Circulation 1995;91(7): 2028–35.

121. Nihill MR OLM, Mullins CE. Effects of atrial septostomy in patients with terminal cor pulmonale due to pulmonary vascular disease. Cathet Cardiovasc Diagn 1991;24: 166–72.

122. Sandoval J, Gaspar J, Pulido T, Bautista E, Martinez-Guerra ML, Zeballos M *et al*. Graded balloon dilation atrial septostomy in severe primary pulmonary hypertension. A therapeutic alternative for patients nonresponsive to vasodilator treatment. J Am Coll Cardiol 1998;32(2): 297–304.

123. Blanc J, Vouhe P, Bonnet D. Potts shunt in patients with pulmonary hypertension. N Engl J Med 2004;350(6):623.

124. Haworth SG. Idiopathic pulmonary arterial hypertension in childhood. Cardiol Rev 2010;18(2):64–6.

125. Haworth SG, Beghetti M. Assessment of endpoints in the pediatric population: congenital heart disease and idiopathic pulmonary arterial hypertension. Curr Opin Pulm Med 2010;16 (Suppl 1):S35–41.

126. Hanna B, Conrad C. Lung transplantation for pediatric pulmonary hypertension. Progr Pediatr Cardiol 2009;27: 49–55.

127. Mallory GB, Spray TL. Paediatric lung transplantation. Eur Resp J 2004;24(5):839–45.

128. Toyoda Y, Thacker J, Santos R, Nguyen D, Bhama J, Bermudez C *et al*. Long-term outcome of lung and heart-lung transplantation for idiopathic pulmonary arterial hypertension. Ann Thorac Surg 2008;86(4):1116–22.

129. Aurora P, Boucek MM, Christie J, Dobbels F, Edwards LB, Keck BM *et al*. Registry of the International Society for Heart and Lung Transplantation: tenth official pediatric lung and heart/lung transplantation report – 2007. J Heart Lung Transplant 2007;26(12):1223–8.

130. Clabby ML, Canter CE, Moller JH, Bridges ND. Hemodynamic data and survival in children with pulmonary hypertension. J Am Coll Cardiol 1997;30(2):554–60.

Persistent pulmonary hypertension of the newborn: Pathophysiology and treatment

STEVEN H ABMAN AND ROBIN H STEINHORN

INTRODUCTION

Oxygenation of the fetus is dependent upon the umbilical circulation and placental function, but at birth, the lung must rapidly assume its role as the organ of gas exchange as it adapts to postnatal conditions. In addition to clearance of fetal lung liquid, establishment of a gas–liquid interface and the onset of ventilation, pulmonary vascular resistance (PVR) must increase nearly 8–10 fold to allow sufficient gas exchange for postnatal survival. Some infants fail to achieve or sustain the normal decrease in PVR at birth, leading to severe hypoxemia, which is known as *persistent pulmonary hypertension of the newborn* (PPHN). PPHN is a syndrome, associated with diverse cardiopulmonary disorders or can be idiopathic, affecting nearly 10 percent of full-term and preterm infants cared for in neonatal intensive care units, causing significant morbidity and mortality (1,2). Newborns with PPHN are at risk for severe asphyxia and its complications, including death, chronic lung disease, neurodevelopmental sequelae, and other problems. This chapter will review normal fetal pulmonary vascular physiology, the pathophysiology of PPHN, and clinical strategies that apply a physiologic approach to the treatment of newborns with severe PPHN.

NORMAL FETAL PULMONARY CIRCULATION

Along with progressive lung vascular growth and structure during development, the normal fetal pulmonary circulation also undergoes maturational changes in function. PVR is high throughout fetal life, especially in comparison with the low resistance of the systemic circulation. As a result, the fetal lung receives less than 3–8 percent of combined ventricular output, with most of the right ventricular output crossing the ductus arteriosus (DA) to the aorta. Pulmonary artery pressure and blood flow progressively increase with advancing gestational age, along with increasing lung vascular growth (1). Despite this increase in vascular surface area, PVR increases with gestational age when corrected for lung or body weight, suggesting increasing vascular tone during late gestation. Studies of the human fetus support these physiologic observations from fetal lambs. Doppler ultrasound measurements of human fetuses suggest that fetal pulmonary artery impedance progressively decreases during the second and early part of the third trimester (2). Pulmonary artery vascular impedance does not decrease further during the latter stage of the third trimester despite ongoing vascular growth.

Several mechanisms contribute to high basal PVR in the fetus, including low oxygen tension, low levels of vasodilator products (such as PgI_2 and NO), increased production of vasoconstrictors (including endothelin-1 (ET-1) or leukotrienes), and altered smooth muscle cell reactivity (such as enhanced myogenic tone) (3–8).

In addition to high PVR, the fetal pulmonary circulation is characterized by maturational changes in responsiveness to vasoconstrictor and vasodilator stimuli. In the ovine fetus, the pulmonary circulation is initially poorly responsive to vasoactive stimuli during the early canalicular period, but vasoreactivity increases during late gestation. For example, the pulmonary vasoconstrictor response to hypoxia, and the vasodilator response to increased fetal PO_2 and acetylcholine increase with gestation (9,10). As observed in the sheep fetus, human studies also demonstrate maturational changes in the fetal pulmonary vascular response to increased PaO_2. Maternal hyperoxia does not increase pulmonary blood flow between 20–26 weeks gestation, but increased PaO_2 caused fetal pulmonary vasodilation at 31–36 weeks (2). These findings suggest that in addition to structural maturation and growth of the developing lung circulation, the vessel wall also undergoes functional maturation, leading to enhanced vasoreactivity during fetal life.

Mechanisms that contribute to pulmonary vasoreactivity during development include maturational changes in endothelial cell function, especially with regard to NO production (11). Lung endothelial NOS (eNOS) mRNA and protein is present in the early fetus and increases with advancing gestation *in utero* and during the early postnatal period in rats and sheep (12–14). The timing of this increase in lung eNOS content immediately precedes and parallels changes in the capacity to respond to endothelium-dependent vasodilators, as assessed by *in vivo* and *in vitro* studies (33,45). The timing of this increase in lung endothelial NOS content coincides with the capacity of the lung vasculature to respond to endothelium-dependent vasodilator stimuli, such as oxygen and acetylcholine (3). In contrast, fetal pulmonary arteries are already quite responsive to exogenous NO much earlier in gestation (15). Thus, the ability of the endothelium to produce or sustain production of NO in response to specific dilator stimuli during maturation, including increased oxygen tension and acetylcholine, lags the capacity of fetal pulmonary smooth muscle to relax to exogenous NO. This may account for clinical observations that extremely premature newborns are highly responsive to inhaled NO despite limited dilation to increased oxygen tension (15).

Endothelial NOS expression and activity are affected by multiple factors, including oxygen tension, hemodynamic forces, hormonal stimuli (e.g. estradiol), paracrine factors (including VEGF), substrate and cofactor availability, superoxide production (which inactivates NO), and others (21–25). Recent studies have shown that estradiol acutely releases NO and upregulates eNOS expression in fetal pulmonary artery endothelial cells. Although estradiol does not cause acute pulmonary vasodilation *in vivo*, prolonged estradiol treatment (over 24–48 hours) causes a delayed but progressive pulmonary vasodilation, which is sustained despite cessation of estradiol infusion. In contrast, VEGF acutely releases NO and causes pulmonary vasodilation *in vivo*. Chronic inhibition of VEGF receptors downregulates eNOS and induces pulmonary hypertension in the late gestation fetus (26). These findings illustrate that diverse hormonal and paracrine factors can regulate eNOS expression and activity during development.

Vascular responsiveness to endogenous or exogenous NO is also dependent upon several smooth muscle cell enzymes, including soluble guanylate cyclase, cGMP-specific phosphodiesterase (PDE5), and cGMP-dependent protein kinase (PKG) (27–30). Several studies have shown that soluble guanylate cyclase, which produces cGMP in response to NO activation, is active before 0.7 of term gestation in the ovine fetal lung. Similarly, PDE5, which limits cGMP-mediated vasodilation by hydrolysis and inactivation of cGMP, is also normally active *in utero*. Infusions of selective PDE5 antagonists cause potent fetal pulmonary vasodilation. In the fetal lung, PDE5 expression has been localized to vascular smooth muscle, and PDE5 activity is high in comparison with the postnatal lung. Thus, PDE5 activity appears to play a critical role in pulmonary vasoregulation during the perinatal period, and must be accounted for in assessing responsiveness to endogenous NO and related vasodilator stimuli.

Functionally, the NO-cGMP cascade plays several important physiologic roles in the regulation of the fetal pulmonary circulation. These include: (1) modulation of basal PVR in the fetus; (2) mediating the vasodilator response to specific physiologic and pharmacologic stimuli; and (3) opposing the strong myogenic tone in the normal fetal lung. Past studies in fetal lambs have demonstrated that intrapulmonary infusions of NOS inhibitors increase basal PVR by 35 percent (21). Since inhibition of NOS increases basal PVR at least as early as 0.75 gestation (112 days) in the fetal lamb, endogenous NOS activity appears to contribute to vasoregulation throughout late gestation.

In addition to high PVR and altered vasoreactivity during development, the fetal lung circulation is further characterized by its ability to oppose sustained pulmonary vasodilation during prolonged exposure to vasodilator stimuli. For example, increased PaO_2 increases fetal pulmonary blood flow during the first hour of treatment; however, blood flow returns toward baseline values over time despite maintaining high PaO_2 (31). Similar responses are observed during acute hemodynamic stress (shear stress) or during infusions of several pharmacologic agents (32,33). These findings suggest that unique mechanisms exist in the fetal pulmonary circulation that oppose vasodilation and maintain high PVR *in utero*, reflecting the presence of an augmented myogenic response within the normal fetal pulmonary circulation.

Recent studies suggest that NO plays an additional role in modulating high intrinsic or *myogenic tone* in the normal fetal pulmonary circulation. The myogenic response is commonly defined by the presence of increased vasoconstriction caused by acute elevation of intravascular pressure or stretch stress (34–37). Past *in vitro* studies have demonstrated the presence of a myogenic response in sheep pulmonary arteries, and that fetal pulmonary arteries have greater myogenic activity than neonatal or adult arteries. More recent studies of intact fetal lambs have demonstrated that high myogenic tone is normally operative in the fetus, and contributes to maintaining high PVR *in utero*. These studies demonstrated that NOS inhibition not only blocks vasodilation to several physiologic stimuli, but acute inhibition of NO production unmasks a potent myogenic response. Decreased NO activity, as observed in experimental pulmonary hypertension, may further enhance myogenic activity, increasing the risk for unopposed vasoconstriction in response to stretch stress at birth. Fasudil, a ROCK inhibitor, causes fetal pulmonary vasodilation and inhibits the myogenic response in fetal sheep (38), suggesting that high ROCK activity opposes pulmonary vasodilation *in utero* and contributes to the myogenic response in the normal fetus.

Other vasodilators, including prostacyclin (PgI$_2$), are released upon stimulation of the fetal lung (for example, increased shear stress), but basal prostaglandin release appears to play a less important role than NO in fetal pulmonary vascular tone (39,40). The physiologic roles of other dilators, including adrenomedullin, adenosine and endothelium-derived hyperpolarizing factor (EDHF), are uncertain. K$^+$-channel activation appears to modulate basal PVR and vasodilator responses to shear stress and increased oxygen tension in the fetal lung, but whether this is partly related to EDHF activity is unknown (41–43).

Several vasodilator products, including lipid mediators (such as thromboxane A$_2$, leukotrienes C$_4$ and D$_4$, and platelet-activating factor) and endothelin-1 (ET-1), have been extensively studied. Thromboxane A$_2$, a potent pulmonary vasoconstrictor that has been implicated in animal models of Group B Streptococcal sepsis, does not appear to influence PVR in the normal fetus. In contrast, inhibition of leukotriene production causes fetal pulmonary vasodilation (44); however, questions have been raised regarding the specificity of the antagonists used in these studies. Similarly, inhibition of platelet-activating factor may influence PVR during the normal transition, but data from recent experimental studies are difficult to interpret due to extensive nonspecific hemodynamic effects.

Endothelin-1 (ET-1), a potent vasoconstrictor and co-mitogen that is produced by vascular endothelium, has been demonstrated to play a key role in fetal pulmonary vasoregulation (45–50). PreproET-1 mRNA (the precursor to ET-1) was identified in fetal rat lung early in gestation, and high circulating ET-1 levels are present in umbilical cord blood. Although ET-1 causes an intense vasoconstrictor response *in vitro*, its effects in the intact pulmonary circulation are complex. Brief infusions of ET-1 cause transient vasodilation, but PVR progressively increases during prolonged treatment. The biphasic pulmonary vascular effects during pharmacologic infusions of ET-1 are explained by the presence of at least two different ET receptors. The ET B receptor, localized to the endothelium in the sheep fetus, mediates the ET-1 vasodilator response through the release of NO. A second receptor, the ET A receptor, is located on vascular smooth muscle, and when activated, causes marked constriction. Although capable of both vasodilator and constrictor responses, ET-1 is more likely to play an important role as a pulmonary vasoconstrictor in the normal fetus. This is suggested in extensive fetal studies that have shown that inhibition of the ET A

receptor decreases basal PVR and augments the vasodilator response to shear stress-induced pulmonary vasodilation. Thus, ET-1 is likely to modulate PVR through the ET A and B receptors, but its predominant role is as a vasoconstrictor through stimulation of the ET A receptor.

PULMONARY CIRCULATION AT BIRTH

Within minutes after delivery, pulmonary artery pressure falls and blood flow increases in response to birth-related stimuli. Mechanisms contributing to the fall in PVR at birth include establishment of an air–liquid interface, rhythmic lung distension, increased oxygen tension, and altered production of vasoactive substances. Physical stimuli, such as increased shear stress, ventilation and increased oxygen, cause pulmonary vasodilation in part by increasing production of vaosodilators, NO and PgI$_2$. Pretreatment with the arginine analog, nitro-L-arginine, blocks NOS activity, and attenuates the decline in PVR after delivery of near term fetal lambs (3). These findings suggest that about 50 percent of the rise in pulmonary blood flow at birth may be directly related to the acute release of NO. Specific mechanisms that cause NO release at birth include the marked rise in shear stress, increased oxygen, and ventilation (5). Increased PaO$_2$ triggers NO release, which augments vasodilation through cGMP kinase-mediated stimulation of K$^+$-channels (51–53). Although the endothelial isoform of NO synthase (type III) has been presumed to be the major contributor of NO at birth, studies suggest that other isoforms (inducible (type II) and neuronal (type I)) may be important sources of NO release *in utero* and at birth as well. Although early studies were performed in term animals, NO also contributes to the rapid decrease in PVR at birth in premature lambs, at least as early as 112–115 days (0.7 term).

Other vasodilator products, including PgI$_2$, also modulate changes in pulmonary vascular tone at birth. Rhythmic lung distension and shear stress stimulate both PgI$_2$ and NO production in the late gestation fetus, but increased O$_2$ tension triggers NO activity and overcomes the effects of prostaglandin inhibition at birth. In addition, the vasodilator effects of exogenous PgI$_2$ are blocked by NO synthase inhibitors, suggesting that NO modulates PgI$_2$ activity in the perinatal lung. Adenosine release may also contribute to the fall in PVR at birth, but its actions may be partly through enhanced production of NO (54).

Thus, although NO does not account for the entire fall in PVR at birth, NOS activity appears important in achieving postnatal adaptation of the lung circulation. Transgenic eNOS knock-out mice successfully make the transition at birth without evidence of PPHN (55,56). This finding suggests that eNOS –/– mice may have adaptive mechanisms, such as a compensatory vasodilator mechanisms (such as up-regulation of other NOS isoforms or dilator prostaglandins) or less constrictor tone. Interestingly, these animals are more sensitive to the development of pulmonary hypertension at relatively mild decreases in PaO_2 and have higher neonatal mortality when exposed to hypoxia after birth (Balasubramaniam; unpublished observations). We speculate that isolated eNOS deficiency alone may not be sufficient for the failure of postnatal adaptation, but that decreased ability to produce NO in the setting of a perinatal stress (such as hypoxia, inflammation, hypertension, or upregulation of vasoconstrictors) may cause PPHN.

Although these studies were performed in term animals, similar mechanisms also contribute to the rapid decrease in PVR at birth in premature lambs (57). The pulmonary vasodilator responses to ventilation with hypoxic gas mixtures (or, rhythmic distension) of the lung or increased PaO_2 are partly due to stimulation of NO release in premature lambs at least as early as 112–115 days (0.7 term) (57). Other vasodilator products, including PgI_2, also modulate changes in pulmonary vascular tone at birth (34,37). Rhythmic lung distension and shear stress stimulate both PgI_2 and NO production in the late gestation fetus; increased O_2 tension triggers NO activity but does not appear to alter PgI_2 production *in vivo*.

ANIMAL MODELS OF PPHN

Mechanisms that lead to the failure of PVR to fall at birth have been pursued in various animal models in order to better understand the pathogenesis and pathophysiology of PPHN. Such models have included exposure to acute or chronic hypoxia after birth, chronic hypoxia *in utero*, placement of meconium into the airways of neonatal animals, sepsis and others. For further details, see refs 58–86.

CLINICAL APPROACH TO PPHN

The first reports of PPHN described term newborns with profound hypoxemia who lacked radiographic evidence of parenchymal lung disease and echocardiographic evidence of structural cardiac disease. In these patients, hypoxemia was caused by marked elevations of PVR leading to right-to-left extrapulmonary shunting of blood across the patent ductus arteriosus (PDA) or foramen ovale (PFO) during the early postnatal period. Due to persistence of high PVR and blood flow through these "fetal shunts," the term "persistent fetal circulation" was originally used to describe this group of patients. Subsequently, it was recognized that this physiologic pattern can complicate the clinical course of neonates with diverse causes of hypoxemic respiratory failure. As a result, the term "PPHN" has been considered as a *syndrome*, and is currently applied more broadly to include neonates that have a similar physiology in association with different cardiopulmonary disorders, such as meconium aspiration, sepsis, pneumonia, asphyxia, congenital diaphragmatic hernia, respiratory distress syndrome (RDS),

and others (87,88). Striking differences exist between these conditions, and mechanisms that contribute to high PVR can vary between these diseases. However, these disorders are included in the syndrome of PPHN due to common pathophysiologic features, including *sustained elevation of PVR leading to hypoxemia due to right-to-left extrapulmonary shunting of blood flow across the ductus arteriosus or foramen ovale*. In many clinical settings, hypoxemic respiratory failure in term newborns is often presumed to be associated with PPHN-type physiology; however, hypoxemic term newborns can lack echocardiographic findings of extrapulmonary shunting across the PDA or PFO. Thus, PPHN should be reserved to describe neonates in whom *extrapulmonary shunting* contributes to hypoxemia and impaired cardiopulmonary function. Recent estimates suggest an incidence for PPHN of 1.9/1000 live births, or an estimated 7400 cases/year (89).

Diseases associated with PPHN are often classified within one of three categories (Table 23.2.1): (i) *maladaptation*: vessels are presumably of normal structural but have abnormal vasoreactivity; (ii) *excessive muscularization*: increased smooth muscle cell thickness and increased distal extension of muscle to vessels which are usually nonmuscular; and (iii) *underdevelopment*: lung hypoplasia associated with decreased pulmonary artery number. This designation is imprecise, however, and high PVR in most patients likely involves overlapping changes among these categories. For more details, see refs 85, 90–92.

CLINICAL EVALUATION

Clinically, PPHN is most often recognized in term or near term neonates, but clearly can occur in premature neonates

Table 23.2.1 Elements of pulmonary vascular disease in PPHN

Elements of pulmonary vascular disease in PPHN

1. Vascular Tone and Reactivity
   - ("maladaptation")
   - imbalance between dilators (NO, pgI_2) and constrictors (ET-1)
   - abnormal smooth muscle cell responsiveness:
     - impaired NO-cGMP signaling (altered sGC, PDE5 activities)
     - high rho kinase activity

2. Vascular Remodeling
   - ("excessive muscularization")
   - smooth muscle cell hyperplasia, fibroblast proliferation, adventitial thickening, occasional thrombosis

3. Vascular Growth
   - ("underdevelopment")
   - impaired angiogenesis, vasculogenesis

as well. PPHN typically presents as respiratory distress and cyanosis within 6–12 hours of birth. While PPHN is often associated with perinatal distress, such as asphyxia, low APGAR scores, meconium staining, and other factors, idiopathic PPHN can present without signs of acute perinatal distress. Laboratory findings can include low glucose, hypocalcemia, hypothermia, polycythemia or thrombocytopenia. Radiographic findings are variable, depending upon the primary disease associated with PPHN. Classically, the chest x-ray in idiopathic PPHN is oligemic, normally or slightly hyperinflated, and lacks parenchymal infiltrates. In general, the degree of hypoxemia is disproportionate to the severity of radiographic evidence of lung disease.

Not all term newborns with hypoxemic respiratory failure have PPHN-type physiology (93). Hypoxemia in the newborn can be due to *extrapulmonary shunt*, as described above, in which high pulmonary artery pressure at systemic levels leads to right-to-left shunting of blood flow across the PDA or PFO. However in many infants *intrapulmonary shunt* or *ventilation-perfusion mismatch*, is the predominant abnormality, in which hypoxemia results from the lack of mixing of blood with aerated lung regions due to parenchymal lung disease, without the shunting of blood flow across the PDA and PFO. In the latter setting, hypoxemia is related to the amount of pulmonary arterial blood that perfuses non-aerated lung regions. Although PVR is often elevated in hypoxemic newborns without PPHN, high PVR does not contribute significantly to hypoxemia in these cases.

Several factors can contribute to high pulmonary artery pressure in neonates with PPHN-type physiology (Figure 23.2.1). Pulmonary hypertension can be due to vasoconstriction or structural vascular lesions that directly increase PVR. Changes in lung volume in neonates with

parenchymal lung disease can also be an important determinant of PVR. PVR increases at low lung volumes due to dense parenchymal infiltrate and poor lung recruitment, or with high lung volumes due to hyperinflation associated with overdistension or gas-trapping. Cardiac disease is also associated with PPHN. High pulmonary venous pressure due to left ventricular dysfunction (e.g. asphyxia or sepsis) can also elevate PAP, causing right-to-left shunting, with little vasoconstriction. In this setting, enhancing cardiac performance and systemic hemodynamics may lower PAP more effectively than promoting pulmonary vasodilation. Thus, understanding cardiopulmonary interactions is central in the successful management of PPHN.

PPHN is characterized by hypoxemia that is poorly responsive to supplemental oxygen. In the presence of right-to-left shunting across the PDA, "differential cyanosis" is often present, which is difficult to detect by physical exam, and is defined by a difference in PaO_2 between right radial artery versus descending aorta values > 10 torr, or an O_2 saturation gradient > 5 percent. However, postductal desaturation can also be found in ductus-dependent cardiac diseases, including hypoplastic left heart syndrome, coarctation of the aorta or interrupted aortic arch. The response to supplemental oxygen can help to distinguish PPHN from primary lung or cardiac disease. Although supplemental oxygen traditionally increases PaO_2 more readily in lung disease than cyanotic heart disease or PPHN, this may not be obvious with more advanced parenchymal lung disease. Marked improvement in SaO_2 (increase to 100 percent) with supplemental oxygen suggests the presence of V/Q mismatch due to lung disease or highly reactive PPHN. Most patients with PPHN have at least a transient improvement in oxygenation in response to interventions such as high inspired oxygen

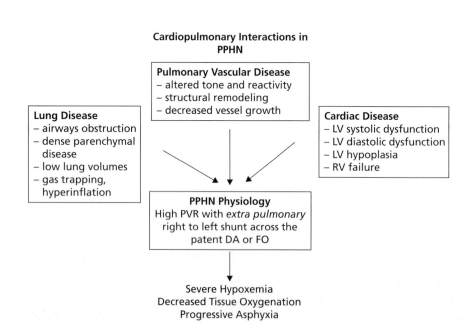

Cardiopulmonary Interactions in PPHN

Pulmonary Vascular Disease
- altered tone and reactivity
- structural remodeling
- decreased vessel growth

Lung Disease
- airways obstruction
- dense parenchymal disease
- low lung volumes
- gas trapping, hyperinflation

Cardiac Disease
- LV systolic dysfunction
- LV diastolic dysfunction
- LV hypoplasia
- RV failure

PPHN Physiology
High PVR with *extra pulmonary* right to left shunt across the patent DA or FO

Severe Hypoxemia
Decreased Tissue Oxygenation
Progressive Asphyxia

Figure 23.2.1 Cardiopulmonary interactions in PPHN. As illustrated, in addition to pulmonary vascular disease, abnormalities of lung and cardiac physiology often contribute to high pulmonary artery pressure or PVR in PPHN. (Abbreviations: LV, left ventricular; RV, right ventricle.)

and/or mechanical ventilation. Acute respiratory alkalosis induced by hyperventilation to achieve $PaCO_2 < 30$ torr and a $pH > 7.50$ may increase $PaO_2 > 50$ torr in PPHN, but rarely in cyanotic heart disease.

The echocardiogram plays an important diagnostic role and is an essential tool for managing newborns with PPHN. The initial echocardiographic evaluation rules out structural heart disease causing hypoxemia or ductal shunting (e.g. coarctation of the aorta and total anomalous pulmonary venous return). Not all term newborns with hypoxemia have PPHN physiology. Although high pulmonary artery pressure is commonly found in association with neonatal lung disease, the diagnosis of PPHN is uncertain without evidence of bidirectional or predominantly right-to-left shunting across the PFO or PDA. Echocardiographic signs suggestive of pulmonary hypertension (e.g. increased right ventricular systolic time intervals and septal flattening) are less helpful. In addition to demonstrating the presence of PPHN physiology, the echocardiogram is critical for the evaluation of left ventricular function and diagnosis of anatomic heart disease, including such "PPHN mimics" as coarctation of the aorta; total anomalous pulmonary venous return; hypoplastic left heart syndrome; and others. Studies should carefully assess the predominant direction of shunting at the PFO as well as the PDA. Although right-to-left shunting at the PDA and PFO is typical for PPHN, predominant right-to-left shunting at the PDA but left-to-right shunt at the PFO may help to identify the important role of *left ventricular dysfunction* to the underlying pathophysiology. In the presence of severe left ventricular dysfunction with pulmonary hypertension, pulmonary vasodilation alone may be ineffective in improving oxygenation. In this setting, efforts to reduce PVR should be accompanied by targeted therapies to increase cardiac performance and decrease left ventricular afterload. In the setting of impaired LV performance, cardiotonic therapies that increase systemic vascular resistance may further worsen LV function and increase pulmonary artery pressure. Thus, careful echocardiographic assessment provides invaluable information about the underlying pathophysiology and will help guide the course of treatment.

TREATMENT OF PPHN

In general, management of the newborn with PPHN includes the treatment and avoidance of hypothermia, hypoglycemia, hypocalcemia, anemia and hypovolemia; correction of metabolic acidosis; diagnostic studies for sepsis; serial monitoring of arterial blood pressure, pulse oximetry (pre- and post-ductal), and transcutaneous PCO_2. Therapy includes optimization of systemic hemodynamics with volume and cardiotonic therapy (dobutamine, dopamine, and milrinone), in order to enhance cardiac output and systemic O_2 transport. Failure to respond to medical management, as evidenced by failure

to sustain improvement in oxygenation with good hemodynamic function, often leads to treatment with extracorporeal membrane oxygenation (ECMO) (94). Although ECMO can be a life-saving therapy, it is costly, labor intensive, and can have severe side effects, such as intracranial hemorrhage. Since arterio-venous ECMO usually involves ligation of the carotid artery, the potential for acute and long-term CNS injuries continues to be a major concern.

The goal of mechanical ventilation is to improve oxygenation, achieve "optimal" lung volume to minimize the adverse effects of high or low lung volumes on PVR, and to minimize the risk for lung injury ("volutrauma"). Mechanical ventilation using inappropriate settings can produce acute lung injury (ventilator-induced lung injury; VILI), causing pulmonary edema, decreased lung compliance and promoting lung inflammation due to increased cytokine production and lung neutrophil accumulation. The development of VILI is an important determinant of clinical course and eventual outcome of newborns with hypoxemic respiratory failure, and postnatal lung injury worsens the degree of pulmonary hypertension (95). On the other hand, failure to achieve adequate lung volumes (functional residual capacity) contributes to hypoxemia and high PVR in newborns with PPHN. Some newborns with parenchymal lung disease with PPHN physiology improve oxygenation and decrease right-to-left extrapulmonary shunting with aggressive lung recruitment during high frequency oscillatory ventilation (96) or with an "open lung approach" of higher positive end-expiratory pressure with low tidal volumes, as more commonly utilized in older patients with ARDS (97).

Past studies have shown that acute hyperventilation can improve PaO_2 in neonates with PPHN, providing a diagnostic test and potential therapeutic strategy. However, there are many issues with the use of hypocarbic alkalosis for prolonged therapy. Depending upon the ventilator strategy and underlying lung disease, hyperventilation is likely to increase VILI, and the ability to sustain decreased PVR during prolonged hyperventilation is unproven. Experimental studies suggest that the response to alkalosis is transient, and that alkalosis may paradoxically worsen pulmonary vascular tone, reactivity and permeability edema (98,99). In addition, prolonged hyperventilation reduces cerebral blood flow and oxygen delivery to the brain, potentially worsening neurodevelopmental outcome.

Additional therapies, including infusions of sodium bicarbonate, surfactant therapy and the use of intravenous vasodilators, are highly variable between centers (100).

Inhaled nitric oxide (iNO) therapy at low doses (5–20 ppm) improves oxygenation and decreases the need for ECMO therapy in patients with diverse causes of PPHN (101–106). Multicenter clinical trials support the use of iNO in near-term (> 34 weeks gestation) and term newborns, although the use of iNO in infants less than 34 weeks gestation remains largely investigational. Studies support the use of iNO in infants who have hypoxemic respiratory failure with evidence of PPHN, who require mechanical ventilation and high inspired oxygen concentrations. The most common criterion employed has been the oxygenation index (OI; mean airway pressure times FiO_2 times 100 divided by PaO_2). Although clinical trials commonly allowed for enrollment with OI levels > 25, the mean OI at study entry in multicenter trials approximated 40. It is unclear whether infants with less severe hypoxemia benefit from iNO therapy (107).

The first studies of iNO treatment in term newborns reported initial doses that ranged from 20 to 80 ppm (103,106). In the former report, rapid improvement in PaO_2 was achieved at low doses (20 ppm) for 4 hours, and this response was sustained with prolonged therapy at 6 ppm. Subsequent multicenter studies confirmed the efficacy of this dosing strategy (101,105), and showed that increasing the dose beyond 20 ppm in non-responders did not improve outcomes. The available evidence, therefore, supports the use of doses of iNO beginning at 20 ppm in term newborns with PPHN, since this strategy decreased ECMO utilization without increasing adverse effects. Although brief exposures to higher doses (40–80 ppm) appear to be safe, sustained treatment with 80 ppm NO increases the risk of methemoglobinemia (102). In our practice, we discontinue iNO if the FiO_2 is < 0.60 and the PaO_2 is > 60 without evidence of "rebound" pulmonary hypertension or an increase in $FiO_2 > 15$ percent after iNO withdrawal. Weaning can generally be accomplished in 4–5 days, and prolonged need for inhaled NO therapy without resolution of disease should lead to a more extensive evaluation to determine whether previously unsuspected anatomic lung or cardiovascular disease is present (for example, pulmonary venous stenosis, alveolar capillary dysplasia, severe lung hypoplasia, or others) (109).

In newborns with severe lung disease, HFOV is frequently used to optimize lung inflation and minimize lung injury. The combination of HFOV with iNO often enhances the improvement in oxygenation in newborns with severe PPHN complicated by diffuse parencyhmal lung disease and underinflation (e.g. RDS, pneumonia). A randomized, multicenter trial of infants with severe PPHN demonstrated that treatment with iNO in combination with HFOV was successful in many patients who failed to respond to HFOV or iNO alone (105). For patients with PPHN complicated by severe lung disease, response rates for HFOV + iNO were better than HFOV alone or iNO with conventional ventilation. In contrast, for patients without significant parenchymal lung disease, both iNO and HFOV + iNO were more effective than HFOV alone. This response to combined treatment with HFOV + iNO likely reflects both improvement in intrapulmonary shunting in patients with severe lung disease and PPHN (using a strategy designed to recruit and sustain lung volume, rather than to hyperventilate) and augmented NO delivery to its site of action. Although iNO may be an effective

treatment for PPHN, it should be considered only as part of an overall clinical strategy that simultaneously addresses the role of parenchymal lung disease, cardiac performance, and systemic hemodynamics.

Although clinical improvement during inhaled NO therapy occurs with many disorders associated with PPHN, not all neonates with acute hypoxemic respiratory failure and pulmonary hypertension respond to iNO. Several mechanisms may explain the clinical variability in responsiveness to iNO therapy. As noted, an inability to deliver NO to the pulmonary circulation due to poor lung inflation is a major cause of poor responsiveness. In addition, poor NO responsiveness may be related to myocardial dysfunction or systemic hypotension, severe pulmonary vascular structural disease, and unsuspected or missed anatomic cardiovascular lesions (such as total anomalous pulmonary venous return, coarctation of the aorta, alveolar capillary dysplasia, pulmonary interstitial glycogenosis, surfactant protein deficiency, and others). Since iNO is usually delivered with high concentrations of oxygen, there is also the potential for enhanced production of reactive oxygen and reactive nitrogen metabolites, both of which may contribute to vasoconstriction and/or inadequate responses to iNO. While hyperoxic ventilation is standard therapy for PPHN, it may be toxic to the developing lung through formation of reactive oxygen species, such as superoxide anions (110). As noted previously, superoxide rapidly combines with and inactivates NO and in the process forms peroxynitrite; both are potent oxidants with the potential to produce vasoconstriction, cytotoxicity, and vascular smooth muscle cell proliferation. Studies in newborn lambs with pharmacologic pulmonary hypertension indicate that iNO responsiveness is significantly blunted after even brief (30 minute) periods of ventilation with 100 percent O_2, and that oxidant stress alters NO responsiveness in part through increasing expression and activity of cGMP-specific phosphodiesterases (82,111).

These and other studies indicate that another important mechanism of poor responsiveness to inhaled NO may be altered smooth muscle cell responsiveness, and there are a number of emerging therapies that take advantage of our increased understanding of the cellular effects of iNO. See refs 112–120 for more details.

Finally, although newer therapies, including HFOV and inhaled NO, have led to a dramatic reduction in the need for ECMO therapy, ECMO remains an effective and potentially life-saving rescue modality for severe PPHN. Current patterns of ECMO use demonstrate persistent use in neonates with congenital diaphragmatic hernia (CDH) and patients with severe hemodynamic instability, with less need for ECMO in meconium aspiration, RDS, idiopathic PPHN and other disorders. Ongoing laboratory and clinical studies are currently exploring newer agents that may have therapeutic roles in PPHN in the near future, such as SOD, sGC activators and stimulators, rho kinase inhibitors and others.

KEY POINTS

- PPHN is a clinical syndrome that is associated with diverse cardiopulmonary diseases, with pathophysiologic mechanisms including pulmonary vascular, cardiac and lung disease.
- Experimental work on basic mechanisms of vascular regulation of the developing lung circulation and models of perinatal pulmonary hypertension has improved our therapeutic approaches to neonates with PPHN.
- Inhaled NO has been shown to be an effective pulmonary vasodilator for infants with PPHN, but successful clinical strategies require meticulous care of associated lung and cardiac disease.
- More work is needed to expand our therapeutic repertoire in order to further improve the outcome of the sick newborn with severe hypoxemia, especially in patients with lung hypoplasia and advanced structural vascular disease.
- Future work is needed to better define basic mechanisms of lung vascular growth and development, which will likely lead to novel therapeutic approaches to diseases associated with impaired vascular growth or pulmonary hypertension.

REFERENCES

1. Heymann MA, Soifer SJ. 1989. Control of fetal and neonatal pulmonary circulation. In: Weir EK Reeves JT (eds). Pulmonary vascular physiology and pathophysiology NY: Marcel-Dekker, 33–50.
2. Rasanen J, Wood DC, Debbs RH, Cohen J, Weiner S, Huhta JC. Reactivity of the human fetal pulmonary circulation to maternal hyperoxygenation increases during the second half of pregnancy. A randomized study. Circulation 1998; 97:257–62.
3. Abman SH, Chatfield BA, Hall SL McMurtry IF. Role of endothelium-derived relaxing factor during transition of pulmonary circulation at birth. Am J Physiol 1990;259: H1921–7.
4. Cassin S. Role of prostaglandins, thromboxanes and leukotrienes in the control of the pulmonary circulation in the fetus and newborn. Semin Perinatol 1987;11:53–63.
5. Cornfield DN, Chatfield BA, McQueston JA et al. Effects of birth-related stimuli on L-arginine-dependent pulmonary vasodilation in the ovine fetus. Am J Physiol 1992;262: H1474–81.
6. Cornfield DN, Reeves HL, Tolarova S et al. Oxygen causes fetal pulmonary vasodilation through activation of a calcium-dependent potassium channel. Proc Natl Acad Sci USA 1996;93:8089–94.
7. Velvis H, Moore P, Heymann MA. Prostaglandin inhibition prevents the fall in pulmonary vascular resistance as the result of rhythmic distension of the lungs in fetal lambs. Pediatric Res 1991;30:62–67.
8. Ivy DD, Kinchella JP, Abman SH. Physiologic characterization of endothelia A and B receptor activity in the ovine fetal lung. J Clin Invest 1994;93:2141–8.
9. Rudolph AM, Heymann MA, Lewis AB. Physiology and pharmacology of the pulmonary circulation in the fetus and newborn. In: Hodson W (ed) Development of the Lung. NY: Marcel Dekker, 1977:497–523.
10. Morin FC, Egan EA, Ferguson W, Lundgren CEG. Development of pulmonary vascular response to oxygen. Am J Physiol 1988;254:H542–6.
11. Abman SH, Chatfield BA, Rodman DM, Hall SL, McMurtry IF. Maturation-related changes in endothelium-dependent relaxation of ovine pulmonary arteries. Am J Physiol 1991;260:L280–5.
12. North AJ, Star RA, Brannon TS, Ujiie K, Wells LB, Lowenstien CJ, Snyder SH, Shaul PW. NO synthase type I and type III gene expression are developmentally regulated in rat lung. Am J Physiol 1994;266:L635–41.
13. Halbower AC, Tuder RM, Franklin WA, Pollock JS, Forstermann U, Abman SH. Maturation-related changes in endothelial NO synthase immunolocalization in the developing ovine lung. Am J Physiol 1994;267:L585–91.
14. Parker TA, Le Cras TD, Kinsella JP, Abman SH. Developmental changes in endothelial NO synthase expression in the ovine fetal lung. Am J Physiol 2000;278:L202–8.
15. Kinsella JP, Ivy DD, Abman SH. Ontogeny of NO activity and response to inhaled NO in the developing ovine pulmonary circulation. Am J Physiol 1994;267:H1955–61.
16. Sherman TS, Chen Z, Yuhanna IS, Lau KS, Margraf LR, Shaul PW. NO synthase isoform expression in the developing lung epithelium. Am J Physiol 1999;276:L383.
17. Rairhig R, Ivy DD, Kinsella JP, Abman SH. Inducible NOS inhibitors increase pulmonary vascular resistance in the late-gestation fetus. J Clin Invest 1998;101:15–21.
18. Tzao C, Nickerson PA, Russell JA, Noble B, Steinhorn RM. Heterogeneous distribution of type I NOS in pulmonary vasculature of ovine fetus. Histochem Cell Biol 2000; 114:421–30.
19. Rairigh RL, Storme L, Parker TA, Le Cras TD, Jakkula M, Abman SH. Role of neuronal nitric oxide synthase in regulation of vascular and ductus arteriosus tone in the ovine fetus. Am J Physiol Lung Cell Mol Physiol 2000;278: L105–10.
20. Rairigh RL, Parker TA, Ivy DD, Kinsella JP, Fan I, Abman SH. Role of inducible nitric oxide synthase in the transition of the pulmonary circulation at birth. Circ Res 2001;88:721–6.
21. Abman SH, Kinsella JP, Parker TA, Storme L, Le Cras TD. Physiologic roles of NO in the perinatal pulmonary circulation. In: Weir EK, Archer SL, Reeves JT. Fetal and Neonatal Pulmonary Circulation. NY: Futura, 1999:239–60.
22. Parker TA, Kinsella JP, Galan HL, Richter G, Abman SH. Prolonged infusions of estradiol dilate the ovine fetal pulmonary circulation. Pediatr Res 2000;47:89–96.
23. Parker TA, Afshar S, Kinsella JP, Ivy DD, Shaul PW, Abman SH. Effects of chronic estrogen receptor blockade on the

pulmonary circulation in the late gestation ovine fetus. Am J Physiol. Heart Circ Physiol 2001;281:H1005–14.

24. MacRitchie AN, Jun SS, Chen Z *et al.* Estrogen upregulates endothelial NO synthase gene expression in fetal pulmonary artery endothelium. Circ Res 1997;81:355–62.

25. Grover TR, Parker TA, Zenge JP, Markham NE, Abman SH. VEGF inhibition impairs endothelial function and causes pulmonary hypertension in the late gestation ovine fetus. Am J Physiol 2002;284:L508–17.

26. Hanson KA, Burns F, Rybalkin SD, Miller J, Beavo J, Clarke WR. Developmental changes in lung cGMP phosphodiesterase-5 activity, protein and message. Am J Resp Crit Care Med 1995;158:279–88.

27. Cohen AH, Hanson K, Morris K, Fouty B, McMurtry IF, Clarke W, Rodman DM. Inhibition of cGMP-specific phosphodiesterase selectively vasodilates the pulmonary circulation in chronically hypoxic rats. J Clin Invest 1996; 97:172–9.

28. Tzao C *et al.* Paracrine role of soluble guanylate cyclase and type III nitric oxide synthase in ovine fetal pulmonary circulation: a double labeling immunohistochemical study. Histochem Cell Biol 2003;119:125–30.

29. Thusu KG, Morin FC, Russell JA *et al.* The cGMP phosphodiesterase inhibitor zaprinast enhances the effect of NO. Am J Respir Crit Care Med 1995;152:1605–10.

30. Ziegler JW, Ivy DD, Fox JJ, Kinsella JP, Clarke WR, Abman SH. Dipyridamole, a cGMP phosphodiesterase inhibitor, causes pulmonary vasodilation in the ovine fetus. Am J Physiol 1995;269:H473.

31. Accurso FJ, Alpert B, Wilkening RB, Petersen RG, Meschia G. Time-dependent response of fetal pulmonary blood flow to an increase in fetal oxygen tension. Respir Physiol 1986; 63:43–52.

32. Abman SH, Accurso FJ. Acute effects of partial compression of the ductus arteriosus on the fetal pulmonary circulation. Am J Physiol 1989;257:H626–34.

33. Abman SH, Accurso FJ. Sustained fetal pulmonary vasodilation during prolonged infusion of atrial natriuretic factor and 8-bromo-guanosine monophosphate. Am J Physiol 1991;260:H183–92.

34. Meininger GA, Davis MJ. Cellular mechanisms involved in the vascular myogenic response. Am J Physiol 1992;263: H647–59.

35. Kulik TJ, Evans JN, Gamble WJ. Stretch-induced contraction in pulmonary arteries. Am J Physiol 1988;255:H1191–8.

36. Belik J, Stephens NL. Developmental differences in vascular smooth muscle mechanics in pulmonary and systemic circulations. J Appl Physiol 1993;74:682–7.

37. Storme L, Rairhig RL, Abman SH. In vivo evidence for a myogenic response in the ovine fetal pulmonary circulation. Pediatr Res 1999;45:425–31.

38. Tourneux P, Chester M, Grover T, Abman SH. Fasudil inhibits the myogenic response in the fetal pulmonary circulation. Am J Physiol 2008;295(4):H1505–13.

39. Leffler CW, Hessler JR, Green RS. Mechanism of stimulation of pulmonary prostacyclin synthesis at birth. Prostaglandins 1984;28:877–87.

40. Leffler CW, Tyler TL, Cassin S. Effect of indomethacin on pulmonary vascular response to ventilation of fetal goats. Am J Physiol 1978;234:H346–51.

41. Campbell WB, Harder DR. Prologue: EDHF what is it? Am J Physiol 2001;280:H2413–6.

42. Storme L, Rairigh RL, Parker TP, Cornfield DN, Kinsella JP, Abman SH. Potassium channel blockade attenuates shear stress-induced pulmonary vasodilation in the ovine fetus. Am J Physiol 1999;276:L220–8.

43. Cornfield DN, Reeves HL, Tolarova S, Weir EK, Archer S. Oxygen causes fetal pulmonary vasodilation through activation of a calcium-dependent potassium channel. Proc Natl Acad Sci USA 1996;93:8089–94.

44. Soifer LTs Soifer SJ, Loitz RD, Roman C, Heymann MA. Leukotriene end organ antagonists increase pulmonary blood flow in fetal lambs. Am J Physiol 1985;249:570.

45. Yanagisawa M, Kurihara H, Kimura S *et al.* A novel potent vasoconstrictor peptide produced by vascular endothelial cells. Nature 1988;332:411–5.

46. Boulanger C, Luscher TF. Release of endothelin from the porcine aorta. Inhibition by endothelium-derived nitric oxide. J Clin Invest 1990;85:587–90.

47. Ivy DD, Abman SH. Role of endothelin in perinatal pulmonary vasoregulation. In: Weir EK, Archer SL, Reeves JT. Fetal and Neonatal Pulmonary Circulation. NY: Futura, 1999:279–302.

48. Chatfield BA, McMurtry IF, Hall SL, Abman SH. Hemodynamic effects of endothelin-1 on the ovine fetal pulmonary circulation. Am J Physiol 1991;261:R182–7.

49. Ivy DD, Kinsella JP, Abman SH. Physiologic characterization of endothelin A and B receptor activity in the ovine fetal lung. J Clin Invest 1996;93:2141–8.

50. Ivy DD, Parker TA, Abman SH. Prolonged endothelin B receptor blockade causes pulmonary hypertension in the ovine fetus. Am J Physiol 2000;279:L758–65.

51. Archer SL, Huang JMC, Hampl V, Nelson DP, Shultz PJ, Weir EK. NO and cGMP cause vasorelaxation by activation of a charybdotoxin-sensitive K channel by cGMP-dependent protein kinase. Proc Natl Acad Sci USA 1994;91:7583–7.

52. Rhodes MT, Porter VA, Saqueton CB, Herron JM, Resnik ER, Cornfield DN. Pulmonary vascular response to normoxia and Kca channel activity is developmentally regulated. Am J Physiol 2001;280:L1250–7.

53. Tristani-Firouzi M, Martin EB, Tolarova S *et al.* Ventilation-induced pulmonary vasodilation at birth is modulated by potassium channel activity. Am J Physiol 1996;271: H2353–9.

54. Konduri GG, Mital S, Gervasio CT, Rotta AT, Forman K. Purine nucleotides contribute to pulmonary vasodilation caused by birth-related stimuli in the ovine fetus. Am J Physiol 1997;272:H2377–84.

55. Fagan KA, Fouty BW, Tyler RC, Morris KG, Helper LK, Sato K, LeCras TD, Abman SH, Weinberger HD, Huang PL, McMurtry IF, Rodman DM. The pulmonary circulation of mice with either homozygous or heterozygous disruption of endothelial NO synthase is hyper-responsive to chronic hypoxia. J Clin Invest 1999;103:291–9.

56. Steudel W, Scherrer-Crosbie M, Bloch KD, Weiman J, Huang PL, Jones RC, Picard MH, Zapol WM. Sustained pulmonary hypertension and right ventricular hypertrophy after chronic hypoxia in mice with congenital deficiency of NOS III. J Clin Invest 1998;101:2468–77.

57. Kinsella JP, McQueston JA, Rosenberg AA, Abman SH. Hemodynamic effects of exogenous nitric oxide in ovine transitional pulmonary circulation. Am J Physiol 1992;263: H875–80.

58. Geggel R, Reid LM. The structural basis for PPHN. Clin Perinatol 1984;11:525–49.

59. Murphy J, Aronovitz M, Reid L. Effects of chronic in utero hypoxia on the pulmonary vasculature of the newborn guinea pig. Pediatr Res 1986;20:292–5.

60. Levin DL, Hyman AI, Heymann MA, Rudolph AM. Fetal hypertension and the development of increased pulmonary vascular smooth muscle: a possible mechanism for persistent pulmonary hypertension of the newborn infant. J Pediatr 1978;92:265–9.

61. Morin III FC, Eagan EA. The effect of closing the ductus arteriosus on the pulmonary circulation of the fetal sheep. J Dev Physiol 1989;11:245–50.

62. Abman SH, Accurso FJ. Acute effects of partial compression of ductus arteriosus on fetal pulmonary circulation. Am J Physiol Heart Circ Physiol 1989;26:H626–34.

63. Storme L, Rairigh RL, Parker TA, Kinsella JP, Abman SH. Acute intrauterine pulmonary hypertension impairs endothelium dependent vasodilation in the ovine fetus. Pediatr Res 1999;45:575–81.

64. Villamor E, LeCras TD, Horan MP, Halbower AC, Tuder RM, Abman SH. Chronic intrauterine pulmonary hypertension impairs endothelial nitric oxide synthase in the ovine fetus. Am J Physiol Lung Cell Mol Physiol 1997;272: L1013–20.

65. Shaul PW, Yuhanna IS, German Z, Chen Z, Steinhorn RH, Morin III FC. Pulmonary endothelial NO synthase gene expression is decreased in fetal lambs with pulmonary hypertension. Am J Physiol Lung Cell Mol Physiol 1997; 272:L1005–12.

66. McQueston JA, Kinsella JP, Ivy DD, McMurtry IF, Abman SH. Chronic pulmonary hypertension in utero impairs endothelium-dependent vasodilation. Am J Physiol Heart Circ Physiol 1995;268:H288–94.

67. Farrow KN, Lakshminrusimha S, Reda WJ, Wedgwood S, Czech L, Gugino SF, Davis JM, Russell JA, Steinhorn RH. Superoxide dismutase restores eNOS expression and function in resistance pulmonary arteries from neonatal lambs with persistent pulmonary hypertension. Am J Physiol Lung Cell Mol Physiol 2008;295(6):L979–87.

68. Hanson KA, Abman SH, Clarke WR. Elevation of pulmonary PDE5-specific activity in an experimental fetal ovine perinatal pulmonary hypertension model. Pediatr Res 1996;39:334A.

69. Steinhorn RH, Russell JA, Morin III FC. Disruption of cyclic GMP production in pulmonary arteries isolated from fetal lambs with pulmonary hypertension. Am J Physiol Heart Circ Physiol 1995;268:H1483–9.

70. Tzao C, Nickerson PA, Russell JA, Gugino SF, Steinhorn RH. Pulmonary hypertension alters soluble guanylate cyclase activity and expression in pulmonary arteries isolated from fetal lambs. Pediatr Pulmonol 2001;31:97–105.

71. Brennan LA, Steinhorn RH, Wedgwood S, Mata-Greenwood E, Roark EA, Russell JA, Black SM. Increased superoxide generation is associated with pulmonary hypertension in fetal lambs. A role for NADPH oxidase. Circ Res 2003; 92:683–91.

72. Rosenberg AA, Kennaugh J, Koppenhafer SL, Loomis M, Chatfield BA, Abman SH. Elevated immunoreactive endothelin-1 levels in newborn infants with persistent pulmonary hypertension. J Pediatr 1993;123:109–14.

73. Ivy DD, Le Cras TD, Horan MP, Abman SH. Increased lung preproET-1 and decreased ETB-receptor gene expression in fetal pulmonary hypertension. Am J Physiol 1998;274 (4 Pt 1):L535–41.

74. Ivy DD, Ziegler JW, Dubus MF, Fox JJ, Kinsella JP, Abman SH. Chronic intrauterine pulmonary hypertension alters endothelin receptor activity in the ovine fetal lung. Pediatr Res 1996;39:435–42.

75. Ivy DD, Parker TA, Ziegler JW, Galan HL, Kinsella JP, Tuder RM, Abman SH. Prolonged endothelin A receptor blockade attenuates pulmonary hypertension in the ovine fetus. J Clin Invest 1997;99:1179–86.

76. Fike CD, Slaughter JC, Kaplowitz MR, Zhang Y, Aschner JL. Reactive oxygen species from NADPH oxidase contribute to altered pulmonary vascular responses in piglets with chronic hypoxia-induced pulmonary hypertension. Am J Physiol Lung Cell Mol Physiol 2008;295(5):L881–8.

77. Konduri GG, Ou J, Shi Y, Pritchard KA, Jr. Decreased association of HSP90 impairs endothelial nitric oxide synthase in fetal lambs with persistent pulmonary hypertension. Am J Physiol Heart Circ Physiol 2003;285(1): H204–11.

78. Wedgwood S, Steinhorn RH, Bunderson M, Wilham J, Lakshminrusimha S, Brennan LA, Black SM. Increased hydrogen peroxide downregulates soluble guanylate cyclase in the lungs of lambs with persistent pulmonary hypertension of the newborn. Am J Physiol Lung Cell Mol Physiol 2005;289(4):L660–66. Epub 2005; Jun 2003.

79. Konduri GG, Bakhutashvili I, Eis A, Pritchard KA. Oxidant stress from uncoupled nitric oxide synthase impairs vasodilation in fetal lambs with persistent pulmonary hypertension. Am J Physiol Heart Circ Physiol 2007;292: H1812–20.

80. Wedgwood S, Black SM. Role of reactive oxygen species in vascular remodeling associated with pulmonary hypertension. Antioxid Redox Signal 2003;5(6):759–69.

81. Lakshminrusimha S, Russell JA, Wedgwood S, Gugino SF, Kazzaz JA, Davis JM, Steinhorn RH. Superoxide dismutase improves oxygenation and reduces oxidation in neonatal pulmonary hypertension. Am J Respir Crit Care Med 2006;174(12):1370–77. Epub 2006; Sep 1328.

82. Farrow KN, Groh BS, Schumacker PT, Lakshminrusimha S, Czech L, Gugino SF, Russell JA, Steinhorn RH. Hyperoxia increases phosphodiesterase 5 expression and activity in

ovine fetal pulmonary artery smooth muscle cells.
Circ Res 2008;102(2):226–33.

83. Faraci F, Didion S. Vascular protection: superoxide
dismutase isoforms in the vessel wall. Arterioscler Thromb
Vasc Biol 2004;24:1367–73.

84. Balasubramaniam V, Le Cras TD, Ivy DD, Kinsella J, Grover
TR, Abman SH. Role of platelet-derived growth factor in
the pathogenesis of perinatal pulmonary hypertension.
Am J Physiol Lung Cell Mol Physiol 2003;284(5):L826–33.

85. Chambers CD, Hernandez-Diaz S, Van Marter LJ, Werler
MM, Louik C, Jones KL, Mitchell AA. Selective serotonin-
reuptake inhibitors and risk of persistent pulmonary
hypertension of the newborn. N Engl J Med 2006;354(6):
579–87.

86. Fornaro E, Li D, Pan J, Belik J. Prenatal exposure to
fluoxetine induces fetal pulmonary hypertension in the rat.
Am J Respir Crit Care Med 2007;176(10):1035–40.

87. Levin DL, Heymann MA, Kitterman JA, Gregory GA, Phibbs
RH, Rudolph AM. Persistent pulmonary hypertension of the
newborn. J Pediatr 1976;89:626–33.

88. Kinsella JP, Abman SH. Recent developments in the
pathophysiology and treatment of persistent pulmonary
hypertension of the newborn. J Pediatr 1995;126(6):853–64.

89. Walsh-Sukys MC, Tyson JE, Wright LL, Bauer CR, Korones
SB, Stevenson DK, Verter J, Stoll BJ, Lemons JA, Papile LA,
Shankaran S, Donovan EF, Oh W, Ehrenkranz RA, Fanaroff
AA. Persistent pulmonary hypertension of the newborn in
the era before nitric oxide: practice variation and
outcomes. Pediatr 2000;105:14–20.

90. Van Marter LJ, Leviton A, Allred EN. PPHN and smoking and
aspirin and nonsteroidal antiinflammatory drug
consumption during pregnancy. Pediatrics 1996;97:658–63.

91. Alano MA, Ngougmna E, Ostrea EM, Jr., Konduri GG. Analysis
of nonsteroidal antiinflammatory drugs in meconium and its
relation to persistent pulmonary hypertension of the
newborn. Pediatrics 2001;107(3):519–23.

92. Pearson DL, Dawling S, Walsh WF, Haines JL, Christman
BW, Bazyk A, Scott N, Summar ML. Neonatal pulmonary
hypertension-urea-cycle intermediates, nitric oxide
production, and carbamoyl-phosphate synthetase function.
N Engl J Med 2001;344(24):1832–8.

93. Abman SH, Kinsella JP. Inhaled nitric oxide for persistent
pulmonary hypertension of the newborn: The physiology
matters. Pediatrics 1995;96:1153–5.

94. UK Collaborative ECMO Trial Group. UK collaborative
randomised trial of neonatal extracorporeal membrane
oxygenation. Lancet 1996;348:75–82.

95. Patterson K, Kapur SP, Chandra RS. PPHN: pulmonary
pathologic effects. In: Rosenberg HS, Berstein J, eds.
Cardiovascular diseases, Perspectives in Pedatric Pathology.
Vol 12. Basel: Karger; 1988:139–154.

96. Kinsella JP, Abman SH. Clinical approach to inhaled NO
therapy in the newborn. J Pediatr 2000;136:717–26.

97. Acute Respiratory Distress Syndrome Network. Ventilation
with lower tidal volumes as compared with traditional tidal
volumes for acute lung injury and the ARDS. N Engl J Med
2000;342:1301–8.

98. Gordon JB, Martinez FR, Keller PA, Tod ML, Madden JA.
Differing effects of acute and prolonged alkalosis on
hypoxic pulmonary vasoconstriction. Am Rev Resp Dis
1993;148:1651–6.

99. Laffey JG, Engelberts D, Kavanaugh BP. Injurious effects of
hypocapnic alkalosis in the isolated lung. Am J Respir Crit
Care Med 2000;162:399–405.

100. Lotze A, Mitchell BR, Bulas DI, Zola EM, Shalwitz RA,
Gunkel JH. Multicenter study of surfactant (beractant) use
in the treatment of term infants with severe respiratory
failure. Survanta in Term Infants Study Group. J Pediatr
1998;132:40–7.

101. Clark RH, Kueser TJ, Walker MW, Southgate WM, Huckaby
JL, Perez JA, Roy BJ, Keszler M, Kinsella JP. Low dose nitric
oxide therapy for persistent pulmonary hypertension of the
newborn. N Engl J Med 2000;342:469–74.

102. Davidson D, Barefield ES, Kattwinkel J, Dudell G, Damask
M, Straube R, Rhines J, Chang C. Inhaled nitric oxide for
the early treatment of persistent pulmonary hypertension
of the term newborn: a randomized, double-masked,
placebo-controlled, dose–response, multicenter study.
Pediatrics 1998;101:325–34.

103. Kinsella JP, Shaffer E, Neish SR, Abman SH. Low-dose
inhalational nitric oxide in persistent pulmonary
hypertension of the newborn. Lancet 1992;340:819–20.

104. Kinsella JP, Truog WE, Walsh WF, Goldberg RN, Bancalari E,
Maylock DE, Redding GJ, deLemos RA, Sardesai S,
McCurnin DC, Moreland SG, Cutter GR, Abman SH.
Randomized, multicenter trial of inhaled nitric oxide and
high–frequency oscillatory ventilation in severe, persistent
pulmonary hypertension of the newborn. J Pediatr
1997;131:55–62.

105. Neonatal Inhaled Nitric Oxide Study Group. Inhaled nitric
oxide in full-term and nearly full-term infants with
hypoxic respiratory failure. N Engl J Med 1997;336:
597–604.

106. Roberts JD, Fineman J, Morin III FC, Shaul PW, Rimar S,
Schreiber MD, Polin RA, Thusu KG, Zayek M, Zwass MS,
Zellers TM, Wylam ME, Gross I, Zapol WM, Heymann MA.
Inhaled nitric oxide and persistent pulmonary hypertension
of the newborn. N Engl J Med 1997;336:605–10.

107. Konduri GG, Solimani A, Sokol GM, Singer J, Ehrenkranz RA,
Singhal N, Wright LL, Van Meurs K, Stork E, Kirpalani H,
Peliowski A, Group NINOS. A randomized trial of early
versus standard inhaled nitric oxide therapy in term and
near–term newborn infants with hypoxic respiratory
failure. Pediatrics 2004;113:559–64.

108. Roberts JD, Polaner DM, Lang P, Zapol WM. Inhaled nitric
oxide in persistent pulmonary hypertension of the
newborn. Lancet 1992;340:818–9.

109. Goldman AP, Tasker RC, Haworth SG, Sigston PE, Macrae
DJ. Four patterns of response to inhaled nitric oxide for
persistent pulmonary hypertension of the newborn.
Pediatrics 1996;98:706–13.

110. Lakshminrusimha S, Russell JA, Steinhorn RH, Ryan RM,
Gugino SF, Morin FC, 3rd, Swartz DD, Kumar VH. Pulmonary
arterial contractility in neonatal lambs increases with

100 percent oxygen resuscitation. Pediatr Res 2006;59(1): 137–41. Epub 2005 Dec 2002.

111. Lakshminrusimha S, Russell JA, Steinhorn RH, Swartz DD, Ryan RM, Gugino SF, Wynn KA, Kumar VH, Mathew B, Kirmani K, Morin FC, 3rd. Pulmonary hemodynamics in neonatal lambs resuscitated with 21 percent, 50 percent, and 100 percent oxygen. Pediatr Res 2007;62:313–8.

112. Ziegler JW, Ivy DD, Wiggins JW, Kinsella JP, Clarke WR, Abman SH. Effects of dipyridamole and inhaled nitric oxide in pediatric patients with pulmonary hypertension. Am J Resp Crit Care Med 1998;158:1388–95.

113. Atz AM, Wessel DL. Sildenafil ameliorates effects of inhaled nitric oxide withdrawal. Anesthesiology 1999;91:307–10.

114. Ichinose F, Erana-Garcia J, Hromi J, Raveh Y, Jones R, Krim L, Clark MWH, Winkler JD, Bloch KD, Zapol WM. Nebulized sildenafil is a selective pulmonary vasodilator in lambs with acute pulmonary hypertension. Crit Care Med 2001;29:1000–5.

115. Weimann J, Ullrich R, Hromi J, Fujino Y, Clark MWH, Bloch KD, Zapol WM. Sildenafil is a pulmonary vasodilator in awake lambs with acute pulmonary hypertension. Anesthesiology 2000;92:1702–12.

116. Shekerdemian L, Ravn H, Penny D. Intravenous sildenafil lowers pulmonary vascular resistance in a model of neonatal pulmonary hypertension. Am J Respir Crit Care Med 2002;165:1098–2002.

117. Shekerdemian LS, Ravn HB, Penny DJ. Interaction between inhaled nitric oxide and intravenous sildenafil in a porcine model of meconium aspiration syndrome. Pediatr Res 2004;55(3):413–8. Epub 2004; Jan 2007.

118. Baquero H, Soliz A, Neira F, Venegas ME, Sola A. Oral sildenafil in infants with persistent pulmonary hypertension of the newborn: a pilot randomized blinded study. Pediatrics 2006;117(4):1077–83.

119. Steinhorn RH, Kinsella JP, Butrous G, Dilleen M, Oakes M, Wessel DL. Open-Label, Multicentre, Pharmacokinetic Study of IV Sildenafil in the Treatment of Neonates With Persistent Pulmonary Hypertension of the Newborn (PPHN). Circulation 2007;116:II-614.

120. Kelly LK, Porta NF, Goodman DM, Carroll CL, Steinhorn RH. Inhaled prostacyclin for term infants with persistent pulmonary hypertension refractory to inhaled nitric oxide. J Pediatr 2002;141:830–2.

121. McNamara PJ, Laique F, Muang-In S, Whyte HE. Milrinone improves oxygenation in neonates with severe persistent pulmonary hypertension of the newborn. J Crit Care 2006;21(2):217–22.

PART 12

PULMONARY CIRCULATION IN CRITICAL CARE

Effects of mechanical ventilation on the pulmonary circulation

MICHAEL R PINSKY

INTRODUCTION

Both spontaneous and positive-pressure ventilation can profoundly alter cardiovascular function, pulmonary blood flow and ultimately gas exchange through processes that are complex and difficult to understand by superficial bedside inspection. However, clinicians usually focus on the immediate hemodynamic effects of initiating mechanical ventilation because the cardiovascular changes often occur rapidly with the institution of mechanical ventilation and serve as the basis for specific treatment algorithms (1).

The hemodynamic effects of positive-pressure ventilation on cardiac output have been known since positive-pressure ventilation was first introduced over sixty years ago (2). However, our understanding of the interactions between ventilation and pulmonary blood flow is still evolving. The boundaries of these interactions are defined by the determinants of both cardiovascular and pulmonary performance.

Positive-pressure breathing alters the pulmonary circulation by two different but related aspects of ventilation, changes in lung volume and changes in ITP. Changes in lung volume appear to be more important for the pulmonary circulation, whereas changes in ITP appear to be more relevant to the systemic circulation. The basic concepts that underpin the effects of mechanical ventilation on the pulmonary circulation are: (1) while lung volume increases primarily during inspiration, it may be kept at a volume greater than normal with the application of increased end-expiratory airway pressure to either recruit collapsed lung units and/or over-distend others; and (2) the increase in

ITP during inspiration produces a decrease in venous return, thereby uncoupling pulmonary blood flow changes with alveolar ventilation. The dynamic changes in lung volume also alter regional pulmonary vascular compliance and resistance. These complex and often counter-balancing effects may seem overwhelming when taken in the aggregate, but if isolated become understandable and allow reconstruction later in different clinical conditions.

RELATION BETWEEN AIRWAY PRESSURE, ALVEOLAR PRESSURE, PLEURAL PRESSURES AND LUNG VOLUME DURING MECHANICAL VENTILATION

Airway and alveolar pressure

The hemodynamic effects of positive-pressure ventilation are often considered relative to changes in Paw (3,4). Lung distention is a function of both increases in the transpulmonary pressure gradient, defined as the difference between P_A and Ppl, and lung compliance, which is both non-linear and non-homogeneous throughout the lung and is subject to rapid change over time. The relation between changes in Paw with changes in both Ppl and lung volume varies as ventilatory patterns, airway resistance and lung compliance change. Additionally, changes in Paw do not accurately reflect changes in Ppc, a primary determinant of transmural LV pressure. With dynamic hyperinflation, end-expiratory Paw will underestimate P_A.

Even stop-flow end-expiratory Paw measures will underestimate P_A if air trapping exists. However, mean Paw is a remarkably good estimate of mean P_A under normal conditions and with acute lung injury, even when airway resistance is increased accordingly (5,6), mean Paw is a useful parameter when determining whether a specific ventilatory pattern is causing lung volume to increase relative to end-expiratory values.

Airway pressure, lung volume and regional pleural pressures

During positive-pressure inspiration, transpulmonary pressure and lung volume increase in parallel with increasing Paw. Since changes in Paw are related to changes in lung volume through the interaction of airway resistance and both lung and chest compliances, directionally similar changes in both Paw and Ppl occur during inspiration.

Lung expansion pushes the chest wall outward, the diaphragm downward and the cardiac fossa in upon itself, increasing lateral wall, diaphragmatic, juxtacardiac Ppl, and Ppc. The degree of increase on each of these surfaces in response to lung expansion will be a function of the compliance and inertance of their opposing structures, specifically the chest wall, diaphragm-abdominal contents, and heart, respectively. Novak et al. (7) demonstrated that the changes in Ppl induced by positive-pressure ventilation are not similar in all regions of the thorax, and increase differently as inspiratory flow rate and frequency increase (Figure 24.1.1). Diaphragmatic Ppl increases least during positive-pressure inspiration, while juxtacardiac Ppl increases most. Since the diaphragm is very compliant, it seems reasonable that diaphragmatic Ppl should increase less than lateral chest wall Ppl with sudden increases in lung volume. However, if abdominal distention develops, as commonly occurs in the setting of sepsis, the diaphragm will become relatively non-compliant because of the increase in abdominal pressure. Under these

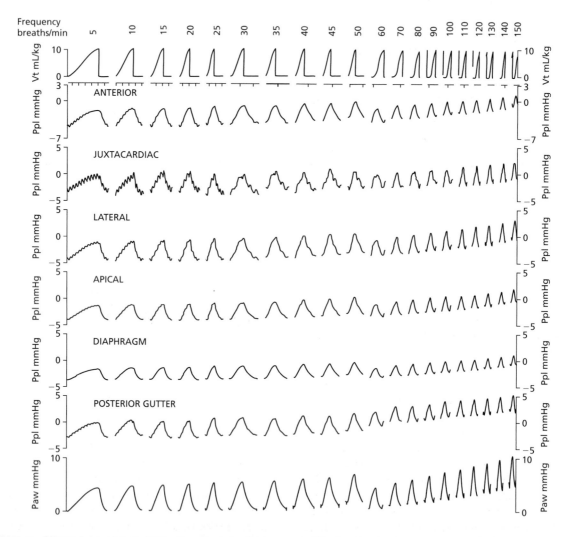

Figure 24.1.1 Effect of changing ventilatory frequency on airway pressure (Paw) and regional pleural pressure (Ppl) at vital volume (Vt) = 10 mL/kg and a 50 percent inspiratory time for one animal. Note that end-expiratory Ppl increases in all regions as frequency increases and that the rate of increase among regions is similar despite their different baseline end-expiratory values. (From Novak et al. J Appl Physiol 1988;65:1314–23.)

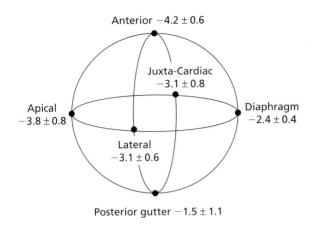

Figure 24.1.2 Apneic pleural pressure (Ppl) (mean ± SE) in Torr for six pleural regions of the right hemithorax of an intact supine canine model: ANT, anterior; AP, apical; PG, posterior gutter; DI, diaphragmatic; JC, juxtacardiac; and LAT, lateral. Ellipses, regional measurements defining three orthogonal planes. (After Novak *et al.* J Appl Physiol 1988;65:1314–23.)

conditions Paw will increase for an unchanged tidal breath, without any change in lung parenchymal compliance (7). This distinction is important because increasing Paw to overcome chest wall stiffness should further increase Ppl, producing greater hemodynamic consequences, but would not improve gas exchange since the alveoli are not damaged nor is the lung over-distended.

In the supine subject, apneic Ppl along the horizontal plane from apex to diaphragm are similar, whereas anterior Ppl is lower and posterior gutter Ppl is greater. This gravitational Ppl gradient is the major reason for the greater distention of non-dependent lung regions compared with dependent regions. P_A is similar in all alveoli, whereas the opposing Ppl varies along its hydrostatic gradient (Figure 24.1.2). Hydrostatic gradients also alter absolute Ppa and Ppv values. Thus, the difference between Ppa and P_A decreases in non-dependent regions, and increases in dependent ones.

Airway pressure, regional pleural pressure and pericardial pressure

Pinsky and Guimond (8) demonstrated that the induction of heart failure was associated with a greater increase in Ppc than in juxtacardiac Ppl. With progressive increases in positive end-expiratory pressure (PEEP) juxtacardiac Ppl increased toward values similar to no PEEP Ppc levels, whereas Ppc initially remained constant. Once these two surface pressures became equal, further increases in PEEP increased both juxtacardiac Ppl and Ppc in parallel (Figure 24.1.3). Thus, if pericardial volume restraint exists, juxtacardiac Ppl will underestimate Ppc and have minimal effects of both pulmonary outflow (pulmonary arterial) and inflow (pulmonary venous) pressures. However, with sustained lung compression of the heart, both juxtacardiac Ppl and Ppc appear to be similar and both pulmonary

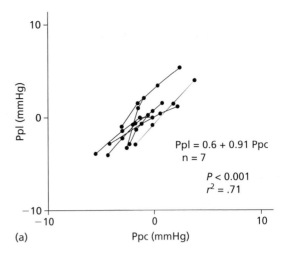

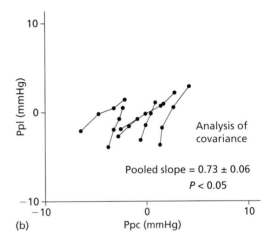

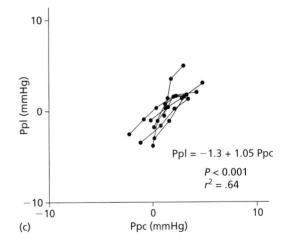

Figure 24.1.3 (a) Shows relationship between Ppc and juxtacardiac Ppl at 0, 5, 10 and 15 cmH$_2$O PEEP in the control condition. Individual data points for the four levels of PEEP in the same dog are connected. (b) Shows the effects of increase in PEEP on the relationship between Ppc and Ppl during acute ventricular failure. (c) Shows the effect of increase in PEEP on the relationship between Ppc and Ppl during acute ventricular failure and lung injury. (Reproduced with permission from Pinsky & Guimond. J Crit Care 1991;6:1–11.)

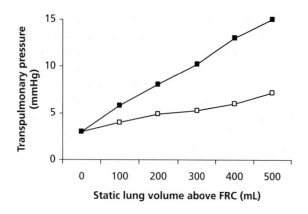

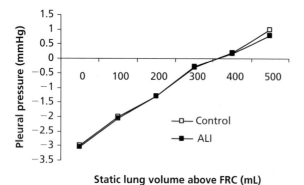

Figure 24.1.4 Relation between airway pressure (Paw) and tidal volume (Vt) and between pleural pressure (Ppl) and Vt in control and oleic acid-induced acute lung injury (ALI) conditions in a canine model. Note that despite greater increases in Paw for the same Vt during ALI as compared to control conditions, Ppl and Ppc increase similarly during both control and ALI conditions for the same increase in Vt. (After Romand J, Shi W, Pinsky MR. Cardiopulmonary effects of positive pressure ventilation during acute lung injury. Chest 1995;108(4):1041–8.)

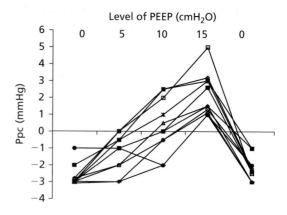

Figure 24.1.5 Relation between pericardial pressure (Ppc) and airway pressure as apneic levels of positive end-expiratory pressure (PEEP) were progressively increased from zero to 15 cmH₂O and then back to zero in 5 cmH₂O increments in patients immediately following open heart surgery. Note that although Ppc increases in all subjects as PEEP is increased from 0 to 15 cmH₂O, the initial Ppc value and the proportional change in Ppc among incremental increases in PEEP are quite different among subject, such that no specific proportion of airway pressure transmission to the pericardial surface can be assumed to occur in all patients. (After Pinsky *et al.* Am Rev Respir Dis 1991;143:25–31.)

arterial and venous pressure increase. For more details, see Figures 24.1.4, 24.1.5 and refs 9–22.

HEMODYNAMIC EFFECTS OF CHANGES IN LUNG VOLUME

Changes in lung volume alter autonomic tone and its influence on pulmonary vascular resistance. Furthermore, at high lung volumes, the expanded lungs mechanically compress the heart in the cardiac fossa limiting cardiac filling. Each of these processes is important in assessing the pulmonary vascular response to mechanical ventilation.

Autonomic tone

The lungs are richly innervated with integrated somatic and autonomic fibers that originate, traverse through, and end in the thorax. These neuronal networks mediate multiple homeostatic processes through the autonomic nervous system.

They alter, for example, both instantaneous cardiovascular function, such as respiratory sinus arrhythmia, and steady-state cardiovascular status, such as anti-diuretic hormone-induced fluid retention. See refs 23–46.

Pulmonary vascular resistance and hypoxic pulmonary vasoconstriction

Lung volume is a major determinant of pulmonary vascular resistance, and extrinsic processes to the lungs, such as a humoral or sympathetic tone changes, are not required to induce the changes in pulmonary vascular resistance seen with ventilation (20,47–51). Lung inflation, independent of changes in ITP, primarily affects the pulmonary circulation by altering both pulmonary vascular resistance and the downstream pressure for pulmonary blood flow (52).

RV afterload is the maximal RV systolic wall stress during contraction (53), which, by the Law of LaPlace, is equal to the radius of curvature of the right ventricle (a function of end-diastolic volume) and transmural pressure (a function of systolic RV pressure) (54). Changes in ITP that occur without changing lung volume, as may occur with occluded respiratory efforts, will not affect the pulmonary vascular resistance since the pressure gradients between the RV and pulmonary artery are not altered.

Since the pulmonary artery resides inside the thorax, actual RV ejection pressure and pulmonary arterial pressure (Ppa) reflect pulmonary arterial intraluminal pressure relative to ITP, referred to as transmural Ppa. Transmural Ppa can increase by one of two mechanisms: (1) an increase in pulmonary arterial pressure without an increase in pulmonary vasomotor tone as may occur with either a marked increase in blood flow (exercise) or an increase in outflow pressure (LV failure, high levels of PEEP), or (2) an increase in pulmonary vascular resistance by either active changes in vasomotor tone or lung inflation. An increase in transmural Ppa during positive-pressure ventilation is due to an increase in pulmonary vascular resistance, since neither instantaneous cardiac output (55) nor LV filling (15) usually increases. However, RV ejection will be impeded if transmural Ppa increases (56). Furthermore, if RV emptying is incomplete, not only will stroke volume decrease (57), but its residual volume will increase and limit subsequent filling (55). If RV dilation persists, RV coronary perfusion cannot be sustained across such high wall stresses, and RV free wall ischemia and infarction can develop (58). Thus, acute cor pulmonale is associated with a profound decrease in cardiac output that is usually resistant to therapies designed to enhance venous return (e.g. fluid challenge).

The mechanisms by which pulmonary vasomotor tone varies during mechanical ventilation are complex and include the effects on hypoxic pulmonary vasoconstriction and the mechanical compression of pulmonary capillaries by lung expansion. During normal end-inspiration, mild hypoxemia ($PaO_2 > 65$ mmHg) and low levels (< 7.5 cmH$_2$O) of PEEP have minimal effects of pulmonary vasomotor tone. If these minimal increases in transmural Ppa are sustained, however, fluid retention occurs and results in an increase in RV end-diastolic volume to maintain cardiac output constant despite the increased pulmonary vasomotor tone (54,59).

Local pulmonary vasomotor tone increases and blood flow decreases when regional alveolar PO_2 (P_AO_2) decreases below 60 mmHg (60). Since lung volume is reduced in acute hypoxemic respiratory failure (61,62), pulmonary vascular resistance is often increased owing to alveolar collapse and the resultant hypoxic pulmonary vasoconstriction.

Mechanical ventilation–induced changes in pulmonary vascular resistance

Mechanical ventilation opens collapsed alveolar units, refreshes alveolar gas with higher FiO$_2$, and reverses respiratory acidosis; as a consequence of these effects, mechanical ventilation may reduce pulmonary vasomotor tone (63–69). These effects do not require positive-pressure breaths as much as expansion of collapsed alveoli (70), which is usually accomplished by the addition of PEEP. The beneficial effect of PEEP on pulmonary vascular resistance is greatest in the neonate, where the vascular response to hypoxia is accentuated.

Changes in lung volume can also profoundly increase pulmonary arterial pressure by passively compressing the alveolar vessels (61,67,68). The pulmonary circulation can be separated into two groups of blood vessels depending on the pressure that surrounds them (67) (Figure 24.1.6). The small pulmonary arterioles, venules, and alveolar capillaries sense alveolar pressure as their surrounding pressure and are referred to as alveolar vessels. The large pulmonary arteries and veins, as well as the heart and intrathoracic great vessels of the systemic circulation, sense interstitial pressure or ITP as their surrounding pressure and can be called extra-alveolar vessels. Since increasing lung volume requires transpulmonary pressure to increase and vice versa, the extravascular pressure gradient between alveolar to extra-alveolar vessels varies with changes in lung volume. The radial interstitial forces of the lung (71,72), act upon the extra-alveolar vessels much as they do on the airways: as lung volume increases, the radial interstitial forces increase, increasing the diameter of both extra-alveolar vessels and airways. Thus, just as airway resistance decreases with lung distention, extra-alveolar vessels dilate (73), causing their capacitance to increase and pooling blood in the pulmonary arteries and veins. The opposite condition occurs during deflation and with sustained decreases in lung volume (63,66). Accordingly, pulmonary vascular resistance is increased at small lung volumes owing to the combined effect of hypoxic pulmonary vasoconstriction and extra-alveolar vessel collapse.

Unlike the extra-alveolar vessels whose resistance decreases during lung inflation, alveolar vessels increase their resistance as lung volume progressively increases to levels above resting lung volume or functional residual

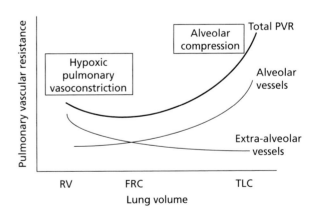

Relation between lung volume and pulmonary vascular resistance

Figure 24.1.6 Schematic diagram of the relation between changes in lung volume and pulmonary vascular resistance, where the extra-alveolar and alveolar vascular components are separated. Note that pulmonary vascular resistance is minimal at resting lung volume or functional residual capacity (FRC). As lung volume increases toward total lung capacity (TLC) or decreases toward residual volume (RV), pulmonary vascular resistance also increases. However, the increase in resistance with hyperinflation is due to increased alveolar vascular resistance, whereas the increase in resistance with lung collapse is due to increased extra-alveolar vessel tone.

capacity (FRC) (63,74). If the cross-sectional area of the pulmonary capillaries is already reduced, the addition of abnormal hyperinflation can create significant pulmonary hypertension and may precipitate acute RV failure (75) and RV ischemia (58). Similarly, if lung volumes are reduced, increasing lung volume back to baseline levels by the use of PEEP decreases pulmonary vascular resistance (76).

PEEP-induced changes in pulmonary blood flow: West zones of the lung and vascular waterfalls

Increases in P_A relative to pulmonary venous pressure also influence pulmonary blood flow. West *et al.* originally described pulmonary blood flow through the alveoli as comprising at least three vascular zones, defined by hydrostatic pressure, vascular pressure and P_A (68) (Figure 24.1.7). When P_A exceeds Ppa there can be no blood flow because downstream pressure exceeds inflow pressure (Zone 1). If Ppa exceeds P_A then blood flow into that region of the lung will occur (Zone 2). Conceptually, one can consider P_A to be the effective backpressure to pulmonary blood flow when $P_A >$ pulmonary venous pressure. This concept has been referred to as the "vascular waterfall" (74) because the flow across these beds will be unaffected by downstream changes in pulmonary venous pressure. However, when pulmonary venous pressure exceeds P_A, the pressure gradient for pulmonary blood flow is defined by the difference between Ppa and pulmonary venous pressure (Zone 3). In the resting supine state with a Ppa of 15/8 mmHg most, if not all of the lung units are in Zone 3 conditions. However, with standing at rest, hyperinflation, or the application of PEEP, Zone 1 and 2 conditions routinely develop (67).

Zone 1 conditions equate to areas of the lung that are ventilated but not perfused. Increasing the amount of lung in Zone 1 conditions increases dead space ventilation,

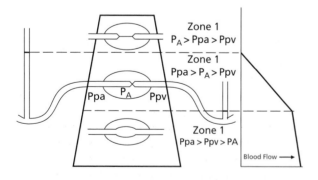

Figure 24.1.7 Schematic representation of the effect of hydrostatic pressure on pulmonary blood flow. Operationally, one can define three unique situations owing to changes in P_A relative to Ppa and Ppv: Zone 1 $P_A >$ Ppa $>$ Ppv, Zone 2 Ppa $> P_A >$ Ppv, Zone 3 Ppa $>$ Ppv $> P_A$. Since these zonal characteristics were first described by West *et al.* they are usually referred to as West Zones, 1, 2 and 3, respectively. (After West *et al.* J Appl Physiol 1964;19:713–24.)

increasing $PaCO_2$ for an unchanged minute ventilation and CO_2 production. This occurs when Ppa decreases, as may occur in hypovolemic shock, or when P_A increases, as would occur with the application of high levels of PEEP. Since an obligatory effect of increasing Zone 1 conditions is to increase $PaCO_2$, a common finding in patients in shock on fixed minute ventilation is hypercarbia. Accordingly, fluid resuscitation by itself often reduces $PaCO_2$, if it results in an increase in pulmonary blood flow and Ppa.

When P_A exceeds pulmonary venous pressure, it becomes the outflow pressure for pulmonary blood flow. Under many clinical conditions P_A may exceed pulmonary venous pressure, as estimated by pulmonary artery occlusion pressure (Ppao). Since the effect of increasing PEEP on pulmonary blood flow is difficult to define in subjects being phasically ventilated and having a phasic RV ejection into the pulmonary circulation, models of isolated perfused lungs allowing one to fix lung distention as various transpulmonary pressures and P_A, as well as constant pulmonary inflow and pulmonary venous pressure levels have been used to simplify this analysis. Lopez-Muniz *et al.* (74) demonstrated in isolated canine lungs with a constant pulmonary inflow rate that increasing pulmonary venous pressure did not alter Ppa until pulmonary venous pressure exceeded P_A, regardless of the level of P_A. Once pulmonary venous pressure exceeded P_A, increases in pulmonary venous pressure further increased Ppa (Figure 24.1.8). Note in Figure 24.1.8 that Ppa is greater than Ppv by an amount equal to the vascular resistance at that moment. As Ppv increases further, the pressure difference between Ppa and Ppv decreases, as more pulmonary vascular units are recruited and pulmonary vascular resistance decreases. Thus, by increasing the outflow pressure, PEEP causes a parallel shift to the left in the pressure flow relationship (Figure 24.1.9). Domino and Pinsky (77) found that the effects of hypoxic pulmonary vasoconstriction and PEEP were complimentary. PEEP did not alter the slope of the pressure flow relation but shifted it leftward. Similarly, hypoxic pulmonary vasoconstriction decreased the slope of the pressure-flow relation but did not alter the zero flow intercept (Figure 24.1.10).

Patients with acute lung injury have complex ventilation-perfusion mismatching due to alveolar flooding, regional hyperinflation and hypoxic pulmonary vasoconstriction. By selectively increasing P_A in aerated lung units, PEEP recruits collapsed lung units by the process of alveolar interdependence. Walther *et al.* (78) demonstrated the application of PEEP in acute lung injury tended to restore a more uniform alveolar ventilation. These data agree with those from chest computed tomography studies (79).

Mechanical ventilation-induced changes in pulmonary vascular capacitance

The lung vasculature is acted upon by a variety of forces which are seldom constant over time. As described above,

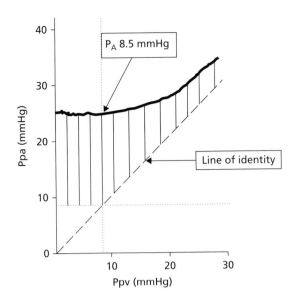

Figure 24.1.8 Effect of increasing Ppv on Ppa at a PEEP of 10 cmH$_2$O in an isolated perfused dog lung at a constant pulmonary flow rate. (After Lopez-Muniz *et al.* J Appl Physiol 1968;24:625–35.)

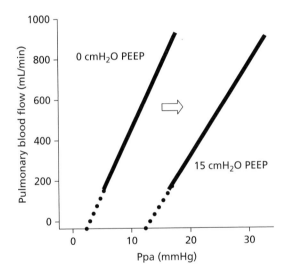

Figure 24.1.9 Effect of 10 cmH$_2$O PEEP the relation between Ppa and pulmonary flow as pulmonary flow is increased. (After data presented in Lopez-Muniz *et al.* J Appl Physiol 1968;24:625–35.)

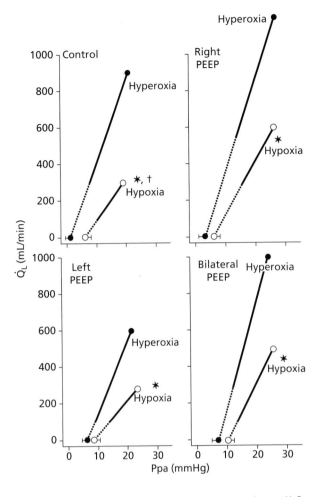

Figure 24.1.10 Effect of unilateral lung hypoxia and 10 cmH$_2$O PEEP on the relation between mean Ppa and pulmonary flow in the dog. (After Domino & Pinsky. Am J Physiol 1990;259:H697–705.)

changes in transpulmonary pressure directly alter the extravascular pressure gradient between alveolar and extra-alveolar vessels. Marked over-distention induces an increased pulmonary vascular resistance due to the increasing transpulmonary pressure relative to pulmonary artery pressure increasing alveolar vessel resistance whereas lung volume collapse by its associated alveolar hypoxia induced extra-alveolar vessel tone to increase by the process of hypoxic pulmonary vasoconstriction. Still, other more dynamic changes in pulmonary vascular state also occur. The effect of changes in lung blood volume during ventilation are considered to be a primary cause of the stroke volume and pulse pressure variation, known as pulsus paradoxus (80,81) and in the evolving role that these changes have in predicting the cardiovascular system's response to volume loading (1,82,83). As lung volume increases owing to the increase in transpulmonary pressure, the radial forces pulling open the airways and making airway resistance low at high lung volumes also increases extra-alveolar vessel radial stretch increasing extra-alveolar vascular capacitance. This must be offset to a certain decrease by the increased transpulmonary pressure causing alveolar capacitance to decrease. Thus, during inspiration (increasing lung volume) pulmonary venous flow may increase, remain constant or decrease depending on the degree to which the alveolar vascular compartments were distended at end-expiration (67). If the alveolar compartments were primarily in Zone 3 conditions, then they would expel their blood into the pulmonary venous circuit. If, however, they were primarily in Zone 2 conditions, then the primary effect of inflation would be to increase extra-alveolar vessel capacitance and pulmonary venous flow would decrease. The documentation of these complex interactions was elegantly described by

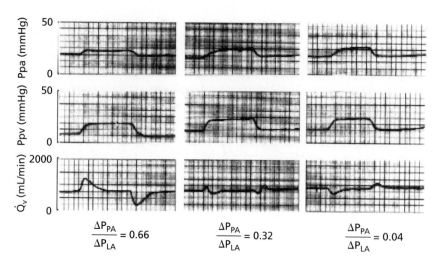

$$\frac{\Delta P_{PA}}{\Delta P_{LA}} = 0.66 \qquad \frac{\Delta P_{PA}}{\Delta P_{LA}} = 0.32 \qquad \frac{\Delta P_{PA}}{\Delta P_{LA}} = 0.04$$

Figure 24.1.11   Representative tracings. Left: inflation in Zone 3 results in a transient increase in Qv. Right: Zone 2 inflation in a transient decrease in Qv. Center: a biphasic change in Qv is observed when lungs are in transition between 2 and 3 Ppa, pulmonary arterial pressure; Palv, alveolar pressure; Qv, pulmonary venous flow; Pla, left atrial pressure. (J Appl Physiol 51985;8:954–63.)

Brower *et al.* (84). Using an isolated canine lung preparation at constant flow, they demonstrated that the global zonal characteristics of the lungs predicted whether pulmonary venous flow increased, remained constant or decreased during inspiration. One can infer the proportion of pulmonary vessels in Zone 3 conditions by examining how inducing a small change in left atrial pressure, estimated by pulmonary artery occlusion pressure causes a similar change in pulmonary artery pressure. If the lung were completely in Zone 3 conditions then all the increase in left atrial pressure would be transmitted to the pulmonary artery pressure. Furthermore, as the amount of Zone 2 conditions increased the degree to which the increase in left atrial pressure increased pulmonary artery pressure would decrease proportionally. An example of the impact of changing Zonal conditions of the dynamic changes in pulmonary venous outflow for a constant tidal volume are illustrated in Figure 24.1.11. Impressively, this dynamic range of flow changes appeared to be linear over the entire range of zonal conditions (Figure 24.1.12).

Ventricular interdependence

Changes in RV output alter LV filling because the two ventricles are linked through the pulmonary vasculature. However, LV preload can also be indirectly altered by changes in RV end-diastolic volume. Similarly, increasing RV outflow impedance will result in a reduced RV stroke volume and RV dilation through an increase in RV end-systolic volume. If RV volume increases, LV diastolic compliance will decrease by the mechanism of ventricular interdependence (85). Increasing RV end-diastolic volume will induce a shift of the intraventricular septum into the LV, thereby decreasing LV diastolic compliance (86) (Figure 24.1.13). Thus, for the same LV filling pressure, LV end-diastolic volume and cardiac output will be decreased. This interaction, known as pulsus paradoxus, is felt to be the major determinant of the phasic changes in arterial pulse pressure and cardiac output seen in cardiac tamponade, and can also be seen in subjects with normal cardiovascular

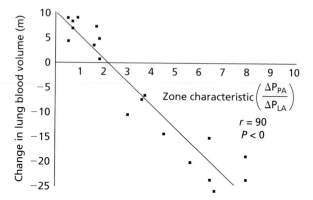

Figure 24.1.12   Series A. Changes in lung blood volume that occurred when lungs were inflated by 10 mmHg. Zone characteristic is an estimate of fraction of lung's alveolar vessels that were in Zone 3; remainder are in Zone 2. Ppa, pulmonary arterial pressure; Pla, left atrial pressure. (J Appl Physiol 1985;58:954–63.)

function during loaded spontaneous inspiration. These phasic changes in LV stroke volume and arterial pulse pressure may reflect ventilation-induced changes in LV filling and can be used to predict preload-responsiveness (1,82,83,87).

By increasing venous return, spontaneous inspiration induces RV dilation that will decrease LV end-diastolic volume. Maintaining a relatively constant rate of venous return, either by volume resuscitation (88), or vasopressor infusion, will minimize this effect. These phasic changes in arterial pressure have also been used as a marker of functional hypovolemia during spontaneous ventilation (1,87).

Mechanical heart–lung interactions

Increases in end-expiratory volume occur in settings of increased expiratory airway resistance such as asthma and chronic obstructive lung disease. Since mechanical ventilation can deliver breaths at almost any Vt, driving pressure and frequency, lung hyperinflation commonly occurs with profound effects on the pulmonary circulation and the heart. The heart can be compressed between the two hyperinflated

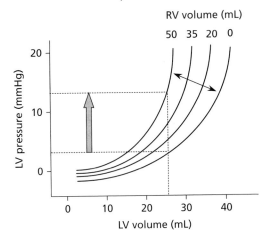

Figure 24.1.13 Schematic diagram of the effect of increasing right ventricular (RV) volumes on the left ventricular (LV) diastolic pressure-volume (filling) relationship. Note that increasing RV volumes decrease LV diastolic compliance, such that a higher filling pressure is required to generate a constant end-diastolic volume. (After Taylor *et al.* Dependence of ventricular distensibility on filling the opposite ventricle. Am J Physiol 1967;213:711–8.)

lungs (89), increasing the pressure surrounding the heart. Since the heart is confined within the cardiac fossa, juxta-cardiac Ppl will increase more than lateral chest-wall or diaphragmatic Ppl (6,17). This compressive effect of the inflated lung can be seen with either spontaneous hyper-inflation (90) or positive-pressure-induced hyperinflation with PEEP (71,72). As Ppc increases, LV distending pressure for a constant LV end-diastolic pressure also decreases. The decrease in "apparent" LV diastolic compliance (88) was previously misinterpreted as impaired LV contractility, because LV stroke work is decreased for a given LV end-diastolic pressure or Ppao (91,92). Numerous studies have shown that when patients are fluid resuscitated to return LV end-diastolic volume to its original level, both LV stroke work and cardiac output also return to their original levels (49,88) despite the continued application of PEEP (93). Takata *et al.* (94) proposed using the terms "coupled" and "uncoupled" pericardial restraint and proposed that peri-cardial stiffness (or elastance) over the right and left ventri-cles is different in constrictive pericarditis but similar in tamponade: in constrictive pericarditis, changes in venous return should selectively alter RV filling, whereas tamponade should alter both RV and LV filling. Using this theoretical framework one may extrapolate to the dynamic effects of ventilation. Tidal increases in lung volume represent "uncou-pled" pericardial restraint because tidal breathing tends to selectively limit RV filling and not LV diastolic compliance. Hyperinflation, however, would produce a "coupled" cardiac fossal restraint. Van den Berg *et al.* (95) found that the instantaneous effect of positive-pressure inspiration was to reduce RV output, while reductions in LV output took several

beats to occur. Sustained increases in Paw induced by apneic PEEP resulted in a parallel reduction in bi-ventricular out-put. Thus, hyperinflation, as occurs in severe asthma and with the use of excessive amounts of PEEP, would produce a clinical picture indistinguishable from tamponade. These findings confirmed those of Rebuck and Read (96) on the hemodynamic effects of severe asthma. Presumably, the shift from "uncoupled" to "coupled" cardiac fossal restraint would occur as absolute lung volume increased, bi-ventricular volume increased, or both. Thus, if cardiac volumes are small and lung inflation does not overdistend the thoracic cage, RV filling will be primarily impeded. However, in congestive heart failure states and with marked lung over distention, both RV and LV filling may be compromised by ventilation.

HEMODYNAMIC EFFECTS OF CHANGES IN INTRATHORACIC PRESSURE

Changes in ITP will affect the pressure gradients for both venous return to the RV and systemic outflow from the LV. Increases in ITP, by increasing right atrial pressure and decreasing transmural LV systolic pressure, will reduce these pressure gradients and thereby decrease intrathoracic blood volume. In the extreme, these spontaneous inspira-tory efforts may precipitate pulmonary edema and arterial hypoxemia. Conversely, decreases in ITP will augment venous return and impede LV ejection, thereby increasing intratho-racic blood volume. In the extreme, these positive-pressure breaths can precipitate hypovolemic cardiovascular collapse.

Systemic venous return

Systemic venous return defines RV filling and is equal to cardiac output in the steady state. As characterized by Guyton *et al.* (97) venous return varies inversely with downstream right atrial pressure in a fashion described by a fixed upstream pressure. Mean circulatory filling pressure is between 7 and 12 mmHg in humans under general anes-thesia (98). Mean systemic pressure does not change rapidly during the ventilatory cycle while right atrial pres-sure (Pra) does, because of the direct influence that con-comitant changes in ITP have on Pra. Accordingly, variations in Pra represent the major factor determining the fluc-tuation in pressure gradient for systemic venous return during ventilation (55,99). Pra increases along with increases in ITP, for example with positive-pressure venti-lation or hyperinflation during mechanical ventilation. As a result, the pressure gradient for systemic venous return decreases, decelerating venous blood flow (57), decreasing RV filling, and consequently, decreasing RV stroke volume (55,57,100–107). During normal spontaneous inspiration, the converse occurs: Pra decreases with decreases in ITP, accelerating venous blood flow and increasing RV filling and RV stroke volume (4,21,57,102,105,108) (Figure 24.1.14).

The decrease in venous return during positive-pressure ventilation may be less than expected based on the above scenario. Since lung volume increase results in diaphragmatic descent, abdominal pressure increases as well. Fessler *et al.* (109) and Takata and Robotham (110) demonstrated in dogs that PEEP-induced increase in abdominal pressure increases the pressure surrounding the intra-abdominal vasculature. Because a large proportion of venous blood is in the abdomen, the net effect of PEEP is to increase both mean systemic pressure and Pra. Accordingly, the pressure gradient for venous return may not be reduced by PEEP, particularly in patients with hypervolemia. Recently, Van den Berg *et al.* demonstrated that the ratio of Pra to abdominal pressure increased little with the application of up to 15 cmH$_2$O PEEP (Figure 24.1.15) (111), and concluded that sustained increases in Paw have minimal effects on venous return when subjects have been adequately fluid resuscitated. With exaggerated swings in ITP, as occur with obstructed inspiratory efforts, venous return behaves as if abdominal pressure is additive to mean systemic pressure in defining total venous blood flow (112–115).

Because inverse ratio ventilation produces substantial degrees of hyperinflation, its hemodynamic effects have been the subject of concern. However, Mang *et al.* (116) found no hemodynamic difference between conventional ventilation and inverse ratio ventilation when total PEEP was similar.

Kim *et al.* (117) recently demonstrated that one could use a sustained end-inspiratory hold maneuver of a small increased airway pressure (e.g. 5 or 10 mmHg) to cause venous return to decrease enough to induce a dynamic decrease in left ventricular end-diastolic volume, thus allowing one to calculate the left ventricular end-systolic pressure-volume relation. Furthermore, Mass *et al.* (118), recently demonstrated that by examining the steady state effects of end-inspiratory hold maneuver, and plotting the new right atrial pressure with the instantaneous steady state cardiac output, one could reconstruct the venous return curve in humans at the bedside with only minimally invasive hemodynamic monitoring (Figure 24.1.16). Thus, these concepts, though described conceptually can more be realized at the bedside of critically ill patients.

Right ventricular filling

Under normal conditions, it is extremely difficult to document that RV filling pressures change as RV filling occurs. When RV filling pressure, defined as Pra minus Ppc, was directly measured in patients undergoing open chest operations, RV filling pressure did not change despite large changes in RV volume (119). Although right atrial pressure increases with volume loading, Ppc also increases and RV filling pressure is unchanged. Similar results are seen when RV volumes are reduced by the application of PEEP in post-operative cardiac patients (120). These data suggest that under normal conditions, RV diastolic compliance is very high and most of the increase in Pra seen during volume loading reflects pericardial compliance and cardiac fossa stiffness rather than changes in RV distending pressure. Presumably, conformational changes in the RV rather than wall stretch are responsible for RV enlargement (16). However, increases in Pra may occur as a result of decreased RV diastolic compliance, increased pericardial compliance, increased end-diastolic volume, or a combination of all three. Since PEEP, and by extension, lung expansion, compresses the heart within the cardiac fossa in a fashion analogous to pericardial tamponade, it is the expanding lungs that increase ITP rather than pericardial restraint, limiting ventricular filling (121,122).

Positive-pressure ventilation impairs normal circulatory adaptive processes operative during spontaneous

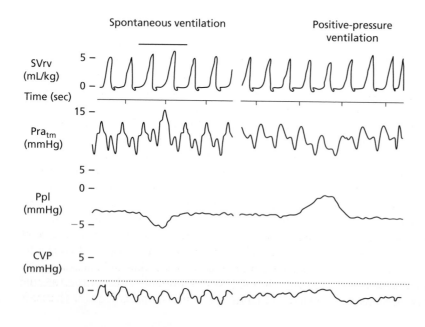

Spontaneous ventilation   Positive-pressure ventilation

SVrv (mL/kg)
Time (sec)
Pra$_{tm}$ (mmHg)
Ppl (mmHg)
CVP (mmHg)

Figure 24.1.14   Continuous trend recording of RV stroke volume (SVrv), transmural Pra, Ppl and Pra during spontaneous ventilation (left panel) and at a similar Vt during positive-pressure ventilation (right panel).

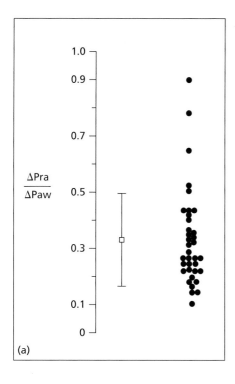

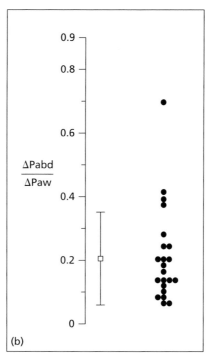

Figure 24.1.15 (a) Relation between change in Pra (ΔPra) to change in Paw (ΔPaw) with the application of 10 cmH$_2$O PEEP. (b) The relation between change in abdominal pressure (ΔPabd) and ΔPaw with the application of 10 cmH$_2$O PEEP. Note that although Paw increases by 10 cmH$_2$O, Pra increases by approximately 70 percent of that value because Pabd increases. (After data reported in Van den Berg P, Jansen JRC, Pinsky MR. The effect of positive-pressure inspiration on venous return in volume loaded post-operative cardiac surgical patients. J Appl Physiol, in press.)

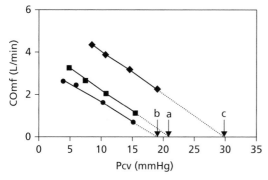

Figure 24.1.16 Assessment of venous return curve and mean systemic filling pressure in postoperative cardiac surgery patients. (Crit Care Med 2009;37:912–8.)

ventilation. Even if one restores the coupling of Pra and RV volume by using partial ventilatory support modes of ventilation, cardiac output will increase only if the RV can convert the increased venous return to forward blood flow. During weaning from mechanical ventilation occult RV failure, manifest by a rapid rise in Pra and a fall in cardiac output, may be exposed. Since the primary effect on normal cardiovascular function of any form of ventilation is to alter RV preload by altering venous return, the detrimental effect of positive-pressure ventilation on cardiac output can be minimized by either fluid resuscitation (4,100,112,113) or by minimizing both mean ITP and swings in lung volume. Prolonging expiratory time, decreasing tidal volume, and avoiding PEEP all minimize the decrease in systemic venous return to the RV (2,55, 102–106,123,124).

Since spontaneous inspiratory efforts increase lung volume by decreasing ITP, one sees an increase in venous

return with spontaneous inspiration owing to the fall in Pra (21,47,103–105). However, this augmentation of venous return is limited (114,115) because if ITP decreases below atmospheric pressure, venous return becomes flow-limited as the large systemic veins collapse upon entering the thorax (97). This venous flow-limitation is a safety valve for the heart because ITP can decrease greatly with obstructive inspiratory efforts (33). If venous return were not flow-limited, the RV could overdistend and fail (125).

LV Preload and ventricular interdependence

In the steady state, changes in venous return must eventually result in directionally similar changes in LV preload, because the two ventricles function in series (126). However, with sustained increases in ITP, only RV output decreases because the intrathoracic blood continues to drain into the left ventricle. This phase delay in changes in output from the RV to the LV is exaggerated if Vt or respiratory rate are increased or intravascular volume is reduced (2,49,50,88,91,92,107,123,127–131). Independent of this series interaction, direct ventricular interdependence can also occur. During positive-pressure ventilation, however, RV volumes are usually decreased, minimizing the influence of ventricular interdependence on LV diastolic performance (85,129–132). Jardin et al. (59,50), using transesophageal echocardiography in ventilator-dependent subjects showed that PEEP did result in some degree of right-to-left intraventricular septal shift, although the amount of this shift was small. Although increases in lung volume during positive-pressure ventilation cause some septal shift, the primary effect of increasing lung volume is to compress the two ventricles into each other, decreasing bi-ventricular volumes (133). Accordingly, the decrease in cardiac output during PEEP is due largely to a decrease in LV end-diastolic volume. Restoration of LV end-diastolic volume by fluid resuscitation returns cardiac output to baseline values (134,135), without any significant change in LV diastolic compliance (88).

LV Afterload

Maximal LV afterload can be equated to the maximal product of LV pressure and volume that represents maximal systolic wall tension. As for the right ventricle, maximal LV wall tension normally occurs at the end of isometric contraction, reflecting both a maximal LV radius of curvature (end-diastolic volume) and aortic pressure (diastolic pressure) product. During ejection, LV volumes decrease rapidly, decreasing LV radius of curvature and LV wall stress. Thus, under normal conditions the left ventricle unloads itself during ejection. When LV dilation exists, as in congestive heart failure, maximal LV wall stress occurs during LV ejection since the maximal product of these two variables occurs later in ejection, owing to the markedly increased radius of curvature and its minimal decrease during ejection. Accordingly, LV afterload varies in its definition depending on the baseline level of cardiac contractility and intravascular volume. See also refs 136–153.

Myocardial energetics and changes in ITP

Increasing LV ejection pressure increases myocardial O_2 demand because stroke work is increased. Since negative swings in ITP increase LV ejection pressure, maneuvers that result in vigorous inspiratory efforts in the setting of airway obstruction (asthma, upper airway obstruction, vocal cord paralysis) or stiff lungs (interstitial lung disease, pulmonary edema and acute lung injury) will selectively increase LV afterload, and have been postulated to be the cause of LV failure and pulmonary edema seen in these conditions (20,33), particularly if LV systolic function is already compromised (154,155). Similarly, removing large negative swings in ITP by either bypassing upper airway obstruction (endotracheal intubation) or instituting mechanical ventilation will selectively reduce LV afterload without significantly decreasing either venous return or cardiac output (4,97,127,156–158). Placing patients in cardiogenic pulmonary edema on mechanical ventilation, for example, will rapidly reverse the pulmonary edema by decreasing intrathoracic blood volume. Furthermore, in the setting of acute cor pulmonale, negative swings in ITP will selectively increase LV afterload without increasing coronary perfusion pressure, setting up a lethal spiral of worsening RV over-distention and ischemia.

HEMODYNAMIC EFFECTS OF VENTILATION BASED ON CARDIOPULMONARY STATUS

Mechanical ventilatory support can be lifesaving for patients with markedly increased work of breathing, hypervolemia, or impaired LV pump function because of its ability to support the cardiovascular system while decreasing global O_2 demand, independent of changes in gas exchange. However, mechanical ventilation may rapidly induce cardiovascular instability by increasing pulmonary vascular resistance and impeding venous return in patients with hypovolemia or a strong tendency to develop hyperinflation. Similarly, withdrawal of ventilatory support can be an exercise stress test in patients with limited cardiovascular reserve (154,155).

The hemodynamic differences between modes of mechanical ventilation at a constant airway pressure and PEEP can be explained solely by their differential effects on lung volume and ITP (159). If two different modes of ventilation induce similar changes in ITP and ventilatory effort, their hemodynamic effects will also be similar despite markedly different airway waveforms. When partial ventilatory support with either IMV or pressure support ventilation were matched for similar Vt in 20 patients following cardiac surgery, the hemodynamic responses were similar (160). Sternberg and Sahebjami (161) showed that switching from assist-control to either IMV and pressure-support ventilation produced similar effects on tissue oxygenation. Finally, high frequency jet ventilation does not affect cardiac output in patients with heart failure, even if the ventilation is delivered synchronous with the cardiac cycle (162).

Acute lung injury

Positive-pressure ventilation decreases intrathoracic blood volume in proportion to the increase in lung volume (103), and PEEP potentiates this effect (120,122) without directly altering LV contractile function (163). Singer et al. (164) demonstrated that the degree of hyperinflation, not mean Paw, determined the decrease in cardiac output in critically ill patients. For more details, see refs 165–176.

One major problem with treating ALI patients with increasing levels of mean Paw is that pulmonary outflow pressure may also increase, impeding RV ejection. Schmitt et al. studied the impact of increasing PEEP on RV outflow impedance (177) the phasic equivalent of pulmonary vasomotor tone that relates dynamic changes in pulmonary inflow (RV stroke volume) to systolic Ppa. Since increasing outflow impedance occurs when pulmonary vasomotor tone increases or greater proportions of the lung are in Zone 2 conditions (increased critical closing pressure), they studied two levels of PEEP in 16 patients with acute lung injury: one level of PEEP equaled the pressure at the lower inflection point, presumably where lung recruitment started, and the other level at a higher level of PEEP associated with the highest lung compliance, presumably where most lung recruitment occurred. They demonstrated that, compared to zero end-expiratory Paw, both levels of PEEP decreased cardiac output and increased RV outflow impedance, but was significantly less when PEEP was titrated upward to the maximal lung compliance level. Thus, lung recruitment and increases in Paw play major roles in determining RV output impedance. Based on this study it appears that increasing PEEP in subjects with acute lung injury may both increase pulmonary input impedance by overdistention of the lung and reduce it by recruiting collapsed alveolar units. Since RV input impedance is a primary determinant of cardiac output, ventilatory strategies that limit its increase would be preferred. Accordingly, pressure-limited ventilatory strategies aimed at ventilating patients from the point of their maximal lung compliance should have the least detrimental effects on hemodynamics while simultaneously improving arterial oxygenation.

Congestive heart failure

As a general rule, when PEEP increases cardiac output, hypoxic pulmonary vasoconstriction has been reversed or LV afterload has been reduced. Clinically, increases in cardiac output with the institution of positive-pressure ventilation suggest the presence of congestive heart failure (158,178). Grace and Greenbaum (156) noted that adding PEEP to patients with heart failure either did not decrease cardiac output or actually increased cardiac output if Ppao exceeded 18 mmHg in patients with cardiogenic pulmonary edema. Unfortunately, PEEP may be detrimental in patients with combined heart failure and acute lung injury, and can result in increased leukocyte retention in human lungs (180) which may reflect endothelial injury (181), or the effects of stasis of pulmonary blood produced by increasing P_A relative to Ppa. For further details, see Figure 24.1.17 and refs 182–191.

Chronic obstructive pulmonary disease

The primary hemodynamic problem seen in patients with chronic airflow obstruction is related to hyperinflation, either due to loss of lung parenchyma or dynamic hyperinflation (intrinsic PEEP) and increased work of breathing. Intrinsic PEEP alters hemodynamic function in a manner similar to extrinsic PEEP. Furthermore, matching intrinsic PEEP with externally applied PEEP has no measurable detrimental hemodynamic effect (192–194) although it decreases the work cost of spontaneous breathing. Furthermore, like PEEP, CPAP has little detrimental effect in these patients when delivered below the intrinsic level of PEEP (195). There is little hemodynamic difference between increasing airway pressure to generate a breath and decreasing extrathoracic pressure (iron lung-negative pressure

ventilation). Ambrosino et al. (196) used negative pressure ventilation to augment ventilation in patients with chronic airflow obstruction and, not surprisingly, found no differences in hemodynamic response with similar Vt levels.

Weaning of patients with chronic airflow obstruction can tax the cardiovascular system because of the increased metabolic demand that spontaneous breathing extracts in these patients. Patients with severe chronic airflow obstruction may go into cardiogenic pulmonary edema during weaning despite adequate weaning parameters (155), owing to both volume overload and reduced LV ejection fraction (197). Mohsenifar et al. assessed the effect of weaning on gastric pHi, as a marker of splanchnic blood flow, in 29 ventilated patients deemed ready for weaning (5). Patients who could not be weaned had a substantially reduced gastric intramucosal pH (pHi) from 7.36 during intermittent positive-pressure ventilation to 7.09 during weaning. Patients who were successfully weaned showed no change in pHi (7.45 to 7.46). Jubran et al. (181) examined the cardiac output and arterio-venous O_2 difference in patients with chronic airflow obstruction during weaning trials. All subjects demonstrated an increase in cardiac output, consistent with the increased metabolic demands of spontaneous ventilation. However, those who failed to wean had an associated increase in the arterio-venous O_2 difference consistent with an impaired circulatory response to the increase metabolic demand. Thus, occult cardiovascular insufficiency may play a major role in the development of failure to wean in critically ill patients (198).

SUMMARY

Positive-pressure breathing alters the pulmonary circulation primarily by two different but related aspects of ventilation, changes in lung volume and changes in ITP. Changes in lung volume appear to be more important for the pulmonary circulation, whereas changes in ITP appear to be more relevant to the system circulation. Increasing lung volume increases pulmonary inflow impedance by increasing Ppa. The primary cause of increasing Ppa during inflation is increased alveolar collapse owing to overdistention pulmonary and increased P_A relative to Ppa. To the extent that recruitment decreases hypoxic pulmonary vasoconstriction, then pulmonary vascular conductance, the reciprocal of vascular resistance, will increase.

The basic concepts that underpin these physiological effects of mechanical ventilation on the pulmonary circulation are: (1) that lung volume increases not only during inspiration, but may be kept at a volume greater than normally existent because of the application of increased end-expiratory airway pressure; and (2) that positive-pressure inspiration is associated with an increase in ITP and its associated decrease in venous return, thus uncoupling pulmonary blood flow changes with alveolar ventilation.

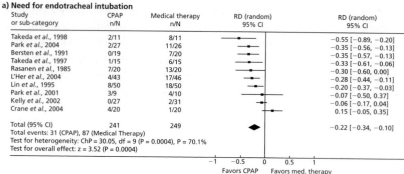

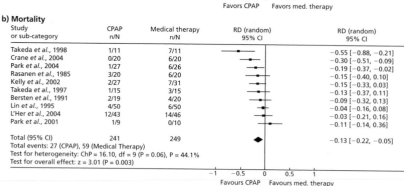

c) Acute myocardial infarction

Study or sub-category	CPAP n/N	Medical therapy n/N	RD (random) 95% CI	RD (random) 95% CI
Crane et al., 2004	3/20	6/20		−0.15 [−0.40, 0.10]
Park et al., 2004	0/27	0/26		0.00 [−0.07, 0.07]
Park et al., 2001	1/9	0/10		0.11 [−0.14, 0.36]
Total (95% CI)	56	56		−0.01 [−0.13, 0.11]

Total events: 27 (CPAP), 59 (Medical Therapy)
Test for heterogeneity: ChP = 2.99, df = 2 (P = 0.22), P = 33.2%
Test for overall effect: z = 0.11 (P = 0.91)

−1   −0.5   0   0.5   1
Favours CPAP   Favours med. therapy

Figure 24.1.17 Efficacy and safety of non-invasive ventilation in the treatment of acute cardiogenic pulmonary edema – a systematic review and meta-analysis. (Crit Care 2006; 10:R69–78.)

KEY POINTS

- End-inspiratory and end-expiratory hold Paw values reflect matched ventilatory cycle P_A values, while mean Paw values reflect mean P_A values.
- It is inaccurate and potentially dangerous to assume a constant fraction of Paw transmission to the pleural surface as a means of calculating Ppl.
- Hyperinflation, as occurs in severe asthma and with the use of excessive amounts of PEEP, may produce a clinical picture indistinguishable from cardiac tamponade.
- Positive-pressure ventilation, by uncoupling Pra from RV filling, impairs the normal adaptive mechanisms by which venous return is coupled to RV output.

REFERENCES

- = Key primary paper
◆ = Major review article
* = Management guideline

•1. Michard F, Chemla D, Richard C, Wysocki M, Pinsky MR, Lecarpentier Y, Teboul JL. Clinical use of respiratory changes in arterial pulse pressure to monitor the hemodynamic effects of PEEP. Am J Respir Crit Care Med 1999;159: 935–9.

*2. Cournaud A, Motley HL, Werko L et al. Physiologic studies of the effect of intermittent positive-pressure breathing on cardiac output in man. Am J Physiol 1948;152:162–74.

*3. Milic-Emili J, Mead J, Turner JM. Improved method for assessing the validity of the esophageal balloon technique. J Appl Physiol 1964;19:207–11.

*4. Braunwald E, Binion JT, Morgan WL, Sarnoff SJ. Alterations in central blood volume and cardiac output induced by positive-pressure breathing and counteracted by metraminol (Aramine). Circ Res 1957;5:670–5.

•5. Kim HK, Alhammouri MT, Mokhtar YM, Pinsky MR. Estimating left ventricular contractility using inspiratory-hold maneuvers. Intensive Care Med 2007;33:181–9.

6. Fuhrman BR, Smith-Wright DL, Venkataraman S, Orr RA, Howland DF. Proximal mean airway pressure: a good estimator of mean alveolar pressure during continuous positive-pressure breathing. Crit Care Med 1989;17: 666–70.

7. Novak RA, Matuschak GM, Pinsky MR. Effect of ventilatory frequency on regional pleural pressure. J Appl Physiol 1988;65:1314–23.

◆8. Pinsky, MR, Guimond JG. The effects of positive end-expiratory pressure on heart–lung interactions. J Crit Care 1991;6:1–11.

9. Romand JA, Shi W, Pinsky MR. Cardiopulmonary effects of positive-pressure ventilation during acute lung injury. Chest 1995;108:1041–8.

•10. O'Quinn RJ, Marini JJ, Culver BH et al. Transmission of airway pressure to pleural pressure during lung edema and chest wall restriction. J Appl Physiol 1985;59:1171–7.

11. Gattinoni, L, Mascheroni D, Torresin A, Fumagalli R, Vesconi S, Rossi GP, Rossi F, Baglioni S, Bassi F, Nastri G, Persenti A. Morphological response to positive end-expiratory pressure in acute respiratory failure. Intensive Care Med 1986;12:137–42.

12. Globits S, Burghuber OC, Koller J, Schenk P, Frank H, Grimm M, End A, Glogar D, Imhof H, Klepetko W. Effect of lung transplantation on right and left ventricular volumes and function measured by magnetic resonance imaging. Am J Respir Crit Care Med 1994;149:1000–4.

13. Scharf SM, Ingram Jr RH. Effects of decreasing lung compliance with oleic acid on the cardiovascular response to PEEP. Am J Physiol 1977;233:H635–41.

14. Pinsky MR, Vincent JL, DeSmet JM. Estimating left ventricular filling pressure during positive end-expiratory pressure in humans. Am Rev Respir Dis 1991;143:25–31.

•15. Buda AJ, Pinsky MR, Ingels NB et al. Effect of intrathoracic pressure on left ventricular performance. N Engl J Med 1979;301:453–9.

16. Kingma I, Smiseth OA, Frais MA, Smith ER, Tyberg JV. Left ventricular external constraint: relationship between pericardial, pleural and esophageal pressures during positive end-expiratory pressure and volume loading in dogs. Ann Biomed Eng 1987;15:331–46.

17. Tsitlik JE, Halperin HR, Guerci AD, Dvorine LS, Popel AS, Siu CO, Yin FCP, Weisfeldt ML. Augmentation of pressure in a vessel indenting the surface of the lung. Ann Biomed Eng 1987;15:259–84.

18. Marini JJ, Rodriguez RM, Lamb V. The inspiratory workload of patient-initiated mechanical ventilation. Am Rev Respir Dis 1986;134:902–9.

•19. Teboul JL, Pinsky MR, Mercat A, Nadia A, Bernardin G, Achard J-M, Boulain T, Richard, C. Estimating cardiac filling pressure in mechanically ventilated patients with hyperinflation. Crit Care Med 2000;28:3631–6.

◆20. Bromberger-Barnea B. Mechanical effects of inspiration on heart functions: a review. Fed Proc 1981;40:2172–7.

◆21. Wise RA, Robotham JL, Summer WR. Effects of spontaneous ventilation on the circulation. Lung 1981;159:175–92.

◆22. Pinsky MR. Breathing as exercise: the cardiovascular response to weaning from mechanical ventilation. Intensive Care Med 2000;26:1164–6.

∗23. Glick G, Wechsler AS, Epstein DE. Reflex cardiovascular depression produced by stimulation of pulmonary stretch receptors in the dog. J Clin Invest 1969;48:467–72.

24. Painal AS. Vagal sensory receptors and their reflex effects. Physiol Rev 1973;53:59–88.

∗25. Anrep GV, Pascual W, Rossler R. Respiratory variations in the heart rate. I. The reflex mechanism of the respiratory arrhythmia. Proc R Soc Lond B Biol Sci 1936;119:191–217.

26. Taha BH, Simon PM, Dempsey JA, Skatrud JB, Iber C. Respiratory sinus arrhythmia in humans: an obligatory role for vagal feedback from the lungs. J Appl Physiol 1995;78:638–45.

27. Bernardi L, Calciati A, Gratarola A, Battistin I, Fratino P, Finardi G. Heart rate-respiration relationship: computerized method for early detection of cardiac autonomic damage in diabetic patients. Acta Cardiol 1986;41:197–206.

28. Bernardi L, Keller F, Sanders M, Reddy PS, Griffith B, Meno F, Pinsky MR. Respiratory sinus arrhythmia in the totally dennervated human heart. J Appl Physiol 1989; 67:1447–55.

29. Persson MG, Lonnqvist PA, Gustafsson LE. Positive end-expiratory pressure ventilation elicits increases in endogenously formed nitric oxide as detected in air exhaled by rabbits. Anesthesiology 1995;82:969–74.

30. Cassidy SS, Eschenbacher WI, Johnson Jr RL. Reflex cardiovascular depression during unilateral lung hyperinflation in the dog. J Clin Invest 1979;64:620–6.

31. Daly MB, Hazzledine JL, Ungar A. The reflex effects of alterations in lung volume on systemic vascular resistance in the dog. J Physiol (London) 1967;188:331–51.

◆32. Shepherd JT. The lungs as receptor sites for cardiovascular regulation. Circulation 1981;63:1–10.

•33. Stalcup SA, Mellins RB. Mechanical forces producing pulmonary edema in acute asthma. N Engl J Med 1977;297:592–6.

34. Vatner SF, Rutherford JD. Control of the myocardial contractile state by carotid chemo- and baroreceptor and pulmonary inflation reflexes in conscious dogs. J Clin Invest 1978;63:1593–601.

35. Pick RA, Handler JB, Murata GH, Friedman AS. The cardiovascular effects of positive end-expiratory pressure. Chest 1982;82:345–50.

36. Said SI, Kitamura S, Vreim C. Prostaglandins: Release from the lung during mechanical ventilation at large tidal ventilation. J Clin Invest 1972;51:83a.

37. Bedetti C, Del Basso P, Argiolas C, Carpi A. Arachidonic acid and pulmonary function in a heart–lung preparation of guinea-pig. Modulation by PCO_2. Arch Int Pharmacodyn Ther 1987;285:98–116.

38. Berend N, Christopher KL, Voelkel NF. Effect of positive end-expiratory pressure on functional residual capacity: Role of prostaglandin production. Am Rev Respir Dis 1982;126:641–7.

39. Pattern MY, Liebman PR, Hetchman HG. Humorally mediated decreases in cardiac output associated with positive end-expiratory pressure. Microvasc Res 1977;13:137–44.

40. Berglund JE, Halden E, Jakobson S, Svensson J. PEEP ventilation does not cause humorally mediated cardiac output depression in pigs. Intensive Care Med 1994;20:360–4.

41. Fuhrman BP, Everitt J, Lock JE. Cardiopulmonary effects of unilateral airway pressure changes in intact infant lambs. J Appl Physiol 1984;56:1439–48.

42. Payen DM, Brun-Buisson CJL, Carli PA, Huet Y, Leviel F, Cinotti L, Chiron B. Hemodynamic, gas exchange, and hormonal consequences of LBPP during PEEP ventilation. J Appl Physiol 1987;62:61–70.

43. Frage D, de la Coussaye JE, Beloucif S, Fratacci MD, Payen DM. Interactions between hormonal modifications during peep-induced antidiuresis and antinatriuresis. Chest 1995;107:1095–100.

44. Frass M, Watschinger B, Traindl O, Popovic R, Podolsky A, Gisslinger H, Flager S, Golden M, Schuster E, Leithner C. Atrial natriuretic peptide release in response to different positive end-expiratory pressure levels. Crit Care Med 1993;21:343–7.

45. Wilkins MA, Su XL, Palayew MD, Yamashiro Y, Bolli P, McKenzie JK, Kryger MH. The effects of posture change and continuous positive airway pressure on cardiac natriuretic peptides in congestive heart failure. Chest 1995;107:909–15.

46. Shirakami G, Magaribuchi T, Shingu K, Suga S, Tamai S, Nakao K, Mori K. Positive end-expiratory pressure ventilation decreases plasma atrial and brain natriuretic peptide levels in humans. Anesth Analg 1993;77:1116–21.

*47. Brecher GA, Hubay CA. Pulmonary blood flow and venous return during spontaneous respiration. Circ Res 1955;3: 210–4.

48. Goldstein JA, Vlahakes GJ, Verrier ED. The role of right ventricular systolic dysfunction and elevated intrapericardial pressures in the genesis of low output in experimental right ventricular infarction. Circulation 1982;65:513–20.

•49. Jardin F, Farcot JC, Boisante L. Influence of positive end-expiratory pressure on left ventricular performance. N Engl J Med 1981;304:387–92.

50. Jardin FF, Farcot JC, Gueret P, Prost JF, Ozier Y, Bourdarias JP. Echocardiographic evaluation of ventricles during continuous positive-pressure breathing. J Appl Physiol 1984;56:619–27.

51. Prec KJ, Cassels DE. Oximeter studies in newborn infants during crying. Pediatrics 1952;9:756–61.

◆52. Luce JM. The cardiovascular effects of mechanical ventilation and positive end-expiratory pressure. J Am Med Assoc 1984;252:807–811.

*53. Maughan WL, Shoukas AA, Sagawa K, Weisfeldt ML. Instantaneous pressure–volume relationships of the canine right ventricle. Circ Res 1979;44:309–15.

54. Sibbald WJ, Driedger AA. Right ventricular function in disease states: pathophysiologic considerations. Crit Care Med 1983;11:339.

55. Pinsky MR. Instantaneous venous return curves in an intact canine preparation. J Appl Physiol 1984;56:765–71.

56. Piene H, Sund T. Does pulmonary impedance constitute the optimal load for the right ventricle? Am J Physiol 1982;242: H154–60.

•57. Pinsky MR. Determinants of pulmonary arterial flow variation during respiration. J Appl Physiol 1984;56:1237–45.

58. Johnston WE, Vinten-Johansen J, Shugart HE, Santamore WP. Positive end-expiratory pressure potentates the severity of canine right ventricular ischemia–reperfusion injury. Am J Physiol 1992;262:H168–76.

59. Sibbald WJ, Calvin J, Driedger AA. Right and left ventricular preload, and diastolic ventricular compliance: implications of therapy in critically ill patients. In: Critical Care State of the Art, Vol. 3. Fullerton, CA: Society of Critical Care, 1982.

60. Madden JA, Dawson CA, Harder DR. Hypoxia-induced activation in small isolated pulmonary arteries from the cat. J Appl Physiol 1985;59:113–18.

*61. Hakim TS, Michel RP, Chang HK. Effect of lung inflation on pulmonary vascular resistance by arterial and venous occlusion. J Appl Physiol 1982;53:1110–15.

62. Quebbeman EJ, Dawson CA. Influence of inflation and atelectasis on the hypoxic pressure response in isolated dog lung lobes. Cardiovas Res 1976;10:672–7.

•63. Hakim TS, Michel RP, Minami H, Chang K. Site of pulmonary hypoxic vasoconstriction studied with arterial and venous occlusion. J Appl Physiol 1983;54:1298–302.

64. Marshall BE, Marshall C. A model for hypoxic constriction of the pulmonary circulation. J Appl Physiol 1988;64:68–77.

*65. Marshall BE, Marshall C. Continuity of response to hypoxic pulmonary vasoconstriction. J Appl Physiol 1980;49:189–96.

66. Dawson CA, Grimm DJ, Linehan JH. Lung inflation and longitudinal distribution of pulmonary vascular resistance during hypoxia. J Appl Physiol 1979;47:532–6.

*67. Howell JBL, Permutt S, Proctor DF et al. Effect of inflation of the lung on different parts of the pulmonary vascular bed. J Appl Physiol 1961;16:71–6.

•68. West JB, Dollery CT, Naimark A. Distribution of blood flow in isolated lung; relation to vascular and alveolar pressures. J Appl Physiol 1964;19:713–24.

69. Fuhrman BP, Smith-Wright DL, Kulik TJ, Lock JE. Effects of static and fluctuating airway pressure on the intact, immature pulmonary circulation. J Appl Physiol 1986;60:114–22.

70. Thorvalson J, Ilebekk A, Kiil F. Determinants of pulmonary blood volume. Effects of acute changes in airway pressure. Acta Physiol Scand 1985;125:471–9.

•71. Hoffman EA, Ritman EL. Heart–lung interaction: effect on regional lung air content and total heart volume. Ann Biomed Eng 1987;15:241–57.

72. Olson LE, Hoffman EA. Heart–lung interactions determined by electron beam X-ray CT in laterally recumbent rabbits. J Appl Physiol 1995;78:417–27.

73. Grant BJB, Lieber BB. Compliance of the main pulmonary artery during the ventilatory cycle. J Appl Physiol 1992; 72:535–42.

•74. Lopez-Muniz R, Stephens NL, Bromberger-Barnea B, Permutt S, Riley RL. Critical closure of pulmonary vessels analyzed in terms of Starling resistor model. J Appl Physiol 1968;24:625–35.

75. Block AJ, Boyson PG, Wynne JW. The origins of cor pulmonale, a hypothesis. Chest 1979;75:109–14.

76. Canada E, Benumnof JL, Tousdale FR. Pulmonary vascular resistance correlated in intact normal and abnormal canine lungs. Crit Care Med 1982;10:719–23.

77. Domino KB, Pinsky MR. Effect of positive end-expiratory pressure on hypoxic pulmonary vasoconstriction in the dog. Am J Physiol 1990;259:H697–705.

78. Walther SM, Domino KB, Glenny RW, Hlasala MP. Positive end-expiratory pressure redistributes perfusion to dependent lung regions in supine but not in prone lambs. Crit Care Med 1999;27:37–45.

♦79. Gattinoni L, Caironi P, Pelosi P, Goodman LR. What has computed tomography taught us about the acute respiratory distress syndrome? Am J Respir Crit Care Med 20001;164:1701–11.

80. Cahoon D, Michael I, Johnson V. Respiratory modifications of the cardiac output. Am J Physiol 1941;133:642–50.

81. Shuler R, Ensor C, Gunning R, Moss W, Johnson V. The differential effects of respiration on the left and right ventricles. Am J Physiol 1942;137:620–7.

•82. Michard F, Boussat S, Chemla D, Anguel N, Mercat A, Lecarpentier Y, Richard C, Pinsky MR, Teboul J-L. Relation between respiratory changes in arterial pulse pressure and fluid responsiveness in septic patients with acute circulatory failure. Am J Respir Crit Care Med 2000;162: 134–8.

83. Monnet X, Rienzo M, Osman D, Anguel N, Richard C, Pinsky MR, Teboul JL. Esophageal Doppler monitoring predicts fluid responsiveness in critically ill ventilated patients. Intensive Care Med 2005;31:1195–201.

•84. Brower R, Wise RA, Hassapoyannes C, Bromberger-Barnea B, Permutt S. Effect of lung inflation on lung blood volume and pulmonary venous flow. J Apply Physiol 1985;58:954–63.

*85. Taylor RR, Corell JW, Sonnenblick EH, Ross Jr J. Dependence of ventricular distensibility on filling the opposite ventricle. Am J Physiol 1967;213:711–8.

86. Brinker JA, Weiss I, Lappe DL et al. Leftward septal displacement during right ventricular loading in man. Circulation 1980;61:626–33.

♦87. Michard F, Teboul JL. Using heart–lung interactions to assess fluid responsiveness during mechanical ventilation. Crit Care 2000;4:282–9.

88. Marini JJ, Culver BN, Butler J. Mechanical effect of lung distention with positive-pressure on cardiac function. Am Rev Respir Dis 1980;124:382–6.

♦89. Butler J. The heart is in good hands. Circulation 1983;67: 1163–8.

90. Cassidy SS, Wead WB, Seibert GB, Ramanathan M. Changes in left ventricular geometry during spontaneous breathing. J Appl Physiol 1987;63:803–11.

91. Cassidy SS, Robertson CH, Pierce AK et al. Cardiovascular effects of positive end-expiratory pressure in dogs. J Appl Physiol 1978;4:743–9.

92. Conway CM. Hemodynamic effects of pulmonary ventilation. Br J Anaesth 1975;47:761–6.

93. Berglund JE, Halden E, Jakobson S, Landelius J. Echocardiographic analysis of cardiac function during high PEEP ventilation. Intensive Care Med 1994;20: 174–80.

94. Takata M, Harasawa Y, Beloucif S, Robotham JL. Coupled vs. uncoupled pericardial restraint: effects on cardiac chamber interactions. J Appl Physiol 1997;83:1799–813.

95. Van den Berg P, Pinsky MR, Grimbergen CA, Spaan JE. Positive-pressure ventilation differentially alters right and left ventricular outputs in post-operative cardiac surgery patients. J Crit Care 1997;12:56–65.

96. Rebuck AS, Read J. Assessment and management of severe asthma. Am J Med 1971;51:788–92.

•97. Guyton AC, Lindsey AW, Abernathy B et al. Venous return at various right atrial pressures and the normal venous return curve. Am J Physiol 1957;189:609–15.

98. Goldberg HS, Rabson J. Control of cardiac output by systemic vessels: circulatory adjustments of acute and chronic respiratory failure and the effects of therapeutic interventions. Am J Cardiol 1981;47:696.

*99. Kilburn KH. Cardiorespiratory effects of large pneumo-thorax in conscious and anesthetized dogs. J Appl Physiol 1963;18:279–83.

100. Chevalier PA, Weber KC, Engle JC et al. Direct measurement of right and left heart outputs in Valsalva-like maneuver in dogs. Proc Soc Exper Biol Med 1972;139:1429–37.

*101. Guntheroth WC, Gould R, Butler J et al. Pulsatile flow in pulmonary artery, capillary and vein in the dog. Cardio-vascular Res 1974;8:330–7.

•102. Guntheroth WG, Morgan BC, Mullins GL. Effect of respiration on venous return and stroke volume in cardiac tamponade. Mechanism of pulsus paradoxus. Circ Res 1967; 20:381–90.

♦103. Guyton AC. Effect of cardiac output by respiration, opening the chest, and cardiac tamponade. In: Circulatory Physiology: Cardiac Output and its Regulation. Philadelphia, PA: Saunders, 1963:378–86.

•104. Holt JP. The effect of positive and negative intrathoracic pressure on cardiac output and venous return in the dog. Am J Physiol 1944;142:594–603.

•105. Morgan BC, Abel FL, Mullins GL et al. Flow patterns in cavae, pulmonary artery, pulmonary vein and aorta in intact dogs. Am J Physiol 1966;210:903–9.

106. Morgan BC, Martin WE, Hornbein TF et al. Hemodynamic effects of intermittent positive-pressure respiration. Anesthesiology 1960;27:584–90.

•107. Scharf SM, Brown R, Saunders N, Green LH. Hemodynamic effects of positive-pressure inflation. J Appl Physiol 1980;49:124–31.

108. Scharf SM, Brown R, Saunders N et al. Effects of normal and loaded spontaneous inspiration on cardiovascular function. J Appl Physiol 1979;47:582–90.

109. Fessler HE, Brower RG, Wise RA, Permutt S. Effects of positive end-expiratory pressure on the canine venous return curve. Am Rev Respir Dis 1992;146:4–10.

110. Takata M, Robotham JL. Effects of inspiratory diaphragmatic descent on inferior vena caval venous return. J Appl Physiol 1992;72:597–607.

111. Van den Berg P, Jansen JRC, Pinsky MR. The effect of positive-pressure inspiration on venous return in volume loaded post-operative cardiac surgical patients. J Appl Physiol 2002;92:1223–31.

112. Magder S, Georgiadis G, Cheong T. Respiratory variation in right atrial pressure predict the response to fluid challenge. J Crit Care 1992;7:76–85.

113. Terada N, Takeuchi T. Postural changes in venous pressure gradients in anesthetized monkeys. Am J Physiol 1993;264: H21–5.

114. Scharf S, Tow DE, Miller MJ, Brown R, McIntyre K, Dilts C. Influence of posture and abdominal pressure on the

hemodynamic effects of Mueller's maneuver. J Crit Care 1989;4:26–34.

115. Tarasiuk A, Scharf SM. Effects of periodic obstructive apneas on venous return in closed-chest dogs. Am Rev Respir Dis 1993;148:323–9.

116. Mang H, Kacmarek RM, Ritz R, Wilson RS, Kimball WP. Cardiorespiratory effects of volume- and pressure-controlled ventilation at various I/E ratios in an acute lung injury model. Am J Respir Crit Care Med 1995; 151:731–6.

117. Kim HK, Alhammouri MT, Mokhtar YM, Pinsky MR. Estimating left ventricular contractility using inspiratory-hold maneuvers. Intensive Care Med 2007;33:181–9.

118. Maas JJ, Geerts BF, de Wilde RBC, van den Berg PCM, Pinsky MR, Jansen JRC. Assessment of venous return curve and mean systemic filling pressure in post-operative cardiac surgery patients. Crit Care Med 2009;37:912–8.

• 119. Tyberg JV, Taichman GC, Smith ER, Douglas NWS, Smiseth OA, Keon WJ. The relationship between pericardial pressure and right atrial pressure: an intraoperative study. Circulation 1986;73:428–32.

120. Pinsky MR, Vincent JL, DeSmet JM. Effect of positive end-expiratory pressure on right ventricular function in man. Am Rev Respir Dis 1992;146:681–7.

121. Shuey CB, Pierce AK, Johnson RL. An evaluation of exercise tests in chronic obstructive lung disease. J Appl Physiol 1969;27:256–61.

122. Jayaweera AR, Ehrlich W. Changes of phasic pleural pressure in awake dogs during exercise: potential effects on cardiac output. Ann Biomed Eng 1987;15:311–8.

♦ 123. Grenvik A. Respiratory, circulatory and metabolic effects of respiratory treatment. Acta Anaesth Scand (Suppl) 1966.

124. Harken AH, Brennan MF, Smith N, Barsamian EM. The hemodynamic response to positive end-expiratory ventilation in hypovolemic patients. Surgery 1974;76:786–93.

125. Lores ME, Keagy BA, Vassiliades T, Henry GW, Lucas CL, Wilcox BR. Cardiovascular effects of positive end-expiratory pressure (PEEP) after pneumonectomy in dogs. Ann Thorac Surg 1985;40:464–73.

• 126. Sharpey-Schaffer EP. Effects of Valsalva maneuver on the normal and failing circulation. Br Med J 1955;1:693–9.

127. Peters J, Kindred MK, Robotham JL. Transient analysis of cardiopulmonary interactions II. Systolic events. J Appl Physiol 1988;64:1518–26.

• 128. Pinsky MR, Matuschak GM, Klain M. Determinants of cardiac augmentation by increases in intrathoracic pressure. J Appl Physiol 1985;58:1189–98.

129. Rankin JS, Olsen CO, Arentzen CE et al. The effects of airway pressure on cardiac function in intact dogs and man. Circulation 1982;66:108–20.

130. Robotham JL, Rabson J, Permutt S, Bromberger-Barnea B. Left ventricular hemodynamics during respiration. J Appl Physiol 1979;47:1295–303.

131. Ruskin J, Bache RJ, Rembert JC, Greenfield Jr. Pressure–flow studies in man: Effect of respiration on left ventricular stroke volume. Circulation 1973;48:79–85.

132. Olsen CO, Tyson GS, Maier GW et al. Dynamic ventricular interaction in the conscious dog. Circ Res 1983;52: 85–104.

133. Bell RC, Robotham JL, Badke FR, Little WC, Kindred MK. Left ventricular geometry during intermittent positive-pressure ventilation in dogs. J Crit Care 1987;2:230–44.

134. Qvist J, Pontoppidan H, Wilson RS, Lowenstein E, Laver MB. Hemodynamic responses to mechanical ventilation with PEEP: the effects of hypovolemia. Anesthesiology 1975;42:45–53.

135. Denault AY, Gorcsan III J, Deneault LG, Pinsky MR. Effect of positive-pressure ventilation on left ventricular pressure-volume relationship. Anesthesiology 1993;79:A315.

136. Beyar R, Goldstein Y. Model studies of the effects of the thoracic pressure on the circulation. Ann Biomed Eng 1987;15:373–83.

137. Pinsky MR, Summer WR, Wise RA, Permutt S, Bromberger-Barnea B. Augmentation of cardiac function by elevation of intrathoracic pressure. J Appl Physiol 1983;54:950–5.

138. Cassidy SA, Wead WB, Seibert GB, Ramanathan M. Geometric left-ventricular responses to interactions between the lung and left ventricle: positive-pressure breathing. Ann Biomed Eng 1987;15:285–95.

139. Scharf SM, Brown R, Warner KG, Khuri S. Intrathoracic pressure and left ventricular configuration with respiratory maneuvers. J Appl Physiol 1989;66:481–91.

140. Pinsky MR, Summer WR. Cardiac augmentation by Phasic High Intrathoracic Support (PHIPS) in man. Chest 1983; 84:370–5.

141. Pinsky MR, Matuschak GM, Itzkoff JM. Respiratory augmentation of left ventricular function during spontaneous ventilation in severe left ventricular failure by grunting: an auto-EPAP effect. Chest 1984;86:267–9.

142. Blaustein AS, Risser TA, Weiss JW, Parker JA, Holman L, McFadden ER. Mechanisms of pulsus paradoxus during resistive respiratory loading and asthma. J Am Coll Cardiol 1986;8:529–36.

143. Strohl KP, Scharf SM, Brown R, Ingram Jr RH. Cardiovascular performance during bronchospasm in dogs. Respiration 1987;51:39–48.

144. Scharf SM, Graver LM, Balaban K. Cardiovascular effects of periodic occlusions of the upper airways in dogs. Am Rev Respir Dis 1992;146:321–9.

145. Viola AR, Puy RJM, Goldman E. Mechanisms of pulsus paradoxus in airway obstruction. J Appl Physiol 1990;68: 1927–31.

146. Scharf SM, Graver LM, Khilnani S, Balaban K. Respiratory phasic effects of inspiratory loading on left ventricular hemodynamics in vagotomized dogs. J Appl Physiol 1992;73:995–1003.

147. Latham RD, Sipkema P, Westerhof N, Rubal BJ. Aortic input impedance during Mueller maneuver: an evaluation of "effective strength". J Appl Physiol 1988;65:1604–10.

148. Virolainen J, Ventila M, Turto H, Kupari M. Effect of negative intrathoracic pressure on left ventricular pressure dynamics and relaxation. J Appl Physiol 1995; 79:455–60.

149. Garpestad E, Parker JA, Katayama H *et al.* Decrease in ventricular stroke volume at apnea termination is independent of oxygen desaturation. J Appl Physiol 1994;77:1602–8.

150. Gomez A, Mink S. Interaction between effects of hypoxia and hypercapnia on altering left ventricular relaxation and chamber stiffness in dogs. Am Rev Respir Dis 1992;146:313–20.

151. Abel FL, Mihailescu LS, Lader AS, Starr RG. Effects of pericardial pressure on systemic and coronary hemodynamics in dogs. Am J Physiol 1995;268:H1593–605.

152. Khilnani S, Graver LM, Balaban K, Scharf SM. Effects of inspiratory loading on left ventricular myocardial blood flow and metabolism. J Appl Physiol 1992;72:1488–92.

153. Satoh S, Watanabe J, Keitoku M, Itoh N, Maruyama Y, Takishima T. Influences of pressure surrounding the heart and intracardiac pressure on the diastolic coronary pressure–flow relation in excised canine heart. Circ Res 1988;63:788–97.

•154. Beach T, Millen E, Grenvik A. Hemodynamic response to discontinuance of mechanical ventilation. Crit Care Med 1973;1:85–90.

•155. Lemaire F, Teboul JL, Cinoti L, Giotto G, Abrouk F, Steg G, Macquin-Mavier I, Zapol WM. Acute left ventricular dysfunction during unsuccessful weaning from mechanical ventilation. Anesthesiology 1988;69:171–9.

156. Grace MP, Greenbaum DM. Cardiac performance in response to PEEP in patients with cardiac dysfunction. Crit Care Med 1982;20:358–60.

157. Rasanen J, Nikki P, Heikkila J. Acute myocardial infarction complicated by respiratory failure. The effects of mechanical ventilation. Chest 1984;85:21–8.

•158. Rasanen J, Vaisanen IT, Heikkila J *et al.* Acute myocardial infarction complicated by left ventricular dysfunction and respiratory failure. The effects of continuous positive airway pressure. Chest 1985;87:156–62.

159. Pinsky MR, Matuschak GM, Bernardi L, Klain M. Hemodynamic effects of cardiac cycle-specific increases in intrathoracic pressure. J Appl Physiol 1986;60:604–12.

160. Dries DJ, Kumar P, Mathru M, Mayer R, Zecca A, Rao TL, Freeark RJ. Hemodynamic effects of pressure support ventilation in cardiac surgery patients. Am Surg 1991;57:122–5.

161. Sternberg R, Sahebjami H. Hemodynamic and oxygen transport characteristics of common ventilatory modes. Chest 1994;105:1798–803.

162. Bayly R, Sladen A, Guntapalli K, Klain M. Synchronous versus nonsynchronous high-frequency jet ventilation: effects on cardiorespiratory variables and airway pressures in postoperative patients. Crit Care Med 1987;15:915–23.

163. Dhainaut JF, Devaux JY, Monsallier JF, Brunet F, Villemant D, Huyghebaert MF. Mechanisms of decreased left ventricular preload during continuous positive-pressure ventilation in ARDS. Chest 1986;90:74–80.

164. Singer M, Vermaat J, Hall G, Latter G, Patel M. Hemodynamic effects of manual hyperinflation in critically ill mechanically ventilated patients. Chest 1994;106:1182–7.

165. Lichtwarck-Aschoff M, Zeravik J, Pfeiffer UJ. Intrathoracic blood volume accurately reflects circulatory volume status in critically ill patients with mechanical ventilation. Intensive Care Med 1992;18142–5.

166. Hartmann M, Rosberg B, Jonsson K. The influence of different levels of PEEP on peripheral tissue perfusion measured by subcutaneous and transcutaneous oxygen tension. Intensive Care Med 1992;18:474–8.

167. Huemer G, Kolev N, Kurz A, Zimpfer M. Influence of positive end-expiratory pressure on right and left ventricular performance assessed by Doppler two-dimensional echocardiography. Chest 1994;106:67–73.

◆168. Jardin F. PEEP and ventricular function. Intensive Care Med 1994;20:169–70.

169. Goetz A, Heinrich H, Winter H, Deller A. Hemodynamic effects of different ventilatory patterns. A prospective clinical trial. Chest 1991;99:1166–71.

170. Gunter JP, deBoisblanc BP, Rust BS, Johnson WD, Summer WR. Effect of synchronized, systolic, lower body, positive-pressure on hemodynamics in human septic shock: a pilot study. Am J Respir Crit Care Med 1995;151:719–23.

171. Schuster S, Erbel R, Weilemann LS, Lu WY, Henkel B, Wellek S, Schinzel H, Meyer J. Hemodynamics during PEEP ventilation in patients with severe left ventricular failure studied by transesophageal echocardiography. Chest 1990;97:1181–9.

172. Lessard MR, Guerot E, Lorini H, Lemaire F, Brochard L. Effects of pressure-controlled with different I:E ratios versus volume-controlled ventilation on respiratory mechanics, gas exchange and hemodynamics in patients with adult respiratory distress syndrome. Anesthesiology 1994;80:983–91.

173. Chan K, Abraham E. Effects of inverse ratio ventilation on cardiorespiratory parameters in severe respiratory failure. Chest 1992;102:1556–61.

174. Abraham E, Yoshihara G. Cardiorespiratory effects of pressure controlled ventilation in severe respiratory failure. Chest 1990;98:1445–9.

175. Poelaert JI, Visser CA, Everaert JA, Koolen JJ, Colardyn FA. Acute hemodynamic changes of pressure-controlled inverse ration ventilation in the adult respiratory distress syndrome. A transesophageal echocardiographic and Doppler study. Chest 1993;104:214–9.

176. Mancini M, Zavala E, Mancebo J, Fernandez C, Barbera JA, Rossi A, Roca J, Rodriguez-Roisin R. Mechanisms of pulmonary gas exchange improvement during a protective ventilatory strategy in acute respiratory distress syndrome. Am J Respir Crit Care Med 2001;164:1448–53.

177. Schmitt JM, Vieillard-Baron A, Augarde R, Prin S, Page B, Jardin F. Positive end-expiratory pressure titration in acute respiratory distress syndrome patients: impact on right ventricular outflow impedance evaluated by pulmonary artery Doppler flow velocity measurements. Crit Care Med 2001;29:1154–8.

178. Abel JG, Salerno TA, Panos A *et al.* Cardiovascular effects of positive-pressure ventilation in humans. Ann Thorac Surg 1987;43:36–43.

179. DeHoyos A, Liu PP, Benard DC, Bradley TD. Haemodynamic effects of continuous positive airway pressure in humans with normal and impaired left ventricular function. Clin Sci Colch 1995;88:173–8.

180. Naughton MT, Rahman MA, Hara K, Flora JS, Bradley TD. Effect of continuous positive airway pressure on intrathoracic and left ventricular transmural pressures in patients with congestive heart failure. Circulation 1995;91:1725–31.

181. Crotti S, Mascheroni D, Caironi P, Pelosi P, Ronzoni G, Mondino M, Marini JJ, Gattinoni L Recruitment and derecruitment during acute respiratory failure. A clinical study. Am J Respir Crit Care Med 2001;164:131–40.

◆182. Rasanen J. Respiratory failure in acute myocardial infarction. Appl Cardiopulm Pathophys 1988;2:271–9.

183. Lin M, Yang YF, Chiang HT, Chang MS, Chiang BN, Cheitlin MD. Reappraisal of continuous positive airway pressure therapy in acute cardiogenic pulmonary edema. Chest 1995;107:1379–86.

184. Buckle P, Millar T, Kryger M. The effect of short-term nasal CPAP on Cheyne–Stokes respiration in congestive heart failure. Chest 1992;102:31–5.

185. Granton JT, Naughton MT, Benard DC, Liu PP, Goldstein RS, Bradley TD. CPAP improves inspiratory muscle strength in patients with heart failure and central sleep apnea. Am J Respir Crit Care Med 1996;153:277–82.

186. Naughton MT, Benard DC, Liu PP, Rutherford R, Rankin F, Bradley TD. Effects of nasal CPAP on sympathetic activity in patients with heart failure and central sleep apnea. Am J Respir Crit Care Med 1995;152:473–9.

187. Yan AT, Bradley TD, Liu PP. The role of continuous positive airway pressure in the treatment of congestive heart failure. Chest 2001;120:1675–85.

188. Baeaussier M, Coriat P, Perel A, Lebret F, Kalfon P, Chemla D, Lienhart A, Viars P. Determinants of systolic pressure variation in patients ventilated after vascular surgery. J Cardiothorac Vasc Anesth 1995;9:547–51.

189. Coriat P, Vrillon M, Perel A, Baron JF, LeBret F, Saada M, Viars P. A comparison of systolic blood pressure variations and echocardiographic estimates of end-diastolic left ventricular size in patients after aortic surgery. Anesth Analg 1994;78:46–53.

•190. Szold A, Pizov R, Segal E, Perel A. The effect of tidal volume and intravascular volume state on systolic pressure variation in ventilated dogs. Intensive Care Med 1989;15:368–71.

191. Winck JC, Azevedo LF, Costa-Pereira A, Antonelli M, Wyatt JC. Efficacy and safety of non-invasive ventilation in the treatment of acute cardiogenic pulmonary edema – a systematic review and meta-analysis. Crit Care 2006;10:R69–78.

192. Ranieri VM, Giuliani R, Cinnella G et al. Physiologic effects of positive end-expiratory pressure in patients with chronic obstructive lung disease during acute ventilatory failure and controlled mechanical ventilation. Am Rev Respir Dis 1993;147:5–13.

193. Baigorri F, De Monte A, Blanch L et al. Hemodynamic response to external counterbalancing of auto–positive end–expiratory pressure in mechanically ventilated patients with chronic obstructive lung disease. Crit Care Med 1994;22:1782–91.

◆194. Pinsky MR. Though the past darkly: Ventilatory management of patients with chronic obstructive pulmonary disease. Crit Care Med 1994;22:1714–7.

195. Ambrosino N, Nava S, Torbicki A, Riccardi G, Fracchia C, Opasich C, Rampulla C. Hemodynamic effects of pressure support and PEEP ventilation by nasal route in patients with stable chronic obstructive pulmonary disease. Thorax 1993;48:523–8.

196. Ambrosino N, Cobelli F, Torbicki A, Opasich C, Pozzoli M, Fracchia C, Rampulla C. Hemodynamic effects of negative-pressure ventilation in patients with COPD. Chest 1990; 97:850–6.

197. Richard C, Teboul JL, Archambaud F, Hebert JL, Michaut P, Auzepy P. Left ventricular function during weaning of patients with chronic obstructive pulmonary disease. Intensive Care Med 1994;20:181–6.

198. Brochard L, Isabey D, Piquet J et al. Reversal of acute exacerbations of chronic obstructive lung disease by inspiratory assistance with a face mask. N Engl J Med 1990;323:1523–30.

Effects of lung injury on the pulmonary circulation

LAURA PRICE, TW EVANS AND S JOHN WORT

INTRODUCTION

The acute respiratory distress syndrome (ARDS) is defined clinically by the rapid-onset of non-cardiogenic pulmonary edema in association with refractory hypoxemia. Since the initial description of ARDS (1), the defining criteria have been revised several times. The most widely used definition in current use is that of the American–European Consensus (AEC) Conference published in 1994, which also defined a less severe form of ARDS, termed acute lung injury (ALI) (2), Table 24.2.1). The AEC definition is fundamentally clinical and descriptive. Although the definitions have facilitated the enrolment of patients with different underlying pathologies into large scale clinical trials, they are inadequate for several reasons. First, they do not take into account the relevance of the precipitating condition to prognosis. Second, the most appropriate system of interpretation of chest radiographs is not defined. Third, they fail to standardize the strategy of mechanical ventilatory support to be used when hypoxemia is quantified.

By contrast, basic research now suggests that ARDS represents the culmination of a process involving cytokine and cell-mediated inflammation; endothelial, epithelial and vascular smooth muscle cell responses; basement membrane and interstitial matrix damage; abnormal coagulation and dysfunctional pulmonary surfactant (3). These processes have profound effects upon the pulmonary vasculature, resulting in abnormal vasomotor control leading to deficiencies in oxygenation and lung metabolic function. In addition, the multiple effects of ventilatory and pharmacological interventions may further exacerbate the inflammatory processes involved in the pathogenesis of ARDS.

Table 24.2.1 The American–European Consensus Conference definitions of acute respiratory distress syndrome (ARDS) and acute lung injury (ALI) (2)

Syndrome	Timing	Oxygenation	Chest x–ray	PAOP
ALI	Acute	$PaO_2/FiO_2 \leq 300\,mmHg$ regardless of PEEP	Bilateral opacities consistent with pulmonary edema	$\leq 18\,mmHg$ if measured or no clinical evidence of left atrial hypertension
ARDS	Acute	$PaO_2/FiO_2 \leq 200\,mmHg$ regardless of PEEP	Bilateral opacities consistent with pulmonary edema	$\leq 18\,mmHg$ if measured or no clinical evidence of left atrial hypertension

PAOP, pulmonary artery occlusion pressure; PaO_2/FiO_2, arterial partial pressure of oxygen/inspired oxygen fraction; PEEP, positive end expiratory pressure.

Table 24.2.2 Common precipitating causes of ARDS

Direct lung injury	Indirect lung injury
Pulmonary infection	Non-pulmonary sepsis
Aspiration	Hemorrhagic shock
Pulmonary contusion	Non-thoracic trauma
Fat embolism	Multiple transfusion
Toxic gas inhalation	Acute pancreatitis
Near drowning	Drug overdose
Oxygen toxicity	Cardiopulmonary bypass
Chemotherapy	Pneumonectomy
Radiotherapy	Pre-eclampsia
Ventilator-induced lung injury	Burns
Lung transplantation	Disseminated intravascular coagulation

ETIOLOGY

The increased alveolar capillary permeability that characterizes ALI/ARDS is associated with many serious medical and surgical conditions, not all of which involve the lung directly (4). Common causes of this unique form of lung injury are listed in Table 24.2.2. The division of causes into direct and indirect injury to the lung is sometimes ill-defined, a well described example being post-pneumonectomy pulmonary edema (5).

INCIDENCE

The 1994 definition for acute lung injury enabled the first estimations of incidence to be made, which range between 4.8 and 34 per 100 000 population a year, with substantial international variability (6,7). However, a prospective study in the United States, including over 1000 patients and performed over 14 months found the incidence of acute lung injury to be higher (78.9 per 100 000 population), suggesting that some 190 600 cases occur in the US each year (8). The incidence of ARDS is influenced by the underlying clinical condition (Table 24.2.2) being highest in patients with sepsis, severe sepsis, and septic shock and lower in patients with trauma (7). Other factors affecting incidence include advanced age and alcohol consumption (9). The extent to which the precipitating condition affects the lung directly or indirectly seems to influence lung compliance and recruitment, appearances on computed tomography, and possibly clinical outcome (10).

TREATMENT

The management of patients with ALI and ARDS is essentially supportive and directed at maintaining adequate systemic oxygen delivery. Mortality has been shown to be decreased significantly by employing a low tidal volume ventilatory strategy aimed at protecting the lung from excessive stretch (11). By contrast, trials of putative therapeutic pharmacologic interventions (vide infra) have not to date improved mortality. Short-term management decisions designed to alter pulmonary perfusion and ventilation to achieve apparently desirable physiological values may not produce a long-term improvement.

MORTALITY

In the United States alone, ALI is associated with 74 500 deaths annually and the care of such patients consumes 3.6 million hospital days (12). Risk factors associated with a poor outcome include advanced age, sepsis, liver disease, and non-pulmonary organ dysfunction (13,14). In Europe, a prospective multinational study has reported crude mortality rates for intensive care units and hospitals of 22.6 percent and 32.7 percent respectively for acute lung injury and 49.4 percent and 57.9 percent respectively for acute respiratory distress syndrome (15). In a UK center a significant reduction in mortality was seen from 66 percent to 34 percent during 1990–97 (16).

PATHOPHYSIOLOGY OF THE PULMONARY CIRCULATION IN ARDS

Pulmonary vascular histopathological evolution in ARDS

The defining histopathological lesion of ARDS involves the alveolar-capillary complex (17,18) in evolving through three successive phases; exudative (week 1), proliferative (weeks 2–3) and fibrotic (week 3 onwards). However, this oversimplifies the evolution of lung injury, in that phases vary in duration and may overlap, recur and resolve, producing a heterogeneous pathological pattern (17,19,20). Pulmonary vascular lesions in ARDS can be placed in a similar temporal distribution to changes in the alveoli (21). Furthermore, ARDS induces changes in the pulmonary vascular tree at all anatomical levels (22).

EXUDATIVE PHASE

Histological studies indicate that endothelial injury is common early in ARDS, as suggested by the early reduction in Vd/Vt (23) and by the release of endothelial biomarkers such as Von Willebrand's factor (VWF) (24). The characteristics of endothelial injury include cellular swelling, the presence of enlarged mitochondria (21), pinocytotic vesicle formation and inter-endothelial cell separation (25,26), and results in increased paracellular permeability (see Figure 24.2.1). Another important early feature of ARDS is microvascular occlusion by platelets,

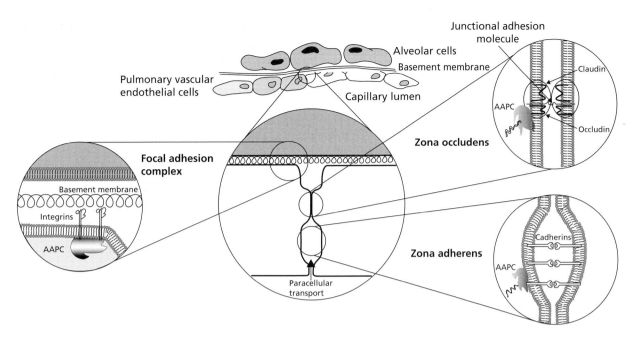

Figure 24.2.1 Examples of endothelial connections modulating paracellular permeability. AAPC, adherence-associated protein complex.

Table 24.2.3 Inflammatory mediators known to modulate capillary permeability

Cytokines	IL-1, IL-2, TNF, IFN-gamma (31)
Growth factors	VEGF (1,32), TGF-beta (33–35)
Clotting factors	thrombin (36)
Complement components	C3a (37,38)
Cell-derived inflammatory mediators	prostanoids (39–41)
	leukotrienes (42)
	platelet-activating factor (43)
	histamine (44)
Neutrophil-derived mediators	superoxide ions
	proteases
	cytokines (45,46)
Bacterial-derived mediators	lipopolysaccharide (LPS) (47)
Redox imbalance	(48)
Oxidative stress	(49)
Ischemia-reperfusion injury	(50,51)

neutrophils and thrombi (27–30), with the resulting inflammatory milieu affecting capillary permeability (Table 24.2.3, refs 31–51).

PROLIFERATIVE PHASE

The proliferative phase affects (a) the capillaries (21,52); (b) the preacinar arteries, veins and lymphatics (21).

FIBROPROLIFERATIVE PHASE

The fibroproliferative phase affects (a) the capillaries (21,53–55); (b) the preacinar arteries (21,56).

PULMONARY VASCULAR METABOLIC FAILURE IN ARDS

The pulmonary endothelium is a site of intense metabolic activity producing transpulmonary concentration differences of bioactive agents (57) (Table 24.2.4). The lung thus reduces recirculation of tissue-derived bioactive substances with usually brief and/or local actions. Models of lung injury demonstrate a fall in the normal pulmonary capacity to remove vasoactive substances. The effect is neither injury- nor substrate-specific. Metabolic dysfunction begins before detectable changes in endothelial permeability and ultrastructure, or the onset of hemodynamic instability (58). A failure in metabolic function may contribute to pulmonary and systemic vasodysregulation in patients with lung injury (59).

Metabolism of 5-hydroxytryptamine and prostaglandin E1 by the lung is impaired in patients with ARDS (60). For amines and prostaglandins, the rate-limiting step is carrier-mediated active transport, rather than enzymatic deactivation. Angiotensin converting enzyme (ACE), which activates angiotensin I and inactivates bradykinin, is present on the pulmonary endothelial surface and intracellular transport is unnecessary. ACE activity measured using a synthetic substrate permits estimations of the perfused capillary surface area in the normal lung (61). This activity decreases early in the course of ARDS and may correlate with severity of lung injury (62). However, plasma angiotensin II levels may actually increase (63).

Endothelin-1 (ET-1) is both cleared from, and released into, plasma by the lung (64). An abnormal pulmonary ET-1 clearance to production ratio develops in ARDS and could contribute to the increase in pulmonary vascular resistance (65,66). Although ET-1 clearance normalizes as

Table 24.2.4 Bioactive compounds normally cleared by the pulmonary circulation

Bioactive compound	% inactivated Amines
5-hydroxytryptamine	65–95%
Norepinephrine	25–50%
Dopamine	30%
Epinephrine	< 10%
Isoproterenol	unaffected
Histamine	unaffected
Prostaglandins	
PGE_1, PGE_2, $PGF_{2\alpha}$, PGD_2	65–98%
Thromboxane	< 10%
PGA	unaffected
Peptides	
Angiotensin I	40–100%
Bradykinin	75–98%
Vasopressin	unaffected

clinical state improves, the mitogenic effect of ET-1 may contribute to pulmonary vascular remodeling.

The removal of other substances, such as propanolol, is affected by lung inflation. However, a ventilatory strategy optimising oxygenation does not improve ACE activity in a model of lung injury (67). Equally, improving hypoxemia by turning patients with ARDS prone does not modify pulmonary angiotensin production nor ET-1 clearance (63). Although maneuvers that improve oxygenation might simultaneously improve the exposed vascular endothelial surface area available for metabolic function, this effect does not appear to be significant.

CLINICAL CORRELATES

Pulmonary hypertension

A mild to moderate level of pulmonary hypertension (mean PAP 25–35 mmHg) is common in ARDS (30). Contributing factors are likely to vary through the time-course of the condition. Early on, these include hypoxic vasoconstriction (HPV) (68,69), vasoactive mediator-induced diffuse vasoconstriction, vascular compression by interstitial edema (70) and early thrombotic processes. In some cases of severe ARDS PH can persist. This is likely to be caused by obstructive and obliterative pulmonary vascular lesions (71), with ongoing microangiopathy and macrothrombosis, as well as later true pulmonary vascular remodeling (72,73).

Since PH was first described in ARDS, its presence, and notably its persistence, has correlated with survival in most studies. An important early study showed that although the presence of raised pulmonary vascular resistance (PVR) or low cardiac index in isolation did not predict mortality, an increase in PVR over the course of the disease

correlated with poor outcome (71). Later studies have confirmed clear outcome associations with the presence of persistent (greater than 7 days) elevated PVR (74–77). More recent studies, following the introduction of protective lung ventilatory strategies, have shown a much lower incidence of PH and acute right ventricular failure, and the association with poor survival is less consistent (78–80). This may relate to several factors including the immediate recognition and treatment of right heart dysfunction leading to bias in these studies (81). The most recent study using invasive hemodynamic data within the first week of ARDS onset in over 450 patients does suggest that the presence of pulmonary vascular dysfunction, as defined by an increased transpulmonary gradient and elevated PVR; does worsen outcomes including 60-day mortality (82).

THE CAUSES OF PULMONARY HYPERTENSION

Disturbed vasomotor control – Imbalance between endogenous vasoconstrictors and vasodilators

Basal pulmonary vascular tone and in particular smooth muscle cell (SMC) and endothelial cell (EC) function is controlled by distinct signaling pathways including the production of nitric oxide (NO), ET-1 and cyclo-oxygenase (COX) products (such as thromboxane A_2 and prostacyclin (PGI_2)) (83). Basal pulmonary vascular tone is further influenced by inflammatory mediators produced by activated endothelium (84). An overall imbalance results in favor of the production of vasoconstrictive mediators (ET-1, angiotensin, thromboxane A_2, reactive oxygen species and serotonin) against vasodilators (NO and PGI_2).

Vascular tone is therefore affected by the following: (i) Nitric oxide (85–89); (ii) ET-1 (90–101); (iii) COX pathway (102–106); (iv) Reactive oxygen species (107–110).

Hypoxic pulmonary vasoconstriction

Hypoxic pulmonary vasoconstriction (HPV), first described in 1946 (111), is a vasoconstrictor response to alveolar hypoxia unique to the pulmonary circulation. Vasoconstriction of the hypoxia-sensitive precapillary resistance pulmonary vessels shunts blood away from poorly oxygenated alveoli (112,113) in an attempt to restore VQ matching and reduce shunt fraction (114). Inhibition of oxygen-sensitive potassium channels (K(v)1.5 and K(v)2.1) on PASMCs occurs, leading to activation of voltage-gated Ca(2+) channels, Ca(2+) influx and vasoconstriction (115). This hypoxic inhibition of K+ currents is not seen in systemic arterial SMCs (116), suggesting it is a property unique to the pulmonary circulation (117). For more details see Table 24.2.5 and refs 118–143.

Pulmonary venoconstriction

The density and variety of receptors on pulmonary veins (144–147) together with their location down-stream of emboli, render them prone to constriction by inflammatory mediators. Pulmonary venous hypertension raises pulmonary capillary pressure and may elevate pulmonary arterial pressures. Although the number of pulmonary

Table 24.2.5 Factors potentially inhibiting hypoxic pulmonary vasoconstriction in ARDS

Pathological	Surgery
	Blunt trauma
	Pneumonia
	Fluid overload
	High pulmonary artery pressure
	High pulmonary venous pressure
Treatment-related	Beta-adrenergic agonists
	Alpha-adrenergic antagonists
	Nitroprusside
	Nitroglycerine
	Calcium channel antagonists
	Prostacyclin
	Dopamine
	Low arterial PCO_2
	High pH
	High mixed venous PO_2
	Low mixed venous PCO_2

angiographic filling defects correlates with pulmonary vascular resistance (148), physical obstruction alone is an unlikely cause of early pulmonary hypertension in ARDS as, to some extent, it is pharmacologically reversible. The comparative potency and local concentration of the transitory mediators is unknown in ARDS, but thromboxane antagonists can reduce the venous component of the rise in pulmonary vascular resistance (149).

Thrombosis

Intravascular macro- and microthromboses consisting of red and white blood cells, hyaline membranes and layered fibrin (21) are seen histologically at all stages of ARDS (21,148), probably due to *in situ* thrombosis rather than from distal emboli (150). The presence of early macrothrombi correlates with increased mortality, and clearing these lesions by thrombolysis improves PVR and oxygenation (150). Activation of coagulation occurs with overactivity of both the extrinsic pathway (mostly due to a reduction in natural anticoagulants and fibrinolytics), and the intrinsic pathway (through local exposure of plasma to tissue factor (TF) on non-vascular tissue or activated ECs) stimulates thrombin generation, controlled by antithrombin and TF pathway inhibitor (TFPI), leading to the intrinsic pathway and amplified thrombin generation and ongoing coagulation (151). During the initial phase of the inflammatory response in ARDS, high levels of proinflammatory cytokines also activate coagulation via TF, and attenuate fibrinolysis by stimulating the release of inhibitors of plasminogen activation (152). Levels of natural anticoagulants including protein C and antithrombin (AT) are low in sepsis (153), due to both decreased production as well as enhanced breakdown (154). The thrombomodulin/protein C axis (155) also contributes to the prothrombotic, antifibrinolytic state. Plasma protein C levels are lower in ALI/ARDS compared with normal controls, associated

with worse clinical outcomes, including death, fewer ventilator-free days, and more non-pulmonary organ failures (156). Further mechanisms may involve high thromboplastin levels. This procoagulant protein is usually maintained at low levels, and increases are seen following stimulation by endotoxin, IL-1 and thrombin (157). Reduced endothelial fibrinolysis (158) and platelet activation may also contribute both to thrombotic and hemorrhagic complications (159).

Inflammation

Neutrophilic inflammation is characteristic of ARDS, with activation of immune, endothelial and epithelial cells leading to tissue damage through the production of free radicals, inflammatory mediators and proteases (160,161), and influencing adherence of neutrophils and their migration through endothelium into the interstitium and alveoli (162). Neutrophilic and platelet activation can injure the endothelium and release mediators that modulate vascular tone (29,163). Other mediators important in vasomotor control also influence inflammation, for example PGI2 reduces cytokine release (164) and suppresses leukocyte activation (165). Neutrophilic deformation is likely to contribute directly to micro-capillary flow obstruction (166,167). Transcription and activation of nuclear factors such as NF-κB occurs (168), with the resulting ongoing inflammation likely to contribute to parenchymal damage even before the fibroproliferative phase (161,169). In PAH, inflammatory vascular injury is thought to be important in some types of PAH with perivascular infiltration of inflammatory cells seen in the complex "plexiform" lesions classical of PAH (170). Although inflammation is prevalent in ARDS, there is no evidence for this extent of vascular remodeling, but inflammatory vascular injury may occur on a smaller scale at the time of parenchymal inflammation.

Hypoxia itself has inflammatory effects further to its vasoconstrictive effects that may be relevant in ARDS. In non-ARDS settings, even moderate and intermittent exposure to hypoxia can lead to increased expression of cytokines, chemokines, adhesion molecules and accumulation of leukocytes in pulmonary vessel walls, and the development of pulmonary vascular remodeling (171). Hypoxic exposure in mice for 48 h leads to perivascular infiltration of neutrophils, macrophages and chemokines including MCP-1, IL1-beta, IL-6, and then also to pulmonary vascular remodeling (172). In humans with HAPE, serum cytokines are elevated and neutrophils and macrophages accumulate in BAL fluid (173), being reversible on return to normoxia. Although these measurements may not be specific to the pulmonary vasculature, they do relate to the changes seen in PVR.

Pulmonary vascular remodeling

Twelve days from the onset of ARDS, a progressive reduction is seen in the internal vascular diameter of arteries in the precapillary bed (21), with an early increased medial wall thickness in the intra-acinar arteries (56). After 18 days, there is histological evidence of local thrombus formation, loss of capillaries, myointimal thickening and tortuous vessel formation (174).

Increased vessel medial wall thickness is thought to reflect neomuscularization, whereby previously non-muscular pre-capillary vessels develop contractile muscle elements and become resistance vessels, leading to an elevation in PVR. This is evidence of proliferating PASMCs and fibroblasts (175,176) that have a reduced level of apoptosis in response to hypoxia; as well as increased extracellular matrix deposition (177). Remodeling appears to start in central vessels and extends to peripheral vessels in later stages of ARDS (56). The vascular remodeling process may be considered adaptive, as it strengthens blood vessels in the face of increasing wall stress (178).

The mechanisms of this process have been studied in non-ARDS models of PH. Increased production of ET-1, and reduced levels of NO and PGI2, together with dysregulated transforming growth factor (TGF) beta and inflammatory pathways lead to a "proliferative vascular cell phenotype". The additional stimulus of hypoxia must be considered (179). Certain smooth muscle cell phenotypes appear to proliferate excessively following a hypoxic stimulus (180–182). Induction of transcription factors, such as HIF-1α by hypoxia, also leads to the transcription of genes important in cell growth and inflammation such as VEGF (183) and ET-1, which both have an important mitogenic influence on smooth muscle cells (184,185). Finally, following bacterial (186) or viral (187) recognition by toll-like receptors (TLR)-3 and 4 respectively, a proliferative and proinflammatory SMC phenotype may be induced.

Hypoxia

Several mechanisms are responsible for the refractory hypoxemia that characterizes ARDS. Lung function tests suggest impaired gas transfer, despite the presence of interstitial edema and intra-alveolar hyaline membranes, is not a principle cause (188) although there is a reduction in accessible capillary blood volume (189). Although alveolar injury may be widespread and even homogeneous, the distribution of the resulting atelectasis and edema within the lungs of supine patients is heterogeneous, as unequivocally demonstrated by computerized tomography (Figure 24.2.2) (190,191). The loss of aeration may be diffuse, patchy or lobar in distribution, but is consistently observed in the lower lobes and extends to the upper lobes in approximately two-thirds of supine patients (192,193). The distribution of aerated and consolidated lung has profound implications for V/Q mismatch in patients with ARDS.

PERFUSION ABNORMALITIES IN ARDS

Computed tomography (CT) has provided a radiological representation of the results of early studies of V/Q mismatch in patients with ARDS that employed the multiple inert gas elimination technique (MIGET). This revealed a bimodal distribution of ventilation–perfusion ratios

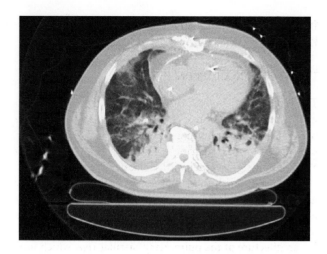

Figure 24.2.2 A computed tomography scan representative of the tissue/air distribution in a patient with acute respiratory distress syndrome (ARDS).

(194,195), approximately half the pulmonary blood flow being distributed to units of normal V/Q ratio. The other half flowed through regions of no ventilation (pure shunt), or units with a very low V/Q ratio. The early increase seen in Vd/Vt fraction is associated with worsened survival (23).

The pulmonary vascular effects of mechanical ventilation in patients with ARDS

Correct ventilatory support in ARDS reduces mortality (196). The reasons for this may be complex. Positive pressure ventilation and the positioning of the patient will have direct and indirect effects on pulmonary blood flow, which will now be discussed.

EFFECTS OF POSITIVE-PRESSURE VENTILATION ON THE DISTRIBUTION OF PERFUSION

In some patients studied using MIGET, the application of positive end expiratory pressure (PEEP) at low levels altered the distribution of blood flow between units of normal and abnormal V/Q, without creating intermediate ratio units (194,197,198). This supports the hypothesis that PEEP physically alters V/Q relationships in a quantal fashion, anatomically represented by the recruitment of collapsed alveolae, reducing shunt and improving arterial oxygenation.

In other patients, PEEP causes a fall in cardiac output, the emergence of units with high V/Q ratios and an increase in physiological dead space (197,198). Despite this, arterial oxygen saturation still sometimes improves with high PEEP because shunt fraction generally decreases as cardiac output falls (199). Improvements in arterial oxygen saturation associated with the application of high PEEP might therefore not improve oxygen delivery. However, in adequately fluid resuscitated patients the reduction in cardiac output induced by PEEP can be small (200–203), confirming that an improvement in arterial oxygenation is produced by improving V/Q matching (198,204).

THE EFFECTS OF THE PRONE POSITION

The vertical distribution of blood flow in the normal lung in the upright position is determined by the relationship between alveolar, pulmonary artery and pulmonary venous pressures (205). Comparing transverse sections of the lung at different heights, gravity influences regional blood flows. However, flow within an individual transverse section or isogravitational plane also forms a heterogeneous pattern not predicted by a gravitational hypothesis (206–208). One factor favoring this uneven distribution is the fractal branching architecture of the pulmonary vascular tree, which produces unequal resistances in diverging vessels (209). Regional differences in vascular resistance related to NO synthesis have also been observed in animals (210). The result of these effects is that perfusion to the dorsal regions of the lung is relatively preserved in comparison to the ventral regions in the prone position in man (211–213).

During mechanical ventilation in the supine position, the majority of studies suggest ventral lung ventilation dominates. By contrast, in the prone position, most investigators demonstrate an even distribution of alveolar ventilation (213). Thus homogeneity in alveolar ventilation with simultaneous preservation of dorsal pulmonary blood flow in the prone position may produce a better correlation of regional alveolar ventilation and pulmonary perfusion (214). The matching of ventilation to perfusion in the prone position during mechanical ventilation explains improvements in oxygenation in some patients with ARDS turned prone (215–217). However, prone positioning has not been shown to afford a survival benefit to patients with ARDS (218).

The improvement in V/Q matching is thought to reduce resistance to blood flow in the lung, a major afterloading factor for the right ventricle during the course of ARDS. A recent study suggests that prone ventilation, through both airway pressure limitation and reduction of hypercapnia, reduces echocardiographic indices of RV dysfunction, at least in a severe subset of ARDS patients (219).

ACUTE COR PULMONALE

During positive pressure ventilation, alveolar pressure becomes the main determinant of transpulmonary pressure (alveolar–pleural pressure) (220), and with these high plateau pressures, transpulmonary pressure may exceed pulmonary venous pressure. This leads to impeded transpulmonary blood flow and an elevation in RV afterload (221,222), inducing acute cor pulmonale (ACP) in some patients with ARDS (223).

In the era before 'lung protective' ventilatory strategies, ACP was seen in up to 61 percent of ARDS cases (224). Lower tidal volumes (reduced from 13 to 6 mL/kg) and reduced PEEP has contributed to the improved ARDS mortality from 40 to 31 percent (225), thought to be related to reduced over-distension of lung units and less injurious alveolar effects. This change in ventilatory practice with a reduction in plateau pressures has also reduced the incidence of ACP to 10–25 percent in post-lung protective era studies (80). A large echocardiographic study of ARDS patients further showed that the incidence of ACP was 56 percent with plateau pressures $> 35\,cmH_2O$, and reduced to 13 percent with pressures $< 27\,cmH_2O$ (220). The hypercapnia tolerated with these ventilatory strategies may, however, adversely affect right heart function (226–228).

Lung hyperinflation following excessive PEEP may induce tricuspid regurgitation by collapsing small pulmonary vessels and increasing right ventricular afterload (229,230). PEEP is useful to splint open dependent or injured alveoli and prevent their de-recruitment at endexpiration, avoiding loss of functional residual capacity (FRC) and reducing further lung injury associated with cyclical over-distension and collapsing of lung units. Without it, loss of lung volume may result, capillaries close and PVR may rise steeply (231), leading to RV dysfunction (232,233). In well-ventilated areas of the lung, PEEP may over-distend and compress capillaries, diverting blood to less well-ventilated areas, with a subsequent increase in intrapulmonary shunt and a reduction in oxygenation (234). Optimal PEEP remains elusive in this setting (235), although the resulting high PVR in the setting of PEEP may be reduced by increasing central blood volume (230).

Recruitment maneuvers, through the application of a short period of sustained lung hyperinflation (236), open collapsed alveoli and restore FRC by manually expanding areas of atelectasis (237). When combined with PEEP, there may be an improvement in oxygenation (236) and reduced ventilator-associated lung injury (238). Recruitment manoeuvres have also been associated with ACP (239–241), with sustained hyperinflation causing leftward shift of the septum and reduced LV cavity size (242).

The effects of pulmonary vasodilators in ARDS

Systemic vasodilators have been prescribed for patients with ARDS first, to reduce pulmonary capillary filtration pressures and thus pulmonary edema formation (243); and second, to reduce pulmonary vascular resistance, thereby increasing the output of the right ventricle and so improving oxygen delivery. Intravenous prostacyclin (244), nitroglycerin (245,246), nitroprusside (247) and diltiazem (248) have been shown to increase cardiac output in ARDS although oxygen delivery may fall because of reduced arterial oxygen saturation, seen also in studies using intravenous (248) and oral (249) sildenafil. This desaturation can be attributed to inhibition of residual HPV in the damaged lung with a consequent increase in heterogeneity of V/Q matching. In addition, increases in shunt fraction and deterioration in oxygenation using intravenous pulmonary vasodilators may risk end-organ ischemia (249).

The administration of inhaled pulmonary vasodilators such as NO and prostacyclins agents can minimize side-effects on the systemic circulation, and in particular systemic hypotension. For example, inhaled NO has been shown to enhance pulmonary vasodilatation in ventilated lung units, reduce V/Q mismatch, and improve oxygenation (250), although, despite this, studies have failed to show a survival benefit (251–267). The findings in trials with prostacyclins yield similar results with improved oxygenation but no outcome benefit (268–272). The use of endothelin receptor antagonists in ARDS remains experimental (273–284). Further to the difficulties in recruiting large numbers, a major limitation to these studies is the lack of trials in the subset of ARDS patients with marked pulmonary vascular dysfunction.

Changes in the pulmonary circulation in survivors of ARDS

Little is known about vascular remodeling in long-term survivors of ARDS (285). Studies of small numbers of survivors have demonstrated variable residual pulmonary vascular effects (286). Extrapolation of early investigations to those performed following publication of the AEC definition and managed using modern techniques is difficult. The etiology of the ARDS, pulmonary or non-pulmonary, may influence mortality but does not alter return of lung function at 6 months (287). Moreover, although between 40 and 80 percent of survivors have abnormal pulmonary function tests 12 months after recovery, their clinical significance may be variable and difficult to ascertain.

A low single-breath carbon monoxide diffusing capacity is a frequent finding (288). The capillary blood volume determinant of the DLCO may be more important to reduced gas transfer than the membrane conductance (289). The DLCO corrected for remaining alveolar volume (KCO) is also commonly reduced. Together with a raised dead space to tidal volume ratio, these results suggest a persistent loss of capillary surface area. This may be secondary to destruction and/or poor perfusion of the remaining capillary bed (289–291). CT appearances 6 months after the acute illness typically show a coarse reticular pattern with distortion of the lung parenchyma, ground-glass opacification and areas of hypo-attenuation dominating the anterior zones (292). This fibrotic appearance with cystic destruction of the lung parenchyma supports a view that collapsed and/or consolidated lung in the acute phase of ARDS is protected from alveolar overdistention during pressure-controlled inverse ratio ventilation. Because arterial and bronchial structures are paired, it is likely that the destruction of the pulmonary vascular bed in patients managed in this way is also localized anteriorly. However, while the extent of the fibrosis on CT is related to loss of lung volume on lung function testing, it is not correlated with loss of gas transfer.

Improvement in pulmonary function tests is usually rapid during the first 3 to 6 months but more gradual subsequently. After 6 months, arterial blood gases at rest are often normal and a shunt fraction characteristic of active ARDS is rare. Significant oxygen desaturation may occasionally still occur on exercise (290,293). Abnormalities persisting for greater than 1 year are unlikely to resolve (294). In general, the relative improvement in lung volumes and restrictive and/or obstructive spirometry is greater than improvement in DLCO, suggesting more permanent destruction or slower useful remodeling of the pulmonary vasculature in comparison to alveolar and airway restoration. Results may be confounded by pre- and post-ARDS lung damage, most commonly the result of smoking, but the majority of the abnormalities in gas transfer are mild at 1 year (286).

Moreover, the degree of abnormality in pulmonary function tests does not correlate with symptoms or quality of life. More than half the survivors of ARDS in some series had persistent pulmonary symptoms 1 year post-discharge although only 12 percent in one study had physical limitations impairing lifestyle (295,296). Health complaints of ARDS survivors at one year are not entirely related to pulmonary factors (297). Nevertheless in comparison to equally injured or ill patients without ARDS, survivors of ARDS do have health-related quality of life indices that reflect pulmonary disease-specific impairments (298). This observation should encourage clinical practice that protects the injured lung with a view to long-term pulmonary outcomes.

KEY POINTS

- Lung injury results in significant changes to the pulmonary circulation.
- The clinical consequence of such pulmonary vascular damage is a rise in pulmonary vascular resistance and hypoxia.
- Pulmonary hypertension is relatively common but generally mild to moderate in severity.
- The presence of pulmonary hypertension is associated with worse outcome, although there is evidence that the use of protective ventilatory strategies is associated with a lower detection rate of pulmonary hypertension.
- ARDS treatment is supportive but should aim to protect the lung and pulmonary vasculature.
- At present there is no evidence that targeting the pulmonary vasculature affects outcome in patients with ARDS.
- Of the 60 percent who survive ARDS, the majority have minor defects in lung function at 1 year, which may reflect persisting vascular damage.

REFERENCES

• = Key primary paper
♦ = Major review article

1. Ashbaugh DG, Bigelow DB, Petty TL, Levine BE. Acute respiratory distress in adults. Lancet 1967;2(7511): 319–23.

•2. Bernard GR, Artigas A, Brigham KL, Carlet J, Falke K, Hudson L *et al.* The American–European Consensus Conference on ARDS. Definitions, mechanisms, relevant outcomes, and clinical trial coordination. Am J Respir Crit Care Med 1994;149(3 Pt 1):818–24.

3. Weinacker AB, Vaszar LT. Acute respiratory distress syndrome: physiology and new management strategies. Annu Rev Med 2001;52:221–37.

4. Brewer L, Burbank B. The "wet-lung" in war casualties. Ann Surg 1946;123:343–62.

5. Jordan S, Mitchell JA, Quinlan GJ, Goldstraw P, Evans TW. The pathogenesis of lung injury following pulmonary resection. Eur Respir J 2000;15(4):790–9.

6. Goss CH, Brower RG, Hudson LD, Rubenfeld GD. Incidence of acute lung injury in the United States. Crit Care Med 2003;31(6):1607–11.

♦7. MacCallum NS, Evans TW. Epidemiology of acute lung injury. Curr Opin Crit Care 2005;11(1):43–9.

8. Gong MN, Thompson BT, Williams P, Pothier L, Boyce PD, Christiani DC. Clinical predictors of and mortality in acute respiratory distress syndrome: potential role of red cell transfusion. Crit Care Med 2005;33(6):1191–8.

9. Wind J, Versteegt J, Twisk J, van der Werf TS, Bindels AJ, Spijkstra JJ *et al.* Epidemiology of acute lung injury and acute respiratory distress syndrome in The Netherlands: a survey. Respir Med 2007;101(10):2091–8.

10. Naeije R. Medical treatment of pulmonary hypertension in acute lung disease. Eur Respir J 1993;6(10):1521–8.

•11. ARDSNetwork. Ventilation with lower tidal volumes as compared with traditional tidal volumes for acute lung injury and the acute respiratory distress syndrome. N Engl J Med 2000;342(18):1301–8.

12. Rubenfeld GD, Caldwell E, Peabody E, Weaver J, Martin DP, Neff M *et al.* Incidence and outcomes of acute lung injury. N Engl J Med 2005;353(16):1685–93.

13. Ely EW, Wheeler AP, Thompson BT, Ancukiewicz M, Steinberg KP, Bernard GR. Recovery rate and prognosis in older persons who develop acute lung injury and the acute respiratory distress syndrome. Ann Intern Med 2002; 136(1):25–36.

14. Ranieri VM, Suter PM, Tortorella C, De Tullio R, Dayer JM, Brienza A *et al.* Effect of mechanical ventilation on inflammatory mediators in patients with acute respiratory distress syndrome: a randomized controlled trial. JAMA 1999;282(1):54–61.

15. Brun-Buisson C, Minelli C, Bertolini G, Brazzi L, Pimentel J, Lewandowski K *et al.* Epidemiology and outcome of acute lung injury in European intensive care units. Results from the ALIVE study. Intensive Care Med 2004;30(1):51–61.

•16. Abel SJ, Finney SJ, Brett SJ, Keogh BF, Morgan CJ, Evans TW. Reduced mortality in association with the acute respiratory distress syndrome (ARDS). Thorax 1998;53(4):292–4.

17. Katzenstein AL, Bloor CM, Leibow AA. Diffuse alveolar damage – the role of oxygen, shock, and related factors. A review. Am J Pathol 1976;85(1):209–28.

18. Bleyl U, Rossner JA. Globular hyaline microthrombi – their nature and morphogenesis. Virchows Arch A Pathol Anat Histol 1976;370(2):113–28.

19. Nash G, Blennerhassett JB, Pontoppidan H. Pulmonary lesions associated with oxygen therapy and artificial ventilation. N Engl J Med 1967;276(7):368–74.

20. Pratt PC, Vollmer RT, Shelburne JD, Crapo JD. Pulmonary morphology in a multihospital collaborative extracorporeal membrane oxygenation project. I. Light microscopy. Am J Pathol 1979;95(1):191–214.

•21. Tomashefski JF, Jr., Davies P, Boggis C, Greene R, Zapol WM, Reid LM. The pulmonary vascular lesions of the adult respiratory distress syndrome. Am J Pathol 1983;112(1): 112–26.

22. Tomashefski JF, Jr. Pulmonary pathology of acute respiratory distress syndrome. Clin Chest Med 2000;21(3):435–66.

•23. Nuckton TJ, Alonso JA, Kallet RH, Daniel BM, Pittet JF, Eisner MD *et al.* Pulmonary dead-space fraction as a risk factor for death in the acute respiratory distress syndrome. N Engl J Med 2002;346(17):1281–6.

24. Rubin DB, Wiener-Kronish JP, Murray JF, Green DR, Turner J, Luce JM *et al.* Elevated von Willebrand factor antigen is an early plasma predictor of acute lung injury in nonpulmonary sepsis syndrome. J Clin Invest 1990;86(2): 474–80.

25. Schnells G, Voigt WH, Redl H, Schlag G, Glatzl A. Electron-microscopic investigation of lung biopsies in patients with post-traumatic respiratory insufficiency. Acta Chir Scand Suppl 1980;499:9–20.

26. Albertine KH. Ultrastructural abnormalities in increased-permeability pulmonary edema. Clin Chest Med 1985;6(3): 345–69.

27. Hechtman HB, Lonergan EA, Shepro D. Platelet and leukocyte lung interactions in patients with respiratory failure. Surgery 1978;83(2):155–63.

28. Warshawski FJ, Sibbald WJ, Driedger AA, Cheung H. Abnormal neutrophil–pulmonary interaction in the adult respiratory distress syndrome. Qualitative and quantitative assessment of pulmonary neutrophil kinetics in humans with in vivo 111indium neutrophil scintigraphy. Am Rev Respir Dis 1986;133(5):797–804.

29. Patterson CE, Barnard JW, Lafuze JE, Hull MT, Baldwin SJ, Rhoades RA. The role of activation of neutrophils and microvascular pressure in acute pulmonary edema. Am Rev Respir Dis 1989;140(4):1052–62.

30. Zapol WM, Jones R. Vascular components of ARDS. Clinical pulmonary hemodynamics and morphology. Am Rev Respir Dis 1987;136(2):471–4.

31. Parsons PE. Mediators and mechanisms of acute lung injury. Clin Chest Med 2000;21(3):467–76.

•32. Thickett DR, Armstrong L, Christie SJ, Millar AB. Vascular endothelial growth factor may contribute to increased vascular permeability in acute respiratory distress syndrome. Am J Respir Crit Care Med 2001;164(9):1601–5.

33. Pittet JF, Griffiths MJ, Geiser T, Kaminski N, Dalton SL, Huang X et al. TGF-beta is a critical mediator of acute lung injury. J Clin Invest 2001;107(12):1537–44.

34. Roupie E. Incidence of ARDS. Intensive Care Med 2000; 26(6):816–7.

35. Lewandowski K, Metz J, Deutschmann C, Preiss H, Kuhlen R, Artigas A et al. Incidence, severity, and mortality of acute respiratory failure in Berlin, Germany. Am J Respir Crit Care Med 1995;151(4):1121–5.

36. Malik AB, Lo SK. Thrombin–endothelial interactions: role in lung vascular permeability. Mol Aspects Med 1985;8(6): 515–54.

37. Hallgren R, Samuelsson T, Modig J. Complement activation and increased alveolar-capillary permeability after major surgery and in adult respiratory distress syndrome. Crit Care Med 1987;15(3):189–93.

38. Roupie E, Lepage E, Wysocki M, Fagon JY, Chastre J, Dreyfuss D et al. Prevalence, etiologies and outcome of the acute respiratory distress syndrome among hypoxemic ventilated patients. SRLF Collaborative Group on Mechanical Ventilation. Societe de Reanimation de Langue Francaise. Intensive Care Med 1999;25(9):920–9.

39. Bernard GR, Brigham KL. Pulmonary edema. Pathophysiologic mechanisms and new approaches to therapy. Chest 1986; 89(4):594–600.

40. Milberg JA, Davis DR, Steinberg KP, Hudson LD. Improved survival of patients with acute respiratory distress syndrome (ARDS): 1983–1993. JAMA 1995;273(4):306–9.

41. Luhr OR, Antonsen K, Karlsson M, Aardal S, Thorsteinsson A, Frostell CG et al. Incidence and mortality after acute respiratory failure and acute respiratory distress syndrome in Sweden, Denmark, and Iceland. The ARF Study Group. Am J Respir Crit Care Med 1999;159(6):1849–61.

42. Matthay MA, Eschenbacher WL, Goetzl EJ. Elevated concentrations of leukotriene D4 in pulmonary edema fluid of patients with the adult respiratory distress syndrome. J Clin Immunol 1984;4(6):479–83.

43. Miotla JM, Jeffery PK, Hellewell PG. Platelet-activating factor plays a pivotal role in the induction of experimental lung injury. Am J Respir Cell Mol Biol 1998;18(2):197–204.

44. Malik AB, Johnson A, Tahamont MV. Mechanisms of lung vascular injury after intravascular coagulation. Ann N Y Acad Sci 1982;384:213–34.

45. Tate RM, Repine JE. Neutrophils and the adult respiratory distress syndrome. Am Rev Respir Dis 1983;128(3):552–9.

ʋ46. Strieter RM, Kunkel SL. Acute lung injury: the role of cytokines in the elicitation of neutrophils. J Investig Med 1994;42(4):640–51.

47. Worthen GS, Haslett C, Rees AJ, Gumbay RS, Henson JE, Henson PM. Neutrophil-mediated pulmonary vascular injury. Synergistic effect of trace amounts of lipopolysaccharide and neutrophil stimuli on vascular permeability and neutrophil sequestration in the lung. Am Rev Respir Dis 1987;136(1):19–28.

48. Zhao X, Alexander JS, Zhang S, Zhu Y, Sieber NJ, Aw TY et al. Redox regulation of endothelial barrier integrity. Am J Physiol Lung Cell Mol Physiol 2001;281(4):L879–86.

49. Lum H, Roebuck KA. Oxidant stress and endothelial cell dysfunction. Am J Physiol Cell Physiol 2001;280(4): C719–41.

50. van Griensven M, Stalp M, Seekamp A. Ischemia-reperfusion directly increases pulmonary endothelial permeability in vitro. Shock 1999;11(4):259–63.

51. Fisher AB, Dodia C, Ayene I, al-Mehdi A. Ischemia-reperfusion injury to the lung. Ann N Y Acad Sci 1994;723:197–207.

52. Bachofen M, Weibel ER. Alterations of the gas exchange apparatus in adult respiratory insufficiency associated with septicemia. Am Rev Respir Dis 1977;116(4):589–615.

53. Burkhardt A. Alveolitis and collapse in the pathogenesis of pulmonary fibrosis. Am Rev Respir Dis 1989;140(2):513–24.

54. Meyrick B. Pathology of the adult respiratory distress syndrome. Crit Care Clin 1986;2(3):405–28.

55. Chang JC, Kathula SK. Various clinical manifestations in patients with thrombotic microangiopathy. J Investig Med 2002;50(3):201–6.

•56. Snow RL, Davies P, Pontoppidan H, Zapol WM, Reid L. Pulmonary vascular remodeling in adult respiratory distress syndrome. Am Rev Respir Dis 1982;126(5):887–92.

57. Wiedemann HP, Gillis CN. Altered metabolic function of the pulmonary microcirculation. Early detection of lung injury and possible functional significance. Crit Care Clin 1986;2(3):497–509.

58. Pitt BR, Lister G. Interpretation of metabolic function of the lung. Influence of perfusion, kinetics, and injury. Clin Chest Med 1989;10(1):1–12.

59. Pitt BR. Metabolic functions of the lung and systemic vasoregulation. Fed Proc 1984;43(11):2574–7.

60. Gillis CN, Pitt BR, Wiedemann HP, Hammond GL. Depressed prostaglandin E1 and 5-hydroxytryptamine removal in patients with adult respiratory distress syndrome. Am Rev Respir Dis 1986;134(4):739–44.

•61. Orfanos SE, Langleben D, Khoury J, Schlesinger RD, Dragatakis L, Roussos C et al. Pulmonary capillary endothelium-bound angiotensin-converting enzyme activity in humans. Circulation 1999;99(12):1593–9.

62. Orfanos SE, Parkerson JB, Chen X, Fisher EL, Glynos C, Papapetropoulos A et al. Reduced lung endothelial angiotensin-converting enzyme activity in Watanabe hyperlipidemic rabbits in vivo. Am J Physiol Lung Cell Mol Physiol 2000;278(6):L1280–8.

63. Wenz M, Hoffmann B, Bohlender J, Kaczmarczyk G. Angiotensin II formation and endothelin clearance in ARDS patients in supine and prone positions. Intensive Care Med 2000;26(3):292–8.

64. Dupuis J, Stewart DJ, Cernacek P, Gosselin G. Human pulmonary circulation is an important site for both clearance and production of endothelin-1. Circulation 1996;94(7):1578–84.

•65. Langleben D, DeMarchie M, Laporta D, Spanier AH, Schlesinger RD, Stewart DJ. Endothelin-1 in acute lung injury and the adult respiratory distress syndrome. Am Rev Respir Dis 1993;148(6 Pt 1):1646–50.

66. Druml W, Steltzer H, Waldhausl W, Lenz K, Hammerle A, Vierhapper H et al. Endothelin-1 in adult respiratory distress syndrome. Am Rev Respir Dis 1993;148(5): 1169–73.

67. Creamer K, McCloud L, Fisher L, Ehrhart I. Optimal positive end-expiratory pressure fails to preserve nonrespiratory lung function in acute lung injury. Chest 1999;116(1 Suppl): 16S–17S.

68. Brimioulle S, LeJeune P, Naeije R. Effects of hypoxic pulmonary vasoconstriction on pulmonary gas exchange. J Appl Physiol 1996;81(4):1535–43.

69. Marshall BE, Marshall C, Frasch F, Hanson CW. Role of hypoxic pulmonary vasoconstriction in pulmonary gas exchange and blood flow distribution. 1. Physiologic concepts. Intensive Care Med 1994;20(4):291–7.

◆70. Moloney ED, Evans TW. Pathophysiology and pharmacological treatment of pulmonary hypertension in acute respiratory distress syndrome. Eur Respir J 2003; 21(4):720–7.

•71. Zapol WM, Snider MT. Pulmonary hypertension in severe acute respiratory failure. N Engl J Med 1977;296(9):476–80.

72. Zapol WM, Kobayashi K, Snider MT, Greene R, Laver MB. Vascular obstruction causes pulmonary hypertension in severe acute respiratory failure. Chest 1977;71(2 suppl): 306–7.

73. Carbone R, Bossone E, Bottino G, Monselise A, Rubenfire M. Secondary pulmonary hypertension – diagnosis and management. Eur Rev Med Pharmacol Sci 2005;9(6): 331–42.

74. Villar J, Blazquez MA, Lubillo S, Quintana J, Manzano JL. Pulmonary hypertension in acute respiratory failure. Crit Care Med 1989;17(6):523–6.

75. Leeman M. Pulmonary hypertension in acute respiratory distress syndrome. Monaldi Arch Chest Dis 1999;54(2): 146–9.

76. Squara P, Dhainaut JF, Artigas A, Carlet J. Hemodynamic profile in severe ARDS: results of the European Collaborative ARDS Study. Intensive Care Med 1998;24(10):1018–28.

77. Sloane PJ, Gee MH, Gottlieb JE, Albertine KH, Peters SP, Burns JR et al. A multicenter registry of patients with acute respiratory distress syndrome. Physiology and outcome. Am Rev Respir Dis 1992;146(2):419–26.

78. Osman D, Monnet X, Castelain V, Anguel N, Warszawski J, Teboul JL et al. Incidence and prognostic value of right ventricular failure in acute respiratory distress syndrome. Intensive Care Med 2009;35(1):69–76.

79. Cepkova M, Kapur V, Ren X, Quinn T, Zhuo H, Foster E et al. Pulmonary dead space fraction and pulmonary artery systolic pressure as early predictors of clinical outcome in acute lung injury. Chest 2007;132(3):836–42.

80. Vieillard-Baron A, Schmitt JM, Augarde R, Fellahi JL, Prin S, Page B et al. Acute cor pulmonale in acute respiratory distress syndrome submitted to protective ventilation: incidence, clinical implications, and prognosis. Crit Care Med 2001; 29(8):1551–5.

81. Vieillard-Baron A. Is right ventricular function the one that matters in ARDS patients? Definitely yes. Intensive Care Med 2009;35(1):4–6.

82. Bull TM, Clark B, McFann K, Moss M. National Institutes of Health/National Heart, Lung, and Blood Institute ARDS Network. Pulmonary vascular dysfunction is associated with poor outcomes in patients with acute lung injury. AM J Respir Crit Care Med 2010;182(9):1123–8.

◆83. Humbert M, Sitbon O, Simonneau G. Treatment of pulmonary arterial hypertension. N Engl J Med 2004;351(14):1425–36.

84. Barnard JW, Patterson CE, Hull MT, Wagner WW, Jr., Rhoades RA. Role of microvascular pressure in reactive oxygen-induced lung edema. J Appl Physiol 1989;66(3): 1486–93.

85. Palmer RM, Ashton DS, Moncada S. Vascular endothelial cells synthesize nitric oxide from L-arginine. Nature 1988; 333(6174):664–6.

86. Pepke-Zaba JMK. Inhaled nitric oxide. In: Pulmonary Circulation, 2004.

◆87. Steudel W, Hurford WE, Zapol WM. Inhaled nitric oxide: basic biology and clinical applications. Anesthesiology 1999;91(4):1090–121.

88. Freeman B. Free radical chemistry of nitric oxide. Looking at the dark side. Chest 1994;105(3 Suppl):79S–84S.

89. Holzmann A, Bloch KD, Sanchez LS, Filippov G, Zapol WM. Hyporesponsiveness to inhaled nitric oxide in isolated, perfused lungs from endotoxin-challenged rats. Am J Physiol 1996;271(6 Pt 1):L981–6.

90. Giaid A, Yanagisawa M, Langleben D, Michel RP, Levy R, Shennib H et al. Expression of endothelin-1 in the lungs of patients with pulmonary hypertension. N Engl J Med 1993;328(24):1732–9.

91. La M, Reid JJ. Endothelin-1 and the regulation of vascular tone. Clin Exp Pharmacol Physiol 1995;22(5):315–23.

92. Dupuis J, Jasmin JF, Prie S, Cernacek P. Importance of local production of endothelin-1 and of the ET(B)Receptor in the regulation of pulmonary vascular tone. Pulm Pharmacol Ther 2000;13(3):135–40.

93. Pittet JF, Morel DR, Hemsen A, Gunning K, Lacroix JS, Suter PM et al. Elevated plasma endothelin-1 concentrations are associated with the severity of illness in patients with sepsis. Ann Surg 1991;213(3):261–4.

94. Michael JR, Markewitz BA, Kohan DE. Oxidant stress regulates basal endothelin-1 production by cultured rat pulmonary endothelial cells. Am J Physiol 1997;273 (4 Pt 1):L768–74.

95. Golden CL, Nick HS, Visner GA. Thrombin regulation of endothelin-1 gene in isolated human pulmonary endothelial cells. Am J Physiol 1998;274(5 Pt 1): L854–63.

96. Langleben D, DeMarchie M, Laporta D, Spanier AH, Schlesinger RD, Stewart DJ. Endothelin-1 in acute lung injury and the adult respiratory distress syndrome. Am Rev Respir Dis 1993;148(6 Pt 1):1646–50.

97. Chen YF, Oparil S. Endothelin and pulmonary hypertension. J Cardiovasc Pharmacol 2000;35(4 Suppl 2):S49–53.

98. Chen SJ, Chen YF, Opgenorth TJ, Wessale JL, Meng QC, Durand J et al. The orally active nonpeptide endothelin A-receptor antagonist A-127722 prevents and reverses hypoxia-induced pulmonary hypertension and pulmonary vascular remodeling in Sprague–Dawley rats. J Cardiovasc Pharmacol 1997;29(6):713–25.

99. Oparil S, Chen SJ, Meng QC, Elton TS, Yano M, Chen YF. Endothelin-A receptor antagonist prevents acute hypoxia-induced pulmonary hypertension in the rat. Am J Physiol 1995;268(1 Pt 1):L95–100.

100. Curzen NP, Kaddoura S, Griffiths MJ, Evans TW. Endothelin-1 in rat endotoxemia: mRNA expression and vasoreactivity in pulmonary and systemic circulations. Am J Physiol 1997;272(5 Pt 2):H2353–60.

101. Guc MO, Furman BL, Parratt JR. Endotoxin-induced impairment of vasopressor and vasodepressor responses in the pithed rat. Br J Pharmacol 1990;101(4):913–9.

102. Tuder RM, Cool CD, Geraci MW, Wang J, Abman SH, Wright L et al. Prostacyclin synthase expression is decreased in lungs from patients with severe pulmonary hypertension. Am J Respir Crit Care Med 1999;159(6):1925–32.

103. Bernard GR, Reines HD, Halushka PV, Higgins SB, Metz CA, Swindell BB et al. Prostacyclin and thromboxane A2 formation is increased in human sepsis syndrome. Effects of cyclooxygenase inhibition. Am Rev Respir Dis 1991; 144(5):1095–101.

104. Hanly PJ, Roberts D, Dobson K, Light RB. Effect of indomethacin on arterial oxygenation in critically ill patients with severe bacterial pneumonia. Lancet 1987; 1(8529):351–4.

105. Bernard GR, Wheeler AP, Russell JA, Schein R, Summer WR, Steinberg KP et al. The effects of ibuprofen on the physiology and survival of patients with sepsis. The Ibuprofen in Sepsis Study Group. N Engl J Med 1997;336(13):912–8.

106. Gust R, Kozlowski JK, Stephenson AH, Schuster DP. Role of cyclooxygenase-2 in oleic acid-induced acute lung injury. Am J Respir Crit Care Med 1999;160(4):1165–70.

107. Vanhoutte PM. Endothelium-derived free radicals: for worse and for better. J Clin Invest 2001;107(1):23–5.

108. Lamb NJ, Quinlan GJ, Westerman ST, Gutteridge JM, Evans TW. Nitration of proteins in bronchoalveolar lavage fluid from patients with acute respiratory distress syndrome receiving inhaled nitric oxide. Am J Respir Crit Care Med 1999;160(3):1031–4.

109. Lamb NJ, Gutteridge JM, Baker C, Evans TW, Quinlan GJ. Oxidative damage to proteins of bronchoalveolar lavage fluid in patients with acute respiratory distress syndrome: evidence for neutrophil-mediated hydroxylation, nitration, and chlorination. Crit Care Med 1999;27(9):1738–44.

110. Rhoades RA, Packer CS, Meiss RA. Pulmonary vascular smooth muscle contractility. Effect of free radicals. Chest 1988;93(3 Suppl):94S–95S.

111. Sill V, Kaukel E, Volkel N, Siemssen S. The significance of cyclic 3′5-AMP for the Euler–Liljestrand mechanism. Pneumonologie 1974;150(2–4):337–44.

112. Hiser W, Penman RW, Reeves JT. Preservation of hypoxic pulmonary pressor response in canine pneumococcal pneumonia. Am Rev Respir Dis 1975;112(6):817–22.

113. Shirai M, Ninomiya I, Sada K. Constrictor response of small pulmonary arteries to acute pulmonary hypertension during left atrial pressure elevation. Jpn J Physiol 1991;41(1): 129–42.

114. Thomas HM, 3rd, Garrett RC. Strength of hypoxic vasoconstriction determines shunt fraction in dogs with atelectasis. J Appl Physiol 1982;53(1):44–51.

115. Yuan XJ, Goldman WF, Tod ML, Rubin LJ, Blaustein MP. Hypoxia reduces potassium currents in cultured rat pulmonary but not mesenteric arterial myocytes. Am J Physiol 1993;264(2 Pt 1):L116–23.

116. Moudgil R, Michelakis ED, Archer SL. The role of K+ channels in determining pulmonary vascular tone, oxygen sensing, cell proliferation, and apoptosis: implications in hypoxic pulmonary vasoconstriction and pulmonary arterial hypertension. Microcirculation 2006;13(8):615–32.

♦117. Moudgil R, Michelakis ED, Archer SL. Hypoxic pulmonary vasoconstriction. J Appl Physiol 2005;98(1):390–403.

118. Ward JP. Curiouser and curiouser: the perplexing conundrum of reactive oxygen species and hypoxic pulmonary vasoconstriction. Exp Physiol 2007;92(5):819–20.

119. Wang Z, Jin N, Ganguli S, Swartz DR, Li L, Rhoades RA. Rho-kinase activation is involved in hypoxia-induced pulmonary vasoconstriction. Am J Respir Cell Mol Biol 2001;25(5):628–35.

120. Liu SF, Crawley DE, Barnes PJ, Evans TW. Endothelium-derived relaxing factor inhibits hypoxic pulmonary vasoconstriction in rats. Am Rev Respir Dis 1991;143(1): 32–7.

121. Groves BM, Droma T, Sutton JR, McCullough RG, McCullough RE, Zhuang J et al. Minimal hypoxic pulmonary hypertension in normal Tibetans at 3,658 m. J Appl Physiol 1993;74(1):312–8.

122. Tucker A, Rhodes J. Role of vascular smooth muscle in the development of high altitude pulmonary hypertension: an interspecies evaluation. High Alt Med Biol 2001;2(2):73–89.

123. Maggiorini M, Leon-Velarde F. High-altitude pulmonary hypertension: a pathophysiological entity to different diseases. Eur Respir J 2003;22(6):1019–25.

124. Bartsch P, Mairbaurl H, Maggiorini M, Swenson ER. Physiological aspects of high-altitude pulmonary edema. J Appl Physiol 2005;98(3):1101–10.

125. West JB. Vulnerability of pulmonary capillaries during severe exercise. Br J Sports Med 2006;40(10):821.

126. Brimioulle S, Julien V, Gust R, Kozlowski JK, Naeije R, Schuster DP. Importance of hypoxic vasoconstriction in maintaining oxygenation during acute lung injury. Crit Care Med 2002;30(4):874–80.

127. Younes M, Bshouty Z, Ali J. Longitudinal distribution of pulmonary vascular resistance with very high pulmonary blood flow. J Appl Physiol 1987;62(1):344–58.

128. Melot C, Naeije R, Hallemans R, Lejeune P, Mols P. Hypoxic pulmonary vasoconstriction and pulmonary gas exchange in normal man. Respir Physiol 1987;68(1):11–27.

129. Schuster DP, Anderson C, Kozlowski J, Lange N. Regional pulmonary perfusion in patients with acute pulmonary edema. J Nucl Med 2002;43(7):863–70.

130. Huttemeier PC, Watkins WD, Peterson MB, Zapol WM. Acute pulmonary hypertension and lung thromboxane release after endotoxin infusion in normal and leukopenic sheep. Circ Res 1982;50(5):688–94.

131. Baraka AS, Taha SK, Yaacoub CI. Alarming hypoxemia during one-lung ventilation in a patient with respiratory bronchiolitis-associated interstitial lung disease. Can J Anaesth 2003;50(4):411–4.

132. Daoud FS, Reeves JT, Schaefer JW. Failure of hypoxic pulmonary vasoconstriction in patients with liver cirrhosis. J Clin Invest 1972;51(5):1076–80.

133. Walther SM, Domino KB, Hlastala MP. Effects of posture on blood flow diversion by hypoxic pulmonary vasoconstriction in dogs. Br J Anaesth 1998;81(3):425–9.

134. Lejeune P, De Smet JM, de Francquen P, Leeman M, Brimioulle S, Hallemans R et al. Inhibition of hypoxic pulmonary vasoconstriction by increased left atrial pressure in dogs. Am J Physiol 1990;259(1 Pt 2):H93–100.

135. Lejeune P, Vachiery JL, De Smet JM, Leeman M, Brimioulle S, Delcroix M et al. PEEP inhibits hypoxic pulmonary vasoconstriction in dogs. J Appl Physiol 1991;70(4):1867–73.

136. Brimioulle S, Lejeune P, Vachiery JL, Leeman M, Melot C, Naeije R. Effects of acidosis and alkalosis on hypoxic pulmonary vasoconstriction in dogs. Am J Physiol 1990;258(2 Pt 2):H347–53.

137. Benumof JL, Wahrenbrock EA. Dependency of hypoxic pulmonary vasoconstriction on temperature. J Appl Physiol 1977;42(1):56–8.

138. Marshall C, Lindgren L, Marshall BE. Effects of halothane, enflurane, and isoflurane on hypoxic pulmonary vasoconstriction in rat lungs in vitro Anesthesiology 1984;60(4):304–8.

139. Kjaeve J, Bjertnaes LJ. Interaction of verapamil and halogenated inhalation anesthetics on hypoxic pulmonary vasoconstriction. Acta Anaesthesiol Scand 1989;33(3):193–8.

140. Johnson D, Hurst T, Mayers I. Insufflated halothane increases venous admixture less than nitroprusside in canine atelectasis. Anesthesiology 1992;77(2):301–8.

141. Nakayama M, Murray PA. Ketamine preserves and propofol potentiates hypoxic pulmonary vasoconstriction compared with the conscious state in chronically instrumented dogs. Anesthesiology 1999;91(3):760–71.

142. Van Keer L, Van Aken H, Vandermeersch E, Vermaut G, Lerut T. Propofol does not inhibit hypoxic pulmonary vasoconstriction in humans. J Clin Anesth 1989;1(4):284–8.

143. Bjertnaes L, Hauge A, Kriz M. Hypoxia-induced pulmonary vasoconstriction: effects of fentanyl following different routes of administration. Acta Anaesthesiol Scand 1980;24(1):53–7.

144. Schellenberg RR, Foster A. Differential activity of leukotrienes upon human pulmonary vein and artery. Prostaglandins 1984;27(3):475–82.

145. Lippton HL, Ohlstein EH, Summer WR, Hyman AL. Analysis of responses to endothelins in the rabbit pulmonary and systemic vascular beds. J Appl Physiol 1991;70(1):331–41.

146. Labat C, Ortiz JL, Norel X, Gorenne I, Verley J, Abram TS et al. A second cysteinyl leukotriene receptor in human lung. J Pharmacol Exp Ther 1992;263(2):800–5.

147. Walch L, de Montpreville V, Brink C, Norel X. Prostanoid EP(1)- and TP-receptors involved in the contraction of human pulmonary veins. Br J Pharmacol 2001;134(8):1671–8.

148. Greene R, Zapol WM, Snider MT, Reid L, Snow R, O'Connell RS et al. Early bedside detection of pulmonary vascular occlusion during acute respiratory failure. Am Rev Respir Dis 1981;124(5):593–601.

149. Schuster DP, Kozlowski JP, Brimioulle S. Effect of thromboxane receptor blockade on pulmonary capillary hypertension in acute lung injury. Am J Respir Crit Care Med 2001;163(5):A820.

•150. Greene R, Lind S, Jantsch H, Wilson R, Lynch K, Jones R et al. Pulmonary vascular obstruction in severe ARDS: angiographic alterations after i.v. fibrinolytic therapy. AJR Am J Roentgenol 1987;148(3):501–8.

◆151. Chambers RC. Procoagulant signaling mechanisms in lung inflammation and fibrosis: novel opportunities for pharmacological intervention? Br J Pharmacol 2008;(153 Suppl 1):S367–78.

152. Levi M, Ten Cate H. Disseminated intravascular coagulation. N Engl J Med 1999;341(8):586–92.

153. Gando S, Kameue T, Matsuda N, Hayakawa M, Morimoto Y, Ishitani T et al. Imbalances between the levels of tissue factor and tissue factor pathway inhibitor in ARDS patients. Thromb Res 2003;109(2–3):119–24.

154. Fourrier F, Chopin C, Goudemand J, Hendrycx S, Caron C, Rime A et al. Septic shock, multiple organ failure, and disseminated intravascular coagulation. Compared patterns of antithrombin III, protein C, and protein S deficiencies. Chest 1992;101(3):816–23.

155. MacGregor IR, Perrie AM, Donnelly SC, Haslett C. Modulation of human endothelial thrombomodulin by neutrophils and their release products. Am J Respir Crit Care Med 1997;155(1):47–52.

◆156. Ware LB, Matthay MA, Parsons PE, Thompson BT, Januzzi JL, Eisner MD. Pathogenetic and prognostic significance of altered coagulation and fibrinolysis in acute lung injury/ acute respiratory distress syndrome. Crit Care Med 2007;35(8):1821–8.

157. Block ER. Pulmonary endothelial cell pathobiology: implications for acute lung injury. Am J Med Sci 1992;304(2):136–44.

158. Grau GE, de Moerloose P, Bulla O, Lou J, Lei Z, Reber G et al. Hemostatic properties of human pulmonary and cerebral microvascular endothelial cells. Thromb Hemost 1997;77(3):585–90.

159. Carvalho AC, Quinn DA, DeMarinis SM, Beitz JG, Zapol WM. Platelet function in acute respiratory failure. Am J Hematol 1987;25(4):377–88.

160. Orfanos SE, Mavrommati I, Korovesi I, Roussos C. Pulmonary endothelium in acute lung injury: from basic science to the critically ill. Intensive Care Med 2004;30(9):1702–14.

161. Bellingan GJ. The pulmonary physician in critical care * 6: The pathogenesis of ALI/ARDS. Thorax 2002;57(6): 540–6.

162. Oberholzer A, Oberholzer C, Moldawer LL. Cytokine signaling – regulation of the immune response in normal and critically ill states. Crit Care Med 2000;28(4 Suppl): N3–12.

163. Heffner JE, Sahn SA, Repine JE. The role of platelets in the adult respiratory distress syndrome. Culprits or bystanders? Am Rev Respir Dis 1987;135(2):482–92.

164. Eisenhut T, Sinha B, Grottrup-Wolfers E, Semmler J, Siess W, Endres S. Prostacyclin analogs suppress the synthesis of tumor necrosis factor-alpha in LPS-stimulated human peripheral blood mononuclear cells. Immunopharmacology 1993;26(3):259–64.

165. Kainoh M, Imai R, Umetsu T, Hattori M, Nishio S. Prostacyclin and beraprost sodium as suppressors of activated rat polymorphonuclear leukocytes. Biochem Pharmacol 1990;39(3):477–84.

166. Doerschuk CM. Mechanisms of leukocyte sequestration in inflamed lungs. Microcirculation 2001;8(2):71–88.

167. Gebb SA, Graham JA, Hanger CC, Godbey PS, Capen RL, Doerschuk CM et al. Sites of leukocyte sequestration in the pulmonary microcirculation. J Appl Physiol 1995; 79(2):493–7.

168. Fan J, Ye RD, Malik AB. Transcriptional mechanisms of acute lung injury. Am J Physiol Lung Cell Mol Physiol 2001;281(5):L1037–50.

169. Pugin J, Verghese G, Widmer MC, Matthay MA. The alveolar space is the site of intense inflammatory and profibrotic reactions in the early phase of acute respiratory distress syndrome. Crit Care Med 1999;27(2):304–12.

170. Dorfmuller P, Perros F, Balabanian K, Humbert M. Inflammation in pulmonary arterial hypertension. Eur Respir J 2003;22(2):358–63.

ʋ171. Stenmark KR, Davie NJ, Reeves JT, Frid MG. Hypoxia, leukocytes, and the pulmonary circulation. J Appl Physiol 2005;98(2):715–21.

172. Minamino T, Christou H, Hsieh CM, Liu Y, Dhawan V, Abraham NG et al. Targeted expression of heme oxygenase-1 prevents the pulmonary inflammatory and vascular responses to hypoxia. Proc Natl Acad Sci USA 2001;98(15):8798–803.

173. Kubo K, Hanaoka M, Yamaguchi S, Hayano T, Hayasaka M, Koizumi T et al. Cytokines in bronchoalveolar lavage fluid in patients with high altitude pulmonary edema at moderate altitude in Japan. Thorax 1996;51(7):739–42.

174. Bachofen M, Weibel ER. Structural alterations of lung parenchyma in the adult respiratory distress syndrome. Clin Chest Med 1982;3(1):35–56.

175. Stenmark KR, Bouchey D, Nemenoff R, Dempsey EC, Das M. Hypoxia-induced pulmonary vascular remodeling: contribution of the adventitial fibroblasts. Physiol Res 2000;49(5):503–17.

176. Stenmark KR, Gerasimovskaya E, Nemenoff RA, Das M. Hypoxic activation of adventitial fibroblasts: role in vascular remodeling. Chest 2002;122(6 Suppl):326S–334S.

177. Maruyama K, Ye CL, Woo M, Venkatacharya H, Lines LD, Silver MM et al. Chronic hypoxic pulmonary hypertension in rats and increased elastolytic activity. Am J Physiol 1991;261(6 Pt 2):H1716–26.

178. Kornecki A, Engelberts D, McNamara P, Jankov RP, McCaul C, Ackerley C et al. Vascular remodeling protects against ventilator-induced lung injury in the in vivo rat. Anesthesiology 2008;108(6):1047–54.

179. Stenmark KR, Fagan KA, Frid MG. Hypoxia-induced pulmonary vascular remodeling: cellular and molecular mechanisms. Circ Res 2006;99(7):675–91.

180. Frid MG, Dempsey EC, Durmowicz AG, Stenmark KR. Smooth muscle cell heterogeneity in pulmonary and systemic vessels. Importance in vascular disease. Arterioscler Thromb Vasc Biol 1997;17(7):1203–9.

181. Xu Y, Stenmark KR, Das M, Walchak SJ, Ruff LJ, Dempsey EC. Pulmonary artery smooth muscle cells from chronically hypoxic neonatal calves retain fetal-like and acquire new growth properties. Am J Physiol 1997;273(1 Pt 1):L234–45.

182. Wohrley JD, Frid MG, Moiseeva EP, Orton EC, Belknap JK, Stenmark KR. Hypoxia selectively induces proliferation in a specific subpopulation of smooth muscle cells in the bovine neonatal pulmonary arterial media. J Clin Invest 1995;96(1):273–81.

183. Nicolls MR, Voelkel NF. Hypoxia and the lung: beyond hypoxic vasoconstriction. Antioxid Redox Signal 2007;9(6):741–3.

184. Aguirre JI, Morrell NW, Long L, Clift P, Upton PD, Polak JM et al. Vascular remodeling and ET-1 expression in rat strains with different responses to chronic hypoxia. Am J Physiol Lung Cell Mol Physiol 2000;278(5):L981–7.

185. Chua BH, Krebs CJ, Chua CC, Diglio CA. Endothelin stimulates protein synthesis in smooth muscle cells. Am J Physiol 1992;262(4 Pt 1):E412–6.

186. Sasu S, LaVerda D, Qureshi N, Golenbock DT, Beasley D. Chlamydia pneumoniae and chlamydial heat shock protein 60 stimulate proliferation of human vascular smooth muscle cells via toll-like receptor 4 and p44/p42 mitogen-activated protein kinase activation. Circ Res 2001;89(3):244–50.

187. Yang X, Murthy V, Schultz K, Tatro JB, Fitzgerald KA, Beasley D. Toll-like receptor 3 signaling evokes a proinflammatory and proliferative phenotype in human vascular smooth muscle cells. Am J Physiol Heart Circ Physiol 2006;291(5):H2334–43.

188. King TK, Weber B, Okinaka A, Friedman SA, Smith JP, Briscoe WA. Oxygen transfer in catastrophic respiratory failure. Chest 1974;(65 Suppl):40S–44S.

189. Macnaughton PD, Evans TW. Measurement of lung volume and DLCO in acute respiratory failure. Am J Respir Crit Care Med 1994;150(3):770–5.

190. Desai SR, Wells AU, Suntharalingam G, Rubens MB, Evans TW, Hansell DM. Acute respiratory distress syndrome caused by pulmonary and extrapulmonary injury: a comparative CT study. Radiology 2001;218(3):689–93.

191. Desai SR, Hansell DM. Lung imaging in the adult respiratory distress syndrome: current practice and new insights. Intensive Care Med 1997;23(1):7–15.

192. Rouby JJ, Puybasset L, Cluzel P, Richecoeur J, Lu Q, Grenier P. Regional distribution of gas and tissue in acute respiratory distress syndrome. II. Physiological correlations and definition of an ARDS Severity Score. CT Scan ARDS Study Group. Intensive Care Med 2000;26(8):1046–56.

193. Puybasset L, Cluzel P, Chao N, Slutsky AS, Coriat P, Rouby JJ. A computed tomography scan assessment of regional lung volume in acute lung injury. The CT Scan ARDS Study Group. Am J Respir Crit Care Med 1998;158(5 Pt 1):1644–55.

194. Dantzker DR, Brook CJ, Dehart P, Lynch JP, Weg JG. Ventilation–perfusion distributions in the adult respiratory distress syndrome. Am Rev Respir Dis 1979;120(5):1039–52.

195. Melot C. Contribution of multiple inert gas elimination technique to pulmonary medicine. 5. Ventilation–perfusion relationships in acute respiratory failure. Thorax 1994;49(12):1251–8.

196. Rasanen J, Vaisanen IT, Heikkila J, Nikki P. Acute myocardial infarction complicated by left ventricular dysfunction and respiratory failure. The effects of continuous positive airway pressure. Chest 1985;87(2):158–62.

•197. Suter PM, Fairley B, Isenberg MD. Optimum end-expiratory airway pressure in patients with acute pulmonary failure. N Engl J Med 1975;292(6):284–9.

198. Ralph DD, Robertson HT, Weaver LJ, Hlastala MP, Carrico CJ, Hudson LD. Distribution of ventilation and perfusion during positive end-expiratory pressure in the adult respiratory distress syndrome. Am Rev Respir Dis 1985;131(1):54–60.

199. Dantzker DR, Lynch JP, Weg JG. Depression of cardiac output is a mechanism of shunt reduction in the therapy of acute respiratory failure. Chest 1980;77(5):636–42.

200. Cheatham ML, Nelson LD, Chang MC, Safcsak K. Right ventricular end-diastolic volume index as a predictor of preload status in patients on positive end-expiratory pressure. Crit Care Med 1998;26(11):1801–6.

•201. Poelaert JI, Visser CA, Everaert JA, Koolen JJ, Colardyn FA. Acute hemodynamic changes of pressure-controlled inverse ratio ventilation in the adult respiratory distress syndrome. A transesophageal echocardiographic and Doppler study. Chest 1993;104(1):214–9.

202. Abraham E, Yoshihara G. Cardiorespiratory effects of pressure controlled inverse ratio ventilation in severe respiratory failure. Chest 1989;96(6):1356–9.

203. Lessard MR, Guerot E, Lorino H, Lemaire F, Brochard L. Effects of pressure-controlled with different I:E ratios versus volume-controlled ventilation on respiratory mechanics, gas exchange, and hemodynamics in patients with adult respiratory distress syndrome. Anesthesiology 1994;80(5):983–91.

204. Matamis D, Lemaire F, Harf A, Teisseire B, Brun-Buisson C. Redistribution of pulmonary blood flow induced by positive end-expiratory pressure and dopamine infusion in acute respiratory failure. Am Rev Respir Dis 1984;129(1):39–44.

•205. West JB, Dollery CT, Naimark A. Distribution of blood flow in isolated lung; relation to vascular and alveolar pressures. J Appl Physiol 1964;19:713–24.

206. Beck KC, Rehder K. Differences in regional vascular conductances in isolated dog lungs. J Appl Physiol 1986;61(2):530–8.

207. Reed JH, Jr., Wood EH. Effect of body position on vertical distribution of pulmonary blood flow. J Appl Physiol 1970;28(3):303–11.

208. Hakim TS, Lisbona R, Dean GW. Gravity-independent inequality in pulmonary blood flow in humans. J Appl Physiol 1987;63(3):1114–21.

209. Glenny RW, Robertson HT. Fractal properties of pulmonary blood flow: characterization of spatial heterogeneity. J Appl Physiol 1990;69(2):532–45.

210. Pelletier N, Robinson NE, Kaiser L, Derksen FJ. Regional differences in endothelial function in horse lungs: possible role in blood flow distribution? J Appl Physiol 1998;85(2):537–42.

211. Nyren S, Mure M, Jacobsson H, Larsson SA, Lindahl SG. Pulmonary perfusion is more uniform in the prone than in the supine position: scintigraphy in healthy humans. J Appl Physiol 1999;86(4):1135–41.

212. Jones AT, Hansell DM, Evans TW. Pulmonary perfusion in supine and prone positions: an electron–beam computed tomography study. J Appl Physiol 2001;90(4):1342–8.

213. Mure M, Lindahl SG. Prone position improves gas exchange – but how? Acta Anaesthesiol Scand 2001;45(2):150–9.

214. Sinclair SE, Albert RK. Altering ventilation–perfusion relationships in ventilated patients with acute lung injury. Intensive Care Med 1997;23(9):942–50.

215. Lamm WJ, Graham MM, Albert RK. Mechanism by which the prone position improves oxygenation in acute lung injury. Am J Respir Crit Care Med 1994;150(1):184–93.

216. Piehl MA, Brown RS. Use of extreme position changes in acute respiratory failure. Crit Care Med 1976;4(1):13–4.

217. Langer M, Mascheroni D, Marcolin R, Gattinoni L. The prone position in ARDS patients. A clinical study. Chest 1988;94(1):103–7.

218. Gattinoni L, Tognoni G, Pesenti A, Taccone P, Mascheroni D, Labarta V et al. Effect of prone positioning on the survival of patients with acute respiratory failure. N Engl J Med 2001;345(8):568–73.

•219. Vieillard-Baron A, Charron C, Caille V, Belliard G, Page B, Jardin F. Prone positioning unloads the right ventricle in severe ARDS. Chest 2007;132(5):1440–6.

220. Jardin F, Vieillard-Baron A. Is there a safe plateau pressure in ARDS? The right heart only knows. Intensive Care Med 2007;33(3):444–7.

221. Jardin F, Brun-Ney D, Cazaux P, Dubourg O, Hardy A, Bourdarias JP. Relation between transpulmonary pressure and right ventricular isovolumetric pressure change during respiratory support. Cathet Cardiovasc Diagn 1989;16(4):215–20.

222. Jullien T, Valtier B, Hongnat JM, Dubourg O, Bourdarias JP, Jardin F. Incidence of tricuspid regurgitation and vena caval backward flow in mechanically ventilated patients. A color Doppler and contrast echocardiographic study. Chest 1995;107(2):488–93.

223. Jardin F, Delorme G, Hardy A, Auvert B, Beauchet A, Bourdarias JP. Reevaluation of hemodynamic consequences of positive pressure ventilation: emphasis on cyclic right ventricular afterloading by mechanical lung inflation. Anesthesiology 1990;72(6):966–70.

•224. Jardin F, Gueret P, Dubourg O, Farcot JC, Margairaz A, Bourdarias JP. Two-dimensional echocardiographic evaluation of right ventricular size and contractility in acute respiratory failure. Crit Care Med 1985; 13(11):952–6.

225. Jardin F, Fellahi JL, Beauchet A, Vieillard-Baron A, Loubieres Y, Page B. Improved prognosis of acute respiratory distress syndrome 15 years on. Intensive Care Med 1999;25(9): 936–41.

226. Balanos GM, Talbot NP, Dorrington KL, Robbins PA. Human pulmonary vascular response to 4 h of hypercapnia and hypocapnia measured using Doppler echocardiography. J Appl Physiol 2003;94(4):1543–51.

227. Eichacker PQ, Gerstenberger EP, Banks SM, Cui X, Natanson C. Meta-analysis of acute lung injury and acute respiratory distress syndrome trials testing low tidal volumes. Am J Respir Crit Care Med 2002;166(11):1510–4.

228. Mekontso Dessap A, Charron C, Devaquet J, Aboab J, Jardin F, Brochard L et al. Impact of acute hypercapnia and augmented positive end-expiratory pressure on right ventricle function in severe acute respiratory distress syndrome. Intensive Care Med 2009;35(11):1850–8.

229. Artucio H, Hurtado J, Zimet L, de Paula J, Beron M. PEEP-induced tricuspid regurgitation. Intensive Care Med 1997;23(8):836–40.

230. Fougeres E, Teboul JL, Richard C, Osman D, Chemla D, Monnet X. Hemodynamic impact of a positive end-expiratory pressure setting in acute respiratory distress syndrome: importance of the volume status. Crit Care Med 2010;38(3):802–7.

231. Murphy DB, Cregg N, Tremblay L, Engelberts D, Laffey JG, Slutsky AS et al. Adverse ventilatory strategy causes pulmonary-to-systemic translocation of endotoxin. Am J Respir Crit Care Med 2000;162(1):27–33.

232. Duggan M, McCaul CL, McNamara PJ, Engelberts D, Ackerley C, Kavanagh BP. Atelectasis causes vascular leak and lethal right ventricular failure in uninjured rat lungs. Am J Respir Crit Care Med 2003;167(12):1633–40.

233. Marshall BE, Marshall C, Magno M, Lilagan P, Pietra GG. Influence of bronchial arterial PO$_2$ on pulmonary vascular resistance. J Appl Physiol 1991;70(1):405–15.

234. Pepe PE, Marini JJ. Occult positive end-expiratory pressure in mechanically ventilated patients with airflow obstruction: the auto-PEEP effect. Am Rev Respir Dis 1982;126(1): 166–70.

235. Levy MM. PEEP in ARDS – how much is enough? N Engl J Med 2004;351(4):389–91.

236. Reis Miranda D, Struijs A, Koetsier P, van Thiel R, Schepp R, Hop W et al. Open lung ventilation improves functional residual capacity after extubation in cardiac surgery. Crit Care Med 2005;33(10):2253–8.

237. Halter JM, Steinberg JM, Schiller HJ, DaSilva M, Gatto LA, Landas S et al. Positive end-expiratory pressure after a recruitment maneuver prevents both alveolar collapse and recruitment/derecruitment. Am J Respir Crit Care Med 2003;167(12):1620–6.

238. Dawson CA, Grimm DJ, Linehan JH. Lung inflation and longitudinal distribution of pulmonary vascular resistance during hypoxia. J Appl Physiol 1979;47(3):532–6.

239. Butler J. The heart is in good hands. Circulation 1983; 67(6):1163–8.

240. Vieillard-Baron A, Charron C, Jardin F. Lung "recruitment" or lung overinflation maneuvers? Intensive Care Med 2006;32(1):177–8.

241. Nielsen J, Ostergaard M, Kjaergaard J, Tingleff J, Berthelsen PG, Nygard E et al. Lung recruitment maneuver depresses central hemodynamics in patients following cardiac surgery. Intensive Care Med 2005;31(9):1189–94.

242. Jardin F. Acute leftward septal shift by lung recruitment maneuver. Intensive Care Med 2005;31(9):1148–9.

243. Benzing A, Mols G, Guttmann J, Kaltofen H, Geiger K. Effect of different doses of inhaled nitric oxide on pulmonary capillary pressure and on longitudinal distribution of pulmonary vascular resistance in ARDS. Br J Anaesth 1998;80(4):440–6.

244. Radermacher P, Santak B, Wust HJ, Tarnow J, Falke KJ. Prostacyclin for the treatment of pulmonary hypertension in the adult respiratory distress syndrome: effects on pulmonary capillary pressure and ventilation–perfusion distributions. Anesthesiology 1990;72(2):238–44.

245. Thompson JS, Kavanagh BP, Pearl RG. Nitroglycerin does not alter pulmonary vascular permeability in isolated rabbit lungs. Anesth Analg 1997;84(2):359–62.

246. Radermacher P, Santak B, Becker H, Falke KJ. Prostaglandin E1 and nitroglycerin reduce pulmonary capillary pressure but worsen ventilation–perfusion distributions in patients with adult respiratory distress syndrome. Anesthesiology 1989;70(4):601–6.

247. Zapol WM, Jones R. Vascular components of ARDS. Clinical pulmonary hemodynamics and morphology. Am Rev Respir Dis 1987;136(2):471–4.

248. Melot C, Naeije R, Mols P, Hallemans R, Lejeune P, Jaspar N. Pulmonary vascular tone improves pulmonary gas exchange in the adult respiratory distress syndrome. Am Rev Respir Dis 1987;136(5):1232–6.

249. Ryhammer PK, Shekerdemian LS, Penny DJ, Ravn HB. Effect of intravenous sildenafil on pulmonary hemodynamics and gas exchange in the presence and absence of acute lung injury in piglets. Pediatr Res 2006;59(6):762–6.

250. Rossaint R, Falke KJ, Lopez F, Slama K, Pison U, Zapol WM. Inhaled nitric oxide for the adult respiratory distress syndrome. N Engl J Med 1993;328(6):399–405.

◆251. Griffiths MJ, Evans TW. Inhaled nitric oxide therapy in adults. N Engl J Med 2005;353(25):2683–95.

252. Garg UC, Hassid A. Inhibition of rat mesangial cell mitogenesis by nitric oxide-generating vasodilators. Am J Physiol 1989;257(1 Pt 2):F60-6.

253. Kouyoumdjian C, Adnot S, Levame M, Eddahibi S, Bousbaa H, Raffestin B. Continuous inhalation of nitric oxide protects against development of pulmonary hypertension in chronically hypoxic rats. J Clin Invest 1994;94(2):578-84.

254. Kubes P, Suzuki M, Granger DN. Nitric oxide: an endogenous modulator of leukocyte adhesion. Proc Natl Acad Sci U S A 1991;88(11):4651-5.

255. Moncada S, Palmer RM, Higgs EA. Nitric oxide: physiology, pathophysiology, and pharmacology. Pharmacol Rev 1991;43(2):109-42.

256. Smith AW, Green J, Eden CE, Watson ML. Nitric oxide-induced potentiation of the killing of Burkholderia cepacia by reactive oxygen species: implications for cystic fibrosis. J Med Microbiol 1999;48(5):419-23.

257. Weitzberg E, Rudehill A, Alving K, Lundberg JM. Nitric oxide inhalation selectively attenuates pulmonary hypertension and arterial hypoxia in porcine endotoxin shock. Acta Physiol Scand 1991;143(4):451-2.

258. Ogura H, Offner PJ, Saitoh D, Jordan BS, Johnson AA, Pruitt BA, Jr. et al. The pulmonary effect of nitric oxide synthase inhibition following endotoxemia in a swine model. Arch Surg 1994;129(12):1233-9.

259. Frostell CG, Blomqvist H, Hedenstierna G, Lundberg J, Zapol WM. Inhaled nitric oxide selectively reverses human hypoxic pulmonary vasoconstriction without causing systemic vasodilation. Anesthesiology 1993;78(3):427-35.

•260. Pepke-Zaba J, Higenbottam TW, Dinh-Xuan AT, Stone D, Wallwork J. Inhaled nitric oxide as a cause of selective pulmonary vasodilatation in pulmonary hypertension. Lancet 1991;338(8776):1173-4.

261. Rich GF, Murphy GD, Jr., Roos CM, Johns RA. Inhaled nitric oxide. Selective pulmonary vasodilation in cardiac surgical patients. Anesthesiology 1993;78(6):1028-35.

262. Macdonald PS, Keogh A, Mundy J, Rogers P, Nicholson A, Harrison G et al. Adjunctive use of inhaled nitric oxide during implantation of a left ventricular assist device. J Heart Lung Transplant 1998;17(3):312-6.

263. Hsu CW, Lee DL, Lin SL, Sun SF, Chang HW. The initial response to inhaled nitric oxide treatment for intensive care unit patients with acute respiratory distress syndrome. Respiration 2008;75(3):288-95.

264. Taylor RW, Zimmerman JL, Dellinger RP, Straube RC, Criner GJ, Davis K, Jr. et al. Low-dose inhaled nitric oxide in patients with acute lung injury: a randomized controlled trial. JAMA 2004;291(13):1603-9.

265. Adhikari NK, Burns KE, Friedrich JO, Granton JT, Cook DJ, Meade MO. Effect of nitric oxide on oxygenation and mortality in acute lung injury: systematic review and meta-analysis. BMJ 2007;334(7597):779.

266. Giacomini M, Borotto E, Bosotti L, Denkewitz T, Reali-Forster C, Carlucci P et al. Vardenafil and weaning from inhaled nitric oxide: effect on pulmonary hypertension in ARDS. Anaesth Intensive Care 2007;35(1):91-3.

267. Ng J, Finney SJ, Shulman R, Bellingan GJ, Singer M, Glynne PA. Treatment of pulmonary hypertension in the general adult intensive care unit: a role for oral sildenafil? Br J Anaesth 2005;94(6):774-7.

268. Walmrath D, Schneider T, Pilch J, Grimminger F, Seeger W. Aerosolised prostacyclin in adult respiratory distress syndrome. Lancet 1993;342(8877):961-2.

269. Zwissler B, Kemming G, Habler O, Kleen M, Merkel M, Haller M et al. Inhaled prostacyclin (PGI2) versus inhaled nitric oxide in adult respiratory distress syndrome. Am J Respir Crit Care Med 1996;154(6 Pt 1):1671-7.

270. van Heerden PV, Barden A, Michalopoulos N, Bulsara MK, Roberts BL. Dose-response to inhaled aerosolized prostacyclin for hypoxemia due to ARDS. Chest 2000; 117(3):819-27.

271. Moncada S, Higgs EA. Metabolism of arachidonic acid. Ann N Y Acad Sci 1988;522:454-63.

272. Geiger R, Kleinsasser A, Meier S, Neu N, Pajk W, Fischer V et al. Intravenous tezosentan improves gas exchange and hemodynamics in acute lung injury secondary to meconium aspiration. Intensive Care Med 2008;34(2):368-76.

273. Hubloue I, Biarent D, Abdel Kafi S, Bejjani G, Melot C, Naeije R et al. Endothelin receptor blockade in canine oleic acid-induced lung injury. Intensive Care Med 2003; 29(6):1003-6.

274. Rubin LJ, Badesch DB, Barst RJ, Galie N, Black CM, Keogh A et al. Bosentan therapy for pulmonary arterial hypertension. N Engl J Med 2002;346(12):896-903.

275. Channick RN, Simonneau G, Sitbon O, Robbins IM, Frost A, Tapson VF et al. Effects of the dual endothelin-receptor antagonist bosentan in patients with pulmonary hypertension: a randomised placebo-controlled study. Lancet 2001;358(9288):1119-23.

276. Galie N, Badesch D, Oudiz R, Simonneau G, McGoon MD, Keogh AM et al. Ambrisentan therapy for pulmonary arterial hypertension. J Am Coll Cardiol 2005;46(3):529-35.

277. Galie N, Olschewski H, Oudiz RJ, Torres F, Frost A, Ghofrani HA et al. Ambrisentan for the treatment of pulmonary arterial hypertension: results of the ambrisentan in pulmonary arterial hypertension, randomized, double-blind, placebo-controlled, multicenter, efficacy (ARIES) study 1 and 2. Circulation 2008;117(23):3010-9.

278. Barst RJ, Langleben D, Frost A, Horn EM, Oudiz R, Shapiro S et al. Sitaxsentan therapy for pulmonary arterial hypertension. Am J Respir Crit Care Med 2004;169(4):441-7.

279. Bohm F, Ahlborg G, Johansson BL, Hansson LO, Pernow J. Combined endothelin receptor blockade evokes enhanced vasodilatation in patients with atherosclerosis. Arterioscler Thromb Vasc Biol 2002;22(4):674-9.

280. Kuklin VN, Kirov MY, Evgenov OV, Sovershaev MA, Sjoberg J, Kirova SS et al. Novel endothelin receptor antagonist attenuates endotoxin-induced lung injury in sheep. Crit Care Med 2004;32(3):766-73.

281. Rossi P, Wanecek M, Konrad D, Oldner A. Tezosentan counteracts endotoxin-induced pulmonary edema and improves gas exchange. Shock 2004;21(6):543-8.

282. Shekerdemian LS, Penny DJ, Ryhammer PK, Reader JA, Ravn HB. Endothelin-A receptor blockade and inhaled nitric oxide in a porcine model of meconium aspiration syndrome. Pediatr Res 2004;56(3):353–8.

282. Cornet AD, Hofstra JJ, Swart EL, Girbes AR, Juffermans NP. Sildenafil attenuates pulmonary arterial pressure but does not improve oxygenation during ARDS. Intensive Care Med 2010;36(5):758–64.

283. Geiger R, Pajk W, Neu N, Maier S, Kleinsasser A, Fratz S et al. Tezosentan decreases pulmonary artery pressure and improves survival rate in an animal model of meconium aspiration. Pediatr Res 2006;59(1):147–50.

284. Rossi P, Persson B, Boels PJ, Arner A, Weitzberg E, Oldner A. Endotoxemic pulmonary hypertension is largely mediated by endothelin-induced venous constriction. Intensive Care Med 2008;34(5):873–80.

285. Ingbar DH. Mechanisms of repair and remodeling following acute lung injury. Clin Chest Med 2000;21(3):589–616.

286. Hert R, Albert RK. Sequelae of the adult respiratory distress syndrome. Thorax 1994;49(1):8–13.

•287. Suntharalingam G, Regan K, Keogh BF, Morgan CJ, Evans TW. Influence of direct and indirect etiology on acute outcome and 6-month functional recovery in acute respiratory distress syndrome. Crit Care Med 2001;29(3):562–6.

288. Luhr O, Aardal S, Nathorst-Westfelt U, Berggren L, Johansson LA, Wahlin L et al. Pulmonary function in adult survivors of severe acute lung injury treated with inhaled nitric oxide. Acta Anaesthesiol Scand 1998;42(4):391–8.

289. Buchser E, Leuenberger P, Chiolero R, Perret C, Freeman J. Reduced pulmonary capillary blood volume as a long-term sequel of ARDS. Chest 1985;87(5):608–11.

290. Elliott CG, Morris AH, Cengiz M. Pulmonary function and exercise gas exchange in survivors of adult respiratory

distress syndrome. Am Rev Respir Dis 1981;123(5): 492–5.

291. Klein JJ, van Haeringen JR, Sluiter HJ, Holloway R, Peset R. Pulmonary function after recovery from the adult respiratory distress syndrome. Chest 1976;69(3): 350–5.

•292. Desai SR, Wells AU, Rubens MB, Evans TW, Hansell DM. Acute respiratory distress syndrome: CT abnormalities at long-term follow-up. Radiology 1999;210(1):29–35.

293. Avdalovic M, Sandrock C, Hoso A, Allen R, Albertson TE. Epoprostenol in pregnant patients with secondary pulmonary hypertension: two case reports and a review of the literature. Treat Respir Med 2004;3(1):29–34.

294. Elliott CG. Pulmonary sequelae in survivors of the adult respiratory distress syndrome. Clin Chest Med 1990;11(4):789–800.

295. Ghio AJ, Elliott CG, Crapo RO, Berlin SL, Jensen RL. Impairment after adult respiratory distress syndrome. An evaluation based on American Thoracic Society recommendations. Am Rev Respir Dis 1989;139(5): 1158–62.

296. Peters JI, Bell RC, Prihoda TJ, Harris G, Andrews C, Johanson WG. Clinical determinants of abnormalities in pulmonary functions in survivors of the adult respiratory distress syndrome. Am Rev Respir Dis 1989;139(5): 1163–8.

297. McHugh LG, Milberg JA, Whitcomb ME, Schoene RB, Maunder RJ, Hudson LD. Recovery of function in survivors of the acute respiratory distress syndrome. Am J Respir Crit Care Med 1994;150(1):90–4.

298. Davidson TA, Caldwell ES, Curtis JR, Hudson LD, Steinberg KP. Reduced quality of life in survivors of acute respiratory distress syndrome compared with critically ill control patients. JAMA 1999;281(4):354–60.

Pharmacological management of pulmonary circulation in critically ill patients

HORST OLSCHEWSKI

INTRODUCTION

Severe pulmonary hypertension may lead to critical illness and eventually death due to progressive right heart failure. This represents an urgent indication for prostanoid therapy, but there are many more constellations involving the pulmonary circulation in critically ill patients. For example, critical illness with de-novo pulmonary hypertension is characterized by right ventricular dilatation and decompensation with moderately elevated pulmonary arterial pressures and critically low systemic pressure. This is typical in acute thromboembolism and sepsis. To make it more complicated, critically ill patients will often present with both an underlying condition and an acute trigger, which is mostly septic, cardiogenic, thromboembolic, or hemorrhagic. Depending on the underlying conditions and concomitant diseases there are multiple scenarios which demand individualized therapy.

DEFINITIONS AND NOMENCLATURE

Right ventricular failure

There is no generally agreed definition for right ventricular failure and decompensation. Here we will understand the term "right ventricular failure" as a condition characterized by elevated right ventricular filling pressure (RAP > 9 mmHg)

and/or diminished cardiac output ($CI < 2.5$ L/min/m^2) at rest resulting from impaired right ventricular function. Reduced right ventricular filling pressure (hypovolemia) must be excluded. The term "right ventricular decompensation" will refer to a condition with manifest right ventricular forward or backward heart failure. The cardiac index in such cases is typically < 1.5 L/min/m^2 and the mixed venous O_2 saturation is < 50 percent while the right atrial pressure is > 18 mmHg. The mixed venous oxygen saturation criterion is only valid when systemic arterial O_2 saturation is > 90 percent (1). Mean life expectancy without disease-targeted therapy is less than a month (2).

Critical illnesses involving the pulmonary circulation with moderately elevated pulmonary arterial pressure

The most common reasons for critical illness are left heart failure and sepsis. They are characterized by elevated pressures in both the post- and precapillary pulmonary vessels. In left heart failure, the pulmonary venous pressure is increased due to increased filling pressures of the left ventricle resulting in elevated pulmonary capillary pressure and pulmonary arterial pressure. In patients with sepsis or SIRS (systemic inflammatory response syndrome), fluid overload due to therapeutic application of large amounts of volume and/or septic heart and renal failure results in elevated pressures ranging from the pulmonary veins to the pulmonary arteries while systemic vascular resistance is decreased resulting in severe systemic hypotension. Pulmonary shunt blood flow can amount to 50 percent of the pulmonary blood flow (3) and leads to severe hypoxemia (Figure 24.3.1). Acute thromboembolism may result in critical illness due to right heart failure from increased afterload and decreased systemic pressure in combination with gas exchange disturbances.

Patients with COPD and lung fibrosis represent a big challenge if they present with critical illness. This is typically triggered by exacerbations but may also be triggered by cardiac events and thromboembolism and frequently entails increased pulmonary vascular resistance and pressure. The same is true if patients with left heart disease develop pneumonia or sepsis or if patients suffer from both severe heart and lung disease. In all these scenarios, the mean pulmonary arterial pressure is below 40 mmHg because the non-adapted right ventricle decompensates before this pressure level is reached. In contrast to these secondary forms of right heart decompensation, primary right heart decompensation with normal or slightly elevated PAP is very rare (Uhl's disease (4)).

Critical illnesses with excessive pulmonary hypertension

Primary right heart decompensation belongs to the rare causes of critical illness. These patients typically present with a mean PAP > 40 mmHg. In PAH patients, hemodynamics are characterized by markedly reduced cardiac output and elevated right atrial pressure while the systemic pressure is significantly decreased. The pulmonary capillary and venous pressures are in the lower normal range. The same is true for CTEPH patients, however, by definition they suffer from pulmonary perfusion heterogeneity and are more prone to hypoxemia in response to vasodilators than PAH patients.

Patients with left heart disease may also present with pulmonary pressures > 40 mmHg. This speaks in favor of an adapted right ventricle due to pre-existing pulmonary hypertension which may be due to excessive increase in precapillary pulmonary resistance in response to chronically increased pulmonary venous pressure ("Kitajev Reflex" (5)) or to any other form of pulmonary hypertension. Patients with chronic lung disease may also present with PAP > 40 mmHg which can be due to chronic hypoxic remodelling of the pulmonary arteries (in 1 percent of COPD patients) but is more often due to other causes of pulmonary hypertension (6).

Critical illness in pulmonary hypertension patients

Often there is a trigger for the decompensation of a pulmonary hypertension patient. Possible causes of decompensation that can be eliminated include non-compliance with medication, overhydration or intercurrent infections or arrhythmias.

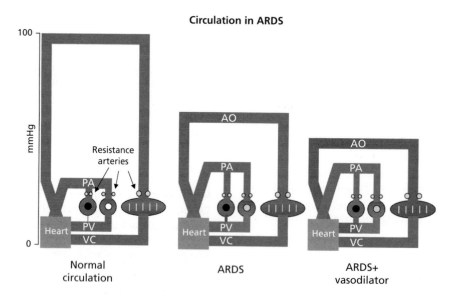

Figure 24.3.1 Vasodilators in ARDS patients. AO, aorta; PA, pulmonary artery; PV, pulmonary vein; VC, vena cava. White, grey, and black circles represent well-ventilated, partly ventilated, and non-ventilated lung areas. Blue vessels indicated deoxygenated and red vessels well-oxygenated blood. In ARDS, systemic pressure is reduced due to reduced systemic vascular resistance and pulmonary pressure is increased due to increased cardiac output and reduction of normally ventilated lung regions and right-to-left shunt blood flow is increased by increase of non-ventilated lung areas, reduced vasoconstrictive tone and increased pulmonary arterial pressure. When a systemic vasodilator is applied, systemic resistance is further decreased and intrapulmonary shunt vessels are opened leading to critical systemic hypotension and hypoxemia.

Except in left heart disease, arrhythmia belongs to the rare triggers of right heart decompensation. However, if arrhythmia occurs in PAH, this represents a life-threatening event (7) and demands immediate aggressive therapy. The best drug is amiodarone because almost all other antiarrythmic drugs have negative inotropic effects. Digoxin may also be helpful in the treatment of atrial fibrillation. Electrical cardioversion is the method of choice in most cases. It is important to ensure that electrolyte and intravascular volume abnormalities are corrected.

As a fundamental rule, infections in the patient with PAH should be treated aggressively with antibiotics, used intravenously if necessary.

Thromboembolic events are rare in PAH and CTEPH because most of these patients are chronically anticoagulated. Patients are at increased risk in periods of cessation of anticoagulation, bed rest, and excessive diuretic therapy.

Acute hemorrhage e.g. due to gastrointestinal bleeding or during surgery is poorly tolerated by PAH patients. Patients need urgent volume or better blood substitution. Oversubstitution is also dangerous because it may cause right heart decompensation.

Pulmonary hemorrhage is always a life-threatening event. Among PAH patients, those with very high PAP (>70 mmHg) and those with preexisting bronchiectasis are more prone to pulmonary hemorrhage. Unfortunately, hemorrhage can also result from acute thromboembolism. This can make therapy decisions very difficult. After optimization of the anticoagulation according to the cause of hemorrhage, persisting significant hemorrhage may necessitate bronchial angiography and embolization or even emergency operation although this confers a high mortality risk.

DIAGNOSTIC STRATEGY

In patients with critical illness it is extremely helpful to compare acute diagnostic results with previous investigations when the patient was clinically stable. In fact this is the only way to fully understand the actual cause of deterioration and the key to successful therapy. Therefore, it is very useful to document echocardiography, chest x-ray and at least one natriuretic peptide during every routine reassessment in patients with severe pulmonary hypertension.

Doppler echocardiography

Among the non-invasive techniques, Doppler echocardiography is the preferred method to detect pulmonary hypertension in critically ill patients. The estimation of systolic pulmonary arterial pressure (SPAP) is assumed to be accurate although invasively controlled prospective studies in a mixed population of ICU patients are missing. Although SPAP is an important indicator of PH, its determination does not help in the prognostic assessment of critically ill patients nor does it explain the underlying cause of pulmonary hypertension. However, echocardiography also contributes to the assessment of right ventricular function which is an important prognostic factor. Among the typical features of pulmonary hypertension, the D-shaped LV, sometimes with paradoxical septal motion due to right ventricular dilatation indicates the severity of disease. Right atrial dilatation and inferior vena caval distension with diminished inspiratory collapse indicate elevated central venous pressure. Longitudinal shortening of the RV contributes significantly to the systolic function of this chamber. This can be assessed by TAPSE (tricuspid annular plane systolic excursion), which correlates with RVEF and is prognostic in patients with heart failure and PAH (8). However, in critically ill patients the prognostic value of this measure has not been evaluated. Apart from right ventricular parameters, echocardiography is indispensable to assess left heart pump and valvular functions in critically ill patients.

Imaging

The chest x-ray is of particular importance in critically ill patients as it allows diagnosis of lung edema and infiltrates as well as exclusion of atelectasis and pneumothorax on a day-to-day basis. The CT-scan is important if thromboembolism, alveolar hemorrhage or PVOD belong in the differential diagnosis.

Biomarkers

Among biochemical measurements, elevated values for natriuretic peptides (BNP, NT-proBNP), uric acid, troponin T, and GDF-15 (9) and lowered sodium levels (10) are of negative prognostic significance. Unfortunately these parameters do not allow differentiation between left and right heart failure.

Right heart catheterization

Right heart catheter examination is disposable if, based on non-invasive examinations, the therapeutic regimen is clear and there are no alternatives. However, in combined conditions including left ventricular failure or septicemia it may be very helpful to analyze the hemodynamic conditions including left ventricular filling pressure, cardiac output and right atrial pressure. For this purpose the Swan–Ganz catheter is the method of choice. If the catheter is in place, pharmacologic testing of the pulmonary vasodilator response may guide the therapeutic approach based on the acute hemodynamic effects which are to be interpreted together with side effects like hypoxemia or systemic pressure drop.

THERAPY

Acute management of decompensated pulmonary arterial hypertension

Patients with acute right ventricular decompensation have not been included in controlled studies. In addition to general therapy recommendations, it is important to search for and eliminate the cause of decompensation, if this is possible, and to transfer the patient to the ICU where vital signs are monitored and an optimized diuretic management, positive inotropes and, in selected cases, mechanical ventilation and immediate cardiopulmonary resuscitation is available.

If right heart decompensation is present, the main circulatory determinants of acute survival are systemic pressure, cardiac output and oxygenation and the management of patients has to consider all these factors and their interaction. Targeted PAH therapy should be introduced promptly and include a prostanoid.

Inotropes

Positive inotropes are indicated when pulmonary vasodilators are not effective enough, when systemic blood pressure is not sufficient, or when critical organ ischemia occurs. Depending on the hemodynamics, epinephrine, dopamine, dobutamine or even norepinephrine may be used, either alone or in combination. Alpha adrenergic agents should be used with great caution in patients who are responsive to vasodilators (responders or previous responders mostly suffer from IPAH (11)) as they may induce excessive pulmonary vasoconstriction and lead to deterioration in right ventricular function as well as impairment of left ventricular filling. Little experience has been reported with levosimendan or phosphodiesterase 3/4 inhibitors such as milrinone and enoximone.

Volume management

Volume management belongs to the most difficult issues in critically ill patients with pulmonary hypertension. Theoretically, the target right atrial pressure is $< 9\,mmHg$, at least in IPAH patients (12). However, in patients with chronically elevated right atrial pressure this would lead to decreased cardiac output and critical systemic hypotension. The same is true in patients with decreased systemic vascular resistance like sepsis or hepatopulmonary syndrome. Therefore, these patients mostly profit from higher central venous pressures around $12\,mmHg$.

In patients with lung fibrosis, the intrathoracic pressure may be $5–10\,mmHg$ lower than in other patients. Accordingly, their target right atrial pressures are lower by the same degree. The opposite is true in COPD patients where an intrinsic PEEP demands higher target right atrial pressures.

In patients with concomitant left heart disease the most important determinant for volume management is the left ventricular filling pressure with a target $< 15\,mmHg$. If no Swan–Ganz catheter for assessment of PAWP is in place, pulmonary volume overload can be assessed by means of the chest x-ray and the degree of hypoxemia. Hyponatriemia should be corrected.

Medications without benefit

Beta-blocking agents are to be avoided by all patients with reduced cardiac output where pulmonary hypertension is not caused by left ventricular failure. Calcium channel blockers (CCB) are not indicated for "non-responders" to pulmonary vasodilators (13). If a clinical long-term CCB responder presents with right heart failure, the CCB should be replaced by a prostanoid. Prostanoids have at least the same pulmonary vasodilatory potency as NO (14) and the NO response is predictive of the CCB response (15). In contrast to CCB, prostanoids have no negative inotropic effects on the right ventricle. ACE inhibitors, angiotensin receptor antagonists, nitrates or molsidomine are not recommended. PAH patients with systemic hypotension generally benefit immediately from the discontinuation of such medications.

Resuscitation

Cardiopulmonary resuscitation is successful only in exceptional cases and then most readily when an acute cause can be quickly identified and treated (7). It has been reported that use of intravenous prostanoids (e.g. iloprost as an intravenous bolus of $10–50\,\mu g$ every $5–10\,min$) during resuscitation has beneficial effects in patients with severe pulmonary hypertension (7).

TARGETED PAH THERAPY

Intravenous prostacyclin

Prostanoids represent the mainstay of therapy of decompensated pulmonary arterial hypertension (16). They primarily target the acutely reversible pulmonary vasoconstriction and right heart function (17,18) and in the long-term also chronic pulmonary vasoconstriction and remodelling by their anti-inflammatory and antiproliferative properties (19) (Figure 24.3.2). Intravenous prostacyclin (Epoprostenol, Flolan®) is used in some countries as standard therapy for decompensated right heart failure but is not available or approved in many other countries. The dose is usually started between 2 and 5 ng/kg/min, and uptitrated as needed and tolerated. In conscious patients the upper dose is mostly limited by subjective side effects like headache and nausea, in mechanically ventilated patients the limiting factors are low systemic pressure due

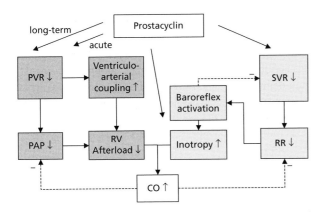

Figure 24.3.2 Hemodynamic effects of systemically applied prostanoids. Within minutes, prostanoids cause vasodilatation, which is more prominent in the systemic than in the pulmonary vessels. This activates the arterial baroreflex which constricts systemic vessels and increases cardiac output by its positive inotropic effects and heart rate increase. Within weeks, the neurohormonal activation increases systemic tone while the slow vasorelaxing effects in the pulmonary arteries cause additional decrease in PVR. Additional positive inotropic effects are caused by interaction with catecholamines and ventriculoarterial coupling.

to systemic vasodilation and poor oxygenation due to increased intrapulmonary shunt blood flow.

Due to its short half-life, epoprostenol is easily handled in the ICU setting. Intravenous treprostinil, a stable prostacyclin analog is an alternative. It has considerable practical advantages due to its chemical stability, for instance in cases of unintentional therapy interruptions. The doses are 1.5–3-fold higher as compared to epoprostenol (20,21). Intravenous iloprost, a stable prostacyclin analog, is an alternative to intravenous epoprostenol despite its low level of evidence. The doses are typically 5–10-fold lower as compared to epoprostenol (22). The infusion is usually started between 0.5 and 1 ng/kg/min, and uptitrated as needed and tolerated.

Inhaled prostacyclin

The inhalative application allows targeting of the pulmonary vessels (pulmonary selectivity) – and the ventilated areas of the lung (intrapulmonary selectivity) (3,23–25). Inhaled iloprost has been used in Germany since the middle of the 1990s for pulmonary hypertension therapy including decompensated right heart failure patients (26,27). One prospective, randomized, double-blind study in Europe (Aerosolized Iloprost Randomized, AIR) involving patients with PAH and CTEPH in functional NYHA Class III–IV confirmed the clinical efficacy and good tolerability of this drug (28). Inhaled treprostinil may induce similar pulmonary vasodilatation but less systemic side effects and a more sustained hemodynamic effect (29). Recently, inhaled treprostinil has been approved for PAH by the FDA.

As general drawbacks to inhalative therapy in critically ill patients there is no EMEA approval for decompensated right heart failure and the application in critically ill patients, particularly on mechanical ventilation, is demanding. The recommended inhaled dose of iloprost is between $6 \times 2.5\,\mu g$ and $9 \times 5\,\mu g$/day but the exact calculation of the dose in a ventilated patient is nearly impossible. Therefore, in such cases, the dose is titrated according to the desired effects (decrease in PVR) and the side effects (systemic pressure drop, oxygenation drop) and repeated every 1–3 hours.

Endothelin receptor antagonists

Endothelin receptor antagonists have been approved for PAH, NYHA class II and III in Europe and class II–IV in the US. In the recommended dose the pulmonary vasodilative effects mostly take several days to occur and there is no convincing evidence that decompensated patients profit from the combination of prostanoids with ERA (30). Nevertheless, it may be helpful to start with an ERA upfront as part of a multimodal therapy strategy.

Phosphodiesterase 5 inhibitors (PDE5i)

Two PDE5i have been approved for PAH, NYHA class II–III in Europe and II–IV in the US. There is some pulmonary and intrapulmonary selectivity of PDE5i (31,32) which results in tolerable side effects in interstitial lung disease (32) as well as non-operable chronic thromboembolic pulmonary hypertension (33). Various case series indicate beneficial effects in combination with prostanoids (34) and one randomized controlled study demonstrated a beneficial effect on top of intravenous prostacyclin (35). Of interest, in this study the most prominent effect of additional sildenafil on mortality was seen in the decompensated patient subgroup. Therefore, a PDE5i in combination with a prostanoid appears as the therapy of choice in decompensated right heart failure.

Other therapeutic measures

ATRIAL SEPTOSTOMY

A congenital shunt connection between the pulmonary and systemic circulation represents a survival advantage in patients with pulmonary hypertension. An iatrogenic atrial septal defect (atrial septostomy) may improve the symptoms and the prognosis in severe PAH (36–38). The procedure is undertaken using transcutaneous catheter technology. A balloon catheter is positioned across the atrial septum and dilated in stages until systemic arterial O_2 saturation falls by a maximum of 10 percent. As a result of atrial septostomy, oxygen transport increases despite the decline in systemic arterial O_2 saturation, and in many cases right ventricular function undergoes long-term improvement. The procedure is high-risk particularly in cases where right ventricular decompensation and a diminished systemic arterial O_2 saturation are already present. Therefore, this procedure is recommended if right heart decompensation cannot be sufficiently improved by prostanoids or prostanoids combined with other targeted therapy. On the other hand, the mortality risk of the procedure is excessively high if right atrial pressure is >20 mmHg, or there is severe pre-existing arterial hypoxemia or renal insufficiency. It may be very difficult to find the optimum time window to perform the procedure.

PERICARDIOCENTESIS

Pericardial effusion is one of the bad prognostic signs in pulmonary hypertension. Unfortunately, pericardiocentesis may have a poor outcome (39) and is only recommended in significant pericardial tamponade.

LUNG TRANSPLANTATION

Lung transplantation continues to play a role for patients who do not respond sufficiently to medical treatment. Transplantation in IPAH has a mortality rate of up to 25 percent during the first weeks after surgery and reaches 35–40 percent after one year. Mean transplantation survival rate is about 4 years and has been improving in recent years.

SPECIAL CONSIDERATIONS IN PATIENTS WITH ASSOCIATED OR CAUSALLY RELATED CONDITIONS

In general, therapy for underlying diseases takes precedence over disease-targeted therapy for pulmonary hypertension and the evidence for disease-targeted therapy for pulmonary hypertension in this situation is low. Practically no evidence-based marketing authorizations by the EMEA or the FDA exist (40).

ASSOCIATED PAH

PAH associated with connective tissue diseases

These patients are similar to IPAH patients, however, their mean age is higher and they more often suffer from concomitant diseases. On average, their PVR is similar to IPAH patients but their mean PAP and cardiac output is lower while the right atrial pressure is higher. Prognosis on medication appears inferior to IPAH patients. Recommendations for targeted therapy do not differ from IPAH patients. Lung transplantation can be considered in patients with scleroderma or SLE associated with pulmonary hypertension that is refractory to therapy, provided there are no contraindications to transplantation and no significant involvement of other internal organs.

PAH with congenital defects

When Eisenmenger patients present with critical illness, this is often triggered by pulmonary hemorrhage or infectious complications (e.g. pneumonia). They are characterized by markedly decreased systemic oxygenation and relatively well-preserved cardiac output. The hemodynamic efficacy of a pulmonary vasodilator can be assessed by simply monitoring the systemic arterial oxygen saturation, provided there is no respiratory disease. If the pulmonary vessels dilate this allows for more pulmonary blood flow compared to the cardiac right-to-left shunt blood flow and increases the oxygenation.

Portopulmonary hypertension (PortoPH) and hepatopulmonary syndrome

On average, these patients present with higher cardiac output and lower systemic vascular resistance as compared to IPAH patients. They are more prone to bleeding complications (gastroesophageal varices, liver failure) and systemic hypotension as well as ascites as compared to IPAH. There are no controlled trials in patients with PortoPH, although various case series indicate acute beneficial effects for prostacyclin, ERA and PDE5i (41). If right heart failure is the leading problem, prostacyclin would be the therapy of choice. If systemic vasodilatation and excessive NO production is a clinical problem, this argues against prostanoids and PDE5i.

PVOD

Pulmonary veno-occlusive disease is characterized by hemodynamics resembling IPAH but patients are prone to lung edema as in left heart disease. This is caused by increased pulmonary capillary pressures (with normal PA wedge pressures!). The thin section CT scan, together with a typical Swan–Ganz catheter result is characteristic and mostly sufficient for a diagnosis of PVOD. Some of these patients respond favorably to vasodilators and decrease their PVR markedly. However, particularly these patients are prone to lung edema formation after application of targeted PAH therapy (42,43). Therefore, it is very important to treat aggressively with diuretics in parallel to vasodilator therapy. If applicable these patients should be listed for lung transplantation because the long-term prognosis with or without PAH therapy is poor.

SPECIAL CONSIDERATIONS IN NON–PAH PH

Left ventricular diseases

No targeted treatment of severely elevated pulmonary vascular resistance has been recommended in left ventricular failure. Even PDE3 inhibitors or dobutamine, which have been used for "bridging" to heart transplantation, do not reliably lower the transpulmonary pressure gradient. Levosimendan and BNP infusions as well as intravenous nitrates may be indicated as they decrease the left ventricular filling pressure together with dilating the pulmonary vessels. Pulmonary selective vasodilators such as NO, ERA, PDE5i or prostanoids are risky because they may increase preload of the left ventricle with consequent pulmonary edema. Long-term application of epoprostenol in left heart patients resulted in detrimental effects on mortality (44). Results might be different in short-term applications and if only patients with severely elevated PVR were selected, but there are no sufficient data to support such an approach.

Chronic lung diseases

In chronic obstructive pulmonary disease continuous (> 16 hours/day) oxygen therapy plays a major therapeutic role. This is the only therapy for which a survival advantage has been demonstrated. COPD should otherwise be treated in accordance with current guidelines. Patients with sleep-related breathing disorders and nocturnal desaturation often benefit from noninvasive home ventilation. The use of vasodilators such as calcium channel blockers, prostanoids, endothelin receptor antagonists and phosphodiesterase inhibitors may be indicated if the lung disease is just a concomitant disease in an IPAH patient. Such patients are characterized by relatively well-preserved lung function and severe pulmonary hypertension.

Chronic thromboembolic pulmonary hypertension (CTEPH)

CTEPH patients may present with critical illness due to primary right heart decompensation but frequently this is triggered by acute events like acute thromboembolism, pneumonia or complications of concomitant diseases. Pulmonary endarterectomy (PEA) is the therapy of choice but this operation is associated with excessive mortality in critically ill patients. Therefore, correction of the right heart failure is the primary therapy goal. In these patients it may be suitable to combine a prostanoid with a low-dose norepinephrine infusion because the pulmonary vessels and the right ventricle may better respond to the prostanoid and the systemic vessels better to the alpha adrenergic agent.

Early postoperative pulmonary arterial hypertension

Shunt defects with pulmonary hypertension and elevated PVR require optimum collaboration between pediatric cardiac surgeons, cardiac anesthetists and pediatric

cardiologists. Hyperventilation as a rapidly available basic measure and inhaled NO (2–80 ppm) are established methods for rapid lowering of pulmonary vascular resistance. The following have been used as experimental treatments in small case series: sildenafil (oral or intravenous), endothelin receptor antagonists (intravenous), iloprost (inhaled or intravenous) and induction of hypometabolism (cooling, relaxation).

Sepsis/ARDS

Patients with sepsis and ARDS are characterized by a lowered systemic vascular resistance and low systemic pressure despite elevated cardiac output. Their pulmonary right to left shunt flow is markedly elevated resulting in severe hypoxemia and pulmonary arterial pressure is moderately increased. The right ventricle may become the limiting factor for oxygen delivery to the peripheral organs. Prostanoids have been advocated to overcome this critical situation, however, they decrease systemic pressure and increase intrapulmonary shunt blood flow (Figure 24.3.1). Inhaled application of prostanoids or NO is better tolerated due to pulmonary and intrapulmonary selectivity (3,23,24). Although oxygenation is acutely improved, inhaled NO has not shown a survival benefit as compared to placebo in ARDS patients (45,46). Inhaled prostanoids have not been formally tested despite their beneficial acute effects.

ACKNOWLEDGMENT

I would like to thank Professor EK Weir, Minneapolis, USA, for critical discussion of the manuscript and his valuable input.

KEY POINTS

- To assess the role of right ventricular function and the pulmonary circulation in critical illness.
- To understand the problems involved in the application of targeted PAH therapy in critically ill patients.
- To appreciate the important role of co-morbidities of the heart and lung.
- To identify the typical triggers for critical illness in severe pulmonary hypertension.
- To foresee the effects and side-effects of PAH therapy in critically ill patients.
- To understand the target values for volume management in critically ill patients.
- To understand the indications for catecholamines, prostanoids, atrial septostomy, and lung transplantation in critically ill PAH patients.

REFERENCES

1. Olschewski H, Hoeper MM, Borst MM *et al.* [Diagnosis and therapy of chronic pulmonary hypertension]. Pneumologie 2006;60:749–71.

2. D'Alonzo GE, Barst RJ, Ayres SM *et al.* Survival in patients with primary pulmonary hypertension. Results from a national prospective registry. Ann Intern Med 1991; 115:343–9.

3. Walmrath D, Schneider T, Pilch J, Grimminger F, Seeger W. Aerosolised prostacyclin in adult respiratory distress syndrome. Lancet 1993;342(8877):961–2.

4. Loire R, Tabib A. [Arrhythmogenic right ventricular dysplasia and Uhl disease. Anatomic study of 100 cases after sudden death]. Ann Pathol 1998;18(3):165–71.

5. Schamarin PI. Über den Kitajew Reflex. Zum Mechanismus der Kompensation des Mitralvitiums. Terapiszeskij Archiv 1952;24:79–85.

6. Chaouat A, Bugnet AS, Kadaoui N, Schott R, Enache I, Ducolone A, Ehrhart M, Kessler R, Weitzenblum E. Severe pulmonary hypertension and chronic obstructive pulmonary disease. Am J Respir Crit Care Med 2005; 172(2):189–94.

7. Hoeper MM, Galie N, Murali S *et al.* Outcome after cardiopulmonary resuscitation in patients with pulmonary arterial hypertension. Am J Respir Crit Care Med 2002;165(3):341–4.

8. Forfia PR, Fisher MR, Mathai SC *et al.* Tricuspid annular displacement predicts survival in pulmonary hypertension. Am J Respir Crit Care Med 2006;174(9):1034–41.

9. Nickel N, Kempf T, Tapken H *et al.* Growth differentiation factor-15 in idiopathic pulmonary arterial hypertension. Am J Respir Crit Care Med 2008;178(5):534–41.

10. Forfia PR, Mathai SC, Fisher MR, Housten-Harris T, Hemnes AR, Champion HC, Girgis RE, Hassoun PM. Hyponatremia predicts right heart failure and poor survival in pulmonary arterial hypertension. Am J Respir Crit Care Med 2008; 177(12):1364–9.

11. Sitbon O, Humbert M, Jais X *et al.* Long-term response to calcium channel blockers in idiopathic pulmonary arterial hypertension. Circulation 2005;111(23):3105–11.

12. Sitbon O, Humbert M, Nunes H, Parent F, Garcia G, Herve P, Rainisio M, Simonneau G. Long-term intravenous epoprostenol infusion in primary pulmonary hypertension: prognostic factors and survival. J Am Coll Cardiol 2002;40(4):780–8.

13. Galie N, Torbicki A, Barst R, D *et al.* Guidelines on diagnosis and treatment of pulmonary arterial hypertension. The Task Force on Diagnosis and Treatment of Pulmonary Arterial Hypertension of the European Society of Cardiology. Eur Heart J 2004;25(24):2243–78.

14. Hoeper MM, Olschewski H, Ghofrani HA *et al.* A comparison of the acute hemodynamic effects of inhaled nitric oxide and aerosolized iloprost in primary pulmonary hypertension. German PPH study group. J Am Coll Cardiol 2000;35(1):176–82.

15. Sitbon O, Humbert M, Jagot JL, Taravella O, Fartoukh M, Parent F, Herve P, Simonneau G. Inhaled nitric oxide as a screening agent for safely identifying responders to oral calcium-channel blockers in primary pulmonary hypertension. Eur Respir J 1998;12(2):265–70.

16. Gomberg-Maitland M, Olschewski H. Prostacyclin therapies for the treatment of pulmonary arterial hypertension. Eur Respir J 2008 Apr;31(4):891–901.

17. Fontana M, Olschewski H, Olschewski A, Schluter KD. Treprostinil potentiates the positive inotropic effect of catecholamines in adult rat ventricular cardiomyocytes. Br J Pharmacol 2007;151(6):779–86.

18. Kerbaul F, Brimioulle S, Rondelet B, Dewachter C, Hubloue I, Naeije R. How prostacyclin improves cardiac output in right heart failure in conjunction with pulmonary hypertension. Am J Respir Crit Care Med 2007;175(8): 846–50.

19. Olschewski H, Rose F, Grunig E *et al.* Cellular pathophysiology and therapy of pulmonary hypertension. J Lab Clin Med 2001;138(6):367–77.

20. Sitbon O, Manes A, Jais X *et al.* Rapid switch from intravenous epoprostenol to intravenous treprostinil in patients with pulmonary arterial hypertension. J Cardiovasc Pharmacol 2007;49(1):1–5.

21. Gomberg-Maitland M, Tapson VF, Benza RL, McLaughlin VV, Krichman A, Widlitz AC, Barst RJ. Transition from intravenous epoprostenol to intravenous treprostinil in pulmonary hypertension. Am J Respir Crit Care Med 2005;172(12):1586–9.

22. Hoeper MM, Gall H, Seyfarth HJ *et al.* Long-term outcome with intravenous iloprost in pulmonary arterial hypertension. Eur Respir J 2009;34(1):132–7.

23. Walmrath D, Schneider T, Schermuly R, Olschewski H, Grimminger F, Seeger W. Direct comparison of inhaled nitric oxide and aerosolized prostacyclin in acute respiratory distress syndrome. Am J Respir Crit Care Med 1996;153(3):991–6.

24. Walmrath D, Schneider T, Pilch J, Schermuly R, Grimminger F, Seeger W. Effects of aerosolized prostacyclin in severe pneumonia. Impact of fibrosis. Am J Respir Crit Care Med 1995;151(3 Pt 1):724–30.

25. Olschewski H, Ghofrani HA, Walmrath D *et al.* Inhaled prostacyclin and iloprost in severe pulmonary hypertension secondary to lung fibrosis. Am J Respir Crit Care Med 1999;160(2):600–7.

26. Olschewski H, Walmrath D, Schermuly R, Ghofrani A, Grimminger F, Seeger W. Aerosolized prostacyclin and iloprost in severe pulmonary hypertension. Ann Intern Med 1996;124(9):820–4.

27. Olschewski H, Ghofrani HA, Schmehl T *et al.* Inhaled iloprost to treat severe pulmonary hypertension. An uncontrolled trial. German PPH Study Group. Ann Intern Med 2000; 132(6):435–43.

28. Olschewski H, Simonneau G, Galie N *et al.* Inhaled iloprost for severe pulmonary hypertension. N Engl J Med 2002; 347(5):322–9.

29. Voswinckel R, Enke B, Reichenberger F et al. Favorable effects of inhaled treprostinil in severe pulmonary hypertension: results from randomized controlled pilot studies. J Am Coll Cardiol 2006;48(8):1672–81.

30. Humbert M, Barst RJ, Robbins IM et al. Combination of bosentan with epoprostenol in pulmonary arterial hypertension: BREATHE-2. Eur Respir J 2004;24(3):353–9.

31. Ghofrani HA, Voswinckel R, Reichenberger F et al. Differences in hemodynamic and oxygenation responses to three different phosphodiesterase-5 inhibitors in patients with pulmonary arterial hypertension: a randomized prospective study. J Am Coll Cardiol 2004;44(7):1488–96.

32. Ghofrani HA, Wiedemann R, Rose F et al. Sildenafil for treatment of lung fibrosis and pulmonary hypertension: a randomised controlled trial. Lancet 2002;360(9337): 895–900.

33. Ghofrani HA, Schermuly RT, Rose F et al. Sildenafil for long-term treatment of nonoperable chronic thromboembolic pulmonary hypertension. Am J Respir Crit Care Med 2003;167(8):1139–41.

34. Ghofrani HA, Rose F, Schermuly RT, et al. Oral sildenafil as long-term adjunct therapy to inhaled iloprost in severe pulmonary arterial hypertension. J Am Coll Cardiol 2003; 42(1):158–64.

35. Simonneau G, Rubin LJ, Galie N, Barst RJ, Fleming TR, Frost AE, Engel PJ, Kramer MR, Burgess G, Collings L, Cossons N, Sitbon O, Badesch DB. Addition of sildenafil to long-term intravenous epoprostenol therapy in patients with pulmonary arterial hypertension: a randomized trial. Ann Intern Med 2008;149(8):521–30.

36. Sandoval J, Rothman A, Pulido T. Atrial septostomy for pulmonary hypertension. Clin Chest Med 2001;22(3):547–60.

37. Reichenberger F, Pepke-Zaba J, McNeil K, Parameshwar J, Shapiro LM. Atrial septostomy in the treatment of severe pulmonary arterial hypertension. Thorax 2003;58(9): 797–800.

38. Kurzyna M, Dabrowski M, Bielecki D et al. Atrial septostomy in treatment of end-stage right heart failure in patients with pulmonary hypertension. Chest 2007;131(4):977–83.

39. Hemnes AR, Gaine SP, Wiener CM. Poor outcomes associated with drainage of pericardial effusions in patients with pulmonary arterial hypertension. South Med J 2008;101(5):490–4.

40. Hoeper MM, Barbera JA, Channick RN et al. Diagnosis, assessment, and treatment of non-pulmonary arterial hypertension pulmonary hypertension. J Am Coll Cardiol 2009;54(1 Suppl):S85–S96.

41. Hoeper MM, Krowka MJ, Strassburg CP. Portopulmonary hypertension and hepatopulmonary syndrome. Lancet 2004;363(9419):1461–8.

42. Rabiller A, Jais X, Hamid A et al. Occult alveolar haemorrhage in pulmonary veno-occlusive disease. Eur Respir J 2006;27(1):108–13.

43. Resten A, Maitre S, Humbert M, Sitbon O, Capron F, Simoneau G, Musset D. Pulmonary arterial hypertension: thin-section CT predictors of epoprostenol therapy failure. Radiology 2002;222(3):782–8.

44. Califf RM, Adams KF, McKenna WJ et al. A randomized controlled trial of epoprostenol therapy for severe congestive heart failure: The Flolan International Randomized Survival Trial (FIRST). Am Heart J 1997;134(1):44–54.

45. Taylor RW, Zimmerman JL, Dellinger RP et al. Low-dose inhaled nitric oxide in patients with acute lung injury: a randomized controlled trial. JAMA 2004;291(13):1603–9.

46. Dupont H, Le CF, Fierobe L, Cheval C, Moine P, Timsit JF. Efficiency of inhaled nitric oxide as rescue therapy during severe ARDS: survival and factors associated with the first response. J Crit Care 1999;14(3):107–13.

PART 13

PULMONARY CIRCULATION IN SPECIAL ENVIRONMENTS

High altitude pulmonary hypertension

DANTE PENALOZA

INTRODUCTION

High altitude pulmonary hypertension (HAPH) is a descriptive term indicating the presence of pulmonary hypertension (PH) in altitudes above 3500 meters. At these altitudes PH is a frequent feature in healthy residents and in people with high altitude diseases. The degree of PH in healthy residents is related to age, level of altitude and altitude ancestry. Healthy highlanders have a mild degree of PH associated with adaptive levels of hypoxemia and polycythemia. After many years of residence at high altitude, some highlanders may lose their adaptation and develop chronic mountain sickness (CMS), a clinical entity associated with marked hypoxemia, exaggerated polycythemia and increased PH, evolving in some cases to heart failure. Chinese and Kyrgyz investigators have described chronic high altitude diseases, with the names high altitude heart disease (HAHD) and high altitude cor pulmonale (HACP) respectively. HAHD and HACP have a clinical picture similar to CMS with lesser degrees of hypoxemia and polycythemia which, however, are often measured at lower levels during recovery. It is highly probable that all these clinical entities are the same disease with different shades. The highest degrees of PH are found in cases with subacute infantile mountain sickness (SIMS) and in people, children or adults, suffering from high altitude pulmonary edema (HAPE). A systematic review of worldwide literature on PH in healthy highlanders and high altitude diseases was undertaken, beginning with the pioneering work done in the Andes several decades ago. The pulmonary hemodynamics, pathological and clinical features of these conditions will be described in this chapter, with the exception of HAPE which is addressed in Chapter 25.2. Then, we propose a reappraisal of the consensus on CMS and SIMS. Finally, the prevention and management of these clinical conditions are outlined.

DEFINITION OF PULMONARY HYPERTENSION

Definition of PH at sea level

PH has been defined as a mean pulmonary arterial pressure (mPAP) >25 mmHg at rest or >30 mmHg with exercise as assessed by right-heart catheterization. This conventional definition remained invariable for more than three decades and was endorsed by the 3rd World Symposium on Pulmonary Arterial Hypertension held in Venice, Italy in 2003 (1).

Recently, Kovacs et al. reviewed the literature searching for the normal range of PAP and identified 47 studies describing 72 populations of healthy volunteers that were submitted to right-heart catheterization during rest and physical exercise (2). The average resting mPAP was 14 ± 3 mmHg, and consequently an upper limit of normal (mean $\pm$ 2 SD) of 20 mmHg for healthy people. Kovacs et al. found that the normal range of resting mPAP is considerably lower than 25 mmHg, usually < 21 mmHg. This observation coincides with the common clinical practice that considers the following levels of PH and the corresponding mPAP values: mild PH, 21 to 30 mmHg, moderate PH, 31 to 40 mmHg and severe PH, over 40 mmHg.

The 4th World Symposium on Pulmonary Hypertension held in Dana Point, California in 2008 (3) and the European (ESC/ERS) Guidelines on Pulmonary Hypertension (2009) (4), include the important contribution of Kovacs *et al.* and propose that a resting mPAP of 8 to 20 mmHg should be considered normal limits, based on available evidence. A resting mPAP ≥ 25 mmHg has been proposed as the threshold for PH. The "grey zone" of mPAP 21 to 24 mmHg for healthy subjects living at sea level probably means a "pre-PH condition." The exercise mPAP is dependent on age and exercise level, and the conventional cutoff value of 30 mmHg is not supported by the current available evidence requiring further studies.

Definition of PH at high altitudes

Definition of PH at altitude is not an easy task. There is a direct relationship between the level of altitude and the degree of mPAP and this relationship is represented by a parabolic line so that above 3500 m it is common to find mild degrees of PH in healthy highlanders (5). Figure 25.1.1 shows this relationship as well as the inverse correlation between mPAP and the degree of hypoxemia. Mild PH in healthy highlanders is a physiological feature and is associated with adaptive levels of hypoxemia and polycythemia. There are available values of mPAP obtained in some groups of healthy subjects at various altitudes (5). There are not registries or clinical trials designed to search for a threshold value of mPAP in different levels of altitude. The purpose to have a unique threshold value resulting from a mixture of pressure values obtained from different altitudes is not acceptable. In this chapter we will follow the commonly used levels of PH at sea level as a reference to appreciate the magnitude of PH in healthy highlanders and patients with high altitude diseases.

CLASSIFICATION OF HIGH ALTITUDE PULMONARY HYPERTENSION

An updated clinical classification of PH was proposed by Simonneau *et al.* during the 4th World Symposium on Pulmonary Arterial Hypertension (6). The chronic exposure to high altitude is included in the group 3.6 of this classification.

PULMONARY HYPERTENSION IN HEALTHY HIGHLANDERS

Asymptomatic postnatal pulmonary hypertension

Peruvian investigators performed pioneering studies with right-cardiac catheterization in healthy highlanders born

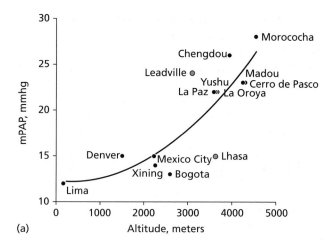

(a)

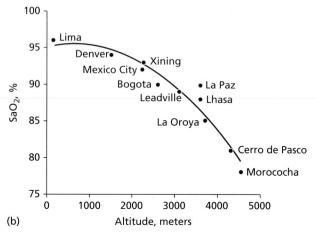

(b)

Figure 25.1.1 (a) Level of altitude as related to mPAP. There is a direct relationship represented by a parabolic line so that, above 3500 m moderate increments in altitude means significant increases in mPAP. There are two exceptions to this correlation (large symbols). mPAP in Leadville, Colorado (3100 m) is greater than expected for this altitude. mPAP in Lhasa, Tibet (3600 m) is lower than expected for this altitude. (b) Level of altitude as related to SaO_2. There is an inverse relationship between these two variables. At high altitudes there are lower values of SaO_2 and higher values of mPAP. Reproduced from Penaloza and Arias-Stella (5) with permission of Lippincott, Williams & Wilkins.

and living at the high altitudes in the Andes. These studies were carried out in children and adults, at an altitude of 4540 m (Morococha, Peru) where the P_B is 445 mmHg and PiO_2 70 mmHg. The mean pulmonary artery pressure (mPAP) in newborns was found to be 60 mmHg, a value similar to that described in sea level newborns (7). After birth, the mPAP decreased slowly at high altitude and persistent pulmonary hypertension of mild or moderate degree was observed in infants, children and adults, in contrast with the fast decline of mPAP described in the postnatal period at sea level (8,9) (Figure 25.1.2). Table 25.1.1 shows pulmonary hemodynamics in children and adults born and living at high altitudes.

The main factor responsible for pulmonary hypertension in healthy high-altitude children is a postnatal delayed remodeling of the distal pulmonary arterial branches and consequently increased amounts of smooth muscle cells (SMC) which increases the pulmonary vascular resistances (PVR) (8–10). The delay of the cardiopulmonary transition in high-altitude infants and children was later confirmed by noninvasive methodology (11,12). The pathogenesis of HAPH has recently been reviewed (5,13).

Combined influence of age and altitude on the pulmonary arterial pressure

For studies on this subject, please see refs 14–17 and Table 25.1.2.

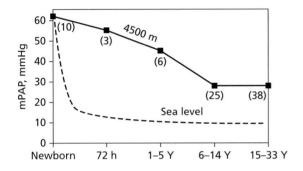

Figure 25.1.2 Relation of mPAP to age in HA natives (4500 m) in comparison to data described at SL. mPAP near 60 mmHg is similar in SL newborns and HA newborns (4540 m). Postnatal changes diverge. mPAP slowly declines in people born at HA, in contrast to the fast decline of mPAP described in subjects born at SL. Numbers in parentheses indicate number of cases. Reproduced from Penaloza and Arias-Stella (5), with permission of Lippincott, Williams & Wilkins.

Pulmonary hypertension as related to high altitude ancestry

In addition to age and altitude, the degree of high altitude ancestry is another factor that affects the pulmonary arterial pressure at high altitude. See refs 19–22.

PULMONARY HYPERTENSION IN CHRONIC MOUNTAIN SICKNESS

Definition and pathogenesis

CMS is a clinical syndrome that occurs in native or long-life residents above 2500 m. It is characterized by excessive erythrocytosis (females Hb ≥19 g/dL; males Hb ≥21 g/dL), severe hypoxemia, and in some cases moderate or severe PH, which may evolve to cor pulmonale, leading to congestive HF. The clinical picture of CMS gradually disappears after descending to low altitude and reappears after returning to HA (23). CMS was first described by Professor Monge who placed emphasis on excessive polycythemia (24). Afterwards, Professor Hurtado pointed out that alveolar hypoventilation is the primary mechanism in CMS leading to severe hypoxemia and hence to exaggerated polycythemia (25). Penaloza et al. were first to describe the evolution from mild-to-physiological PH of healthy highlanders to moderate-to-severe PH seen in patients with CMS who may develop chronic cor pulmonale and HF as a consequence of loss of altitude adaptation (26,27). Recent reviews on pulmonary circulation in CMS have been published (5,28,29).

CMS is a variety of chronic alveolar hypoventilation that results in a complex syndrome integrating four main components. Respiratory features are characterized by alveolar hypoventilation, relative hypercapnea, V/Q mismatch, widened (A-a) PO_2 gradient and increased hypoxemia.

Table 25.1.1 Hemodynamic values in healthy highlanders by comparison with SL residents studied at their respective locations

	HA children 1 to 5 years old (n = 7)	HA children 6 to 14 years old (n = 32)	HA adults 18 to 33 years old (n = 38)	SL adults 17 to 23 years old (n = 25)	P HA adults vs. SL adults
Hct (%)	43.9 ± 3.87	48.0 ± 3.25	59.1 ± 7.20	44.1 ± 2.59	<0.001
Hb (g/dL)	14.1 ± 0.66	15.7 ± 1.07	19.5 ± 1.97	14.7 ± 0.88	<0.001
SaO_2 (%)	78.2 ± 2.76	77.3 ± 5.76	78.4 ± 4.81	95.7 ± 2.07	<0.001
CI (L min m^{-2})	4.4 ± 0.60	4.5 ± 1.39	3.7 ± 1.64	3.9 ± 0.97	NS
RAP (mmHg)	2.8 ± 1.57	1.8 ± 1.46	2.6 ± 1.69	2.6 ± 1.31	NS
mPAP (mmHg)	45 ± 16.6	28 ± 10.2	28 ± 10.5	12 ± 2.2	<0.001
PWP (mmHg)	6.7 ± 2.21	5.0 ± 1.00	5.4 ± 1.96	6.2 ± 1.71	NS
PVR (dyne s cm^{-5})	–	459 ± 273.7	332 ± 212.6	69 ± 25.3	<0.001

Values are mean ± SD. CI indicates cardiac index; RAP, right atrial pressure; mPAP, mean value of PAP; PWP, pulmonary wedge pressure; PVR, pulmonary vascular resistance; and NS, not significant. Data derived from Sime et al. (8) and Penaloza et al. (9). Reproduced from Penaloza and Arias-Stella (5), with permission of Lippincott, Williams & Wilkins.

Table 25.1.2   Combined effect of age and the level of altitude on the right ventricular hypertrophy assessed by ECG (ÂQRS >90°)

Altitude	Newborn	1 week 3 months	4–11 months	1–5 years	6–14 years	15–20 years	21–40 years	41–60 years
LIMA (sea level)	**145 ± 20.1**	**110 ± 27.2**	65 ± 22.3	51 ± 27.4	57 ± 27.7	55 ± 22.3	45 ± 32.4	30 ± 32.7
AREQUIPA (2400 m)	**149 ± 25.2**	**124 ± 23.1**	88 ± 34.1**	52 ± 26.3	64 ± 18.9	56 ± 31.1	47 ± 9.8	44 ± 29.2*
HUANCAYO (3200 m)	**148 ± 28.5**	**145 ± 29.3**	**129 ± 47.1**	74 ± 37.3*	73 ± 18.8**	75 ± 34.5**	54 ± 36.8	52 ± 29.8*
LA OROYA (3700 m)	**150 ± 22.3**	**147 ± 31.0**	**141 ± 34.1**	**97 ± 31.2**	85 ± 33.4**	68 ± 35.3*	45 ± 40.2	49 ± 39.0*
CERRO DE PASCO (4300 m)	**142 ± 24.1**	**147 ± 30.3**	**156 ± 41.3**	**132 ± 39.7**	**102 ± 21.3**	**97 ± 36.8**	81 ± 39.1**	79 ± 69.1**
MOROCOCHA (4540 m)	**133 ± 28.5**	**152 ± 32.1**	**155 ± 38.1**	**155 ± 44.9**	**137 ± 46.2**	**125 ± 46.1**	**105 ± 70.2**	**108 ± 78.5**

ÂQRS° values are mean ± SD. Figures in bold mean ÂQRS > 90°. The statistical significance between the altitude places and sea level is shown for each group of age.

*$P < 0.01$; **$P < 0.001$. Lima (sea level) n = 550. MorocOcha (4540 m) n = 400. Other levels, n = 550. Data from Penaloza *et al.* (15) and Penaloza *et al.* Reproduced from Penaloza *et al.* (17) with permission of Mary Ann Liebert, Inc. publishers.

Hematological features are excessive polycythemia, increased blood viscosity and expanded total and lung blood volume. Cardiopulmonary abnormalities include moderate or severe PH and RVH, which may evolve to hypoxic cor pulmonale and HF. Neuropsychic symptoms include sleep disorders, headaches, dizziness and mental fatigue (5,27).

CMS may be classified as primary, without identified cause, or secondary due to underlying conditions. The **primary type of CMS** is diagnosed after exclusion of lung diseases by pulmonary function testing. The **secondary variety of CMS** is associated with lung diseases, neuromuscular disorders or chest wall deformities. However, most cases represent unrecognized respiratory abnormalities because it is not easy to rule out the influence of smoking and environmental pollution, factors often mentioned in papers dealing with CMS (5,27).

Clinical picture

Peruvian investigators carried out pioneering cardio-pulmonary studies in 10 male patients with CMS, from 22 to 51 years of age, who were born and lived around Cerro de Pasco (4340 m). They did not have any history of pulmonary diseases and had never worked in mines or in any other dusty occupation. Clinical and hemodynamic studies were done in these patients and the results were compared with a group of healthy natives residing at the same altitude (26,27). In recent decades Asian investigators studied patients with CMS and described a clinical picture (30,31) which closely resembles the classic description by Peruvian investigators.

Frequent symptoms in patients with CMS are decreased exercise tolerance, sleep disorders, headaches, dizziness, tinnitus, paresthesias, physical weakness and mental fatigue.

Physical examination shows that the ruddy or erythremic color usually seen in healthy highlanders becomes cyanotic. Cyanosis is of variable degree and particularly visible at the nail beds, ears and lips. In some cases the face is almost black and the mucosa and conjunctiva dark red. Clubbing of fingers is a frequent finding. The pulmonary second sound is increased and often associated with a soft mid-systolic ejection murmur. Signs of mild or moderate HF are found in some cases. The systemic diastolic blood pressure is often increased, which has been related to excessive polycythemia (26,27).

Heart size is significantly increased on chest x-rays as compared with healthy highlanders, and this feature is due to increased size of the right chambers. Prominence of the main pulmonary artery is found in all patients and pulmonary vascular markings are accentuated in the central and peripheral regions of the lung fields. All these findings are indicative of PH and RVH (26,27,30,31). A direct relationship between mPAP and the heart size has been demonstrated (26).

The electrocardiogram often shows peaked P waves with increased voltage in leads II, III and aVF as well as in the right precordial leads. A right ÂQRS° deviation is often observed. An rS pattern in the right precordial leads and complexes of RS or rS type in the left precordial leads are common findings. Negative T waves over the right precordial leads are also common. These findings are indicative of RVH and overload of the right heart chambers as consequence of increased PH (26,27,30,31). A direct relationship between mPAP and right ÂQRS° deviation has been demonstrated (26).

In summary, there is clinical, radiological and electrocardiographic evidence of moderate to severe PH which, in some cases, may evolve to chronic cor pulmonale and HF. When patients with CMS are moved to sea level, symptoms and signs improve promptly while the electrocardiographic

Table 25.1.3 Pulmonary arterial pressure in chronic mountain sickness. Data obtained by cardiac catheterization at the altitude of residence

First author (Ref.)	Location	Altitude (m)	Hemoglobin (g/dL) (n)	mPAP (mmHg) (n)
Rotta (32)	Morococha Peru	4540	26 (1)	35 (1)
Penaloza (26)	Cerro de Pasco Peru	4340	25 ± 2 (10)	47 ± 17 (10)
Ergueta (33)	La Paz Bolivia	3600	26 (2)	51 (2)
Manier (34)	La Paz Bolivia	3600	21 ± 2 (8)	27 ± 10 (8)
Pei (30)	Lhasa Tibet	3600	23 ± 2 (5)	40 ± 11 (5)
Yang Z (36)	Chengdou Qinghai, China	3950	22 (6)	31 (6)

Values for mPAP are mean or mean ± SD. Reproduced from Penaloza (64) with permission of Springer.

Table 25.1.4 Hemodynamic values in CMS in comparison with healthy highlanders and SL subjects

	SL controls (n = 25; age 17 to 23 years)	Healthy highlanders controls (n = 12; age 19 to 38 years)	CMS subjects (n = 10; age 22 to 51 years)	P CMS vs. healthy highlanders
Hb (g/dL)	14.7 ± 0.88	20.1 ± 1.69	24.7 ± 2.36	<0.001
Hct (%)	44.1 ± 2.59	59.4 ± 5.4	79.3 ± 4.2	<0.001
SaO_2 (%)	95.7 ± 2.07	81.1 ± 4.61	69.6 ± 4.92	<0.001
RAP (mmHg)	2.6 ± 1.31	2.9 ± 1.4	3.9 ± 1.8	NS
mPAP (mmHg)	12 ± 2.2	23 ± 5.1	47 ± 17.7	<0.001
PWP (mmHg)	6.2 ± 1.71	6.9 ± 1.4	5.7 ± 2.3	NS
PVR (dynes cm^{-5})	69 ± 25.3	197 ± 57.6	527 ± 218.1	<0.001
CI (L min^{-1} m^{-2})	3.9 ± 0.97	3.8 ± 0.62	4.0 ± 0.93	NS

Values are mean ± SD. Hct indicates hematocrit; RAP, right atrial pressure; PWP, pulmonary wedge pressure; CI, Cardiac Index; and NS, non-significant. Data derived from Penaloza et al. (9) and Penaloza and Sime (26). Reproduced from Penaloza and Arias-Stella (5) with permission of Lippincott, Williams & Wilkins.

and radiographic evidence of PH and RVH decreases, the greatest changes occurring in patients with the longest residence at sea level (26,27).

Pulmonary hemodynamics

HEMODYNAMIC STUDIES OF CMS AT THE ALTITUDE OF RESIDENCE

Studies with cardiac catheterization in patients with CMS at the altitude of their residence have been carried out in Peru (26,27,32), Bolivia (33,34) and China (30,35,36). See Tables 25.1.3, 25.1.4 and Figure 25.1.3.

HEMODYNAMIC STUDIES OF CMS AT THE RECOVERY PERIOD IN LOWER PLACES

There are two Chinese studies in patients with CMS from the Guolok area (3700–4200 m) and Xining (2100 m). One of the studies was carried out with cardiac catheterization and the mPAP was 18 mmHg, an unexpectedly low value which is incompatible with the evidence of RVH found by ECG and chest x-ray in the same patients. The authors ascribed the low mPAP value to the lower altitude where the study was undertaken (37). The second study was

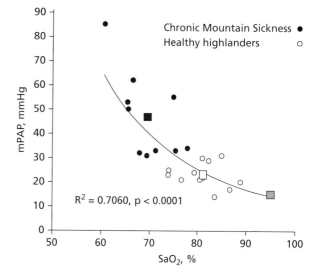

Figure 25.1.3 mPAP as related to SaO_2 in patients with CMS. There is an inverse relationship between these two variables. As SaO_2 decreases mPAP increases and the patient with the lowest SaO_2 has the highest mPAP (filled circles). By comparison, values in healthy highlanders are shown (open circles). The average values of mPAP for CMS, healthy highlanders and for SL residents are also shown (square symbols). Data derived from Penaloza and Sime (26) and Penaloza et al. (27) Reproduced from Penaloza and Arias-Stella (5) with permission of Lippincott, Williams & Wilkins.

performed with a non-invasive procedure ("an equation related to the alveolar air") and the calculated mPAP was 39 mmHg (38). There is an unexplained discrepancy between both studies carried out by the same research group in patients who came from the same HA and studied at the same lower place.

HEMODYNAMIC STUDIES OF CMS WITH DOPPLER–ECHOCARDIOGRAPHY

These investigations were carried out in La Paz, Bolivia (3600 m) and the results are shown in Table 25.1.5. From systolic PAP (sPAP) values reported in these publications we calculated the corresponding mPAP values by using new formulas (39,40). Antezana *et al.* studied a group of patients with an average age of 40 years and excessive polycythemia (Hb 22 g/dL), and the mPAP was 26 mmHg (sPAP 42 mmHg) (41). Vargas and Spielvogel studied two groups of patients with CMS, old and young patients, with Hb values of 24 and 19 g/dL, respectively. The mPAP value in both groups was 22 mmHg (sPAP 35 mmHg), a value similar to the mPAP of healthy people living in La Paz. This result in CMS patients is incompatible with the finding in the same patients of moderate or definite RVH (42). Maignan *et al.* (43) studied a group of patients with CMS with an average age of 45 years with excessive polycythemia (Hb 23 g/dL) and a calculated mPAP of 25 mmHg (sPAP 39 mmHg calculated from TR 34 mmHg + 5 mmHg of assumed RA pressure). Most studies with Doppler-echocardiography show lower mPAP values than those previously obtained with right-cardiac catheterization in patients with CMS living in laPaz (33,34). A recent prospective study demonstrates discrepancies between both methodologies indicating that Doppler-echocardiography frequently underestimates PAP in patients with PH (44).

An unexpected finding in these studies from Bolivia was the discrepancy of mPAP values amongst control groups (normocythemic and asymptomatic subjects). The mPAP value was 27 mmHg in the first study (41) and 18/19 mmHg in the other two studies (42,43). The mPAP of 27 mmHg is too high and mPAP values of 18/19 m Hg are lower in comparison with an mPAP of 22 mmHg found in healthy people of La Paz in several cardiac catheterization studies, as reported by Vargas and Spielvogel (42). The mPAP of 27 mmHg is found in healthy people living above 4000 m and is usually associated with definite signs of RVH in the ECG which was recorded but not described by Antezana *et al.* (41). On the other hand, mPAP values such 18 or 19 mmHg are found in healthy people living below 3000 m of altitude. These discrepancies may be ascribed to inaccuracies of sPAP values obtained with Doppler-echocardiography. It is well known that the tricuspid regurgitant jet is frequently trace or mild in healthy subjects and is not easily recorded (45).

PULMONARY HYPERTENSION IN HIGH ALTITUDE HEART DISEASE (CHINA)

Definition and clinical picture

A clinical picture named high altitude heart disease (HAHD) was described by Wu *et al.* in 1965 (46). The same investigators were also the authors of the last original paper on this clinical entity published in 1990 (47). Chinese authors describe the adult type of HAHD as a chronic disease characterized by clinical evidence of PH, RVH and in some cases heart failure, in absence of accentuated hypoxemia and polycythemia. However, the initial descriptions of adult HAHD were confused and there was a great overlapping with the polycythemic variety of high altitude chronic disease (CMS). Most publications on HAHD show a variable degree of polycythemia. The original description included 22 cases with average values of Hb 21.1 g/dL and Hct 73 percent (46) and the last original publication recorded 202 cases with an average Hb of 23.3 g/dL (47). Wu *et al.* have recognized that publications on adult HAHD, most of them from their own group, actually correspond to CMS (38).

Table 25.1.5 Pulmonary arterial pressure in CMS vs. controls. Data obtained by Doppler-echocardiography at the altitude of residence, La Paz, Bolivia (3600 m)

First author (Ref.)	Group P vs. N	Number of cases	Age (y)	Hemoglobin (g/dL)	sPAP (mmHg)	mPAP* (mmHg)
Antezana (41)	**P (old)**	**17**	**40**	**22**	**42**	**26**
	N (young)	14	28	17	43	27
Vargas (42)	**P (old)**	**28**	**47**	**24**	**35**	**22**
	N (old)	27	43	17	29	18
	P (young)	**30**	**22**	**19**	**35**	**22**
	N (young)	30	22	17	28	18
Maignan (43)	**P (old)**	**55**	**45**	**23**	**39[†]**	**25**
	N (old)	15	44	16.5	29[†]	18

P, polycythemia; N, normocythemia.
*Calculated mPAP values.
[†]Calculated sPAP value: Tricuspid regurgitation + 5 mmHg (assumed right auricle pressure).

Pulmonary hemodynamics

There are no measurements of PAP obtained by cardiac catheterization in the so-called adult HAHD. Review of the literature only found two reports of PAP obtained by Doppler-echocardiography after one week of residence at the lower altitude of Xining (2261 m). The calculated mPAP values in these studies were 36 ± 3 and 28 ± 4 mmHg, respectively, values similar or somewhat lower than most of those reported in CMS (47,48) (Table 25.1.6). In concordance, the ECG, VCG and chest x-ray findings described in patients with adult HAHD are similar to those described in patients with CMS in Peru (26,27) and China (30,31). In short, as asserted by Wu, the adult type of HAHD actually corresponds to CMS, and the lesser degrees of hypoxemia and polycythemia are ascribed to the lower altitudes where the patients were studied.

PULMONARY HYPERTENSION IN HIGH ALTITUDE COR PULMONALE (KYRGYZSTAN)

Definition and clinical picture

Kyrgyzian investigators do not have publications with the name CMS. Several decades ago they described a clinical picture named high altitude pulmonary hypertension (HAPH) that may evolve to high altitude cor pulmonale (HACP) and heart failure. Following the pioneering research of Peruvian investigators, Mirrakhimov was second to use the concept of chronic cor pulmonale as a consequence of loss of altitude adaptation (49). This clinical entity is observed in people living at the high altitudes of the Tien-Shan and Pamir Mountains (2800–4200 m) and its prevalence is 4.6 percent in the male population. HACP is characterized by a variable degree of PH, RVH and HF in the absence of significant hypoxemia and polycythemia (50,51). Cardiac auscultation and the findings obtained by ECG and chest-x ray resemble those found in patients with CMS (26,27,30,31) and the so-called adult HAHD (46,47).

Pulmonary hemodynamics

From 1989 to 1999 cardiac catheterization studies were carried out in 136 symptomatic highlanders (2800–3600 m) and resting PH with an mPAP value of 37 ± 3 mmHg was found in 27 subjects (20 percent) (50). Sarybaev and Mirrakhimov found a mPAP of 38 ± 3.2 mmHg in a group of patients with HACP living at 3200–4200 m (51). Recently, Aldashev et al. reported a mPAP of 32 ± 4 mmHg (range 20–64 mmHg) in 11 subjects with HACP living at 2800–3100 m (50). It should be noted that all cardiac catheterization studies reported by Kyrgyzian investigators were performed after one week of residence at low altitude (Bishkek, 750 m) (Table 25.1.6), which may explain the absence of significant hypoxemia and polycythemia. There is little data on SaO_2, Hb and Hct in Kyrgyzian investigations. SaO_2 improves promptly after descending to low levels and becomes normal or near normal in reported cases (50). There is enough evidence to postulate that HACP is actually a variety of CMS.

PULMONARY HYPERTENSION IN SUBACUTE MOUNTAIN SICKNESS

Definition and pathogenesis

Five decades ago Chinese investigators described in humans the counterpart of cattle brisket disease with the name HAHD of pediatric type (52). This clinical picture is mainly observed in infants of Chinese Han origin who are born at low altitude and then brought to high altitude where they develop pulmonary hypertension and heart failure within a few weeks or months, with a fatal outcome if the infants are not moved down to lower places. Occasionally, this entity might occur among infants born at altitude but usually of low-altitude ancestry. It is also observed in children from 2 to 14 years of age but the prevalence is lower than in infants. Prevalence of pediatric HAHD is higher in Han infants than in Tibetan infants (53).

Table 25.1.6 Pulmonary arterial pressure in high altitude heart disease (HAHD) and high cor altitude cor pulmonale (HACP) obtained during recovery at lower places

First author (Ref.)	Diagnosis	Location	Altitude of residence (m)	Altitude of study (m)	mPAP, mmHg(n)
Wu (47)	HAHD	Qinghai–Tibetan Plateau, China[†]	3000–5000	2260	36 ± 3 (108)
Cheng (48)	HAHD	Qinghai–Tibetan Plateau, China[†]	3000–5000	2260	28 ± 4 (10)
Saryvaeb (51)	HACP	Tien-Shan & Pamir Mountains, Kyrgyzstan[‡]	3200–4200	760	38 ± 3 (8)
Aldashev (50)	HACP	Tien-Shan & Pamir Mountains, Kyrgyzstan[‡]	2800–3100	760	32 ± 4 (11)

Values for mPAP are mean ± SD. Reproduced from Penaloza (64) with permission of Springer.
[†]Doppler echocardiography in Xining, 2260 m
[‡]Cardiac catheterization in Bishkek, 760 m

The mechanism of this clinical entity is ascribed to exaggerated hypoxic pulmonary reactivity of distal pulmonary arterial branches which are muscularized in excess.

Pulmonary hemodynamics and pathology

In 1963, Khoury and Hawes reported their findings in 11 infants from 6 to 23 months living in Leadville, Colorado (3100 m), with a clinical picture diagnosed as "primary pulmonary hypertension." Five of the infants were moved to Denver, Colorado (1500 m) and had cardiac catheterization with an average mPAP of 44 mmHg and a range of 28–72 mmHg (Table 25.1.7). Post-mortem studies in two patients showed severe RVH and distal pulmonary arteries with marked hypertrophy of the medial muscular coat and intimal proliferation, but no occlusive lesions (54).

Three years later, Tibetan investigators described similar pathological findings in 57 infants who died with the diagnosis of pediatric HAHD and subsequently, these authors extended their pathological investigations to 100 infants with HAHD (55,56). Lin and Wu published their clinical observations in 286 cases of pediatric HAHD (57).

The first report in English with the name subacute infantile mountain sickness (SIMS) was published in 1988 by Asian and British investigators who placed emphasis on the subacute evolution of this disease and reported the post-mortem findings in 15 infants. Extreme medial hypertrophy of the small pulmonary arteries and massive hypertrophy and dilatation of the right ventricle were the main findings (18).

Some hemodynamic studies have been undertaken in SIMS. Wu and Miao reported an average mPAP of 33 mmHg in eight infants living at 3000–4000 m and recovering from SIMS in Xining (2261 m) (58). A moderate-to-severe pulmonary hypertension with a mPAP of 72 mmHg was assessed by Doppler-echocardiography in 55 infants coming from high altitudes and recovering from SIMS in Xining (59). Recently the cardiac structure and function in 10 infants with SIMS was studied with magnetic resonance imaging and Doppler-echocardiography and the mPAP was 63 mmHg (60) (Table 25.1.7). SIMS is not frequent in the Andes but some observational cases have been described in Peru and Bolivia (5,61,62). A rare variety of subacute mountain sickness in adults has been described in Indian soldiers patrolling at very high altitudes of the Himalayan Mountains with prompt recovery after returning to lower altitude (63).

HIGH ALTITUDE PULMONARY HYPERTENSION: A DISTINCTIVE FEATURE OF HEALTHY HIGHLANDERS AND HIGH ALTITUDE DISEASES

We envisage HAPH as a true pathophysiological spectrum. At one end of the spectrum there are healthy highlanders with mild PH and at the other end of the spectrum there are pediatric patients with subacute infantile mountain sickness (SIMS or pediatric HAHD) who have severe PH. High altitude pulmonary edema (HAPE), an acute HA disease, is frequently at this end of the spectrum. In the middle of the spectrum are chronic high altitude diseases: CMS, HAHD, described in China and HACP, described in Kyrgyzstan.

A systematic review of worldwide literature regarding pulmonary hemodynamics in healthy highlanders and high altitude diseases has demonstrated that PH, in different magnitude, is a distinctive feature of these conditions. The analysis based on current evidence may be summarized as follows:

- **Healthy highlanders.** There are several studies with cardiac catheterization performed in Peru, Bolivia and China. People native to these altitudes have mild PH, with mPAP range from 22 to near 30 mmHg (Table 25.1.1). At the highest altitudes some individual cases may have moderate PH and even values of mPAP greater than 40 mmHg (9).
- **Chronic mountain sickness.** There are six studies with cardiac catheterization carried out at the altitude of residence. The average value of mPAP is 39 mmHg with a range from 27 to 51 mmHg. The degree of PH is mild in one study, moderate in two studies and severe in three studies (Table 25.1.4).
- **Other chronic high-altitude diseases.** There is high evidence that HAHD, described in China, and HACP, described in Kyrgyzstan, are varieties of CMS with lesser degrees of hypoxemia and polycythemia. There are four

Table 25.1.7 Pulmonary arterial pressure in infants with subacute mountain sickness while recovering at lower places

First author (Ref.)	Location	Altitude of residence (m)	Altitude of study (m)	mPAP, mmHg (n)
Khoury (54)	Leadville Colorado[‡]	3100	1500	44 (5)
Wu (58)	Qinghai–Tibetan Plateau, China[†]	3000–4200	2260	33 ± 11 (8)
Ma Ru-Yan (59)	Qinghai–Tibetan Plateau, China[†]	2440–3700	2260	72 ± 17 (55)
Ge Ri-Li (60)	Qinghai–Tibetan Plateau, China[†]	3600–4600	2260	67 ± 7 (10)

Values for mPAP are mean or mean ± SD.
[†]Doppler echocardiography in Xining, 2260 m.
[‡]Cardiac catheterization in Denver, 1500 m.

studies, all of them undertaken at low altitudes. The average mPAP is 33.5 mmHg with a range from 28 to 38 mmHg. The degree of PH is mild in one study and moderate in three. No study with severe PH has been reported (Table 25.1.6).

- **Subacute infantile mountain sickness.** There are four hemodynamic studies in infants coming from HA and studied during recovery at lower places. Average mPAP is 54 mmHg with a range from 33 to 72 mmHg. The degree of PH was moderate in one study and severe in three (Table 25.1.7).

REAPPRAISAL OF THE CONSENSUS ON CHRONIC AND SUBACUTE HIGH ALTITUDE DISEASES

Background

During the VI World Congress on Mountain Medicine and High Altitude Physiology which was held in Xining, Qinghai, China in 2004 a Consensus Statement on Chronic and Subacute High Altitude Diseases was attained by an ad hoc committee of the International Society for Mountain Medicine (ISMM). The Consensus Statement was published in 2005 and a cautious warning was mentioned on the possible evolution of this consensus as result of further research (23). Reappraisal of this document has recently been proposed (64).

Classification of high altitude diseases (Consensus Group, 2004)

The Consensus recognizes two main groups of high altitude diseases. (A) Chronic mountain sickness (CMS) and (B) high altitude pulmonary hypertension (HAPH) which includes several entities: adult HAHD, HACP and SIMS (or infantile HAHD). The main rationale for this classification was the assumption that PH was always present in diseases of group B, in contrast to CMS.

This classification, excluding CMS from the group of diseases associated with HAPH, does not concur with the analysis based on current evidence nor with expert opinion. There are no data in the current literature indicating that CMS is not associated with PH of variable magnitude and there are no data demonstrating that the so-called adult HAHD and HACP have greater degrees of PH than CMS. Differences of mPAP amongst these diseases are not significant; however, the evidence demonstrates that mPAP in CMS is somewhat greater than in HAHD and HACP and severe degrees of PH have only been reported

in CMS. It is surprising that in the Consensus Statement there are no references to original research dealing with PH in HAHD. There are ten references from Wu et al. and none of them deals with PH in HAHD.

Chronic HA diseases (CMS, HAHD, HACP) and subacute HA diseases are associated with PH in different magnitude. Therefore, the presence or absence of PH should not be the rationale for a classification of HA diseases. Instead the time course of the disease, following a chronic, subacute or acute evolution, should be the natural and logical criterion for any classification of HA diseases. Chronic HA diseases, all of them associated with PH, should be integrated in one group. It is highly probable that CMS, HAHD and HACP are the same disease with different tints. SMS and HAPE should be considered separately.

Scoring system for diagnosis of chronic mountain sickness

In the last two decades, epidemiological studies of CMS have been performed in Peru, China and Kyrgyzstan and several scoring systems for its diagnosis have been proposed. However, it is not easy to develop a unique scoring system because of individual characteristics (ethnicity, gender, age) and dissimilar geographical areas and altitudes.

The Qinghai score proposed by Chinese investigators was approved by the CMS Consensus Group during the VI World Congress on Mountain Medicine (Xining, China, 2004) (23).** This score system is somewhat empiric and has some limitations. Therefore, some comments are pertinent (65).

HEMOGLOBIN THRESHOLD VALUES

The Hb threshold value of 21 g/dl, selected at 4340 m, in a mining city of Peru, may not be valid for lower altitudes and the diagnosis of CMS may be missed. A review of the epidemiological Chinese study in more than 5000 subjects at three levels of altitude demonstrates that the Hb values significantly vary according to the level of altitude and ethnicity and consequently the threshold values are not the same (66). Similar reasoning may be applicable to the range of altitudes between 2500 m and 4500 m in Peru and Bolivia.

HYPOXEMIA LEVELS

This key feature of CMS was not included in the scoring system despite it being proposed in previous scoring systems. Variable threshold values for SaO_2 as < 82 percent, < 85 percent and < 90 percent were proposed by Peruvian, Chinese and Kyrgyzian investigators, respectively. These values could be scored as 3, 2 and 1, respectively.

**The Qinghai score system is based on the level of Hb ≥21 for men and ≥19 for females, the presence of cyanosis and subjective symptoms such as breathlessness, sleep disorders, headache, tinnitus and paresthesias. Each symptom is scored as 0, 1, 2, 3 based on absent, mild, moderate and severe symptoms, respectively. Hb is scored 3 if it equals or exceeds the limits pointed out. According to the overall scoring, CMS is defined as follows: absent (0–5), mild (6–11), moderate (10–14) and severe (>15) (23).

PULMONARY HYPERTENSION

PH, a major component of CMS, was mentioned in most previous scoring systems; however, it was not included in the approved scoring system. The exclusion of CMS from the group of diseases associated with PH is disconcerting in an era when PH is the target of recent clinical trials for the management of CMS. The clinical evidence of PH assessed by auscultation, chest x-ray and ECG, has been advised as the initial methodology for diagnosis of PH (1,67). The clinical evidence of PH in CMS could be scored as 1 (mild), 2 (moderate) and 3 (severe), based on simple objective diagnostic procedures (ECG, chest x-ray) and the clinical signs. Quantification of PH by Doppler-echocardiography or right-heart catheterization could be carried out in selected cases of CMS when these procedures are available in the altitude of residence (65).

LIMITATIONS AND EXPANSION OF THE SCORING SYSTEM FOR DIAGNOSIS OF CHRONIC MOUNTAIN SICKNESS

The scoring system should not be limited to CMS and should be extended to other chronic high altitude diseases such as HAHD and HACP since PH is a common feature to all of them, without significant differences. Moreover, most of the symptoms and signs are also similar with the exception of the levels of hemoglobin and hypoxemia which, however, should be considered at the place of residence and not during the recovery at lower places. On the other hand, SIMS and HAPE are clinical entities associated with moderate or severe PH but with a distinct time course. Therefore, these diseases should be out of the scope of the scoring system for CMS.

PREVENTION AND TREATMENT OF CHRONIC MOUNTAIN SICKNESS

CMS is a public health problem for the populations living in the mountainous regions of the world. Therefore, the dissemination of the preventive measures should be emphasized, particularly those measures directed toward modifiable risk factors of the secondary variety of CMS, such as smoking, obesity, domestic and industrial air pollution and lung diseases.

The traditional and definitive treatment of CMS is descending to lower altitudes or SL. Following this, a prompt improvement of the subjective symptoms and sleep disorders is observed. Alveolar hypoxia, hypoxemia and cyanosis disappear. Polycythemia decreases and after a few weeks or months Hb and Hct return to SL values. PH and RVH regress gradually and disappear after one or two years (26,27).

Bloodletting alone or isovolemic hemodilution are palliative procedures to reduce the exaggerated polycythemia with partial improvement of signs and symptoms (68).

Other procedures are directed to improve ventilation by using stimulant drugs such as acetozolamide. The increased ventilation reduces hypoxemia and hematocrit and as a consequence improves symptomatology (69).

Vasodilators are being tested to reduce high-altitude PH. Calcium-channel blockers such as Nifedipine, already used for treatment and prevention of high-altitude pulmonary edema (HAPE), have also been tested in CMS, resulting in transient and partial reduction of PH (41). Selective pulmonary vasodilators, currently used for idiopathic pulmonary arterial hypertension (IPAH), are being tried for long-term treatment of high-altitude PH. Sildenafil, a phosphodiesterase-5 inhibitor, has been tested on symptomatic highlanders with PH and after several months improvement in pulmonary hemodynamics and exercise tolerance was observed (70). Further information regarding the pharmacological basis for the vasodilator therapy in PH is addressed in Part 5 of this book.

KEY POINTS

- HAPH is a distinctive feature, in variable magnitude, of healthy highlanders and high altitude diseases.
- Healthy highlanders have a mild and asymptomatic PH associated with adaptive levels of hypoxemia and polycythemia. PH is related to age, level of altitude and altitude ancestry.
- CMS patients have accentuated hypoxemia and exaggerated polycythemia associated with moderate or severe PH which, in some cases, may evolve to chronic cor pulmonale and heart failure.
- HAHD, described in China, and HACP, described in Kyrgyzstan, have a clinical picture similar to CMS with lesser degrees of hypoxemia and polycythemia. These patients are generally studied during the recovery period at lower altitudes.
- CMS, HAHD and HACP are actually the same chronic high altitude disease, with different shades. These clinical entities develop when the altitude adaptation is lost.
- SIMS is a subacute disease described in infants of Chinese Han origin who are born at low altitude and then brought to HA. They develop severe degree of PH and heart failure with fatal outcome if are not moved to lower places.
- Chronic high altitude diseases (CMS, HAHD and HACP) are a public health problem in mountainous regions of the world and, therefore, preventive and therapeutic measures should be disseminated.

REFERENCES

• = Key primary paper
◆ = Major review article

1. Barst RJ, McGoon M, Torbicki A et al. Diagnosis and differential assessment of pulmonary arterial hypertension. J Am Coll Cardiol 2004;43:40S–47S.

2. Kovacs G, Berghold A, Scheidl S et al. Pulmonary arterial pressure during rest and exercise in healthy control subjects: a systematic review. Eur Respir J 2009;34:888–94.

3. Badesch DB, Champion HC, Gomez Sanchez MA et al. Diagnosis and assessment of pulmonary arterial hypertension. J Am Coll Cardiol 2009;54:55S–66S.

4. Galie N, Hoeper MM, Humbert M et al. ESC/ERS Guidelines for the diagnosis and treatment of pulmonary hypertension. Eur Respir J 2009;34:1219–63.

◆5. Penaloza D, Arias-Stella J. The heart and pulmonary circulation at high altitude. Healthy highlanders and chronic mountain sickness. Circulation 2007;115:1132–46.

6. Simmoneau G, Robbins IM, Beghetti M et al. Updated clinical classification of pulmonary hypertension. J Am Coll Cardiol 2009;54:43S–54S.

7. Gamboa R, Marticorena E. Presión arterial pulmonar en el recién nacido en la grandes alturas. Arch Inst Biol Andina 1971;4:55–66.

•8. Sime F, Banchero N, Penaloza D et al. Pulmonary hypertension in children born and living at high altitudes. Am J Cardiol 1963;11:143–9.

•9. Penaloza D, Sime F, Banchero N et al. Pulmonary hypertension in healthy men born and living at high altitudes. Am J Cardiol 1963;11:150–7.

•10. Arias Stella J, Saldaña M. The terminal portion of the pulmonary arterial tree in people native to high altitude. Circulation 1963;28:915–25.

11. Niermeyer S. Cardiopulmonary transition in the high altitude infant. High Alt Med Biol 2003;4:225–39.

12. Aparicio O, Romero F, Harris P et al. Echocardiography shows persistent thickness of the wall of the right ventricle in infants at high altitude. Cardioscience 1991;2:63–8.

13. Reeves JT, Grover RF. Insights by Peruvian scientists into the pathogenesis of human chronic hypoxic pulmonary hypertension. J Appl Physiol 2005;98:384–9.

14. Pang Y, Ma RY, Qi HY, Sun K. Comparative study of the indexes of pulmonary arterial pressure of healthy children at different altitudes by Doppler echocardiography. Zhonghua Er Ke Za Zhi 2004;42:595–9.

•15. Penaloza D, Gamboa R, Dyer J et al. The influence of high altitudes on the electrical activity of the heart. Electrocardiographic and vectorcardiographic observations in the newborn, infants and children. Am Heart J 1960;59:111–28.

•16. Penaloza D, Gamboa R, Marticorena E et al. The influence of high altitudes of the electrical activity of the heart. Electrocardiographic and vectorcardiographic observations in adolescence and adulthood. Am Heart J 1961;61:101–15.

◆17. Penaloza D, Sime F, Ruiz L. Pulmonary hemodynamics in children living at high altitudes. High Alt Med Biol 2008;9:199–207.

•18. Sui GJ, Liu YH, Cheng XS, Anand IS et al. Subacute infantile mountain sickness. J Pathol 1988;155:161–70.

19. Groves BM, Droma T, Sutton JR et al. Minimal hypoxic pulmonary hypertension in normal Tibetans at 3658 m. J Appl Physiol 1993;74:312–8.

20. Grover RF. Chronic hypoxic pulmonary hypertension. In: Fishman AP (ed.) The Pulmonary Circulation: Normal and Abnormal. Philadelphia, PA: University of Pennsylvania, 1990:283–99.

21. Huicho L, Niermeyer S. Cardiopulmonary pathology among children resident at high altitude in Tintaya, Peru: a cross-sectional study. High Alt Med Biol 2006;7:168–79.

22. Huicho L. Postnatal cardiopulmonary adaptations at high altitude. Respir Physiol Neurobiol 2007;158:190–203.

23. León-Velarde F, Maggiorini M, Reeves JT et al. Consensus statement on chronic and subacute high altitude diseases. High Alt Med Biol 2005;6:147–57.

•24. Monge MC. La Enfermedad de los Andes. Síndromes eritrémicos. Anal Fac Med Lima, Peru, 1929.

•25. Hurtado A. Animals in high altitude: Resident man. In: Handbook of Physiology. (Section 4, Volume 1). Chapter 54: Adaptation to the Environment. Washington DC: Am Physiol Soc 1964:843–60.

•26. Penaloza D, Sime F. Chronic cor pulmonale due to loss of altitude acclimatization (chronic mountain sickness). Am J Med 1971;50:728–43.

•27. Penaloza D, Sime F, Ruiz L. Cor pulmonale in chronic mountain sickness: present concept of Monge's disease. In: Porter R, Knight J, eds. High Altitude Physiology: Cardiac and Respiratory Aspects. Edinburgh and London: Churchill Livingstone, 1971:41–60.

28. Penaloza D, Sime F. Pulmonary hypertension in chronic mountain sickness. In: Humbert M and Lynch III JP (eds). Pulmonary Hypertension. Paris, Los Angeles: Informa Healthcare, 2009:292–304.

29. Richalet JP, Rivera M, Maignan, M et al. Pulmonary hypertension and Monge's disease. PVRI Rev 2009;1:114–9.

30. Pei SX, Chen XJ, Si Ren BZ et al. Chronic mountain sickness in Tibet. QJ Med 1989;266:555–74.

31. Wu TY. Chronic mountain sickness on the Qinghai–Tibetan plateau. Chinese Med J 2005;118:161–8.

32. Rotta A, Cánepa A, Hurtado A et al. Pulmonary circulation at sea level and at high altitude. J Appl Physiol 1956;9:328–36.

33. Ergueta J, Spielvogel H, Cudkowitz L. Cardio-respiratory studies in chronic mountain sickness (Monge's syndrome). Respiration 1979;28:485–517.

34. Manier G, Guénard H, Castaing Y, Varene N, Vargas E. Pulmonary gas exchange in Andean natives with excessive polycythemia – effect of hemodilution. J Appl Physiol 1988;65:2107–17.

35. Wu TY, Li W, Li Y et al. Epidemiology of chronic mountain sickness: ten year's study in Qinghai–Tibet. In: Ohno H, Kobayashi T, Masuyama S, Nakashima M (eds). Progress in

Mountain Medicine and High Altitude Physiology. Matsumoto, Japan: Dogura & Co., 1998:120–5.

36. Yang Z, He ZQ, Liu XL. Pulmonary hypertension and high altitude. Chin Cardiovasc Dis 1985;13:32–4.

37. Wu TY, Miao CY, Li WS et al. Studies on high altitude pulmonary hypertension. Chin J High Alt Med 1999;9:1–8.

38. Wu TY, Zhang Q, Jin B et al. Chronic mountain sickness (Monge's disease): An observation in Qinghai–Tibet Plateau. In: Ueda G, Reeves JT, Sekiguchi M (eds). High Altitude Medicine, Matsumoto. Japan: Shinshu University Press, 1992:314–24.

39. Chemla D, Castelain V, Provencher S et al. Evaluation of various empirical formulas for estimating mean pulmonary artery pressure by using systolic pulmonary artery pressure in adults. Chest 2009;135:760–8.

40. Syyed R, Reeves JT, Welsh D et al. The relationship between the components of pulmonary artery pressure remains constant under all conditions in both health and disease. Chest 2008;133:633–9.

41. Antezana AM, Antezana G, Aparicio O et al. Pulmonary hypertension in high-altitude chronic hypoxia: response to nifedipine. Eur Respir J 1998;12:1181–5.

42. Vargas E, Spielvogel H. Chronic mountain sickness, optimal hemoglobin and heart disease. High Alt Med Biol 2006;7: 138–49.

43. Maignan M, Rivera M, Privat, C et al. Pulmonary pressure and cardiac function in chronic mountain sickness. Chest 2009;135:499–504.

44. Fisher MR, Forfia PR, Chamera E et al. Accuracy of Doppler echocardiography in the hemodynamic assessment of pulmonary hypertension. Am J Respir Crit Care Med 2009;179:615–21.

45. McQuillan BM, Picard MH, Leavitt M et al. Clinical correlates and reference intervals for pulmonary artery systolic pressure among echocardiographically normal subjects. Circulation 2001;104:2797–802.

46. Wu TY, Li CH, Wang ZW. Adult high altitude heart disease; an analysis of 22 cases. Chin Int Med J 1965;13:700–2.

47. Wu TY, Jing BS, Xu FD, Cheng QH. Clinical features of adult high altitude heart disease. An analysis of 202 cases [In Chinese with English abstract]. Acta Cardiovasc Pulm Dis 1990;9:32–5.

48. Cheng DS, Yang YX, Bian HP et al. A study on altitude hypoxic pulmonary hypertension by Doppler echocardiography. Chin J High Alt Med 1996;6:28–31 [In Chinese with English abstract].

49. Mirrakhimov MM. Chronic high-altitude cor pulmonale. In: Transactions of the International Symposium on Pulmonary Arterial Hypertension. Frunze, Kyrgyzstan: Kyrgyz Institute of Cardiology, 1985:267–87.

50. Aldashev A, Sarybaev AS, Sydkykov AS et al. Characterization of high-altitude pulmonary hypertension in the Kyrgyz: Association with angiotensin-converting enzyme genotype. Am J Respir Crit Care Med 2002;166:1396–402.

51. Sarybaeb A, Mirrakhimov M. Prevalence and natural course of high altitude pulmonary hypertension and high altitude cor pulmonale. In: Ohno H, Kobayashi T, Masuyama S, Nakashima M (eds). Progress in Mountain Medicine and High Altitude Physiology. Matsumoto. Japan: Dogura & Co., 1998:126–31.

52. Wu DC, Liu YR. High altitude heart disease. Chin J Pediat 1955;6:348–50 [In Chinese].

53. Wu TY, Die TF, Huo KS et al. An epidemiological study on high altitude heart disease at Qinghai–Tibetan Plateau. Chin J Epidemiol 1987;8:65–9 [In Chinese with English abstract].

54. Khoury GH, Hawes CR. Primary pulmonary hypertension in children living at high altitude. J Pediatrics 1963;62:177–85.

55. Li JB, Wang IY. Infantile malacclimatized to high altitude. A pathologic observation. Chin J Pathol 1966;10:98–9. [In Chinese]

56. Li JB, Sui GJ. Pathological findings in high altitude heart disease. In: Applied High Altitude Medicine. Lhasa, Tibet: Tibet Press, 1984:288–305.

57. Lin CP, Wu TY. Clinical analysis of 286 cases of pediatric high altitude heart disease. Chin Med J 1974;54:99–100. [English supplement to No. 6]

58. Wu TY, Miao CY. High altitude heart disease in children in Tibet. High Alt Med Biol 2002;3:323–5.

59. Ma Ru-Ya., Pang Y, Ge Ri-Li. Clinical study of 55 cases of high altitude heart disease in children in Qinghai. (Abstract). High Alt Med Biol 2004;5:259.

60. Ri.Li Ge, Ma Ru-yan, Bao Hai-hua et al. Changes of cardiac structure and function in pediatric patients with high altitude pulmonary hypertension. High Alt Med Biol 2009;10:247–52.

61. Hurtado GL, Calderon RG. Hipoxia de altura en la insuficiencia cardiaca del lactante. Bol Soc Boliv Pediatr 1965;9:11–23.

62. Penaloza D. Mal de montaña subagudo. En: El Reto de Vivir en los Andes. Monge C, León Velarde F (eds). IFEA-UPCH, Lima, Peru, 2003:399–408.

63. Anand IS, Malhotra R, Chandershekhar T et al. Adult subacute mountain sickness. A syndrome of congestive heart failure in man at very high altitude. Lancet 1990;335:561–5.

64. Penaloza D. High altitude pulmonary hypertension and chronic mountain sickness – Reappraisal of the consensus on chronic and subacute high altitude diseases. In: Aldashev A and Naeije R (eds). Problems of High Altitude Medicine and Biology. NATO Series A: Chemistry and Biology. Dordrecht, The Netherlands: Springer, 2007:11–37.

65. Penaloza D. Chronic mountain sickness: an open debate of scoring systems used for its diagnosis. J Qinghai Med Coll 2004;25:248–55.

66. Wu TY, Li W, Wei L et al. A preliminary study on the diagnosis of chronic mountain sickness in Tibetan populations. In: Ohno H, Kobayashi T, Masuyama S, Nakashima M (eds). Progress in Mountain Medicine and High Altitude Physiology. Matsumoto, Japan: Dogura & Co., 1998:337–42.

67. McGoon M, Gutterman D, Steen V *et al.* Screening, early detection and diagnosis of pulmonary arterial hypertension. ACCP Evidence-Based Clinical Practice Guidelines. Chest 2004;126:14S–34S.

68. Winslow RM, Monge CC, Brown EG *et al.* Effects of hemodilution on O_2 transport in high altitude polycythemia. J Appl Physiol 1985;59:1495–502.

69. Richalet JP, Rivera M, Maignan M *et al.* Acetozolamide for Monge's disease. Efficiency and tolerance of 6-month treatment. Am J Respir Crit Care Med 2008;177: 1370–6.

70. Aldashev AA, Kojonorazov BK, Amatov *et al.* Phosphodiesterase type 5 and high altitude pulmonary hypertension. Thorax 2005;60:683–7.

High altitude pulmonary edema

MARCO MAGGIORINI AND PETER BÂRTSCH

INTRODUCTION

The physiological relevance of hypoxic pulmonary vaso-constriction (HPV) in healthy humans moving to altitude has not yet been fully understood. Mechanistically thinking we could assume that moderately elevated pulmonary artery pressures (Ppa) optimize oxygen delivery by recruiting ventilated but not blood-perfused lung areas. However, an excessive rise of Ppa may harm and lead either to high altitude pulmonary edema (HAPE) (1,2), an illness that can occur after rapid ascent without proper acclimatization, or within weeks or months to congestive right heart failure of high altitude also named subacute mountain sickness (3,4). This latter disease, which might more appropriately be termed "cor pulmonale" or "right heart failure of high altitude," was first discovered in cattle in Colorado and named "Brisket Disease" (5). Brisket is the depending part of the neck where edema accumulates.

It is one of the most exciting and challenging goals to unravel the genetic basis of HPV and its inter-individual variability. There is convincing evidence of a genetic basis in animals and humans. Excessive HPV and thus susceptibility to brisket disease has been bred out in Colorado cattle (6) and in Tibetans, the best-adapted human population to high altitude, HPV has virtually vanished (7). Furthermore, in the Andes it was shown that susceptibility to HAPE runs in families (8). This observation, if confirmed in a larger number, not only underlines the genetic basis of HPV, but suggests also that hypoxic vasoconstriction of pulmonary arterioles may be a disadvantage when living at high altitude. In addition, it shows that HPV is not of vital importance since it appears to have vanished due to evolutionary adaptation to high altitude in Tibetans.

PULMONARY HYPERTENSION IN LOWLANDERS AT HIGH ALTITUDE

The physiological response of pulmonary circulation to hypobaric and normobaric hypoxia is to increase pulmonary arteriolar resistance. The magnitude of hypoxic pulmonary vasoconstriction is highly variable between humans. Sites of hypoxic pulmonary vasoconstriction are small pulmonary arterioles and veins of a diameter less than $900\,\mu m$, the veins accounting approximately for 20 percent of the total increase in pulmonary vascular resistance caused by hypoxia (9,10). The structural differences at the site of hypoxic pulmonary vasoconstriction within humans appear to reflect a genetically determined and adaptive process (7,11).

In healthy lowlanders at altitudes between 3800 and 4600 m, invasively assessed resting mean pulmonary artery pressure (Ppa) ranges between 15 and 35 mmHg (average 25 mmHg) and the systolic Ppa between 27 and 48 mmHg (average 37 mmHg) (12–14) (Figure 25.2.1). Mean Ppa at altitudes above 5000 m during exposure in a barochamber (Operation Everest II) in healthy and partially acclimatized volunteers was 24 mmHg at 6100 m (barometric pressure 347 mmHg) and 34 mmHg at 7620 m (282 mmHg). At both altitudes physical exercise significantly increased mean Ppa to 41 and 54 mmHg, respectively (15).

Abnormal rise of Ppa is associated with life-threatening diseases in newcomers to high altitude. Individuals susceptible to HAPE had a mean Ppa of 39 mmHg (range 22–47) at 3100 m (16) and of 38 mmHg (31 and 51 mmHg) at an altitude of 4559 m (14) (Figure 25.2.1). Indirect evidence of abnormally high Ppa was reported after prolonged stay at high altitude. Right heart failure associated with congestion

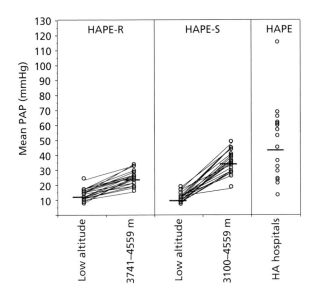

Figure 25.2.1 The figure shows individual pulmonary artery pressure (Ppa) values reported at low and approximately 24 hours after ascent at high altitude using a right heart catheter in high-altitude pulmonary edema resistant (HAPE-R) (12,13) and susceptible subjects (HAPE-S) (14,16), and mean Ppa values reported in subjects with HAPE after hospital admission (47,48,50,51). The figure illustrates that in ~50% of the HAPE-susceptible subjects mean Ppa exceeds the 40 mmHg mark. The horizontal bars indicate median Ppa value for each group of subjects.

has been described in infants of Han descent born at low altitude brought to reside in Lhasa (3) and Indian soldiers who failed to acclimatize at the extreme altitude of 5800–6700 m (4). This syndrome, which appears after an exposure of several weeks or months at high altitude, has been named infantile and adult subacute mountain sickness, respectively. Cases of severe pulmonary hypertension with chronic congestive right heart failure were described in an immigrant Han population after an average of 15 years of residence (17). Subacute and chronic mountain sickness will be discussed in Chapter 25.1 of this book.

HIGH ALTITUDE PULMONARY EDEMA

Epidemiology

There are two typical settings for HAPE, a condition that occurs within a few days of arrival at high altitude. The first setting involves high altitude dwellers who return from a sojourn at low altitude (8,18,19) and the second involves unacclimatized lowlanders (20). The first two publications suggesting that HAPE is a non-cardiogenic pulmonary edema were from Peru 1955 (reentry HAPE) by Lizzarraga (18) and from the Rocky Mountains 1960 (unacclimatized lowlanders) by Houston (20). Altitude, rate of ascent and, most importantly, individual susceptibility are the major determinants of HAPE in mountaineers and trekkers. The estimated incidence in visitors to ski resorts in the Rocky

Mountains of Colorado is 0.01–0.1 percent (18,21). The prevalence of HAPE is < 0.2 percent in a general alpine mountaineering population when ascent occurs in three and more days to an altitude of 4559 m (22). When the same altitude is reached within 22 hours, the incidence increases to 7 percent in mountaineers without and to 62 percent in mountaineers with a history of radiographically documented HAPE (23). The incidence of HAPE also increases from 2.5 to 15.5 percent when an altitude of 5500 m is reached by airlift (24) as opposed to trekking over 4–6 days (25). Women may be less susceptible to HAPE than men (22,26).

Signs and symptoms

HAPE presents within 2–5 days after arrival at high altitude (24). It is rarely observed below altitudes of 2500–3000 m and after 1 week of acclimatization at a particular altitude. In most cases, it is preceded by symptoms of acute mountain sickness (AMS). Early symptoms of HAPE include exertional dyspnea, cough and reduced exercise performance. As edema progresses, cough worsens and breathlessness at rest and sometimes orthopnea occur. Gurgling in the chest and pink frothy sputum indicate advanced cases.

The clinical examination reveals cyanosis, tachypnea, tachycardia and elevated body temperature, which generally does not exceed 38.5°C. Râles are discrete at the beginning, typically located over the middle lung fields. Often, there is a discrepancy between the minor findings at auscultation compared with the widespread disease on the chest radiograph. In advanced cases, signs of concomitant cerebral edema, such as ataxia and decreased levels of consciousness are frequent findings.

Laboratory evaluation

There are no characteristic findings in common laboratory examinations (27). Abnormal results may be due to accompanying dehydration, stress and preceding exercise. Arterial blood gas measurements of four cases of advanced HAPE at 4559 m demonstrate the severity of this illness (28) (Table 25.2.1). In early cases values around 30 mmHg for PO_2 and 70 percent for SaO_2 are observed at this altitude. Chest radiographs and CT-scans of early HAPE cases show a patchy, peripheral distribution of edema as shown in Figure 25.2.2 (29). The radiographic appearance of HAPE is more homogeneous and diffuse in advanced cases and during recovery (30). Autopsies showed distended pulmonary arteries and diffuse pulmonary edema with bloody foamy fluid present in the airways but no evidence of left ventricular failure (31).

Prevention

Slow ascent is the major measure of prevention that is effective even in susceptible individuals. Personal observations

Table 25.2.1   Arterial blood gas analysis at 4559 m

	PaO_2 (mmHg)	$PaCO_2$ (mmHg)	SaO_2 (%)
Controls ($n = 22$)	40 ± 5	30 ± 5	78 ± 7
HAPE ($n = 4$)	23 ± 3	28 ± 4	48 ± 8
P	< 0.001	NS	< 0.001

Mean values $\pm$ SD. $PaCO_2/PaO_2$, arterial partial pressure of CO_2/O_2; SaO_2, arterial oxygen saturation.

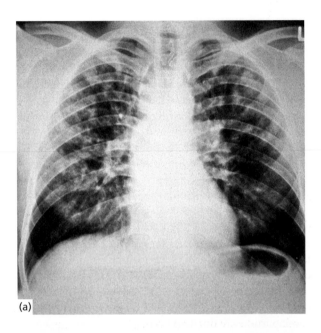
(a)

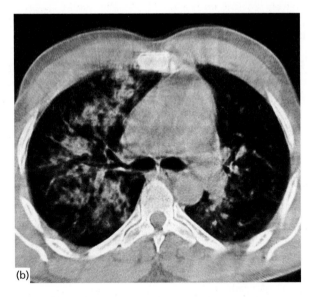
(b)

Figure 25.2.2   Radiograph of a female patient with HAPE, predominantly in the lower lung quadrants (a). The CT of the same patient shows a patchy distribution of edema, which is more severe in the anterior parts (b). (These illustrations were kindly provided by Dr. H. Fischer, Regionalspital Visp, Switzerland.)

of nine ascents in seven mountaineers, who all developed HAPE more than once upon rapid ascent in the Alps, indicate that altitudes up to 7000 m can be reached by these individuals without medical problems when the average daily ascent rate above 2000 m does not exceed 350–400 m per day or with staged ascent. People should be advised not to ascend further with any symptoms of AMS or beginning HAPE and to avoid vigorous exercise during the first days of altitude exposure, since exercise-induced circulatory changes may enhance or cause pulmonary edema (32). Furthermore, susceptibility to HAPE may be increased during and shortly after infection (33).

Prophylaxis with nifedipine can be recommended for individuals with a history of unquestionable HAPE when slow ascent is not possible (34). Sixty mg daily of a slow-release formulation should be given starting with the ascent and ending on the third or fourth day after arrival at the final altitude in the case of a prolonged stay or after returning to an altitude below 3000 m or to an altitude to which the individual is acclimatized. Ten mg of tadalafil or 8 mg dexamethasone, both twice daily, were also shown to prevent HAPE in susceptible individuals ascending within 2 days to 4559 m (35). It should be emphasized that nifedipine and tadalafil help to avoid HAPE and that they are not effective for preventing AMS (35,36), while dexamethasone is known to reduce or prevent symptoms of AMS (37).

Treatment

Immediate improvement of oxygenation is the treatment of choice. Specific recommendations on how to obtain this goal depend on where HAPE occurs. For the mountaineer in a remote area without medical care descent has first priority while the tourist with HAPE in a resort in the Rocky Mountains may stay at altitude if the arterial oxygen saturation can be kept above 90 percent with low-flow oxygen (2–4 L/min) and monitoring by family or friends is guaranteed. Relief of symptoms is achieved within hours and complete clinical recovery usually occurs within 2–3 days. Although intermittent continuous positive end-expiratory airway pressure has been shown to improve SaO_2 in subjects with HAPE by 10–20 percent (38,39), its use is not recommended because it may cause high altitude cerebral edema (HACE) by decreasing venous return (40).

When descent is impossible and supplemental oxygen is not available, portable hyperbaric chambers (41,42) and treatment with nifedipine (20 mg slow release formulation every 6 h) should be initiated until descent is possible. In mountaineers with HAPE at 4559 m persistent relief of symptoms, improvement of gas exchange and radiographical appearance were documented over 34 h with 20 mg nifedipine every six hours (43). Recently, some patients with HAPE were successfully treated with sildenafil (44). However, to prove efficacy and safety a randomized controlled trial is warranted.

Pathophysiology of high altitude edema

PULMONARY ARTERY PRESSURE

Since the first hemodynamic measurements performed in patients with HAPE admitted to the hospital with HAPE it has been shown that this condition is associated with elevated pulmonary artery pressure (27,45–49). In a prospective hemodynamic evaluation of HAPE-susceptible subjects after rapid ascent to 4559 m within 24 hours, it has been shown recently that mean Ppa was elevated on average to 42 mmHg (range 36–51 mmHg) in those subjects who developed pulmonary edema during their stay at high altitude (14). All these hemodynamic studies consistently show that in HAPE left atrial pressure, as assessed by occluded (or wedged) Ppa, right atrial pressure and cardiac output are normal. Invasive hemodynamic evaluations at low and high altitude show that excessive reactivity of the pulmonary vessels is the mechanism leading to pulmonary hypertension of high altitude (12–14,16) (Figure 25.2.1). Additionally, the key role of elevated Ppa in the pathogenesis of HAPE was demonstrated by the data showing that this condition is prevented or improved by the use of pulmonary vasodilators (34,35,43,50). Interestingly, dexamethasone might also prevent HAPE predominantly by lowering PAP (Figure 25.2.3, neu), since it was as effective as tadalafil in lowering PAP in HAPE susceptible individuals (35).

The pathophysiological mechanism of high altitude-associated pulmonary hypertension has only been incompletely understood. Inhibition of voltage dependent potassium channels by PO_2 might be crucial (51). However, other endothelium based humoral mechanisms such as the synthesis of nitric oxide and endothelin may contribute to the mechanisms leading to excessive hypoxic pulmonary vasoconstriction. This notion is supported by lower levels of exhaled NO in hypoxia (52,53) by lower nitrate and nitrite concentrations in bronchoalveolar lavage fluid (ref 72) and by endothelial dysfunction in the forearm circulation under hypoxia (54) in HAPE susceptible vs. non-susceptible individuals. Furthermore, pulmonary artery pressure rises higher in HAPE susceptible individuals compared with non-susceptible controls not only in hypoxia but also during exercise in normoxia (55–57). This could be explained by an impaired NO release in response to increased blood flow in the pulmonary circulation and point to decreased NO bioavailability in HAPE susceptible individuals in hypoxia and during exercise. The role of the autonomic nervous system in the initiation and progress of pulmonary edema in this particular setting remains to be determined. Compared to non-HAPE susceptibles, persons prone to the disease present with an enhanced sympathetic activity (58). Dexamethasone may favorably modulate adrenal medullary (59) and heart rate response to altitude exposure (35,59). Blockage of epinephrine excretion and sympathetic activity by dexamethasone may contribute to decrease post pulmonary capillary resistance and hence

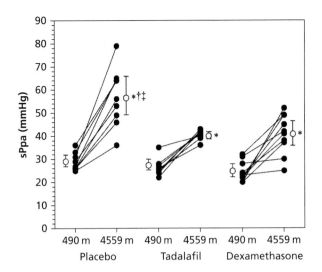

Figure 25.2.3 Increase in systolic pulmonary artery pressure upon ascent to high altitude. Seven of the nine participants on placebo developed HAPE, whereas only 1 of 8 on tadalafil and none of those on dexamethasone had HAPE. Mean values (95% CI) of sPpa at 490 m and 4559 m. $*P < 0.001$ for the difference between 490 m and 4559 m, $^{†}P = 0.012$ for the difference between dexamethasone and placebo, $^{‡}I = 0.005$ for the difference between tadalafil and placebo.

pulmonary edema formation in HAPE susceptible persons taking it as a prophylaxis (35). Interestingly, dexamethasone is known to decrease alcohol and insulin mediated sympathetic activation and vasodilation (60,61).

It should, however, be pointed out that not all subjects with high altitude associated pulmonary hypertension develop HAPE. About 40 percent of the HAPE susceptible subjects do not re-develop HAPE after rapid ascent to 4559 m (62). Invasive hemodynamic measurements showed that Ppa was on average lower in HAPE susceptible subjects who did not develop HAPE than in those who did (14). However, 10 young healthy adults with enhanced hypoxic pulmonary vasoreactivity following transient perinatal hypoxemia did not develop HAPE during an observation period of 72 hours after rapid ascent to 4559 m in spite of an elevated systolic Ppa pressure (62 mmHg; echocardiography) (63).

PULMONARY CAPILLARY PRESSURE

Using the arterial occlusion method, which is likely to measure pressures in vessels close to 100 μm in diameter (64), it has been demonstrated recently that the pulmonary capillary pressure (Pc) is elevated in HAPE. Pc was on average 16 mmHg (range 14–18 mmHg) in HAPE susceptible subjects without pulmonary edema and 22 mmHg (range 20–26 mmHg) in those who developed HAPE (14). These results suggest that the Pc threshold value for edema formation in this setting is 20 mmHg (Figure 25.2.4). This is in keeping with previous experimental observations in dogs of a PO_2-independent critical capillary pressure of

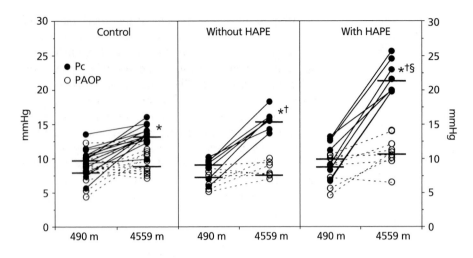

Figure 25.2.4 Individual pulmonary capillary pressure (Pc (filled circles)) and pulmonary artery occluded pressure (Ppao, or wedge pressure (open circles)), assessed using the arterial occlusion technique, in controls, HAPE susceptible subjects without and with pulmonary edema (14). The figure shows that in subjects who develop HAPE Pc was higher than 19 mmHg, and that the increase in Ppao, though significant, is minimal.

17 to 24 mmHg, above which the lungs continuously gain weight (65,66).

The question arises how increased arteriolar vasoconstriction causes an abnormal rise in capillary pressure in subjects susceptible to HAPE. The two most likely explanations inhomogeneous hypoxic vasoconstriction causing regional over-perfusion of capillaries in areas with the least arterial vasoconstriction (67) or hypoxic constriction occurring at the level of the pulmonary veins (50). Lung perfusion imaging by MRI provides evidence that hypoxic pulmonary vasoconstriction is inhomogeneous in humans and particularly in HAPE susceptible individuals (68,69) and can explain the patchy distribution of edema as we observe it on chest radiographs and CT scans (Figure 25.2.2). There also is evidence that the small arterioles can be the site of transvascular leakage in the presence of markedly increased Ppa in hypoxia (70) and that pulmonary veins contract in response to hypoxia (71,72) increasing the resistance downstream of the region of fluid filtration (73) suggesting that in addition to inhomogeneous vasoconstriction constriction of pulmonary veins contributes to the elevated vascular pressures following excessive hypoxic vasoconstriction.

There are data which suggest that in normoxia and hypoxia the increase in Ppa during strenuous exercise is essentially related to the upstream transmission of increased left atrial pressure, the increase in pulmonary vascular resistance being less important (74,75). Furthermore, it has been reported that in HAPE susceptible subjects Ppa and Ppao increased more during exercise than in HAPE-resistant subjects (32). This could be at least in part attributed to an impaired left ventricular filling, because of the dilation of the right ventricle and bulging of the septum to the left side (76).

It has been suggested that pulmonary capillary hypertension may lead to increased hoop tension of the capillary wall, and hence stress failure of the blood–gas barrier (77,78). However, the rapid regression of the leak after initiation of a vasodilator therapy (43) and the lack of an activation of the coagulation cascade in early HAPE (28) give some indirect evidence against this mechanisms in humans.

PERMEABILITY OF BLOOD–GAS BARRIER

Bronchoalveolar lavage (BAL) performed within a day after ascent to 4559 m revealed elevated red blood cell counts and serum derived protein concentration in their BAL fluid both in subjects with HAPE and in those who developed HAPE within the next 24 hours (79). There was, however, no increase in alveolar macrophages and neutrophiles, nor in the concentration of pro-inflammatory mediators (interleukin-1 (IL-1), TNF-alpha, IL-8, thromboxane, prostaglandin E2 and leukotriene B4) at high altitude and there was no difference between HAPE-resistant and susceptible individuals. Interestingly, the albumin concentration and the number of red blood cells in the BAL fluid were significantly correlated with systolic Ppa measured by echocardiography, the threshold for albumin being at a systolic Ppa around 40 mmHg and for red blood cells around 60 mmHg (Figure 25.2.5). This fits well with the clinical observation of pink, frothy sputum in advanced HAPE (24).

Analysis of bronchoalveolar lavage (BAL) fluid of mountaineers with HAPE on Mount McKinley (80) and in hospitalized patients with HAPE (81) showed, however, in many but not all cases high concentrations of proteins, cytokines, leukotriene B$_4$ and increased granulocytes. Furthermore, urinary leukotriene E$_4$ excretion was increased in patients with HAPE reporting to clinics in the Rocky Mountains (82). These observations suggest that in more advanced cases of HAPE inflammation may occur and contribute to enhance the permeability of pulmonary capillaries.

Exposure of pulmonary endothelial cells and alveolar epithelial cells to hypoxia induces profound alteration of cells' cytoskeleton organization (83,84) hence dysfunction and leakage of the blood–gas barrier. In endothelial cells hypoxia activates MAPK-activated protein kinase MK2 in connection with HSP27 phosphorylation and reorganization of the actin cytoskeleton. Interestingly, delivery of nitric oxide and treatment with sildenafil and cyclic guanosine monophosphate analogs recovers endothelial cells from hypoxia-induced leakiness by reorganizing the actin based cytoskeleton and by reducing hypoxia-induced membrane

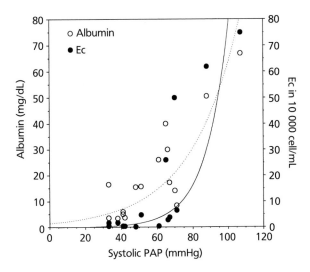

Figure 25.2.5 Individual bronchoalveolar lavage (BAL) red blood cells and albumin concentration plotted against systolic pulmonary artery pressure (sPpa) at high altitude (4559 m). The figure shows that the threshold sPpa for the appearance in the BAL fluid of albumin was 35 mmHg and the one for red blood cells > 60 mmHg (72).

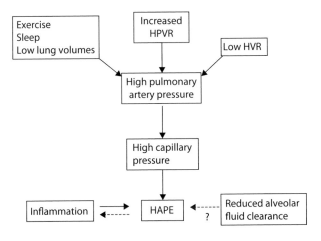

Figure 25.2.6 The hallmark of the pathogenesis of high-altitude pulmonary edema (HAPE) is excessive hypoxic pulmonary vasoconstriction leading initially to an increased pulmonary capillary pressure. However, as shown in the figure, other factors may add to increase pulmonary capillary pressure or pulmonary capillary permeability.

tension (85). Thus, it is likely that low nitric oxide availability in HAPE susceptibles not only contributes to increase pulmonary vascular tone but also leakiness of endothelial cells. Similarly, hypoxia disrupts cytoskeleton and tight junction organization in alveolar epithelial cells, which participates at least in part to hypoxia-induced decrease of transepithelial sodium transport (86).

In conclusion, all these recent results suggest that HAPE is initially a hydrostatic pulmonary edema, its pathophysiological mechanism being an excessive hypoxic pulmonary vasoconstriction of small arteries and veins, leading

probably to an over-distension of the vessel wall, which together with hypoxia-induced unfavorable cytoskeleton rearrangement of both endothelial and epithelial cells opens intercellular junctions and possibly causes stress failure of the alveolo-capillary membrane. Signs of inflammation found in the BAL fluid of patients with advanced HAPE are thus a secondary event, which may further add to increase the permeability of pulmonary capillaries, hence alveolar edema formation. Other non-hemodynamic factors that add to increase the risk for HAPE are discussed in the next section. The concept of the interaction of these various hemodynamic and non-hemodynamic elements is illustrated in Figure 25.2.6.

NON-HEMODYNAMIC RISK FACTORS

Behavioral and constitutional risk factors

Both, a low hypoxic ventilatory drive, leading to increased pulmonary vasoconstriction (87–89) and a smaller lung in relation to body size (decreased pulmonary vascular cross-sectional area) (90,91) are factors known to increase pulmonary artery pressure and hence susceptibility to HAPE.

However, the considerable overlap for both factors between HAPE-susceptible and resistant individuals, suggest that they are at best permissive but not compulsory regarding susceptibility to HAPE.

Congenital anomalies of the large pulmonary arteries (92,93) have been reported to be associated with an increased risk to develop HAPE already at an altitude of about 2000 m.

Increased permeability

It is conceivable that any process enhancing the permeability of the alveolar-capillary barrier would lower the pressure required for generating edema. Increased fluid accumulation during hypoxic exposure after priming by endotoxins or viruses in animals (94) and the association of preceding viral infections (predominantly of the upper respiratory tract), with HAPE in children visiting Colorado (33) support the concept shown in Figure 25.2.7. Under conditions of increased permeability HAPE may also occur in individuals with normal hypoxic pulmonary vascular response.

Reduced fluid clearance from the alveolar space

Investigations obtained in cell cultures and animal models suggest that impairment of fluid clearance from the alveoli may be involved in the pathophysiology of HAPE. The water and sodium transport across type II pneumocytes is shown in Figure 25.2.8. Hypoxia decreases the transepithelial sodium transport (95) and accounts for decreased fluid clearance from the alveoli of hypoxic rats at an FIO_2 of 8 percent (83,96). Mice partially deficient in the epithelial sodium channel show greater accumulation of lung water in hypoxia (97). Transalveolar sodium transport can be

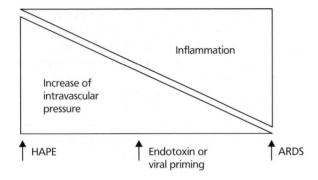

Figure 25.2.7 Tentatively, the high pressure leak of pulmonary capillaries in HAPE contrasts with the inflammation-mediated low-pressure leak occurring in the acute respiratory distress syndrome (ARDS). It is conceivable that in some cases of HAPE enhancement of capillary permeability by endotoxin or viral priming (systemic inflammation) lowers the pulmonary capillary pressure threshold for edema formation.

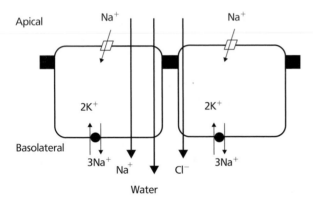

Figure 25.2.8 Alveolar epithelial apical and baso-lateral membrane ion channels and exchangers involved in active transepithelial sodium and water absorption. There is an active re-absorption of sodium; water and chloride follow passively. Acute hypoxia reduces alveolar fluid clearance by inhibition of apical sodium entry pathways and baso-lateral Na^+/K^+-ATPase activity. (Figure kindly provided by H. Mairbäurl.)

stimulated by beta-2 receptors (96), glucocorticoids (98) and the endothelin-1 dual receptor antagonist bosentan (99). It was reported that HAPE incidence could be significantly decreased by the inhalation of salmeterol, a beta-2 agonist. Because of multiple actions of this drug, like lowering pulmonary artery pressure, increasing ventilatory response to hypoxia and tightening cell-to-cell contacts, we need more specific drugs for a precise evaluation of the role of alveolar fluid clearance from the alveoli for the pathophysiology of HAPE.

GENETICS OF HAPE

Familial clusters have been reported for re-entry HAPE in the Andes (19,100,101). No cases with familial clustering have been reported so far in low land dwellers. In this latter population, however, identification of the phenotype "susceptibility to HAPE" is often not possible in most members of a family because of lack of an altitude exposure that can cause the disease. Nevertheless, anecdotal evidence in re-entry HAPE may also be relevant for HAPE of the low altitude populations and may point to a contribution of genetics for susceptibility of HAPE.

Earlier in this chapter we have summarized the evidence for excessive hypoxic pulmonary vasoconstriction (HPV) being the hallmark of susceptibility to HAPE. Several observations suggest that HPV is under genetic control. HPV is considerably reduced or almost abandoned (7,102) in Tibetans. This finding is explained by genetic adaptation of the Tibetan population to high altitude. Furthermore, abnormally high HPV is also found in some cattle and was identified as the cause of Brisket disease (103), an illness for which a genetic basis was demonstrated (104). HAPE susceptible individuals do not only have an abnormal rise in pulmonary artery pressure in hypoxia but also during exercise in normoxia. This pattern of response is also found in asymptomatic gene carriers of familial or idiopathic pulmonary arterial hypertension (105) suggesting that the abnormal response of pulmonary artery pressure to exercise in HAPE susceptibles may be genetically determined. Since these family members of patients with familial or pulmonary arterial hypertension had never exposed themselves rapidly to high altitude it is not known whether they are susceptible of HAPE.

Because of the crucial role of an excessive HPV in HAPE gene polymorphisms of candidate genes that might contribute to such a phenotype were investigated in several association studies, which have been summarized recently (106). Various polymorphisms of the following genes that might modify HPV were investigated: endothelial NO synthase, angiotensin converting enzyme, angiotensin receptor-1 and 2, and endothelin-1. Furthermore, polymorphisms of genes encoding for surfactant protein A1 and A2, thyrosin hydroxylase, human leukocyte antigens and most recently also vascular endothelial growth factor (107) were examined. All these studies involved only small samples of at best 50–70 HAPE susceptible individuals and as many control subjects. When more than one study of a particular polymorphism was published, no clear concept evolved since results were usually contradictory (106). In addition the mutation of the BMPR-2 gene found in familial pulmonary arterial hypertension was not found in 10 HAPE susceptible individuals (published as abstract only (108)).

If excessive HPV and more so susceptibility to HAPE is predominantly genetically determined, a large variety of genes might contribute to the phenotype. Around 1000 or more persons and as many controls would be necessary to have enough statistical power for detecting small effects. In addition replication studies are needed to confirm initial findings. Therefore it is unlikely that association studies of polymorphisms of single candidate genes will help to unravel the genetic basis of HAPE unless this disease can be attributed to one or very few gene polymorphisms. A combined effort of various research groups and a more sophisticated approach are needed to improve our knowledge in the field.

KEY POINTS

Pulmonary circulation at altitude

- Normal mean Ppa in newcomers at altitudes between 3000 and 4500 m ranges from 20 and 30 mmHg.
- Excessive hypoxic pulmonary vasoconstriction, leading to a mean Ppa which mostly exceeds 40 mmHg, is the hallmark of maladaptation to high altitude in acute, prolonged, and most likely also chronic exposure.

High altitude pulmonary edema

- HAPE develops subjects within 2 to 5 days after acute exposure to high altitude. Typical symptoms and signs are: dyspnea at rest, incapacitating weakness, cough, tachycardia, hypoxemia and pulmonary râles.
- A high recurrence rate in individuals with a history of HAPE indicates particular susceptibility of certain individuals for this disease.
- HAPE is caused by elevated pressures in leaky pulmonary arterioles (~100 µm) and capillaries as a consequence of an excessive hypoxic and presumably inhomogeneous constriction of small arteries or veins, or both.
- In early HAPE edema fluid is rich in albumin and contains red blood cells but there are no markers of an inflammatory response. Markers of inflammation are found in edema fluid of advanced HAPE indicating that inflammation is a secondary event in more severe cases and is likely to enhance the leak.
- Additional factors such as exhaustive physical exercise, hypoxia-induced neurohumoral activation, impaired transepithelial sodium transport and viral infections may contribute to the development of HAPE.
- Pulmonary vasodilators, such as calcium-channel blockers are the drug of choice for prevention or treatment of HAPE.

REFERENCES

1. Bärtsch P. High altitude pulmonary edema. Med Sci Sports Exerc 1999;31:S23–S27.
2. Schoene RB, Swenson ER, Hultgren HN. High-altitude pulmonary edema. In: Hornbein TF, Schoene R (eds). High altitude – an exploration of human adaptation. New York: Marcel Dekker Inc 2001;161:777–814.
3. Sui GJ, Liu YH, Cheng XS, Anand IS, Harris E, Harris P, Heath D. Subacute infantile mountain sickness. J Pathol 1988;155:161–70.
4. Anand IS, Malhotra RM, Chandrashekhar Y, Bali HK, Chauhan SS, Jindal SK, Bhandari RK, Wahi PL. Adult subacute mountain sickness – A syndrome of congestive heart failure in man at very high altitude. Lancet 1990;335:561–5.
5. Hecht HH, Kuida H, Lange RL, Thorne JL, Brown AM, Carlisle R, Ruby A, Ukradyha F. Brisket disease. II. Clinical features and hemodynamic observations in altitude-dependent right heart failure of cattle. Am J Med 1962;32:171–83.
6. Fagan KA, Weil JV. Potential genetic contributions to control of the pulmonary circulation and ventilation at high altitude. High Alt Med Biol 2001;2:165–71.
7. Groves BM, Droma T, Sutton JR et al. Minimal hypoxic pulmonary hypertension in normal Tibetans at 3,658 m. J Appl Physiol 1993;74:312–8.
8. Hultgren HN, Marticorena EA. High altitude pulmonary edema. Epidemiologic observations in Peru. Chest 1978;74:372–6.
9. Hakim TS, Michel RP, Minami H, Chang HK. Site of pulmonary hypoxic vasoconstriction studied with arterial and venous occlusion. J Appl Physiol 1983;54:1298–302.
10. Audi SH, Dawson DA, Rickaby A, Linehan JH. Localization of the sites of pulmonary vasomotion by use of arterial and venous occlusion. J Appl Physiol 1991;70:2126–36.
11. Moore LG. Human genetic adaptation to high altitude. High Alt Med Biol 2001;2:257–79.
12. Kronenberg RS, Safar P, Lee J et al. Pulmonary artery pressure and alveolar gas exchange in man during acclimatization to 12,470 ft. J Clin Invest 1971;50:827–37.
13. Vogel JHK, Goss GE, Mori M, Brammell HL. Pulmonary circulation in normal man with acute exposure to high altitude (14,260 feet). Circulation 1966;34:III-233.
14. Maggiorini M, Mélot C, Pierre S et al. High-altitude pulmonary edema is initially caused by an increase in capillary pressure. Circulation 2001;103:2078–83.
15. Groves BM, Reeves JT, Sutton JR, et al. Operation Everest II: elevated high-altitude pulmonary resistance unresponsive to oxygen. J Appl Physiol 1987;63:521–30.
16. Hultgren HN, Grover RF, Hartley LH. Abnormal circulatory responses to high altitude in subjects with a previous history of high-altitude pulmonary edema. Circulation 1971;44:759–70.
17. Pei SX, Chen XJ, Si Ren BZ, Liu YH, Cheng XS, Harris EM, Anand IS, Harris PC. Chronic mountain sickness in Tibet. Q J Med 1989;71:555–74.
18. Lizarraga L. Soroche agudo: Edema agudo del pulmón. An Fac Med (San Marco, Lima) 1955;38:244–74.
19. Scoggin CH, Hyers TM, Reeves JT, Grover RF. High-altitude pulmonary edema in the children and young adults of Leadville, Colorado. N Engl J Med 1977;297:1269–72.
20. Houston CS. Acute pulmonary edema of high altitude. N Engl J Med 1960;263:478–80.

21. Sophocles AM Jr. High-altitude pulmonary edema in Vail, Colorado, 1975–1982. West J Med 1986;144:569–73.

22. Hochstrasser J, Nanzer A, Oelz O. Altitude edema in the Swiss Alps. Observations on the incidence and clinical course in 50 patients 1980–1984. Schweiz Med Wochenschr 1986;116:866–73.

23. Bärtsch P, Maggiorini M, Mairbäurl H, Vock P, Swenson E. Pulmonary extravascular fluid accumulation in climbers. Lancet 2002;360:571.

24. Singh I, Roy SB. High altitude pulmonary edema: clinical, hemodynamic, and pathologic studies. In: Biomedicine of high terrestrial elevation problems. Washington D.C.: U.S. Army Research and Development Command; 1969, pp. 108–120.

25. Hackett PH, Rennie D, Levine HD. The incidence, importance, and prophylaxis of acute mountain sickness. Lancet 1976;II(Nov. 27):1149–54.

26. Hultgren HN, Honigman B, Theis K, Nicholas D. High-altitude pulmonary edema at a ski resort. West J Med 1996;164:222–7.

27. Kobayashi T, Koyama S, Kubo K, Fukushima M, Kusama S. Clinical features of patients with high-altitude pulmonary edema in Japan. Chest 1987;92:814–21.

28. Bärtsch P, Waber U, Haeberli A, Maggiorini M, Kriemler S, Oelz O, Straub WP. Enhanced fibrin formation in high-altitude pulmonary edema. J Appl Physiol 1987;63:752–7.

29. Vock P, Fretz C, Franciolli M, Bärtsch P. High-altitude pulmonary edema: findings at high-altitude chest radiography and physical examination. Radiology 1989;170:661–6.

30. Vock P, Brutsche MH, Nanzer A, Bartsch P. variable radiomorphologic data of high altitude pulmonary edema – features from 60 patients. Chest 1991; 100:1306–11.

31. Nayak NC, Roy S, Narayanan TK. Pathologic features of altitude sickness. Am J Pathol 1964;45:381–91.

32. Eldridge MW, Podolsky A, Richardson RS et al. Pulmonary hemodynamic response to exercise in subjects with prior high-altitude pulmonary edema. J Appl Physiol 1996;81:911–21.

33. Durmowicz AG, Nooordeweir E, Nicholas R, Reeves JT. Inflammatory processes may predispose children to develop high altitude pulmonary edema. J Pediatr 1997;130:838–40.

34. Bärtsch P, Maggiorini M, Ritter M, Noti C, Vock P, Oelz O. Prevention of high-altitude pulmonary edema by nifedipine. N Engl J Med 1991;325:1284–9.

35. Maggiorini M, Brunner-La Rocca H-P, Peth S et al. Both tadalafil and dexamethasone may reduce the incidence of high-altitude pulmonary edema. Ann Intern Med 2006;145:497–506.

36. Hohenhaus E, Niroomand F, Goerre S, Vock P, Oelz O, Bärtsch P. Nifedipine does not prevent acute mountain sickness. Am J Respir Crit Care Med 1994;150:857–60.

37. Luks AM, Swenson E. Medication and dosage considerations in the prophylaxis and treatment of high-altitude illness. Chest 2008;133:744–55.

38. Schoene RB, Roach RC, Hackett PH, Harrison G, Mills WJ. High altitude pulmonary edema and exercise at 4400 meters on Mount McKinley: effect of expiratory positive airway pressure. Chest 1985;87:330–3.

39. Larson EB. Positive airway pressure for high-altitude pulmonary edema. Lancet 1985;I(8425):371–3.

40. Oelz O. High altitude cerebral edema after positive airway pressure breathing at high altitude. Lancet 1983;II(8359):1148.

41. King SJ, Greenlee RR. Successful use of the Gamow Hyperbaric Bag in the treatment of altitude illness at Mount Everest. J Wildern Med 1990;1:193–202.

42. Taber RL. Protocols for the use of portable hyperbaric chamber for the treatment of high altitude disorders. J Wildern Med 1990;1:181–92.

43. Oelz O, Ritter M, Jenni R, Maggiorini M, Waber U, Vock P, Bärtsch P. Nifedipine for high altitude pulmonary edema. Lancet 1989;2(8674):1241–4.

44. Fagenholz PJ, Gutmann JA, Murray AF, Harris NS. Treatment of high altitude pulmonary edema at 4240 m in Nepal. High Alt Med Biol 2007;8:139–46.

45. Antezana G, Leguia G, Morales Guzman A et al. Hemodynamic study of high altitude pulmonary edema (12,200 ft). In: Brendel W, Zink RA (eds). High altitude physiology and medicine. New York: Springer, 1982:232–41.

46. Hultgren HN, Lopez CE, Lundberg E, Miller H. Physiologic studies of pulmonary edema at high altitude. Circulation 1964;29:393–408.

47. Koizumi T, Kawashima A, Kubo K, Kobayashi T, Sekiguchi M. Radiographic and hemodynamic changes during recovery from high-altitude pulmonary edema. Intern Med 1994;33:525–8.

48. Roy SB, Guleria JS, Khanna PK, Manchanda SC, Pande JN, Subba PS. Haemodynamic studies in high altitude pulmonary edema. Br Heart J 1969;31:52–8.

49. Penaloza D, Sime F. Circulatory dynamics during high altitude pulmonary edema. Am J Cardiol 1969;23:369–78.

50. Hackett PH, Roach RC, Hartig GS, Greene ER, Levine BD. The effect of vasodilatators on pulmonary hemodynamics in high altitude pulmonary edema: a comparison. Int J Sports Med 1992;13:S68–S71.

51. Weir EK, Archer SL. The mechanism of acute hypoxic pulmonary vasoconstriction: the tale of two channels. FASEB J 1995;9:183–9.

52. Duplain H, Sartori C, Lepori M, Egli M, Allemann Y, Nicod P, Scherrer U. Exhaled nitric oxide in high-altitude pulmonary edema: role in the regulation of pulmonary vascular tone and evidence for a role against inflammation. Am J Resp Crit Care Med 2000;162:221–4.

53. Busch T, Bärtsch P, Pappert D, Grünig E, Elser H, Falke KJ, Swenson ER. Hypoxia decreases exhaled nitric oxide in mountaineers susceptible to high altitude pulmonary edema. Am J Respir Crit Care Med 2001;163:368–73.

54. Berger M, Hesse C, Dehnert C et al. Hypoxia impairs systemic endothelial function in individuals prone to high-altitude pulmonary edema. Am J Respir Crit Care Med 2005;172:763–7.

55. Kawashima A, Kubo K, Kobayashi T, Sekiguchi M. Hemodynamic responses to acute hypoxia, hypobaria, and exercise in subjects susceptible to high-altitude pulmonary edema. J Appl Physiol 1989;67:1982–9.

56. Eldridge MW, Braun RK, Yoneda KY, Walby WF. Effects of altitude and exercise on pulmonary capillary integrity: evidence for subclinical high-altitude pulmonary edema. J Appl Physiol 2006;100:972–80.

57. Grünig E, Mereles D, Hildebrandt W, Swenson ER, Kübler W, Kuecherer H, Bärtsch P. Stress Doppler echocardiography for identification of susceptibility to high altitude pulmonary edema. J Am Coll Cardiol 2000;35:980–7.

58. Duplain H, Vollenweider L, Delabays A, Nicod P, Bärtsch P, Scherrer U. Augmented sympathetic activation during short-term hypoxia and high-altitude exposure in subjects susceptible to high-altitude pulmonary edema. Circulation 1999;99:1713–8.

59. Johnson TS, Rock PB, Young JB, Fulco CS, Trad LA. Hemodynamic and sympathoadrenal responses to altitude in humans: effect of dexamethasone. Aviat Space Environ Med 1988;59:208–12.

60. Randin D, Vollenweider P, Tappy L, Jéquier E, Nicod P, Scherrer U. Suppression of alcohol-induced hypertension by dexamethasone. New Engl J Med 1995;332:1733–7.

61. Scherrer U, Vollenweider P, Randin D, Jéquier E, Nicod P, Tappy L. Suppression of insulin-induced sympathetic activation and vasodilation by dexamethasone in humans. Circulation 1993;88:388–94.

62. Bärtsch P, Vock P, Maggiorini M et al. Respiratory symptoms, radiographic and physiologic correlations at high altitude. In: Sutton JR, Coates G, Remmers JE (eds). Hypoxia: The Adaptations. Toronto, Philadelphia: BC Decker Inc, 1990:241–5.

63. Sartori C, Allemann Y, Trueb L, Delabays A, Nicod P, Scherrer U. Augmented vasoreactivity in adult life associated with perinatal vascular insult. Lancet 1999;353:2205–7.

64. Hakim TS, Kelly S. Occlusion pressures vs. micropipette pressures in the pulmonary circulation. J Appl Physiol 1989;67:1277–85.

65. Homik LA, Bshouty RB, Light RB, Younes M. Effect of alveolar hypoxia on pulmonary fluid filtration in in situ dog lungs. J Appl Physiol 1988;65:46–52.

66. Drake RE, Smith JH, Gabel JC. Estimation of the filtration coefficient in intact dog lungs. Am J Physiol Heart Circ Physiol 1980;238:H430–H438.

67. Hultgren HN. High altitude pulmonary edema. In: Staub NC, ed. Lung Water and Solute Exchange. New York: Marcel Dekker, 1978:437–64.

68. Hopkins SR, Garg J, Bolar DS, Balouch J, Levin DL. Pulmonary blood flow heterogeneity during hypoxia and high altitude pulmonary edema. Am J Respir Crit Care Med 2005;171:83–7.

69. Dehnert C, Risse F, Ley S et al. Magnetic resonance imaging of uneven pulmonary perfusion in hypoxia in humans. Am J Respir Crit Care Med 2006;174:1132–8.

70. Whayne TF Jr, Severinghaus JW. Experimental hypoxic pulmonary edema in the rat. J Appl Physiol 1968;25:729–32.

71. Raj JU, Chen P. Micropuncture measurement of microvascular pressures in isolated lamb lungs during hypoxia. Circ Res 1986;59:398–404.

72. Zhao Y, Packer CS, Rhoades RA. Pulmonary vein contracts in response to hypoxia. Am J Physiol 1993;265:L87–L92.

73. Mitzner W, Sylvester JT. Hypoxic vasoconstriction and fluid filtration in pig lungs. J Appl Physiol 1981; 51:1065–71.

74. Naeije R, Mélot C, Niset G, Delacroix M, Wagner PD. Mechanisms of improved arterial oxygenation after peripheral chemoreceptor stimulation during hypoxic exercise. J Appl Physiol 1993;74:1666–71.

75. Reeves JT, Dempsey JA, Grover RF. Pulmonary circulation during exercise. In: Weir E, K, Reeves JT (eds). Pulmonary Vascular Physiology and Pathophysiology. New York: Marcel Dekker, 1989:107–33.

76. Ritter M, Jenni R, Maggiorini M, Grimm J, Oelz O. Abnormal left ventricular diastolic filling patterns in acute hypoxic pulmonary hypertension at high altitude. Am J Noninvas Cardiol 1993;7:33–8.

77. West JB, Tsukimoto K, Mathieu-Costello O, Prediletto R. Stress failure in pulmonary capillaries. J Appl Physiol 1991;70:1731–42.

78. West JB, Colice GL, Lee Y-J, Namba Y, Kurdak SS, Fu Z, Ou L-C, Mathieu-Costello O. Pathogenesis of high-altitude pulmonary edema: Direct evidence of stress failure of pulmonary capillaries. Eur Respir J 1995;8:523–9.

79. Swenson ER, Maggiorini M, Mongovin S, Gibbs JSR, Greve I, Mairbäurl H, Bärtsch P. Pathogenesis of high-altitude pulmonary edema: Inflammation is not an etiologic factor. JAMA 2002;287:2228–35.

80. Schoene RB, Swenson ER, Pizzo CJ, Hackett PH, Roach RC, Mills WJ, Henderson WR, Martin TR. The lung at high altitude: bronchoalveolar lavage in acute mountain sickness and pulmonary edema. J Appl Physiol 1988;64:2605–13.

81. Kubo K, Hanaoka M, Yamaguchi S et al. Cytokines in bronchoalveolar lavage fluid in patients with high altitude pulmonary edema at moderate altitude in Japan. Thorax 1996;51:739–42.

82. Kaminsky DA, Jones K, Schoene RB, Voelkel NF. Urinary leuktriene E (4) levels in high-altitude pulmonary edema: A possible role for inflammation. Chest 1996;110:939–45.

83. Kayyali US, Pennella CM, Trujillo C, Villa O, Gaestel M, Hassoun PM. Cytoskeletal changes in hypoxic pulmonary endothelial cells are dependent on MAPK-activated protein kinase MK2. J Biol Chem 2002;277:42596–602.

84. Bouvry D, Planès C, Malbert-Colas L, Escabasse V, Clerici C. Hypoxia-induced cytoskeleton disruption in alveolar epithelial cells. Am J Respir Cell Mol Biol 2006;35:519–27.

85. Kolluru GK, Tamilarasan KP, Rajkumar AS, et al. Nitric oxide/cGMP protects endothelial cells from hypoxia-mediated leakiness. Eur J Cell Biol 2008;87:147–61.

86. An SS, Pennella CM, Gonnabathula A et al. Hypoxia alters biophysical properties of endothelial cells vie p38 MAPK- and Rho kinase-dependent pathways. Am J Physiol Cell Physiol 2005;289:C521–30.

87. Hackett PH, Roach RC, Schoene RB, Harrison GL, Mills WJ. Abnormal control of ventilation in high-altitude pulmonary edema. J Appl Physiol 1988;64:1268–72.

88. Matsuzawa Y, Fujimoto K, Kobayashi T et al. Blunted hypoxic ventilatory drive in subjects susceptible to high-altitude pulmonary edema. J Appl Physiol 1989;66:1152–7.

89. Hohenhaus E, Paul A, McCullough RE, Kücherer H, Bärtsch P. Ventilatory and pulmonary vascular response to hypoxia and susceptibility to high altitude pulmonary edema. Eur Respir J 1995;8:1825–33.

90. Viswanathan R, Jain SK, Subramanian S, Subramanian TAV, Dua GL, Giri J. Pulmonary edema of high altitude II. Clinical, aerohemodynamic, and biochemical studies in a group with history of pulmonary edema of high altitude. Am Rev Respir Dis 1969;100:334–41.

91. Podolsky A, Eldridge MW, Richardson RS et al. Exercise-induced VA/Q inequality in subjects with prior high-altitude pulmonary edema. J Appl Physiol 1996;81:922–32.

92. Fiorenzano G, Rastelli V, Greco V, Di Stefano A, Dottorini M. Unilateral high-altitude pulmonary edema in a subject with right artery hypoplasia. Respiration 1994;61:51–4.

93. Hackett PH, Creagh CE, Grover RF et al. High altitude pulmonary edema in persons without the right pulmonary artery. N Engl J Med 1980;302:1070–73.

94. Carpenter TD, Reeves JT, Durmowicz AG. Viral respiratory infection increases susceptibility of young rats to hypoxia-induced pulmonary edema. J Appl Physiol 1998;84:1048–54.

95. Wodopia R, Ko HS, Billian J, Wiesner R, Bärtsch P, Mairbäurl H. Hypoxia decreases proteins involved in epithelial electrolyte transport in A549 cells and rat lung. Am J Physiol Lung Cell Mol Physiol 2000;279:L1110–L1119.

96. Vivona ML, Matthay M, Chabaud MB, Friedlander G, Clerici C. Hypoxia reduces alveolar epithelial sodium and fluid transport in rats: reversal by beta-adrenergic agonist treatment. Am J Respir Cell Mol Biol 2001;25:554–61.

97. Scherrer U, Sartori C, Lepori M, Allemann Y, Duplain H, Trueb L, Nicod P. High altitude pulmonary edema: from exaggerated pulmonary hypertension to a defect in transepithelial sodium transport. Adv Exp Med Biol 1999;474:93–107.

98. Matthay MA, Clerici C, Saumon C. Active fluid clearance from distal airspaces of the lung. J Appl Physiol 2002;93:1533–41.

99. Bergermm, Rozendahl CS, Schieber C, Dehler M, Zügel S, Bardenheuer HJ, Bärtsch P, Mairbäurl H. The effect of endothelin-1 on alveolar fluid clearance and pulmonary edema formation in the rat. Anesth Analg 2009;108:225–31.

100. Hultgren HN, Spickard WB, Hellriegel K, Houston CS. High altitude pulmonary edema. Medicine (Baltimore) 1961;40:289–313.

101. Fred HL, Schmidt AM, Bates T, Hecht HH. Acute pulmonary edema of altitude. Clinical and physiologic observations. Circulation 1962;25:929–37.

102. Hoit BD, Dalton ND, Erzurum SC, Laskowski D, Strohl KP, Beall CM. Nitric oxide and cardiopulmonary hemodynamics in Tibetan highlanders. J Appl Physiol 2005;99:1796–801.

103. Hecht HH, Lange RL, Carnes WH, Kuida H, Blake J. Brisket disease: general aspects of pulmonary hypertensive heart disease in cattle. Trans Assoc Am Physicians 1959;72:157–72.

104. Weir EK, Tucker A, Reeves JT, Will DH, Grover RF. The genetic factor influencing pulmonary hypertension in cattle at high altitude. Cardiovasc Res 1974;8:745–9.

105. Grünig E, Dehnert C, Mereles D, Koehler R, Olschweski H, Bärtsch P, Janssen B. Enhanced hypoxic pulmonary vasoconstriction in families of adults or children with idiopathic pulmonary arterial hypertension. Chest 2005;128:630S–633S.

106. Rupert JL, Koehle MS. Evidence for a genetic basis for altitude-related illnesses. High Alt Med Biol 2006;7:150–67.

107. Hanaoka M, Droma Y, Ota M, Ito M, Katsuyama Y, Kubo K. Polymorphisms of human vascular endothelial growth factor gene in high-altitude pulmonary edema susceptible subjects. Respirology 2009;14:46–52.

108. Dehnert C, Miltenberger-Miltenyi G, Grünig E, Bärtsch P. Normal BMPR-2 gene in individuals susceptible to high altitude pulmonary edema. High Alt Med Biol 2002;3:100.

The pulmonary circulation and the underwater environment

STEPHEN J WATT

INTRODUCTION

During diving, the principle environmental change underwater is a substantial increase in ambient pressure. This results in important physiological effects on ventilation, the handling of gases in tissues and the circulation. The distinction between disturbed physiology and the onset of pathology is blurred, but diving is associated with specific illnesses such as decompression sickness and barotrauma. The pulmonary circulation is important in enabling a return to normal environmental conditions after underwater exposure without pathological result, thereby protecting man from some adverse effects of pressure exposure. Knowledge of the role of the pulmonary circulation during diving is restricted by the difficulties of human investigation at pressure and we remain heavily dependent on animal data.

Diving techniques vary from simple breath-hold diving at shallow depth (less than 30 meters of seawater [msw]) carried out by snorkel divers or the pearl diving Ama of Korea (female divers renowned for their courage and stamina), to deep saturation dives lasting several weeks now regularly conducted at depths of 350 msw.

Breath-hold diving is normally conducted from the surface but may be from a submerged air source such as the diving bell designed by Sir Edmund Halley in 1716. To remain under the water for more than a minute or two, a supply of breathing gas is necessary. This can be provided from the surface by a hose or umbilical or from a cylinder containing compressed gas carried by the diver.

The breathing apparatus may be a ventilated helmet, a demand valve system or a closed circuit rebreathing system. Whatever the technique, the diver is subject to the effects of pressure and the gas laws immediately on entering the water.

PHYSICAL PROPERTIES OF THE ENVIRONMENT

Underwater, ambient hydrostatic pressure increases in a linear fashion by 1 atmosphere absolute (ATA) for every 10 meters increase in depth of seawater. Hence, in addition to being a measure of depth, meters of seawater (msw) may also be used as a unit of pressure. The scale of pressure change contrasts with changes on ascent to altitude, which are non-linear and where pressure reduces by only 0.5 ATA on ascent to 5500 meters.

The gas laws define the important physical concepts. Boyle's Law states, "that for a fixed mass of gas at constant temperature the pressure is inversely proportional to the volume," i.e. a one liter balloon of gas at 1 ATA pressure (sea level) will contain 500 mL at 2 atmospheres, 250 mL at 4 ATA, etc. This has important implications for the gas containing spaces within the body. Dalton's Law states, "in a mixture of gases, the pressure exerted by one of the gases is the same as it would exert if it alone occupied the same volume." Hence the total pressure exerted by a gas mixture is the sum of the partial pressures of the constituents, e.g. in air at 1 atmosphere the pressure comprises the sum of partial pressures of approximately 0.79 ATA nitrogen and

0.21 ATA oxygen with minor contributions from other gases. Finally, Henry's Law states, "that at constant temperature, the amount of gas which dissolves in a liquid, with which it is in contact, is proportional to the partial pressure of that gas." A direct consequence is that the amount of nitrogen dissolved in body tissues at sea level relates to both the 0.79 ATA partial pressure of nitrogen in air and the solubility of nitrogen in body tissues. When a man breathing an air environment (79 percent nitrogen) is exposed to a change in pressure, the amount of nitrogen absorbed or released will relate to the change in total pressure.

Underwater the partial pressure of nitrogen in the lungs increases and more dissolves in body tissues. On ascent, pressure falls and this additional dissolved gas must be released gradually to prevent the formation of excessive gas bubbles, which places the diver at risk of decompression illness.

The important implications of diving for the pulmonary circulation relate to the following three main factors:

- Hydrostatic pressure resulting from **immersion**.
- Gas bubbles in tissue formed from dissolved gas which may result in **decompression illness**.
- Exposure to high partial pressures of oxygen which may result in **pulmonary oxygen toxicity**.

IMMERSION

Immersion affects the circulation through three major mechanisms, hydrostatic pressure, temperature, and the diving reflex. The effects of hydrostatic pressure have usually been studied in human subjects during immersion up to the neck (head out) in water. Immersed up to the neck in water the pressure differential from neck to feet is approximately 150 cm H_2O in the upright position. This hydrostatic pressure forces blood from the lower extremities upwards and increases the intrathoracic blood volume and hence the pulmonary blood volume. During head out immersion Arborelius et al. observed rises in right atrial pressure and pulmonary arterial pressure of approximately 15 mmHg (1). There was an associated 30 percent increase in cardiac output without any change in heart rate and calculated central blood volume increased by 700 m (1). Immersion reduces functional residual capacity and the engorgement of the pulmonary capillary circulation contributes to a reduction in lung volumes (2,3) and results in a degree of air trapping (4) demonstrated by an increase in closing volume. The increase in right atrial pressure results in diuresis. Immersion is frequently associated with cold and the resultant cutaneous vasoconstriction also contributes to a shift of blood volume (5). Cold together with immersion contribute to an acute rise in pulmonary blood volume which may result in acute pulmonary edema (6). The cardiovascular effects of hydrostatic pressure and cold are modified by the diving reflex which is stimulated by immersion of the head or face in water (7) and is more marked in cold water (7,8). It results in bradycardia and some depression of myocardial contractility (9) but the reflex is poorly developed in man compared with other diving mammals.

Ventilation-perfusion relationships are altered as the distribution of perfusion of the lung becomes more even during immersion (1,10). However, gas exchange is impaired as a result of increased intrapulmonary shunt (11) and there is a reduction in diffusing capacity partly related to reduction in lung volume (11).

The impact of these physiological effects on the free swimming diver is difficult to assess. The time course of effects on the pulmonary circulation is unclear as most studies have involved a stabilization period of 15–20 minutes of immersion and the immediate effects are variable (1). The hydrostatic pressure differential between chest and legs varies as the diver may stand upright, swim horizontally or even head down, reversing the gradient. These rapid changes in differential hydrostatic pressure are likely to have marked effects on venous return and may be important in the pathogenesis of transient syncope underwater as well as decompression illness.

PULMONARY EDEMA

Pulmonary edema may result from the acute lung injury associated with water inhalation or near drowning (12) and is a common finding in diving fatalities (13). However, acute pulmonary edema provoked by immersion may occur in divers (6,14) and is regarded as a rare but well recognized complication of diving. It frequently recurs with further dives and susceptible individuals are often hypertensive and may have an enhanced vasoconstrictor response to cold (6). However, it may also occur in warm water or in divers using adequate thermal protection (14). Pulmonary edema has also been reported in swimmers when working hard (15). More recent reports of this condition have demonstrated that it has a tendency to occur in middle-aged divers (16,17) although in a review of cases occurring after both scuba diving and surface swimming, the association with hypertension was less apparent (18).

The mechanism of pulmonary edema occurring during scuba-diving remains unclear, but contributing factors may be the acute fluid shifts induced by immersion associated with pulmonary vascular hypertension possibly resulting in acute stress failure of pulmonary capillaries (17). However, other cardiovascular effects of diving probably induced by decompression may be contributory (19,20).

Symptoms of cough, breathlessness and chest pain usually present during the dive and deteriorate until the dive ends when hemoptysis may be observed. Since symptoms often lead to the dive being aborted and an unplanned or rapid ascent, the deterioration during ascent can readily be mistakenly attributed to decompression illness. Recovery after termination of the dive usually occurs over a short period but despite this, episodes are a serious threat to diver safety because symptoms of breathlessness are exacerbated by the use of breathing apparatus and increased gas density while in the water. Furthermore, if symptoms are attributed to pulmonary decompression illness, the problems of breathing apparatus and increased gas density may be imposed again during recompression treatment.

Some divers experience multiple episodes which may become increasingly severe. Anecdotally these individuals are more likely to be older and have hypertension. Advising divers who have had an episode is difficult, but the recurrent nature of episodes and the potential severity of outcome suggests that these individuals should be advised not to risk further events (21) although some divers have successfully returned to diving (17).

DECOMPRESSION ILLNESS

Decompression illness can be divided into two main types according to the pathological causation. Barotrauma is direct tissue injury associated with the change in volume of enclosed gas containing spaces within or surrounding the body. The lungs represent an enclosed gas space when the mouth or glottis is closed or when a peripheral airway is obstructed; hence in a breath-hold dive, the volume of the lung will reduce during descent and will increase again on ascent. A diver breathing a gas supply at ambient pressure maintains near normal lung volumes. On ascent, gas within the lungs expands and must be exhaled or the lung may burst. Such episodes of pulmonary barotrauma may result from failure to breathe out on ascent or from local pathological abnormality leading to gas trapping (22,23). Air trapping resulting from increased pulmonary blood volume may be relevant to the pathogenesis of pulmonary barotrauma which has occasionally been reported after breath-hold dives (24,25). Lung rupture occurs at alveolar level, and expanding extra alveolar gas may track through the hilum to the mediastinum, rupture into the pleural cavity or burst into the pulmonary venous system. Both transpulmonary pressure gradient and differential pressure between the airways and the left atrium appear important factors in the development of air embolism (26). In this situation the pulmonary circulation provides a route for gas passing to the heart resulting in cerebral air embolism.

Decompression sickness results from gas bubbles forming in body tissues from excess gas dissolved during prior exposure at higher pressure. The precise mechanisms causing the variety of clinical symptoms remain inadequately understood, but the pulmonary circulation is of considerable importance in one major mechanism.

The risk of decompression illness relates to the duration of exposure and depth (pressure) of the preceding dive or dives. Greater depth results in more inert gas dissolving in body tissues. Decompression procedures are based on dive depth and duration to take account of the inert gas load

and are designed to provide a slow ascent in stages to permit excess gas to be expired. Originally these procedures were designed to avoid bubble formation, but the development of Doppler ultrasonic bubble detectors (27) has established that bubbles are formed during or after safe and symptom free dives (28–30). The amount of bubbles produced after a dive varies considerably both between and within individuals for reasons unknown, but a bout of aerobic exercise has recently been shown to protect against both bubble formation and death from decompression illness in a rat model (31). Many such factors may contribute to the unpredictable nature of decompression illness.

Bubbles form in many body tissues and may cause local pathology or pass through the peripheral venous system to the major veins and right heart (32). Gas bubbles are not inert; the bubbles' surface is active and stimulates coagulation so that the bubble becomes a bubble-protein-platelet complex. As bubbles pass through the circulation they have important effects on the endothelium which relate to the number of bubbles (31). The number of bubble echoes seen increases with limited exertion such as a knee bend maneuver. Despite bubbles being readily detected in the right heart, very few are seen normally in the left heart or arterial circulation as the pulmonary circulation acts as a filter for bubble complexes and protects from arterial embolization. Clinical episodes of decompression sickness are associated with high bubble scores in the right heart (33) and with appearance of arterial or left heart bubbles.

The role of the pulmonary circulation in trapping venous gas emboli has been extensively studied in animal models. The pulmonary vasculature of dogs traps polystyrene microspheres injected into the pulmonary artery with increasing efficiency as the diameter increases with only a small percentage of spheres greater than $8\,\mu m$ reaching the arterial circulation. However, efficiency is affected by vasoactive drugs and by phase of respiration (34). Bubbles formed during decompression of dogs have been found to range in size from $19–700\,\mu m$ (35) but unlike microspheres, gas bubbles may deform in transit through vessels. The studies of Butler and Hills (36) suggested that the threshold diameter for passage of bubbles through the lung must be less than $22\,\mu m$, but also demonstrated that infused microbubbles of much larger diameter (up to $130\,\mu m$) would escape entrapment and appear in the systemic circulation following treatment with aminophylline. The same authors demonstrated a progressive elevation of pulmonary arterial pressure and pulmonary vascular resistance with continued air embolization and an apparent threshold effect for appearance of arterial bubbles at a pulmonary vascular pressure gradient of $34\,mmHg$ (37). This suggests that large volumes of gas bubbles can overload the circulation and open shunts for bubbles to access the systemic circulation. They also demonstrated that the appearance of arterial bubbles could be induced when pulmonary arterial pressure was elevated by diverting pulmonary blood flow from one lung to the other prior to air embolization (38). However, in this case the transit of bubbles may be related either to the pressure per se or to the increase in pulmonary blood volume in one lung.

These findings are consistent with the common clinical observation of transitory respiratory symptoms prior to the development of serious neurological decompression illness. Pulmonary decompression sickness, known as "the chokes" is rare, but a serious form of the disease is associated with massive bubble formation which leads to cough, hemoptysis and dyspnea with clinical evidence of pulmonary edema. Such patients almost inevitably develop neurological abnormality and may progress to circulatory collapse.

The entrapment of bubbles within the pulmonary circulation may have long-term effects. Divers exposed to deep saturation dives have been shown to have abnormal lung function post-dive with reduced dynamic volumes and diffusing capacity (39,40). These effects reverse slowly but some divers may sustain a permanent reduction in function. This has been attributed to both oxygen toxicity and to repeated episodes of micro-embolization during prolonged decompressions (41). Significant reductions in diffusing capacity have been reported after single brief air dives (42) but appear to be completely reversible.

Sustained experimental air embolism in sheep results in a large and sustained rise in pulmonary vascular resistance and pulmonary arterial pressure (43) which is associated with increased vasoreactivity. Ultrastructural studies have shown that the air emboli attract clumps of neutrophils and damage the microvaculature by inducing gaps between endothelial cells with damage to the basement membrane and some associated edema (44). This microvascular injury may be mediated by oxygen free radicals as it can be prevented by administration of catalase or superoxide dismutase (45). One study has suggested that the abnormal lung function seen in saturation divers is a result of oxygen toxicity (46); this does not explain all of the abnormality observed. In addition in a recent deep dive abnormal lung function appeared to be related to right heart bubble counts and the occurrence of decompression sickness (47).

The appearance of bubbles in the pulmonary circulation may have greater effects than previously suspected. Echocardiographic studies before and after a single air dive to 30 msw have demonstrated a significant increase in pulmonary arterial pressure (19) with associated right ventricular dysfunction, which may result from alterations in endothelial function and these changes may persist for 48 hours (20). It remains unclear whether these changes are related to bubble embolization or to the impact of immersion since the effect does not appear to occur during decompression without immersion (48,49).

The recognition that cardiac shunts (50) and the presence of patent foramen ovale are a risk factor for neurological decompression sickness has thrown further light on the role of the pulmonary circulation. Two studies (51,52) have demonstrated that the prevalence of patent foramen ovale is much greater in patients with neurological decompression sickness (approximately 65 percent) compared to the prevalence in the normal population or asymptomatic divers of 20–25 percent (53–55). Patent foramen ovale can be demonstrated by contrast echocardiography using agitated normal saline to provide bubbles as contrast (53). If the passage of bubbles from the right to left atrium cannot be seen after an initial injection, further injections following head-down tilt or Valsalva maneuver may provoke shunting across the foramen (53). These maneuvers are frequently mimicked in diving by the changes in hydrostatic pressure and the need to equalize middle ear pressure on ascent (56). The presence of patent foramen ovale may be more than double a diver's risk of decompression illness (57,58). The more widespread use of transesophageal echo cardiography and also of transcranial Doppler examination of the cerebral arterial tree has expanded the understanding of this problem (59). The appearance of contrast bubbles in the cerebral circulation after intravenous injection indicates the presence of right to left shunting. Echocardiography may confirm the presence of an intracardiac shunt but where this is not detected, intrapulmonary shunt appears the likely explanation. This is consistent with Wilmshurst's investigation of explanatory factors for decompression illness in which abnormal lung function was commonly found in the absence of intracardiac shunt (60). Investigation for the presence of right-to-left shunt is helpful in patients who have sustained neurological or cutaneous decompression illness to advise on the risk of future diving. Closure of a patent foramen ovale can now be carried out using a closed technique (61). It is commonly offered to divers who have experienced an episode of neurological decompression illness and are demonstrated to have a patent foramen with the intention of protecting them from future episodes. A small but significant number of divers who have had patent foramen ovale closure have experienced further episodes of decompression illness. This may reflect the multifactorial causation of decompression illness, and the high prevalence of patent foramen ovale but no studies demonstrating the efficacy of closure for this purpose are available.

Exercise after diving may increase bubble counts in the venous circulation (32) and is often considered to be a risk for decompression illness. Intrapulmonary shunting has been demonstrated to occur during light exercise (62) but one study has failed to demonstrate that exercise affects the appearance of bubbles in the arterial system following an open sea dive (63).

Factors which disturb the pulmonary circulation in a way that increases the risk of right-to-left intrapulmonary shunting, are also likely to increase the risk of decompression illness. Asthma has previously been regarded as a significant potential risk factor for pulmonary barotrauma and hence a contraindication to diving. However, some asthmatics do dive and it has proved difficult to prove this risk. One study (64) suggested that asthmatics do appear to have an increased risk of diving related illness, but not of barotrauma. This may reflect an increased risk of decompression sickness. Potential causes for venous bubbles reaching the arterial circulation in this situation include local disturbance of the pulmonary circulation with right-to-left shunt secondary to uneven ventilation, the possible distension of the pulmonary capillary bed secondary to increased negative transpulmonary pressure or the use of bronchodilators. Other pulmonary conditions may also carry an increased risk, for example, decompression sickness has been reported in association with a unilateral proximal occlusion of a pulmonary artery (65). Smoking also appears to be a risk factor (60).

OXYGEN TOXICITY

Diving normally involves exposure to breathing gas with an elevated partial pressure of oxygen. During a scuba dive to 50 msw breathing compressed air, the partial pressure of oxygen is 1.2 ATA. Short exposures at higher partial pressures occur during nitrox diving (up to 1.5 ATA), during decompression breathing oxygen (up to 2.5 ATA), and prolonged exposures at low pressure (0.4 ATA) occur during saturation diving. Oxygen exposure at a relatively high dose (2–3 ATA) is part of the standard and effective therapy for decompression illness and is occasionally associated with minor symptoms of toxicity.

The pathogenesis of pulmonary oxygen toxicity has been extensively reviewed (66). The pulmonary capillary endothelium appears the most sensitive tissue within the lung. This has been demonstrated both histologically (67,68) and by use of biochemical markers of endothelial cell function in animal models (69,70). Although there is some difference in species response to oxygen, histological studies from patients ventilated with high concentrations of oxygen suggest that the histological pattern of human oxygen toxicity is similar to that in animals (71). Pulmonary oxygen toxicity has previously been assumed to have a threshold pressure for onset of 0.5 ATA (72), but significant effects are observed below this pressure (46,73). The pathological mechanism may not be the same at all pressures as animal data suggest that endothelial cell dysfunction may be less important at higher pressures (74).

In the diving situation acute pulmonary oxygen toxicity is characterized clinically by central chest discomfort and pain, cough and dyspnea. These symptoms reverse gradually over hours following exposure. Lung function tests have consistently demonstrated a reduction in vital capacity and of diffusing capacity (66). Measurement of the pulmonary capillary blood volume and diffusing capacity of the alveolar membrane in volunteer studies (75) have indicated a reduction in pulmonary capillary blood volume, but more detailed information on the circulatory effects of developing oxygen toxicity are lacking.

The implications are perhaps most important because of the potential for interaction with other effects such as gas bubble injury to endothelium, water inhalation, pulmonary edema of immersion and the efficiency of the pulmonary vasculature to remove bubbles from the circulation.

CONCLUSIONS

During diving, the pulmonary circulation has an important role in preventing gas bubbles produced in peripheral tissues from gaining access to the arterial circulation, where they may generate the pathological sequence of decompression illness. Unfortunately its ability to achieve this is readily compromised by other diving-induced insults such as the hydrostatic pressure of immersion, cold, oxygen exposure, water inhalation and transthoracic pressure. Knowledge of these effects and their interaction is valuable in the evaluation of diving casualties. Greater understanding of the formation of gas bubbles and the mechanisms which provide protection, principally the pulmonary circulation, might allow diving safety to be enhanced.

CASES

Patent foramen ovale

A 35-year-old diver conducted a single uneventful dive to 24 msw for 32 minutes. Five minutes after surfacing she developed abdominal discomfort followed by paresthesiae of both legs distal to the thigh and both arms distal to the elbow. By the time of arrival at hospital, symptoms had improved spontaneously with only abdominal discomfort and tiredness persisting. All symptoms resolved during recompression therapy. Contrast echocardiography at a later date confirmed the presence of patent foramen ovale.

Comment

The early onset of neurological illness, which may be transient, after a non-provocative dive is strongly associated with right-to-left shunt.

Pulmonary edema

While diving to 23 msw, a diver noted inhalation of seawater spray from a leaking demand valve. During the ascent, chest tightness and breathlessness occurred. After surfacing, a pronounced cough with watery secretions persisted for almost 24 hours. A dive to 39 msw later the following day was uneventful until the ascent phase when breathlessness recurred. Increasing distress with chest pain occurred during the staged ascent, ultimately necessitating assistance from the water. Cough recurred with pink frothy sputum and hemoptysis. The patient was immediately taken to a recompression chamber where a diagnosis of pulmonary decompression sickness was made. Recompression in a small chamber necessitated lying flat and breathing oxygen through a demand valve. This exacerbated symptoms, though some improvement occurred towards the end of the 5-hour treatment. On exit from the chamber, chest radiography in hospital confirmed bilateral alveolar edema, which resolved over the next 24 hours.

Comment

A minor degree of sea water inhalation almost certainly induced significant alveolar injury and increased susceptibility to immersion-induced pulmonary edema. The rapid recovery despite ventilatory impediment is consistent with this diagnosis. Although inhalation injury might impair the pulmonary circulation's ability to filter bubbles, the absence of any other manifestations of decompression illness make this diagnosis unlikely.

KEY POINTS

- Underwater, ambient hydrostatic pressure increases in a linear fashion by 1 atmosphere absolute (ATA) for every 10 meters increase in depth of seawater (msw).
- The important implications of diving for the pulmonary circulation relate to the following three main factors:

    (i) hydrostatic pressure resulting from immersion;
    (ii) gas bubbles in tissues formed from dissolved gas, which pass through the system venous and pulmonary arterial trees and which may result in decompression illness;
    (iii) exposure to high partial pressures of oxygen which may result in pulmonary oxygen toxicity.

- Immersion affects the circulation through three major mechanisms; hydrostatic pressure, temperature and the diving reflexes.
- The prevalence of patent foramen ovale is much greater in patients with neurological decompression illness (approximately 65 percent) compared with the prevalence in the normal population or asymptomatic divers (20–25 percent).
- The pulmonary capillary endothelium appears the most sensitive tissue within the lung to oxygen toxicity.
- During diving the pulmonary circulation has an important role in preventing bubbles, produced in peripheral tissues, from gaining access to the arterial circulation.

REFERENCES

1. Arborelius M, Balldin UI, Lilja B, Lundgren CEG. Hemodynamic changes in man during immersion with the head above water. Aerospace Med 1972;43:592–8.
2. Prefaut C, Lupich E, Anthonisen NR. Human lung mechanics during water immersion. J Appl Physiol 1976;40:320–3.
3. Robertson CH, Engle CM, Bradley ME. Lung volumes in man immersed to the neck; dilution and plethysmographic techniques. J Appl Physiol 1978;44:679–82.
4. Lanphier EH, Rahn H. Alveolar gas exchange during breath-hold diving. J Appl Physiol 1963;18:471–7.
5. Glasser EM, Berridge FR. Effects of heat and cold on the distribution of blood within the human body. Clin Sci 1950;9:181–8.
6. Wilmshurst PT, Crowther A, Nuri M, Webb-Peploe MM. Cold-induced pulmonary edema in scuba divers and swimmers and subsequent development of hypertension. Lancet 1989;1:62–5.
7. Song SH, Lee WK, Chung YA, Hong SK. Mechanism of apneic bradycardia in man. J Appl Physiol 1969;27:323–7.
8. Sterba JA, Lundgren CEG. Diving bradycardia and breath-holding time in man. Undersea Biomed Res 1985;12:139–50.
9. Frey MAB, Kenney RA. Changes in left ventricular activity during apnoea and face immersion. Undersea Biomed Res 1977;4:27–37.
10. Lopez-Majano V, Data PG, Martignoni R, Lossredo B, Arborelius M. Pulmonary blood flow distribution in erect man in air and during breath-hold diving. Aviat Space Environ Med 1990;61:1107–15.
11. Lollgren H, Von Neiding G, Krekeler H, Smidt U, Koppenhagen K, Frank H. Respiratory gas exchange and lung perfusion in man during and after head-out water immersion. Undersea Biomed Res 1976;3:49–56.
12. Modell JH. Drowning. New Eng J Med 1993;328:253–6.
13. Edmonds C, Lowry C, Pennefather UJ, Walker R (eds). Drowning syndromes: why divers drown. In: Diving and Subaquatic Medicine, 4th edn. London: Arnold, 2002; Chapter 25:277–84.
14. Hampson NB, Dunford RG. Pulmonary edema of scuba divers. Undersea Hyperbaric Med 1997;24(1):29–33.
15. Shupak A, Weiler-Ramell D, Adir Y, Daskalovic YI, Ramon Y, Kerem D. Pulmonary edema induced by strenuous swimming – a field study. Respir Physiol 2000;121:25–31.
16. Pons M, Blickenstorfer D, Oechslin E, Hold G, Greminger P, Franzeck UK, Russi EW. Pulmonary edema in healthy persons during scuba-diving and swimming. Eur Respir J 1995;8:762–7.
17. Slade JB, Hattori T, Ray CS, Bove AA, Cianci P. Pulmonary edema associated with scuba diving. Chest 2001;120:1686–94.
18. Koehle MS, Lepawsky M, McKenzie DC. Pulmonary edema of immersion. Sports Med 2005;35:183–90.
19. Dujic Z, Obad A, Palada I, Valic Z, Brubakk AO. A single open sea air dive increases pulmonary artery pressure and reduces right ventricular function in professional divers. Eur J Physiol 2006;97:478–85.
20. Obada A, Palada I, Valic Z, Ivancev V, Bakovic D, Wisloff U, Bribakk AO, Dujic Z. The effects of oral antioxidants on diving-induced alterations in human cardiovascular function. J Physiol 2007;578:859–70.
21. BTS Fitness to dive group. British Thoracic Society guidelines on respiratory aspects of fitness to dive. Thorax 2003;58:3–13.
22. Calder IM. Autopsy and experimental observations on factors leading to barotrauma in man. Undersea Biomed Res 1985;12:165–82.

23. Maklem H, Emhjellen S, Horgen O. Pulmonary barotrauma and arterial gas embolism caused by an emphysematous bulla in a scuba diver. Aviat Space Environ Med 1990;61:559-62.

24. Kol S, Weisz G, Melamed Y. Pulmonary barotrauma after a free dive – a possible mechanism. Aviat Space Environ Med 1993;64:236-7.

25. Bayne CG, Wurzbacher T. Can pulmonary barotrauma cause cerebral air embolism in a non-diver. Chest 1982;81:648-50.

26. Schaeffer KE, McNulty WP, Carey C, Liebow A. Mechanisms in development of interstitial emphysema and air embolism on decompression from depth. J Appl Physiol 1958;13:15-29.

27. Smith KH, Spencer MP. Doppler indices of decompression sickness: their evaluation and use. Aerospace Med 1970;41:1396-400.

28. Masurel G, Gardette B, Comet M, Kisman K, Guillerm R. Ultrasonic detection of circulating bubbles during Janus IV excursion dives at sea to 460 and 501 msw. Undersea Biomed Res 1978;5(Suppl):29.

29. Brubakk AO, Petersen R, Grip A, Holand B, Onarheim J, Segedal K, Kunkle TD, Tonjum S. Gas bubbles in the circulation of divers after ascending excursions from 300-250 msw. J Appl Physiol 1986;60:45-51.

30. Spencer MP, Clarke HF. Precordial monitoring of pulmonary gas embolism and decompression bubbles. Aerospace Med 1972;43:762-7.

31. Nossum V, Koteng S, Brubakk AO. Endothelial damage by bubbles in the pulmonary artery of the pig. Undersea Hyperbaric Med 1999;26(1):1-8.

32. Nishi RY, Bennett PB, Elliott DH (eds). Doppler and ultrasonic bubble detection. In: The Physiology and Medicine of Diving, 4th edn. London: W.B. Saunders, 1993;15:433-53.

33. Eatock BC. Correspondence between intravascular bubbles and symptoms of decompression sickness. Undersea Biomed Res 1984;11:326-9.

34. Ring GC, Blum AS, Kurbatov T, Moss WG, Smith W. Size of microspheres passing through pulmonary circuit in the dog. Am J Physiol 1961;200:1191-6.

35. Hills BA, Butler BD. Size distribution of intravascular air emboli produced by decompression. Undersea Biomed Res 1981;8:163-70.

36. Butler BD, Hills BA. The lung as a filter for microbubbles. J Appl Physiol 1979;47:537-43.

37. Butler BD, Hills BA. Transpulmonary passage of venous air emboli. J Appl Physiol 1985;59:543-7.

38. Butler BD, Katz J. Vascular pressures and passage of gas emboli through the pulmonary circulation. Undersea Biomed Res 1988;15:203-9.

39. Cotes JE, Davey IS, Reed JW, Rooks M. Respiratory effects of a single saturation dive to 300 meters. Br J Indus Med 1987;44:76-82.

40. Thorsen E, Hjelle J, Segedal K, Gulsvik A. Exercise tolerance and pulmonary gas exchange after deep saturation dives. J Appl Physiol 1990;68:1809-14.

41. Thorsen E, Segedal K, Myrseth E, Pasche A, Gulsvik A. Pulmonary mechanical function and diffusion capacity after deep saturation dives. Br J Indus Med 1990;47:242-7.

42. Dujic Z, Eterovic D, Denoble P, Krstacic G, Tocilj J, Gosovic S. Effect of a single air dive on pulmonary diffusing capacity in professional divers. J Appl Physiol 1993;74:55-61.

43. Perkett EA, Brigham KL, Meyrick B. Continuous air embolisation into sheep causes sustained pulmonary hypertension and increased pulmonary vasoactivity. Am J Path 1988;132:444-54.

44. Albertine KH, Weiner-Kronish JP, Koike K, Staub N. Quantification of damage by air emboli to lung microvessels in anaesthetized sheep. J Appl Physiol 1984;57:1360-8.

45. Flick MR, Milligan SA, Hoeffel JM, Goldstein IM. Catalase prevents increased lung vascular permeability during air emboli in unanesthetized sheep. J Appl Physiol 1988;64:929-35.

46. Thorsen E, Segedal K, Reed J et al. Effects of raised partial pressure of oxygen on pulmonary function in saturation diving. Bergen, Norwegian Underwater Technology Centre, 1992.

47. Watt SJ, Ross JAS. Health and Safety during Aurora 93. Aurora 93 Dive Report. Aberdeen. National Hyperbaric Centre Ltd, 1993.

48. Valic Z, Duplancic D, Bakovic D, Ivancev V, Eterovic D, Wisloff U, Brubakk AO, Dujic Z. Diving-induced venous gas emboli do not increase pulmonary artery pressure. Int J Sports Med 2005;26:626-31.

49. Diesel DD, Ryles MT, Pilmanis AA, Balldin UI. Non-invasive measurement of pulmonary artery pressure in humans with simulated altitude induced venous gas emboli. Aviat Space Environ Med 2002;73:128-33.

50. Wilmshurst PT, Ellis BG, Jenkins BS. Paradoxical gas embolism in a scuba diver with an atrial septal defect. Br Med J 1986;293:1277.

51. Moon RE, Camporesi EM, Kisslo JA. Patent foramen ovale and decompression sickness in divers. Lancet 1989;1:513-4.

52. Wilmshurst PT, Byrne JC, Webb-Peploe MM. Relation between interatrial shunts and decompression sickness in divers. Lancet 1989;2:1302-6.

53. Lynch JJ, Schuchard GH, Gross CM, Wann LS. Prevalence of right-to-left atrial shunting in a healthy population: detection by Valsalva maneuver contrast echocardiography. Am J Cardiol 1984;53:1478-80.

54. Hagen PT, Scholz DG, Edwards WD. Incidence and size of patent foramen ovale during the first 10 decades of life: an autopsy study of 965 normal hearts. Mayo Clin Proc 1984;59:17-20.

55. Cross SJ, Evans SA, Thomson LF, Lee HS, Jennings KP, Shields TG. Safety of subaqua diving with a patent foramen ovale. Br Med J 1992;304:481-2.

56. Balestra C, Germonpre P, Marroni A. Intrathoracic pressure changes after Valsalva strain and other manoeuvres: implications for divers with patent foramen ovale. Undersea Hyperbaric Med 1998;25(3):171-4.

57. Bove AA. Risk of decompression sickness with patent foramen ovale. Undersea Hyperbaric Med 1998;25(3):175-8.

58. Torti SR, Billinger M, Schwerzmann M, Vogel R, Zbinden R, Windecker S, Seiler C. Risk of decompression illness among 230 divers in relation to the presence and size of patent foramen ovale. Eur Heart J 2004;25:1014–20.

59. Glen S, Georgiadis D, Grosset DG, Douglas JD, Lees KR. Transcranial Doppler ultrasound in commercial air divers: a field study including cases with right to left shunting. Undersea Hyperbaric Med 1995;22(2):129–35.

60. Wilmshurst PT, Davidson C, O'Connell G, Byrne C. Role of cardiorespiratory abnormalities, smoking and dive characteristics in the manifestations of neurological decompression illness. Clin Sci 1994;86:297–303.

61. Wahl A, Meier B. Patent foramen ovale and ventricular septal defect closure. Heart 2009;95:70–82.

62. Eldridge MW, Dempsey JA, Havenkamp HC, Lovering AT, Hokansen JS. Exercise-induced intrapulmonary arteriovenous shunting in healthy humans. J Appl Physiol 2004;97:797–805.

63. Dujic Z, Palada I, Obad A, Duplancic D, Brubakk AO, Valic Z. Exercise induced intrapulmonary shunting of venous gas emboli does not occur after open-sea diving. J Appl Physiol 2005;99:944–9.

64. Corson KS, Dovenbarger JA, Moon RE, Hodder S, Bennett PB. Risk assessment of asthma for decompression illness. Undersea Biomed Res 1991;18(Suppl):16–7.

65. Debatin JF, Moon RE, Spritzer CE, McFall J, Sosman HD. MRI of absent left pulmonary artery. Journal of Computer Assisted Tomography 1992;16:641–5.

66. Clark JM, Bennett PB, Elliott DH, eds. Oxygen toxicity. In: The Physiology and Medicine of Diving, 4th edn. London: W.B. Saunders, 1993;6:121–69.

67. Kistler GS, Caldwell PRB, Weibel ER. Development of fine ultra-structural damage to alveolar and capillary ling cells in oxygen poisoned rats. J Cell Biol 1967;33:605–28.

68. Crapo JD, Barry BE, Foscue HA, Shelburne J. Structural and Biochemical changes in rat lungs occurring during exposures to lethal and adaptive doses of oxygen. Am Rev Resp Dis 1980;122:123–43.

69. Block ER, Fisher AB. Depression of serotonin clearance by rat lungs during oxygen exposure. J Appl Physiol 1977;42:33–8.

70. Dobuler KJ, Catravas JD, Gillis NC. Early detection of oxygen-induced lung injury in conscious rabbits. Am Rev Resp Dis 1982;126:534–9.

71. Nash G, Blennerhasset JB, Pontoppidan H. Pulmonary lesions associated with oxygen therapy and artificial ventilation. N Engl J Med 1967;279:368–74.

72. Clark JM, Bennett PB, Elliott DH, eds. Oxygen toxicity. In: The Physiology and Medicine of Diving, 3rd edn. London: Bailliere Tindall, 1982;9:200–38.

73. Bruce Davis W, Rennard SI, Bitterman PB, Crystal RG. Pulmonary oxygen toxicity – early reversible changes in human alveolar structures induced by hyperoxia. N Engl J Med 1983;309:878–83.

74. Allen MC, Watt SJ. Effect of hyperbaric and normobaric oxygen on pulmonary endothelial cell function. Undersea Hyperbaric Med 1993;20:39–48.

75. Puy RJM, Hyde RW, Fisher AB, Clark JM, Dickson J, Lambertson CJ. Alterations in the pulmonary capillary bed during early oxygen toxicity in man. J Appl Physiol 1968;24:537–43.

PART 14

DISORDERS CAUSING INTRAPULMONARY SHUNT

Hepatopulmonary syndrome

MICHAEL J KROWKA

INTRODUCTION

In an 1884 German publication, Dr M. Fluckiger described a 37-year-old woman with profound cyanosis and digital clubbing who died following an episode of hematemesis and probable hepatic coma. A postmortem examination conducted by Professor v. Recklinghausen demonstrated cirrhosis, enlarged twisted veins around the esophagus and abnormally dilated pulmonary vessels (1). Approximately 75 years later, in a 1959 case report describing the death of a 17-year-old male with severe hypoxemia and juvenile cirrhosis, Rydell and Hoffbauer emphasized the dramatic clinical relationship between hypoxemia and hepatic dysfunction. Their postmortem study described both precapillary dilatations and direct arteriovenous communications as demonstrated by vascular injections of the pulmonary arteries with a plastic vinyl acetate solution (2). Berthelot and colleagues from England confirmed these pulmonary vascular observations in their 1969 autopsy study of 12 patients with microscopic "lung spiders" that complicated advanced liver disease (3). The entity of hypoxemia due to such pulmonary vascular abnormalities in the setting of liver disease was later termed "hepatopulmonary syndrome" by Knudsen and Kennedy in 1979 (4). Over the last 30 years the international importance of and intrigue surrounding the hepatopulmonary syndrome (HPS) has steadily unfolded as a consequence of the clinical experiences during pre and post liver transplant evaluations.

The spectrum of pulmonary vascular pathology that can occur in the setting of liver disease is shown in Figure 26.1.1 (5). It is hypothesized that the pulmonary arterial and capillary beds experience the "downstream" effects of circulating vascular mediators that exist due to hepatic dysfunction. Such effects may be due to the absence of essential vasomediators emanating from the hepatic veins or within the pulmonary endothelium (prostacyclin synthase), the *excess/existence* of vascular modulating factors due to effects of portal hypertension (endothelin-1), and/or the abnormal regulation of pulmonary vasomediating receptors (endothelin A and B), all in genetically susceptible patients (6).

This chapter will focus on the concept of pulmonary vascular dilatation that causes arterial hypoxemia in the setting of liver and portal circulation dysfunction HPS is

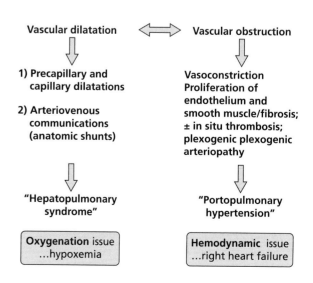

Figure 26.1.1 Spectrum of pulmonary vascular abnormalities in advanced liver disease.

distinct from portopulmonary hypertension, the other major insult to the pulmonary circulation associated with liver disease (discussed in Chapter 15.5).

DIAGNOSTIC CRITERIA

The triad of hepatic dysfunction, pulmonary vascular dilatation and arterial hypoxemia characterizes HPS (4,6). Specific diagnostic criteria currently followed by most clinical investigators are summarized in Table 26.1.1.

Hepatic dysfunction

Pediatric and adult patients with HPS most commonly have chronic liver disease (cirrhosis) with portal hypertension (7,8). However, HPS has been reported in the setting of noncirrhotic portal hypertension and ischemic hepatitis (9,10). In addition, pulmonary vascular dilatations have been demonstrated at autopsy in the setting of fulminant hepatic failure (11). Severity of liver disease characterized by the Child–Pugh classification (based upon ascites, encephalopathy, bilirubin, albumin and prothrombin time) or the Model for End Stage Liver Disease score (MELD – a function of INR, serum bilirubin and serum creatinine) correlates poorly with the severity of hypoxemia (6,12,13).

Pulmonary vascular dilatation

Noninvasive diagnosis of pulmonary vascular dilatations rests upon detecting the abnormal passage of microbubbles (Figure 26.1.2) or technetium radiolabeled macroaggregated albumin (^{99m}TcMAA – Figure 26.1.3) through dilated capillary beds or discrete arteriovenous communications (14,15). Normally, microbubbles (>10 microns) or ^{99m}TcMAA (20–60 microns) are absorbed or trapped, respectively, and do not pass through capillaries (<8 microns in diameter). ^{99m}TcMAA lung scanning offers the advantage

of quantifying the degree of pulmonary vascular dilatation by measuring brain versus lung uptake. Neither method, however, can distinguish between diffuse vascular dilatations and discrete arteriovenous communications (16).

The chest radiograph is frequently unremarkable; patterns consistent with lower lung field "interstitial lung disease" may be reported, but on occasion a distinct abnormality may be seen. Subsequent chest CT scanning can reveal both distinct and diffusely dilated vessels (Figure 26.1.4). Pulmonary angiography confirms at least two types of vascular abnormality that characterize HPS (17,18). The more common Type I pattern is characterized by a normal to diffuse spongy/blush appearance during the

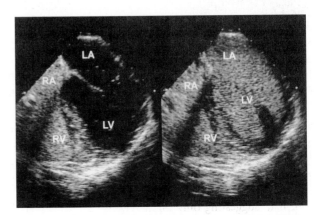

Figure 26.1.2 Transthoracic echocardiogram demonstrating: RA, right atrium; RV, right ventricle; LA, left ventricle; and LV, left ventricle. Left panel: Right heart chamber opacification following peripheral vein injection of agitated saline; Right panel: Left heart chamber opacification 4–6 cardiac cycles later due to abnormal intrapulmonary passage of microbubbles through dilated precapillary and capillary vessels.

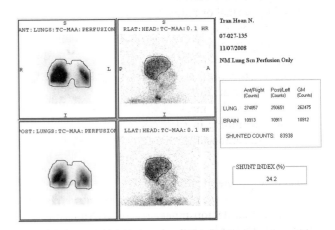

Figure 26.1.3 ^{99m}TcMAA brain and lung perfusion scan demonstrating a 24.2% brain uptake (normal $<6\%$) in a patient with nodular regenerative hyperplasia, portal hypertension and severe hepatopulmonary syndrome.

Table 26.1.1 Hepatopulmonary syndrome diagnostic criteria

1. Liver disease
   - Cirrhosis with portal hypertension (any cause)
   - Non-cirrhotic portal hypertension
2. Hypoxemia
   - $PaO_2 < 70$ mmHg; or
   - Alveolar-arterial (A-a) oxygen gradient > 20 mmHg
3. Pulmonary vascular dilatation
   - "Positive" contrast-enhanced echocardiogram showing microbubble opacification in the left atrium > 3 cardiac cycles after right ventricular opacification; or
   - ^{99m}TcMAA brain uptake $> 6\%$ following lung perfusion scanning

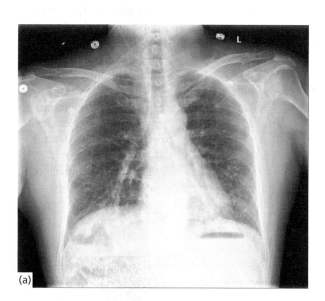 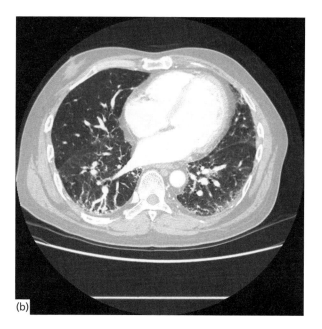

Figure 26.1.4   Chest imaging in HPS: abnormal chest radiograph showing dilated vessels especially in right lower lobe; and chest computed tomography in the same patient demonstrating both discrete and diffuse arteriovenous communications in the lung bases.

arterial phase of imaging. The rare Type II lesions are seen as discrete arteriovenous communications (which may be amenable to coil embolotherapy to improve oxygenation and reduce the risk of brain embolic events). It is not uncommon for the angiogram images to be reported as "normal," suggesting only rapid venous filling (17). HPS patients with $PaO_2 > 300\,mmHg$ breathing 100 percent oxygen are unlikely to have clinically significant lesions demonstrated by pulmonary angiography (13). Overall, pulmonary angiography should be conducted in a select group of HPS patients and only if coil embolotherapy is to be considered.

Unlike portopulmonary hypertension associated with vasoconstriction and obstruction to pulmonary blood flow, the pulmonary vascular dilatations in HPS are characterized by normal or reduced pulmonary vascular resistance measured during right heart catheterization (5). Cardiac outputs may be quite high due to the hyperdynamic circulatory state created by portal hypertension. Pulmonary artery pressures may be increased in HPS due to the high flow state through the pulmonary vascular bed, but rarely does the mean pulmonary arterial pressure exceed 40–45 mmHg in such cases; pulmonary vascular resistance calculations in such cases are normal.

Arterial hypoxemia

A schematic that demonstrates precapillary/capillary dilatation and anatomic shunt pathophysiology associated with HPS is shown in Figure 26.1.5. Such pathology causes arterial hypoxemia from three mechanisms; low ventilation-perfusion (V/Q) ratio due to excess perfusion (Q) to a given area of ventilation (V); impaired diffusion of oxygen

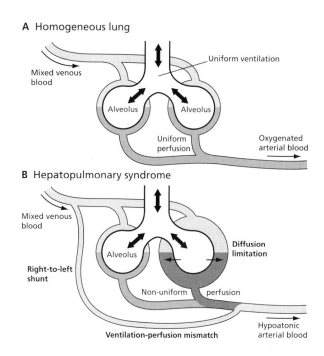

Figure 26.1.5   The schematic of abnormal physiology associated with dilated precapillary/capillary vessels and direct arteriovenous communications.

molecules through dilated peri-alveolar vessels (a diffusion-perfusion defect) and true anatomic (intrapulmonary) right-to-left shunt (6,19–22).

The multiple inert gas elimination technique (MIGET) has been the gold standard in studying the physiology of hypoxemia in the presence of pulmonary vascular dilations (19,20). Following a venous infusion of inert gases with varying solubilities, exhalation and arterial concentrations allow numerical approximations of pulmonary ventilation/perfusion relationships The dramatic response to 100 percent inspired oxygen in the setting of severe hypoxemia breathing room air argues against the existence of a clinically significant right-to-left anatomic shunt in most patients with HPS (19). The accuracy and interpretation of MIGET in the setting of severe hypoxemia due to diffuse vascular dilatation (not distinct arteriovenous communications) has been questioned (21).

Clinically, many patients with HPS have near normal PaO_2 (>500 mmHg) when breathing 100 percent oxygen (13). High concentrations of alveolar O_2 are able to completely penetrate dilated capillary channels and thus PaO_2 improves. For this reason it is *unlikely* that most cases of HPS involve true "shunt." Worsening of arterial oxygenation when moving from the supine to standing position (orthodeoxia) has been documented in HPS (22). Orthodeoxia has been attributed to the predominance of vascular dilatations in the lung bases, effects of gravity on blood flow and reduced cardiac output when standing.

The severity of arterial hypoxemia breathing room air correlates modestly with 100 percent inspired oxygen and ^{99m}TcMAA lung scanning (Figure 26.1.6). Indeed, multiple reasons for hypoxemia (lung atelectasis caused by hepatic hydrothorax, effects of massive ascites upon the diaphragms, chronic obstructive lung disease and interstitial lung disease) may exist in approximately 20–30 percent of patients with pulmonary vascular dilatations (23). Hypoxemia due to HPS may worsen significantly with sleep (24).

SCREENING AND DIAGNOSTIC ALGORITHM

Screening for hypoxemia

Oxyhemoglobin saturation (SaO_2) measured by pulse oximetry, arterial partial pressure of oxygen (PaO_2) and the alveolar-arterial (A-a) oxygen gradient characterize the degree of hypoxemia in patients with liver disease (25). The obvious advantage of pulse oximetry is that the measurement is non-invasive. However, this method has been reported to overestimate oxyhemoglobin saturations obtained via arterial puncture and blood gas analysis by approximately 4 percent (26). Pulse oximetry ($SpO_2 < 94$ percent) detected all subjects with a $PaO_2 < 60$ mmHg in the same study.

Indeed, PaO_2 and A-a oxygen gradient determinations require arterial puncture, but this method can be safely accomplished by experienced individuals even in the setting of thrombocytopenia and coagulopathy due to liver disease. Due to hyperventilation, which accompanies liver disease, most investigators concur that PaO_2 values < 70 mmHg should be considered abnormal (6,13,25). Determination of the (A-a) oxygen gradient, which takes into consideration not only the PaO_2, but also the $PaCO_2$ effect on oxygenation, provides the most sensitive assessment of abnormal arterial oxygenation. Normal (A-a) oxygen gradient is age dependent, but usually considered abnormal if greater than 20 mmHg (5). The measurement of the (A-a) oxygen gradient, however, must take into consideration the daily barometric pressure in calculating the alveolar partial pressure of oxygen. Although hypoxemia is common in liver disease and not necessarily due to HPS, patients with severe hypoxemia ($PaO_2 < 50$ mmHg) should be considered to have hepatopulmonary syndrome until proven otherwise.

Screening for pulmonary vascular dilatations

Most centers screen for pulmonary vascular dilatation using transthoracic, contrast-enhanced echocardiography (27–29). If necessary, contrast transesophageal echocardiography can distinguish between intracardiac shunts and intrapulmonary vascular dilatations by direct imaging of the intraatrial septum and pulmonary veins, respectively (16). ^{99m}TcMAA lung scanning should be accomplished if the screening PaO_2 (and contrast echocardiography) suggest HPS. Brain uptake (normal less than 6 percent) following lung perfusion adds an additional measure of quantifying HPS (15).

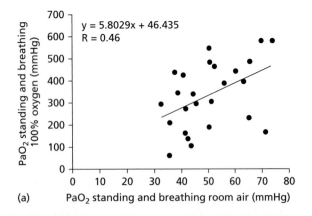

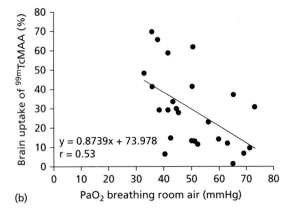

Figure 26.1.6 Oxygenation relations in HPS: (a) Relationships between oxygenation (breathing room air versus 100% inspired oxygen); and (b) ^{99m}TcMAA lung scanning with brain uptake versus room air PaO_2).

The HPS screening and diagnostic algorithm followed at the Mayo Clinic is shown in Figure 26.1.7.

INCIDENCE

The frequency of transthoracic echo-detected pulmonary vascular dilatation associated with liver disease has ranged from 7 to 47 percent. Hypoxemia was reported in 32–65 percent of those with "positive" contrast-enhanced echocardiograms and in 5–17 percent of all patients screened (5,14,28). A subclinical or *forme fruste* aspect of HPS may exist which, over time, results in progressive hypoxemia (5).

PATHOPHYSIOLOGY

Circulating vasomediators that result in diffuse vascular dilatations, discrete arteriovenous communications, and possible angiogenesis, have not been identified in humans. Increased levels of exhaled nitric oxide (NO) have been documented in HPS with resolution of such findings and hypoxemia following successful LT (6,30–33). However, the administration of L-NAME (L-arginine methyl ester) which can block production of exhaled NO in humans has *not* been shown to improve arterial oxygenation (32). Recently, animal models have provided links between hepatic dysfunction and the pulmonary endothelium (33,34). Common bile duct ligation models of cirrhosis in the rat have been developed to study the circulating levels of endothelin-1 and the over production of nitric oxide (33). Increased levels of endothelin-1 (originating from the liver) may interact with endothelin A and endothelin B receptors in the pulmonary vascular bed (34). These receptors normally cause vasodilation (endothelin B receptors on the luminal side of the endothelium) and vasoconstriction (endothelin A and B receptors on smooth muscle which surround the vessels). An up-regulation of the endothelin B receptors has been demonstrated in the animal model of HPS (34).

Angiogenesis and the role of vascular endothelial growth factor (VEGF) remain interesting hypotheses in the evolution of HPS. Indeed, autopsy descriptions have documented an apparent increase in the number of peri-alveolar vessels compared to controls (3). No human studies have confirmed an increase in VEGF in HPS to date.

There appear to be remarkable similarities (angiography and mechanisms of hypoxemia) between the pulmonary vascular abnormalities documented in HPS, those acquired following pediatric post cavopulmonary shunt surgery for tricuspid atresia (35,36), and lesions demonstrated in HHT (hemorrhagic hereditary telangiectasia (37).

CLINICAL PRESENTATION AND NATURAL HISTORY

The natural history of HPS has been poorly defined and complicated by the advent of successful liver transplantation as a method to treat this syndrome (16,29,38,39). HPS appears to develop slowly over months to years after the onset of hepatic dysfunction and its presence portends an independent, adverse prognosis (40). Young children, as well as adults, may have profound presentations of cyanosis due to HPS (7). Clubbing, cyanosis and spider angiomas of the skin in the setting of liver disease strongly suggest the existence of pulmonary vascular dilatations. Correlation with the stage of liver disease (as documented by the Child–Pugh classification or with the existence of esophageal varices) and MELD scores (serum bilirubin, serum creatinine and INR) is poor (6,13).

Patients with HPS awaiting liver transplantation tend to have a slowly progressive, symptomatic deterioration in PaO_2, averaging approximately 5 mmHg per year (39). Rarely, HPS can resolve spontaneously, especially in the setting of alcoholic cirrhosis and subsequent alcohol abstention.

TREATMENT OPTIONS

By definition HPS patients are hypoxemic at rest. This may worsen with changing position (from supine to standing – "orthodeoxia"), exercise and sleep (6). Most patients respond well to low flow oxygen (1–5 L/min) via nasal cannula (6).

Pharmacologic

Most medication approaches have been disappointing in providing a consistent and reproducible improvement in the hypoxemia associated with HPS. Small series have involved the open label use of vascular mediators such as almitrine bismesylate, somatostatin analog, high-dose aspirin, intravenous methylene blue, and garlic preparation; except

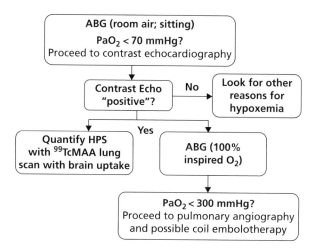

Figure 26.1.7 Hepatopulmonary syndrome "Screening and Diagnostic Algorithm" currently followed at the Mayo Clinic.

for long-term use of pentoxifylline (41) in a pilot study of mild HPS, significant improvement in PaO_2 could not be consistently demonstrated in these studies (5,6).

Recent case reports have documented a successful role for pulmonary vasodilators (oral sildenafil, inhaled nitric oxide and inhaled prostacyclin) as a means to redistribute pulmonary blood flow away from pulmonary vascular dilatations, thus improving ventilation-perfusion matching and increasing PaO_2 (36,42).

Interventional radiology

The placement of TIPS (transjugular intrahepatic portosystemic shunting) to improve hypoxemia due to HPS remains controversial and cannot be advised at this time without further prospective study (43,44). Coil embolotherapy to occlude discrete arteriovenous communications in patients with severe hypoxemia and type II HPS lesions that did not change after liver transplantation has resulted in significant increases in PaO_2 (45,46).

Liver transplantation

The existence of HPS has evolved from an "absolute" or "relative" contraindication to "indication" for liver transplantation in the majority of patients with this syndrome (5,47–54). No intraoperative deaths directly related to this syndrome have been reported, but post-transplant hospitalization mortality may still approach 16 percent (51). Complete resolution of hepatopulmonary syndrome, even in the setting of severe hypoxemia ($PaO_2 < 50\,mmHg$), has been well documented in both children and adults (39,48,49,52–54). However time to resolution of HPS following LT and mortality following LT in patients with HPS has been related to the severity of pre-transplant hypoxemia measured by PaO_2 ($< 50\,mmHg$) and the degree of brain uptake (> 20 percent) as quantitated by ^{99m}TcMAA lung perfusion scanning (49,50). In the largest single institution series from the Mayo Clinic, the 5-year survival following cadaveric LT was 76 percent (Figure 26.1.8). From this series, the natural history of this syndrome *without* LT demonstrated only a 5-year 23 percent survival. For these reasons patients with HPS associated with $PaO_2 < 60\,mmHg$ has been granted higher priority for LT (transplant to be accomplished approximately within 3 months), in the United States organ transplant system (55).

Of interest is the rare development of pulmonary hypertension following the resolution of HPS (56). This observation suggests the co-existence of pulmonary vascular pathologies, with post-LT resolution of vascular dilatation and manifestation of pulmonary vascular obstruction. Use of extracorporal support has been used to treat severe

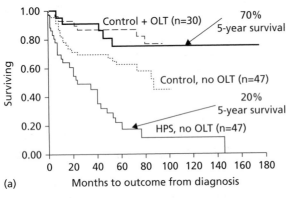

(a)

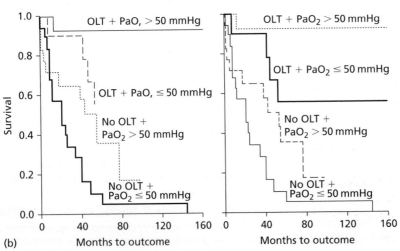

(b)

Figure 26.1.8 (a) Long-term survival in the presence of HPS (with and without liver transplant) versus matched controls. (b) Long-term survival categorized by initial PaO_2 values. (With permission from Hepatology 2005;41:1122–9, Fig. 1).

Table 26.1.2 Outcomes following liver transplantation (LT) in hepatopulmonary syndrome (HPS)

An indication for LT per pediatric and adult UNOS criteria in the United States.

Increased transplant priority if $PaO_2 < 60\,mmHg$ (breathing room air/sitting).

Resolution of the syndrome in 62–82% (usually 3–15 months).

Mortality ranges from 16 to 38% within one year post-transplant.

Pretransplant risk factors for increased mortality within 90 days of transplant:

- $PaO_2 < 50\,mmHg$.
- $^{99m}TcMAA$ brain uptake $> 20\%$.

Prolonged intubation/mechanical ventilation (4–77 days) in 22%.

Resolution of syndrome post-LT related to severity of pre-LT hypoxemia.

Recurrence of HPS following LT extremely rare.

UNOS, United Network for Organ Sharing.

hypoxemia post-LT with success (57). Recurrence of HPS following successful LT is very uncommon (58,59). Key clinical observations in HPS patients who have undergone LT are summarized in Table 26.1.2.

Other non-medical options

Cavoplasty in Budd–Chiari syndrome (60) and surgical ligation of portosystemic shunts have been reported to correct hypoxemia in highly selected HPS cases (61,62).

FUTURE DIRECTIONS

Detection of the circulating vascular mediators and identifying genetic predispositions associated with the pulmonary vascular remodeling associated with HPS remain high priorities for clinical investigation. Efforts continue to select pharmacologic means that would significantly and consistently improve hypoxemia due to HPS.

KEY POINTS

- The clinical triad of hepatic dysfunction, pulmonary vascular dilatation and arterial hypoxemia characterizes hepatopulmonary syndrome (HPS).
- Pulmonary vascular pathology documented in HPS includes diffuse precapillary/capillary dilatations, discrete arteriovenous communications and possible angiogenesis.
- Arterial hypoxemia may be severe and is caused by excess perfusion to ventilation ratios, diffusion-perfusion impairment and anatomic right to left shunts.

- Hypoxemia associated with HPS is usually progressive and correlates poorly with severity of liver disease with an untreated (no transplant) 5-year survival of approximately 23 percent.
- Liver transplantation frequently results in complete resolution of arterial hypoxemia caused by HPS; however, post-transplant mortality and time until syndrome resolution are strongly correlated to the severity of pre-transplant PaO_2.
- 5-year 76 percent survival in HPS patients following LT is well documented.

REFERENCES

- $\bullet$ = Key primary paper
- $\blacklozenge$ = Major review article
- $*$ = Management guideline

1. Fluckiger M. Vorkommen von trommelschlagelformigen fingerendphalangen ohne chronische veriinderungen an den lungen oder am herzen. Wiener Medizinische Wochenschrift, 1884;49:1457–8.
- •2. Rydell R, Hoffbauer FW. Multiple pulmonary arteriovenous fistulae in juvenile cirrhosis. Am J Med 1956;21:450–9.
- •3. Berthelot P, Walker JG, Sherlock S. Arterial changes in the lungs in cirrhosis of the liver: lung spider nevi. N Engl J Med 1966;274:291–8.
4. Kennedy TC, Knudsen RJ. Exercise-aggravated hypoxemia and orthodeoxia in cirrhosis. Chest 1977;72:305–9.
- ◆5. Rodriguez-Roisin R, Krowka MJ, Herve P, Fallon MB. Pulmonary-hepatic vascular disorders: consensus from a task force. Eur Respir J 2004;24:861–80.
- ◆6. Rodriguez-Roisin R, Krowka MJ. Hepatopulmonary syndrome: a liver-induced lung vascular disorder. N Engl J Med 2008;358:2378–87.
7. Noli K, Solomon M, Golding F, Charron M, Ling SC. Prevalence of hepatopulmonary syndrome in children. Pediatrics 2008:e522–e527.
8. Fallon MB, Krowka MJ, Brown RS, Trotter JF, Zacks S, Roberts K et al. Impact of hepatopulmonary syndrome on quality if life and survival in liver transplant candidates. Gastroenterology 2008;135:1168–75.
9. Kaymakoglu S, Kahraman T, Kudat H, Demir K, Cakaloglu Y, Adalet I et al. Hepatopulmonary syndrome noncirrhotic portal hypertensive patients. Dig Dis Sci 2003;48:556–60.
10. Fuhrmann V, Madl C, Mueller C, Holzinger U, Kitzberger R, Funk GC, Schenk P. Hepatopulmonary syndrome in patients with hypoxic hepatitis. Gastroenterology 2006; 131:69–75.
11. Williams A, Trewby P, Williams R. Structural alterations to the pulmonary circulation in fulminant hepatic failure. Thorax 1979;34:447–53.
12. Wiesner RH, Lake JR, Freeman RB, Gish RG. Model for end-stage liver disease (MELD) exception guidelines. Liver Transpl 2006;12:S85–87.

*13. Krowka MJ, Wiseman GA, Burnett OL. Hepatopulmonary syndrome: a prospective study of relationships between severity of liver disease, PaO₂ response to 100% oxygen, and brain uptake after ⁹⁹ᵐTcMAA lung scanning. Chest 2000;118:815–24.

•14. Krowka MJ, Tajik AJ, Dickson ER. Intrapulmonary vascular dilatations (IPVD) in liver transplant candidates. Chest 1990;97:1165–70.

•15. Abrams GA, Nanda NC, Dubovsky EV. Use of macroaggregated lung perfusion scan to diagnose hepatopulmonary syndrome: a new approach. Gastroenterology 1998;114:305–10.

16. Vedrinne JM, Duperret S, Bizollon T. Comparison of transesophageal and transthoracic contrast echocardiography for the detection of intrapulmonary shunt in liver disease. Chest, 1997;111:1236–40.

17. Lee KN, Lee HJ, Shin WW et al. Hypoxemia and liver cirrhosis (hepatopulmonary syndrome) in eight patients: comparison of the central and peripheral pulmonary vasculature. Radiology 1999;211:549–53.

18. Koksal D, Kacar S, Koksal AS, Tufekcioglu O, Kucvukay F, Okten S et al. Evaluation of intrapulmonary vascular dilations with high resolution computed thorax tomography in patients with hepatopulmonary syndrome. J Clin Gastroenterol 2006;40:77–83.

19. Edell ES, Cortese DA, Krowka MJ et al. Severe hypoxemia and liver disease. Am Rev Respir Dis 1989;140:1631–5.

20. Thorens JB, Junod AF. Hypoxemia and liver cirrhosis: a new argument in favor of a "diffusion–perfusion" defect". Eur Respir J 1992;5:754–6.

21. Crawford ABH, Regnis J, Laks L et al. Pulmonary vascular dilatation and diffusion-dependent impairment of gas exchange in liver cirrhosis. Eur Respir J 1995;8:2015–21.

22. Gomez FP, Martinez-Palli G, Barbera JA, Roca J, Navasa M, Rodriguez-Roisin R. Gas exchange mechanism of orthodeoxia in hepatopulmonary syndrome. Hepatology 2004;40:660–6.

•23. Martinez G, Barbaera JA, Navasa M et al. Hepatopulmonary syndrome associated with cardiorespiratory disease. J Hepatol 1999;30:882–9.

24. Palma DT, Philips GM, Arguedas MR, Harding SM, Fallon MB. Oxygen desaturation during sleep in hepatopulmonary syndrome. Hepatology 2008;47:1257–63.

25. Schenk P, Fuhrmann V, Madl C, Funk G, Lehr S, Kandel O, Muller C. Hepatopulmonary syndrome: prevalence and predictive value of various cutoffs for arterial oxygenation and their clinical consequences. Gut 2002;51:853–9.

*26. Abrams GA, Sanders MK, Fallon MB. Utility of pulse oximetry in the detection of arterial hypoxemia in liver transplant patients. Liver Transpl 2002;8:391–6.

27. Roberts DN, Arguedas MR, Fallon MB. Cost-effectiveness of screening for hepatopulmonary syndrome in liver transplant candidates. Liver Transpl 2007;13:206–14.

28. Hopkins WE Waggoner AD, Barzilai B. Frequency and significance of intrapulmonary right-to-left shunt in end-stage hepatic disease. Am J Cardiol 1992;70:516–9.

*29. Fallon MB, Mulligan DC, Gish RG, Krowka MJ. Model for end-stage liver disease (MELD) exception for hepatopulmonary syndrome. Liver Transpl 2006;12:S105–S107.

•30. Cremona G, Higenbottam TW, Mayoral V et al. Elevated exhaled nitric oxide in patients with hepatopulmonary syndrome. Eur Respir J 1995;8:1883–5.

31. Rolla G, Brussino L, Colagrande P et al. Exhaled nitric oxide and oxygenation abnormalities in hepatic cirrhosis. Hepatology 1997;27:842–7.

•32. Gomez FP, Barbera JA, Roca J, Burgos F, Gistau C, Rodriguez-Roisin R. Effects of nebulized N(G)-nitro-L-arginine methyl ester in patients with hepatopulmonary syndrome. Hepatology 2006;43:1084–91.

33. Luo B, Tang L, Wang Z, Zhang J, Ling Y, Feng W et al. Cholangiocyte endothelin 1 and transforming growth factor beta1 production in rat experimental hepatopulmonary syndrome. Gastroenterology 2005;129:682–95.

34. Tang L, Luo B, Patel RP, Ling Y, Zhang J, Fallon MB. Modulation of pulmonary endothelial endothelin B receptor expression and signaling: implications for experimental hepatopulmonary syndrome. Am J Physiol Lung Cell Mol Physiol 2007;292:L1467–72.

35. Duncan BW, Desai S. Pulmonary arteriovenous malformations after cavopulmonary anastomosis. Ann Thor Surg 2003;76:1759–66.

36. Bhate S, Rossiter-Thorton M, Cooper SG, Gillis J, Cole AD, Sholler GS et al. Use of sildenafil and nitric oxide in the management of hypoxemia owing to pulmonary arteriovenous venous fistulas after total cavopulmonary connection. J Thor Cardio Vasc Surg 2008;135:446–8.

37. Pierucci P, Murphy J, Henderson KJ, Chynn D, White RI. New definition and natural history of patients with diffuse pulmonary arteriovenous malformations. Chest 2008;133:653–61.

38. Krowka MJ, Dickson ER, Cortese DA. Hepatopulmonary syndrome: clinical observations and lack of therapeutic response to somatostatin analogue. Chest 1993;104:515–21.

•39. Swanson KL, Wiesner RH, Krowka MJ. Natural history of hepatopulmonary syndrome: impact of liver transplantation. Hepatology 2005;41:1122–9.

•40. Schenk P, Schoniger-Hekele M, Fuhrmann V, Madl C, Silberhumer G, Muller C. Prognostic significance of the hepatopulmonary syndrome in patients with cirrhosis. Gastroenterology 2003;125:1042–52.

41. Gupta LB, Kumar A, Jaiswal A, Yusaf J, Mehta V, Tyagi S et al. Pentoxyfylline therapy for hepatopulmonary syndrome: a pilot study. Arch Intern Med 2008;168:1820–24.

42. Krug S, Seyfarth HJ, Hagendorff A, Wirtz H. Inhaled iloprost for hepatopulmonary syndrome: improvement in hypoxemia. Eur J Gastro Hepatol 2007;19:1140–3.

43. Corley DA, Scharschmidt B, Bass N et al. Lack of efficacy of TIPS for hepatopulmonary syndrome. Gastroenterology 1997;113:728–31.

44. Lasch HM, Fried MW, Zacks SL, Odell P, Johnson MW, Gerber DA et al. Use of transjugular intrahepatic portosystemic shunt as a bridge to liver transplantation in a patient with severe hepatopulmonary syndrome. Liver Transpl 2001;7:147–9.

*45. Poterucha JJ, Krowka MJ, Dickson ER *et al.* Failure of hepatopulmonary syndrome to resolve after liver transplantation and successful treatment with embolotherapy. Hepatology 1995;21:96–100.

46. Saad NAE, Lee DE, Waldman DL, Saad WAE. Pulmonary arterial coil embolization for the management of persistent type I hepatopulmonary syndrome after liver transplantation. J Vasc Interv Radioli 2007;18:1576–80.

◆*47. Krowka MJ, Porayko MK, Plevak DJ et al. Hepatopulmonary syndrome with progressive hypoxemia as an indication for liver transplantation: case reports and literature review. Mayo Clin Proc 1996;72:44–53.

48. Egawa H, Hasahara M, Inomata Y *et al.* Long-term outcome of living related liver transplantation for patients with intrapulmonary shunting and strategy for complications. Transplantation 1999;67:712–7.

49. Taille C, Cadranel J, Bellocq A, Thabut G, Soubrane O, Durand F, Ichai P, Duvoux C, Belghiti J, Calmus Y, Mal H. Liver transplantation for hepatopulmonary syndrome: a ten-year experience in Paris, France. Transplantation 2003;75:1482–9.

50. Arguedas MR, Abrams GA, Krowka MJ, Fallon MB. Prospective evaluation of outcomes and predictors of mortality in patients with hepatopulmonary syndrome undergoing liver transplantation. Hepatology 2003; 37:192–7.

●51. Krowka MJ, Mandell MS, Ramsay MA, Kawut SM, Fallon MB, Manzarbeitia C *et al.* Hepatopulmonary syndrome and portopulmonary hypertension: a report of the multicenter liver transplant database. Liver Transpl 2004; 10:174–82.

52. Collisson EA, Nourmand H, Fraiman MH, Cooper CB, Bellamy PE, Farmer DG *et al.* Retrospective analysis of the results of liver transplantation for adults with severe hepatopulmonary syndrome. Liver Transpl 2002;8:925–31.

53. Schiffer E, Majno P, Mentha G, Giostra, Burri H, Klopfenstein CE *et al.* Hepatopulmonary syndrome increases the postoperative mortality rate following liver transplantation: a prospective study in 90 patients. Am J Transplant 2006;6:1430–7.

54. Tumgor G, Arikan C, Yuksekkaya H, Cakir M, Levent E, Yagci RV *et al.* Childhood cirrhosis, hepatopulmonary syndrome, and liver transplantation. Pediatr Transplant 2008;12:353–7.

*55. Fallon MB, Mulligan DC, Gish RB, Krowka MJ. Model for end-stage liver disease (MELD) exception for hepatopulmonary syndrome. Liver Transpl 2006;12: S105–107.

◆56. Aucejo F, Miller C, Vogt D, Eghesad B, Nakagawa S, Stoller JK. Pulmonary hypertension after liver transplantation in patients with antecedent hepatopulmonary syndrome: cases and review of the literature. Liver Transpl 2006; 12:1278–82.

57. Fleming GM, Cornell TT, Welling TH, Magee JC, Annich GM. Hepatopulmonary syndrome: use of extracorporeal life support for life-threatening hypoxia following liver transplantation. Liver Transplant 2008;14:966–70.

58. Krowka MJ, Wiseman GA, Steers JL. Late recurrence and rapid evolution of severe hepatopulmonary syndrome after liver transplantation. Liver Transpl 1999;5:451–3.

59. Jonas MM. Krawczuk LE. Kim HB. Lillehei C. Perez-Atayde A. Rapid recurrence of nonalcoholic fatty liver disease after transplantation in a child with hypopituitarism and hepatopulmonary syndrome. Liver Transpl 2005;11:108–10.

60. De BK, Sen S, Biswas PK, Mandal SK, Das D, Das U, Guru S, Bandyopadhyay K. Occurrence of hepatopulmonary syndrome in Budd–Chiari syndrome and the role of venous decompression. Gastroenterology 2002;122:897–903.

61. Morikawa N, Honna T, Kuroda T, Kitano Y, Fuchimoto Y, Kawashima N *et al.* Resolution of hepatopulmonary syndrome after ligation of a portosystemic shunt in Abernethy malformation. J Pediatr Surg 2008;43:E35–8.

62. Tercier S, DeLarue A, Rouaulkt F, Roman C, Breaud, Petit P. Congential portocaval fistula associated with hepatopulmonary syndrome: ligation vs liver transplantation. J Pediatr Surg 2006;41:E1–3.

Pulmonary arteriovenous malformations

CLAIRE L SHOVLIN AND JAMES E JACKSON

INTRODUCTION

Historical overview

Pulmonary arteriovenous malformations (PAVMs) are abnormal vascular structures that provide a direct capillary-free communication between the pulmonary and systemic circulations. First described at post mortem (1), affected individuals were subsequently recognized exhibiting the physiological consequences of a massive right to left shunt (dyspnea, cyanosis, clubbing and polycythemia). Some also manifest the consequences of paradoxical emboli through the shunts with the development of brain abscess (2).

Soon after PAVMs were first described during life, a link with the inherited condition hereditary hemorrhagic telangiectasia (HHT, Osler–Weber–Rendu syndrome) was appreciated (3). Approximately 90 percent of PAVMs are now known to be due to HHT, the majority of the remainder being attributed to sporadic disease. With the introduction of surgical treatments for cyanotic congenital heart disease in the 1960s, a further type of PAVM became apparent, as PAVMs developed in the lung not receiving inferior caval blood via surgically generated cavopulmonary or atriopulmonary shunts (4). The associations of PAVMs with the two disease processes HHT and cavopulmonary shunts have led to important breakthroughs in our understanding of their pathogenesis.

The clinical picture of PAVMs

It is often assumed that all patients with clinically significant PAVMs will have prominent respiratory symptoms: pulmonary arterial blood passing through these right-to-left (R-L) shunts cannot be oxygenated leading to hypoxemia. Unexplained and often profound hypoxemia is the hallmark of large PAVMs, but most patients with clinically significant PAVMs do not have respiratory symptoms or profound hypoxemia (Table 26.2.1).

In such patients, PAVMs are not benign. The absence of a filtering capillary bed allows particulate matter to reach the systemic circulation where it impacts in other capillary beds, including the cerebral circulation resulting in embolic

Table 26.2.1 Clinical features of PAVMs on presentation

	Published series		
	Mean (%)	Range	N
Respiratory			
Asymptomatic	49	25–58	260
Dyspnea	50	27–71	685
Chest pain	12	6–18	390
Hemoptysis	11	4–18	671
Hemothorax	1	0–2	258
Cyanosis	27	9–73	467
Clubbing	28	6–68	459
Bruit	31	3–58	455
Embolic phenomena			
Cerebral abscess	12.9	0–25	635
CVA/TIA	27	11–55	401
CVA	13.7	9.5–18	262
TIA	22.1	6.3–36	262
Migraine	44.7	38–57	266

Data from studies in ref 6, and refs 7–10.

cerebrovascular accidents (CVA) and brain abscesses. The incidence of major, usually neurological complications approaches 50 percent (Table 26.2.1) with 10 percent cerebral abscess and 27 percent embolic stroke or transient ischemic attack recorded in all series. Recent data demonstrate that these risks are essentially independent of PAVM size and symptoms (5). Additional complications of PAVMs include hemorrhage (which may be life-threatening, particularly in pregnancy and in the setting of elevated PAVM sac perfusion pressures), and migraine.

PAVM complications can be limited if the condition is recognized and treated. Treatment of the asymptomatic patient was advocated as early as 1950 (11), but the benefits of intervention were mitigated by the significant morbidity associated with surgical resection. With the advent of embolization therapy in the late 1970s (12), a parenchymal-sparing treatment regime became available for patients. Embolization using metal coils or plug devices is now the treatment of choice for almost all patients. In experienced centers, there are proven long-term benefits of embolization, with excellent safety profiles, and this has supported the trend towards earlier treatment of the asymptomatic patient, accompanied by clinical screening of high risk groups.

Significant clinical concerns remain however. First, many PAVM patients remain under regular follow-up in respiratory units without consideration of intervention: in a recent series the average delay to treatment was 6.8 years (95 percent CI 4.1–9.5 years) for patients with respiratory symptoms, compared to 1.1 to 1.7 years for patients diagnosed either by post stroke/abscess investigation or by screening programs (5). Second, published and anecdotal data suggest higher rates of complications in inexperienced hands. These include peri-procedural events and long-term development of systemic arterial feeders to the sac resulting in catastrophic hemorrhage (13), but this is not widely recognized. Third, there are clinical scenarios such as severe pulmonary hypertension which modify risk benefit analyses almost always in favour of non intervention (14), and again this is poorly recognized. Finally, modern detection methods reveal more disease than is treatable with today's technologies and much of current management lies in the long-term prevention of cerebral embolic events in patients with residual disease following maximal embolotherapy.

DEFINITIONS

- **Pulmonary arteriovenous malformations (PAVMs)** are abnormal vessels replacing the pulmonary capillary bed between the pulmonary arterial and venous circulations. PAVMs range in size from communications within the microvasculature (telangiectases (15)) to large complex structures consisting of a bulbous aneurysmal sac between dilated feeding arteries and draining veins (16) (Figure 26.2.1). Approximately 70 percent of PAVMs are basally situated (17–20). Dilated feeding

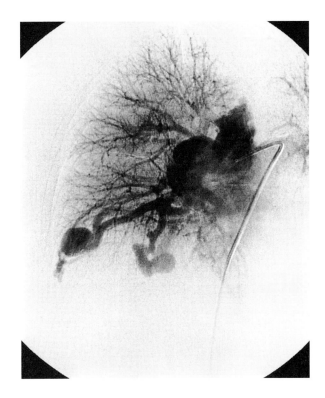

Figure 26.2.1   Non-selective pulmonary angiographic appearances of a single large PAVM.

arteries and dilated veins are characterized by walls of varying degrees of thickness even over relatively short segments, with disorganized adventitia. Medial thinning is observed, but also prominent are areas of focal thickening with abundant elastin tissue and a varying contribution of smooth muscle cells (15,21,22). Diffuse PAVMs have been defined as multiple small PAVMs affecting every segment of one or more lobes (23) or a single segment (24) (Figure 26.2.2).

- **Right to left shunts:** PAVMs result in a right to left shunt because they allow blood to flow directly from the right to left side of the circulation. In normal individuals, the anatomical shunt is less than 2 percent of the cardiac output, ascribed to the post-pulmonary drainage of bronchial veins into the pulmonary vein and thebesian vessels into the left atrium. PAVMs provide a low resistance shunt pathway, with the fraction of the cardiac output flowing through the fistula varying according to the relative vascular resistances of the shunt and normal lung. Where PAVMs are present in dependent portions of the lung, gravitational forces will increase flow through these shunts, a phenomenon first noted by auscultation, and more recently quantitated. As the majority of PAVMs are at the lung bases, orthodeoxia (desaturation on standing) is frequently found.
- **Pulmonary hemodynamics:** In the absence of coexisting pathologies resulting in pulmonary hypertension, in chronically adapted patients, there is a reduced total pulmonary vascular resistance (PVR), low-normal mean pulmonary arterial pressure (PAP), and increased

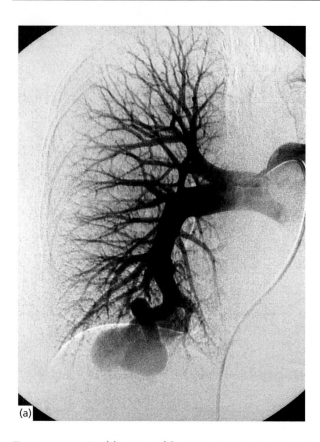

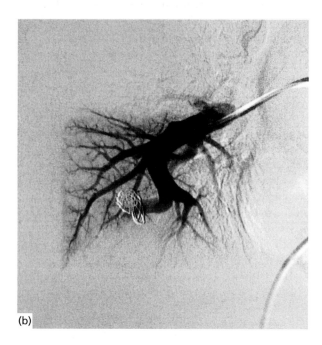

Figure 26.2.2   Pre (a) and post (b) embolization chest radiographs of a patient with PAVMs.

cardiac output (Qt) (25). Reduced PVR in the uninvolved lung (25) is likely to have reflected the presence of undetected microvascular PAVMs in the apparently normal lung, though there are also data from an acute dog model of PAVMs that would support the presence of significant vasodilatory stimuli (26). In later studies of patients with smaller mean R–L shunt fractions (8.5–11.5 percent) mean pulmonary systolic and diastolic pressures have been in the normal range (27–29), and recent studies have focussed on the occasional presence of coexisting pulmonary hypertension (see below).

- **Distinction from hepatopulmonary syndrome:** The true anatomical shunts of PAVMs are usually distinguished from the diffusion–perfusion defects that arise in patients with intrapulmonary vascular dilatations secondary to the hepatopulmonary syndrome (HPS). First described in 1884 as a triad of features (cirrhosis, clubbing, and cyanosis) associated with normal heart and lungs (30), HPS results in hypoxemia in 30–70 percent of cirrhotic patients (31). The syndrome is defined by the presence of liver disease, an increased $P(A\text{-}a)O_2$ breathing room air, and evidence of intrapulmonary vascular dilatations (32). The anatomical basis appears to be due to smaller vessels than usually discussed as representing PAVMs (20 μm, ref 31), and in contrast to PAVMs, as this produces a physiological not anatomical shunt, most patients respond to 100 percent oxygen (33). The hypoxemia and impaired gas transfer (and DL_{CO}) recover post liver transplantation (34,35).

INCIDENCE/EPIDEMIOLOGY

There have been no studies to assess the incidence of PAVMs in the general population, but due to the association with other diseases, an estimate may be made.

The majority of PAVMs occur in individuals affected by hereditary hemorrhagic telangiectasia (HHT). In one series of 219 consecutive PAVM patients, a clinical diagnosis of HHT could be established in 93.6 percent of cases (5). Careful epidemiological surveys suggest HHT incidences far in excess of previously quoted figures, including greater than 1 in 2500 in the Jura Valley in France (36) and the Dutch Antilles (37), 1 in 6400 in Denmark (38) and 1 in 5–8000 in Japan (39). PAVMs affect almost 50 percent of HHT patients (40). Assuming a conservative HHT prevalence of 1 in 8000, then for the UK population of 60 million, there will be 3–4000 HHT-associated PAVM cases, and for the US population of 300 million, 15–20 000 cases. The majority of these will be undiagnosed. These prevalence estimates do not include further PAVMs resulting from surgical cavopulmonary and atriopulmonary shunts, sporadic disease, and rare traumatic aetiologies.

PAVMs can develop in the pre- or perinatal period and in these there is a 2:1 male:female predominence in contrast to the female preponderance of approximately 1.6:1 seen in teenagers and adults (6). Screening of individuals over a period of years shows that PAVMs can develop in adult life in radiologically and/or physiologically normal vessels, although it is likely that functional changes at a cellular or microscopic level predate the development of the macro-scopic lesions. There are few data available regarding growth of PAVMs once present, but proven times of growth include puberty, pregnancy (41); and in the setting of pul-monary venous hypertension secondary to mitral stenosis or left ventricular dysfunction (42). On rare occasions, spontaneous regression has been described (43).

ETIOLOGY

Macroscopic PAVMs may develop idiopathically, post-trauma, in association with hereditary hemorrhagic tel-angiectasia (the majority), and following surgery for congenital heart disease. In the absence of any previous car-diac surgery, a very careful search for HHT in the patient and their family is warranted, due to the importance of presymp-tomatic screening and treatment for other family members.

Hereditary hemorrhagic telangiectasia (HHT) and PAVMs

HHT is a disorder of vascular development inherited as an autosomal dominant trait. It is usually recognized by physi-cians due to the consequences of abnormal dilated vessels developing in the systemic circulation, leading to epistaxes (nose bleeds), mucocutaneous telangiectasia and iron defi-ciency anaemia secondary to chronic gastrointestinal and/or nasal hemorrhage (Table 26.2.2). Pulmonary AVMs are now estimated to affect at least 48 percent of HHT patients (40), when they are often multiple. Large arteriovenous malforma-tions also occur in several systemic vascular beds such as the cerebral, spinal, and hepatic circulations. In contrast to cere-bral AVMs that are thought to develop perinatally, the major-ity of abnormal vessels in HHT, including PAVMs, develop postnatally. As a result, HHT exhibits age-dependent pene-trance, with most index patients presenting in early to mid-adulthood. The diagnosis of HHT is frequently not known to the affected individual. In one recent series 59 percent (95 percent confidence intervals 52.2; 65.5 percent; 121/205) of

consecutive PAVM patients with HHT were unaware they had HHT when their PAVMs were diagnosed (5).

MOLECULAR BASIS OF HHT

HHT is inherited as an autosomal dominant trait. Three disease genes have been identified. See refs 44–51.

PHENOTYPE–GENOTYPE CORRELATIONS

See refs 52–58.

TRIGGERS FOR VASCULAR DEFECTS IN HHT

In any one individual with HHT, however severe, the majority of vascular beds develop normally with macro-scopic malformations developing in only a small fraction. A characteristic finding is that different affected members of the same HHT family display highly disparate pheno-types, which may range from life-threatening events in childhood to non-penetrance. Different patterns of disease are also observed in mouse models of the same causative mutation suggesting that other genetic and environmental influences modify the HHT phenotype.

PULMONARY HYPERTENSION (PH) ASSOCIATED WITH HHT

PH has been recognized in a number of HHT patients (42,59–64). As recently reviewed (29), the causes of PH in HHT are diverse, as in the normal population. Two forms of PH predominate in HHT, true pulmonary arterial hyper-tension (PAH) phenotypes (62,63,65), and a post-capillary PH occurring in the context of high output cardiac failure secondary to hepatic AVMs, a potentially reversible form of PH (66). Mixed pictures are also observed (29).

The overall prevalence of PH in HHT is low. Catheter-based studies in a group of 143 PAVM/HHT patients, mean age 47 (range 8–78) years undergoing PAVM embolization identified median (interquartile range) mmHg values for PAP as 23 (19–27) systolic; 7 (5–9) diastolic; and 13 (11–16)

Table 26.2.2 Clinical features of hereditary hemorrhagic telangiectasia (HHT)

Feature	Overall frequency	Approximate penetrance at age (years)				
		0	15	25	45	90
Epistaxes (nose bleeds)	>90%	0%	40%	60%	90%	97%
Mucocutaneous telangiectasia	75%	0%	11%	30%	50%	75%
Chronic GI hemorrhage	25%					
Pulmonary AVMs (PAVMs)	50%					
Hepatic AVMs*	30%					
Cerebral AVMs (CAVMs)	15%					
Spinal AVMs	>2%					

Data on age-related penetrance data adapted from 324 patients reviewed in ref 111.

mean compared with normal values of 13–26, 6–16 and 7–19 mmHg, respectively (29). There was a significant increase in PAP with age (29). While PAP mean exceeded 20 mmHg in 9/143 (6%), only two patients referred from services other than specialized pulmonary hypertension units had PAP mean exceeding 35 mmHg (29). In an echocardiographic study of 68 HHT patients mean age 51 (range 19–84) years, from a separate HHT population, estimated systolic PAP were above the normal range in 9 (20.5%), in whom ePASP ranged from 40 to 58 mmHg (67).

The frequency of pulmonary hypertension (PH), and hepatic AVMs differs with HHT genotype: PAH phenotypes and hepatic AVMs are more common in HHT type 2 due to *ACVRL1* mutations than HHT type 1 due to *ENG* mutations (53,63,65,68). While in HHT, PAH was initially considered attributable solely to *ACVRL1* mutations, there are now rare reports of PAH associated with *ENG* mutations, and both genes are to be included in the latest WHO classification of PAH.

Sporadic PAVMs

Sporadic PAVMs occur, though many are in fact due to underlying, undiagnosed HHT since the diagnosis of HHT is more difficult to make than textbooks suggest, and the majority of HHT patients worldwide are probably undiagnosed. Sporadic PAVMs are usually single, and multiple PAVMs should raise particular suspicion that there is underlying HHT (5,19,69,70). These considerations are particularly pertinent for children presenting with PAVMs (71).

Cavopulmonary shunts

Surgical treatments of several forms of complex cyanotic congenital heart disease rely on the establishment of anastomoses between the vena cavae and pulmonary arteries. In non-HHT patients, cavopulmonary and atriopulmonary shunts result in PAVMs macroscopically indistinguishable from sporadic and HHT-associated macroscopic PAVMs. In one study, 31 percent of patients developed angiographically detectable PAVMs after a mean follow-up of 6.8 years (4). It has been suggested that following superior bidirectional cavopulmonary anastomosis (BCPA), the development of functional intrapulmonary shunts (detectable by perfusion scans using technetium-99m (99^{m}Tc)-labeled albumin macroaggregates) may be universal (72). In another study, 17 patients post-BCPA had shunts ranging from 11 percent to 64 percent of the cardiac output, compared to 3–8 percent in controls (72), and < 3.5 percent in normal adults (73).

The key pathogenic feature appears to be the route taken by hepatic venous effluent: First, PAVMs are found in the lung which receives no or minimal hepatic venous return (74,75). Secondly, these PAVMs can be treated by restoring hepatic venous return to the affected pulmonary circulation either by rerouting the hepatic veins to the pulmonary arteries (76); reconnecting the pulmonary arteries (77); or incorporating the hepatic vein into the cavopulmonary system (78). These observations, and data from hepatopulmonary syndrome (Chapter 26.1) (31), highlight the role of hepatic metabolism in influencing dilatation and/or remodelling of the pulmonary vascular bed. Whether there will be common underlying mechanisms between PAVMs developing in the setting of cavopulmonary shunts and HHT is unclear.

CLINICAL PRESENTATION OF PAVMS

In spite of the significant hazards of untreated PAVMs, approximately 50 percent of patients have no respiratory symptoms at the time of presentation, even with physical signs such as cyanosis, clubbing, or a vascular bruit, or abnormal chest radiographs. It is particularly important to recognize patients with paroxysmal neurological symptoms that may be attributable to transient ischemic attacks secondary to paradoxical emboli. As noted below, these are not necessarily the more severely affected as judged by respiratory symptoms or signs. Table 26.2.1 summarizes presentation patterns.

Respiratory symptoms

- **Dyspnea.** Dyspnea is the respiratory symptom most commonly reported by PAVM patients, but may not be appreciated until after the condition has been treated. One recent series of 219 consecutive PAVM patients stratified the proportion of dyspnoeic patients according to the degree of hypoxemia, and indicated that PAVMs generally result in symptomatic dyspnea only when resting arterial oxygen saturations are below 80 percent (5,14).
- **Hemorrhage.** Hemoptysis and hemothorax are relatively rare features for PAVMs, with three important exceptions: (1) spontaneous and post-embolization systemic arterial blood supply to PAVM sacs (13,24); (2) pulmonary hypertension; and (3) pregnancy-associated changes (22). These conditions place patients at higher risk of hemorrhage from PAVMs, which may be massive and life-threatening.
- **Chest pain.** Pleuritic chest pain of uncertain aetiology is reported to occur in up to 10 percent of PAVM patients. Such figures are likely to be overestimated however, in series which do not correct for ascertainment bias of incidental PAVM detection following protocol-driven CT scans for patients with chest pain investigated for suspected pulmonary embolism.

Neurological features

- **Strokes and cerebral abscess.** Ischaemic strokes and brain abscess, each attributed to paradoxical emboli through PAVMs were reported in high proportions of patients in historical series. Correcting for ascertainment bias (that is, diagnosis of PAVMs because of a stroke/abscess), in a recent series of 219 PAVM patients the respective rates were 9% for cerebral abscess and 11.3% for ischemic stroke (5). Relative risks compared with control populations were particularly high in young adults (5). The risks of stroke/abscess for PAVM patients are however poorly recognized, and were not mentioned in a recent authoritative set of guidelines for stroke prevention (79). Although univariate analyses in small studies had suggested that neurologic complications were more common in patients with more severe (7) or diffuse PAVMs (24), a recent cohort study of 219 consecutive PAVM patients utilizing the Anderson Gill extension of Cox proportional hazards models indicated that there was no clear relationship between the risk of ischemic stroke or cerebral abscess with any of six markers of PAVM severity (symptoms, arterial oxygen saturation, R-L shunt, PAVM multiplicity, diameter of largest feeding vessel, or presence of small untreatable PAVMs) (5). In this study, ischemic stroke risk was also unrelated to conventional neurovascular risk factors such as smoking, hypertension, diabetes mellitus, atrial fibrillation, and hypercholesterolemia. There was a very strong association between ischemic stroke and low PAP mean (hazard ratio 0.89 [95% Cl 0.83–0.95] per mmHg increase, $p < 0.0001$), as well as strong associations between cerebral abscess and male gender and dental microorganisms (5).

- **Migraines** (8,9,80).

Pregnancy

PAVM hemorrhage and PAVM growth have been reported during pregnancy (see for example, refs 41,81). A recent study of 484 pregnancies in women with HHT and PAVMs demonstrated that 1.0 percent (95 percent Cl 0.1–1.9 percent) of pregnancies resulted in a major PAVM bleed; and that such events often occurred in the setting of small PAVMs and no evidence of pulmonary hypertension (22).

INVESTIGATIONS FOR PAVMS

Many PAVM patients are diagnosed as a result of a chest radiograph or thoracic CT scan obtained for investigation of respiratory symptoms such as dyspnea, hemoptysis or chest pain, or incidentally due to investigations performed for other reasons. In other cases, PAVM screening in an at-risk population will be required in order to confirm or refute the diagnosis of PAVMs.

The overall incidence of PAVMs in the general population is so low (< 0.01 percent) that targeted screening protocols are required. Suitable populations to screen would be patients with HHT, patients with cerebral abscesses, and any young patient with an embolic CVA, even if an apparent alternative cause is present. The high proportions of HHT/PAVM patients undiagnosed at the time of their PAVM-induced ischemic stroke (66.7 percent) or cerebral abscess (64.3 percent) highlight the importance of robust PAVM screening programs for the HHT population (5). Screening HHT patients poses a particular difficulty as most individuals with HHT are unaware they have the disease.

PAVM centers differ in the exact screening modalities employed, according to the particular expertise of the institution. Common to all programs are the policies of minimizing the radiation burden in an often young population; having a sensitive screen to detect all clinically significant PAVMs; and concern to avoid missing any treatable PAVMs. Figure 26.2.3 delineates two commonly used approaches. Some centers will use pulmonary angiography as a tool to confirm the diagnosis, but in order to reduce the radiation burden, we prefer to restrict angiography to therapeutic embolization sessions.

The optimal screening intervals are unknown. Current recommendations are to screen every five to ten years, or if the patient is approaching a period known to be associated with PAVM enlargement and rupture such as puberty or pregnancy. Given the development of lesions over a two to three-year period, even these rarely instituted regimes may be insufficient. It is particularly important to screen prior to pregnancy, in view of the maternal risks of PAVMs (22,81).

Specific investigations

IMPAIRED OXYGENATION ON ROOM AIR

The simplest method for detecting the right-to-left shunt of a PAVM is the demonstration of hypoxemia breathing room air, but the differential diagnosis of hypoxemia is wide, and additional investigations are required to suggest that this is due to PAVMs rather than other etiologies. Further desaturation on assuming the upright posture, orthodeoxia, may be useful supporting evidence as the majority of PAVMs are in the lower lobes. The detection of hypoxemia alone, either by age-defined PaO_2, or SaO_2 from pulse oximetry is insufficiently sensitive to be used as a single diagnostic test (82).

RADIOLOGY INVESTIGATIONS

These include:

- **Chest radiographs.**
- **Thoracic CT scanning.**
- **MRI** (83).

CONTRAST ECHOCARDIOGRAPHY

There has also been significant interest in contrast echocardiography (CE) due to the absence of radiation exposure. For more details see refs 84–88D, and Figure 26.2.3.

OTHER METHODS TO DETECT AND QUANTIFY THE RIGHT-TO-LEFT SHUNTS

These include:

- **Impaired oxygenation following 100 percent O_2 re-breathing** (28).
- **Radionuclide scanning** (28,73,89).

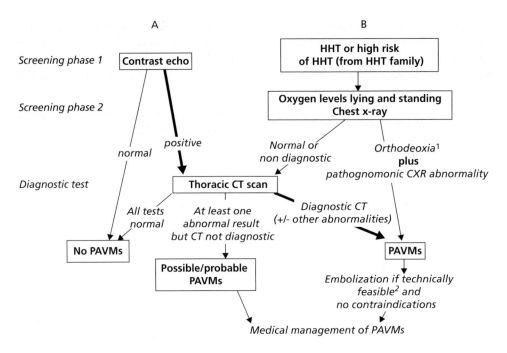

A

B

Figure 26.2.3 Alternate algorithms for screening for PAVMs: (A) As recommended in ref 88D (before data in ref 88B suggesting may not be cost efficient in HHT families). (B) PAVM screening protocols employed in our institution (note HHT family history is equivalent to a first screening step, ref 88E). Note: Protocols do not refer to patients being investigated for possible PAVM in the setting of respiratory or neurological symptoms, although similar investigations will be used. 1. Other indicator of right to left shunting could be used here (e.g. contrast echocardiogram, bubble study, technetium scan). 2. Determined by CT (may be performed for first time here), and not angiography which due to radiation burden, should be reserved for therapeutic procedures.

TREATMENT/MANAGEMENT

Expectant management is indicated only when physician and patient are fully informed of the risks of leaving PAVMs untreated – PAVMs are not benign lesions that can be safely ignored.

Management modalities

EMBOLIZATION

During embolization (the mainstay of treatment), the feeding vessels of the AVMs are usually embolized with detachable metallic coils or plugs depending on the size and blood supply of the malformation. Occluding devices must be placed as close as possible to the neck of the malformation in an attempt to avoid the occlusion of normal pulmonary artery branches and to reduce the risk of the development of a bronchial arterial collateral supply to the sac. Other techniques such as packing the venous sac with coils may be required if the anatomy of the PAVMs precludes "conventional" embolization.

Embolization series published to date provide clear evidence for regression of the PAVM sac (90), and substantial improvement in oxygenation for patients with pre-embolization hypoxemia (see for example, refs 27, 29, 91, 92). The majority of patients however, will notice little improvement in dyspnea or exercise tolerance as most PAVMs are not associated with substantial R-L shunts and hypoxemia. Two recent studies have now demonstrated the clinical efficacy of embolization in improving stroke/abscess risk (5), and reducing the prevalence of migraine (93).

SURGERY

Embolization has generally supplanted surgical procedures, due to reduced periprocedural risks; parenchymal sparing in patients at risk of recurrent disease; and the documented benefits. Surgical resection of PAVMs may be useful in two settings. Surgery can be a useful adjunctive therapy for highly selective cases where (further) embolization is not feasible, but PAVMs are sufficiently localized for thoracoscopic resection. At our institution, we reserve elective surgical approaches for highly selected patients with ongoing ischemic strokes, transient ischemic attacks, or significant respiratory symptoms following maximal embolization. In emergency situations, particularly associated with massive hemoptysis, lobectomy or pneumonectomy may be appropriate (22,94).

ACCESSORY MANAGEMENT MODALITIES

Although formal treatment of PAVMs either by angiographic embolization techniques or by surgery is required to radically alter the long-term prognosis, several medical maneuvers are recommended in patients suspected of having PAVMs. Such maneuvers are also important in many treated patients since postembolization, residual shunting through untreatable (< 2 mm diameter) arterial feeding vessels is common.

Dental issues

Until recently, due to the links between oral bacteria and cerebral abscess, antibiotic prophylaxis before dental and surgical procedures was recommended for patients with PAVMs and HHT, based on the endocarditis paradigm. As is now well recognized, the American Heart Association (95) and British NICE guideline committee (96) have both stated that antibiotic prophylaxis is no longer required for most patients with structural heart disease. PAVM/HHT patients did not fall into the groups considered by AHA/NICE however (97), and are at higher individual risk (5), with strengthened evidence for an association between oral microorganisms and brain abscess (5). As a result, a recent article providing recommendations for PAVM/HHT patients to reduce the risk of dental bacteraemias, included the use of antibiotic prophylaxis prior to dental procedures (97).

Thromboembolic risks

There are no data on maneuvers to reduce thromboembolic risks, but based on the high frequency of cerebral thromboembolic complications in these patients, and evidence that many have a prothrombotic state we have suggested that options such as cessation of hormonal therapy, or antiplatelet therapy, should be considered on a case-by-case basis for patients experiencing transient ischemic attacks, even if there is underlying HHT (98).

Air emboli

Recent guidelines have highlighted the importance of ensuring that when intravenous access is in place, extra care is required to avoid air bubbles entering the venous circulation (88D). The same guidelines also recommend avoidance of SCUBA diving (88D). At our institution, we discourage individuals with PAVMs from taking up scuba diving. For existing divers however, we inform of the potential increased risk of decompression illness, and allow the individual to make an educated decision about whether to continue diving, by following dive profiles and breathing gas mixtures that are known to avoid venous bubble liberation, guided by a physician knowledgeable in diving medicine.

Importance of regular follow-up with shunt assessments

Following initially complete embolization or surgical resection, residual macroscopic disease may develop several months after treatment, following a period of vascular remodeling. It is well recognized that removal of a low resistance shunt can unmask or provoke the development of additional PAVMs elsewhere in the pulmonary circulation,

and occasionally, new pulmonary artery feeder vessels to the treated lesion. As a result, review of all patients and right-to-left shunt measurement after several months is generally recommended, and a series of treatments may be needed.

Detection of underlying HHT and family screening of PAVM patients

Diagnosis and treatment of any PAVM is only one part of the management of a PAVM patients. It is crucial that the physician is alert to the possibility of HHT in the patient and therefore other family members. PAVMs may be the first sign of HHT in the presenting patient, and may be the only feature of HHT evident in patients through their thirties, forties, fifties and beyond. (The mean penetrance of HHT reaches 95 percent by 40 years of age, but is only 62 percent by 16 years (Table 26.2.2)). Mucocutaneous telangiectasia are often subtle. Furthermore, the majority of patients will not volunteer a personal or family history of nosebleeds unless specifically asked, and allowed time to check with relatives.

Current clinical diagnostic criteria for a definitive diagnosis of HHT require the presence of three out of four key features, namely (1) spontaneous recurrent epistaxis; (2) telangiectases at characteristic sites; (3) a visceral manifestation; and (4) an affected first degree relative (99). For more details see refs 88D, 95, 96, 100–104. Families can be provided with information about HHT patient self-help groups, such as HHT Foundation International (http://www.hht.org) and the UK Telangiectasia Self-Help Group (http://www.telangiectasia.co.uk).

COMPLICATIONS OF PAVM TREATMENT

In expert hands, embolization is efficacious, and complications are rare, though the procedure is not without risk. Successive series highlight a learning curve and smaller series have higher complication rates. The most common complication is of transient pleurisy in up to 10 percent of patients, particularly those with peripheral PAVMs. Higher rates are seen for patients with diffuse PAVMs (24). The mechanism for the pleurisy is unknown but it appears unrelated to pulmonary infarction. Angina, due to transient air bubble emboli, has been reduced by the technical advances reported in later series. There are occasional reports of long-term neurological complications following paradoxical emboli.

Development of systemic arterial supply

Recanalization by further pulmonary arterial feeders may result in requirements for further embolization, but it is the risk of recanalization by systemic arterial feeders that poses the greater potential risk to patients. The risk of massive hemoptysis from PAVM sacs that persist postembolization and that acquire a systemic arterial collateral blood supply was first highlighted in a small series published in 1998 (13) and is discussed in detail elsewhere (105). Development of systemic collaterals post PAVM embolization may affect significant proportions of patients (106) but is of consequence only if the fragile PAVM sac persists, a consequence of embolization technique. None of the cases in series (106) experienced hemoptysis, in contrast to the majority of those in a smaller series (13).

Development of pulmonary hypertension

PAVM embolization may be expected to elevate PAP, because PAVMs provide low resistance pathways for pulmonary blood flow. Data on PAP measurements pre- and post-embolization were scarce, with anecdotal reports of increasing PAP post-embolization (66,62). PAP measurements pre- and post-successful PAVM embolization, as demonstrated by improved arterial oxygen saturation, were recently reported for 35 patients with measurements from two or more consecutive embolization sessions, and for eight patients in whom PAP measurements were repeated at the end of embolization in the same session due to higher baseline PAP; there was no evidence of a sustained or acute change in PAP in the majority of patients, and in half, embolization led to a fall in PAP (29). Nevertheless, PAP did rise in occasional individuals (29).

Displacement of embolic device

Paradoxical emboli could result in tissue infarction, potentially most severe in cerebral and coronary circulations. This has been a well-recognized risk of pulmonary angiography and embolization, and great care is taken to avoid this possibility. It is instructive therefore, to compare the low rates in PAVM treatment series to the 35 percent incidence of pulmonary emboli of cyanoacrylate or platinum coils following embolization of cerebral AVMs (107). For PAVMs, in addition to embolization of coils or plugs, any thrombus which forms in the embolized sac has the potential to embolize prior to organization, and there are some data to suggest this may be the case particularly when there is a persistent feeder, as in one individual treated by an experienced center (108). Avoidance of strenuous exercise in the week following embolization, as suggested by this group (108) may be appropriate.

Consideration of treatments in special circumstances

MANAGEMENT STRATEGY FOR PREGNANT PATIENTS

In view of the risks of PAVM growth and rupture during pregnancy, female patients should be advised to defer pregnancy pending formal PAVM assessment and treatment. Pregnancies should be managed with close liaison between obstetricians, pulmonologists and interventional radiologists, using appropriate "high-risk" obstetric management strategies (22). Patients and their medical practitioners should be alerted to the possibility of hemoptysis or sudden severe dyspnea that requires urgent admission and management: embolization in the second and third trimesters is feasible and safe (22,109). The question of whether PAVM embolization should be offered to asymptomatic pregnant women differs between countries; at our institution it is not performed (22).

MANAGEMENT IN PRESENCE OF PRE-EXISTING PULMONARY HYPERTENSION

Should embolization of PAVMs be performed in patients with severe pre-existing pulmonary hypertension? This question was specifically addressed in ref 14, evaluating risk-benefits in the light of new data regarding stroke risk (5), the known risks of PAVMs in the setting of PH, and data that test balloon occlusion did not predict subsequent rise in PAP following definitive embolization (29). We concluded that for patients with pre-existing severe pulmonary hypertension, the risks of pulmonary AVM embolization generally outweigh potential benefits (14), recognizing that the most difficult judgements relate to individuals with severe pulmonary hypertension and major active hemoptysis.

SEVERE DIFFUSE DISEASE: A ROLE FOR LUNG TRANSPLANTATION?

Lung transplantation has been undertaken in a few patients with severe hypoxemia secondary to diffuse disease (see for example ref 110). Transplantation-associated morbidity and mortality however, are likely in most cases to exceed the long-term risks of PAVMs. Three PAVM patients in our clinic (one male, two female) who elected not to proceed with transplantation after discussion of the risks at two different UK transplant centers have remained stable over the subsequent 15, 17, and 21 years, respectively, and one patient has had three successful pregnancies. In a retrospective series of 36 patients with diffuse PAVMs for whom follow-up data were available for a mean of 8.5 years (range 0.12–26 years), 24 of the 27 survivors were working or studying full time, and one of the deaths was transplantation-associated (24).

FUTURE DIRECTIONS OF THERAPY

We suspect that in expert hands, transcatheter embolization techniques may have reached potential technical limits: it is doubtful that advances will permit routine embolization of feeding vessels of less than 2 mm in diameter. We would suggest that new medical therapeutic modalities developed from a clear understanding of the pathogenic basis of PAVMs are likely to provide the next significant advance. The importance of such manoeuvres will depend on elucidation of the true natural history of the smaller shunt vessels.

KEY POINTS

- **50 percent of patients with PAVMs are asymptomatic, but:**
- All patients with PAVMs are at risk of stroke and cerebral abscess due to paradoxical emboli through the right-to-left shunt.
- PAVMs can be readily detected by noninvasive methods, and safely treated.
- **Treatment should be considered for all patients to limit complications from PAVMs:**
- Embolization is the treatment of choice, and can be repeated
- Surgery should be only rarely undertaken because of the likelihood of extensive or recurrent disease.
- All patients with PAVMs should receive antibiotic prophylaxis for dental or surgical procedures.
- **90 percent of PAVM patients will have hereditary hemorrhagic telangiectasia and an "at-risk" family:**
- All PAVM patients with HHT need long-term follow-up to assess for growth of new PAVMs.
- No relatives of patients with PAVMs should be allowed to present with catastrophic consequences of a cerebral abscess.

REFERENCES

• seminal primary article
◆ key review paper
* first formal publication of a management guideline

1. Churton TL, communicated by J Branthwaite. Multiple aneurysm of pulmonary artery. Br Med J 1897;1:1223.
2. Reading B. A case of congenital telangiectasia of the lung complicated by brain abscess. Texas State J Med 1932;23:462.
3. Rundles RW. Hemorrhagic telangiectasia with pulmonary artery aneurysm: Case report. Am J Med Sci 1945;210: 76–81.
4. Kopf G, Laks H, Stansel H et al. Thirty-year follow-up of superior vena cava-pulmonary artery (Glenn) shunts. J Thoracic Cardiovasc Surg 1990;100:662–71.
•*5. Shovlin CL, Jackson JE, Bamford KB et al. Primary determinants of ischemic stroke/brain abscess risk are independent of severity of pulmonary arteriovenous malformations in hereditary hemorrhagic telangiectasia. Thorax 2008;63(3):259–66.
◆6. Shovlin CL, Letarte M. Hereditary hemorrhagic telangiectasia and pulmonary arteriovenous

malformations: issues in clinical management and review of pathogenic mechanisms. Thorax 1999;54:714–29.
•7. Moussouttas M, Fayad P, Rosenblatt M et al. Pulmonary arteriovenous malformations. Cerebral ischemia and neurologic manifestations. Neurology 2000;55:959–64.
•8. Post MC, Letteboer TG, Mager JJ et al. A pulmonary right-to-left shunt in patients with hereditary hemorrhagic telangiectasia is associated with an increased prevalence of migraine. Chest 2005;128:2485–9.
9. Thenganatt J, Schneiderman J, Hyland RH et al. Migraines linked to intrapulmonary right-to-left shunt. Headache 2006;46:439–43.
10. Cottin V Chinet T, Lavolé A et al. Pulmonary arteriovenous malformations in hereditary hemorrhagic telangiectasia patients: a series of 126 patients. Medicine (Baltimore) 2007;86(1):1–17.
11. Lindskog G, Liebow A, Kausel H, Janzen A. Pulmonary arteriovenous aneurysm. Ann Surg 1950;132:591–610.
•12. Porstmann W. Therapeutic embolization of arteriovenous pulmonary fistulas by catheter technique. In: Kelop O, ed. Current concepts in pediatric radiology. Berlin: Springer 1977:23–31.
13. Sagara K, Miyazono N, Inoue H et al. Recanalization after coil embolotherapy of pulmonary arteriovenous malformations: study of long-term outcome and mechanism for recanalization. Am J Roent 1998;170:727–30.
14. Shovlin CL, Gibbs JSR, Jackson JE. Management of pulmonary arteriovenous malformations in pulmonary hypertensive patients. A pressure to embolise? Eur Respir Rev. Eur Respir Rev 2008;18(111):4–6.
15. Hales M. Multiple small arteriovenous fistulas of the lungs. Am J Path 1956;32:927–37.
16. Anabtawi IA, Ellison RG, Ellison LT. Pulmonary arteriovenous aneurysms and fistulas. Ann Thorac Surg 1965;1:277–85.
17. Bosher L, Blake A, Byrd B. An analysis of the pathologic anatomy of pulmonary arteriovenous aneurysms with particular reference to the applicability of local excision. Surgery 1959;45:91–104.
18. Shumacker H, Waldhausen J. Pulmonary arteriovenous fistulas in children. Ann Surg 1963;158:713–20.
19. White RIJ, Lynch-Nylan A, Terry P et al. Pulmonary arteriovenous malformations: Techniques and long-term outcomes of embolotherapy. Radiology 1988;169:663–9.
•20. Dutton JAE, Jackson JE, Hughes JMB et al. Pulmonary arteriovenous malformations: results of treatment with coil embolization in 53 patients. Am J Roent 1995;165: 1119–25.
•21. Bourdeau A, Cymerman U, Paquet M-E et al. Endoglin expression is reduced on normal vessels but still detectable in arteriovenous malformations of patients with hereditary hemorrhagic telangiectasia type I. Am J Pathol 2000;156:911–23.
•*22. Shovlin CL, Sodhi V, McCarthy A et al. Estimates of maternal risks of pregnancy for women with hereditary hemorrhagic telangiectasia: suggested approach for obstetric services. BJOG 2008;115(9):1108–15.

23. Faughnan ME, Lui YW, Wirth JA *et al.* Diffuse pulmonary arteriovenous malformations. Characteristics and prognosis. Chest 2000;117:31–8.

●24. Pierucci P MJ, Henderson KJ, Chyun DA, White RI Jr. New definition and natural history of patients with diffuse pulmonary arteriovenous malformations: twenty-seven-year experience. Chest 2008;133:653–61.

●25. Whyte MKB, Hughes JMB, Jackson JE *et al.* Cardiopulmonary response to exercise in patients with intrapulmonary vascular shunts. J Appl Physiol 1993;75(1):321–8.

26. Waldhausen J, Abel F. The circulatory effects of pulmonary arteriovenous fistulas. Surgery 1966;59:76–80.

●27. Gupta P, Mordin C, Curtis J *et al.* Pulmonary arteriovenous malformations: Effect of embolization on right-to-left shunt, hypoxaemia and exercise tolerance in 66 patients. Am J Roent 2002;179:347–55.

●28. Mager JJ, Zanen P, Verzijbergen F *et al.* Quantification of right-to-left shunt with (99m)Tc-labelled albumin macroaggregates and 100% oxygen in patients with hereditary hemorrhagic telangiectasia. Clinical Science (London) 2002;102:127–34.

●*29. Shovlin CL, Tighe HC, Davies RJ *et al.* Embolization of pulmonary arteriovenous malformations: no consistent effect on pulmonary artery pressure. Eur Resp J 2008;32(1):162–9.

30. Fluckiger M. Vorkommen von trommelschlagelformigen Finger und Phalanger ohne chronische Veranderunger an den Lungen oder am Herzen. Wien Wochenschr 1884;34:1457.

31. Schraufnagel D, Kay J. Structure and pathological changes in the lung vasculature in chronic liver disease. Clin Chest Med 1996;17(1 The Lung in Liver Disease):1–15.

32. Krowka M, Cortese D. Hepatopulmonary syndrome. Current concepts in diagnostic and therapeutic considerations. Chest 1994;105:1528–37.

33. Castro M, Krowka M. Hepatopulmonary syndrome: A pulmonary vascular complication of liver disease. Clin Chest Med 1996;17(1 The Lung in Liver Disease):35–48.

34. Agusti A, Roca J, Rodriguez-Roisin R. Mechanisms of gas exchange in patients with liver cirrhosis. Clinics in Chest Medicine 1996;17(1 The Lung in Liver Disease):49–66.

35. Krowka M. Recent pulmonary observations in a1-antitrypsin deficiency, primary biliary cirrhosis, chronic hepatatis C, and other hepatic problems. Clin Chest Med 1996;17(1 The Lung in Liver Disease):67–82.

●36. Bideau A, Brunet G, Heyer E *et al.* An abnormal concentration of cases of Rendu–Osler disease in the Valserine valley of the French Jura: a geneological and demographic study. Ann Human Biol 1992;19:233–47.

37. Jessuron GA, Kamphuis DJ, Zande FHvd, Nossent JC. Cerebral arteriovenous malformations in the Netherlands Antilles. High prevalence of hereditary hemorrhagic telangiectasia-related single and multiple cerebral arteriovenous malformations. Clin Neurol Neurosurg 1993;95(3):193–8.

●38. Kjeldsen AD, Vase P, Green A. Hereditary hemorrhagic telangiectasia: a population–based study of prevalence and mortality in Danish patients. J Intern Med 1999;245:31–9.

39. Dakeishi M, Shioya T, Wada Y *et al.* Genetic epidemiology of hereditary hemorrhagic telangiectasia in a local community in the northern part of Japan. Hum Mut 2002;19:140–8.

●40. Cottin V, Plauchu H, Bayle J-Y *et al.* Pulmonary arteriovenous malformations in patients with hereditary hemorrhagic telangiectasia. Am J Respir Crit Care Med 2004;169(9):994–1000.

41. Shovlin CL, Winstock AR, Peters AM *et al.* Medical complications of pregnancy in hereditary hemorrhagic telangiectasia. Quart J Med 1995;88:879–87.

42. Chow LT, Chow WH, Ma KF. Pulmonary arteriovenous malformation. Progressive enlargement with replacement of the entire right middle lobe in a patient with concomitant mitral stenosis. Med J Aus 1993;158:632–4.

43. Vase P, Holm M, Arendrup H. Pulmonary arteriovenous fistulas in hereditary hemorrhagic telangiectasia. Acta Med Scand 1985;218(1):105–9.

●44. McAllister KA, Grogg KM, Johnson DW *et al.* Endoglin, a TGF-β binding protein of endothelial cells, is the gene for hereditary hemorrhagic telangiectasia type 1. Nature Genet 1994;8:345–51.

●45. Johnson DW, Berg JN, Baldwin MA *et al.* Mutations in the activin receptor-like kinase 1 gene in hereditary hemorrhagic telangiectasia type 2. Nature Genet 1996;13:189–95.

●46. Gallione C, Repetto GM, Legius E *et al.* A combined syndrome of juvenile polyposis and hereditary hemorrhagic telangiectasia is associated with mutations in MADH4 (SMAD4). Lancet 2004;363:852–9.

47. Cole SG, Begbie ME, Wallace GMF, Shovlin CL. A new locus for hereditary hemorrhagic telangiactasia (HHT3) maps to chromosome 5. J Med Genet 2005;42:577–82.

48. Bayrak-Toydemir P, McDonald J, Akarsu N *et al.* A fourth locus for hereditary hemorrhagic telangiectasia maps to chromosome 7. Am J Med Genet 2006;140:2155–62.

◆49a. Shovlin CL. Hereditary hemorrhagic telangiectasia: pathophysiology, diagnosis and treatment. Blood Rev 2010;24(6):203–19.

49b. Park S, Wankhede M *et al.* Real-time imaging of de novo arteriovenous malformation in a mouse model of hereditary hemorrhagic telangiectasia. Nat Med 2010;16:420–8.

49c. Mahmoud M, Allinson K, Zhai Z *et al.* Pathogenesis of arteriovenous malformations in the absence of endoglin. Circ Res 2010;106(8):1425–33.

49d. Lebrin F, Srun S, Raymond K *et al.* Thalidomide stimulates vessel maturation and reduces epistaxis in individuals with hereditary hemorrhagic telangiectasia. Nat Med 2010;16:420–8.

50. Cymerman U, Vera S, Pece-Barbara N *et al.* Identification of hereditary hemorrhagic telangiectasia type I in newborns by protein expression and mutation analysis of endoglin. Pediatric Res 2000;47:24–35.

51. Abdalla S, Pece-Barbara N, Vera S *et al.* Analysis of ALK-1 and endoglin in newborns from families with hereditary hemorrhagic telangiectasia type 2. Hum Mol Genet 2000;9:1227–37.

52. Kjeldsen AD, Moller TR, Brusgaard K *et al.* Clinical symptoms according to genotype amongst patients with hereditary hemorrhagic telangiectasia. J Int Med 2005;258:349–55.

•53. Letteboer TG, Mager H, Snijder RJ *et al.* Genotype–phenotype relationship in hereditary hemorrhagic telangiectasia. J Med Genet 2006;43:371–7.

54. Bossler AD, Richards J, George C *et al.* Novel mutations in ENG and ACVRL1 identified in a series of 200 individuals undergoing clinical genetic testing for hereditary hemorrhagic telangiectasia (HHT): correlation of genotype with phenotype. Hum Mutat 2006;27:667–75.

55. Bayrak-Toydemir P, McDonald J, Markewitz B *et al.* Genotype–phenotype correlation in hereditary hemorrhagic telangiectasia. Am J Med Genet 2006;140A:463–70.

56. Sabba C, Pasculli G, Lenato GM *et al.* Hereditary hemorrhagic telangiectasia: clinical features in ENG and ALK1 mutation carriers. J Thromb Hemost 2007;5:1149–57.

57. Lesca G, Olivieri C, Burnichon N, *et al.* Genotype–phenotype correlations in hereditary hemorrhagic telangiectasia: data from the French–Italian HHT network. Genet Med 2007;9:14–22.

58. Berg JN, Porteous MEM, Reinhardt D *et al.* Hereditary hemorrhagic telangiectasia: a questionnaire based study to delineate the different phenotypes caused by endoglin and ALK 1 mutations. J Med Genet 2003;40:585–90.

59. Sapru R, Hutchison D, Hall J. Pulmonary hypertension in patients with pulmonary arteriovenous fistulae. Br Heart J 1968;31:559.

60. le Roux B, Gibb B, Wainwright J. Pulmonary arteriovenous fistula with bilharzial pulmonary hypertension. Br Heart J 1970;32:571–4.

61. Trell E, Johansson BW, Linell F, Ripa J. Familial pulmonary hypertension and multiple abnormalities of large systemic arteries in Osler's disease. Am J Med 1972;53:50–63.

62. Pennington D, Gold W, Gordon R *et al.* Treatment of pulmonary arteriovenous malformations by therapeutic embolization. Am Rev Resp Dis 1992;145:1047–51.

•63. Trembath R, Thomson J, Machado R *et al.* Clinical and molecular features of pulmonary hypertension in patients with hereditary hemorrhagic telangiectasia. N Engl J Med 2001;345:325–34.

•64. Olivieri C, Lanzarini L, Pagella F *et al.* Echocardiographic screening discloses increased values of pulmonary artery systolic pressure in 9 of 68 unselected patients affected with hereditary hemorrhagic telangiectasia. Genet Med 2006;8:183–90.

65. Harrison RE, Flanagan JA, Sankelo M *et al.* Molecular and functional analysis identifies ALK-1 as the predominant cause of pulmonary hypertension related to hereditary hemorrhagic telangiectasia. J Med Genet 2003;40: 865–71.

66. Haitjema T, ten Berg J, Overtoom TT *et al.* Unusual complications after embolization of a pulmonary arteriovenous malformation. Chest 1996;109:1401–4.

67. Olivieri C Lanzarini L, Pagella F *et al.* Echocardiographic screening discloses increased values of pulmonary artery systolic pressure in 9 of 68 unselected patients affected

with hereditary hemorrhagic telangiectasia. Genet Med 2006;8:183–90.

68. Chaouat A, Coulet F, Favre C *et al.* Endoglin germline mutation in a patient with hereditary hemorrhagic telangiectasia and dexfenfluramine associated pulmonary arterial hypertension. Thorax 2004;59:446–8.

69. Dines DE, Arms RA, Bernatz PE, Gomes MR. Pulmonary arteriovenous fistulas. Mayo Clin Proc 1974;49:460–5.

70. Dines DE, Steward JB, Bernatz PE. Pulmonary arteriovenous fistulas. Mayo Clin Proc 1983;58:176–81.

71. Curie, Lesca G, Cottin V et al. Long-term follow-up in 12 children with pulmonary arteriovenous malformations: confirmation of hereditary hemorrhagic telangiectasia in all cases. J Pediatr Surg 2007;151:299–306.

72. Vettukattil J, Slavik Z, Monro J *et al.* Intrapulmonary arteriovenous shunting may be a universal phenomenon in patients with the superior cavopulmonary anastemosis. Heart 2000;83:425–8.

73. Thompson RD, Jackson J, Peters AM *et al.* Sensitivity and specificity of radioisotope right–left shunt measurements and pulse oximetry for the early detection of pulmonary arteriovenous malformations. Chest 1999;115:109–13.

74. Srivastava D, Preminger T, Lock JE *et al.* Hepatic venous blood and the development of pulmonary arteriovenous malformations in congenital heart disease. Circulation 1995;92:1217–22.

75. Larsson E, Solymar L, Eriksson B *et al.* Bubble contrast echocardiography in detecting pulmonary arteriovenous malformations after modified Fontan operations. Cardiol Young 2001;11:505–11.

76. Agnoletti G, Borghi A, Annecchino F, Crupi G. Regression of pulmonary venous fistulas in congenital heart disease after redirection of hepatic venous flow to the lungs. Ann Thorac Surg 2001;72:909–11.

77. Aboul Hosn J Danon S, Levi D, *et al.* Regression of pulmonary arteriovenous malformations after transcatheter reconnection of the pulmonary arteries in patients with unidirectional Fontan. Congenit Heart Dis 2007;2:179–84.

78. McElhinney DB Kreutzer J, Lang P, *et al.* Incorporation of the hepatic veins into the cavopulmonary circulation in patients with heterotaxy and pulmonary arteriovenous malformations after a Kawashima procedure. Ann Thorac Surg 2005;80:1597–603.

79. Sacco RL, Adams R, Albers G *et al.* Guidelines for prevention of stroke in patients with ischemic stroke or transient ischemic attack: a statement for healthcare professionals from the American Heart Association/ American Stroke Association Council on Stroke. Circulation 2006;113:e409–e49.

80. Marziniak M, Jung A, Guralnik V *et al.* An association of migraine with hereditary hemorrhagic telangiectasia independently of pulmonary right-to-left shunts. Cephalalgia. 2008; (in press).

81. Ference BA, Shannon TM, White RI *et al.* Life threatening pulmonary hemorrhage with pulmonary arteriovenous malformations and hereditary hemorrhagic telangiectasia. Chest 1994;106:1387–92.

82. Haitjema T, Disch F, Overtoom TTC *et al*. Screening family members of patients with hereditary hemorrhagic telangiectasia. Am J Med 1995;99:519–24.

83. Gutierrez F, Glazer H, Levitt R, Moran J. NMR imaging of pulmonary arteriovenous fistulae. J Comput Assist Tomogr 1984;8:750–2.

84. Zukotynski K Chan R, Chow CM *et al*. Contrast echocardiography grading predicts pulmonary arteriovenous malformations on CT. Chest 2007; 132:18–23.

85. Feinstein J, Moore P, Rosenthal D *et al*. Comparison of contrast echocardiography versus cardiac catheterization for detection of pulmonary arteriovenous malformations. Am J Cardiol 2002;89:281–5.

86. Gazzangia P Buscarini E, Leandro G *et al*. Contrast echocardiography for pulmonary arteriovenous malformations (PAVMs) screening: Does any bubble matter? Eur J Echocardiogr 2009;10(4):513–8. Epub 2008 Dec 17.

87. Nanthakumar K, Graham A, Robinson T *et al*. Contrast echocardiography for detection of pulmonary arteriovenous malformations. Am Heart J 2001;141:243–6.

88. van Gent MW Post M, Luermans JG *et al*. Screening for pulmonary arteriovenous malformations using transthoracic contrast echocardiography: a prospective study. Eur Respir J 2009;33(1):85–91. Epub 2008 Sep 17.

88a. van Gent MW, Post MC, Snijder RJ, Swaans MJ, Plokker HW, Westermann CJ, Overtoom TT, Mager JJ. Grading of pulmonary right-to-left shunt with transthoracic contrast echocardiography: does it predict the indication for embolotherapy? Chest. 2009 May;135(5):1288–92. Epub 2008 Dec 31.

•88b. van Gent MW, Post MC, Snijder RJ, Westermann CJ, Plokker HW, Mager JJ. Real prevalence of pulmonary right-to-left shunt according to genotype in patients with hereditary hemorrhagic telangiectasia: a transthoracic contrast echocardiography study. Chest 2010 Feb 12. [Epub ahead of print].

88c. Parra JA, Bueno J, Zarauza J, Fariñas-Alvarez MC, Cuesta JM, Ortiz P, Zarrabeitia R, Del Molino AP, Bustamante M, Botella LM, Delgado MT. Graded contrast echocardiography in pulmonary arteriovenous malformations. Eur Respir J 2009 Dec 8. [Epub ahead of print].

88d. Faughnan ME, Palda VA, Garcia-Tsao G, Geisthoff UW, McDonald J, Proctor DD, Spears J, Brown DH, Buscarini E, Chesnutt MS, Cottin V, Ganguly A, Gossage JR, Guttmacher AE, Hyland RH, Kennedy SJ, Korzenik J, Mager JJ, Ozanne AP, Piccirillo JF, Picus D, Plauchu H, Porteous ME, Pyeritz RE, Ross DA, Sabba C, Swanson K, Terry P, Wallace MC, Westermann CJ, White RI, Young LH, Zarrabeitia R. International Guidelines for the Diagnosis and Management of Hereditary Hemorrhagic Telangiectasia. J Med Genet 2009 Jun 29 [Epub ahead of print].

89. Chilvers ER, Peters AM, George P *et al*. Quantification of right to left shunt through pulmonary arteriovenous malformations using 99Tc^m albumin microspheres. Clin Radiol 1989;39:611–4.

•90. Remy-Jardin M, Dumont P, Brillet PY *et al*. Pulmonary arteriovenous malformations treated with embolotherapy: helical CT evaluation of long-term effectiveness after 2–21-year follow-up. Radiology 2006;239:576–85.

91. Haitjema TJ, Overtoom TTC, Westermann CJJ, Lammers JWJ. Embolization of pulmonary arteriovenous malformations: results and follow-up in 32 patients. Thorax 1995;50: 719–23.

92. Lee D, White R, Egglin T *et al*. Embolotherapy of large pulmonary arteriovenous malformation: long term results. AnnThor Surg 1997;64:930–40.

93. Post MC Thijs V, Schonewille WJ et al Embolization of pulmonary arteriovenous malformations and decrease in prevalence of migraine. Neurology 2006;66:202–5.

94. Ravasse P, Maragnes P, Petit T, Laloum D. Total pneumonectomy as a salvage procedure for pulmonary arteriovenous malformation in a newborn: Report of one case. J Pediatr Surg 2003;38:254–5.

∗95. Wilson W, Taubert K, Gewitz M *et al*. Prevention of infective endocarditis: guidelines from the American Heart Association: a guideline from the American Heart Association Rheumatic Fever, Endocarditis and Kawasaki Disease Committee, Council on Cardiovascular Disease in the Young, and the Council on Clinical Cardiology, Council on Cardiovascular Surgery and Anesthesia, and the Quality of Care and Outcomes Research Interdisciplinary Working Group. J Am Dent Assoc 2008;138:739–45;47–60.

∗96. Wray D RF, Richey R, Stokes T. Guideline Development Group. Prophylaxis against infective endocarditis for dental procedures – summary of the NICE guideline. Br Dental J 2008;204:555–7.

∗97. Shovlin CL, Bamford KB, Wray D. Post NICE: Antibiotic prophylaxis prior to dental procedures for patients with pulmonary arteriovenous malformations (PAVMs) and hereditary hemorrhagic telangiectasia. Br Dent J 2008; (in press).

•98. Shovlin CL, Sulainam NL, Govani FS *et al*. Elevated Factor VIII in hereditary hemorrhagic telangiectasia (HHT): association with venous thromboembolism. Thromb Hemostas 2007;98(5):1031–9.

◆99. Shovlin CL, Guttmacher AE, Buscarini E *et al*. Diagnostic criteria for hereditary hemorrhagic telangiectasia (Rendu–Osler–Weber syndrome). Am J Med Genet 2000;91:66–7.

•100. Lerut J, Orlando G, Adam R *et al*. Liver transplantation for hereditary hemorrhagic telangiectasia: Report of the European liver transplant registry. Ann Surg 2006;244: 854–62.

∗101. Buscarini E, Plauchu H, Garcia Tsao G *et al*. Liver involvement in hereditary hemorrhagic telangiectasia: consensus recommendations. Liver Internat 2006;26:1040–6.

◆102. Bayrak-Toydemir P Mao R, Lewin S, McDonald J. Hereditary hemorrhagic telangiectasia: an overview of diagnosis and management in the molecular era for clinicians. Genet Med 2004;6:175–91.

◆103. Sabba C. A rare and misdiagnosed bleeding disorder: hereditary hemorrhagic telangiectasia. J Thromb Hemost 2005;3:2201–10.

◆104. Govani FS, Shovlin CL. Hereditary hemorrhagic telangiectasia: A clinical and scientific review. Eur J Hum Genet 2009;17:7;860–71.

◆105. Shovlin CL, Jackson JE. Pulmonary arteriovenous malformations and other pulmonary–vascular abnormalities. In: Mason B, Murray, Nadel, eds. Murray and Nadel's Textbook of Respiratory Medicine, 5th edn. Pennsylvania: Elsevier–Saunders 2009 (in press).

106. Brillet PY Dumont P, Bouaziz N et al. Pulmonary arteriovenous malformation treated with embolotherapy: systemic collateral supply at multidetector CT angiography after 2–20-year follow-up. Radiology 2007;242:267–76.

107. Kjellin I, Boechat MI, Vinuela F et al. Pulmonary emboli following therapeutic embolization of cerebral arteriovenous malformations in children. Paediatr Radiol 2000;30:279–83.

∗108. Mager J, Overtoom T, Mauser H, Westermann CJJ. Early cerebral infarction after embolotherapy of a pulmonary arteriovenous malformation. J Vasc Intervent Radiol 2001;12:122–3.

109. Gershon A, Faughnan M, Chon K et al. Transcatheter embolotherapy of maternal pulmonary arteriovenous malformations during pregnancy. Chest 2001;119:470–7.

110. Reynaud-Gaubert M, Thomas P, Gaubert J-Y et al. Pulmonary arteriovenous malformations: lung transplantation as a therapeutic option. European Respiratory Journal 1999;14:1425–8.

●111. Plauchu H, de Chadarévian J-P, Bideau A, Robert J-M. Age-related clinical profile of hereditary hemorrhagic telangiectasia in an epidemiologically recruited population. Am J Med Genet 1989;32:291–7.

Index